A Textbook of Epilepsy

Edited by

John Laidlaw F.R.C.P. (Edin)

Consultant Physician to Epilepsy Centre, Quarrier's Homes,
Bridge of Weir.
Formerly Physician in charge of the National Hospitals –
Chalfont Centre for Epilepsy and Honorary Consultant to the
National Hospitals.

Alan Richens Ph.D., F.R.C.P.

Formerly Professor of Clinical Pharmacology, Institute of
Neurology, The National Hospitals, London; Honorary
Consultant, The National Hospitals – Chalfont Centre for
Epilepsy.
Professor of Pharmacology and Materia Medica, Welsh
National School of Medicine, Cardiff.

Foreword by **Denis Williams**

Introduction by **Maurice Parsonage**

SECOND EDITION

CHURCHILL LIVINGSTONE
EDINBURGH LONDON MELBOURNE AND NEW YORK 1982

CHURCHILL LIVINGSTONE
Medical Division of Longman Group Limited

Distributed in the United States of America by Churchill
Livingstone Inc., 19 West 44th Street, New York, N.Y.
10036, and by associated companies, branches and
representatives throughout the world.

First edition 1976
Second edition 1982

ISBN 0 443 02039 6

British Library Cataloguing in Publication Data
Laidlaw, J.
    A textbook of epilepsy. – 2nd ed.
    1. Epilepsy
    I. Title   II. Richens, Alan
    616.8'53   RC372

Library of Congress Catalog Card Number 81-10031

Printed in Hong Kong by
Wilture Enterprises (International) Ltd.

A Textbook of Epilepsy

Foreword

The epilepsies have been classified and reclassified upon the basis of each of their attributes – seizure pattern, temporal occurrence, aetiology and accompaniments. There are quite clearly as many classifications as there are needs to classify. Although this volume deals with all aspects of epilepsy, its authors have managed to conceal the classifications in the logical framework of their chapters; and yet this division of the subject is inevitable, for the epilepsies involve so much of the whole person and his whole life. This is part of their fascination to the neurologist.

The polymorphous nature of the subject is seen also in the evolution of our knowledge of it. First, there was the description of the observed and sensed events of the ictus itself, which slowly changed epilepsy into the epilepsies, and which so blurred its boundaries that physiogenesis and psychogenesis became indistinguishable. Later there was the identification of the ictal events with cerebral morphology, and consequently with recognised disease forms. This was encouraged by the sequential gain in knowledge of cerebral function. Encouragement of specific research into the nature of epilepsy seemed to be unnecessary, for the disease itself was the research tool for the early neurophysiologists.

Then with the advent of controlled anaesthesia the advance in knowledge was in the hands of physiologically orientated neurosurgeons, working mainly in North America, but following the English tradition of identification of the site of the epileptogenic lesion. This work was much helped by the development of the electroencephalogram shortly before World War II, and afterwards by electrophysiological ways of recording from the surface of the exposed human brain, and later within its depth. At this time, provision was not made for research into epilepsy as such, because the ictus, since it was a research tool, was a model of the behaviour of that part of the cortex – albeit a caricature of the function involved. Still, it was a tiny window into the brain which gave a view of its function. This, of course, was distorted by circumstance, for which the observer had to allow, both at the time of his observations and later in the holistic deductions he drew from them.

Neurosurgery taught us much about the focal fit, something about the general epilepsies, and furthered knowledge of cerebral function. The unfortunate genitor of the attacks may have had rather less attention though, as has the patient who is regarded by his physician as 'an interesting case'. Simultaneously, by good fortunate, the drug treatment of epilepsy was advanced by the use of the hydantoins for major epilepsy, and the diones for minor. But a third of a century had to pass before the pharmacology of these drugs began to be understood, and a wider variety of antiepileptic drugs became available. This delay on both sides of the Atlantic was caused mainly by the war: not merely the five years of war but the length of time it took afterwards for a new generation to emerge from training to ask themselves: why? This trend is pari passu with the enormous increase in knowledge in neurochemistry. In this subject, epilepsy is no longer the tool as it was for the neurophysiologist, but it is the object towards which the advances of neurochemistry itself are directed.

The fit itself continues to fascinate physiologists as well as clinicians, not so much for its pattern but for the circumstances of its occurrence, why it starts at all (for it must always have a final precipitant, the reflex epilepsies being exceptional stereotyped examples), and why it stops spontaneously, which is more important to the therapist.

There is so much to intrigue everyone in the very occurrence of epilepsy that scientific enquiry generates itself. But there has been a major change in attitude to the epilepsies in our own time, a change fostered by those who live with people with epilepsy, in the home, in society at large, in clinics and hospitals, and in special centres. This change is reflected in booklets for the layman, in special societies, in congresses, in the social services, and in scientific publications such as this. It consists of putting the person with epilepsy before his handicap. The change is worldwide and pervades the whole of the society which is involved in the problem of epilepsy. It is epitomised in the British Government's report *People With Epilepsy* (HMSO, 1969) and is reflected in its title. The people precede the epilepsy. This may be partly because now we are in general more liberal; we are certainly more egalitarian; we may have, as a whole society, more regard for the handicapped; and clearly we have greater material resources and knowledge. We also have a limitless capacity for communication through the community so that education in the home is commonplace. More than all these, we who work in the field of epilepsy have come to learn that regard for the personal problems of the patient and knowledge of the psychological consequences of the affliction (caused both by disordered brain and disquiet mind) are of first importance in treatment. After our scientific enquiry into the physical causes of the epilepsy, we use medical methods of treat-

ment, and perhaps later on may use surgical procedures, but throughout we attend to the needs of the whole person, the person with epilepsy.

I was honoured to be asked six years ago to write the Foreword to the first edition of this textbook, which has become a best seller in this particularly wide field of medicine – a field which demands the labour and the love of people from several disparate scientific disciplines. That is not surprising, for after all the brain, to which the disability epilepsy is unique, pervades every aspect of living. Communally, it dominates society too, or should.

So in these six years, the authors have faced up to the task of casting their net more widely to include our recently won knowledge, as you will see from the many new authors. The titles of sections shows that they have also used a finer mesh to enable them to include such diverse topics as traumatic and photosensitive epilepsy, telemetry, adverse therapeutic effects, and cerebellar stimulation. The first edition came to be used as a standard work of reference, as well as of education. Now the informed can take the second edition from its shelf with some confidence when searching for the up-to-date or the more esoteric topics. The introduction of so much which is new mirrors the change that there can be in modern medicine, even in six short years – a change in the depth of understanding as well as in the breadth of knowledge.

1982   D.W.

Preface to the Second Edition

This edition has been expanded considerably. There has been a major revision and updating of the original chapters and nearly all of our original authors have contributed again. Mr Richardson was not able to revise his chapter on Neurosurgery and we have been very fortunate in being able to include a completely new and stimulating chapter by Mr Polkey.

The first edition was essentially a British textbook, with comments by two American authors. Advisedly, this second edition is more international. We have introduced sub-sections to the main chapters by those with specialised experience and we have included new chapters on subjects such as: Epidemiology, Neuropsychology, Epilepsy in Developing Countries, Epilepsy and Work, and Dental Problems.

In the first edition the chapter on Psychiatry was a combination of the views of Dr Betts and Dr Merskey and Professor Pond. In this edition Dr Betts is responsible for the main section of the chapter with special sections by Professor Sir Desmond Pond and Dr Trimble. Again, the original chapter by Dr Meldrum on Neuropathology and Pathophysiology has been split up with a new section by Professor Mathieson on Pathology and a revised section by Dr Meldrum on Pathophysiology.

With such a larger book and with so many new contributors, it is inevitable that some differences of opinion or emphasis should appear. As editors, we have not in any way tried to introduce conformity to a single viewpoint. There is still so much to be learnt about epilepsy that it is sensible to offer alternative ideas, if only to stimulate further thought. Our original intention was to offer a Textbook of Epilepsy, so that those involved in different disciplines should be able to appreciate the work being done by those in disciplines other than their own. It is our hope that this larger second edition will still meet this need.

With so many contributors we have had even greater problems in keeping to deadlines – keeping the interval between receipt of typescripts and publication as short as possible. Although we may not have been altogether successful, we have done our best. As before, we would like to acknowledge the invaluable help of our secretaries, Mrs Dunbar (JL) and Miss Jones (AR) and in particular Mrs Dunbar, to whom was delegated the unenviable job of keeping authors up to schedule.

1982

J.L.
A.R.

Preface to the First Edition

An essential function of a textbook of epilepsy is to record the present state of our knowledge of all the various aspects of epilepsy. However, there is a serious danger that accumulated information in different fields might prove so extensive and often so recondite that its usefulness can be appreciated only by specialists in their respective disciplines, and might not be intelligible readily to the doctor who has the primary responsibility for the patient, whether he be general practitioner, neurologist, psychiatrist or neurosurgeon. The fundamental concept of this book is that our contributors, well known in their own specialties, should present their experience in such a way that those in other disciplines should be able to understand fully what they are reading. If we have achieved our aim, most of this book should be intelligible and of considerable value to any intelligent educated non-medical person with a particular interest in epilepsy, whether professional or personal. Naturally, experts want to write, in part, for others working in the same field. When this has been done in a manner intelligible and interesting to others, the material has been included in the body of the chapter, but whenever possible technicalities of limited interest have been included in appendices or referred to by reference to the literature.

We have broadened the scope of this essentially British textbook by including, free from editorial interference, contributions from two distinguished physicians from the United States.

We have tried to collect in a coherent whole the very considerable present understanding of epilepsy. Nonetheless, if, from our vantage point as editors, we survey this island of knowledge, we see inevitably that it is compassed by a vast uncharted sea of ignorance. In the Introduction, we will consider briefly some of the fundamental questions about epilepsy which are as yet not answered. The chapters which follow may offer some clues, but, if this book is to serve its real purpose of helping the patient, it will do so by stimulating others to seek answers to those questions, helped we would hope by the knowledge presented in this book.

We would like to thank all those who have made the production of this book possible. Firstly, our contributors who have put up with incessant nagging to achieve the impossible deadlines which we set them. Secondly, our publishers who accepted with equanimity when the impossible could not be achieved. Thirdly, our secretaries Mrs Thrift and Mrs Wilmot (JL) and Miss Hazel Boughton (AR) who, as all authors must know, do the really hard work. Finally, we would like to acknowledge all that we have learnt from the very many people with epilepsy under our care and express the hope that this book may help their doctors the better to help them with knowledge and understanding to overcome a disability which they face with such courage.

1975 J.L.
A.R.

Contributors

Jean Aicardi M.D.
Maître de Recherche, Institut National de la Santé et de la Recherche Medicale, Hôpital des Enfants Malades, Paris, France

T.A. Betts M.B., Ch.B., D.P.M., M.R.C.Psych
Senior Lecturer in Psychiatry, University of Birmingham. Consultant Psychiatrist to the Queen Elizabeth and the General Hospitals, Birmingham

W.T. Blume M.D., F.R.C.P.(C).
Associate Professor, Department of Clinical Neurological Sciences and Paediatrics, University of Western Ontario, London, Ontario. Co-director, Epilepsy Unit, University Hospital, London, Ontario

J. Keith Brown M.B., F.R.C.P., D.C.H.
Consultant Paediatric Neurologist, RHSC, Edinburgh. Senior Lecturer, Department Child Life and Health, University of Edinburgh

Benjamin Chandra M.D., Ph.D.
Professor and Head of Department of Neurology, University of Airlangga, Surabaya

R.E. Cull B.Sc. (Hons Physiol), Ph.D., M.B., Ch.B., M.R.C.P.(UK)
Lecturer in Clinical Neurology, The National Hospitals, London

David D. Daly M.D., Ph.D.
Professor of Neurology, Health Science Center, University of Texas South-western Medical School, Dallas, U.S.A.

M. Dam M.D.
Associate Professor, University Clinic of Neurology, Hvidovre Hospital, Hvidovre, Denmark

Carl B. Dodrill M.D., Ph.D.
Associate Professor of Neurological Surgery, University of Washington School of Medicine, Seattle, Washington, U.S.A.

M.V. Driver M.B., B.S., Ph.D., M.R.C. Psych.
Consultant Neurophysiologist, Bethlem Royal and Maudsley Hospitals, London

R.W. Gilliatt D.M., F.R.C.P.
Professor of Clinical Neurology, The National Hospitals, London

John P. Girvin M.D., Ph.D., F.R.C.S.(C).
Associate Professor, Department of Clinical Neurological Sciences and Physiology, University of Western Ontario, London, Ontario. Co-director, Epilepsy Unit, University Hospital, London, Ontario

Peter M. Jeavons M.A., F.R.C.P., F.R.C. Psych.
Honorary Visiting Professor, Clinical Neurophysiology Unit, Department of Ophthalmic Optics, Aston University in Birmingham

Bryan Jennett M.D., F.R.C.S.
Professor of Neurosurgery, Institute of Neurological Sciences, Glasgow.

B.E. Kendall F.R.C.P., F.R.C.R.
Consultant Radiologist, National Hospitals for Nervous Diseases, Hospital for Sick Children and Middlesex Hospital, London

John Laidlaw F.R.C.P. (Edin)
Consultant Physician to Epilepsy Centre, Quarrier's Homes, Bridge of Weir, Scotland. Formerly Physician in charge, Chalfont Centre for Epilepsy

Mary V. Laidlaw S.R.N.
Rehabilitation Adviser to Epilepsy Centre, Quarrier's Homes, Bridge of Weir, Scotland. Formerly at Chalfont Centre for Epilepsy

Margaret A. Lennox-Buchthal B.A., M.D., Dr. Med.
Associate Professor, Institute of Neurophysiology, University of Copenhagen, Denmark

Michael Linnett O.B.E., M.B., B.S., F.R.C.G.P.
General Practitioner, Sloane Street, London

B.B. McGillivray B.Sc., M.B., F.R.C.P.
Consultant in Clinical Neurophysiology, National Hospitals and the Royal Free Hospital, London

C.D. Marsden M.Sc., F.R.C.P., M.R.C. Psych.
Professor of Neurology, Institute of Psychiatry, King's
College Hospital Medical School, London

B.S. Meldrum M.A., M.B., B.Chir., Ph.D.
Senior Lecturer, Department of Neurology, Institute of
Psychiatry, London

Gordon Mathieson M.B., Ch.B., M.Sc., F.R.C.P. (C)
Professor of Pathology, Memorial University of
Newfoundland, Canada

Maurice Parsonage B.Sc., M.B., F.R.C.P., D.C.H.
Director of the Neuropsychiatric Unit and Special
Centre for Epilepsy, Bootham Park Hospital, York

Emilio Perucca M.D. (It), Ph.D.
Lecturer, Clinical Pharmacology Unit, Institute of
Medical Pharmacology, University of Pavia, Pavia, Italy

C.E. Polkey M.D., F.R.C.S.
Consultant Neurosurgeon, Bethlem Royal Hospital and
Maudsley Hospital, London

Sir Desmond Pond M.A., M.D., F.R.C.P.,
F.R.C.Psych., F.B.P.S.(Hon)
Professor of Psychiatry, The London Hospital Medical
College, London

R. Quy Ph.D.
Research Assistant, Department of Neurology, The
National Hospitals, London

E.H. Reynolds M.D., F.R.C.P.
Consultant Neurologist, Bethlem Royal, Maudsley and
King's College Hospitals. Honorary Senior Lecturer,
University Department of Neurology, Institute of
Psychiatry and King's College Hospital Medical School,
London

A. Richens M.B., B.S., B.Sc., Ph.D., F.R.C.P.
Professor of Pharmacology and Materia Medica, Welsh
National School of Medicine, Cardiff; Consultant
Physician, Llandough Hospital, Cardiff

Ernst A. Rodin M.D.
Professor of Neurology, Wayne State University,
Detroit. Director of EEG and Epilepsy Program,
Henry Ford Hospital, Detroit. Medical Director,
Epilepsy Center of Michigan, Detroit, Michigan

Michael Trimble M.B., B.Sc., M.Phil., M.R.C.P.,
M.R.C. Psych.
Consultant Physician, National Hospitals, London.
Senior Lecturer in Behavioural Neurology, Institute of
Neurology, University of London

Adrian R.M. Upton M.A., M.B., B.Chir., F.R.C.P.(C)
Professor of Medicine, Head Division of Neurology,
Director, Diagnostic Neurophysiology, Visiting
Professor, New York Medical College, New York

Peter Westphal D.D.S.
Chief Dental Officer, Stockholm

Denis Williams, C.B.E., M.D., D.Sc., F.R.C.P.
Honorary Consulting Physician, the National Hospitals,
London. Honorary Consulting Neurologist, St George's
Hospital, London. The Clinical Consultant Neurologist,
the Royal Air Force

R.G. Willison D.M., F.R.C.P.(E)
Consultant Neurophysiologist, University Department
of Neurology, The National Hospitals, London

J.J. Zielinsky M.D., D.Sc.
Associate Professor in Neurology, Psychoneurological
Institute, Warsaw, Poland. The National Hospitals –
Chalfont Centre for Epilepsy, Chalfont St Peter, Bucks

Contents

Introduction

THE CLASSIFICATION OF THE EPILEPSIES

The clinical manifestations of epilepsy in the human subject are multitudinous and the terminologies used to describe them have become so varied and confused that the need to draw up a generally acceptable classification has become increasingly pressing in recent years. The growth of knowledge has tended to encourage the creation of classifications of increasing complexity which have not endeared themselves either to clinicians or to experimental workers. Undoubtedly, the main obstacle in the construction of an adequate classification stems not so much from the extent but the incompleteness of our understanding of epileptic phenomena. At the present time we can therefore only do the best we can with what knowledge we have in the hope that, as understanding increases, our attempts at classification will improve accordingly.

The essential need is a classification which not only embodies all currently available knowledge but which also combines sufficient clarity and simplicity to make it generally acceptable. Such a classification would help to improve communication in the field of epilepsy. This is particularly important now that there are so many workers in so many allied disciplines and the need to establish a common language has never been greater than it is now.

As a basis to any discussion on the classification of epileptic phenomena we need to be clear in our minds about the distinctions between classifications of epileptic seizures as opposed to those which apply to the epilepsies themselves. With seizures we are primarily concerned with clinical manifestations and with their neurophysiological basis, whereas with the epilepsies we are more concerned with groupings of seizures or syndromes, their natural histories and their underlying causes. Failure to observe these distinctions has often led to confusion in the past and still seems to be doing so at the present time.

Classification of epileptic seizures

It is now more than ten years since the publication of a scheme for the classification of seizures recommended by the International League Against Epilepsy (Gastaut, 1969). This is reproduced in full on pages xviii–xxiv. Despite its imperfections it has been widely used and I believe it has much to commend it, as a careful study of it will show.

Three main categories of seizure are recognised in the International Classification, namely, *partial* (*I*), *generalised* (*II*), and *unilateral* (*III*), with a fourth category for those which cannot yet be classified. In all categories the basic criteria are fourfold – clinical, EEG (ictal and interictal), aetiological and chronological in that order.

The subdivision of partial seizures into those with *elementary* (*simple*) and those with *complex symptomatology* is based on the assumption that the latter arise in areas of 'higher' cerebral organisation and are generally associated with impairment of consciousness. In addition, there is recognition of the fact that all partial seizures may become *secondarily generalised*, a phenomenon which sometimes occurs so rapidly as to obscure any focal features. Such generalisation most commonly takes the form of tonic-clonic (grand mal) seizures, although sometimes there may be either tonic or clonic manifestations alone.

The subdivision of *simple partial seizures* into motor, sensory, autonomic and compound forms has not been seriously challenged over the years and requires no further comment here.

There have however been objections to some of the sub-categories of *complex partial seizures*. For example, a complex partial seizure characterized only by impaired consciousness has been criticized as a rather doubtful entity; indeed, the frequent association of other features, such as psychosensory, affective or psychomotor manifestations, would often enable them to be placed in other categories (Gastaut & Broughton, 1972). However, it must be pointed out that Gloor et al (1980) have recently reported instances of seizures of temporal lobe origin in which loss of consciousness (defined as unresponsiveness) was virtually the only clinical sign. Nevertheless, in the vast majority of the seizures studied by these observers the accompanying epileptic seizure discharges involved both temporal lobes widely as well as limbic and neocortical structures; there was however one instance in which there appeared to be only minimal limbic involvement. Nevertheless the inclusion of such seizures under the term 'partial' does seem questionable if there is strict adherence to the definition laid down in the International Classification. It may also be argued that the term 'focal' is hardly applicable to any seizure in which there is impairment of consciousness, since the latter is a phenomenon which appears to be dependent upon the integrity of function in both cortical and brain stem structures. Furthermore, if impairment or loss of consciousness be equated with unresponsiveness, as may be observed in association with some partial seizures, some would maintain that such a state might more properly be regarded as inattentiveness or diminished vigilance.

It has also been questioned (Parsonage, 1979) as to whether seizures with 'psychomotor' symptomatology (automatisms) should properly be regarded as 'partial' as defined in the International Classification. Such seizures seem to be most commonly associated with widespread discharges involving cortical and diencephalic structures (see Fenton, 1980); moreover, they resemble absences in many respects and they may even sometimes be generalised from the onset. On these grounds it could be argued that they should really be regarded as generalised seizures.

The International Classification of *generalised seizures* seems to have been widely accepted and has been subjected to only minor criticisms. Thus, it has been said that the subdivision of absences into numerous sub-varieties is needlessly complicated and of academic rather than practical value; however, I think that there is some justification for this even if only on the grounds of the variable responsiveness to treatment of the various sub-varieties. It has also been advocated that so-called akinetic seizures might be jettisoned from the list as a somewhat doubtful entity.

The designation of *unilateral or predominantly unilateral seizures* as a separate group has not perhaps been universally accepted but I believe it can be justified on the grounds of the variable features and age-dependence which they show.

Classification of the epilepsies

Up to the present time there has never been an officially recommended international classification of the epilepsies. Gastaut (1969) made a valiant attempt to create one but in view of the many criticisms to which it was subjected he concluded that his proposals could best be regarded as a basis for discussion directed towards constructing a more satisfactory classification in the future.

Gastaut proposed that the epilepsies be subdivided into two main groups – the *generalised* and the *partial (focal)*. It has, of course, been pointed out that they can be classified in other ways with varying emphasis on such basic criteria as aetiology, type of seizure and anatomical localisation. Even so, I believe there is still much to be said for Gastaut's proposed basic sub-division, although some might feel that the use of the terms 'generalised' and 'partial' in this context also could be a source of confusion.

The *generalised epilepsies* can be further subdivided into primary and secondary varieties. The *primary generalised epilepsies* are manifested by seizures which are invariably generalised from their onset, are usually unassociated with neuropsychiatric disorders and are generally considered to have a predominantly genetic basis. The *secondary generalised epilepsies*, on the other hand, give rise to seizures which may be either generalised from the start or secondarily generalised from a focal source which is not apparent; furthermore, such epilepsies can often be ascribed, but by no means always, to diffuse or multi-focal cerebral lesions and are frequently associated with other neuropsychiatric disorders. West's syndrome, the Lennox-Gastaut syndrome and the progressive myoclonus epilepsies are important members of this group. Nevertheless, it must be recognized that the distinctions between these two major subdivisions are not absolute. Rather is it better to regard the generalised epilepsies as a large group embodying a wide range of disorders in which there are forms which are intermediate between the two extremes as well as others which show features common to both.

In contrast, the *partial (focal) epilepsies* are associated with cortical seizure discharges which are either localised or diffuse, even generalised. The patterns of the seizures themselves are determined by the site of origin of the discharges, having a characteristic local onset often leading to secondary generalisation in the form of tonic-clonic seizures. These epilepsies are typically associated with a 'more or less evident organic aetiology' (trauma, tumour, etc.) and may be further subdivided on a topographical basis into frontal lobe, temporal lobe epilepsies, etc. They may also be classified in accordance with their predominant type of seizure; for example, simple, complex, psychomotor epilepsies, etc.

GENERAL COMMENTS ON TERMINOLOGY

Perusal of the various chapters of this textbook will make it clear that there has not been unqualified acceptance of the International Classification of epileptic seizures. Indeed, their contents reflect commonly held individual views and an understandable desire to retain familiar terms in accordance with their original usage. Certainly, some degree of flexibility in this situation is both desirable and inevitable and it now only remains for me to make some attempt at collation in order to try and remove at least some of the possible sources of confusion.

Partial seizures

Despite the now widespread application of the term 'partial' to seizures of localised origin the term 'focal' continues to be used as an acceptable alternative. It is, after all, deeply ingrained in the minds of many and it effectively embodies a widely recognised concept despite the objection that some seizures, especially those arising in the temporal lobes, have too diffuse an origin to be regarded as focal in nature.

There are evident differences of view about the criteria for subdividing partial seizures into those with simple and those with complex symptomatology. As stated earlier, in the International Classification this is based on whether the lower or higher levels of cerebral organisation are involved in the seizure process, the associated maintenance or impairment of consciousness being a secondary consideration. As an alternative method of subdivision the preservation or loss of consciousness has been used as a primary criterion (see Table 4.1, p. 99). As discussed earlier, this could give rise to difficulties with regard to a different use of the terms 'partial' and 'complex' and also with regard to problems related to the definition of what is meant by unconsciousness.

In accordance with the definition of simple partial seizures used in the International Classification there seems to be general acceptance of their subdivision into those with motor, sensory (including special sensory) and autonomic features. It is however perhaps noteworthy that there is nowadays a much wider use of the term 'Jacksonian' which is applied to both motor and sensory seizures of local origin. Indeed, it could also be applied to complex seizures involving affect, cognition, etc., although not so readily in view of our less complete knowledge of their neurophysiology. Even so, this usage of the term signifies the widely recognized tendency of partial seizures to exhibit a 'march' of events in accordance with anatomico-physiological organization.

A further problem with regard to the classification of those partial seizures characterised by what may be termed psychic or psychological experiences is highlighted in Parts one and two of Chapter 4. In Part two of this chapter there is strict adherence to the International Classification and it will be noted that those seizures causing altered perception of surroundings (déjà vu, etc.) are here classified as disturbances of cognitive function with dysmnesic features and not as illusions of perception (Gastaut & Broughton, 1972). There is also recognition of the usual subdivision of psychosensory seizures into two types – firstly, illusions of perception (distortions of vision, hearing and bodily configuration) and, secondly, those which give rise to highly organized hallucinatory experiences related to vision, hearing, etc. It should however be remembered that the latter are to be distinguished from those types of simple partial seizure in which sensory and autonomic functions are involved at a comparatively low level of organization; for example, simple, undifferentiated sounds or smells in auditory and olfactory seizures respectively.

On the basis of the recommendation in Chapter 4, Part one (see Table 4.1) that partial seizures be subdivided in accordance with whether or not consciousness is impaired it will be seen that what would be regarded as either cognitive or affective features in the International Classification now come under the heading of complex partial seizures with 'psychic' symptoms. The latter category includes both 'thought disturbances' (déjà vu, etc.), 'perceptual disturbances' (hallucinations, distorted perceptions) and 'emotional experiences' (fear, etc.). Finally, it will be noted that seizures with automatisms are designated as belonging solely to those of the complex partial variety.

The recognition of a type of complex partial seizure characterised by impairment of consciousness alone, as in the International Classification, is not a subject of specific discussion in this volume and need not be referred to again. On the other hand reference is made to the well recognized fact that seizures with psychomotor symptomatology are a common manifestation of temporal lobe epilepsy, although it is recognized that the two terms are not interchangeable. Indeed, it has rightly been pointed out that such seizures may arise from sources other than the temporal lobes and may sometimes be apparently generalized from the onset. That they have many features in common with absences with automatisms has also been rightly emphasized (see Ch. 4, Part two), and I would once again express doubts about the correctness of classifying seizures with psycho-motor symptomatology (automatisms) as partial in type. Loss of consciousness associated with automatic actions and subsequent amnesia must surely reflect widespread and not localised disturbance of cerebral function.

Generalised seizures

The use of terminology with regard to generalised seizures does not pose any great problems, although there are a few interchangeable terms which deserve brief mention.

The term 'absence' has come into very general use in recent years, although some still may prefer to retain the familiar synonym 'petit mal'. The latter has acquired a lack of precision in that it has been applied to almost any type of seizure short of a generalised convulsion and calls to mind the use of 'minor' and 'major' in this context. The term 'absence' therefore seems preferable both descriptively and because it has been clearly defined in both clinical and EEG terms. Perhaps therefore it might be more usefully applied to that variety of generalised epilepsy of which absences are the sole manifestation. The term 'atypical absence' has now replaced its forerunner 'petit mal variant'.

With regard to generalised seizures with predominantly motor manifestations, 'myoclonic jerks' is an alternative term to 'bilateral massive epileptic myoclonus' and 'epileptic drop attacks' is an acceptable alternative to atonic seizures of brief duration. Some may wish to retain the terms 'myoclonic-atonic' or 'myoclonic-astatic' for those atonic seizures in which myoclonic and atonic components are combined and there are still some who prefer the term 'grand mal' to tonic-clonic seizure for a generalised convulsion. Perhaps however it might nowadays be better to use this term to designate that form of generalised epilepsy giving rise only to tonic-clonic convulsive attacks in a way comparable to the suggested use of the term 'petit mal'.

The epilepsies

Epilepsy of temporal lobe origin figures largely among the *partial epilepsies* in view of its commonness and the widespread interest which its manifestations and associated disorders have generated over so many years. Indeed, little or nothing is heard of such terms as frontal or parietal lobe epilepsy and the tendency seems to be to designate epilepsies of such origin in accordance with the type of seizure to which they predominantly give rise. A welcome trend is the growing recognition of benign centrotemporal (Rolandic) epilepsy of childhood as a unique variety of partial epilepsy in view of its benign course and its probable genetic origin (O'Donoghue, 1980).

The subdivision of the *generalised epilepsies* into primary and secondary varieties seems to be recognized as useful, although there are differences in detail with regard to the terminology used in this context. Thus, the *primary variety* is variously referred to as 'essential', 'idiopathic' or 'cryptogenic' epilepsy, and may be further divided into such sub-varieties as petit mal epilepsy (pyknolepsy), juvenile myoclonic or impulsive petit mal epilepsy (Janz, 1973), petit mal–grand mal epilepsy and grand mal epilepsy. The *secondary varieties* embody a wider range of manifestations and include such important sub-varieties as the syndromes of West (infantile spasms) and of Lennox-Gastaut, the latter being a welcome alternative to the cumbersome term 'epileptic encephalopathy with diffuse sharp and slow wave discharges' despite disagreement about its precise definition (see Ch. 3, Part three).

Problems with regard to the classification of the myoclonic and other types of childhood epilepsy not included in the already recognized syndromes are discussed in Chapter 3, Part three. In general, it seems wise to adapt a classification in accordance with the predominant type of seizure. In conclusion, it seems hardly possible yet to make a satisfactory classification of those episodic disorders thought to be or suspected of being epileptic in nature, and apparently arising in the brain stem or basal ganglia (see Ch. 3, Part one), until they are better understood.

CONCLUSION

The subject of the classification of epileptic disorders is one which will clearly need to be debated for a long time to come. This should however give continuing impetus to the quest for new knowledge which will throw more light on the many dark areas waiting to be illuminated. Inevitably, I have not been able to do more than scant justice to so great a problem in this introduction since it is surely not the place for lengthy discussions. As a final note I would again make a plea for simplicity rather than complexity in the creation of future classifications. There are already foreshadowings of a trend towards the unification of epileptic phenomena (Gloor, 1979) and this is surely a trend that we should welcome.

Clinical and electroencephalographic classification of epileptic seizures recommended by the *International League against Epilepsy*, the *World Federation of Neurology*, the *World Federation of Neurosurgical Societies* and the *International Federation of Societies for Electroencephalography and Clinical Neurophysiology*

Clinical seizure type	Electroencephalographic seizure type	Electroencephalographic interictal expression*	Anatomical substrate	Etiology	Age

I. PARTIAL SEIZURES OR SEIZURES BEGINNING LOCALLY

Seizures in which the first clinical changes indicate activation of an anatomical and/or functional system of neurones limited to a part of a single hemisphere; in which the inconsistently present electrographic seizure patterns are restricted, at least at their onset, to one region of the scalp (the area corresponding to the cortical representation of the system involved); and in which the initial neuronal discharge usually originates in a narrowly limited or even quite diffuse cortical (the most accessible and vulnerable) part of such a system.

Clinical seizure type	Electroencephalographic seizure type	Electroencephalographic interictal expression*	Anatomical substrate	Etiology	Age
Elementary or complex symptomatology depending on the discharge of a system localized in one or, sometimes, both hemispheres	Rhythmic discharge of spikes and/or of more or less slow waves more or less localized over one or, sometimes, both hemispheres	Intermittent local discharges, generally over one hemisphere only	Various cortical and/or subcortical regions corresponding with functional representation in one hemisphere	Usually related to a wide variety of local brain lesions (cause known, suspected or unknown). Constitutional factors may be important	Possible at all ages but more frequent with increasing age·
A. Partial seizures with elementary symptomatology (generally without impairment of consciousness)	local contralateral discharge starting over the corresponding area of cortical representation (not always recorded on the scalp)	local contralateral discharges	usually in the cortical region of one hemisphere corresponding to functional representation	as above	as above

1. *With motor symptoms*
    (i) focal motor (without march), including localized epileptic myoclonus
    (ii) jacksonian
    (iii) versive (generally contraversive)
    (iv) postural
    (v) somatic inhibitory(?)
    (vi) aphasic
    (vii) phonatory (vocalization and arrest of speech)

* The incidence of interictal abnormalities varies; they may be absent.

Clinical seizure type	Electroencephalographic seizure type	Electroencephalographic interictal expression	Anatomical substrate	Etiology	Age
2. *With special sensory or somatosensory symptoms* (i) somato-sensory (ii) visual (iii) auditory (iv) olfactory (v) gustatory (vi) vertiginous					
3. *With automic symptoms*					
4. *Compound forms*****					
B. Partial seizures with complex symptomatology***** (generally with impairment of consciousness; may sometimes begin with elementary symptomatology)	unilateral or bilateral discharge, diffuse, or focal in temporal or fronto-temporal regions	unilateral or bilateral, generally asynchronous, focus; usually in the temporal region(s)	usually cortical and/or subcortical temporal or fronto-temporal regions (including rhinencephalic structures), unilateral or bilateral	as above	as above
1. With impaired consciousness alone					
2. With cognitive symptomatology (i) with dysmnesic disturbances (conscious amnesia, 'déjà vu', 'déjà vécu") (ii) with ideational disturbances (including 'forced thinking', dreamy state...)					

** Compound implies a joining together of elementary or (and/or) complex symptoms.

*** Complex vs. elementary, implies an organized, high-level cerebral activity.

Clinical seizure type	Electroencephalographic seizure type	Electroencephalographic interictal expression	Anatomical substrate	Etiology	Age
3. *With affective symptomatology*					
4. *With 'psychosensory' symptomatology* (i) illusions (*e.g.* macropsia, metamorphopsia) (ii) hallucinations					
5. *With 'psychomotor' symptomatology* (automatisms)					
6. *Compound forms*					
C. Partial seizures secondarily generalized (all forms of partial seizures, with elementary or complex symptomatology, can develop into generalized seizures, sometimes so rapidly that the focal features may be unobservable. These generalized seizures may be symmetrical or asymmetrical, tonic or clonic, but most often tonic-clonic in type)	above discharge becomes secondarily and rapidly generalized		⟶ refer to partial seizures in general ───────		

II. GENERALIZED SEIZURES, BILATERAL SYMMETRICAL SEIZURES OR SEIZURES WITHOUT LOCAL ONSET

Seizures in which the clinical features do not include any sign or symptom referable to an anatomical and/or functional system localized in one hemisphere, and usually consist of initial impairment of consciousness, motor changes which are generalized or at least bilateral and more or less symmetrical and may be accompanied by an "en masse" autonomic discharge; in which the electroencephalographic patterns from the start are bilateral, grossly synchronous and symmetrical over the two hemispheres; and in which the responsible neuronal discharge takes place, if not throughout the entire grey matter, then at least in the greater part of it and simultaneously on both sides.

Clinical seizure type	Electroencephalographic seizure type	Electroencephalographic interictal expression	Anatomical substrate	Etiology	Age
Convulsive or non-convulsive symptomatology, without sign referable to a unilateral system localized in one hemisphere	Bilateral, essentially synchronous and symmetrical discharge from the start	Bilateral, essentially synchronous and usually symmetrical discharges	Unlocalized (? meso-diencephalon)	No cause found or: (i) diffuse or multiple bilateral lesions, and/or: (ii) toxic and/or metabolic disturbances, and/or: (iii) constitutional, often genetic factors (epileptic predisposition)	All ages
1. Absences (a) Simple absences, with impairment of consciousness only	1. with rhythmic 3 c/s spike and wave discharge ('petit mal' or typical absence)	spike and waves and/or polyspike and wave discharges	as above	as above (organic etiology is unusual)	especially in children
	2. without 3 c/s spike and wave (variant of 'petit mal' or atypical absence) (i) low-voltage fast activity or rhythmic discharge at 10 or more c/s, or (ii) more or less rhythmic discharge of sharp and slow waves, sometimes asymmetrical	more or less rhythmic discharges of sharp and slow waves, sometimes asymmetrical	as above	as above(organic etiology is usual; cerebral metabolic disturbances superimposed on previous brain lesion may be important)	especially in children
(b) Complex absences, with other phenomena associated with impairment of consciousness (i) with mild clonic components (myoclonic absences)			as above	as above	as above

Clinical seizure type	Electroencephalographic seizure type	Electroencephalographic interictal expression	Anatomical substrate	Etiology	Age
(ii) with increase of postural tone (retropulsive absences)					
(iii) with diminution or abolition of postural tone (atonic absences)					
(iv) with automatisms (automatic absences)					
(v) with autonomic phenomena (*e.g.* enuretic absences)					
(vi) as mixed forms					
2. *Bilateral massive epileptic myoclonus* (myoclonic jerks)	polyspike and waves or, sometimes, spike and waves or sharp and slow waves	polyspike and waves, or spike and waves, sometimes sharp and slow waves	as above	as above	all ages
3. *Infantile spasms*	flattening of the hypsarhythmia during the spasm, or exceptionally more prominent spikes and slow waves	hypsarhythmia	as above	as above (cerebral metabolic disturbances superimposed on previous brain lesion may be important)	infants only
4. *Clonic seizures*	mixture of fast (10 c/s or more) and slow waves with occasional spike and wave patterns	spike and waves and/or polyspike and wave discharges	as above	as above	especially in children

Clinical seizure type	Electroencephalographic seizure type	Electroencephalographic interictal expression	Anatomical substrate	Etiology	Age
5. *Tonic seizures*	low voltage fast activity or a fast rhythm (10 c/s or more) decreasing in frequency and increasing in amplitude	more or less rhythmic discharges of sharp and slow waves, sometimes asymmetrical	as above	as above (organic etiology is usual)	especially in children
6. *Tonic-clonic seizures* ('grand mal' seizures)	rhythm at 10 or more c/s, decreasing in frequency and increasing in amplitude during the tonic phase, interrupted by slow waves during the clonic phase	polyspike and waves and/or spike and waves or, sometimes, sharp and slow wave discharges	as above	as above	less frequent in young children than other forms of generalized seizures. All ages except infancy
7. *Atomic seizures* sometimes associated with myoclonic jerks (myoclonic-atonic seizures)			as above	as above (organic etiology is usual)	especially in children
(a) of very brief duration (epileptic drop attacks)	polyspike and waves (more waves than in the myoclonic polyspike and wave)	polyspike and wave			
(b) of longer duration (including atonic absences)	rhythmic spike and wave (3 to 1 c/s) or mixture of fast and slow waves with occasional spike and wave patterns	polyspike and waves and/or spike and waves or, sometimes, sharp and slow wave discharges			
8. *Akinetic seizures* (loss of movement without atonia)	rhythmic spike and wave (3 to 1 c/s) or mixture of fast and slow waves with occasional spike and wave patterns	polyspike and waves and/or spike and waves or, sometimes, sharp and slow wave discharges	as above	as above	especially in children

III. UNILATERAL OR PREDOMINANTLY UNILATERAL SEIZURES

Seizures in which the clinical and electrographic aspects are analogous to those of the preceding group (II), except that the clinical signs are restricted principally, if not exclusively, to one side of the body and the electrographic discharges are recorded over the contralateral hemisphere. Such seizures apparently depend upon a generalized or at least very diffuse neuronal discharge which predominates in, or is restricted to, a single hemisphere and its subcortical connections.

Clinical seizure type	Electroencephalographic seizure type	Electroencephalographic interictal expression	Anatomical substrate	Etiology	Age
A. Characterised by clonic, tonic or tonic-clonic convulsions, with or without an impairment of consciousness, expressed only or predominantly in one side. Such seizures sometimes shift from one side to the other but usually do not become symmetrical	(i) partial discharge very rapidly spreading over only one hemisphere (corresponding with only contralateral seizures), or:	focal contralateral discharges	cortical and/or subcortical region in one hemisphere	wide variety of focal, unilateral lesions, generally in immature brain (constitutional factors may be important)	almost exclusively in very young children
	(ii) discharges generalised from the start but considerably predominant over one hemisphere, susceptible to change from one side to the other at different moments (corresponding to alternating seizures)	bilateral and synchronous symmetrical or asymmetrical discharges of spike and waves and/or polyspike and waves	unlocalized (? mesodiencephalon)	no cause found, or: (i) diffuse or multiple bilateral lesions, and/or: (ii) toxic metabolic perturbations, and/or: (iii) constitutional, often genetic factors (epileptic predisposition), generally in immature brain	almost exclusively in very young children
	(iii) partial discharge, susceptible to change, from time to time, in morphology and topography (from area to area and, sometimes, from one side to the other)	focal discharges, susceptible to change, from time to time, in morphology and topography	cortical and/or subcortical region in one or both hemispheres, or unlocalized	focal or diffuse lesions of diverse etiology or metabolic and/or toxic. Constitutional factors and cerebral immaturity are important	limited virtually to the new-born

IV. UNCLASSIFIED EPILEPTIC SEIZURES

Includes all seizures which cannot be classified because of inadequate or incomplete data.

ADDENDUM

Epileptic seizures have been considered in the light of clinical, electroencephalographic, anatomical and etiological factors. They may also be classified according to their frequency:

(1) Isolated epileptic seizures: epileptic seizures that occur only once. They are usually generalized tonic-clonic seizures provoked by some accidental cause in subjects predisposed to convulsions, but they may be spontaneous epileptic seizures of any other type. A subject who shows an isolated epileptic seizure is not to be regarded as an epileptic.

(2) Repeated epileptic seizures occur under a variety of circumstances:

(i) as fortuitous attacks, coming unexpectedly and without any apparent provocation;

(ii) as cyclic attacks, at more or less regular intervals (*e.g.*, in relation to the menstrual cycle, or the sleep-waking cycle);

(iii) as attacks provoked by: (a) non-sensory factors (fatigue, alcohol, emotion, etc.) or (b) sensory factors, and sometimes referred to as 'reflex seizures'.

(3) Prolonged or repetitive seizures (status epilepticus). The term 'status epilepticus' is used whenever a seizure persists for a sufficient length of time or is repeated frequently enough to produce a fixed and enduring epileptic condition. ('Status' implies a fixed or enduring state). Status epilepticus may be divided into partial (*e.g.* jacksonian), or generalized (*e.g.* absence status or tonic-clonic status), or unilateral (*e.g.* hemiclonic) types.

REFERENCES

Fenton, G.W. (1980) Epilepsy and automatism. In Symposium on Recent Advances in Epilepsy. Supplement, *Irish Medical Journal*, **73**, No. 10, pp. 11–19.

Gastaut, H. (1969) Classification of the epilepsies. Supplement, *Epilepsia*, **10**, S14.

Gastaut, H. (1969) Clinical and electroencephalographical classification of epileptic seizures. International League Against Epilepsy. Supplement, *Epilepsia*, **10**, S2–S13.

Gastaut, H. & Broughton, R. (1972) In *Epileptic Seizures – Clinical and Electrographic Features, Diagnosis and Treatment*. Springfield: Thomas.

Gloor, P. (1979) Generalised epilepsy with spike-and-wave discharge – a re-interpretation of its electrographic and clinical manifestations. *Epilepsia*, **20**, 571.

Gloor, P., Olivier, A. & Ives, J. (1980) Loss of consciousness in temporal lobe seizures; observations obtained with stereotaxic depth electrode recordings and stimulations. In Canger, R., Angelen, F. & Penry, J.K. (eds) *Advances in Epileptology. XIth Epilepsy International Symposium*, pp. 349–353. New York: Raven Press.

Janz, D. (1973) The natural history of primary generalised epilepsies with sporadic myoclonias of the 'impulsive petit mal' type. In Lugaresi, E., Pazzaglia, P. & Tassinari, C.A. (eds) *Evolution and Prognosis of Epilepsies*, pp. 55–72. Milan: Italseber Farmaceutici.

O'Donohue, N.V. (1980) Benign focal epilepsy of childhood. Supplement, *Irish Medical Journal*, **73**, No. 10, 62.

Parsonage, M.J. (1979) In *Aspects of Epilepsy. Proceedings of the Oxford Scientific Meeting of the International League Against Epilepsy (British Branch)*, pp. 17–25. MCS Consultants.

Penfield, W. (1958) Discussion. In Baldwin, M. & Bailey, P. (eds) *Temporal Lobe Epilepsy*, pp. 26–32. Springfield: Thomas.

Penfield, W. (1969) Epilepsy, Neurophysiology and some Brain Mechanisms related to Consciousness. In Jaspar, H.H., Ward, A.A. & Pope, A. (eds) *Basic Mechanisms of the Epilepsies*, Ch. 29, pp. 791–805. London: Churchill.

1

People with epilepsy – the burden of epilepsy

M.J. Linnett

We are concerned in this book to explore every area of knowledge and every modern technique that can help the person with epilepsy, and it is appropriate that a general practitioner with a special interest in the disease should have been invited to write the opening chapter of a book of which the greater part is by specialists in their various fields. For the initial diagnosis of epilepsy is often not in serious doubt, as its general characteristics are well described and documented, although the exceptions may present diagnostic problems of great interest; but in the management of epilepsy the successful treatment of the patient and his family is particularly dependent on the interplay of the expertise of the specialist and the personal knowledge and experience of the family doctor.

Although the condition is common, there are relatively few people with epilepsy in the care of any one family doctor. Nevertheless, he has the responsibility for taking most of the decisions which may affect profoundly the patient and his family. The extent to which he is able to advise such a family will, of course, depend on his experience of the condition and his knowledge of the special problems that arise when an otherwise normal individual is subject to unpredictable episodes of unconsciousness for shorter or longer periods. But when all the investigations have been done, and all the specialists have given their views, it will be the family's own doctor who will explain and interpret the opinions that have been given, and who will adapt them to the special needs of that family, modifying them where necessary as time passes. The concept of continuous care and support by the general practitioner over a considerable length of time is crucial to the proper treatment and management of epilepsy, however many other medical disciplines, social workers, or other members of the health team may from time to time be asked for advice.

In this chapter I will describe the initial impact of epilepsy on the family, and the first involvement of the family doctor. I will refer to the various forms of epilepsy as they present in general practice, although a detailed analysis will be given in later chapters. Emphasis will be placed on the continuing need for explanation, and the need to adapt it to the powers of comprehension of the patient and his family, at every stage of investigation and treatment. The latter part of the chapter will consider problems that arise in the everyday life and family setting of the patient, and the help that the family doctor can give in solving them.

A surprising number of doctors and nurses have never seen a major epileptic attack, so it seems appropriate to begin with short narratives, written by a patient and by a member of his family, which show in a personal way what it means to have an attack, and what it means to a family to witness one.

THE ATTACK

This description of his attack was written by an 18-year-old as soon as he had recovered:

'Have I? Yes I have. I must have done otherwise the light wouldn't be up there. I wish somebody would turn the bloody thing off. Give me a spit bowl, I want to spit.'
There then issued from his mouth the gurgling noise indicative of someone about to relieve themselves of excess mucus and sputum. Some deep instinct, rather than any conscious thought, forced him on to his feet. Standing up was difficult as it entailed putting all his twelve stone weight on to one chair, which he remembered even in his groggy

state, was fragile at the best of times. As he struggled to get up, a faint but perceptible whiff of burnt steak drifted into his nostrils.

This was the only means he had of knowing what he had been doing thirty seconds, two minutes or even twenty-four hours previously. The time lag was unimportant because as far as he was concerned it did not exist – only the sight of flames shooting out in luminous streaks from beneath the grill. Consciously galvanizing himself into activity he blew out the flames and turned on the extractor fan. In so doing he almost lost his balance once again, and found himself looking down at the frying pan full of boiling fat with which he had almost steadied himself.

He then sat down to enjoy a couple of aspirins as an aperitif to his carboniferous steak and chips. He felt the large bump developing on his forehead, wondering which shade of glorious technicolour it would be next morning. It also occurred to him that three fits in two weeks was unusual – possibly due to exam strain. Well, it would be nice to think so anyhow.

Only he now knew that a minute before he had been prostrate on the kitchen floor, to all intents and purposes dead, at any rate from his point of view. This, however, introduced an element of the melodramatic into the subject which he dismissed as being alien and indeed contrary to the truth of the matter.

Half an hour after the fit no evidence of what had happened remained except for the bump and an odd taste of nothing in particular in his mouth which he knew from experience would take several hours to disappear. The slight numbness in the head, which was also felt, and the odd indefinable taste were, although impossible to describe fully, sensations which could never be forgotten.

A parent describes the first time his family saw one of his son's attacks:

It was Christmas morning and the children had come into our room to open presents. They sat all three bouncing around on the foot of our bed, the younger girl in the middle, Jonathan and his older sister on each side.

Suddenly one of them shouted 'Mummy, something's wrong with Jonathan,' and we all looked at him. He sat quite still, with a fixed stare in his eyes. Slowly his head turned to the left and his eyes moved sideways. His body stiffened, and as he began to slide off the bed I jumped out and supported him. For seconds he seemed to get tighter and tighter, and his colour became pallid and then a horrible blue. Then small convulsive movements began in his arms and legs, which although they were not violent were very forceful and not to be restrained. He grunted, as if he were making a great physical effort with each jerk. This seemed to go on for an eternity, although it cannot have been much more than half a minute, with his colour getting worse all the time.

Then it stopped, fairly quickly, and he lay there with his eyes turned up, once again motionless, not even seeming to breathe. I felt for his pulse and it was still there. As I held his wrist, Jonathan gave a few deep gasping breaths, and his colour began to come back, and the blueness disappeared. He coughed and spat, and my wife wiped his lips with a handkerchief because he seemed to have much more saliva than usual.

When he was breathing normally again, and murmuring to us, we carried him back to his bed, where he slept for a quarter of an hour. When he got up, he was a bit tired and silent, but he was soon back to normal, and returned to his very subdued sisters for more opening of presents.

I suppose the whole incident could only have lasted less than half an hour, but those thirty minutes changed our family life.

These narratives describe, from different points of view, typical grand mal attacks of so-called idiopathic epilepsy. They are quoted as accounts by those who experienced them, of events which will be described in clinical terms in later chapters; the intense emotions, which their restrained wording does not completely conceal, are common to all people with epilepsy, in whichever of its varieties it may present, and to all families who have to live with it.

THE INITIAL IMPACT ON THE FAMILY

The reaction of a family to the appearance of fits in one of its members will vary with the type of fit, the way in which it declares itself, and the age of the patient; and the reaction will differ between parents and brothers and sisters, husband or wife.

Infantile convulsions, even when they occur with a fever, can cause great anxiety, especially when there is a history of febrile convulsions in one or other parent; there is intense concern over the management of the fit, and the likelihood of recurrence or brain damage. It is usually possible, however, by explanation and practical reassurance to allay fears for the future, and unless there are several attacks it may be wiser not to pursue immediately more complex forms of investigation which are likely to prove unprofitable.

In early childhood the onset of petit mal attacks may pass unnoticed at first, until it is realized that the child is having frequent *dreamy* attacks, in which he either stops whatever he is doing, or makes only vaguely purposeful movements while he seems to be staring into the distance, unapproachable. When this has happened a few times, the parents usually will realise that there is something abnormal, and will take the child to their doctor. If a good history can be obtained, it is possible in most cases to make the diagnosis at once, whether or not an attack occurs during the consultation. Petit mal is very much less alarming than a generalized convulsion, although if parents are aware of the possible implications there may be great anxiety.

The first grand mal attack of adolescence is of course the most shattering for the family. It may occur on the way to school, when the child is seen to have a fit in the street, the ambulance is sent for, and he is taken to hospital. Or the police may be involved and the first news the parents receive is their child's appearance at the front door, supported by two policemen. Or the attack may occur at school, when it may well cause more alarm to the teaching staff than to the pupils, who seem to take such matters remarkably calmly, and will usually refrain from the more damaging forms of first aid. In whatever way the attack is announced, but especially if it happens at home in front of brothers or sisters, the reaction will be one of intense alarm, dismay and anxiety, amounting often to a sense of disaster, since in the post-clonic phase the child may literally look like death. The doctor will be summoned as a matter of urgency, and the way in which he deals with this family crisis may be crucial in determining for years ahead the pattern of that family's reaction to its new burden.

Reactions to major epileptic attacks occurring for the first time in adults are curiously variable. If the attack is post-traumatic, the fact that there is an obvious explanation may make the situation less intolerable: many patients and their families will be aware of this complication of head injury, and will regard it as something that can be controlled and is likely eventually to disappear. The immediate implications for driving a motor vehicle and for employment will be worrying and frustrating to the patient, but symptoms for which there is an obvious reason and a reasonable hope of control may not be especially frightening. The fit that appears without obvious cause and is perhaps the first symptom of serious intracranial disease can be much more alarming: the patient will only know that he had a lapse of consciousness, but his relatives will have found the sequence of events in a full grand mal attack very disturbing. Focal or Jacksonian attacks however, which at first can be relatively trivial, may not cause enough disquiet to prompt consulting the doctor until the pattern is further developed; a delay in investigation and treatment which may be of considerable importance.

THE FIRST APPEAL TO THE FAMILY DOCTOR

The realization that there is something abnormal about their child's behaviour, the occurrence of a convulsion in an infant or in an adult, will usually prompt relatives, full of anxiety for the future, to consult their family doctor. He will need to listen with care and sympathy to the narrative and to take a careful history on which he can base a provisional diagnosis. He can then when necessary initiate investigations and obtain specialist advice which may produce a more accurate diagnosis and make possible the planning of treatment. At each stage he must be ready to explain what he has learnt, what it means, what can be done, and what is implied for the future, and all those factors will vary as the child grows up, or as the observation and investigation of an adult progresses.

What has happened?

In a survey of the epilepsies in general practice by the Research Committee of the Royal College of General Practitioners (1960), the following definition was suggested by Denis Williams:

> Epilepsy for our purpose will include all attacks primarily cerebral in origin in which there is disturbance of *movement*, *feeling* or *consciousness*.

Although this definition exactly served the purpose of the survey, it referred only to clinical manifestations, and was not intended to take any account of the fundamental neuronal disturbances which produce them. It is possible to postulate and often to demonstrate in the laboratory the kind of neuronal discharge, localized or progressive, which will produce an epileptic phenomenon, to detect the type of brain damage which may be expected to provoke the attack, and to offer suggestions about the relationship between the two. From our knowledge of the primary lesion, when it is detectable, we may even be able to forecast the nature of the attacks and the anatomical area which will be affected, but however detailed our knowledge of the neuropathology one question has so far seemed unanswerable. Why exactly did this person have an attack of this particular type, at this moment, on this particular day? It is our inability to answer that question, and all that this failure implies, that explains our relatively low success rate in treating some of the epilepsies.

Incidence

The incidence of epilepsy in this country has been variously estimated. Cohen (1956) wrote that the incidence of epilepsy was between two and four per 1000 of the population, so that he estimated that there were in Great Britain between 100 000 and 200 000 epileptics. The RCGP Survey of the Epilepsies (1960) put the overall figure at 4.82 per 1000, while the Research Committee Report of 1962 put the figure at 3.3 persons per 1000 at risk. The Reid report (1969) suggests that the population with epilepsy includes some 190 000 adults and some 100 000 children of 16 and under. The prevalence of epilepsy amongst school children is around eight per 1000, representing some 60 000 in England and Wales, while there are probably around 91 000 people with epilepsy among the working population, less than 19 000 of whom are registered as disabled.

In practical terms, probably one person in 20 has a fit of some sort during his life, most often during the pre-school years. The incidence of fits rises slightly in the 15–24 age group, and later in the 65-plus group, especially in men (RCGP Survey 1960). Although statistics are small comfort to a family which is confronted with this problem, they will sometimes help to put the first incident in proportion, both in their minds and in that of their doctor. It is important, especially with idiopathic epilepsy in children and young people, that from the outset everyone should understand that this is not an uncommon condition, that it can be treated, and that there may well be no need to impose more than a few, if any, limitations on the life of the patient.

Presentation

Detailed classifications of the many forms that epilepsy may take are considered in detail in the Introduction and Chapter 4: the family doctor will bear in mind a simple clinical classification which, as patients are presented to him, will help determine the direction and extent of his investigations and treatment.

Idiopathic epilepsy

Petit mal attacks may be difficult to identify unless the history is clear, or an attack is actually seen by the doctor. They start commonly in early childhood, when the break in consciousness is brief and may appear to be incomplete or even interruptable. Slight bilateral movements may camouflage the absence of attention, as the patient rarely falls and may even continue walking in an indeterminate fashion. A child may have so many such attacks during a day that they interfere considerably with school work, and are clearly identifiable during a visit to the surgery, or they may be so infrequent that diagnosis may only be made when the characteristic 3 per second spike and wave pattern is seen on an EEG.

Although the diagnosis of grand mal is generally evident, the taking of a careful history may be necessary to differentiate it from a syncopal attack. In syncope there is usually an evident cause, some warning of the attack, and absence of tonic-clonic movements. For the grand mal seizure of idiopathic epilepsy, there is usually no apparent cause, neither is there any warning, although, occasionally, attacks may be precipitated by visual stimuli, such as flickering lights, or auditory stimuli, such as certain forms of music. The attacks recur at varying intervals until controlled. The first major fit in a child who has previously suffered from petit mal attacks commonly occurs in the middle or late teens, at a time when the acquisition of increasing independence by the burgeoning personality is so very important. Generalised attacks without convulsive movements, so-called akinetic attacks, are fairly common in the 10–15 age group.

Symptomatic epilepsy

The diagnosis of idiopathic epilepsy in the adult usually depends on the history alone, unless a fit is seen by the doctor, but a careful examination is essential in order not to miss a clinically obvious cause for the seizure.

Although most commonly related to feverish infections, infantile convulsions, if they continue, cannot be assumed to be transitory. They may in fact be the first sign of brain damage, either congenital, or the result of an apparently minor birth injury.

Baby B was born normally, although his head size was at the lower limit of normal. He developed normally until the age of three months, when he had a spasm, so little marked that the mother doubted whether the behaviour was really unusual. Within a week he was having frequent spasms, and was admitted for investigation, when eventually brain scan revealed cortical atrophy.

The occurrence of a focal or generalised fit in an otherwise healthy adult with no history of cranial injury should be presumed to be due to an intracranial lesion unless full investigation fails to reveal a cause; and even then the presence of a space-occupying lesion cannot be ruled out.

Mrs M.L. aged 54, a heavy smoker, reported spasms of tingling in her right arm over the past four months, progressing to involuntary movements of increasing frequency. Clinical examination between attacks was normal, as was the plain chest and skull X-ray. Brain scan, however, suggested a lesion in the area of the left central sulcus, with a smaller area on the right side of the brain. A later burr-hole biopsy revealed a secondary adenocarcinomatous deposit.

The first signs of symptomatic epilepsy may be behavioural, suggesting a temporal lobe focus, before proceeding to a full motor attack.

Mrs B. complained that her husband, aged 46, had changed his attitude to her, and exploded into paroxysms of rage, in one of which he had pushed her downstairs. In between attacks he was his normal self. Examination by a neurologist, including plain skull X-ray and EEG proved normal. Six months later, having left his wife and his job, he had his first grand mal attack, and was subsequently found to have an inoperable glioblastoma.

As these examples show, the range of symptoms and pathology responsible for the presentation of a person with epilepsy to his doctor is extremely variable. The family doctor's first inquiry of his neurological colleague will be whether the fit is attributable to a specific cause, and if so, can this be treated, or whether it is idiopathic, and if so, how can it best be controlled.

How far should investigations go?

Although on medical grounds it might seem obvious that every new case of epilepsy, no matter which type, should be referred to a neurologist for full investigation before a course of treatment is planned, in practice this may not always happen. It is certain, for example, that many mothers may not summon the doctor when their baby has a single febrile convulsion, a symptom that is known to be quite common. If he is asked to see the child, the doctor may decide that, provided there is an obvious precipitating factor and the attacks are not repetitive, the anxiety generated by referral to a paediatrician or a neurologist is likely to be greater than the benefits to be gained. It is equally true that there are adults who suffer from bizarre behavioural attacks which are never brought to the notice of a doctor. If they are seen, moreover, the true nature of the phenomenon may not be appreciated, and may be thought to be psychosomatic and treated without seeking the help of a neurologist.

The RCGP survey (1960) suggested that one-half of first fits which are major attacks are not referred to a specialist, although most of these were febrile convulsions in children. Repeated fits tend to be referred more often, and the survey showed that 60 per cent were seen by a consultant. But the surprising estimate that not more than three-quarters of all patients suffering from epilepsy are passed on to the specialist points to the need for more study of the disease at general practitioner level, where the majority of cases are first seen.

In this chapter, epilepsy has been regarded as a family problem which, however it develops, will modify in varying degrees the lives of all its members. Therefore, the over-riding responsibility of the family doctor, must be first to arrive at an accurate clinical assessment of the symptoms and their possible cause. If he decides that the help of the specialist is needed, he will be able to discuss with him the history and results of investigations so that plans for future treatment and care can be made. All this must be explained to members of the family in terms they can understand, and he must discuss with them how this will affect their lives in the future.

Childhood epilepsy

The simple febrile convulsion has been referred to above, and in most cases the level of parental anxiety and the confidence they have in their family doctor will determine whether referral and further investigation is required. But a history of recurrence will dictate further investigation.

A.M., aged 2, a normal small boy subject to frequent upper respiratory tract infections with high fevers, had a convulsion during one of these attacks. The doctor saw him, and decided that this was a febrile convulsion. Three weeks later, after recovery, there was another convulsion, and a week later, during which he had seemed perfectly well, a third attack, after which the mother brought the child to the doctor again. The seizure was described as of sudden onset, with clonic movements and a period of sleepiness afterwards. The boy was sent to a paediatrician, who, after discussing the problem with the family doctor, arranged for an EEG which, however, was normal.

In childhood epilepsy, as a general rule, investigations should be kept to the minimum, consistent with the making of a firm diagnosis and the exclusion of treatable causes. A small child with petit mal attacks may only become aware that something unusual is happening in his life because of the behaviour of those around him, parents, brothers or sisters, or the school teacher, and his reactions are likely to take colour from theirs. This is even more true of grand mal attacks since, as the 18-year-old on page 1 was at pains to point out, he will be aware of nothing during the attack itself, and his reactions will be dictated by the circumstances in which he finds himself on recovery. If his parents can successfully disguise their anxiety, he is likely to take a visit to the paediatrician or the neurologist with relative equanimity or even frank interest, even if this means a skull X-ray or an EEG. The older he is, however, the more his questions will be to the point, and they will need answering in terms he can understand. With the average family in this predicament, there is every advantage to be gained by fuller investigation so that they can be brought to accept a firm diagnosis, arrived at in full and evident consultation between themselves, their doctor and the specialist.

There is therefore, in the investigation of childhood epilepsy, a delicate balance to be maintained between adding to parental anxiety by subjecting their child to a battery of interviews, tests and complex investigations, and the need to establish a firm diagnosis whereby anxiety can be made less dreadful and formless in the relief of knowing what it is they have to face.

Adult epilepsy

The extent of investigation of adult epilepsy is governed by rather different considerations. Although in grand mal seizures it remains true that the sufferer is only aware of his situation on recovery, he is more likely to be conscious of the implications of such an attack for the future. If he depends on his car for his work, for example, or if his work is of a nature that such lapses of consciousness involve danger to himself or to others, he will be anxious to find out exactly what has happened and how to stop it. On the other hand, people have been known to keep quiet about first attacks, where they have occurred without witnesses, out of fear of losing their driving licence or their job, or of fear of the implications for the future. In any event, when the doctor is consulted, it will be essential to investigate the attack by every relevant method, since the sudden onset of epilepsy in adult life in an apparently normal person will commonly be due to a specific, even localized cause for which there may be a permanent cure.

Control of attacks

First aid treatment

In dealing with a grand mal attack there are only two essentials. Firstly, the patient must be protected from harming himself, and secondly, the airway must be protected. Unless he is in a position of physical danger, the patient should not be moved. His collar should be loosened. It is seldom possible to put anything between the teeth and the patient will not be grateful if he recovers to find the crown of a tooth broken yet again by the efforts of a well-intentioned onlooker, nor is he pleased by abrasions caused by efforts to move him to a more suitable place. When he stops convulsing, he can be rolled on to his side to aid expulsion of saliva and to keep clear the airway: it will be necessary to watch for evidence of incontinence. With recovering consciousness he can be helped to a more convenient place, where he can rest until the post-ictal state wears off.

Long-term treatment

The treatment of symptomatic epilepsy is of course primarily the treatment of the cause, although anticonvulsant drugs may have to be used to control fits until the cause can be dealt with. Where the fits are due to a medical cause, such as meningitis, encephalitis, or uraemia, for example, the treatment of the infection, or of the metabolic defect will be primary, and will usually take place in hospital, with intensive investigation and monitoring. Surgical causes, such as abscesses, neoplasms and some types of vascular lesions will also be dealt with in hospital, although there may be long periods of home care when seizures may need to be controlled as far as possible by the use of drugs.

It has been well said that in general it is rarely the fit that is dangerous, but rather the place where it happens. Attacks of idiopathic epilepsy are more frequent at the beginning of the day, during the first waking hour when, as it were, the brain is changing from a sleeping to a waking rhythm, and at the end of the day. Even if complete remission from fits cannot be induced, it may be possible largely to avoid exposure to potentially dangerous surroundings at times of maximum risk: thus, for example, it may be wiser to take a bath on return from work or school rather than first thing in the morning or late at night. Those who live with people with epilepsy need to be as aware as the patients themselves of the added risks at such times.

Medication

Anticonvulsant drugs are used with the aim of producing complete remission from attacks, so that both the patient and his family can live a normal life, free of special limitations and without the anxiety that the continual thought of an impending fit will produce. So complete a control as this is frequently difficult, if not impossible, and many doctors and their patients, faced with a situation so difficult to judge, will need further advice on the principles to be followed. Laurence (1973) sums up the results of drug treatment by saying that up to half the patients are completely relieved of fits, of whom one in five may be able to give up drugs after three years, without recurrence. About a third of all patients are only partially relieved and the remainder are not helped at all.

The range of anticonvulsant drugs available has, unlike some other groups of drugs, expanded relatively slowly over the years and this may reflect our lack of understanding of their mode of action and the apparent variability of their effect on the patient. It is widely recognized that some anticonvulsants are more effective in certain forms of epilepsy than others, and although there are several schemes of drug regimes hallowed by time and experience, it remains unclear why there should be so large a complete or partial failure rate in the treatment of idiopathic epilepsy. To stand any chance of success, however, it is essential that medication should be continuous, and supervised at regular intervals. The rate at which anticonvulsant drugs are metabolized, and the variations in serum levels that are found in different individuals at different times can now be measured, and patients whose attacks respond poorly to treatment can sometimes be referred by their general practitioner to centres where such estimations can be done. In this way more accurate control can be exercised over drug dosage, and it is to be hoped that as such facilities become more widely available it may become possible for doctors to treat epilepsy with greater understanding of the effects of the drugs they prescribe.

In practice, especially among developing children, it may be necessary to resist the temptation to increase the dose and types of drugs used in a vain attempt to stop the attacks entirely, because of the disadvantages of their side effects on awareness and concentration in school or university work. Considerable risks may be courted by the long-term use of drugs whose unwanted effects are unpleasant or even serious, and it is not uncommon to find patients whose attacks are difficult to control and who are more disabled by the toxic effects of their medication than by their epilepsy.

The life situation

There seems to be another series of factors, other than medication, which govern the frequency of attacks in children, and in planning drug treatment, appreciation of their existence may avert a tendency to over-frequent changes of drug regime. These factors are related to the life situation of the child.

The family doctor, if he has been involved in

the situation from the beginning and knows the family, with its infinitely variable pattern of stresses and emotional interplay, will become aware that the frequency of the child's attacks, and even their nature, will often alter according to family attitudes and pressures, and to educational and social circumstances. A child with petit mal, for example, became so worried about his progress at his junior school and his chances of entry to senior school, that from having four or five attacks a day, he had such showers of attacks during lessons that his concentration and absorption were seriously interfered with. After consulting the parents, the headmaster took the boy on one side and explained to him firmly but without rancour that there was no doubt of his ability to do the work, and that if he were to try to concentrate harder, the attacks might be less frequent. The master followed this up shortly by making him head boy, and the petit mal attacks subsided to below their previous normal level with an obvious increase in the boy's self-confidence. There was no change of medication throughout this episode.

The same child as he grew older, noticed that his petit mal changed in intensity. Whereas previously there was complete absence of recall, he was now dimly aware of things going on in his environment during an attack, although if asked a question before recovery he was unable to answer coherently: his impression was that he was more easily rousable by a firm command, or a gentle shake. The absence of recall became more complete again when he was under stress, such as when working for an examination, or when he was anxious or frustrated by the limitations which might have to be imposed on his future plans. Incidentally, he reported that after he had developed grand mal, a shower of petit mal attacks was often the precursor of a major seizure.

Grand mal attacks seem also to be in part related to factors other than medication or pathophysiological variation. The RCGP survey (1960), already quoted, found that 40 per cent of all epileptics had more than one fit a year, and an adolescent, in his most formative years when he and his family are most anxious to be able to plan for his future, may have ten or a dozen fits a year while living a full life at home and at school. These attacks may cluster at times of maximum stress, they may occur when the patient is most anxious, frustrated and depressed by his future prospects and by the degree of restraint which even the most apparently understanding parents must from time to time impose; and they may disappear for months at a time in the summer holidays when life seems straightforward and the future can be for the moment forgotten.

Psychiatric help

This variability may seem both incomprehensible and the sign of medical ineptitude to the parents, who, however well they appear to conceal it, are bound to be full of apprehension about every aspect of their child's present and future life. Small wonder, therefore, that in dealing with the developing situation in a family containing one member with epilepsy, the family doctor may in more complex cases seek the advice of a psychiatrist. The latter should be experienced in the stresses and conflicts that may arise in the mind of a patient, in the group of which he is a member, and during childhood, in those who are responsible for bringing him up. It may be possible with the psychiatrist's help to enable the growing child with unresponsive epilepsy, and his family, to understand better the problems they have to face, and to realize what goes to make up the tangled web of anxiety, fear, guilt, depression and despair, which may from time to time overwhelm them. Education adapted to the needs and capabilities of the child will encourage a more positive attitude to the disability, and at least temper the emotions of the patient and his family, even though only a complete remission could allay them completely.

THE EXPERIENCE OF THE SUFFERER

The 18-year-old whose account of an attack opened this chapter had these comments to make on the general problems of having epilepsy:

It is difficult to convey to anyone who has never experienced an epileptic fit the complete and utter insignificance of the attack to the afflicted, although it may be a drama the beholder will never be able to forget. Epilepsy, however, does not leave the epileptic unscathed. His freedom, a gift which is never fully appreciated until people are themselves deprived of it, is greatly limited. This cannot entirely be attributed to the illness but more to the demands of society. It would be easier to carry on life as if nothing had happened, but this is impossible because of the responsibility of a man to his fellow beings, be it in the capacity of father, husband, son, friend or whoever. Further, the law, quite sensibly, prevents epileptics from driving and flying and it is often found that many outdoor activities such as diving are made difficult. However, if he is to survive, the epileptic must accept these limitations as being so, and carry on in spite of them with the air of living a normal useful life . . .

Those who, for various reasons, need special long-term help and care with their epilepsy will be considered in Chapter 15; they will include those whose fits have, for complex reasons involving environmental problems, not yet been effectively controlled, and those who because of intellectual inadequacy require medical supervision under everyday living conditions or in a work setting (Reid, 1969).

In most of the rest of this chapter we shall be considering the problems facing a young person who has grown up with idiopathic epilepsy, at first petit mal, and later grand mal; for it is such people, and their families, who frequently have the greatest and most long-lasting burden to bear.

Child with petit mal

It is likely that a child who starts petit mal attacks at the age of 4 is unaware of them until some time after they have been noticed by others. The first time he is aware that something odd has happened may be when he hears a brother or sister saying, as he recovers 'Look, Jonathan's dreaming again.' He will slowly come to realize that there are lapses of time in his life when things seem to have happened in a flash, without his realizing it, and in infancy and early childhood this may not disturb him. In the home, if the parents are understanding, he is to some extent cushioned from the more hurtful results of his absences; but at school he may be teased by his friends, and worse, may attract the displeasure of his teachers for reasons which seem to him both inexplicable and unjust. Thus not only will his scholastic performance fail to reflect his true intellectual standard, but the first realization that there is something odd about himself which can get him into trouble can lead to an attitude of withdrawal from his world. It can indeed often result in emotional instability or aggressiveness in a child who had previously been

normally confident of his place in the scheme of things and of the affection of his family.

It is often at this stage necessary for the parents to tell him in very simple terms that he has these attacks for which every family will coin its own name such as, for example, 'dreams', and that they are not his fault, and nobody is cross with him for them. He should be told that it is only if other people do not understand that they will be puzzled, and that if he feels he has had a *dream* and missed what has been going on, he must not be afraid to ask. Children being children, they have been known to seem to turn their absences to good effect in avoiding situations with which they feel themselves inadequate to cope, as in the example quoted on page 8, but realization of what is happening by parents or teacher will, with wise handling, resolve this kind of reaction.

Petit mal is predominantly a condition of childhood, and attacks tend to diminish in frequency after the age of 14: it is rare to see petit mal in adults over 30 years old. In early school years, when life is normally supervised fairly closely, the child will not necessarily experience the frustrating restrictions which can, necessarily or unnecessarily, be imposed upon his life later on. If drug therapy is successful, he may live through his petit mal with minimal disturbance.

Adolescent with grand mal

As the patient gets older, however, grand mal attacks may appear, and that is the time at which the seeds of emotional reactions of great importance for the future may be sown. The first attack is always puzzling though not necessarily alarming. As far as the patient is concerned, from carrying on some quite normal activity, he suddenly finds himself with no warning, lying in a peculiar position, dazed, stiff, unsteady, unable to talk coherently or clearly, and surrounded by people whose concern and alarm is both evident and intense. Furthermore, he feels incapable of impressing on them that given time he will recover completely, and willy-nilly finds himself in an ambulance on the way to hospital. On arrival, although feeling quite well apart from a slight headache, he finds he cannot be allowed to go home until his parents have been summoned to fetch him. And because he has been feeling quite normal and was following his ordinary pursuits, all this is to him quite inexplicable.

Because something so unusual has happened he is taken to his doctor and then to the neurologist; X-rays and an EEG are done, and finally he learns that he has something called epilepsy, which will mean taking tablets regularly, and the imposition of certain restrictions on what he can be allowed to do by himself. From what is *not* said he will sense the concern of his parents, however much they may attempt to conceal it.

The threat to independence

As he grows older the patient who continues to have attacks may come to resent, although he may try to understand, his parents' suggestion that he should always let them know where he is going and how long he will be out, and their inevitable anxiety when he comes in late. If attacks are frequent, the number and amount of drugs he must remember to take will irritate him, and their side effects may affect his personality to a variable degree. His performance at school may begin to suffer, and the contribution that can be made by an enlightened staff in unobtrusively making sure that he takes the fullest possible part in every school activity can hardly be overestimated. As attack succeeds attack, perhaps after a long interval when he had begun to hope they had stopped, or after a shorter time when he felt he couldn't be due for another one yet, and always with the implied failure of his medication, he comes to realize that his disability, however well he is between attacks, is bound to limit his choice of job or his entry to a career in which he is passionately interested.

Emotional reactions

It is small wonder therefore that such a patient may come to look upon himself as a second-class citizen, prevented from living a normal life through no fault of his own, and with his independence, the most treasured acquisition of the adolescent, threatened or curtailed. The way in which he deals with his resentment will vary

enormously. He may decide that medication has failed him, and abandon it. His despair may lead him to leave his home and family and seek to make a life for himself amongst other friends, sometimes bizarre and irresponsible people. The irregular life and infrequent medication will encourage more fits, which will in turn add to his desperation. If on the other hand his family remains the firm basis of his life he may bury his resentment in apparently firm self-control, and will deny that his fits are anything but a passing annoyance which do not fundamentally concern him. This can even amount to a gay amenable insouciance which conceals emotions so strong that the very normality of his behaviour is in reality neurotic. At either extreme, the emotional reaction may occasionally be so intense as to lead to attempted suicide.

It is hard enough for an adult to learn that there is no easy path to equanimity in the face of continuing adversity: the adolescent needs all the help he can be given in order to arrive at a reasonable acceptance of the changed circumstances of his life. Because he has had to grow up in an atmosphere of family concern, it is likely that he will turn to someone outside the family to whom he can unburden himself. This may be a friend, a respected relative, or perhaps the family doctor, whom he may regard as a sufficiently uninvolved expert to be able to help. It should be one of the prime duties of the general practitioner always to be prepared to allow time for such talking out of emotions.

If he can be guided wisely through this difficult adolescent phase, there is no reason why an otherwise healthy young adult, provided his attacks are not too frequent, should not enter training for a job, or go to university to start a career. The fact that he has an occasional fit is often taken with surprising composure by his fellow-students, and need in no wise limit his activities. In fact, one student with epilepsy returned from a rugger practice highly amused because, he said, he'd had a petit mal in the middle of the match, turned round and put down the ball over his own goal line. His choice of occupation will, of course, be governed by whether or not his fits are completely controlled, and it will greatly add to this burden if he is unable to drive a car, or manipulate potentially dangerous machinery.

In fact, as he grows up, his anxieties assume more and more a concern for the future – what is the likelihood of his becoming free from attacks, and can such an event be predicted with any certainty; how are his attacks likely to affect his job, his freedom of movement, his wife, his children? The answer to all these questions, where an answer is possible, depends upon the complex problems which are considered in later chapters of this book.

THE BURDEN ON THE FAMILY

First reactions

When a child first shows signs of epilepsy, and particularly with the appearance of grand mal attacks, the shock to the family, and especially to the parents, is profound. The appearance of such a dramatically threatening sequence of events which they may never have seen before, and which is quite unheralded, induces a sudden acute anxiety which may be momentarily overwhelming. There is apparently no cause over which they can have any control, and they are quite unable to influence in any way the inevitable progress of the attack. The anxiety is, of course, usually canalised into seeking the help of their doctor, and the subsequent chain of specialist examination and investigation carries the expectation of control; but where the attacks continue despite treatment it is hard for parents not to view each succeeding attack with a desperation that may be deceptively concealed beneath a disciplined exterior.

It is often held that the immediate response of parents to a child with epilepsy is one of rejection which is followed by an over-compensatory concern. This may be true in families where there is little understanding of illness, casual bonds between parents and children, and an inability, either emotionally or intellectually, to face the reorientation which the onset of epilepsy implies. But in a family where bonds are close and understanding is implicit, rejection in the ordinary or in the psychiatric sense must be rare, and the intense concern springs more from a normal protective instinct and an ever-present dread of what might happen to harm the child.

Explanation

Their first need will be a firm diagnosis. A simple explanation of what happens when their child has a fit, and of what happens within the brain to cause it, is an essential start to their understanding of the condition. It should be explained that all movement and all activity in the nervous system is initiated by electrical discharges within the brain, but that in most people the excitability of the nerve cells is controlled by an intricate system of checks and balances so that it never gets out of control. There is, however, a level at which these controls cease to operate, and an uncontrolled discharge produces a fit. In some people this level is lower than in others, and even varies at different times, for example early in the morning or during the night, or in different circumstances such as illness, fatigue or emotional stress. The parents have to be told that their child is such a person, but that the chances of controlling the attacks are good, given the right medicaments and the avoidance, as far as is consistent with a normal life, of those situations likely to favour an attack. The general trend, moreover, is likely to be of improvement as the child grows up and there may well be no impairment of intellectual capacity; but it is often wise to face at the outset the fact that it is impossible to be certain that attacks will not continue for many years, with or without the use of anticonvulsant drugs.

The extent to which these details are discussed will depend on the family doctor's knowledge of the parents' reaction to the illness and of their powers of comprehension; but in one form or another some basic understanding of the reasons for the attacks is essential if the child's future is to be planned intelligently.

Treatment

If the attacks continue at intervals despite treatment, the parents will often press for increased doses, or a change of drugs, and it may be difficult to explain to them that neither is necessarily likely to improve their child's condition. An inquiry into the problems the child has to face at home or at school, whether he seems to be content, with normal and predictable emotional responses, or whether he has been unwell, miserable or obviously worried about his performance in class, may yield valuable clues to suggest the reason for the apparently inadequate control of his epilepsy.

Planning activities

Parents will want to know what limitations they should impose, for his protection, on their child's activities, and the question at the back of their minds, spoken or unspoken, is always, 'Is he likely to die in an attack?' The answer to this question must be a firm assurance that death in an ordinary epileptic attack is very rare, and when it occurs it is a result rather of the circumstances in which the attack occurs, than from the attack itself. Every doctor knows of instances where a person with epilepsy has had an attack in the bath and drowned, or even died of suffocation in bed, face-downward on a saliva-soaked pillow, but such events are happily uncommon enough for the parents not to have their anxieties compounded by such detailed descriptions of possibilities.

The extent of limitations is of more immediate importance and it is in this field that the parents have to be made aware of the balance of anxieties within the family. They cannot fail to feel concern for the safety of their child all the time, whereas the child's main emotion will be of frustration at limitations of any kind and, however reasonable he seems to be, of resentment at what he sees as excessive parental fuss, supervision and control. He will often say, as he grows up, that it is after all *his* life, and the extent to which he chooses to take risks should be entirely his own concern. There must therefore be a balance between his acceptance of certain rules of life which should be kept as few and as simple as possible, and the parents' burden of anxiety about risks that have to be accepted if their child is to live as free a life as possible. The achievement of such a balance is essential if the child is to develop naturally, and to avoid deeper embedded resentments which will colour his adult life.

The restrictions to be applied should therefore be few, and might include merely a ban on cycling on the road, on swimming alone, climbing, and on going on holidays or long cross-country treks without a friend. These measures need not be too

tiresome for the growing child or adolescent, and many children with epilepsy take their full part in school games, athletics, football and even competitive swimming as long as the school staff are aware of the problem and have been properly briefed. It is always important, in fact, to keep the school informed about the state of the child's health. Schools nowadays are for the most part enlightened and helpful, and provided they are fully informed about the nature of the epileptic attack, and know what to do (or perhaps more to the point, what *not* to do) if an attack occurs, they willingly accept the responsibilities of the child's disability, and the need to keep him involved fully in all school activities.

Education

Parents and teachers will often wish to know whether the child's intellectual development is likely to suffer as a result of the disease. The consensus of opinion would be that if attacks are not too frequent, intellectual impairment does not occur, but that if a child has frequent clusters of grand mal attacks he may become less capable as times goes on. This may be due to brain damage secondary to frequent periods of neuronal hyperactivity followed by anoxia, but also to the interruption of learning and study by the attacks and their sequelae. A child may, for example, pass through a period when there are so many petit mal attacks that it is impossible for him to maintain his concentration on the lesson: if this is repeated he will fall behind the rest of the class and his performance compared with his peers will be substandard.

This can lead later to the problem of how far a child with recurring seizures should be encouraged to follow an academic course of studies. Because his interests or inclinations lie that way, because all his friends are going on to further study, or because he thinks family traditions demand it of him, a boy may seek to prove to himself and to the world that nothing is going to prevent him living up to the standards he has set himself. His condition or his capabilities may make this difficult or impossible to attain, and parents will need to be very cautious in the way they discuss their child's ideas about his future with him, neither discouraging enterprise nor encouraging plans for which he may not be equipped. The ideal career is one which engages his interest and follows his natural gifts without risking too many disappointments during the acquisition of basic knowledge and skills.

The way parents learn to live with this burden is often truly remarkable. They may manage the family life by virtually ignoring the problem and treating it purely episodically; or they may allow it to dominate every aspect of family life, to the detriment of brothers and sisters whose own lives and attitudes may become considerably modified by the constant need to be on watch. But with help, parents, family and patient alike will often come to accept attacks as part of life which should cause as little interruption as possible to normal activities, even though this is achieved at the cost of disciplined repression of any outward signs of anxiety.

Deep anxiety is always there however, and has to be accepted as a normal and natural response to adversity. To identify it in terms of psychological reaction patterns does not make it any less real, nor do attempts to explain and rationalise it cause it to disappear. Concern for their young and their protection is part of the fundamental pattern of normal animal behaviour, and often the greatest help that can be offered to the parents of a disabled child is the sharing of their problem with a sympathetic friend who is both less involved and better informed than they are.

THE RESPONSIBILITY OF THE DOCTOR

In ideal circumstances, and in fact more frequently than not, the role of the sympathetic friend will be played by the family doctor, a role which, in turn, imposes on him a special burden of responsibility. The family doctor will be aware of the limitations and the risks in the life of a person with epilepsy, but he will also know the importance to the parents and to the patient of living a normal family life.

The family

He must, in fact, accept the responsibility of being, for the parents, the means of lessening their own feeling of total responsibility; of removing their fear, at times almost overwhelming, that should their decisions be wrong, or should disaster occur, it will have been entirely their fault. The parental sense of guilt may stem from happenings before the child was born; the child's later affliction may, for example, be wrongly attributed to an attack of 'flu, to self medication, or to undue activity during pregnancy. The guilt is transformed, as time goes on, to an ever-present sense of concern and responsibility for the child's activities and welfare, and part of this burden can be eased from parents if their doctor is prepared to discuss with them how far it is reasonable for them to agonise over the origin and extent of their child's disabilities, and to advise them responsibly what he should be allowed to do. Where risks may have to be taken, he must, in fact, be prepared to bear the responsibility of encouraging or confirming the parents' decisions, which they may have taken after much heart-searching. Equally important, he can with the knowledge he has gained from the specialist fields he has drawn upon, help them by making a series of informed estimates about the future.

The patient

For the patient, especially as he grows up, the family doctor may be the one person with whom he can discuss his treatment, his problems at school, at work and in the family circle. When the limitations imposed on his developing individuality seem to him intolerable, the doctor, being uninvolved, can often explain, from a fresh and detached viewpoint, the inevitability of parental concern, and how, though it may seem irksome, it has its uses, and that its significance is usually for the good. The doctor may often be able to smooth areas of friction by a suitable word dropped to either side.

Driving

As he gets older, the young man with epilepsy will wish to know his legal position about driving. Whatever the position of the individual, the doctor must explain to the sufferer the implications of driving for himself, for his passengers, and for other road users. This is considered further in Chapter 15.

Marriage and children

As the boy or girl with epilepsy grows up, they will naturally form friendships with the opposite sex, which will eventually ripen into deeper relationships. As thoughts of marriage arise, the effect of epilepsy on the future will cause concern. How frankly should the situation and the future be discussed before becoming engaged, and how far is the family doctor justified in discussing the confidential details of the sufferer's health with his fiancée? If attacks are infrequent, how will the young bride react the first time her husband has a fit? Can the man be sure that his fits are infrequent enough, and sufficiently well controlled, to make sure that they will not prevent him earning enough to support his family? Is the girl with epilepsy capable of running a home without danger to herself or to any children who may arrive? Should they in fact have children at all?

My personal view is that if one of the partners has well-controlled epilepsy, obstacles should not be put in the way of their marriage, for the stability and self-confidence which will be gained by the intimate love and respect of the other will tend to lessen the likelihood of continuing attacks. And this happy state will be more likely if the family doctor is able to discuss frankly with the man and woman, together, the problems that may arise, the attitude they should take to them, and the ways in which they can deal with them. Everything is to be gained by giving them every opportunity to ask questions and seek advice about any detail of their life together, and they should at the same time be encouraged to plan and live a completely normal life.

It has been said that the only important advice about marriage that should be given to a person with epilepsy is not to marry someone with a family history of epilepsy, but that if he does, he should take care to avoid having children.

Marriage will bring inevitable inquiries about the likelihood of the disease being transmitted to the children of a person with epilepsy, and expert genetic counselling may be necessary for a reasonably valid estimate of probability. Emery (1974) quotes the risk of a parent with *idiopathic* epilepsy having an affected child as 1 in 20. Such figures may not be an easy basis for a decision to marry or to have children; but it will be for the family doctor, with the aid of the geneticist, to help the young couple to the right decision.

Throughout this chapter I have used the adjective idiopathic in its true sense of meaning *for which no cause is apparent*. Modern thinking no longer draws a sharp distinction between idiopathic and symptomatic epilepsy: potentially all cases of idiopathic epilepsy may have a pathophysiological cause, if only it could be found; not all patients who have apparently similar lesions have fits, and it is necessary to postulate that those who do must have been born with a greater tendency to have them, whether or not genetically determined. Therefore, it is no longer possible to reassure that those with symptomatic epilepsy carry no genetic trait. However, in our present state of knowledge, it would be reasonable to suggest that, if there is an obvious causative lesion, which is known to be highly epileptogenic, there is less need to adduce an important genetic contribution to the production of epilepsy. An important corollary of this proposition is that a family history of epilepsy does not mean that there may not be an underlying lesion. There are still doctors who feel that, if there is a family history, investigations to exclude remediable causative lesions are not necessary. This error may be very dangerous.

The general practitioner, who has the responsibility for the management of epilepsy within the setting of ordinary family life, has to rely on the skills and knowledge of specialists in other disciplines. The chapters which follow should help him to be able to ease the burden of epilepsy.

REFERENCES

Cohen (1956) Medical Care of Epileptics, *Report of Cohen Sub-committee*. London: HMSO.

Emery, A.E.H. (1974) *Practitioner*, **213**, 643.

Laurence, D.R. (1973) *Clinical Pharmacology*, 4th edition. Edinburgh: Churchill Livingstone.

Reid (1969) People with Epilepsy, *Report of Central Health Services Council*. London: HMSO.

Research Committee of College of General Practitioners (1960) Survey of the Epilepsies in General Practice. *British Medical Journal*, **ii**, 416.

Research Committee of College of General Practitioners (1962) Morbidity Statistics from General Practice 3, *Disease in General Practice*. London: HMSO.

2

Epidemiology

J.J. Zielinsky

GENERAL INTRODUCTION

The aims and scope of epidemiology have expanded greatly over recent decades. At first it was concerned mainly with infectious diseases and their spread through a community. Nowadays it has extended to cover all diseases and pathological processes. Hence, epidemiology may be defined as a branch of medicine concerned with the frequency and distribution of disabilities, diseases and deaths in human populations and with factors causing them or influencing their natural history. Over the years epidemiology has not only made important contributions to research but also has been of great value in practical medicine. John Snow in London in the 1840s was able to show how cholera was spread and to recommend preventative measures long before the discovery of the causative vibrio (after Schoenberg, Mann & Kurland, 1974). Later using epidemiological methods Fletcher (1907) found the cause of and inferred ways of preventing beri-beri, and Goldberger (1914) pellagra, many years before the identification of thiamine and nicotonic acid.

Over the last 30 years many epidemiological studies of epilepsy have been published and they have increased significantly our knowledge of the condition. Before a detailed consideration of these studies, the basic methodology of epidemiology will be reviewed.

BASIC EPIDEMIOLOGICAL METHODS

Descriptive epidemiology analyses the frequency of health phenomena in populations defined in terms of variables such as sex, age, race, occupation and residence (urban or rural). Use is made of routine records, for examples: death certificates, sick-leave certificates and the files of insurance companies. Frequencies of the phenomena in different populations and at different times may be compared, and hypotheses may be proposed concerning the influence of a particular factor or complex of factors on these frequencies.

Analytical epidemiology verifies such hypotheses and it is usually necessary to devise special retrospective or prospective studies.

Experimental epidemiology considers the introduction of some new factor in the course of a prospective study. For example: the effect of immunization on the incidence of an infectious disease, or of a recently established speed limit on the number of cases of post-traumatic epilepsy following road traffic accidents.

The usefulness of epidemiology in clinical medicine

The records of the medical practitioner provide one of the most important sources of information for the epidemiologist. The results of the epidemiologist's field surveys, in return, are of value to the practitioner in many ways. They help to: determine the natural course of a disorder; develop and test clinical hypotheses of aetiology; improve the precision of diagnosis as based for examples on medical history or an EEG; check clinical assessments of long-term prognosis; recognise the social and environmental implications of diseases; and improve the organization of treatment and management.

Basic epidemiological measurements

A. Morbidity rates measure the frequency of the disorder within a population which is defined and with the time and place specified.

Incidence (I) is the rate at which new cases of a disease occur. For epilepsy the average annual incidence is usually calculated per 100 000 according to the formula:

$$I = \frac{\text{number of new cases within a given period (e.g. 1 year)}}{\text{population at the middle of the period}} \times 100\,000$$

Since the estimate is based on the number of first cases of epilepsy diagnosed, the rate would be described better as the 'first attendance rate' or 'accession rate'. Several years may elapse between the first seizure and the actual diagnosis of epilepsy (Zielinski, 1974a; Hauser & Kurland, 1975) and there are other patients who never consult a doctor or who remain undiagnosed (Zielinski, 1975). It follows that the 'accession rate' may fall well below the real rate, particularly if calculated over a short period. *Prevalence* (P) describes the frequency of all current cases of a disease and for epilepsy is usually estimated per 1000 according to the formula:

$$P = \frac{\text{number of epileptic people (in population at any given time)}}{\text{population}} \times 1000$$

The number of cases in a population on a particular day is the point-prevalence rate and is most often used.

Prevalence varies as the product of time and incidence. With a chronic condition like epilepsy the number of patients accumulates with time and so the prevalence is high although the incidence rates are low. The so-called 'life-time' or 'total' prevalence can be calculated when the numerator is the number of people who have ever suffered from recurrent seizures. The 'accumulated incidence' (Juul-Jensen & Ipsen, 1976; Hauser, 1978) seems, however, an even better method of estimating the risk of contracting epilepsy during a lifetime. It is calculated by adding the incidence rates for different age groups. For example, if the annual incidence rates for the 0–4 year age group and the 5–9 age group are 80 and 50 respectively, then the total number of patients at the end of the first decade would be some 650 per 100 000 or 0.6 per cent.

B Mortality rates measure the frequency of deaths within the defined population. The 'cause-specific death rate' is that due to a specific disorder and is calculated per 100 000 according to the formula:

$$\text{cause-specific death rate} = \frac{\text{number of deaths assigned to a specific cause in a given time interval}}{\text{mid-interval population}} \times 100\,000$$

The case-fatality rate or ratio (CFR) gives another measure where:

$$\text{CFR} = \frac{\text{number of deaths assigned to a specific disease during a given time interval}}{\text{number of cases of that disease during the same time interval}} \times 100$$

All the above rates can be calculated for specific groups defined by age, sex, race and so forth.

The estimation and interpretation of both CFR and cause-specific rates are often difficult in epilepsy. Epileptic patients seldom die of epilepsy. Thus, when estimating the CFR only deaths due to epilepsy should be entered in the numerator, while the denominator includes cases of 'active' epilepsy or all known cases. Mortality rates most usually are calculated as a proportion of all deaths of persons with diagnosed epilepsy to the mid-interval general population.

Case-ascertainment methods

It would be the epidemiologist's dream that every person contracting a disease should immediately consult his doctor and that the diagnosis should be recorded at once. Unfortunately just the opposite happens. Many patients do not notice their symptoms or dismiss them as unimportant (Zielinski, 1976). In a sample from 17 general practices in Metropolitan London only a fifth of patients with epilepsy had suspected the diagnosis before they decided to consult their doctor (Hopkins & Scambler, 1977). Another serious problem is caused by patients who decide to give up treatment after a time, stop going to the doctor and so drop out of medical files (Zielinski, 1974a). Twenty to 25 per cent of children in Newcastle upon Tyne suffering from various types of seizures never sought medical advice (Miller et al, 1960) and similar figures were found in Warsaw.

One of the oldest and most popular methods of case-finding is to review medical and other records in a selected area to find those which have any mention of the diagnosis of epilepsy or of an epileptic seizure. This method may be supplemented by a medical re-examination of all patients, or of a random sample, to verify the accuracy of the original diagnosis (Gudmundsson, 1966; Zielinski, 1974a). Another method is to compile a register to which data on new cases of epilepsy in a population are added as they are diagnosed. This method increases the chance of an accurate estimate by bringing together information about the same patient from different sources.* A register of patients with epilepsy, suspected epilepsy and febrile convulsions since 1945 for the population of Rochester was compiled from the medical files of the Mayo Clinic (Kurland, 1959; Hauser & Kurland, 1975). A similar register has been introduced recently in Aarhus, Denmark (Juul-Jensen & Ipsen, 1975).

Another approach is a specially designed study of chosen populations or random samples of them. Such studies have been carried out in Guam, Carlisle, Warsaw and Bogota. In Carlisle and Warsaw medical files were surveyed as well. Some workers limit their survey to more selected population groups because of a better chance of a more nearly complete identification of cases. For examples: workers' sick-fund policy holders (Wajsbort, Haral & Alfandary, 1967), mine workers (Bird, Heinz & Klintworth, 1962) and army draftees (Bayley et al, Edwards et al, after Lennox, 1960).

There have been a number of community or births-cohort studies of children (Kuran, 1975; Rose et al, 1973; Rutter et al, 1972; Meighan, Queener & Weitman, 1978; Milleretal, 1960; Cooper, 1965; Van den Bergh & Yerusalmy, 1969; Gates, 1972; Blom, Heijbel & Bergfors, 1978). The main difficulty in comparing the results of

different surveys is the use of different diagnostic criteria or even a lack of a precise definition of epilepsy. Gastaut's (1973) definition* is not always applicable to epidemiological field surveys because it may not be possible to carry out medical or EEG examinations.

The term 'chronic disorder' may be ambiguous. During the discussion on the definitions and classifications of epilepsy for epidemiological purposes as proposed by Alter et al (1972) it was agreed that cases with a single seizure, including a febrile convulsion and those due to an acute cause (illness, trauma, intoxication)† should be considered separately in epidemiological studies.

There is further disagreement about the length of time free of seizures before a patient may be considered as 'cured' of epilepsy, or whether it should be thought 'once epileptic, always epileptic' (Lennox, 1960). To get over this difficulty some authors define the proportions of 'active' and 'non-active' epilepsy in the material of their study. The 'non-active' group includes those who have been free of seizures for usually five, sometimes two, years. Patients who have had a long remission but who are still on antiepileptic drugs are considered as having 'active epilepsy' (Grudzinska, 1974; Gudmundsson, 1966; Hauser & Kurland, 1975; Nowak, 1972; Zielinski, 1966; Zielinski, 1974a). Some authors exclude cases of symptomatic epilepsy from their estimates (Brewis et al, 1966; Leibowitz & Alter, 1968).

These sources of inaccuracy have concerned the numerator of the formulae. The denominator seldom causes difficulty. The size of the population and its demographic and socioeconomic characteristics are usually obtained from the census. However, sometimes the denominator is the population of patients in general practices or the number of people seen by doctors. In such cases if there is an age bias there may be too high an incidence rate if it is young, or too high a mortality rate if the population is older.

---

*During the review of medical records in Warsaw it was found that information about 30 per cent of cases was discovered independently in at least two files. This was also found by Gudmundsson (1966) and Rutter, Graham & Yule (1972).

*A chronic brain disorder of various aetiologies characterised by recurrent seizures due to excessive discharge of cerebral neurones . . . Single or occasional epileptic seizures as well as those occuring during an acute illness should not be classified as epilepsy'.

†An acute episode is defined as lasting less than 72 hours.

Table 2.1 Incidence rates for epilepsy review of selected studies

Country author	Case ascertainment method	Population studied	Annual incidence per 100 000	Definition, comment
Denmark, Juul-Jensen & Ipsen, 1976	Medical records, 'Epilepsy Register'	Aarhus, Denmark	30	Including 'Observation for epilepsy'
Great Britain, Crombie et al, 1960	Information from general practitioners	Population of 67 practices, England and Wales	63	Included single and febrile seizures
Great Britain, Pond et al, 1960	Review of records of general practitioners	Population of 14 practices, SE England	70	First diagnoses of epilepsy
Great Britain, Brewis et al, 1966	Review of medical records, central register of patients	Carlisle, England	30	Symptomatic epilepsy not included, recurrent seizures only
Guam, Stanhope et al, 1972	Records of neurological clinic	Guam	23	More than one seizure
Guam, Stanhope et al, 1972	Field survey	Guam, same area	46	Definition as above; age-adjusted rate for US population = 35, including 23 for idiopatic epilepsy
Iceland, Gudmundsson, 1966	Review of medical records, re-examination	Iceland	26	Clinical diagnosis of epilepsy
Japan, Sato, 1964	Medical records	Niigata	17	Symptomatic seizures excluded
Norway, Krohn, 1961	Review of medical records	Northern Norway	11	Recurrent seizures only
Norway, De Graaf, 1974	Records of neurological and EEG services	Subarctic Norway	33	Patients of general practitioners not included, large area, difficult travelling
Poland, Grudzińska, 1974	Records of Epilepsy Clinic	Industrialized urban area, Zabrze	22	First attendance, clinical diagnosis
Poland, Zieliński, 1974a	Records of neurological and psychiatric services	Warsaw	20	First attendance, recurrent seizures, febrile fits excluded
Sweden, Blom et al, 1978	Follow-up of children after first seizure	Swedish county, children up to 16	82	Recurrent, afebrile seizures only. Highest incidence /140/ in age 1–4. Rates for primary generalised — 23, benign Rolandic epilepsy – 21
USA, Kurland, 1959	Review of the Mayo Clinic medical records	Rochester, Minn.	30	More than one afebrile seizure
USA, Hauser & Kurland, 1975	Records of Mayo Clinic	Rochester, Minn. 1955–1964 1965–1967 1935–1967	54 46 49	As above

INCIDENCE OF EPILEPSY

Table 2.1 shows that, although different methodology may be used, most studies give incidence rates from 20 to 50 per 100 000. The rather higher rates from the British authors (Crombie et al, 1960; Pond, Bidwell & Stein, 1960) seem to be due to the inclusion of patients with single seizures and with febrile convulsions. The incidence rates, however, approach the combined incidence rates of isolated and recurrent seizures in Rochester (Hauser & Kurland, 1975). The Guam results show that the incidence estimated by the more complete case finding method of field survey may be twice as high as that based on medical records only (Stanhope, Brody & Brink, 1972). According to the results of the Rochester study the combined annual incidence rates for recurrent and single seizures as well as for febrile fits reach almost 120 per 100 000 (Hauser & Kurland, 1975). Even so, the incidence of the two latter groups seems still to be underestimated. However, these incidence rates make it possible to estimate the number of people who will need medical advice each year because of the occurrence of their first seizure.

Sex and age specific incidence

Most authors have found higher incidence rates in males although Pond's study showed a higher rate for females. There is a general consensus of opinion concerning age-specific rates (Table 2.2). The rates are higher within the first decade, and within this decade in the first year of life, somewhat lower in the second decade, and thereafter they become low. However, there are obvious differences between the studies, particularly in the figures for those of 60 and above. In Iceland, Carlisle and Greater Aarhus these rates are the lowest while in Rochester and Warsaw there is a marked increase in the oldest age group. This increase may be due to more effective case finding methods in these two studies. According to Hauser and Kurland (1975) an increased rate in the elderly does not necessarily reflect a higher incidence of brain tumours or cerebrovascular disease since in 70 per cent of new cases over 60 no clear aetiological factor could be found.

Prevalence of epilepsy

The literature contains a considerable number of studies devoted to estimating the prevalence of epilepsy in different countries. Many of them include more or less detailed descriptions of the method employed, definitions of the cases examined, and characteristics of the population studied. The results of the relevant epidemiological studies are given in Table 2.3.

The overall prevalence rates per 1000 of the general population vary from 1.3 in Formosa (Lin, 1953) and 1.5. in Niigata, Japan (Sato, 1964) to 9.2 in Warsaw (Zielinski, 1974a) and as high as 19.5 in Bogota, Colombia (Gomez, Arciniegas & Torres, 1978). In over half of the studies the rates

Table 2.2 Proportions of age-specific incidence rates for epilepsy (average annual incidence rate for all ages = 1.00)

Age	Rochester Minn. 1945–1954	Carlisle England 1955–1961	Iceland 1959–1964	Rochester Minn. 1935–1964	Warsaw Poland 1970–1972	Greater Aarhus Denmark 1960–1972
All ages = 1.00	30	28	33	45	20	30
0– 9	3.40	2.03	1.87	1.88	2.28	2.38
10–19	0.70	1.71	1.78	0.80	1.18	1.62
20–29	0.13	0.78	0.69	0.51	0.64	0.63
30–39	0.70	0.57	0.54	0.60	0.74	0.59
40–49	0.33	0.78	0.42	0.62	0.77	0.60
50–59	0.60	0.75	0.33	0.82	0.69	0.52
60 and above	0.70	0.42	0.18	1.33	0.93	

Table 2.3 Prevalence rates for epilepsy

Country, area studied	Author/s/	Case ascertainment method*	Rate per 1000	Comment*
Chile, Melipilla	Chiofale et al., 1979	SP, Itv + ME of selected sample	27.6 Range 21.1–31.9	Children aged 9, method and definition similar to Washington County study of Rose et al. (see below)
Colombia, Bogota	Gomez et al., 1978	SP, Itv + ME	19.5	Fs, Ss not included
Denmark, Aarhus	Juul-Jensen & Ipsen, 1976	ER	6.9	Including 1.1 for 'observation of epilepsy'
Formosa	Lin, 1953	RMR + ME	1.3	No definition. Study aimed toward epidemiology of mental disorders
Great Britain: England and Wales	Logan & Cushion, 1958	Information from 106 general practices	3.3	Epilepsy as diagnosed by GPs, annual attendance 1954/55
England and Wales	Crombie et al., 1960	Information from GPs, 67 practices	4.2	Epilepsy as diagnosed by GPs; 'non-active' cases not included
England	Pond et al., 1960	RMR in 14 general practices + Itv	6.2	Ss included, epilepsy as diagnosed by GPs, prev. per practice ranged 3.0–12.9; prev. of 'chronic epilepsy' – 4.2'
Carlisle	Brewis et al., 1966	RMR, including kind of ER, SP: Itv + ME	5.5 6.0	'lifetime'; Fs, Ss and symptomatic epilepsy not included
Isle of Wight	Rutter et al., 1972	ME of cohort of children aged 5–14	7.2	including 5.4 for 'uncomplicated' epilepsy
	Pless & Graham, 1970	as above, children aged 10–12	8.9	including 6.4 for 'uncomplicated' epilepsy and 4.9 for having fits in last year
Iceland	Schleisner, 1849 (after Gudmundsson, 1966)	RMR in 1847	5.8	After Gudmundsson
	Gudmundsson, 1966	RMR + ME	3.4 – for 'active' 5.2 – 'lifetime'	Fs and Ss cases excluded
Israel	Wajsbort et al., 1967	RMR of representation of insured in Workers Sick Fund	2.3	'Chronic epilepsy' 1.3 for inhabitants of Afro-Asian origine, 3.1 – European-American and 2.5 – Israel
Jerusalem	Leibowitz & Alter, 1968	RMR	4.1	Cases of Fs and Ss not included, unknown etiology only
Japan Niigata City	Sato, 1964	RMR	1.5	All symptomatic seizures excluded
Mariana Islands Guam	Lessel, Torres & Kurland, 1962	SP, Itv + ME	3.7	Afebrile Ss included

Country, area studied	Author/s/	Case ascertainment method*	Rate per 1000	Comment*
	Mathai et al., 1968	SP, Itv + ME	2.3– for 'active epilepsy 4.4– total	Fs and Ss cases not included
	Stanhope et al., 1972	SP, Itv + ME RMR only	5.3 3.1	Fs and Ss excluded 'active' cases only. High proportion of symptomatic epilepsy
Mexico Mexico City	Olivares, 1972	RMR of government employees	3.5	
Netherlands Zeeland	Bongers et al., 1976	Information from GPs	2.9	Epilepsy as diagnosed by interviewed GPs, prevalence per practice ranged 1.0–7.0
Nigeria Lagos	Dada, 1968	SP, Itv + ME apartmental area	3.1	Cit. Dada, 1976
Norway Northern	de Graaf, 1974	RMR of neurological and EEG services	3.5	Subarctic large area, difficult travelling
Poland: Pruszków	Zieliński, 1966	RMR + ME	4.3	Urban area, Fs and Ss not included, population aged 16 and above
Kielce	Nowak, 1972	RMR + ME + active case finding in rural area	4.9 – urban area 2.9 – rural area	Fs and Ss not included Pop'n aged 16 and above
Pruszków	Kuran, 1975	RMR and school files review, ME	6.7	School children aged 7–14
Zabrze	Grudzińska, 1974	ER + ME	3.4	Fs and Ss not included, highly industrialized urban area
Warsaw	Zieliński, 1974a	RMR + ME of random sample SP, Itv + ME	4.3 7.8 – 'active' 9.2 – 'lifetime'	Cases of Fs and Ss not included
Sampled areas all over Poland	Zieliński, 1975	Information from all medical services	2.8	Epilepsy as diagnosed by interviewed doctors, one year attendance
Romania	Milea & Tudor, 1969	RMR	3.9	No definition, children up till 15
South Africa	Bird et al., 1962	RMR	3.7	Male mine-workers aged 15–55 Bantu African people
USA: Rochester Minn.	Kurland, 1959	RMR of Mayo Clinic	3.6	Fs and Ss not included
	Hauser & Kurland, 1975 after Hauser, 1978	as above	5.3 for 1950 6.2 for 1960 5.7 for 1965	Recurrent, afebrile seizures; 'active' cases of epilepsy existent (whether diagnosed or not) on January 1 in various years

Country, area studied	Author/s/	Case ascertainment method*	Rate per 1000	Comment*
	Annegers & Hauser, 1977	as above	6.5 for 1970	as above
Washington County, Md	Rose et al., 1973	SP, Itv + ME of selected sample	18.6 Range 14.1–20.1	3rd grade school children aged 8–9; included cases of Fs and Ss with eeg changes or positive family history of epilepsy; response rate 91%
Multnomah County, Ore	Meighan et al., 1976	as above	9.7 Range 7.8–12.8	population and definition of 'a case' as above, response rate 76%

*RMR – Review of medical records in area studied,
ER – Epilepsy Register, continuous collection of data in area studied,
SP – Study based on general population or a sample of it,
Itv – Interview of inhabitants in population or its sample,
ME – Medical examination or re-examination of epileptic individuals or cases suspected of epilepsy,
GPs – General practitioners,
Fs – cases of febrile seizures,
Ss – cases with single afebrile seizure

lie between 4 and 10 per 1000. In most of the studies where the rate was lower than 4 per 1000 information was obtained solely from a review of medical records or from general practitioners. This includes the Polish survey which relied upon the total number of medical attendances in randomly sampled geographical areas (Zielinski, 1975). The necessary incompleteness of such data is shown by the results of the Guam and Warsaw studies (Stanhope et al, 1972; Zielinski, 1974a). The prevalence rates estimated on the basis of a population survey appeared to be higher by 70 per cent in the former and more than 100 per cent in the latter study. The differences between the rates in the Carlisle study, where they were founded both on medical files and on a house to house survey, were minimal. This was probably because only a single question was asked: 'Have you ever-suffered from attacks of loss of consciousness?' Moreover the prevalence in the last year of the Warsaw study, which was based only on cases attending the medical services, was lower by a third at 2.6 per 1000. This shows that the longer the period of study or the more intensive the case-finding method, the higher the probability of finding a larger number of affected people in the population. It is also worth noting that the prevalence of 'active' cases of epilepsy seems to be quite close in several studies: 2.3 in Guam (Mathai et al,

1968), 3.4 in Iceland (Gudmundsson, 1966), 5.7 or 6.5 in Rochester (Hauser & Kurland, 1975, Hauser, Annegers & Kurland, 1977) and 7.8 in Warsaw (Zielinski, 1974a).

'Lifetime' or 'total' prevalence

The estimate of this rate is founded on the determination of the number of people within a population who have ever suffered from epileptic seizures. It is difficult, if not virtually impossible, to discover all such cases. This is because of the varying clinical presentations of seizures, long term remissions and of the case-finding problems which have been described. The problem may be illustrated by the Warsaw study during which there was a review of medical and social services, a random sample of the epileptic patients being examined, and also a field survey of a sample of the population of Warsaw. The case-finding method in the field survey was in four stages. Firstly, an interview with a questionnaire covering six points about possible epileptic seizures or any other form of paroxysmal events, whether in the present or the past. Secondly, an independent evaluation of this information by two neurologists and a psychiatrist. Thirdly, a medical interview with those people whose past or present history suggested some form of epileptic seizure. And fourthly, a detailed comprehensive examination of those suspected of suffering from epilepsy. Finally, two groups are compared: those known to the medical and social services (group K) and those found in the population survey (group F). According to the distribution of basic clinical variables in these two groups, the following prevalence rates per 1000 population were estimated:

	Group K	Group F
Cases of epilepsy = total	4.3	9.2*
Seizures during past 5 years	4.2	7.8
Ever on medication	3.9	5.2
On medication when examined	3.3	3.2
6 years free of seizures	0.5	1.4

*If the expected number of people with epilepsy among those respondents who refused the questionnaire is included the rate would rise to 10.4.

It is clear that almost all the K group are cases of active epilepsy. Over 90 per cent took antiepileptic drugs regularly in the past and over 75 per cent were on medication when examined. The prevalence rates of those on medication are almost exactly the same in the two groups, although only some 35 per cent of group F were on drugs. Furthermore of the group F patients, over 35 per cent have never been on medication and some 25 per cent have never consulted a doctor because of their seizure disorder. The percentage of group F patients in the Warsaw study who have never been treated is very close to the 32 per cent found in Iceland. In both studies long term remission is significantly more frequent among these subjects than average. Thus milder and non-active epilepsy appears to be much commoner among undiagnosed and untreated cases. This seems to confirm the opinion of Rodin (1968) that the majority of patients who attend clinics regularly do so because their seizures are not satisfactorily controlled. Juul-Jensen & Ipsen (1976) also point out that a large number of patients become free of seizures and so are not included in the Epilepsy Register.

Incidence and prevalence rates based on data from medical records can thus be severely underestimated. The proportion of cases overlooked decreases when a field survey method is used, but even then some patients may refuse to disclose their epilepsy to the interviewer. In the Warsaw field survey patients whose names were known from medical files refused to complete the questionnaire more often than the rest of the sampled population (8.0 per cent v. 1.4 per cent).

The overall prognosis as estimated from relatively unselected groups of subjects seems to be far better than is expected generally. In the Rochester series, 20 years after the diagnosis of epilepsy was made, 40 per cent of patients had been free of seizures for at least 10 years, and 55 per cent for at least two years (Hauser & Kurland, 1975). On follow-up of the Warsaw patients, 37 per cent had been seizure-free for six years or more and 60 per cent for at least two years. It is worth emphasising that in our experience patients who have been free of seizures for a long time are unwilling to give information at follow-up examination and may even refuse to do so. They consider themselves cured and often state that they do not want to be reminded of their past illness (Zielinski, Kuran & Witkowska-Olearska, 1978). This explains why the more benign forms of epilepsy are under-represented in the medical case series. Therefore, it should be pointed out again that the 'accumulated incidence' seems to be the most precise tool to estimate the lifetime risk of epilepsy. Thus Hauser and Kurland (1975, assuming that the average life expectancy of a Rochester resident was 70 years, estimated that about six per cent of the total population may be expected to suffer from at least a single non-febrile epileptic seizure, whilst almost four per cent will have had recurrent seizures at some period of their lives.

Sex and age specific prevalence rates for epilepsy

In the vast majority of the studies quoted in Table 2.3, males tend to predominate and only in Juul-Jensen's and one of Pond's studies were there more females. Several authors have suggested that the high male rate is due to more frequent head injuries. Indeed in a random sample of the Warsaw population some 2.2 per cent of children and 4 per cent of adults reported at least one admission to hospital because of a head injury. Further, head injury prior to the onset of seizures was noted nearly twice as often in males (30 per cent v. 16 per cent). The prevalence rates of post-traumatic epilepsy were estimated in the study at 1.0–1.5 per thousand (Zielinski, 1977).

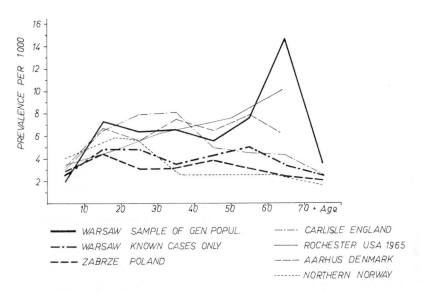

AGE - SPECIFIC PREVALENCE RATES OF EPILEPSY PER 1000
ACCORDING TO RESULTS OF SELECTED COMMUNITY SURVEYS

——— WARSAW SAMPLE OF GEN. POPUL.   —·— CARLISLE ENGLAND
—·— WARSAW KNOWN CASES ONLY   ——— ROCHESTER USA 1965
— — ZABRZE POLAND   ——— AARHUS DENMARK
                                     ········ NORTHERN NORWAY

Fig. 2.1 Age-specific prevalence rates of epilepsy per 1000 according to results of selected community surveys

Age specific prevalence rates from several studies are shown in Figure 2.1. In most studies the
rates which were based on medical services case
series show a very similar pattern. The lowest
rates, which usually occur in the first decade,
increase in the older age groups and then show a
marked drop after 50. Only in Rochester and
Warsaw were there high prevalences at older ages,
and in Aarhus during the sixth decade. This rise
in prevalence rates in the elderly seems to be due
to more effective case-finding methods showing up
the accumulation of cases.

Prevalence in children

Several studies estimate the prevalence in the
youngest age groups in which the chance of seizures occurring is greatest. On follow-up of a
cohort of children born in Newcastle upon Tyne,
Miller et al (1960) found that before the age of five
one or more seizures occurred in seven per cent of
subjects, and of these two per cent had recurrent
seizures. Cooper (1965) during a British national
survey of 5000 births estimated that over two per
cent of children experienced at least one seizure
before the age of two. According to reports of

school medical officers, based chiefly on information from parents, 7–8 per thousand of school
children between the ages of six and fifteen had
had some kind of fit during the previous year.
McDonald (1961) estimated that 1.5 per cent of
school children had a positive history of seizures.
Similarly, Van den Bergh & Yerushalmy (1969)
found in a cohort of children born in the San
Francisco area that one per cent had had afebrile
seizures before the end of their fifth year, usually
early in life. Similarly, according to Gates (1972)
3.4 per cent of a cohort of children born in New
York experienced at least one afebrile seizure
before the age of eight. Studies of school children
in Poland yielded similar results: 6.7 per thousand,
aged 7–8, had repeated seizures, including 5.2
with seizures during the previous two years
(Kuran, 1975). Studies of Rose et al (1973),
Meighan et al (1976), and Chiofale et al (1979)
used the same methodological approach and a
wide definition of epilepsy which included febrile
fits and single seizures with EEG signs or a positive family history of epilepsy. Although in Multnomah County the response rate was lower than in
Washington County, the results of these two
studies estimate the prevalence of epilepsy among

Table 2.4 Relative frequency of generalised and partial seizures in case – series of epileptic patients found during selected epidemiological studies (percentage)

Type of seizure	a Rochester (1960)	b Warsaw		c Bogota	d Large epileptic out-patients population (non epidemiological study)
		Known cases	Field survey		
Generalised	34	48	35	73	38
Partial	66	52	65	27	62
Including temporal lobe	27	34	43		40

a Hauser & Kurland, 1975
b Zieliński, 1974a
c Gomez et al, 1978
d Gastaut et al, 1975

third grade children at about 1–2 per cent, while in the Chilean town of Melipilla it was nearly three per cent.

Seizure type

The frequency of various types of seizures has usually been analysed in selected out- and in-patient case series. Gastaut et al (1975) calculated the relative distribution in a series of 4590 private patients. Unfortunately, only very few epidemiologists have reported comparable data.

Table 2.4 shows that the distribution of patients with primary generalised seizures as contrasted with partial seizures is similar in the Rochester and Warsaw Group F studies (field survey), close to Gastaut's series but very different to that from Bogota. The percentage for temporal lobe epilepsy is a good deal higher in the Warsaw Group F and from Gastaut than in the Rochester series. The difference in the frequency of partial seizures between Warsaw Groups K and F is due to the patients with complex partial seizures without secondary generalization – 12 per cent in Group F and 4 per cent in Group K, $p < 0.01$. Secondary generalised temporal lobe seizures at 30 per cent were equally frequent in each group. This shows that some types of fits, particularly those which do not develop to major convulsions, are either ignored by patients or considered as some natural phenomenon of rather minor importance. Most patients do not consider that such problems need medical treatment.

Frequency of chronic institutionalized cases of epilepsy

The percentage of chronic inpatients with epilepsy in mental hospitals and long-stay care institutions in Poland has been estimated at three per cent of all patients with epilepsy known to the medical services. In all these cases severe mental, intellectual or neurological handicap seemed to be responsible for institutionalization (Zielinski, 1972; Zielinski, Okolowicz-Zielinska & Kuligowski, 1973). This agrees with Pond & Burden (1963) and Janz (1972) in their estimates for Great Britain and the Federal Republic of Germany.

Time trends

Time trends for incidence and prevalence rates have only been given in one study, that of Rochester which covers 40 years. The average annual incidence rates calculated since 1935 for three 10-year periods and for the final three-year period 1965–1967 showed a substantial increase from 35 per 100 000 in 1935–1944 to 54 per 100 000 during the next two periods. In the last three years, however, the rate dropped down to 46. These changes were seen most dramatically for the rates during the first year of life: 111, to 250 and 138 with a drop to 73. Prevalence rates estimated on January 1st of the years 1940, 1950, 1960 and 1970 showed less variation at 3.7, 5.3, 6.2, and 5.7 per thousand (Hauser & Kurland, 1975). Recently Hauser et al (1977) found a further fall in the annual incidence rate in Rochester during the period 1965–1974 to 33 per 100 000. The fall was particularly marked in the young and was thought to be due to starting treatment more often after a single seizure. This hypothesis should be tested carefully since many clinicians are not convinced that a single fit is a sufficient indication for initiating treatment. On the other hand, it should be stressed that the same authors also established a decrease in the incidence rates of single seizures. This might be due to various factors including better pre-, perinatal and obstetric care with more effective prevention of brain infections or trauma.

MORTALITY RATES FOR EPILEPSY

Studies on mortality and the causes of death are usually based on death certificates and special analyses of selected groups of patients. Some of the methodological difficulties have been discussed already. There is also a difference between the terms 'death due to epilepsy' and 'death of a person with epilepsy'. If a patient dies in status epilepticus, then death is obviously due to epilepsy. However, in cases of symptomatic epilepsy the death certificates will state the diagnosis of the underlying condition: e.g. head injury or brain tumour. Further, in cases of non-active epilepsy it is unlikely that the diagnosis of epilepsy

will appear on the certificates. On the other hand, even if death is due directly to epilepsy as for example from an accident during a seizure, the diagnosis of epilepsy will not appear if the certifying doctor does not happen to know that the victim suffered from epilepsy. Thus the broader and less specific category 'death of a person with epilepsy' cannot be estimated accurately from an analysis of death certificates.

Mortality statistics based on death certificates

Although only a fraction of all people with epilepsy who die can be identified through death certificates, routine mortality statistics are the only ready source of data with which to compare deaths due to epilepsy in different countries and at different times. Figure 2.2 shows age-adjusted annual death rates for epilepsy in different mainly European countries. In two thirds of the 32 selected countries the rates were between 1.1 and 2.0 per 100 000. The rank order of the countries with the highest rates was virtually the same in the years 1951 to 1958 (Goldberg & Kursland, 1962) as in the years 1974 to 1976. The differences between countries might be due to local methods of filling in death certificates. This hypothesis would be supported by the fact that the countries with the highest rates were also those in which epilepsy was most often certified as the underlying cause of

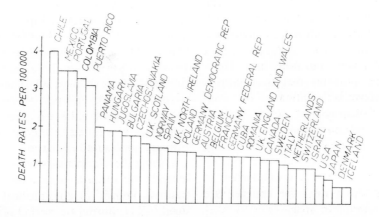

Fig. 2.2 Age-adjusted annual death rates for epilepsy per 100 000 population in selected countries, 1974–1976

death. This ratio varies between 1.0 and 2.0 per 1000 deaths, except in Chile and Colombia where it is 3.0 and over. It may be noted that recent epidemiological surveys in these countries have shown high prevalence rates for epilepsy (Gomez et al, 1978; Chiofale et al, 1979), and epilepsy may indeed be a more frequent underlying cause of death. In the USA the annual death rates for epilepsy tended to decline from 1939 to 1967, whereas in Poland they remained fairly stable between 1960 and 1975 (Kurtzke, 1972; Zielinski, 1978).

Sex and age specific death rates

In most countries the death rates are higher for males than for females. Age specific rates are usually high in the first year of life, and then stay low until they rise again in the fifth and sixth decades.

Death rates according to race, marital status and domicile

A detailed analysis of deaths due to epilepsy in the USA (Kurtzke, 1972; Kurtzke et al, 1973) reveals that the rates are significantly higher for non-whites. This applies particularly to males for whom the rates are three times as high as those for whites, and five or more times as high between the ages of 25 and 55. This may be due either to fatal cases of epilepsy being more common or to there being a greater chance of epilepsy being listed on the death certificate of a non-white person.

Death rates are significantly higher for the single than the married. Kurtzke considers that this reflects a more regular life with more reliable taking of medication among married people with a lesser risk of head injury and alcoholism. However, it seems more probable that those factors which have an unfavourable influence on prognosis in epilepsy, (neurological deficit, mental changes, frequent and uncontrollable seizures), also tend to lessen a person's chance of getting married.

Some studies, including those conducted in Poland, claim that death rates for epilepsy are higher in rural than in urban areas.

Special studies on mortality and survivorship in epilepsy

There are very few studies founded on observation of large and relatively unselected groups of patients. Henriksen, Juul-Jensen and Lund (1967) carried out a follow-up of Danish epileptic patients between 15 and 59, the majority being examined in neurological departments. Those with epilepsy due to tumours or cerebrovascular malformations were excluded. The authors believed that milder cases were only slightly under-represented although they did not try to prove this. Holders of a life insurance policy acted as controls. They found the death rates for the epileptic patients to be 2.9 times higher than controls. The excess was 3.7 times for males and 2.2 for females and it was noted particularly in the fourth and fifth decades. If cases with more frequent seizures were excluded, the excess fell to 2.0.

Hauser and Kurland (1975) carried out an analysis of all deaths among those in Rochester with epilepsy which occurred during the 20 years after the diagnosis was made. These authors claimed that the 'survivorship ratio' – the ratio of survivals among patients to survivals among matched controls – seemed to be more useful than the 'mortality ratio' – the ratio of deaths between the two groups. The survivorship ratio for Rochester epileptic patients was 91 per cent at five years, 85 per cent at 10, and 83 per cent at 15 years after diagnosis. Thus the greatest difference between the groups occurred during the first few years after the diagnosis. Thereafter the rate of decline of the survivorship is much the same although the survival curve for the patients is of course lower. The survivorship ratio is better for females and worse for those diagnosed during the first year of life or between 20 and 59. It is lower in patients with epilepsy of suspected aetiology than in those of unknown origin. No significant difference was found in the ratios for partial and primary generalised epilepsy.

During the Warsaw survey (Zielinski, 1974b) an attempt was made to analyse mortality in epileptic patients known to the medical services. Total deaths (TD) during the period of study were 218.

If symptomatic cases with brain tumours or cerebrovascular malformations were excluded – the same criteria as were used by Henriksen et al (1967) – a subgroup (A) had 120 deaths. Only 10 per cent of deaths were of patients within the first three decades, whereas 50 per cent were of patients over 60. The average age at death in group TD was 55 years, contrasted with 47 years in group A. For the last year of the study the annual case fatality ratio in known epileptic patients reached almost 1.6 per cent. While the total observed death rate among patients was only 1.8 times the expected, for those who died before the age of 50 the ratio was as high as 3.5. This would support the hypothesis that younger epileptic patients particularly run a greater than expected risk of death.

Causes of death in epileptic patients

There is a number of papers on causes of death among epileptic out- and more especially in-patients. Unfortunately most of the groups are highly selected.

Hauser and Kurland (1975) found that, apart from an excess due to brain tumour, the rank order by cause of death among Rochester patients with epilepsy was the same as for the general population.

During the Warsaw survey, Table 2.5, the cause of death in each case was reviewed in the light of information from all available sources, including death certificates, medical and police records, and interviews with the family and general practitioners. Comparable data was obtained on the causes of death for 97 chronic epileptic patients from one of Poland's mental hospitals (Kahl-Kunstetter & Zielinski, 1972). It will be seen that in the whole group of 218 (TD) heart disease and brain tumour were the commonest causes of death with epilepsy coming third. In four out of the nine (4.1 per cent) accidents not related to seizures there was a high blood alcohol level. The miscellaneous causes include 27 strokes and seven acute alcoholic deaths in patients who before death presented severe behavioural problems due to an organic brain syndrome. In group A epilepsy followed by suicide were the two commonest causes of death.

In the highly selected group of patients dying in a mental hospital there were very high percentages of deaths from status epilepticus and pneumonia. This agrees with the results of Krohn (1963), Neploch (1965) and Penning, Muller and Ciompi (1969) who reported on similar populations.

Thus it will be seen that the frequencies of different causes of death depend on the epileptic population surveyed.

Table 2.5 Verified causes of death in epileptic patients known to Warsaw medical services, and in chronic mental hospital patients with epilepsy (percentage; N = 100%)

| | Percentage of patients | | |
| | Warsaw known cases | | Mental hospital |
Cause of death	Total TD N = 218	Group A (symptomatic epilepsy excluded) N = 120	MH N = 97
Status epilepticus	3.2	5.8	17.5
Death during or after seizure	3.2	5.8	2.1
Sudden unexplained death	4.2	7.5	1.0
Fatal accident due to seizure	3.2	5.0	0
Epilepsy, subtotal	13.8	24.1	20.6
Brain tumour	15.1	0	5.2
Heart disease	16.1	8.3	19.6
Tumour not involving brain	8.7	11.7	2.0
Pneumonia	7.8	9.2	24.7
Suicide	7.3	11.7	3.1
Accident not due to seizure	4.1	7.5	0
Miscellaneous	27.1	27.5	24.8

Table 2.6 Causes of death of epileptic patients (percentage)

Cause of death	Zieliński 1974a (group A) POLAND	Haltrich FRG	Henriksen et al. 1967 DENMARK
Status epilepticus	6	10	—
Sudden death	13	6	—
Accident due to seizure	5	8	—
Epilepsy total	24	24	26
Suicide	12	10	22
Accident not due to seizure	7	3	11
Heart diseases	8	9	11
Carcinoma	12	10	6
Miscellaneous	27	18	17

Because group A was selected according to the same criteria as Henricksen's series, and, with the exception of vascular malformations, to Haltrich's (after Janz, 1969), the results of the three studies comparable are shown (Table 2.6). It will be seen that the mortality rates for different causes, and particularly for epilepsy, are very similar in each series. It would seem therefore that each study reviewed similar epileptic populations, in which, as in the Warsaw survey, milder cases were greatly under-represented.

Suicides accounted for about 10 per cent of deaths in Poland and West Germany but for twice as many in Denmark. In Poland suicides in epileptic males were five times as high as in the general population and for females twice. This excess was particularly marked in group A patients and in the younger age groups. It should be remembered that the frequency of attempted suicide in the general population is highest in the young, and yet among such cases only 2.5 per cent of males and 0.7 per cent of females were diagnosed as having epilepsy (Kostrzewa et al, 1972).

Frequency of the diagnosis of epilepsy on death certificates

During the Warsaw study it was found that epilepsy as the underlying cause of death or as an associated condition appeared on 63 (29 per cent) of the 218 certificates of people who for one to four years before their death had attended doctors because of epilepsy.

Table 2.7 Place of death and diagnosis of epilepsy (as underlying or associated disease) in death certificates of 218 epileptic patients*

Place of death	No.† of deaths (= 100%)	Percentage of death certificates containing diagnosis of epilepsy
Neurological or neurosurgical department	59	37.3
Mental hospital	16	75.0
Other hospital departments	46	15.2
Other places	16	43.8
Total	218	28.9

*From Zieliński, 1974b

†In this table as in Table 2.8 the percentage in the right hand column relates to the number in the middle column. For example: of the 59 patients who died in neurological or neurosurgical departments, 22 or 37.3% had a death certificate containing the diagnosis of epilepsy.

The data in Tables 2.7 and 2.8 illustrate the probability of finding the diagnosis of epilepsy on death certificates according to where the patient died and the underlying cause of death. It will be seen that these factors influence significantly the estimates of routinely calculated death rates for epilepsy. For instance, the annual mortality rate for known epilepsy in Warsaw was 7.8 per 100 000 in 1969. When the rate was calculated on

Table 2.8 Verified cause of death and diagnosis of epilepsy (as underlying or associated disease) in death certificates of 218 epileptic patients*

Cause of death (re-evaluated) – verified	No. of deaths (100%)	Percentage of death certificates containing the diagnosis of epilepsy
Epilepsy†	23	73.9
Accident due to seizure	7	42.8
Epilepsy, subtotal	30	66.6
Heart disease	35	28.6
Brain tumour	33	39.4
Stroke	27	14.8
Tumour not involving brain	19	10.5
Pneumonia	19	52.6
Suicide	16	6.3
Accident not due to seizure	9	0
Miscellaneous	30	10.0
Total	218	28.9

the basis of death certificates that reported epilepsy as a diagnosis it dropped to 2.4, and when based only on death certificates in which epilepsy as a diagnosis, it dropped to 2.4, and death it fell as low as 1.0 per 100 000, a figure comparable to the epilepsy mortality rate given for the US population (Kurtzke et al, 1973). It seems, therefore, that the results of the many studies of mortality rates are useful for determining the fraction of people with epilepsy who die rather than for evaluating the prognosis in epilepsy.

THE NATURE OF POPULATIONS OF PEOPLE WITH EPILEPSY

Because patients conceal their epilepsy and because others ignore certain types of seizures, even the most sophisticated field survey methods are bound to miss some patients, and it may be assumed that most of these will be the milder cases. According to the Warsaw study the variable 'under medication at the time of the examination' correlated highly with frequent major convulsions, lack of remission, as well as with neurological and psychiatric evidence of brain damage. These variables also correlated highly with each other as well as with variables such as a low socioeconomic status as evidenced by a low level of education, lack of professional qualifications and a poor work record. This complex of specific interrelated traits encompasses the group presenting medical and social problems. It is obvious that this group, which requires special medical and social care, will be over-represented among the population known to the medical and social services as contrasted with their representation in the epileptic population found in a general survey. This must be remembered when trying to generalise from the results of studies on selected case series. On the other hand, an epidemiological study based on medical records would be likely to give a relatively accurate estimate of the size of the epileptic population which needs special medical and social care.

Personal situation 1

M.S., a 32-year-old female, at questionnaire responded to the question: 'Have you had a feeling of momentary absent-mindedness?'. On this basis two out of three experts rated her as 'slightly suspect of having epilepsy'.

She was the second of a twin delivery and heard from her mother that she was cyanosed at birth and did not breathe spontaneously. Her later physical and intellectual development was normal and after leaving secondary school she worked as a teller. She married and had one healthy child.

Since the age of 20 she has experienced episodes of momentary loss of consciousness, sometimes preceded by brief dizziness. She has never collapsed but occasionally she would drop some object she was holding. Automatic movements of varying complexity had been noticed. After the attack she usually felt slightly confused. She was aware that she had had a blackout. These paroxysmal episodes were always the same and appeared for no apparent reason. They occurred about once a month and they had been less frequent in the year before the interview. She did not think that her symptoms were due to any disease and observed: 'I imagine anyone may feel like that at times'.

No abnormalities were found on neurological or psychiatric examination, and her IQ on the WAIS was 100. On her EEG slow waves at 5 to 6 Hz were seen over both temporal areas and on over-breathing paroxysmal discharges of sharp waves appeared over the same areas with a tendency to generalisation.

About five years later on a follow-up examination it was found that she had been free of attacks for three years. The patient was never treated for her fits and had refused such an opportunity when she had been first examined.

Personal situation 2

J.C. was a 13-year-old secondary school boy. At questionnaire his mother affirmed 'Episodes of sudden loss of consciousness' and 'Convulsions'. She said that her son had had a single febrile convulsion at the age of four and that since then he had been in good health although he had had infrequent headaches and had had some difficulties at school. However, there had been no behavioural problems.

On neurological examination the boy admitted that at least once a month he experienced a momentary feeling of confusion when he could not understand what people were talking about and that he was then briefly unconscious. He could not remember for how long he had had these attacks. He thought that they were quite natural and they did not worry him. He never told his mother or anyone else about them. He himself did not know about the febrile convulsion he had had when he was young. Neurological examination was normal. Psychiatric testing showed some evidence of immaturity although his intelligence was normal. His EEG series showed sharp waves and high amplitude theta activity over the right temporal area.

He refused both treatment and further examination. On follow-up five years later, the only information which could be obtained was that he had had no blackouts during the past two years.

REFERENCES

Alter, M., Masland, R.L., Kurtzke, J.F. & Reed, D.M. (1972) Proposed definitions and classifications of epilepsy for epidemiological purposes. In *The Epidemiology of Epilepsy: a Workshop*, eds Hauser, W.A., Alter, M., NINDS Monograph No. 14, pp. 147–148, Washington DC: USDHEW.

Bird, A.V., Heinz, H.J. & Klintworth, G. (1962) Convulsive disorders in Bantu mine workers, *Epilepsia*, **3**, 175.

Blom, S., Heijbel, J., Bergfors, P.G. (1978) Incidence of epilepsy in children: a follow-up study three years after the first seizure. *Epilepsia*, **19**, 343.

Bongers, E., Coppoolse, J., Meinardi, H., Posthuma, E.P.S. & VanZijl, C.H.W. (1976) *A survey of epilepsy in Zealand, the Netherlands*. Heemstede Instituut voor Epilepsiebestrijding, Meer en Bosch.

Brewis, M., Poskanzer, D., Rolland, C. & Miller, H. (1966) Neurological disease in an English city. *Acta Neurologica Scandinavica*, **42**, Supplement 24.

Chiofale, N., Kirschbaum, A., Fuantes, A., Cordero, M.L. & Madsen, J. (1979) Prevalence of epilepsy in children of Melipilla, Chile. *Epilepsia*, **20**, 262.

Cooper, J.E. (1965) Epilepsy in a longitudinal survey of 5000 children. *British Medical Journal*, **1**, 1020.

Crombie, D.L., Cross, K.W., Fry, J., Pinsent, R.J. & Watts, C.A. (1960) A survey of the epilepsies in general practice. A report by the Research Committee of College of General Practitioners. *British Medical Journal*, **2**, 416–422.

Dada, T.O. (1976) The epilepsies: their incidence and causation in Nigeria. In *Epileptology. Proceedings of the Seventh International Symposium on Epilepsy, Berlin, 1975*, ed. Janz, D., p. 24. Stuttgart: Georg Thieme Publishers.

De Graaf, A.S., (1974) Epidemiological aspects of epilepsy in Northern Norway. *Epilepsia*, **15**, 291–299.

Fletcher, W. (1907) Rice and beri-beri: preliminary report of an experiment conducted at the Kuala Lumpur Lunatic Asylum. *Lancet*, **1**, 1776–1779.

Gastaut, H. (1973) *Dictionary of epilepsy*. Part I: Definitions. Geneva: WHO.

Gastaut, H., Gastaut, J.L., Goncalves e Silva, G.E. & Fernandez Sanohez, G.R. (1975) Relative frequency of different types of epilepsy: a study employing the classification of the International League Against Epilepsy. *Epilepsia*, **16**, 457.

Gates, M.J. (1972) Age: risk of seizure in infants. *The Epidemiology of Epilepsy: a Workshop*, eds Hauser, W.A. & Alter, M. NIND Monograph No. 14, p. 75, Washington, D.C.: USDHEW.

Goldberger, J. (1914) The etiology of pellagra. The significance of certain epidemiological observations with respect hereto. *Public Health Reports*, **29**, 1683.

Goldberg, I.D. & Kurland, L.T. (1962) Mortality in 33 countries from diseases of the nervous system. *World Neurology*, **3**, 444.

Gomez, J.G., Arciniegas, E. & Torres, J. (1978) Prevalence of epilepsy in Bogota, Colombia. *Neurology*, **28**, 90.

Grudzińska, B. (1974) Epidemiology of epilepsy in population of a large industrial city. Incidence and prevalence (in Polish). *Neurologia Neurochirurgia Polska*, **8**, 175.

Gudmundsson, G. (1966) Epilepsy in Iceland. *Acta Neurologica Scandinavica*, **43**, Supplement 25.

Hauser, W.A. (1978) Epidemiology of epilepsy. *In Advance in Neurology*, Vol. 19, Neurological Epidemiology: Principles and Clinical Applications, ed. Schoenberg, B.S., pp. 313, New York: Raven Press.

Hauser, W.A. & Kurland, L.T. (1975) The epidemiology of epilepsy in Rochester, Minnesota, 1935 through 1967. *Epilepsia*, **16**, 1.

Hauser, W.A., Annegers, J.F. & Kurland, L.T. (1977) Is incidence of epilepsy declining? *American Journal of Epidemiology*, **106**, 246 (Abstract).

Henriksen, P.B., Juul-Jensen, P. & Lund, M. (1967) The mortality of epileptics. *Epilepsy and Insurance. Social Studies in Epilepsy*, No. 5. London: International Bureau for Epilepsy.

Hopkins, A., Scambler, G. (1977) How doctors deal with epilepsy. *Lancet*, **1**, 183.

Janz, D. (1969) *Die Epilepsien*. Stuttgart: Georg Thieme Verlag.

Janz, D. (1972) Social prognosis in epilepsy especially in regard to social status and the necessity for institutionalization. *Epilepsia*, **13**, 141.

Juul-Jensen, P. & Ipsen, J. (1975) Prevalence and incidence of epilepsy in Greater Aarhus. *Ugeskrift for Laeger*, **137**, 2380.

Juul-Jensen, P., Ipsen, J. (1976) Prevalence and incidence of epilepsy in Greater Aarhus. *Epileptology. Proceedings of the Seventh International Symposium on Epilepsy*. Berlin/West June 1975, ed. Janz, D., p. 10. Stuttgart: Georg Thieme Publishers.

Kahl-Kunstetter, J., Zieliński, J.J. (1972) Causes of deaths of epileptic patients-inmates of a mental hospital. (in Polish) *Neurologia Neurochirurgia Polska*, **22**, 6, 847.

Kostrzewa, T., Mijal, K., Pańków, T., Pluzek, Z. & Wilk, Z. (1972) Attempts of suicide in Kraków, in 1962, 1966, 1967 and 1969. (in Polish). *Psychiatria Polska*, **6**, 299.

Krohn, W. (1961) A study of epilepsy in northern Norway, its frequency and character. *Acta Psychiatrica Scandinavica*, **36**, Suppl. 150.

Krohn, W. (1963) Causes of death among epileptics. *Epilepsia*, **4**, 315.

Kuran, W. (1975) Epidemiology of epilepsy in school children in two small towns. (in Polish). *Neurologia Neurochirurgia Polska*, **9**, 57.

Kurland, L.T. (1959) The incidence and prevalence of convulsive disorders in a small urban community. *Epilepsia*, **1**, 143.

Kurtzke, J.F. (1972) Mortality and morbidity data on epilepsy. *The Epidemiology of Epilepsy: a Workshop*, ed. Milton, A., Hauser, W.A. pp. 21, NINDS Monograph No. 14. Washington, D.C.: DHEW.

Kurtzke, J.F., Kurland, L.T., Goldberg, I.D., Won Choi, N. & Reeder, F.A. (1973) Convulsive disorders. *Epidemiology of Neurologic and Sense Organ Disorders*, ed. Kurland, L.T., APHA Monograph, Cambridge, Massachusetts: Harvard University Press.

Leibowitz, M. & Alter, M. (1968) Epilepsy in Jerusalem, Israel. *Epilepsia*, **9**, 87.

Lennox, W.G. (1960) *Epilepsy and related disorders*. London: Churchill.

Lessel, S. Torres, I.M. & Kurland, L.T. (1962) Seizure disorders in a Guamanian village. *Archives of Neurology*, **7**, 37.

Lin, T. (1953) A study of the incidence of mental disorders in Chinese and other cultures. *Psychiatry*, **16**, 313.

Logan, W.P.D. & Cushion, A.A. (1958) Studies on medical and population subjects, *No 14. Morbidity Statistics from*

General Practice, I, pp. 174. London: Her Majesty's Stationery Office.

Mathai, K.V., Dunn, D.P., Kurland, L.T. & Reeder, F.A. (1968) Convulsive disorders in the Mariana Islands, Epilepsia, 9, 77.

McDonald, A. (1961) Maternal health in early pregnancy and congenital defect. Final report on a prospective inquiry. British Journal of preventive and social Medicine, 15, 154.

Meighan, S.S., Queener, L. & Weitman, M. (1976) Prevalence of epilepsy in children of Multnomah County, Oregon. Epilepsia, 17, 245.

Milea, S. & Tudor, I. (1969) Epilepsy in children in a middle city. (in Rumanian). Neurologia (Bucuresti), 14, 63.

Miller, F.J., Court, S.D., Walton, W.S. & Knox, E.G. (1960) Growing up in Newcastle upon Tyne. A continuing study of health and illness in young children with their families. London/New York: Oxford University Press.

Neploch, I. (1965) Causes of death in epilepsy. (in Russian). Zhurnal Nevropatologii i Psikhiatrii im. Korsakova, 65, 1383.

Nowak, S. (1972) Epidemiology and social-medical aspects of epilepsy in a rural and city communities. (in Polish). Neurolog Neurochirurgia Polska, 6, 369.

Olivares, L. (1972) Epilepsy in Mexico: a population study. The Epidemiology of Epilepsy: a Workshop, ed. Milton, A. & Hauser, W.A. pp. 53, NINDS Monograph N° 14. Washington: DHEW.

Penning, R., Muller, C. & Ciompi, L. (1969) Mortality and cause of death in epileptics. (in French). Psychiatria Clinica (Basel) 2, 85.

Pless, B. & Graham, P. (1970) Epidemiology of physical disorder. Education, Health and Behaviour, ed. Rutter, M., Tizard, J., Whitmore, K. pp. 285. London: Longman.

Pond, D.A., Bidwell, B.H. & Stein, L. (1960) A survey of epilepsy in fourteen general practices. I demographic and medical data. Psychiatria, Neurologia, Neurochirurgia, 63, 217.

Pond, D.A. & Burden, G.S. (1963) Review of the social and medical services for the epileptic patient in England and Wales. Epilepsia, 4, 77.

Rodin, E.A. (1968) The prognosis of patients with epilepsy. Springfield, Illinois, USA: Thomas.

Rose, S.W., Penry, J.K., Markush, R.E., Radloff, L.A. & Putnam, P.L. (1973) Prevalence of epilepsy in children. Epilepsia, 14, 133.

Rutter, M., Graham, P. & Yule, W. (1972) A neuropsychiatric study in childhood. London: Spastics International Medical Publication in association with William Heinemann Medical Books.

Sato, S. (1964) An epidemiologic and clinicostatistical study of epilepsy in Niigata City. Epidemiologic study. (in Japanese). Clinical Neurology, 4, 413.

Schoenberg, B.S., Mann, R.J. & Kurland, L.T. (1974) Snow on the water of London. Mayo Clinic Proceedings, 49, 680.

Stanhope, J.M., Brody, J.A. & Brink, E. (1972) Convulsions among the Chamorro people of Guam, Mariana Islands. I. Seizure disorders. American Journal of Epidemiology, 95, 292.

Van den Berg, B.J. & Yerushalmy, J. (1969) Studies on convulsive disorders in young children, Part I (Incidence of febrile and nonfebrile convulsions by age and other factors). Pediatric Research, 3, 298.

Wajsbort, J. Haral, N. & Alfandary, I. (1967) A study of the epidemiology of chronic epilepsy in Northern Israel. Epilepsia, 8, 105.

Zieliński, J.J. (1966) Epileptic patients in the district city population. (in Polish). Neurologia, Neurochirurgia Polska, 16, 511.

Zieliński, J.J. (1972) Social prognosis in epilepsy. Epilepsia, 13, 133.

Zieliński, J.J. (1974a) Epidemiology and medical-social problems of epilepsy in Warsaw. Warsaw: Psychoneurological Institute.

Zieliński, J.J. (1974b) Epilepsy and mortality rates and cause of death. Epilepsia, 15, 191.

Zieliński, J.J. (1975) Epidemiology of epilepsy in Poland on the basis of visits to physicians. (in Polish). Przeglad Epidemiologiczny, 29, 123.

Zieliński, J.J. (1976) People with epilepsy who do not attend doctors. Epileptology. Proceedings of the Seventh International Symposium on Epilepsy, Berlin (West), June 1975, ed. Janz, pp. 18. Stuttgart: Georg Thieme.

Zieliński, J.J. (1977) Frequency of head trauma and posttraumatic epilepsy in Warsaw population. Posttraumatic Epilepsy and Pharmacological Prophylaxis. Proceedings of First European Regional Conference on Epilepsy, Warsaw, June 1976, ed. Majkowski, J. pp. 30. Warsaw: Polish Chapter of the ILAE.

Zieliński, J.J. (1978) Neurologic diseases and syndromes in Poland, 1960–1970. (in Polish). Poland 2000: Presence and future of frequent diseases in Poland, ed. Kopczyński, J., Korzybski, T. & Sawicki, T. pp. 174–192. Wroclaw: Zaklad Narodowy im. Ossolińskich.

Zieliński, J.J., Kuran, W. & Witkowska-Olearska, K. (1978) The course of epilepsy and drug taking in randomly selected groups of patients in the light of 5-year follow-up. (in Polish). Polski Tygodnik Lekarski, 33, 1927.

Zieliński, J.J., Okolowicz-Zielińska, I. & Kuligowski, Z.W. (1973) Long-term epileptic patients of psychiatric hospitals and nursing care institutions. (in Polish). Neurologia, Neurochirurgia Polska, 7, 514.

3

Fits in children

PART ONE

J.K. Brown

GENERAL INTRODUCTION

A fit is probably the commonest neurological disorder seen in the neonate and preschool child. Fits are commoner at this time of life than at any other with a combined incidence of up to 60 per 1000, and 85 per cent of cases of status epilepticus occur in this age group. The brain in the preschool child is growing rapidly and so a fit may have a more profound effect on subsequent brain development. It is known that antiepileptic drugs may cause congenital abnormalities by affecting the fetus in utero but there is also the danger that they may interfere with brain growth, a risk to which the mature adult brain is not exposed. Brain damage may be produced by perinatal events complicated by fits or by prolonged febrile convulsions. Therefore many cases of adult epilepsy are due to potentially preventable causes in infancy and early childhood.

Definition

Fits are 'dysrhythmias of the nervous system' and should be regarded in a similar way to cardiac dysrhythmias. Fits may occur as the first sign of acute disease and may be single, multiple or status and may occur only in the acute phase or persist for the rest of the patient's life. They may be due to actual pathology of the brain or be part of general-

ised systemic disorders such as poisoning, septicaemia or metabolic diseases. Drugs used in cardiac dysrhythmias such as lignocaine, procainamide, or phenytoin have ionotropic effects and also are antiepileptic. Digoxin used to be given to treat epilepsy. Hypocalcaemia in small preterm infants whose brain is too immature to convulse at a particular calcium level may present as a cardiac dysrhythmia. Drugs which cause cardiac dysrhythmias such as tricyclic antidepressants may also cause fatal status epilepticus. Little is gained in paediatric practice by trying to guess if a neonate in status epilepticus following asphyxia or a child with status from a pyrexial convulsion has 'epilepsy'; he has an acute cerebral dysrhythmia and needs urgent treatment or he will certainly develop a chronic recurrent dysrhythmia. Pyrexial convulsions have been described by adult orientated epileptologists in the past as 'banal' or 'not epilepsy'. The many adults with chronic epilepsy attributable to badly treated febrile convulsions are not likely to agree. Again, if we follow through with the simile, cardiac dysrhythmias may occur in a perfectly normal healthy heart as in isolated paroxysmal supraventricular tachycardia or in a failing heart with chronic structural disease. The cerebral dysrhythmias may also occur with a normal intelligence or may be associated with mental retardation, dementia, cerebral palsy, learning disorders and organic behaviour problems. Cardiac dysrhythmias will decompensate grossly a failing heart and cerebral dysrhythmias can increase the risk of permanent brain damage in any encephalopathy. Elaborate classifications depending upon descriptions of individual seizure types are necessary to compare therapies and to ensure people are comparing like to like. How-

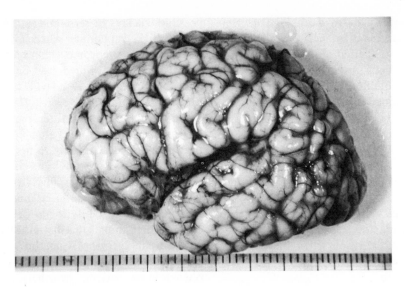

Fig. 3.1 The brain

ever, they may produce a communication block. As a result of some recent systems of classifications, half the medical profession do not understand what neurologists are talking about. In children a description of the fit itself may help guide therapy, but the type of fit changes from year to year so that it is not a good guide to any permanent classification of the acute and chronic cerebral dysrhythmias of infancy and childhood.

Brain maturation

The brain at birth weighs some 350 g and by 4 years 1350 g, and this rapid brain growth is a continuation of the rapid differentiation which was occurring especially in the cerebral cortex in the last trimester of pregnancy (Fig. 3.1). The rapidly growing brain is more susceptible to certain diseases than the less dynamic mature brain, e.g. metabolic disease (phenylketonuria), endocrine disease (hypothyroidism) or the pattern of response to asphyxia.

Myogenic movements can be seen when the limb buds appear about 6 weeks after fertilization. By 12 weeks, the foetus is in a state of flexion and adduction with well-developed flexor muscle tone, flexor withdrawal reflexes and dermatome to myotome responses over flexor and adductor surfaces. Grasp reflexes, head turning and mouth opening can also be obtained by dermatome stimu-

lation. The peripheral nerves, muscle spindles and anterior horn cells are well developed. The cerebral cortex is a thin layer of undifferentiated neuroblasts with a thick subependymal matrix still extremely active mitotically. There are no basal ganglia, thalami, or mid-brain nuclei. This is the stage of spinal integration. The only myelin in the central nervous system (CNS) is a little in the posterior columns. There is, however, electrical activity in the pons which is affected by cutaneous stimulation over the trigeminal area (Bergstrom, 1969).

In the period from about 18 to 28 weeks a further change takes place. Flexor tone is inhibited, brain stem extensor reflexes (asymmetrical tonic neck reflexes, trunk incurvation reflexes and the Moro reflex) appear and stimulation of the snout of perineum causes brisk extension of the limbs with spontaneous Babinski responses. Spontaneous sucking, grasping and limb movements are now more common with cycling and doggy paddling. This is the stage of mainly brain stem maturation, that is, physiological decerebration. Anencephalic foetuses show all these movements. Twenty weeks before birth the EEG is now recorded easily, and yet in the cerebral cortex there are no dendrites, no myelin and very little differentiation of cortical layers. It seems clear that the rhythms must be originating from the brain stem.

The last trimester (28–40 weeks) is the time which the premature baby may spend in the incubator. This is the period of mid-brain maturation with the development of pupil responses, eye movements and the establishment of homeostasis. Gradually the infant resumes the flexed position so that at full term he is again tightly flexed and adducted. At the time of full term birth the thalami and basal ganglia are well developed anatomically. Some myelin appears in the pyramidal tracts during the last few weeks of normal pregnancy. However, dendritic connections are sparse in the cortex and there is no myelin in any commissure. During the last trimester there is a further spurt of cell division when the oligodendroglia differentiate before the rapid post-natal phase of myelination.

The brain continues to mature and by six weeks after full term the infant has lost his flexed position and again is in extension with brisk extensor reflexes. By six months he has lost these obligatory responses and muscle tone becomes increasingly dependent on learned responses.

Dendritic spine maturation and a large increase in neuronal surface area occurs also in the last trimester with the spurt in ganglioside production at about 36 weeks which corresponds to the time when the cortical type of clonic seizure is first seen. Myelination, increase in Nissl substance and the formation of commissural and association fibres is not complete until 16 years of age. Brain maturation is always slower in boys than girls so pyrexial convulsions occur at a younger age in girls than boys.

The anatomical maturation of the brain must be paralleled by physiological and biochemical maturation. Certain biochemical features such as the appearance of glia specific protein, the ganglioside spurt, the appearance of enzymes such as succinic dehydrogenase have been well studied (Brown, 1980). What is not so well understood is the maturation of the different amine and transmitter systems. Cholinesterase concentrations in developing brain do not seem to correspond at all to the development of brain synapses. Dopamine systems depend upon the supply of tyrosine from the substantia nigra which only becomes pigmented at the end of the first year. The totally different sleep patterns of the newborn suggest possible changes in serotonin and amine development. 50H tryptamine when given to children with Down's syndrome can precipitate infantile spasms. Carbonic anhydrase concentrations alter with maturation and so will affect convulsive thresholds (Millichap, 1965). It is important to understand these transmitter substances and the development of synapses better in order to explain the changing susceptibility to fits with age and to develop models to study the effect of drugs or even fits themselves on this susceptibility. The immature brain appears to be more liable to damage from fits. Certainly it has been shown in the experimental animal that fits in infancy will arrest future brain growth (Waterlain, 1978). There is room for worry about the effects of drugs such as phenytoin on synaptic growth.

The effects of brain maturation upon fits

Fits may arise in two ways. Firstly, a focal discharge causes local stimulation of surrounding brain and the symptomatology arises from the function of the stimulated area, e.g. jargon speech, hallucination, motor or sensory phenomenon. Secondly, there may be a widespread secondary discharge which paralyses an extensive volume of brain with positive symptoms due to the release of lower centres. There may be loss of consciousness, loss of posture, release of decerebration (tonic phase of grand mal) release of sucking, cycling, grasping, Moro or startle reflexes (infantile spasms), asymmetric tonic neck reflexes (adversive seizure), central neurogenic hyperventilation, athetoid movements, ballismic movements, or rotatory nystagmus. It is relatively easy to realise that when a three-year-old child's head rotates to the right, his right arm and leg extend, he rotates to the right and falls suddenly, then he is having a seizure of some kind. However, when a one-month-old infant has a seizure with severe discharges in one hemisphere, this may present as a tonic neck reflex posture (Fig. 3.2). This is less easy to recognize. The same is true of sudden sucking, nystagmus, hyperventilation, cycling and startles which may represent fits in the newborn but which may occur also (but not obligatorily or continuously) in the normal newborn.

The type of fit changes with age so that the

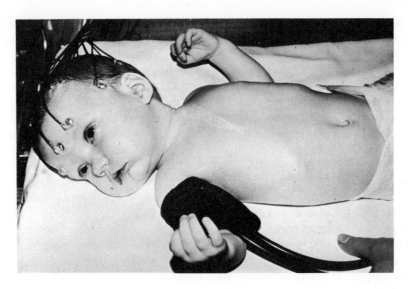

Fig. 3.2 Tonic neck reflex posture

small premature infant usually has tonic seizures or fragmentary episodes of brain stem reflex release as described above. The full term infant has focal clonic seizures at a rate of one or three per second which may remain localised or spread first of all to the vertex of the same side and then to the opposite vertex and opposite hemisphere when consciousness is lost, feeding ceases, and there is interference with respiration and cyanoisis. The resistance to fits in the first year of life is very high and so it takes quite a severe insult such as non-accidental injury, meningitis, encephalitis (e.g. with cytomegalic virus, or CMV), anatomical abnormality (e.g. tuberous sclerosis), or severe brain damage from birth, to produce a fit. The anatomical and physiological maturation is such that the fit produced is often of infantile spasm type. Because of the severe nature of the pathology, not the type of fit, the long term prognosis is poor. Genetic factors are not important; less than 5 per cent have a positive family history. From one to four years resistance to seizures is very low, especially if we add to a physiologically vulnerable period of brain development a genetically low threshold (50 per cent of those having fits have a positive family history). Trivial virus infections may then precipitate fits which can be major tonic-clonic or focal motor in nature, i.e. a pyrexial convulsion. After four years resistance is again high so that fits tend to occur in already

brain damaged children. This is the age of the 'Lennox-Gastaut Syndrome' when fits take on the form of stare, jerk and fall seizures, with interspersed major tonic-clonic seizures, and long periods of pseudodementia and ataxia due to a continuing electrical encephalopathy. Idiopathic epilepsy tends to appear around seven-plus years and again when the convulsive threshold is at its lowest next around the prepubertal growth spurt. A child who has had birth trauma or has mesial temporal sclerosis secondary to severe pyrexial convulsions as a toddler, may have remained well for many years only for fits to return at puberty.

Although the genetic predisposition influences the susceptibility to fits the age-dependent threshold change must be determined by brain maturation and the balance between inhibitory and excitatory systems. The aetiological factor, the focus of brain damage, remains constant throughout the growing period and so this is not what determines when fits will occur. Anatomical maturation will affect the type and spread of the seizure. This developmental outlook on seizures in children is the only way we can explain why, for example, a child has multiple fits at birth, is normal for the first year of life with no seizures at all, then presents with fits at eighteen months, with pyrexia precipitated epilepsy rather than pyrexial convulsions (Livingston, 1972). He may have several episodes as a toddler and is then again clear of fits until ten years of age, a freedom which is thought wrongly to be due to treatment with anti-epileptic drugs. Another child who suffered from severe asphyxia at birth, will have developed slowly. At six months he starts to have infantile spasms which by the age of four merge into the stare jerk and fall pattern of the Lennox-Gastaut Syndrome. The same child when he is seven may have focal Jacksonian motor seizures.

Maturation of the EEG

This will be considered in detail elsewhere. The EEG is measurable as a potential difference between the primitive hemispheres from about 12 weeks gestation but slow rhythmic activity within a hemisphere only appears at about 18 weeks. By 20 weeks a lot of rhythmic and paroxysmal activity in the 4–7 Hz (theta) range is seen which increases over the next ten weeks. Gradually the rhythmic paroxysmal activity becomes confined to sleep and the waking record becomes progressively more inhibited and flat so that the featureless recording of the alert newborn at term could be misinterpreted as underdeveloped. However, spike wave paroxysms can be very pronounced at this time during non-eye movement sleep. Over the first few months after birth the pattern changes and the episodic activity disappears in normal sleep but may reappear in deep anaesthesia or when there is severe cortical damage, as in the prehypsarrhythmia or burst-suppression encephalopathies of infants. Sleep spindles normally appear when episodic sleep activity becomes suppressed. A posterior rhythm blocking on eye opening appears during the first year, increasing considerably in frequency over the next few years. It may be asymmetrical at first and this is of no significance. There is also more alpha rhythm on the right and theta rhythm on the left by six years of age. Prominent runs of temporal theta, especially with the eyes closed, are also common at this age. Vertex sharp waves (up to seven years) or 14 and 22 second fast waves all represent different phases of maturation of the EEG, as does the slow or sharp and slow wave response to hyperventilation (Eeg Oloffson, 1970). This brief account is given simply to illustrate further the concept of the brain as in a constant state of flux in the young child with a continuously changing EEG patttern which must be considered in attempting to interpret EEGs in children. The different significance of EEG signs such as spikes in neonatal sleep, vertex sharp waves, exaggerated hyperventilation responses, and wave spike runs during early school years emphasize the added importance in children of only interpreting EEGs in relation to the clinical position.

GENETICS

It is necessary to draw together several points to explain another developmental phenomenon. In order to do this it is easier to consider a typical case. A child with a strong family history of epilepsy but where the pregnancy and delivery were normal had at eighteen months a prolonged tonic-clonic pyrexial convulsion lasting 45 minutes, followed by two briefer episodes over the next year from which he appeared to recover completely. At six years he presented with typical absences and a three per second spike and wave EEG which responded to ethosuximide or sodium valproate. When he was ten he began to have attacks with grasping movements of his hands, mouthing and occasionally incontinence or falling. His EEG showed a definite temporal lobe spike. It is not possible to think in terms of grand mal, petit mal or temporal lobe epilepsy, nor of primary and secondary generalised seizures. This child has had them all.

The genetics of epilepsy need to be considered from two points of view: genetically transmitted 'disease' which may cause fits such as tuberous sclerosis, neurofibromatosis and dominantly inherited neonatal fits as opposed to the dominantly inherited proclivity to fits.

Classical tuberous sclerosis with adenoma sebaceum, mental retardation, and fits is relatively uncommon. However, Langhans giant cells have been found in lobectomy specimens from those with temporal lobe epilepsy and it may be that formes frustes of tuberous sclerosis might be considered wrongly as cases of dominantly inherited epilepsy. One of the most useful clinical markers has been the recognition of the significance of depigmented macules in the skin as an aid to diagnosis. These are more easily seen after exposure to sun or by using an ultra violet lamp. Small areas of scalp depigmentation may show a small tuft of white hair. The use of CT scanning is now able to show the presence of calcified lesions or tubers to prove the diagnosis (Gastaut et al, 1978). The incomplete penetrance of tuberous sclerosis, which is characteristic of many dominantly inherited conditions, may account for many more cases than we used to recognise. It seems that in such dominant hereditary disorders the infant may be affected more severely when the mother rather than the father carries the trait. In tuberous sclerosis there is a defect in the migration of cells in the developing cortex resulting in areas of heterotopia. If this is severe, there may be fits at birth or infantile spasms at six months with a continuing problem of intractable seizures. However, milder cases may present as simple seizures with a familial history. It is important to appreciate that these are due to the underlying disease and not to a genetic proclivity. Other metabolic diseases such as those affecting the urea cycle may cause fits in several members of a family. Hereditary coproporphyria is being recognised as presenting in children without the severe generalised manifestations of the more common porphyrias. There are a group of disorders classified as Leigh's encephalopathy in which trivial infections may precipitate episodes of acute necrotising encephalopathy and these may be thought to be status epilepticus due to a 'pyrexial convulsion' or an unspecified encephalitis. The dominantly inherited proclivity to fits needs to be differentiated from actual genetic disease. It appears that the trait which results in the three second spike and wave complex on the EEG is what is inherited (p. 52). Studies of this inherited pattern have also shown that the EEG does not necessarily parallel the clinical seizure disorder. The EEG pattern is rare under three years and yet it is exactly in this group that the genetic predisposition appears to summate with the physiologically low threshold to give pyrexial convulsions. On the other hand the EEG pattern may occur in these same children when they are totally asymptomatic three years later (Lennox-Buchtal, 1973). The genetic predisposition may of itself be the sole cause of the primary generalised epilepsies which usually appear about seven years of age with a second peak at puberty. However, spike and wave complexes on hyperventilation or after photic stimulation can occur in children who are otherwise absolutely normal (Doose et al, 1969). Although a spike discharge must accompany a cortical fit, the presence of spike wave complexes in the EEG does not mean clinical 'epilepsy'. They may occur in normal children carrying the trait, or in children who have stopped having fits.

Our understanding of epilepsy in children has changed totally over recent years. The same child may have different types of fit depending on the state of brain maturation. We can no longer consider children as suffering from grand mal, petit mal, primary or secondary generalised seizures, West's syndrome, or Lennox-Gastaut syndrome as though they were disease entities. Effort should not be wasted on bigger and more exhaustive classifications but should concentrate on studying human brain development and the biochemical basis of day to day changes in threshold. Substances such as ACTH, which used to be thought of only as a stimulator of cortisol production by the adrenals, are now known to be present in particular parts of the brain and may possibly act as neurotransmitters. This might suggest a rationale for the use of ACTH in the treatment of infantile spasms, and a biochemical basis for the occurrence of hypsarrhythmia. The endorphins used to be thought to be concerned only with pain mechanisms. However, in an animal experimental model gammahydroxybutyrate has been shown to produce a generalised spike wave abnormality in the EEG, associated with impaired consciousness and responsive to ethosuximide (Snead, 1978). This response can be blocked by beta-endorphin antagonists such as Naloxone. This model is particularly interesting to paediatric neurologists since the epileptic response to gamma hydroxybutyrate is age dependent. Therefore, any genetic abnormality in these systems would only show up at certain stages of brain maturation and might offer a possible explanation of genetic/developmental interaction.

GENERAL CONSIDERATION OF FITS IN CHILDREN

Incidence

Livingston (1972) gives an overall incidence for epilepsy of 1 per cent. The incidence for army recruits has been given as 5/1000 but this excludes young adults of the same age who are physically or mentally ill in hospitals or institutions. Our own figures from Edinburgh (Brown, Cockburn & Forfar, 1972) for the newborn period were 12/1000. This figure is now halved (Brown, 1980). Thom found from 6 to 7 per cent of an unselected group of children had had a fit before five years of age (Thom, 1942), and almost exactly the same figure was found in the Newcastle family study (Miller *et al.*, 1960). Studies of the childhood population in the Isle of Wight gave an incidence at school age of 7/1000 (Rutter, Graham & Yule, 1970). Some of these figures are compared in Table 3.1 with the incidence of other handicaps in children.

Table 3.1 Incidence of fits at different ages and other handicaps in children

	Number per 10 000	Reference
Fits		
Newborn	60	Brown et al, 1979
Toddler	500	Miller et al, 1960
School age	70	Rutter et al, 1970
Army recruits	50	W.H.O., 1957
Other handicaps		
Spina bifida	25	
Cerebral palsy	25	
Mental handicap	300	
Profound mental handicap	35	
Autism	1	
Deafness	10	
Severe blindness	10	
Muscular dystrophy	8	

Classification of epilepsy

The classification used in this book is based on the international one put forward by Gastaut and discussed on page xiii. This is a classification which is ideal for comparing data between different centres but paediatricians only witness the onset of a minority of seizures; even fewer are recorded on the EEG. A child cannot describe the aura, so whether the seizures starts focally or generally is often not known. 70 per cent of fits in the newborn are reported by skilled nursing staff as generalised and yet 95 per cent have a focal onset on the EEG. This sophisticated classification is not understood by general paediatricians, nurses or general practitioners, who have been brought up on grand mal and petit mal, and so an unnecessary communications barrier is raised. A generalised insult, e.g. hypocalcaemia, hypomagnesaemia, hypoglycaemia, asphyxia, or pyrexial convulsions may all cause focal fits and therefore a motor Jacksonian seizure does not necessarily mean a focal pathology. We now recognise, as has already been described, that the type of fit may change with age so that although we may use phenytoin for grand mal, carbamazepine for focal seizures, ACTH for infantile spasms, a benzodiazepine for minor motor seizures and valproate for petit mal the same child may have all types and may correctly have been on all these medications at some time in his life. What in theory appears to be clear cut and scientific is still in practice an art. The more seizures one witnesses personally, and documents accurately, the more one appreciates that in children only a very general classification is meaningful.

AETIOLOGY OF FITS

Primary cryptogenic epilepsy

By definition these children will have been born by normal delivery after an uneventful pregnancy and will have had normal development and intellect. Their seizure pattern will be primary generalised: grand mal or petit mal. Conditions such as neonatal seizures, infantile spasms and the Lennox-Gastaut syndrome, have a very low genetic predisposition of the order of five per cent, and can only be considered as 'idiopathic' in the sense that the responsible causative condition has not been identified. The advent of the CT scan has shown pathology in many cases previously thought to be idiopathic, and present day epidemiological studies of primary idiopathic epilepsy should include a CT scan. Idiopathic epilepsy has a peak age of onset around seven years (Livingston, 1972) and around 50 per cent have a positive family history. If we were to exclude pathology with more sophisticated means, e.g. CT scans, and if we could get accurate genetic history, e.g. EEGs with activation in all members of the family between 3 and 15 years, then we would probably find a pure cohort of primary genetic epilepsy inherited in a dominant manner, but with incomplete penetrance.

Congenital structural brain damage

It is important to remember that in cases of hydrocephalus there may be fluctuations in intracranial pressure, often with a rise when going off to sleep which may cause tonic seizures or attacks of apnoea with myoclonus. The treatment of these is to relieve the raised intracranial pressure urgently and not to give antiepileptic drugs. When the hydrocephalus has been shunted the cannula may cause a traumatic focus in the cortex. If now there is a rise in pressure the tract may be distended with a pseudoporencephaly which may produce seizures. Intracranial pressure must be monitored, since it is only when it is not raised that the appropriate treatment is with antiepileptic drugs.

Absence of the corpus callosum itself is usually asymptomatic, but when associated with cortical and retinal dysplasia in the Aicardi syndrome there is a high incidence of fits, especially infantile spasms. Structural derangement of the cortex occurs in tuberous sclerosis, neurofibromatosis, Zellwegger's cerebro-hepato-renal syndrome, associated with anophthalmia or colobomas and in the fetal alcohol syndrome, and in chromosome disorders, e.g. of 8 and 13. The severity of the dysplasia determines the extent of any associated mental defect and whether fits start in the immediate neonatal period or later. In the Sturge Weber syndrome the cerebral naevus is associated with dysplasia of the underlying cortex. Facial naevi may occur without any cerebral naevus. On the other hand a cerebral naevus may cause intractable seizures leading to hemiplegia and increasing brain damage without there being any facial naevus to see. Brain growth is affected by most of the congenital dysplasias and may show as microencephaly or megalencephaly. Fits may be of any type, neonatal, infantile spasms, Lennox-Gastaut, partial or generalised. 10 per cent of infantile spasms were thought to be due to congenital structural malformations by Rukonen and Donner (1979).

Infections

Bacterial meningitis may present in the first 24 hours of life and even be fatal within this period. Fits are often present in neonatal meningitis. In older children it is particularly with infection due to haemophilus influenzae (which causes a bacterial encephalitis as well as meningitis) that fits may be intractable and the presenting feature. Intrauterine infection with rubella, cytomegalovirus or toxoplasmosis may cause an antenatal encephalitis with periventriculitis and calcification with fits in the newborn period and continuing epilepsy for the rest of the child's life. Toxoplasmosis and cytomegalovirus may be acquired after birth and present at any age with an encephalitic illness in which fits, often of infantile spasm type, are usually prominent. Toxocara canis is another acquired infection which may present as epilepsy in childhood. Fits may be due to an acute encephalitis caused by viruses such as echo or herpes simplex. The latter is thought to cause specific temporal lobe damage which may not always be of the acute necrotising type but may take the form of a more insidious temporal lobe syndrome. On the other hand, virus infections may trigger off other reactions such as: parainfectious demyelination, Reye's syndrome, haemolytic uraemic syndrome. They may provoke pyrexial convulsions, unmask inborn errors of metabolism or act as a slow virus causing a sub-acute sclerosing encephalitis. Fits may be due to metabolic disorders secondary to infections. For example typhoid and shigella, causing gastroenteritis, produce neurotoxins. Infections may cause hyponatraemia, hypernatraemia, hypocalcaemia, hypomagnesaemia, disseminated intravascular coagulation, or hypoglycaemia, all of which may precipitate fits. It is worth emphasizing yet again that it is essential to seek the cause of a fit occurring in a child. Merely to give antiepileptic drugs without treating the real cause is to invite the disaster of permanent brain damage and later epilepsy.

Acquired brain damage

Head injury is the most obvious way in which the brain is injured and this may be due to birth injury, the battered baby syndrome or road traffic or other accidents in later childhood. Probably more important than actual trauma is anoxic ischaemic brain damage due to impaired respiration, blocked airways, shock or impaired cerebral circulation secondary to raised intracranial pressure which may complicate the trauma. Asphyxia itself may cause brain damage and may be due to neonatal asphyxia, poisoning (e.g. methadone, barbiturates), cardiac by-pass surgery, cardiac arrests (e.g. anaesthetic accidents) or to prolonged status epilepticus itself.

The importance of status epilepticus in causing mesial temporal sclerosis and permanent epilepsy is reviewed on page 477. Uncontrolled seizures may occur in most encephalopathies and are important in increasing the amount of brain damage. Improved control of neonatal seizures has lessened the morbidity in the long term of asphyxiated newborn infants. The best way to prevent adult epilepsy is to prevent or treat vigorously anoxic ischaemic episodes in the infant and child. The damage done by severe status epilepticus to the immature brain has been highlighted by the recent investigation into brain damage supposed to be due to pertussis immunization. Those children left with profound mental handicap and epilepsy were those who had had a sudden episode of status, whether or not this was precipitated by the immunization. Intracranial haemorrhage in children is much more common in the first week of life than in the next 20 years. Birth trauma may cause subdural and subarachnoid haemorrhage. Intraventricular haemorrhage is likely to occur in the premature infant. Cerebellar haemorrhage due to occipital bone compression fractures is seen more often now than in the past. Intracerebral haemorrhage was thought to be very uncommon in the neonate unless there was bleeding into an infarcted area. It has now been shown by CT scans that primary intracerebral bleeding may occur in the neonate and be a cause of fits. Intracranial bleeding in later childhood may be secondary to a bleeding diathesis. It is rare but may be seen in haemophilia, haemorrhagic disease of the newborn or thrombocytopenias. It is more common in those cases of thrombocytopenia due to marrow replacement or aplasia than in the commoner idiopathic thrombocytopenic purpura or the thrombocytopenia secondary to infections such as rubella.

Permanent brain damage resulting in cerebral palsy, mental defect and epilepsy is most likely to be due to prematurity or asphyxia, causing subependymal bleeding or cerebral infarction. It is also possible to get brain damage due to perinatal strokes which are commoner in the small-for-dates infants. Whether these are due to the marked polycythaemia or to placental emboli is not yet known. About 33 per cent of all children suffering from cerebral palsy (35 per cent of hemiplegias, 56 per cent of tetraplegias) have associated epilepsy (Ingram, 1974). Fits are much more common when asphyxia rather than prematurity is the cause, and in the spastic rather than the ataxic or dyskinetic types of cerebral palsy.

Tumours and degenerative diseases

There is a significant number of children presenting with fits who are found to have a glioma. Although posterior fossa tumours are the most frequent in children, and although the focal seizure does not have the same significance in a child as an adult, one must still be wary of cerebral neoplasms as a cause of fits. Fits may be of any type and a hemisphere tumour may cause classical infantile spasms. The diagnosis has been aided greatly by the availability of CT scans. Arteriovenous (AV) malformations are more difficult to diagnose and although most greater than 1.0 cm show on a CT scan, especially if associated with calcification, it is still occasionally necessary to resort to angiography in order to be sure that a child with intractable focal seizures does not have an AV malformation. Unless a child has a severe seizure disorder or has bled, it is difficult to justify surgery and so except in these cases it is our usual policy to rely on CT scanning.

The leukaemias are the commonest type of malignancy met with in children. These children can now be kept alive and increasingly one is asked to see them with seizure problems. The CSF pathway is an immunologically privileged site and so drugs may not penetrate. Cells may arise in the CSF spontaneously or be implanted by lumbar puncture. Fits may be due to CNS leukaemia and perivascular deposits may occur in the brain itself as well as on the surface. Bleeding and brain deposits can result in extensive intracerebral calcification and so true epilepsy may result even though the malignant disease is under control. Treatment by radiation and intrathecal drugs, especially methotrexate and cytosine, can cause a toxic encephalopathy and intractable seizures. The immunosuppressive effects of therapy also means that opportunist infections such as cytomegalovirus, toxoplasmosis and Listeria monocytogenes may occur or slow virus infections with papova, measles or rubella virus may cause a subacute encephalitis.

The number of possible degenerative diseases in children, both enzyme positive (Tay Sach's, Niemann Pick, Krabbe, GMI, Gaucher's etc.) and enzyme negative (Batten's, Alper's Alexander's disease, Addisonian Schilder, Canavan's, Unverricht etc) is enormous and discussion outwith the scope of this book (Brown, 1978). Nevertheless, difficulties arise in children with what may appear to be an intractable seizure problem and deterioration when an underlying degenerative disease may not be apparent. The greatest worry to paediatricians in this respect is in the Lennox-Gastaut syndrome when periods of ataxia, pseudo-dementia, recurrent falls and minor status may gradually merge so that deterioration is thought to be due to the fits. Some paediatric neurologists feel that an underlying disorder of a progressive nature similar to Batten's late infantile disease may be present in some of these cases.

Biochemical causes

Early in my own interest in epilepsy I found two people who between them had spent over 30 years in an 'epileptic colony', one with hypoparathyroidism and one with recurrent hypoglycaemia. Nearly every case of hypoparathyroidism, porphyria, adrenal hypoplasia, or ketotic hypoglycaemia that one sees has been diagnosed at some stage as simple epilepsy. Seizures are such a social and personal disaster for the patient and his family that to record miles of EEG but fail to exclude simple curable conditions is indefensible. Many of the metabolic disorders are in themselves rare, but any person who sees large numbers of children with seizures is likely to see every one of the conditions listed in Table 3.2 during his career. Some are more common in children than adults, for

Table 3.2 Metabolic conditions which may present with fits in children

(1) Hypocalcaemia
(2) Hypomagnesaemia (including magnesium malabsorbtion syndrome)
(3) Hypoglycaemia (including galactosaemia, glycogenoses, etc.)
(4) Hyponatraemia
(5) Hypernatraemia
(6) Water intoxication
(7) Inappropriate ADH secretion
(8) Diabetes Insipidus
(9) Hyperbilirubinaemia
(10) Alkalosis (hyperventilation, pyloric stenosis)
(11) Vitamin B6 deficiency, dependancy
(12) Porphyria
(13) Uraemia
(14) Cholaemia
(15) Toxins – exogenous, e.g. lead, drugs, plants
(16) Aminoacidurias – phenylketonuria, maple syrup urine disease, hypermethioninaemia, hyperglycinaemia, argininuria, hyperkynureninuria, urea cycle abnormalities, malignant hyperphenylalaninaemia
(17) Familial metabolic acidoses – lactic, methylmalonic, proprionic, Leigh's encephalopathy
(18) Neurolipidoses – GM1, GM2, Gaucher's, Niemann Pick, etc.

example, hypocalcaemia and hypernatraemia used to be very common causes of fits. I personally have seen over 200 infants with hypocalcaemic fits. By recognising the metabolic basis of these conditions prevention is now possible. We used to treat children with phenylketonuria as 'mentally retarded epileptics' until the basic biochemistry was discovered and it has become possible to avoid these disasters now. Further research has revealed more new variants such as the malignant hyperphenylalaninaemias when severe recurrent fits and an intractable downward course are the usual clinical presentation.

Hypocalcaemia and hypomagnesaemia

The conduction of a nerve impulse depends upon the inward movement of sodium ions and the outward movement of potassium ions across the neural membranes. The ions probably pass through channels which are the hydrophilic pores in the membrane. Sodium and potassium appear to pass through different channels, sodium ions being controlled by carboxyl and potassium by phosphate groups (Freeman & Lietman, 1973). Calcium has an effect upon ion movements; a low calcium concentration allowing more sodium into the cell. Calcium itself is an extracellular ion and magnesium an intracellular one. Depolarisation depends upon the influx of sodium and so a low calcium concentration can result in spontaneous depolarisation. The potassium is kept in the cell and the sodium out by the energy of the cells' ionic pumps. A failure of energy may result in an influx of sodium and calcium and efflux of potassium and magnesium. It can be seen that a defect in sodium, calcium, magnesium, potassium, glucose or oxygen availability would all result in changes in membrane permeability, depolarisation and so ease of firing. It is thought that the astrocyte may also play a part in controlling extracellular ion concentration by mopping up excess potassium. Calcium and magnesium have complex effects on muscle contraction, the neuromuscular junction, axonal conduction and midbrain function. Some of the effects oppose each other and so the net clinical result depends on the balance. There may be fits, tetany, decerebration, sunsetting or neuromuscular hyperexcitability. Profound hypocalcaemia and hypermagnesaemia have a blocking effect on neuromuscular transmission and so may block seizures effectively. The total serum calcium consists of the amount of bound calcium attached to plasma protein, the non-dialysable fraction, and the ionized fraction (active calcium). The degree of ionization depends upon pH. Alkalosis may provoke tetany by its effect in decreasing the ionization of the calcium. The effect of a low serum calcium will also depend upon the serum potassium and magnesium concentrations. Whether a particular level of total serum calcium causes symptoms will, therefore, depend upon several factors; the serum protein, pH, serum potassium, serum magnesium and the health of the ionic pumps. In severe asphyxia, for example, when the ionic pumps fail the calcium may become intracellular and acute hypocalcaemia will result. It is for these reasons that there is no absolute total serum calcium concentration at which convulsions always occur. As mentioned on page 57 hypocalcaemia and hypomagnesaemia with a combined incidence of 1.2 per cent were in the past an extremely important cause of convulsions in the newborn period (Brown et al, 1972).

Primary hypocalcaemic tetany. Primary hypocal-caemic or neonatal tetany is a condition with well-defined clinical criteria. It occurs in full term infants of normal birth weight who have had uncomplicated births. Typically it starts, after a period of normal behaviour and feeding, between the 5th and 7th day after birth. There is a seasonal incidence, it being commoner in the spring months, and it occurs in infants on artificial feeds, particularly evaporated milks. It is rare in breast fed infants and uncommon in those fed with the more modern modified milks.

The mother often notices the first convulsion while the infant is feeding. The fit is at first multifocal and the infant continues to feed, cyanosis occurring only when it becomes generalised. There may be a single episode or more than 50. They are true convulsions and the EEG shows epileptic spike activity during the ictus. The baby is alert or sometimes more than usually alert and his behaviour is commensurate with his gestational age. He may be jittery with exaggerated phasic reflexes, and various types of clonus. If he is hyperalert, he may show rapid feeding reflexes and brisk progression reflexes such as cycling, walking or crawling. There is often increased extensor type muscle tone with strong extensor reflexes such as the asymmetrical tonic neck reflex. Head control is unusually advanced when lying prone and the legs may be extended at the hip or the knee rather than showing the usual right angled flexion. Generalised hypotonia is not seen and in fact tone is often completely normal. About a third show no neurological abnormality at any time. However, a Todd's paresis may follow a fit when a hypotonic hemisyndrome may be seen (Cockburn et al., 1973). Diagnosis is confirmed by the laboratory findings of a serum calcium of less than 7.4, a phosphorus of over 8.2 and a magnesium below 1.4 mg per cent.

Various hypotheses have been suggested to explain the condition but these have not yet been able to be accepted as a wholly acceptable theory. Immature renal function may impair phosphorus excretion. The parathyroids may be merely immature, or they may have been suppressed as a result of a relative hyperparathyroidism in the mother. It has been suggested that vitamin D deficiency in the mother may be a cause of this secondary hyperparathyroidism, and there is some biochemical support for this. The concentration of vitamin D measured as 25 OH cholecalciferol is lower in mothers whose infants have fits, and there is a marked seasonal variation in plasma vitamin D corresponding to the seasonal incidence in the babies. Administration of vitamin D to mothers reduces significantly the incidence of fits in their babies even though they may still be fed on a high phosphate milk. Measurement of the actual vitamin D content of diets during pregnancy suggests many are markedly deficient. It has also been suggested that the infants show enamel hypoplasia of the teeth and this may have occurred during the last trimester when the foetal calcium demands may be as high as 200 mg per day (Purvis et al., 1973). The condition increases with parity and low social class. There would appear, therefore, to be a predisposition to hypocalcaemia which may be precipitated by certain post-natal stresses, such as a high phosphate and fat content of milk causing a further loss of calcium as soap in the stools and an abnormal magnesium-calcium ratio. It is also important to note that hypomagnesaemia is present in 52 per cent of infants with primary hypocalcaemia; this is not usually a feature of hypoparathyroidism. Cows may develop grass tetany with hypocalcaemia convulsions and hypomagnesaemia. Calves fed solely on their mother's milk may also develop hypocalcaemic and hypomagnesaemic convulsions. It has been suggested that electrolyte imbalance in grass due to modern fertilizers may be responsible. The associated hypomagnesaemia appears to be an important feature of neonatal tetany and any theory which is finally developed must explain this as well (Forfar, Cockburn & Brown, 1972).

It does appear however, that to ensure exposure to sunshine, an adequate oral vitamin D intake for the mother, and a low phosphate milk for the baby can reduce very significantly the incidence of hypocalcaemic fits in the newborn.

The treatment has changed over recent years and if the infant has hypocalcaemic fits in spite of the measures outlined above the treatment of choice is intramuscular magnesium sulphate in a dose of 0.2 ml/kg given twice. This is usually enough and more should not be given until the serum magnesium concentration has been measured. In refractory cases maternal calcium, mag-

nesium and phosphate must be measured as hypoparathyroidism and hyperparathyroidism in the mother may result in chronic hypocalcaemia in the infant. Oral calcium gluconate 10 ml 10 per cent solution is often given before the feed but is not particularly effective in raising serum calcium. Calcium chloride provides more ionic calcium but is irritant to the gastro-intestinal tract. Intravenous calcium is dangerous, causing cardiac arrhythmias, and only a very transient effect unless given by continuous infusion with a glucose electrolyte cocktail as in the treatment of secondary hypocalcaemia. The long-term prognosis is excellent.

Secondary hypocalcaemia. Hypocalcaemia may occur in a large number of other conditions in the newborn baby although these are much less common; for example, in asphyxiated infants, as a result of birth trauma, following exchange transfusion, after a period of artificial ventilation or as a result of operative stress. Most of these cases occur in the first 48 hours unless they are due to later associated disease, operation or injury. In most cases the phosphate will be normal or low and the magnesium will usually be normal. The infant may be breast fed. It is important in these secondary conditions to emphasize the necessity for checking for hypocalcaemia in an ill infant with fits. In contrast to primary hypocalcaemic tetany, the prognosis in these secondary cases is much more guarded.

Hypoglycaemia

Hypoglycaemia is common in the neonatal period. It may be seen in the preterm or small-for-dates infant, or the child of a diabetic mother. It occurs with severe hydrops, hypothermia, or with inborn errors of metabolism such as galactosaemia, glycogenoses or maple syrup urine disease. It may be a cause of convulsions in any young child, but those infants with convulsions who have been admitted to a Special Care Unit should have routine monitoring of blood glucose by dextrostix estimation every three or four hours. In most neonatal units a glucose infusion will be given if the blood glucose falls below 20 mg per cent. Brain damage itself may cause hypoglycaemia and it may be difficult to know whether the hypoglycaemic episode is the result or the cause of brain damage. In the past, severe prolonged hypoglycaemia was fairly common and there is no doubt that in many cases it caused brain damage (Anderson, Millner & Strich, 1967). The fits which occur may take various forms and are accompanied by cyanotic attacks, apathy or hypotonia with loss of progression and feeding reflexes. Treatment is by intravenous glucose either as a single dose of 2 ml/kg of 50 per cent glucose, or an intravenous infusion of 10 per cent dextrose in a dose of 65 ml/kg every 24 hours.

Hypoglycaemia may be a cause of fits at any age, especially from hyperinsulinism secondary to pancreatic islet cell hyperplasia. Certain metabolic disorders such as leucine hypersensitivity or fructose intolerance may cause a reactive hypoglycaemia and this is not easily diagnosed by measuring fasting blood sugars. A dextrostix estimation should be done on all children at the time of their first fit. The co-existence of diabetes and epilepsy is not too uncommon and then the effect of hypoglycaemia in precipitating fits may be extremely difficult to evaluate. Nowadays, most parents are shown how to administer intramuscular glucagon in children at risk of hypoglycaemic fits. Hyperglycaemia occurs in stage one of status epilepticus but in stage two with decompensation hypoglycaemia can be due to the fits themselves.

Pyridoxine deficiency and dependency

Pyridoxine is essential as a part of the coenzyme system for a wide variety of enzyme reactions, particularly those involved in amino acid metabolism. It is essential for the formation of GABA in the brain and a deficiency may result in low levels of this natural anticonvulsant and so result in convulsions. This deficiency may result from lack of the vitamin in the diet, as may happen with the processing of certain milk feeds if there is no added vitamin, or in malnutrition, malabsorption conditions, or it may be due to an interference with its metabolism by other compounds such as isoniazid. In these cases GABA is low in the brain and rises back to normal when pyridoxine is administered (Richter, 1960). If this type of deficiency occurs it may be corrected by means of a physiological dose of 5 mg of the vitamin a day.

There may also be a disturbance of vitamin B_6 metabolism in the case of pyridoxine dependency. There is no reduction in the blood level of pyridoxal phosphate and it has been suggested that there may be a defect in certain enzyme systems which can be corrected by supplying large doses of coenzyme B_6. This condition is genetically determined and although the mode of inheritance is not clearly defined, it has been described in siblings (Bejsovec, Kulenda & Ponca, 1967). There may be convulsions in utero when the mother will be aware of abnormal movements which may be stopped by giving her pyridoxine. If untreated, the infant will have focal and generalised convulsions within the first 24 hours of life. He will also be very irritable, show increased startle responses to noise, be jittery, with brisk reflexes and hypotonia, and may die with an unknown encephalopathy or survive with later mental defect. This condition is treated by pharmacological doses of pyridoxine of at least 100 mg a day. There is no specific test which can be applied in the newborn period to diagnose pyridoxine dependency and it is usually necessary to give a trial of pyridoxine in any convulsive state which is resistant to conventional treatment or for which no cause has been found. The EEG is usually abnormal but will become normal purely if treatment is given and will relapse as soon as the treatment is withdrawn.

There seems to be a non-specific response to B_6 in older children with epilepsy when a reduction in fits may be seen (Hansson, 1968). Pyridoxine is also useful in convulsions associated with other rare inherited metabolic diseases such as cystathioninuria and hydroxykynureninuria.

Abnormalities of sodium metabolism

Hyponatraemia may occur due to sodium loss in gastroenteritis, salt losing nephropathies and congenital adrenal hypo/hyperplasias, but hyponatraemia in infants and children is more often of dilutional type due to an increase in plasma water rather than serious diminution in total body sodium. Any child with an acute neurological disease such as trauma, meningitis, encephalitis or asphyxia has an impaired ability to excrete a water load and may easily get waterlogged with resultant cerebral oedema decerebration and fits. This may occur in the small infant simply due to an overload with intravenous 5 per cent dextrose fluids. The syndrome of inappropriate antiduretic hormone secretion will also aggravate the condition if it is not the prime cause of it. Hyponatraemia is especially likely to cause severe fits when the plasma sodium concentration falls below 120 mEq/1.

Theoretically, hypernatraemia should not be associated with fits but in fact fits are one of the commonest accompaniments of hypernatraemic dehydration in young infants. However they are more likely to occur during treatment, especially if the sodium concentration is reduced too rapidly when fits and rebound brain swelling may be fatal. In the acute stage, before treatment, extreme jitteriness with brisk reflexes, ankle clonus and muscular rigidity, especially of the legs, may make one suspect that the child has cerebral palsy. These neurological findings are reversed by therapy. Hypernatraemia is also suggested as a cause of intraventricular haemorrhage in the preterm infant. It is certainly associated with intracranial haemorrhage in the older child but this is usually secondary to massive venous infarction. Hypernatraemia may arise in several ways. It may complicate diabetes insipidus, be due to excess salt intake as can occur using older non-modified milk, to confusing sugar and salt, using oral sodium bicarbonate for wind, as a complication of diarrhoea if a high salt feed is maintained, or be due to high doses of intravenous sodium bicarbonate used in treating acidosis.

Miscellaneous metabolic diseases

A vast number of inborn errors of metabolism may be associated with fits in children (Table 3.2). There may be disturbance of carbohydrate metabolism as in galactosaemia or the glycogenoses, of amino acids metabolism as in phenylketonuria, maple syrup disease, malignant hyperphenylalaninaemia or hyperammonaemias, and of organic acids metabolism such as proprionic acidaemia, methylmalonic acidaemia, as well as such metabolic diseases as the porphyrias. One of the constant worries of the paediatric neurologist is how far to investigate a child with fits. There is no doubt that the more laboratory-minded the

physician the more exotic diseases he will pick up in what would otherwise be classified as the 'epilepsies', 'cerebral palsies' or 'mental handicaps'. We are trying to dispel the concept of 'cerebral palsy' as a disease and get it accepted as the motor manifestation of brain damage and there is a danger that thinking of 'epilepsy' as a disease rather than a cerebral dysrhythmia also inhibits thought and prevents further investigation.

Iatrogenic and pharmacologically provoked seizures

The reticular formation is thought to be the neuronal network which is responsible for cortical arousal and inhibition. There is normally a balance with the cortex. However, pathological processes such as asphyxia may effect one system more than the other so that after a period of total depression the arousal system is left relatively uninhibited, and fits, tremor, irritability or extensor hypertonus may appear. Abnormalities of blood pressure and respiration may also be found.

Certain drugs may cause inbalance and therefore fits in two ways. Firstly, some compounds such as the phenothiazines and lomotil have antitransmitter effects. Actual anticholinesterases or transmitter substances themselves, like 5 hydroxytryptamine, have an obvious direct effect. Secondly, drugs such as the barbiturates and benzodiazepines will cause a chronic decrease in cortical arousal and when suddenly discontinued may leave inbalance with a relative excess of excitation and it may take several days for the balance to be restored. So-called withdrawal fits may occur in otherwise normal people at this time. Infants born to mothers taking barbiturates during pregnancy may be extremely irritable, hyperexcitable, with severe jitteriness and fits which may persist for several weeks. A similar picture is seen in infants of mothers who are narcotic addicts.

Certain other drugs, especially analeptics such as leptazol, nikethamide, and bemegride, are used specially to arouse and try and provoke fits. Fits may occur as a side effect from a number of other drugs, such as cycloserine or metronidazole.

Intrathecal injections of drugs such as methotrexate and cytosine have already been mentioned as a cause of fits, but one of the most potent is an overdose of intrathecal penicillin which can provoke fatal intractable status epilepticus. Penicillin may also cause seizures when given intravenously if there is an impairment of the blood-brain barrier, as after cardiac by-pass surgery.

Poisoning with overdose of drugs, as opposed to side effects occurring at therapeutic doses, is mainly a problem with tricyclic antidepressants, but other drugs, e.g. aminophylline, may also provoke severe fits. Antiepileptic drugs such as carbamazepine and phenytoin in high concentration, e.g. blood levels over 120μ mol/1 of phenytoin, will also cause fits and nitrazepam may occa-

sionally precipitate tonic-clonic status (Hagberg, 1968).

Chronic poisoning with exogenous compounds such as lead are well recognised. It should be remembered that we are surrounded by such potentially toxic compounds in food additives, preservatives and colouring agents. The difficulty in recognising the dangers of such compounds was exemplified by the toxicity to the brain of hexachlorophane antiseptic used to bath premature babies. There is a great concern in North America about the possible neurotoxicity of certain red food dyes.

Table 3.3 Causes of fits in children

Causes of fits in the first forty-eight hours of life
(1) Hypoxia – asphyxia
(2) Birth trauma
(3) Intracranial haemorrhage
(4) Hypoglycaemia
(5) Water intoxication
(6) Hypocalcaemia (normophosphataemic)
(7) B_6 dependancy
(8) Hyponatraemia (adrenal hypo/hyperplasia)
(9) Cortical dysplasia

Causes of fits at end of first week
(1) Hypocalcaemia (hyperphosphataemic)
(2) Hypomagnesaemia
(3) Infective – meningitis, septicaemia with disseminated intravascular coagulation, encephalitis, rubella, toxoplasmosis, herpes simplex, cytomegalovirus
(4) Genetic – familial neonatal fits, tuberous sclerosis, Von Recklinghausen's incontinentia pigmentii, 13/15 trisomy, ectodermal dysplasia, Alpers disease
(5) Metabolic causes – hyperammoniaemia – parenteral feeding, hexachlorophene, hypernatraemia, aminoacidurias
(6) Kernicterus
(7) Galactosaemia

Causes of fits after neonatal period
(1) Battered baby syndrome
(2) Meningitis especially haemophilus influenzal
(3) Herpes simplex encephalitis
(4) Reye's syndrome
(5) Post-immunization encephalopathy
(6) Hypernatraemic dehydration
(7) Septicaemia – biochemical and vascular
(8) Cryptogenic infantile spasms
(9) Symptomatic infantile spasms syndrome
(10) Cerebral palsy
(11) Menkes kinky hair syndrome
(12) Aicardi syndrome
(13) Tay Sach's disease
(14) Niemann Pick
(15) Gaucher's disease – infantile
(16) Haemolytic uraemic syndrome
(17) Aminoacidurias

(18) Hypoglycaemia – pancreatic, ketotic, reactive to leucine, fructose, hepatic, etc.
(19) Hypocalcaemia – coeliac, parathyroid, renal failure
(20) Toxoplasmosis, toxocariasis, rubella, cytomegalovirus
(21) Virus encephalitis

Convulsions in the toddler – over one year
(1) Pyrexial convulsions syndrome
(2) Petit mal
(3) Idiopathic epilepsy
(4) Cerebral palsy
(5) Neonatal brain damage
(6) Meningitis (haemophilus influenzal, TB)
(7) Encephalitis – Herpes simplex, and all common viruses, acquired toxoplasmosis, toxocariasis, Q fever
   – para-infectious encephalomyelitis
   – specific exanthemata, measles
(8) Battered baby syndrome
(9) Reye's syndrome
(10) Drug intoxication – tricyclic antidepressants
(11) Lead poisoning
(12) Scalds encephalopathy
(13) Acute nephritis
(14) Degenerative diseases – neurolipidoses, etc.
(15) Carotid arteritis HHE syndrome
(16) Subacute sclerosing panencephalitis
(17) Brain tumour
(18) Cerebral leukaemia, retinoblastoma, neuroblastoma
(19) Metabolic diseases – aminoacidurias, intermittent hyperammonaemias
(20) Hypoglycaemia, metabolic diseases listed plus salicylate or alcohol ingestion, post-insulin, etc.
(21) Hypocalcaemia – familial hypoparathyroidism
(22) Arteriovenous cerebral malformation
(23) Neurodermatoses – Sturge-Weber, tuberous sclerosis, Von Recklinghausen's
(24) Post-head injury – accidental
(25) Hydrocephalus – shunt trauma, pseudoporencephaly
(26) Intracranial haemorrhage – phaeochromocytoma, idiopathic thrombocytopenic purpura, haemophilia, leukaemia, consumption coagulopathy, acute nephritis
(27) Inappropriate ADH water intoxication
(28) B_6 deficiency – dietary, isoniazid

Finally, it is important to consider the age of the child when he first presents with fits, as this does help to suggest the possibilities most likely statistically (see Table 3.3).

DIFFERENTIAL DIAGNOSIS OF EPILEPSY

One can parody Dubowitz's aphorism that 'all that waddles is not dystrophy' by 'all that convulses is not epilepsy'. It is easy enough to recognise that a single episode of convulsions, even with multiple attacks, is due to an underlying acute disorder. However, it may be much more difficult to make the diagnosis when the parent describes recurrent attacks which sound epileptic and which are not associated with fever of any apparent acute illness.

Syncopal attacks in children have many causes (Table 3.4), and they may present as recurrent

Table 3.4 Differential diagnosis of fits in children

A. Syncope (Anoxic/Ischaemic attacks)
  1. Vasovagal attacks
  2. Paroxysmal tachycardia
  3. Sick sinus syndrome
  4. Atrial myxoma
  5. Congenital heart block
  6. Reflex anoxic seizures
  7. Breath holding attacks
  8. Migraine
  9. Acute asphyxiating asthma
B. Rage reactions, panic attacks
C. Masturbation
D. Tic convulsif
E. Myoclonic encephalopathy of infancy (dancing eyes syndrome)
F. Toxic confusional state, e.g. hyoscine or laburnum ingestion
G. Night terrors
H. Inappropriate emotional outbursts (Sydenham's chorea, other extrapyramidal syndromes)
I. Paroxysmal familial choreas

major seizures. Episodes of paroxysmal supraventricular tachycardia may each be associated with a major seizure at the onset, and in an infant it may take some time to recognise the true underlying nature of the disorder. The same is true of the sick sinus syndrome in which tonic-clonic seizures or drop attacks may follow exercise when the heart cannot increase its rate and so its output. It is seen in the deaf child with the Lange Nielsen syndrome. Vasovagal attacks may cause a major con-

vulsion at any age but this has been highlighted recently by the studies in Glasgow of Stephenson (1978) on what he has termed reflex anoxic seizures. Young children in the first four years of life can respond to a sudden unexpected bump, bang, surprise or fright by either reflex apnoea or reflex asystole. In a typical 'blue breath holding attack', or episode of reflex apnoea, consciousness is lost when the child cries, stops in mid-expiration, and goes apnoeic. Cyanosis comes on quickly and in about five per cent of children may be very severe. If the attack is protracted, it may end with the eyes rolling up, stiffening of all four limbs and sometimes clonic movements of the arms. Alternatively there may be a period of reflex cardiac standstill lasting 20 seconds or more. This can be seen on the ECG as cardiac asystole and may be produced in the EEG laboratory by steady pressure over the eyeball for 10 seconds. The EEG usually flattens and again there is a tonic seizure with extension and abduction followed by adduction of the arms. These attacks may be precipitated repeatedly by minor trauma and may easily be mistaken for epilepsy or even febrile seizures. Reflex apnoea has been recognised for a long time but it has only been appreciated recently that reflex asystole may be much commoner than used to be thought.

Another condition which may cause marked clinical confusion is migraine. This is a common condition and about 10 per cent of ten year olds have recurrent headache. About 17 per cent of children with migraine have associated epileptic manifestations (Prensky, 1976) and no paediatric neurologist will be in doubt about the epilepsy/migraine syndrome, even though it is sometimes denied in adults. The situation is further compounded by the descriptions of headache as a sole manifestation of a seizure disorder (Swaiman, 1979; Millichap, 1978). The vasoconstrictive phase of migraine is commoner in children especially in the preschool period and neurological abnormalities may not be directly associated with headache at this stage. Basilar migraine in the young child may present as recurrent vertigo; the child simply staggers and drops down and he may not be able to give an account of any rotation (Golden & French, 1975; Hockaday, 1979). Classical temporal lobe syndromes due to ischaemia may result in behaviour changes, hallucinations, déjà vu and fait or speech disturbances such as jargon dysphasia (Brown, 1977). At times it may be impossible to distinguish migraine from complex partial seizures. There may be further diagnostic difficulty since migraine may be associated with other conditions found in normal children such as travel sickness and sleep disturbances. A child of eight or nine often presents with a history of awakening screaming in the night, confused, unable to recognise his parents, and then wandering around, mumbling incomprehensibly, and hallucinated with his hands grasping for invisible objects in front of him. This is more likely to be a simple so-called night terror than a nocturnal complex partial seizure. It is often necessary to do repeated EEG studies, chlorpromazine stimulated EEGs or all night recordings, and even then one may have to resort occasionally to treating the child with carbamazepine without a sure diagnosis of epilepsy. In most children the episodes disappear after puberty. Sleep can also further confuse the issue in certain children as it is well known that fits are especially liable to occur on going off to sleep or upon awakening. What is less well known is that intracranial pressure is also most likely to rise at these times in pathological states and the fit may be the only sign of dangerously raised intracranial pressure and not simple epilepsy (Minns & Brown, 1978). Myoclonic jerks, tremor and apnoea on going off to sleep are often pronounced in the presence of raised intracranial pressure and these again may be confused with simple benign hypnogogic myoclonus, or a fit.

Finally, there is a miscellaneous group of disorders which may cause difficulty. Young infants may present with multiple myoclonic jerks often precipitated by movement and sometimes looking choreic, and the eyes show opsoclonus hence the name 'dancing eyes syndrome'. This may vary from hour to hour and may strongly suggest an epileptic basis. The EEG is always normal and there is such a strong association with neuroblastoma that even in the presence of normal VMA (vanillylmandefic acid) estimations a CT body scan of the adrenals should be performed to exclude a maturing ganglioneuroma (Watters 1979).

Masturbation is quoted in all the paediatric textbooks as a condition to be considered in the differential diagnosis of fits and yet it is still assumed that a child must be handling his genitals. Young toddlers may simply rock, go flushed, stare unblinkingly into space and may appear not 'with it'. Certain metabolic disorders may cause repeated seizures before the underlying basic defect is recognised. Hypoparathyroidism may present simply as recurrent seizures in a toddler with no other clinical suggestion of tetany. Recurrent hypoglycaemia may again be easily missed if a dextrostix blood sugar estimation is not performed on every child at the time he has his fit. Ketotic hypoglycaemia is one of the more common types and may be precipitated by infection when a 'pyrexial convulsion' is easily misdiagnosed.

PARTICULAR TYPES OF FIT IN CHILDREN

One of the problems in classification is that some groups of seizures are really an aetiological grouping, e.g. pyrexial convulsions, when the presenting type of fit may be generalised, partial with simple symptomatology or status epilepticus. Others depend upon the stage of maturation of the brain such as infantile spasms when the aetiology can include every major group, congenital, traumatic, infective agent, or even cerebral tumours. Neonatal fits tend to be separated because babies are in maternity hospitals and whilst most adult orientated epileptologists would try their hand at a six-year-old they would not at a six-hour-old.

Grand mal fits

A major convulsion may take the form of an aura followed by a tonic and then clonic phase with cyanosis, incontinence and a post-ictal state as described for the adult in Chapter 4. It can be the result of an acute or chronic disorder and there is no difference in the actual fit itself.

In neonates a major seizure may have only a tonic phase, or there may be a generalised spread from a focal Jacksonian type of seizure and in this case the convulsion will be clonic without any tonic component. The EEG commonly shows a focal onset for both the tonic and clonic types of major neonatal seizures, and both types may be followed by a unilateral Todd's paresis. A generalised major tonic-clonic convulsion may be seen in any of the acute childhood encephalopathies, meningitides, Reye's syndrome, hypoglycaemia, inborn errors of metabolism, post-traumatic seizures or the encephalitides. Most pyrexial convulsions are of a generalised tonic-clonic type.

Idiopathic grand mal epilepsy (primary major generalised seizures) is a disorder of early life, the great majority of cases occurring before the age of 20 years. The peak age of onset is about seven years. In order to make the diagnosis, it is necessary to exclude all known causes of epilepsy, and it seems probable that the group will become smaller and smaller with further knowledge and fuller investigation (90 per cent have normal CT scans, Gastaut and Gastaut, 1977). Some authorities would suggest that idiopathic epilepsy (epilepsy of unknown origin) wil disappear eventually as the presently unknown causes are discovered. Nevertheless, there is a group of patients, in whom there is no evidence of brain damage, who have normal intelligence and have developed normally. In this group it is assumed that there is an important genetic influence.

Grand mal convulsions are found in a number of types of symptomatic epilepsy in children. They occur in children with perinatal brain damage from birth injury or asphyxia, and are often associated with cerebral palsy. The majority of severely mentally handicapped children with associated behaviour disorders, who require institutional care, have major fits. Those who have suffered from the myoclonic encephalopathies as infants or toddlers, may have grand mal in their school years. Reflex epilepsy, such as that induced by television, is usually of grand mal type. Infections such as toxoplasmosis, toxocariasis, or cytomegalovirus, apart from causing brain damage as an intrauterine infection, may give rise later to a subacute encephalitis with major fits.

The clinical features of a major fit in a child are similar to those in the adult, although a child may often have even more difficulty in describing the aura, saying only, 'There is a funny feeling in my head (or tummy).' Most children do not go through the post-ictal phase of coma, confusion, headache and sleep, but usually recover completely within minutes. Even a child who is found immediately after his first fit with fixed pupils, unconscious and unresponsive, whose condition may be mistaken for the result of a severe head injury, usually recovers rapidly within half an hour.

Treatment is considered in Chapter 8. However, phenobarbitone, a safe and valuable drug, is liable to cause irritability and hyperkinesis so phenytoin or sodium valproate are the usual drugs of first choice for primary generalised seizures or carbamazepine if there is a known focal origin with secondary generalised spread.

Petit mal

An immense amount of confusion surrounds the term 'petit mal' as many use it synonymously with all forms of minor epilepsy. Others use it specifically to mean an absence seizure of idiopathic or genetic aetiology associated with a three per second symmetrical generalised spike and wave discharge. Absence seizures may occur in the so-called petit mal variant or Lennox-Gastaut syndrome associated with a wide range of different pathologies. They may occur in degenerative brain disease such as Batten's disease, tuberous sclerosis or even be associated with cerebral tumours and brain damage (Millichap & Aymat, 1967). Clinically identical absences occur with complex partial seizures and whilst on some occasions they may be accompanied by other motor phenomena such as sniffing, sucking, pulling at clothes or incontinence, they may at other times be clinically identical to classical petit mal absences.

The EEG abnormality arises from normal background activity, is synchronous and symmetrical and in most cases is aggravated by hyperventilation. It may be seen after as few as ten breaths before a significant fall in pCO_2 or alkalosis could develop or there could be any significant change in cerebral blood flow. Normal children of the same age as those with petit mal often develop a marked slow wave response at about three cycles per second in response to hyperventilation. The discharges may also be produced by photic stimulation and sleep or provoked by leptazol, methohexitone and hypoglycaemia. Although often now classed as a primary generalised epilepsy it may have a definite focal onset with secondary generalised spread. The 2½ per second less synchronous spike and wave of petit mal variant may also be associated with classical absences.

Petit mal in a pure setting is relatively rare. Livingston gives an incidence in his specialist epilepsy clinic of 2.5 per cent while this may reflect a low rate due to referral policy since it is one of the easier forms of seizure to treat, it is not as common as is often imagined. Although a high percentage of children with febrile convulsions develop the spike and wave pattern on the EEG, relatively few develop true petit mal and those who do often progress to more complicated symptomatology which merges into minor complex partial seizures over the years.

Twin studies have shown a concordance rate as high as 75 per cent (Lennox, 1960). The incidence of a positive family history varies with the selection of cases from 16 to 43 per cent (Millichap & Aymat, 1967). The concordance rate for twins with fast spike and wave EEG discharges has been put even higher at 84 per cent, and it has been suggested that a third of all cases have a family history of epilepsy (Lennox, 1960).

Classically the child, slightly more often a girl, between 3 and 15 years with a peak between 6 and 8, starts to have blank spells, petits, or absences. There is a momentary vacant look when the eyes stare in an unseeing affectless way. The child stops whatever she is doing. The whole episode lasts less than 30 seconds, and is usually about 15 seconds. The eyelids may flutter at the rate of about three times a second, other muscles of the neck or even a limb may be involved, and the eyes may deviate. There is no loss of posture, no incontinence, and no disturbance of breathing and so no cyanosis. The episode may not be obvious and may easily be mistaken for day dreaming or some tic or habit. The frequency varies from one or two to several hundred a day and the attacks tend to continue and not to show the periodicity of minor complex partial seizures. Typically, there is no history of febrile convulsions, the child is of normal intelligence with no neurological signs. It has been suggested that children with petit mal, as opposed to minor complex partial seizures, are nice and passive and do not present behaviour problems. After the attack there is never any post-ictal paresis, the child returns quickly to her normal self and is usually unaware that anything untoward has happened. The attacks tend to cease after adolescence and it is often quoted that as many as 50 per cent progress to grand mal seizures. This has been disputed by Sato, Dreifuss and Penry (1976), who found that absence seizures had an excellent prognosis, 90 per cent stopped, if there was a negative family history, normal intelligence, no other form of seizure and a normal background EEG.

Treatment with sodium valproate or ethosuximide is considered in Chapter 8. These drugs are thought to act on thalamo/cortical excitatory pathways and have little effect on focal cortical lesions (Nowack et al, 1979).

Complex partial seizures

Complex partial seizures are not synonymous with temporal lobe epilepsy. The latter is an EEG diagnosis, whereas a complex partial seizure is a clinical one, and attacks may occur with foci in the frontal lobes or elsewhere.

Ounsted's work in the field of temporal lobe epilepsy in children is outstanding and his 1966 clinic has not been rivalled (Ounsted, Lindsay & Norman, 1966). In his 100 cases of temporal lobe epilepsy he found that one third were due to known disease, another third to the febrile convulsion-mesial temporal sclerosis syndrome, and for the remaining third no cause could be found. Corsellis (1970) has shown that lobectomy specimens may show hamartomas, possible tuberous sclerosis cells, gliomas in situ, or infarcts. Some of these pathological changes might well have been present in Ounsted's one third of unknown aetiology. Other important causes of temporal lobe damage are the trauma of birth injury, the battered baby syndrome or road traffic accidents. In these cases the brain damage may well have been caused by coning consequent upon brain swelling. Among infections, which may cause local temporal lobe damage, may be noted herpes simplex encephalitis, focal cortical thrombophlebitis, and suppurative encephalitis or frank abscess from the middle ear infections. Cocksackie B5 may cause a limbic encephalitis. Cells looking like tuberous sclerosis giant cells have been found in lobectomy specimens, and these might suggest that formes frustes of this condition may have been undiagnosed and may account for some of the strongly familial cases.

The pathogenesis of mesial temporal lobe sclerosis will be considered in Chapter 11. It is a common finding in patients with epilepsy, and even some who have never had fits, and is particularly common in those who die in institutions. Margerison and Corsellis (1966) found it in 66 per cent of 55 epileptic patients. Gastaut (1957) has opposed the idea that a fit can cause long-term brain damage. However, there is a widespread view, propounded particularly by Ounsted, that in some cases febrile convulsions, largely genetically determined, may result in brain damage to the temporal lobes which causes established epilepsy in later life. Certainly there is sufficient evidence that severe status epilepticus in very young children may predispose to later epilepsy, to make it mandatory to treat this medical emergency strenuously, not only to save life acutely, but to avoid the development of a lifelong disability.

In the preschool child, unless there is evidence of fear, laughter, autonomic features or automatisms, it may be difficult to make the diagnosis, since the younger the child the more primitive the pattern of the fit.

Grand mal fits are common in children with temporal lobe epilepsy. They may be preceded by affective auras or automatisms, and may be followed by automatisms. It has been reported that 65 per cent of children had grand mal fits before the development of psychomotor attacks (Lennox, 1960).

Absences clinically similar to petit mal may occur, or they may be accompanied by muttering, lip smacking, grunting, hissing, drooling, sniffing, pulling at clothing, or adversive head movements. Sometimes in the absence of a complex partial seizure the child may raise his arms or pass urine.

The characteristic motor phenomenon is a fugue-like state. In this the child wanders away and may do complex things like getting on a bus, paying the fare, and later getting off again, to find himself, when he recovers consciousness fully, sitting on a wall. Walking away is very common and the child may go long distances, the police having been alerted that he has been abducted. Sometimes behaviour is stereotyped as with the child who invariably climbed a tree during his attack and could easily be found sitting on the same branch of the same tree. In many cases behaviour is superficially normal but no memory store is being laid down and the child has no recollection of what has happened. In other cases there is obviously abnormal behaviour, the child muttering rubbish, undressing, or appearing wide eyed and terrified. Sometimes the behaviour is determined by the child's hallucinations. There may be cursive behaviour of running up and down or round and round in circles.

Speech is often affected and may take many forms: unintelligible muttering, speaking backwards, or sentences apparently formed but with no meaning. During the fugue state the child may be able to reply to a question but usually does not understand and often his reply is quite inappropriate. He may repeat prelearned material, count or repeat his name.

There may be distortion of vision with or without hallucinations. Hallucinations are common in school age children. It used to be said that the child remembers the hallucinations of migraine but not of temporal lobe epilepsy. This is not true. However, the child may be very frightened by his hallucinations and be afraid that he is going mad and will be taken away from his parents. If he is reassured and encouraged not to hide his experiences, it is surprising how often stories are heard such as of seeing monsters, being chased by witches, of the mother changing in werewolf fashion, people stabbing mother, or giant rulers rising from the floor to squash him. He may be in a car and see his mother's ear getting bigger and bigger to fill the whole car. Everyone, including himself, may be speaking at a very slow rate. He may feel that he is a puppet on a string with giant teeth fruitlessly trying to bite the string. Hallucinations of taste or smell may show up as lip smacking or sniffing. At other times the hallucinations may be pleasant and the child will sit in obvious pleasure staring at what he calls his beautiful scenes. The content of the hallucinations will reflect the child's age, his past learning and experiences, and the fears and stresses to which he has been subject. The 'psychotic' component may cause difficulty in diagnosis unless prolonged EEG monitoring is available (Gladwell, Kaufman & Driver, 1979).

Fear or wild panic are common and there may be aggression with destructive violence. Gelastic seizures of continuous laughing are comparatively common (Gascon & Lombroso, 1971). A few children describe angor animi with a vivid fear of impending death.

The sensations or déjà vu, déjà fait, and the feelings of depersonalisation described by adults are seldom put into words by children. More often they complain they are feeling funny or that the inside of their head is peculiar.

Although paroxysms of bilateral wave and spike EEG discharges may be found in association with the absences, which may be found in some children with complex partial seizures, the essential EEG diagnostic criterion is the finding of a focal discharge of spikes or spikes and slow waves. However, in children the focus may be variable and migrate with age and maturation. Activation or overbreathing, photic stimulation or sleep may be helpful but sphenoidal leads or leptazol activation are seldom contributory.

Behavioural abnormalities are three times as common in children with complex partial seizures as in other forms of epilepsy (Rutter et al, 1970) and the hyperkinetic syndrome occurs probably in about a quarter of these children and is a major problem, being more likely than their fits to cause exclusion from ordinary schools. Behaviour problems are more likely in boys with left-sided lesions. It is more common in those children whose temporal lobe epilepsy is due to mesial temporal sclerosis. However, since it occurs in children with other forms of epilepsy it is considered later under the general management of the child with epilepsy. It has been reported that 36 per cent of children with temporal lobe epilepsy, apart from hyperkinesis, have episodes of cataclysmic rage (Ounsted, 1971).

The antiepileptic drug treatment of this group of children using carbamazepine and phenytoin is essentially the same as that of adults, and is dealt with in Chapter 8. However, it might be emphasised that more children are excluded from school on account of their behaviour than of their fits, and therefore particular care needs to be taken in using phenobarbitone which is liable in children to exacerbate hyperirritability.

Falconer is an advocate of temporal lobectomy at an early age in those with complex partial seizures due to a focal lesion in one temporal lobe (Falconer, 1970). The hyperkinetic behaviour disorder, although disabling, is not an indication for surgery as it may be due to more diffuse brain damage. In assessing the indications for surgery it is important to remember the tendency to improve when adolescence is established and the fact that at 18 years, there are fewer people having fits than at nine years (Table 3.1). On the other hand, prospective studies are needed of the natural history of complex partial seizures, and in particular, the likelihood of mirror foci developing in the contralateral temporal lobe, if surgery is withheld. The ten year follow-up studies of the Oxford Group suggest that approximately 33 per cent are seizure free and independent, 33 per cent are independent but require continuing antiepileptic drugs and 33 per cent die in institutions or continue to be dependent upon their parents (Lindsay, Ounsted & Richards, 1979).

Focal fits

Most fits in the newborn are focal, although they are often reported by the nursing staff as being generalised. If carefully watched, probably at least 25 per cent of febrile convulsions have a focal origin. Generalised provocations such as asphyxia or hypocalcaemia may cause focal seizures in infancy and childhood. As might be expected, fits following hemiplegic cerebral palsy, birth injury and the battered baby syndrome are commonly focal. A focal fit occurring during the course of meningitis does not mean that an abscess has formed.

Focal seizures in a young child do not have the same significance as they do in an adult or older child, and focal fits with febrile convulsions do not have a worse prognosis than generalised ones. The focal fit carries the risk associated with its cause, but there is not the strong indication for neurological investigation that there is in the adult. This applies to fits which occur during the pubertal growth spurt which may have clinical and EEG focal features. A neoplasm is a very rare cause of fits in the child. However, if there are any lateralising signs then a CT scan is indicated.

Brain stem epilepsy

Brain stem fits are quite common in children with an acute neurological disease but are rare as a manifestation of a chronic epileptic disorder. They are seen in children without raised intracranial pressure in rhombencephalitis, pontine gliomas and the kinked brainstem of the well controlled hydrocephalic. There may be signs of sudden rotatory nystagmus, alternating dilatation and constriction of the pupils, salivation, bronchorrhoea, hypertension, hyperglycaemia, hyperventilation or respiratory arrhythmia with cyanosis, borborygmi, defaecation, sudden bradycardia of 30 or tachycardia of over 200 per minute. There may be motor phenomena such as cycling or doggy paddle movements of the arms and vigorous sucking. The tongue and the palate may show sudden bursts of rhythmic myoclonus or tongue rolling and the vocal cords may be affected so that the child is breathing against a closed glottis during the attack. In the latter condition, since there is no loss of consciousness, the child will be intensely anxious. The hypertension referred to may be severe and since it is paroxysmal may mimic a phaeochromocytoma. Familial paroxysmal choreoathetosis which responds to anti-epileptic drugs may be considered as a fit of basal ganglia origin (Hudgins & Corbin, 1966).

Reflex epilepsies

The reflex epilepsies which are precipitated by a definite environmental stimulus, although they are rare and often bizarre, have always aroused great interest. They are also discussed in Chapters 4 and 6. Many examples have been described in children: the child in whom a tap on the head always makes his head go nid nod, or children who have a convulsion when undressed or placed in bath water. Olfactory stimuli may provoke seizures, as with the child who has a fit whenever he goes into the chemistry laboratory at school. Music is a well-known precipitant of attacks. A curious form of epilepsy precipitated by reading (Oettinger, Nekowiski & Pitt, 1967) has been described and has caused much interest but it is probably an extremely rare cause of reading retardation. It is thought that reading induces a cerebral dysrhythmia which blocks the comprehension of the meaning of the print which had been read, and this may have a dominant familial inheritance (McKusick, 1971). Reading epilepsy may be similar to pattern-evoked fits when EEG seizure discharges can be produced repeatedly by looking at certain patterns. Episodes of staring triggered by vertical lines such as striped or corduroy trousers, absences precipitated by other vertical lines such as air vents, tiles or bed spreads have been reported (Chatrian et al, 1970). These attacks respond better to antiepileptic drugs than local measures such as special spectacles.

Keith (1963) described children who would stand in the sun waving their fingers in front of their eyes to produce what must have been a very pleasurable trance-like state. Sometimes this may produce petit mal attacks. There is also another group of children in whom it appears that it is the intensity of the light rather than the flicker which provokes the attack. In these cases the seizure may take various forms such as an absence, adversive seizure, confusional state, jerking of the head and arms, or even a major attack. These children are usually of normal intelligence with no neurological signs. In Keith's 27 cases the EEG usually showed a spike and wave pattern, either that typical of petit mal or an atypical form. There is a very rare form of genetic photogenic epilepsy associated with deafness and diabetes, and another with mental retardation and spastic diplegia. When attacks are precipitated by bright light they are better treated by using polaroid glasses with side shades than by antiepileptic drugs. Similarly, television-induced seizures are best treated by practical measures such as keeping away from a flickering set, having a colour rather than black and white set, not looking at the screen when trying to adjust it and sitting level with the screen with a light on top of the set. If the child feels that he is going to have a fit he can often avoid the attack simply by covering one eye. The images on the cinema screen are usually at too high a frequency to induce fits.

Post-traumatic epilepsy in children

Jennett (1973) analysed 282 cases of post-traumatic epilepsy in children under 16 years. Some 10 per cent of children admitted to hospital with a significant head injury have a fit during the first week. However, only about 20 per cent of these will go on to have later established epilepsy, a figure very similar to that found after birth injury. Fits are commoner when the .injury is penetrating, especially when the motor area is affected, and when there is a depressed fracture and intracranial haematoma. The risk is also increased if post-traumatic amnesia lasts more than 24 hours or if there are focal signs. Of post-traumatic epilepsies 50 per cent occur during the first year. Of those who are going to have fits, 70 per cent will have had them by the end of the second year. The worst prognosis therefore for epilepsy is a post-traumatic amnesia over 24 hours, a dural tear, a depressed fracture, and a fit in the acute stage. In such cases the risk may be as high as 50 per cent.

Table 3.5 The causes of convulsions in the first month of life

A. Metabolic
1. Asphyxia
2. Alkalosis
3. Hypocalcaemia
4. Hypomagnesaemia
5. Hypoglycaemia
6. Hyponatraemia
7. Water Intoxication
8. Hypernatraemia
9. Hyperbilirubinaemia
10. Pyridoxine deficiency
11. Pyridoxine dependency
12. Neurolipidoses
13. Organic acidurias
14. Galactosaemia
15. Hyperammonaemia
16. Aminoacidopathies

B. Intracranial Haemorrhage
1. Traumatic asphyxia
2. Birth trauma (subdural and subarachnoid)
3. Intraventricular haemorrhage – low birth weight – asphyxia
4. Asphyxia – consumption coagulopathy – secondary haemorrhagic disease
5. Haemorrhagic disease of the newborn (Vit. K deficiency)
6. Arteriovenous malformations
7. Berry aneurysms (with coarctation aorta)
8. Battered baby syndrome (subdural and subarachnoid)
9. Hypernatraemic dehydration
10. Thrombocytopenia (drugs to mother, idiopathic thrombocytopenic purpura mother, consumption and disseminated intravascular coagulation (DIC), rhesus, intrauterine infection)
11. Idiopathic subarachnoid haemorrhage
12. Dissecting subependymal haemorrhage – low birth weight

C. Infections
1. Meningitis
2. Encephalitis
3. Abscess or subdural empyema
4. Rubella encephalitis
5. Congenital toxoplasmosis
6. Cytomegalic inclusion disease
7. Septicaemia with D.I.C.
8. Gastroenteritis (biochemical)

D. Genetic
1. Familial neonatal convulsions
2. Neurodermatoses, neurofibromatosis, incontinentia pigmentii, tuberous sclerosis
3. 13/15 trisomy
4. Congenital cerebral malformations and dysplasias
5. Alpers cortical degeneration of infancy
6. Degenerative disease (Gaucher's, Krabbe, leucodystrophy, Niemann Pick disease)

E. Miscellaneous
1. Narcotic withdrawal
2. Compression head injury without haemorrhage
3. Neoplasm

Fits in the newborn

Fits are the commonest neurological abnormality in the newborn period, but over recent years, with improvements in obstetrics and changes in infant feeding, the incidence has halved from 12/1000 to between 4 and 6/1000 live births. In the past a fit especially if due to perinatal asphyxia carried a high mortality and up to 50 per cent morbidity. Again with changes in obstetrics and neonatal paediatrics the morbidity has been drastically reduced to less than a third of this figure. About 1/1000 of these infants went on to long-term epilepsy and the control of neonatal seizures could theoretically reduce the later incidence of epilepsy. Over 90 per cent of neonatal seizures are due to asphyxia, trauma, hypocalcaemia, hypomagnesaemia or hypoglycaemia. Infections and the cortical dysplasias make up most of the rest but as asphyxia, trauma and hypocalcaemia are now better controlled these other disorders are becoming more important (Table 3.5). The subject of neonatal seizures has recently been extensively reviewed (Brown, 1980) and will not be considered in detail here.

MANAGEMENT OF THE EPILEPTIC CHILD

Is hospital referral necessary?

The G.P. has to decide whether to refer a child who has had his first fit to hospital immediately, or, if not, whether he needs to be sent for an outpatient appointment or whether he can be treated at home by the primary care team. In Edinburgh we suggest that a G.P. called to a toddler with what appears to be a febrile convulsion should ask himself the following questions:

1. Is the diagnosis definite or is there the suspicion that there might be a haemophilus influenzae meningitis or encephalitis (neck stiffness need not be present), or even some condition like poisoning with a tricyclic antidepressant? If brain damage results from a delay in diagnosing a haemophilus infection the child may be left with disastrous permanent disabilities, which, incidentally, would justify very heavy damages.
2. Can I be back within 10–15 minutes at any

time during the next 24 hours should the child develop status or have further fits?
3. Do I feel confident to treat a podgy toddler with no visible veins with intravenous diazepam or have I got paraldehyde always with me in my bag?
4. What are the social circumstances? Will the mother know if the child convulses in the night? Is a telephone available or are they all vandalised?

Admission to hospital in this example has the advantages that: there are facilities for a lumbar puncture, continuous nursing observation is available, and a resident paediatrician can be called within minutes.

In other cases it is usually as well to refer a child to a paediatric or paediatric neurological department for further investigation because of the large number of conditions, which have already been mentioned, of which a fit may be a symptom. It has been emphasised that idiopathic epilepsy is a diagnosis by exclusion, and more and more often it is being excluded.

When a child has been referred after his first fit to the outpatient clinic, the first line investigations would be a full neurological examination, skull x-ray, EEG, estimation of serum calcium and glucose and a full blood count. A blood count is useful since many viral infections, such as glandular fever, may present with a fit without any other obvious signs, and an eosinophilia may point to such uncommon conditions as toxocariasis. If the first line investigations are negative or confirm petit mal absences, all that is necessary will be observation of fit frequency and appropriate adjustment of medication. If there are neurological signs, focal EEG abnormalities, biochemical changes, calcification or sprung sutures on x-ray, further investigation will be necessary. The extent of these investigations will depend to some extent on the age of the child. For the neonate, biochemical investigations are particularly important. Nowadays every child with infantile spasms should have a CT scan, as should any child with intractable or focal seizures.

Does the child need treatment?

In most centres it is not usual practice to treat first

single fits. If, however, the child presents for the first time in status, or if the fit is complicated by persistent hemiplegia or other focal neurological signs, treatment is often started because there would be a risk of permanent serious brain damage should there be further fits.

Antiepileptic drugs are not always the treatment of choice. If a child has reflex epilepsy, it is more important to take steps to avoid the trigger mechanism, for example to wear polaroid spectacles, or to cover one eye or sit well away from the television set in a well lighted room. Antiepileptic drugs will not help and may make worse fits due to biochemical disorders. When there is a chronic persisting infection – toxoplasmosis or toxocariasis – the infection and not the fits should be treated. Children with myoclonic epilepsies are often refractory to antiepileptic drugs and they are at serious risk of chronic toxicity from polypharmacy. It is sometimes better to accept his stare-jerk-fall seizures and simply give him a small dose of an antiepileptic drug to prevent status.

Drug medication

The hope for the future is that with improved drug treatment it will be possible for the child with epilepsy to live a normal life at a normal school provided that he takes his antiepileptic drugs regularly. To an appreciable extent this aim has been achieved in petit mal and in many cases of grand mal epilepsy. However, the myoclonic epilepsies on the whole remain refractory to treatment. With further progress in the understanding of neonatal medicine and of the pathophysiology of febrile convulsions, many cases (?4/1000) of epilepsy in children may be able to be prevented altogether.

The aim of treatment is to prevent status epilepticus, to avoid further brain damage or the development of secondary foci and, above all, to reduce the severe social handicap of recurrent seizures. A further reason for treatment is that it has been shown in experimental animals with both leptazol and electrically-induced seizures that there appears to be a lowering of the threshold as the result of fits (Friedlander, 1973). Assuming that this is so, if seizures are not controlled, the more they recur the more likely it is that epilepsy will become established. It has been shown that, if

one stops a child's treatment and fits return, the same dose of the same antiepileptic drugs will not reestablish control. On the other hand, the better seizures are controlled, the more likely it is that epilepsy will not become established and that eventually it will be possible to withdraw drug treatment altogether. The essential question is not whether epilepsy needs to be treated but rather whether treatment is proving effective and whether the price paid in side effects is too high for the measure of control achieved.

If long-term medication is considered necessary the benefits must be explained to the parents and the child and they must be convinced of the importance of taking tablets regularly. In particular, without engendering undue alarm, they must be told of the dangers of precipitating severe status epilepticus if treatment is stopped suddenly. On the other hand, most of the major antiepileptic drugs have long half-lives and they must be reassured not to panic if one lunch-time tablet is forgotten.

For how long treatment needs to be continued depends on the age of the child. Neonatal seizures may prove intractable for the first 48 hours and the child may have 100 or more. However, unless they are due to cortical dysplasia, it is rarely necessary to continue treatment for more than three weeks.

If antiepileptic drugs have been given prophylactically to prevent the recurrence of febrile convulsions, these should be stopped before the child goes to school at five. It is usually suggested that after two years clear of fits it is possible to start reducing the dose. However, this reduction is not wise during the prepubertal period when fits are particularly likely to recur. Equally, if fits start at this age, treatment should be continued until the patient has passed through adolescence, and, in the case of girls, until the menstrual rhythm is established.

Because fits in children may be due to such a variety of causes as hypocalcaemia and hypomagnesaemia, pyridoxine deficiency or dependency, and those causing infantile spasms, many drugs other than the antiepileptic ones used for adult epilepsy may be indicated. The latter are considered in Chapter 8.

It is important to remember that a child's brain

increases by 1000 gm during the first four years and that little is known of the effect of antiepileptic drugs on brain growth. The breakdown epoxides from phenytoin bind to RNA and have antimetabolic effects. Whilst a teratogenic effect is recognised an effect on brain development must also be considered. This is clearly a field where much research is necessary. The potential dangers in the use of antiepileptic drugs must be balanced against the known risks of status epilepticus and the great susceptibility of the immature brain to permanent damage as a result of fits (Waterlain, 1978). Seizures themselves may have an effect on brain growth.

When treating the school age child it must be appreciated that may of the antiepileptic drugs interfere with learning and may aggravate existing school problems. Therefore, they must never be given lightly or when there is doubt about the diagnosis. The dose used should be the smallest necessary to control seizures and not that required to produce a so-called therapeutic blood level. The physician should try to keep to drugs with which he is familiar, and, except in unusual cases, restrict himself to one or at most two drugs. If multiple drug combinations, or the use of second-line drugs such as sulthiame, have been resorted to, the epilepsy is probably drug resistant and would be likely to have no more seizures on no drugs at all.

Most drugs are given at least twice a day: the once daily dose often used for adults may cause gastric upset, and the rapid rate of metabolism of the small child may mean that adequate serum levels would not be maintained. For example in the newborn, phenytoin may need to be repeated after an hour and the dose needed to achieve a serum concentration of $20\,\mu$mol/l may vary between 3 and 25 mg/kg, and may alter from week to week. $20\,\mu$mol/l appears to be the lower limit for phenytoin to be effective, and to be of use huge doses may be necessary to keep the serum level in the adult range of $40-80\,\mu$mol/l. Even mild viral infection may upset hepatocyte function, reduce the rate of metabolism and result in acute toxicity. Severe myoclonic seizures which are sensitive to a benzodiazepine may need a small dose to be given every two hours if they are to be controlled.

Apart from phenytoin, serum levels are of more value for checking compliance than for adjusting treatment. We are not absolutely sure that the so-called therapeutic levels are the same for the young child as for the adult. After all, it is the brain concentration which matters and this can be influenced by different rates of hydroxylation, variations in albumin binding, and the state of the blood-brain barrier. For example, one might expect that premature infants might have a poorly developed barrier and so have a higher brain level for a given serum concentration. This may well not be true; it is known that CNS infections can cause a very high brain level of drugs with a quite low serum concentration.

Signs of toxicity such as ataxia and gum hyperplasia cannot be used as a guide in the small child, and, as with adults, high doses may result in an increase in fits. Because of the difficulty of venepuncture in these small children, some people are tempted to try to manage without measuring serum levels. This is indefensible and in the newborn with intractable seizures daily levels are often necessary. It has not, however, been shown that csf estimations are any better than serum levels to assess brain concentration. The possibility of using salivary levels in order to avoid repeated venepuncture should be explored (Rylance, Moreland & Butcher, 1979).

The management of the attack

Although the physician may be faced very rarely with a sudden unexpected death in a fit for which no cause can be found at autopsy (Hirsch & Martin, 1971), it is important to reassure the parents that, even if they do nothing, the child will not die in a single fit. They must be told that the fit cannot be stopped by trying to restrict the child's movements. It is usually too late to try to get anything between the teeth and, if attempts are made, lacerations to the gums and bleeding are likely and may obstruct the airway. The parents should be shown how to place the child in the three-quarter prone position and to wipe the inside of the cheek with a finger or a handkerchief. In hypotonic attacks it is necessary to support the jaw. Tight clothing around the neck, which might interfere with the venous return, should be loosened. The child need not be moved unless he is in danger, for example, in the road, or if he is likely to bang himself against metal or concrete objects. If there are repeated severe seizures with salivation and cyanosis, the parents should be given an infant mucus extractor in order to clear the airway. In hospitals and special schools with children with intractable fits, a Guidal anaesthetic airway is the best method of keeping the tongue out of the way and the airway clear. Some children have an aura and they should be told how to move to somewhere safe and sit down. Children with akinetic seizures and atypical petit mal often fall repeatedly on the same place, usually the occiput, forehead or chin. After a while, the skin is so scarred from repeated suturing that either it will not heal or it breaks down with the least trauma. These attacks come without warning, are highly resistant to treatment, and some form of protection is often necessary. The main problem is not to devise the protection but to make sure that it is sufficiently attractive to persuade the child to wear it. Surprisingly little work has been done in this direction.

Personal restrictions

All children are subject to risks in their everyday lives, in crossing the road, climbing stairs and lighting the gas. These have to be accepted. For the child with epilepsy these are greater, but it is of the utmost importance that he should live as normal a life as possible. It is sometimes more difficult to know whether to restrict non-essential pleasurable pastimes such as games, P.T. swimming or riding. There is, of course, an added risk which should not be hidden from the parents; a number of children with epilepsy are still drowned (Sillanpaa, 1973). At the same time, if we make a child different from his siblings, friends and classmates, so that he always stands out as peculiar and abnormal, this is the best way of producing neurotic reactions and possibly the so-called epileptic personality. If the fits can be well controlled, then apart from boxing, lone canoeing, high diving, and rock climbing, no restrictions should really be necessary. The child who has only one fit every few months should be allowed complete freedom for most normal school activities provided that the teachers understand the situa-

tion. Swimming should be allowed in the swimming bath but should be discouraged alone with other young children in a remote loch. A responsible person should be present and should keep an eye out for any difficulties which may occur. In fact, fits seldom occur while swimming, even in special schools for children with epilepsy. However, if they do, it is important to avoid panic. The child should simply be turned on his back and the jaw supported. It is very difficult to drag a convulsing child up the side of a swimming pool and efforts to do so may be disastrous. Horse riding has contributed much to the lives of children with cerebral palsy and mental handicap whose seizures are controlled. Bicycle riding is less of a problem than it used to be, since nowadays the roads are so busy that many parents do not allow any child to ride on main roads but restrict them to the park or back streets. Football, cricket, and physical education under a trained instructor do not present any problems. Although hyperventilation may increase the susceptibility to fits by producing an alkalosis, this does not occur with vigorous exercise since the breathlessness is due to a lactate/pyruvate acidosis which, in fact, is likely to inhibit an attack. A fit is much more likely to occur during a long and boring church or kirk sermon!

Naturally the great majority of parents are anxious to do the best possible for their children and particularly for one disadvantaged by epilepsy. It is important to reassure them that love, a stable home, exercise, fresh air, sunshine, and a normal diet are as essential as for any child, and in most cases are all that is required. The doctor, whether general practitioner or specialist, must spend time to explain that the very slight dangers inherent in allowing the child to lead as normal a life as possible, are less than the subsequent disasters which may accrue from over-restriction or over-protection which may build up deep-seated resentments and a lasting distortion of his personality.

Parental attitudes

The approach to the parents of a child with febrile convulsions, or the infant with fits at birth, poses a special problem and I will consider only the child with established epilepsy. It is of paramount importance to gain the confidence of the parents. Despite the initial shock, nothing is to be gained by refraining from using the word epilepsy. If circumlocutions are used, confidence will be lost and it will be much more difficult to reassure them later that the child does not have a brain tumour or some degenerative disease. At some stage the doctor will need to discuss the varying types and degrees of severity of epilepsy, and his informed discussion is likely to be much less frightening than tittle-tattle from a neighbour who knows of a tetraplegic ament with epilepsy or someone whose great-aunt Martha died suddenly in a fit. It is often helpful to give the parents an appointment a week later and to ask them to put down on paper a list of their worries. After the diagnosis has been given, the sudden shock may block completely the assimilation of any further information. Parents will often believe emotionally what they want to believe and this may bear little relationship to what they have been told. At the second meeting it may be useful to ask them to tell you what they understand about their child's condition. However carefully the facts are explained, it must be appreciated that what is accepted as fact may not be accepted at an emotional level, particularly by the father. Probably nearly half of the parents will try to hide from their neighbours and friends the fact that their child has epilepsy. It requires little imagination to appreciate the immense complications which this reticence may produce both within the family and, more importantly, on the child himself. The social effects of epilepsy depend very largely upon how well the fits are controlled (Ward & Bower, 1978).

When epilepsy is due to a genetically determined disorder, genetic counselling must be given. However, this must be done with the greatest delicacy in order to avoid feelings of parental guilt.

The doctor has to steer a delicate course; on the one hand, reassuring the parents and preventing unnecessary alarm and despondency and, on the other hand, convincing them of the importance of adequate treatment. The side effects of antiepileptic drugs must be explained but the importance of continued treatment emphasised. Much publicity has been given in the mass media to the effect of drugs and it is important for the practitioner to be able to discuss this problem with the parents in an informed manner. The British, and other Epilepsy Associations have done a great deal of good work in public education. It is unfortunate that this has not been appreciated as widely as it should have been. In a school for children with epilepsy the parents of only one child had ever heard of the British Epilepsy Association (McGrath, 1972).

Faced with any handicap, the reaction of parents depends, firstly, upon the handicap, whether there are associated mental, physical or behavioural problems, or whether special schooling or particular restrictions on normal activities are required; and secondly, upon the parents' personality, their own life experience, prejudices, religious beliefs, but not upon their intelligence. The reaction of parents to the diagnosis of epilepsy, often considered so disastrous, is comparable to that of a person told that he has a fatal illness and is going to die. Four stages of reaction can be recognised: denial, aggression, mourning and peace (Kubler-Ross, 1969). Similar reactions are seen in the parents of handicapped children. Some parents, possibly only a few, achieve peace and accept the handicap of their child, but others arrest at different stages of reaction. This may explain why different parents assimilate varying amounts of what they are told by their doctor. In the stage of denial, they will believe little of what they are told, whilst in the aggressive phase they need something or someone to blame. This may be the medication, the physician, the obstetrician, the educational psychologist, the school teacher, or anyone directly involved with the child: any or all of whom may be accused of inefficiency for their failure to effect a cure. At this stage they may well go from one doctor to another seeking second, third or fourth opinions, or even resort to paramedical advice. Much is heard of social work support but there is no firm evidence that this helps parents to accept the situation. Unfortunately, relatives often exacerbate the situation. The parents are told horrifying stories of death and disaster. Close friends and relatives may refuse to baby sit, or run from the room when a fit occurs. It is not uncommon to hear the accusation from grandparents that 'of course, the fits do not come from our side of the family'. Such attitudes may aggravate greatly the feelings of guilt, despair and desertion that the parents already feel. The support which parents need so desperately must not be looked for from the hospital, local authority or the social work department but must depend on the stability of the home, immediate family and friends, and the good family doctor is probably in the best position to nurture this support. In the literature of those organisations emphasising the normality, or even the special attributes, of people with epilepsy, it is common to point out that Caesar, Handel, Mohammed and Alexander the Great all suffered from epilepsy. Or, again, that when one walks down the street doing one's Christmas shopping, there are a score of other people in the same street who may suddenly, at any time, have a fit. All these facts may be a great comfort to the parents. However, basically, parents will reflect the attitude of their family doctor to their child with epilepsy and his problems: this places upon him a very great responsibility.

EDUCATION

The School

In the past there has been a tendency to set up special schools for handicapped children, not because they had a particular educational need but because they had a particular handicap. There is no doubt that certain groups do have special needs: deaf, blind or mentally handicapped children. However, it is highly desirable that other handicapped children should be integrated into ordinary schools and not segregated just because they have a handicap. Certainly children with epilepsy should not be excluded from normal schools because of prejudice against their having fits. Children with epilepsy at the two extremes of the epilepsy spectrum do not present any difficulty. A child with normal IQ and behaviour, without any physical handicap or social problems, who can keep up with his peers at the local school should obviously be there, and any efforts to exclude him should be resisted strenuously. At the other end of the spectrum are those children with intractable epilepsy, who are likely to be brain-damaged and severely mentally retarded, and who

will need the services of the schools for the mentally handicapped. There are also those with severe behavioural and social problems and these account for the one per cent of children in Britain who are in the special schools for epilepsy: six in England and one in Scotland. These schools have an additional advantage for deprived and handicapped children since apart from formal education they have ancilliary workers such as physiotherapists, speech therapists and occupational therapists. They help deprived children to become personally and socially independent: to care for their immediate personal needs, to shop, cook, use the telephone and so on. However, our present state of knowledge is uncertain, and there are probably other children with epilepsy who present special educational problems related to their epilepsy. Some of these problems will be considered later, and it will need to be decided whether they can be helped better by a short period in a highly specialised school or whether it may be possible to help them adequately by giving special training to certain teachers in ordinary schools.

The teacher

It is very important that teachers in training should learn about disorders such as epilepsy which may affect a child's attainment in class or relationship with other pupils. This is also the function of the School Health Service, and the School Medical Officer should explain to the teacher the particular problems of any epileptic child in her class. For example: how to deal with particular types of fit, strange behaviour or automatisms which might occur during or after an attack, that there is no need to send a child to the rest room after every minor seizure or when there has been full recovery from a major fit. Livingston (1972) makes the point that the teacher must explain to the class that epilepsy is not contagious, must not convey prejudice and must give a simple explanation to the other children about the nature of fits. It is notable how well other children will accept epilepsy if the general attitude is sensible. It is essential that the same normal discipline should apply to the epileptic child as to the rest of the class. In its broadest sense school is a training for later life and society will not accept a different standard of behaviour just because a person has epilepsy. A child will quickly come to dominate the class situation if he knows he will not be punished like the other children. There are physicians who still make the excuse that a child cannot help his behaviour because he has epilepsy. This may sometimes be true but this attitude is responsible for some secondary personality disturbances.

The child

The reasons for the epileptic child having problems at school are listed in Table 3.6.

Table 3.6 Causes of schooling problems in epileptic children

1. Associated mental handicap
2. Defect in concentration
3. Specific learning defects
4. Left-sided epileptic foci
5. Subclinical seizures
6. Antiepileptic drug toxicity
7. Effects of lack of understanding or boredom
8. Lack of expectation
9. Reading epilepsy
10. Absence from school due to fits
11. Anxiety due to stress at home (effect of fits upon family)

The child with epilepsy must have a full educational assessment. It is not adequate simply to perform a battery of I.Q. tests. The varying concentration span, subclinical discharges and the effect of antiepileptic drugs mean that a single I.Q. estimation, particularly if low, must be interpreted with caution. It has been shown that the I.Q. in children with epilepsy is not constant but varies in an unpredictable way (Ounsted, 1971). Rutter and his colleagues (1970) in their Isle of Wight survey showed that the mean I.Q. of uncomplicated epilepsy was 102 on the Wechsler scale. Twin studies have shown that if one twin has had a febrile convulsion he does not have an I.Q. significantly different from the other although the child who had the fit underachieves (Christenson & Bruhn, 1973). Yule (1973) has stressed the importance of measuring attainment as well as intelligence, since many epileptic children underachieve in learning to read, and this cannot be accounted for by absences from school. Ounsted (1971) has shown that 25 per cent of children with

temporal lobe epilepsy have slow speech development. It is now well established that specific reading retardation at school is much more common in children who had difficulty in acquiring speech in the pre-school years (Ingram, 1963).

An estimated 33 per cent of all epileptic children are in fact also mentally retarded as a result of the brain damage which caused the epilepsy (Sillanpaa, 1973). There is therefore a global impairment in cognitive function and in particular in the use of symbols (phonemes, graphemes, musical, arithmetic, chemical, electronic) to code information and allow thought and reasoning. Mental handicap is a disorder of the brain's learning ability (Brown, 1978). About 33 per cent of epileptic children who are of normal intelligence have learning difficulty in particular areas. There may be a specific learning difficulty which shows as reading retardation. There may be special difficulty with mental arithmetic since they cannot hold numbers in their heads and manipulate them although they can manage with concrete materials such as rods, blocks or fingers. We have already said that, excluding those children who require special schooling because of associated cerebral palsy and mental handicap, most children with epilepsy should attend normal schools. This has been official policy for over 20 years, but it is alarming that until the study of Holdsworth and Whitmore (1974), the learning problems of these epileptic children in normal schools were not realised and so the necessary remedial education was not forthcoming; in fact, 40 per cent had not even been assessed by an educational psychologist.

Learning may be disrupted in various other ways. Focal seizures arising in the dominant hemisphere appear to be associated with specific schooling problems (Stores, 1976, 1978). As with any child, the parents' attitude to education and the child's motivation to learn are of paramount importance. Teachers often report that concentration is poor and yet formal measurements of attention do not often show this. There is no doubt, however, that some severely hyperactive children with temporal lobe damage may have a specific attention disorder. Attention may be affected if the child is anxious whether about his fits, unrecognised specific learning problems, or problems of a broken or turbulent home. Drugs such as phenobarbitone, ethosuximide or clonazepam may seriously disrupt attention (Guey, 1967). If the child does not understand what the teacher is trying to teach, his concentration span will be reduced because of lack of comprehension. It is often postulated that poor concentration is due to brain damage. However, this should not be accepted glibly as the cause of school failure until other remediable causes have been excluded.

Fits themselves may interfere with learning due to multiple absences, post-ictal confusion or after repeated minor complex partial seizures when periods of pseudodementia, i.e. epileptic encephalopathy, may be prolonged. Subclinical fits as shown by paroxysms of spike and wave discharges on the EEG may interfere with learning (Geller & Geller, 1970). Ounsted (1971) described petit mal as 'peppering the child's learning with small gaps'. If the child is bored or not understanding the lesson then the amount of abnormal electrical discharge on the EEG increases. Guey et al (1967) showed when telemetering the EEG that comprehension and enjoyment were associated with fewer spike wave paroxysms than when the child was bored.

Drugs used to control seizures may interfere with learning in several ways. They may disrupt attention, cause drowsiness, slow down reaction times and possibly interfere with brain growth or the metabolic basis of memory (Guey et al, 1967). Improvement in seizure control will improve learning and so apparently paradoxically even drugs such as phenobarbitone may occasionally improve learning (Hutt et al, 1968). Mental deterioration, i.e. dementia, can occur in epileptic children and may show first of all as school failure. Repeated anoxic episodes especially from nocturnal seizures, repeated severe head bangs from falling, a bout of status epilepticus, may cause mental deterioration as a result of the seizures themselves. Phenytoin may cause a severe dementia in chronic overdose which resembles degenerative brain disease; this may be related in part to its antifolate effect (Vallarta, Bell & Reichest, 1974). Progressive brain disease may not have been suspected as a cause of the fits; this most often presents as the dilemma in severe Lennox Gastaut syndrome. Mentally handicapped children often appear to reach a ceiling in ability around seven

years and the failure thereafter to make further progress results in an apparent falling off in I.Q.

BEHAVIOUR PROBLEMS

The parents of all children with epilepsy have many burdens to bear; anxiety about the fits themselves, feelings of guilt, the fear of social embarrassments or sudden death in an attack. However, some parents have another and often intolerable burden, that of an associated behavioural abnormality in their child. I have already touched on some of the secondary disorders of the personality which may accrue from faulty management. These and other disturbances of behaviour are considered further in Chapter 6. However, I will consider in detail one condition peculiar to children; the hyperkinetic behaviour disturbance.

Hyperkinetic behaviour disturbance

Over-activity may result from anxiety, or simply because the child does not understand the environment, as is the case with autistic or mentally handicapped children. The fundamental defect in the hyperkinetic syndrome is in focusing the attention and maintaining concentration. The child sees but does not look, hears but does not listen. He may wander around touching everything, taps, toilet, or power sockets, with a complete lack of awareness. He will not settle to play, watch television, or sit at a meal table for more than a few minutes. The anxious child with specific learning disorders such as dyspraxia, dyslexia, dysgraphia or dysphasia only shows his abnormal behaviour when the area of disability is under stress and his concentration span is good when he is succeeding. The child who is hyperkinetic from brain damage may be upset by his inability to control his attention and to select what is relevant from the mass of information provided by his senses. He may be relieved to go into a corner, behind the shutters or under the bed for a sensory rest. Sometimes perseveration occurs and repetitive activities such as trampolining or running round and round in circles may appear to relax the child. Sleep disturbances are the earliest manifestation of the hyperkinetic disorder and, if it is due to perinatal brain damage, the problem may present as early as four months of age. The older child may get up at six o'clock in the morning and wreck the house. Sleep studies of infants in the pre-hyperkinetic state would be useful.

Attacks of catastrophic rage over minor frustrations are common, although these may occur in brain-damaged children without the hyperkinesis. These reactions might be considered as reflex fits associated with a low frustration threshold. The child loses control and goes berserk, screams, spits, kicks, swears and is aggressive and destructive. Cruelty to animals seems to be a particularly unpleasant and common manifestation and we have had children who have bitten the dog, painted the dog, eaten the gold-fish, squeezed the budgie to death or tried to break the tortoise with a coal hammer.

Hyperkinetic children are extremely resistant to hypnotics. Phenobarbitone, primidone and some benzodiazepines may make the child irritable and decrease the concentration span even more.

The full hyperkinetic syndrome consists of poor concentration, over-activity, rage reactions, early morning wakening and an abnormal pharmacological response. Some children may not have all these features. The hyperkinetic syndrome is much more common in boys than in girls and tends to be associated with brain damage, particularly if diffuse, occurring before the age of three years. It is interesting to note, in passing, that the severe behaviour disturbances which followed outbreaks of encephalitis lethargica were four times as common in boys (Stevens, Sachder & Milstein, 1968). When hyperkinesis is due to temporal lobe epilepsy it is much more likely to occur in those with mesial temporal sclerosis following status epilepticus than in those with a discreet temporal lobe lesion. The intellectual ability of hyperkinetic children is significantly retarded when compared with other children with temporal lobe epilepsy (Ounsted et al, 1966).

The difficulty of trying to bring up a child with a hyperkinetic disorder requires patience and self-control which may be greater than many normal parents possess. They may feel that the child always gets the better of them, and if they try to avoid rage reactions the other siblings may resent different standards of discipline. Inevitably there are occasions when parents lose their self-control and attempt to discipline the child by physical means, only to feel intensely guilty afterwards. It is cruel to insinuate that good parents who have been able to deal with normal children are in any way at fault because of their failure to deal with a problem which is often quite intractable and requires hospital admission, residential schooling or institutional care. The control of fits will not necessarily control behaviour and may in fact make them worse. Drugs such as phenobarbitone, primidone, or the benzodiazepines may make the behaviour worse or intolerable. It has been suggested that sulthiame or carbamazepine may be helpful. Although phenothiazines tend to aggravate fits, occasionally they may help behaviour. If the seizures are well controlled and behaviour is still a major problem then a trial with sympathomimetic amines such as methylphenidate is justified (Millichap & Fowler, 1967). This is usually given in one dose first thing in the morning, or in two doses in the morning and at lunchtime; later doses should be used very cautiously as sleep may be interfered with. It is usual to start with 5 mg which may be increased to 25 mg. Blood concentrations of 'Ritalinic acid' show that absorption and metabolism vary and failure to control behaviour may be due to an inadequate blood level of the drug. Some doctors use 40 mg or more but anorexia, nervousness, tics and sleep disturbances occur at this dose level and these very large doses rarely give dramatic relief. If the child is sensitive to methylphenidate, the response is usually very good in a few days. If there has been no response, there is no purpose in continuing the drug for longer periods.

It is important to talk to the parents and to reassure them that this is a well-known behaviour problem which is in no way due to any failure on their part. They should be offered an emergency placement to which they can take their child at any time of the day or night, if they feel they cannot manage any longer. In this way it should be possible for them to have the child back home again when he has settled. Psychotherapy is rarely of any help and it has even been suggested that it may increase later psychopathology (Stevens et al, 1968). In severe cases it is necessary to place the child in an environment where there is as little distraction as possible, and where he can have individual teaching and therapy sessions. Psychosurgery has little to offer and occasionally results in even more socially unacceptable behaviour, such as hypersexuality. However, if there is a clear temporal lobe focus and a severe seizure disorder, temporal lobectomy will be indicated and occasionally may help the behaviour disturbance.

SUMMARY

The field of epilepsy has made quite dramatic strides over the last ten years. We are now in a position to understand fits against a background of physiological change and know that fits which were regarded as disease entities, e.g. infantile spasms, are no different from any other cerebral dysrhythmia. The advent of newer antiepileptic drugs and the recognition of the feedback effects of environmental stresses in the educational problems common with epileptic children has meant that we can help more children suffering from epilepsy than in the past. The possible prevention of epilepsy has become a reality with greatly improved perinatal care and the recognition that pyrexial convulsions may have long term effects. Hopefully the next ten years may be even more exciting if we can show that substances such as the beta-endorphins or brain hormones like ACTH are involved in the developing systems which under genetic control are responsible for the changing types and incidence of fits in the child's growing brain

REFERENCES

Anderson, J.M., Milner, R.D.G. & Strich, S.J. (1967) Effects of neonatal hypoglycaemia on the nervous system. *Journal of Neurology, Neurosurgery and Psychiatry*, **30**, 295.

Bejsovec, M.R., Kulenda, Z. & Ponca, E. (1967) Familial intra-uterine convulsions in pyridoxine dependency. *Archives of Diseases in Childhood*, **42**, 201.

Bergstrom, R.M. (1969) Electrical parameters of the brain during ontogeny. In Robinson, R.J. (ed.) *Brain and Early Behaviour*, p. 15. London & New York: Academic Press.

Brown, J.K. (1977) Migraine and migraine equivalents in children. *Developmental Medicine and Child Neurology*, **19**, 683.

Brown, J.K. (1978) Mental handicap and degenerative encephalopathies. In Forfar, J.O. & Arneil, G. (eds.) *Textbook of Paediatrics*. Edinburgh: Churchill Livingstone.

Brown, J.K. (1979) Foetal brain development and phenylketonuria. Sardawalla, I. (ed.), *Symposium on P.K.U.*, Bristol, S.S.I.E.M. Lancaster: M.T.P. Press.

Brown, J.K. (1980) Neonatal fits. In Tyrer, J (ed.) *The Treatment of Epilepsy*. Lancaster: M.T.P. Press.

Brown, J.K., Cockburn, F. & Forfar, J.O. (1972) Clinical and chemical correlates in convulsions in the newborn. *Lancet*, **1**, 135.

Chatrian, G.E., Lettich, E., Miller, L.H. & Green, J.R. (1970) Pattern-sensitive epilepsy, part 1. *Epilepsia* (Amsterdam) **11**, 125.

Christensen, E.S. & Bruhn, P. (1973) Intelligence, behaviour, and scholastic achievement subsequent to febrile convulsions. *Developmental Medicine and Child Neurology*, **15**, 565.

Cockburn, F., Brown, J.K., Belton, N.R. & Forfar, J.O. (1973) Neonatal convulsions associated with primary disturbance of calcium, phosphorus, and magnesium metabolism. *Archives of Diseases in Childhood*, **48**, 99.

Corsellis, J.A.N. (1970) The neuropathology of temporal lobe epilepsy. In Williams, D. (ed.) *Modern Trends in Neurology*, **5**, p. 254. London: Butterworths.

Doose, H., Gerken, H., Hien-volpel, K.F. & Volzke, E. (1969). Genetics of photosensitive epilepsy. *Neuropadiatrie*, **1**, 56.

Eeg-Olofsson, O. (1970) The development of the EEG in normal children and adolescents from the age of 1 through 21 years. *Acta Paediatrica Scandinavica*, Supplement, **208**.

Falconer, M.A. (1970) Significance of surgery for temporal lobe epilepsy in childhood and adolescence. *Journal of Neurosurgery*, **33**, 233.

Forfar, J.O., Cockburn, F. & Brown, J.K. (1972) The role of disturbed magnesium metabolism in neonatal convulsions. *Proceedings of the 1st Symposium on Magnesium deficit in human pathology*, p. 269, Paris 1972.

Freeman, J.M. & Lietman, P.S. (1973) A basic approach to the understanding of seizures and the mechanism of action and metabolism of anticonvulsants. *Advances in Paediatrics*, vol. 20, p. 291. Chicago: Year Book Publishers.

Friedlander, W.J. (1973) Review of epilepsy. *In Progress in Neurology and Psychiatry*. Edit. Spiegel, **28**. New York & London: Grune and Stratten.

Gascon, G.G. & Lombroso, C.T. (1971) Epileptic (gelastic) laughter. *Epilepsia* (Amsterdam) **12**, 63.

Gastaut, H. (1957) Etiology, pathology and pathogenesis of temporal lobe epilepsy. In Merlis, J.K. (ed.) *Epilepsia* (Amsterdam), Newsletter, 15

Gastaut, H. et al (1978) Computerised tomography in the study of West's syndrome. *Developmental Medicine and Child Neurology*, **20**, 21.

Geller, M. & Geller, G. (1970) Brief amnestic effects of spike-wave discharges. *Neurology* (Minneapolis), **20**, 1089.

Gladwell, S.R.F., Kaufman, K.R. & Driver, M.V. (1979) Psychosis or epilepsy; differentiation of a complex case. *Developmental Medicine and Child Neurology*, **21**, 95.

Golden, G.S. & French, J.H. (1975) Basilar migraine in young children. *Pediatries*, **56**, 722.

Guey, J., Charles C., Coquery, C., Roger, J. & Soulayrol, R. (1967). Study of psychological effects of ethosuximide

(Zarontin) on twenty-five children suffering from petit mal epilepsy. *Epilepsia* (Amsterdam), **8**, 129.

Hagberg, B. (1968) The chlordiazepoxide analogue nitrazepam in the treatment of epileptic children. *Developmental Medicine and Child Neurology*, **10**, 302.

Hansson, O. (1968) Studies of tryptophan load test and pyridoxine treatment in children with epilepsy. *Abstracts of Uppsala Dissertations in Medicine*, University Hospital, Uppsala.

Hirsch, C.S. & Martin, D.L. (1971) Unexpected death in young epileptics. *Neurology* (Minneapolis), **21**, 682.

Hockaday, J. (1979) Basilar migraine in childhood. *Developmental Medicine and Child Neurology*, **21**, 455.

Holdsworth, L. & Whitmore, K. (1974) A study of children with epilepsy attending ordinary schools. *Developmental Medicine and Child Neurology*, **16**, 746.

Hudgins, R.L. & Corbin, K.B. (1966) An uncommon seizure disorder: familial paroxysmal choreoathetosis. *Brain*, **89**, 199.

Hutt, S.J., Jackson, P.M., Belsham, A. & Higgins, G. (1968) Perceptual-motor behaviour in relation to blood phenobarbitone level. *Development Medicine and Child Neurology*, **10**, 626.

Ingram, T.T.S. (1963) *Paediatric aspects of cerebral palsy*. Edinburgh: Livingstone.

Ingram, T.T.S. (1974) *Paediatric aspects of cerebral palsy*. Edinburgh: Churchill Livingstone.

Jennett, B. (1973) Trauma as a cause of epilepsy in childhood. *Developmental Medicine and Child Neurology*, **15**, 56.

Keith, H.M. (1963) *Convulsive disorders in children with reference to treatment with ketogenic diet*. Boston: Little, Brown & Co.

Kubler-Ross, E. (1969) *On death and dying*. New York: Macmillan.

Lennox, W.G. (1960) *Epilepsy and related disorders*. London: Little, Brown & Co., J. & A. Churchill Ltd.

Lennox-Buchthal, M.A. (1973) *Febrile convulsions*. Amsterdam: Elsevier Publishing Co.

Lindsay, J., Ounsted, C. & Richards, P. (1979) Longterm outcome in children with temporal lobe seizures. *Developmental Medicine and Child Neurology*, **21**, 285.

Livingston, S. (1972) *Comprehensive management of epilepsy in infancy, childhood and adolescence*. Springfield, Illinois: C.C. Thomas.

Margerison, J.H. & Corsellis, J.A.N. (1966) Epilepsy and the temporal lobes. *Brain*, **89**, 499.

McGrath, A.P. (1972) The epileptic child and his family. *Special Education*, **61**, 23.

McKusick (1971) *Mendelian Inheritance in Man*. Baltimore & London: Johns Hopkins Press.

Miller, F.J.W., Court S.D.M., Walton, W.S. & Knox, E.J. (1960) *Growing up in Newcastle upon Tyne: a continuing study of health and illness in young children within their families*. London: Oxford University Press.

Millichap, J.G. (1965) Anticonvulsant drugs. In Root, W.S. & Hogman, F.G. (eds) *Physiological Pharmacology*, vol. ii, part B, p. 97. New York: Academic Press.

Millichap, J.G. (1978) Recurrent headaches in 100 children. *Child's Brain*, **4**, 95.

Millichap, J.G. & Aymat, F. (1967) Treatment and prognosis of petit mal epilepsy. Paediatric clinics of North America. *Paediatric Neurology*, **14**, 905.

Millichap, J.G. & Fowler, G.W. (1967) Treatment of the minimal brain dysfunction syndrome. Paediatric clinics of North America, *Paediatric Neurology*, **14**, 767.

Minns, R.A. & Brown, J.K. (1978) Intracranial pressure

changes associated with childhood seizures. *Developmental Medicine and Child Neurology*, **20**, 561.

Nowack, W.G., Johnson R.N., Englander, R.N. & Hanna, G.R. (1979) Effects of valproate and ethosuximide on thalamocortical excitability. *Neurology*, **29**, 96.

Oettinger, L., Nekowishi, H. & Gill, I.G. (1967) Cerebral dysrhythmia induced by reading. *Developmental Medicine and Child Neurology*, **9**, 191.

Ounsted, C. (1971) Some aspects of seizure disorders. In Gairdner, D. & Hull, D. (eds) *Recent advances in Paediatrics*, p. 363. London: Churchill.

Ounsted, C., Lindsay, J.M. & Norman, R.M. (1966) Biological factors in temporal lobe epilepsy. *Clinics in Developmental Medicine*, No. 22. London: Heinemann.

Prensky, A.L. (1976) Migraine and migrainous variants in pediatric patients. *In Pediatric Clinics of North America*, vol. **23**, No. 3, p. 461.

Purvis, R.J., Mackay, G.S., Cockburn, F., Barrie, W.J., Wilkinson, E.M., Belton, N.R. & Forfar, J.O. (1973) Enamel hypoplasia of the teeth associated with neonatal tetany. *Lancet*, **2**, 811.

Richter, D. (1960) Epilepsy and convulsive states. In Cummings, J.N. (ed) *Modern Scientific Aspects of Neurology*, p. 314. London: Arnold Ltd.

Rukonen, R. & Donner, M. (1979) Incidence and aetiology of infantile spasms from 1960–76. *Developmental Medicine and Child Neurology*, **21**, 333.

Rutter, M., Graham, P. & Yule, W. (1970) A neuropsychiatric study in childhood. *Clinics in Developmental Medicine*, No. 35–36. London: Heinemann.

Rylance, G.W., Moreland, T.A. & Butcher, G.M. (1979) Carbamazepine dose – frequency requirement in children. *Archives of diseases in childhood*, **54**, 193.

Sato, S., Dreifuss, F.E. & Penry, J.C. (1976) Prognostic factors in absence seizures. *Neurology* **26**, 788.

Sillanpaa, M. (1973) Medico-social prognosis of children with epilepsy. *Acta Paediatrica Scandinavica*. Supplement, **237**.

Snead, O.C. (1978) Gamma hydroxybutyrate in the monkey. *Neurology*, **28**, 636.

Stephenson, J.P.B. (1978) Reflex anoxic seizures. *Archives of Diseases in Childhood*, **53**, 193.

Stevens, J.R., Sachdev, K. & Milstein, V. (1968) Behaviour disorders of childhood and the electroencephalogram. *Archives of Neurology* (Chicago), **18**, 160.

Stores, G. (1976) The investigation and management of school children with epilepsy. *Public Health, London*, **90**, 171.

Stores, G. (1978) School children with epilepsy at risk for learning and behaviour problems. *Developmental Medicine and Child Neurology*, **20**, 502.

Thom, D.A. (1942) Convulsions of early life and their relation to chronic convulsive disorders and mental defect. *American Journal Psychiatry*, **98**, 574.

Vallarta, J.M., Bell, D.B. & Reichert, A. (1974) Progressive encephalopathy due to chronic hydantoin intoxication. *American Journal of Disease in Childhood*, **128**, 27.

Ward, F. & Bower, B.D. (1978) A study of certain social aspects of epilepsy in childhood. *S.I.M.P.* No. **39** supplement, vol. 20, No. 1.

Waterlain, C.G. (1978) Neonatal seizures and brain growth. *Neuropadiatrie*, **9**, 213.

Watters, G. (1979) Body scanning in the diagnosis of adrenal tumours presenting with 'dancing eyes'. Canadian Association of Neurological Sciences Meeting. Halifax, Nova Scotia.

Yule, W. (1973) Epilepsy – education and enigma. *Special Education*, **62**, 16.

PART TWO
FEBRILE CONVULSIONS

M.A. Lennox-Buchthal

The syndrome of febrile convulsions has fortunately attracted a great deal of interest and study in recent years. It was first mentioned in the Babylonian code of Hammurabi in 2080 B.C. (Rossiter *et al.*, 1977). The syndrome was clearly described in the Hippocratic corpus, which goes back to the 5th century B.C. These writings showed great clinical acumen, since the temperature could not at that time be measured. 'Convulsions occur to children if acute fever be present...most readily up to their seventh year. Older children and adults are not equally liable to be seized with convulsions in fevers, unless some of the strongest and worst symptoms precede' (Adams' translation, 1939, p. 212). This clinical acuity is the more extraordinary since convulsions in infancy can be caused by illnesses that could not then be differentiated such as birth injury, meningitis and tetany. Willis (1685) excelled some of our modern clinicians in recognising that the syndrome cannot be related to developmental factors common to children in general. 'For as much as Children, who fall into Fevers about the time of breeding of Teeth, are not all tormented with Convulsions, it therefore follows that some disposition to this disease, either innate or acquired, doth proceed...' (cited in Lennox, 1960).

The recent keen interest is due not only to the fascination of unravelling the causes of the peculiar syndrome, but also to the size of the problem and to the occasional tragic consequences. About 5 per cent of children have at least one convulsion in the first 5 years of life, and more than half of them are febrile convulsions. It is as well to recognise at the outset that fevers run high not only in the affected children, but also (figuratively speaking) in those who investigate them. That is to say, there are wide and sometimes inexplicable differences of opinion. Some are due to differences in the populations studied, or in the manner of

study. Whatever the cause, opinions are generally hotly defended.

THE SYNDROME OF FEBRILE CONVULSIONS[*]

Fever

The prime determinant of febrile convulsions is by definition fever. A temperature of 38°C is accepted as the lower limit, but it is usually higher: 75 per cent of the children have a rectal temperature of 39.2°C or more, and 25 per cent have 40.2°C or more (Herlitz, 1941).

Age

The second invariable feature of the syndrome is the young age. The age of highest incidence is 9–20 months when more than half the initial convulsions occur. They are so rare before the age of 6 months and after 5 years that reports of febrile convulsions in adults (Bird, Heinz & Klintworth, 1962; Osuntokun & Odeku, 1970) are met with some scepticism. The peak age at onset is in the second year of life, when close to half of all initial convulsions occur. The age predilection is a true factor of age, and not an artefact of the susceptibility to infectious diseases (Lennox-Buchthal, 1973).

Inheritance

The third determinant of the syndrome is as Willis (1685) surmised, genetic predisposition. The incidence of 'occasional convulsions' (infantile, febrile or single convulsions) in relatives is high – as high as 30–35 per cent in some studies, and even up to 40–50 per cent, and the incidence of 'epilepsy' (recurrent spontaneous convulsions) as high as 20–25 per cent (Lennox-Buchthal, 1973). It is plain that the incidence in relatives depends to a high degree on how detailed and specific the questions are. It also depends on how frank the popular attitudes are with respect to convulsions. In

---

[*]Readers are referred to the previous review of the subject for detailed documentation (Lennox-Buchthal, 1973). Here I shall cite reports mainly published since 1973, and those that were overlooked in the previous review, called 'the Gentofte series' in the text.

any case, more positive family histories are obtained when the questions are put both initially and later, when the parents have had time in their turn to question their parents and other members of the family about the occurrence of convulsions in themselves and their descendents (Frantzen *et al.*, 1970).

Although the high incidence of a family history of epilepsy may at first sight seem to connect the two convulsive disorders, the relation is much more tenuous, indeed it is highly doubtful when one considers the histories more closely. Febrile convulsions occur mainly in close relatives (95 per cent in parents, sibs, parents' sibs or their children) whereas epilepsy is reported mainly in more distant relatives (72 per cent, Frantzen *et al.*, 1970). Moreover the 'epilepsy' of some affected relatives may have been due to severe febrile convulsions, and this relation may have been forgotten or overlooked. In the main, then, the genetic traits determining febrile convulsions and epilepsy seem to be distinct. Analysis of the incidence of febrile convulsions in parents and sibs strongly suggests that the specific trait, susceptibility to febrile convulsions, is transmitted by a single dominant gene with incomplete penetrance (Ounsted, 1951, 1952, 1970a; Frantzen *et al.*, 1970).

Although 'epilepsy' in general seems not to be genetically related to febrile convulsions, there does seem to be some genetic relation to nocturnal convulsions. The relation is evidenced in two ways. Firstly, febrile convulsions often occur as the child is falling asleep, is asleep or is awakening. Secondly, when two monozygotic twins had substantially the same intelligence, and the proband had febrile convulsions, 80 per cent of the co-twins had febrile convulsions, and the remaining 20 per cent had nocturnal convulsions (Lennox-Buchthal, 1971). There seems, however, to be a quantitative difference. The convulsions in the relatives of twins with febrile and with nocturnal convulsions were similar, but the incidence was half as great in the relatives of twins with nocturnal convulsions.

I have no explanation of the difference between the twins I reported (collected by W.G. Lennox over about 20 years and reported by him and his collaborators: Collins & Lennox, 1947; W.G. Lennox, 1947, 1960; Lennox & Jolly, 1954) and the twins reported by Schiøttz-Christensen and his colleagues (Schiøttz-Christensen, 1972; Schiøttz-Christensen & Hammerberg, 1975). Whereas the monozygotic pairs of twins collected by W.G. Lennox were 100 per cent concordant for seizures (when the intelligence of the two twins was no more than 20 I.Q. points apart), those collected by Schiøttz-Christensen were mainly discordant (8 monozygotic pairs concordant for febrile seizures and 15 discordant, none with nocturnal seizures). Either the history taking of Schiøttz-Christensen was grossly in error, and that it could have been so faulty seems doubtful; or the twins collected by Lennox were unrepresentative, since all were referred to him because of a convulsive disorder in the proband. That this fact could have made the results so different seems doubtful, since Schiøttz-Christensen also sought his twin pairs out by finding the proband with febrile seizures. Finally, the births of Lennox's twins seem to have been more often abnormal, since 26 of the 38 monozygotic twin pairs had evidence of possible or certain brain damage, related to birth in 21, congenital mental defect in four, and severe illness at one year in one. This fact, too, seems unlikely as a possible explanation of the different findings in the two series, and it must be left as one of the inexplicable discrepancies between series of patients reported in the literature.

Sex

Sex seems to be a factor in the manifestation of febrile convulsions. Boys outnumber girls by a mean of 1.4 to 1 (Millichap, 1968). Just why boys should be more often affected is still one of the puzzles about the syndrome. Ounsted (1953) made the astute observation that the excess of boys was due entirely to an excess of boys from one-sex sibships. The boy to girl ratio in mixed sibships was 95 to 100; whereas in one-sex sibships there were 160 boys to 100 girls. I found nearly precisely the same figures in 205 children with febrile convulsions: the boy to girl ratio was 105 to 100 in mixed sibships, whereas in one-sex sibships there were 152 boys to 100 girls (1973). So far there has been no satisfactory explanation of this curious gender difference (*see* Taylor & Ounsted, 1972, for another opinion).

The convulsions

Febrile convulsions are usually defined as a convulsion, i.e. loss of consciousness with tonic, clonic or rarely atonic motor phenomena with a rectal temperature over 38°C. Although most of the convulsions are brief, even extremely brief, the range is in fact wide, and the convulsion may last over 30 minutes, when it is usually classified as severe and, if not stopped by adequate medication, prolonged convulsions lasting hours do occur. They are now fortunately rare, since intravenous or intrarectal diazepam can stop the convulsion promptly. Though the convulsions are generalised as a rule, some – especially the long ones – may be unilateral or show focal features. The distracted parents often describe the convulsion as generalised, but the physician who sees the convulsion is apt to detect lateralising features (Aicardi & Chevrie, 1970). There seems no reason to exclude these occasional long or lateralised convulsions from the group of febrile convulsions.

As a rule, a single convulsion occurs as the temperature is rapidly approaching its peak, and the fever subsides after the convulsion (Fig. 3.3). There are, however, many exceptions to the rule (Fig. 3.4). In Figure 3.4A the child had multiple convulsions as the temperature was falling; in

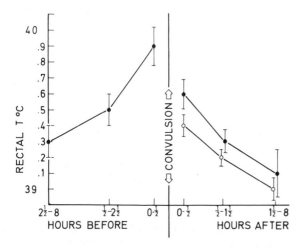

Fig. 3.3 The mean rectal temperature within the given times before and after a febrile convulsion. The vertical bars give the mean error. Closed circles: the temperature in those children whose temperature was measured both before and after the convulsion (drawn from Table 6 in Herlitz, 1941). Open circles: the mean temperature of all 725 children in his series (Table 5 in Herlitz, 1941) (from Lennox-Buchthal, 1973)

Figure 3.4B there were several convulsions with a lower temperature than the initial one, and no new convulsion with a higher temperature some 18 hours later. Such exceptions as these make one believe that it is not the fever *per se* that sets off the convulsion, but that fever initiates some process, which in its turn sets off the convulsion.

Several factors are related to severe (long or lateralised) convulsions. The most important is age: in the 'Gentofte series' the proportion of severe convulsions was about 30 per cent when the age was 3 to 13 months[*], half that at 14 to 18 months, and the proportion diminished gradually to nine per cent above the age of three years. The precise age limits differ somewhat in different series, but there is nearly universal agreement that infants in the first 1.5–2 years of life are more apt to have severe convulsions than children three years old and older.

Some people seem to think that if the first convulsion was severe, subsequent convulsions may also be severe and that they should therefore be prevented. There was no basis for that belief in the 'Gentofte series' nor in that of Aicardi and Chevrie (1970). In the 'Gentofte series', 40 children had a severe convulsion. Of these, 32 had an episode of status initially: 26 had no more seizures, five had subsequent mild ones, and only one child had first and second severe seizures and then recurrent afebrile convulsions. On the other hand, eight of the 40 children had initial brief seizures and subsequent severe ones, one ending fatally. In fact, as the number of convulsions increased, the proportion of severe convulsions rose sharply (Fig. 3.5), even though the child was getting older and so coming into the age when severe convulsions are rare.

Thirdly, long seizures tend to become lateralised; and for this reason focal seizures are much more apt to be long lasting than generalised ones. The same phenomenon was described in adolescent baboons (Meldrum & Horton, 1973).

Cause of the fever

The cause of the fever is, in Western countries at

[*]The difference below and above 14 months is highly significant (p < 0.001); the difference below and above 18 months is significant (p < 0.01). From Table 32 in Lennox-Buchthal, 1973.

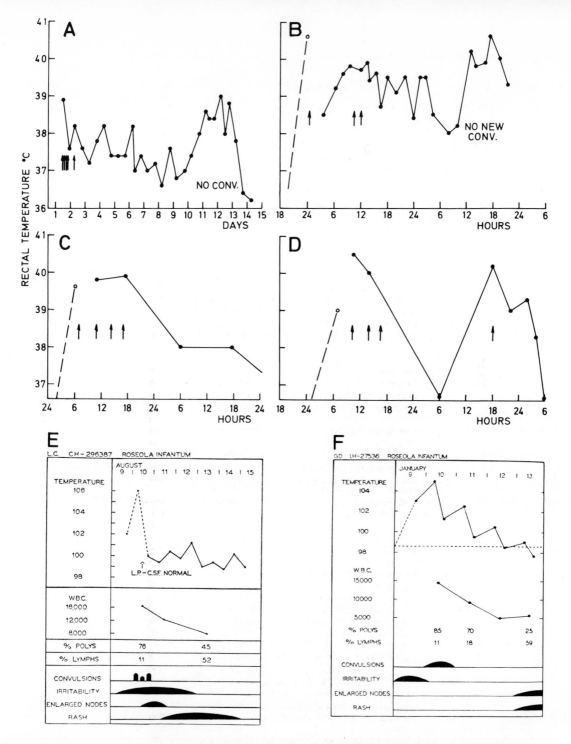

Fig. 3.4 Exceptions to the rule that the convulsion occurs as the temperature is increasing rapidly to its peak. The rectal temperature (C) is shown on the ordinate, time on the abscissa. The convulsions are indicated by arrows. A – The only convulsions of a girl at the age of eight months. No more convulsions in spite of higher fever two weeks and two and four months later; last seen at the age of seven. EEG at three years and nine months showed 3/sec spike-wave paroxysms. Mother has epilepsy. B – The only convulsions of a 3-year-old boy, first with T. 40.6°C, repeated with T. 39.8°C, and no further convulsions in spite of a new elevation to 40.6°C. Family history negative. Later developed 3/sec spike-wave paroxysms in the EEG. Last seen at the age of seven. C and D – The two febrile convulsive episodes of a boy at 16 and 17 months of age. Family history negative. EEG normal. Last seen at the age of four years. (The above patients are in the Gentofte series). E and F – Convulsions and fever in two children with exanthem subitum (from Berenberg *et al.*, 1949) (from Lennox-Buchthal, 1973)

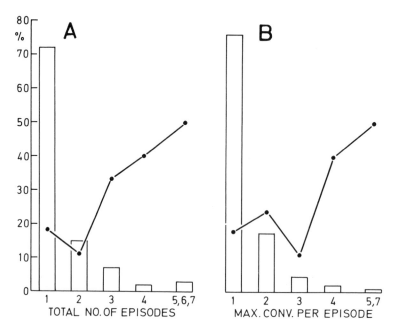

Fig. 3.5 The filled circles give the proportion of severe convulsions (ordinate) as a function of the number of convulsions (abscissa). The columns give the number of episodes (A) and of convulsions in an episode (B) as per cent in 218 consecutive children with febrile convulsions (Gentofte series, Lennox-Buchthal, 1973)

least, most often an upper respiratory tract infection or bronchitis. However, these illnesses are common in young children, and the incidence of febrile convulsions is in fact on the low side – 5–7/1000 (Table 3.7). Less frequent illnesses – gastroenteritis, pneumonia, exanthem subitum (*roseola infantum*) – have a higher rate of febrile convulsions as complicating factor – 13/1000 to as

Table 3.7 Incidence of convulsions during infective illnesses in the first 5 years (data in Miller *et al.*, 1960).

Rate 1000	Illnesses in 847 children	Number	Convulsions	FC per 1000 illnesses
Low				
	Undiff. resp. infections	584	0	0
	Severe colds	1619	4	3
	Mumps	113	1	
	Chicken pox	240	0	
	Rubella	134	0	
	Pertussis	392	1 + 1 hemiplegia	
5 to 7				
	Tonsillitis, otitis	847	5	6
	Bronchitis	624	3	5
	Measles	540	4	7
High				
	Gastroenteritis (first 3 years)	546	7(2)*	13
	Pneumonia + Møller's cases	253	4	16
	Unknown	184	5	27
	Exanthem subitum			14–20†
CNS infections				
	Tb. Meningitis	5	3 (4)	
	Probable encephalitis after vaccination.	1	1	

* Numbers in parentheses indicate number of patients who died.

† From the literature.

From Lennox-Buchthal, 1973

high as 27/1000 (Table 3.7). Of course central nervous system infections have a high rate of complicating convulsions (Ounsted, 1951; Miller et al., 1960), and the common infectious diseases of childhood (measles, mumps, whooping cough, chicken pox) seem to have a low rate. Pyelitis is a rare cause of febrile convulsions because it is not frequent in the susceptible age (Kastrup, 1971).

These data were gathered before rapid typing of viruses was available. More recent evidence suggests that virus illnesses may be the main cause of febrile convulsions. Wallace and Zealley (1970) found that half of 53 children admitted for their first febrile convulsion had a viral illness – but three-quarters of children admitted for a febrile illness without convulsions also had a viral disease. Wallace and Zealley stressed that children with viral illnesses, whether with or without convulsions, were much more apt to have neurological sequelae than children with non-viral febrile illnesses. The viruses tested for included some not known to attack the nervous system*.

Later studies have not confirmed the high rate of neurological sequelae in children with viral illnesses, but they have confirmed the high rate of viral infections in children with febrile convulsions: half of the children hospitalized for febrile convulsions on whom material was taken for viral typing had a viral illness (Regnard et al., 1972; Stokes et al., 1977). The viruses found by Stokes et al. (1977) are listed in Table 3.8. Since the faeces were not examined, a viral aetiology was probably more frequent than these figures indicate. There was no difference between children who were positive for virus and those who were negative: severe convulsions were equally frequent and the groups were not different in age, sex, family history, previous history of seizures or neurological abnormalities. The discrepancy from the findings of Wallace and Zealley (1970) is one of the many puzzling ones in the literature on febrile convulsions. The groups of children studied were plainly different, but where the difference lay is not apparent.

During an epidemic of Influenza A infections,

*The following antigens were used: Influenza A, B and C, Sendai, parainfluenza 1, 2 and 3, adenovirus, respiratory syncytial virus (RSV), mumps, measles, psittacosis, *Coxiella burnettii*, and *Mycoplasma pneumoniæ*.

Table 3.8 Viruses identified from 276 children admitted with febrile convulsions

Influenza A	35
Influenza B	5
Parainfluenza 1	4
Parainfluenza 2	1
Parainfluenza 3	9
Parainfluenza 4A	4
Parainfluenza 4B	2
Respiratory syncytial virus	20
Rhinoviruses	3
Adenoviruses	26
Coxsackie B	14
Echoviruses	9
Measles	3
Mumps	2
Herpesvirus hominis	12
Total	149*

*The number of children in whom a virus was identified was 136 (49 per cent); 13 children had two virus types identified simultaneously, one of which was usually herpesvirus or an adenovirus.
From Stokes et al., 1977

40 per cent of the children had a febrile convulsion – a high rate presumably due to the fact that most of the children (58 per cent) were in the first two years of life, the older children having retained immunity from a previous epidemic (Brockelbank et al., 1972). Parainfluenza is also a frequent cause of febrile convulsions (Downham, McQuillin & Gardner, 1974), the incidence varying from 7 per cent with Para 1 to 62 per cent with Para 4 b.

Since there is still controversy as to the role of immunization in the causation of febrile convulsions, the findings of Harker (1977) are pertinent. The incidence of febrile convulsions after primary immunization was a good deal lower than the general incidence, and the conclusion was drawn that febrile convulsions after immunization occur by chance and are due to age. In Oxford the incidence of febrile convulsions is 30/1000, whereas in the 28 days after immunization febrile convulsions occurred in 0.09/1000 after triple vaccine (diphtheria, pertussis and tetanus), in 0.6/1000 after polio and in 0.9/1000 after measles immunization.

In Africa the causative infections are more numerous than, and are of course different to, those in Western countries. For example, malaria is a frequent cause, as is septicemia (Patel, 1971; Familusi et al., 1972).

Exanthem subitum must be a common cause of febrile convulsions since the epidemiology of the disease indicates that it must be a universal infection in the first five – particularly in the first two – years of life, and that immunity acquired from the early infection must account for the virtual absence of the disease in children over five years old and in adults. Möller (1956) and Broberger (1958) saw many frank cases and said that many children with febrile convulsions had a fever curve and blood picture like that of exanthem subitum but had no rash.

I followed this suggestion up, and found that half of the children with febrile convulsions had a total neutrophil count of less than 2000/mm³ (Lennox-Buchthal, 1972). Of course only those children were considered whose differential white count was obtained on the day before, on the day of, or the day after defervescence, since neutropenia on the day the temperature falls to normal is one of the hallmarks of the disease. When more than one blood count was taken, the neutrophil count usually rose abruptly after defervescence, but neutropenia could still be present for at least 10 days, as in exanthem subitum. One quarter of the children with neutropenia were diagnosed clinically as having exanthem subitum. Presumably the three quarters not so diagnosed had an illness caused by the same virus. If so, the findings support Zahorsky's (1947) statement that 'we ought to accept that *roseola* (exanthem subitum) *sine eruptione* is a common malady'. It is therefore puzzling that in no instance was exanthem subitum diagnosed in the large consecutive series of Miller *et al.* (1960) and none in the large group of Stokes *et al.* (1977), both from Newcastle upon Tyne. Stokes *et al.* found only few children with neutropenia, but they do not say on what day the blood count was obtained. The controversy will not be settled until it is possible to identify the virus that causes exanthem subitum, as it is now possible to identify many other viruses.

Is it important to identify those children who have neutropenia (less than 2000/mm³) on the day of defervescence, or is the question of purely academic interest? The only previous report (Lennox-Buchthal, 1972) found that those children with neutropenia had significantly more severe convulsions (more than 30 minutes or focal) than children without neutropenia. If these findings could be confirmed in a larger series of

children, there would be added impetus to identify the virus and to include it among the viruses now tested for as part of the routine investigation of children with febrile convulsions.

DIAGNOSIS AND LABORATORY INVESTIGATION

Meningitis, encephalitis, lumbar puncture

The main differential dilemma facing the physician is whether the convulsion is attributable to the fever *per se*, or whether the child may have meningitis or encephalitis. In other words, should the child with the first (or a subsequent, for that matter) febrile convulsion have a lumbar puncture?

Rutter and Smales (1976) found that infants presenting with their first febrile convulsion could have meningitis without specific clinical evidence of it, and they recommend routine lumbar puncture in infants under the age of 18 months. Of 314 children presenting with their first febrile convulsion and with no meningeal signs, routine lumbar puncture revealed four with unsuspected meningitis, three viral and one bacterial. The lumbar puncture was repeated later in two children and demonstrated meningococcal meningitis. All the children with meningitis over the age of three years had positive clinical signs.

Samson, Apthorp and Finley (1969) also found clinical signs of meningitis to be lacking in 11 of 27 children admitted with their first febrile convulsion, and four of them had evidence of other infection, though all had purulent meningitis. All those with no clinical signs were in the age group 16 months or less, those with meningeal signs were 3½–9 years old. Nonetheless, of the 27 children with meningitis and convulsions, 16 had no stiff neck, 20 had no Brudzinski's sign, 14 had no impairment of consciousness, and 16 had no bulging fontanelle.

Of the other routine laboratory tests (Rutter & Smales, 1976), haemoglobin in 309 revealed two children to be anaemic. The white count was of little value for treatment, though of value for diagnosis. I agree, but I believe that a white and differential white count on admission and on the day of defervescence are indicated. Blood glucose in 269 children showed hyperglycemia (transient) in 14 per cent, half of them with glucose levels over 11.1 mmol/l (200 mg per cent) (Rutter & Smales, 1976). The elevation is presumably due to the muscular exertion during the convulsion and does not require treatment (Spirer *et al.*, 1974). Of our 200 consecutive children with febrile convulsions, one had repeated episodes of hypoglycemia with convulsions, which were not however related to his febrile convulsions. Routine blood calcium rarely shows a low value, of the order of 1/200 in Western countries at least, and routine blood calcium seems of dubious necessity unless there are clinical signs. When rickets was common, there was a great deal of speculation, especially in the German literature, as to the role of spasmophilia in febrile convulsions. Routine magnesium levels were normal both in the blood and in the spinal fluid in all of 75 consecutively admitted children with febrile convulsions (Rutter & Smales, 1976), whereas half of Indian children with febrile convulsions had low serum magnesium and two thirds had low CSF magnesium (Chhaparawal *et al.*, 1971). Mild hyponatremia is, on the other hand, a frequent finding (Rutter & O'Callaghan, 1978), occurring in about one third of the children. Although it does not cause the febrile convulsion, it may contribute to recurrent convulsions and does require treatment.

Of other routine tests, ophthalmological examination is not contributory, unless severe brain damage is suspected (Sørensen, 1977). Routine skull X-rays are unnecessary (Berman & Johnson, 1977). It would be enlightening to know how often cerebral oedema occurs in febrile convulsions, information presumably only obtainable by a CT scan. In my experience routine electroencephalography is more misleading than helpful in diagnosis and prognosis, its only value being for research purposes (Frantzen, Lennox-Buchtal Nygaard, 1968).

Electroencephalography

Since electroencephalography has been rather widely misused, especially for prognosis and treatment, I shall document my mistrust of it, though I recognise its value as a research tool. The most frequently heard misconceptions are: (1) that the child whose EEG is abnormal after the first week should not be considered to have true (or some use the expression 'benign') febrile convulsions; and (2) that the child with a paroxysmal EEG should be treated prophylactically with anticonvulsants for at least two years. Both these assumptions are false. I have reviewed the subject (Lennox-Buchthal, 1973), and base my opinion mainly on the EEG findings in 218 children admit-

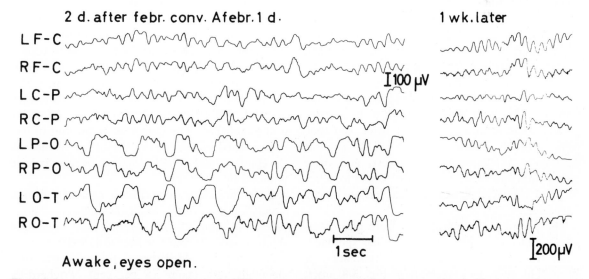

Fig. 3.6 An example (left) of acute slowing in the EEG, most marked in the occipital and temporal leads. The boy was three years and two months old and had four convulsions hours apart, lasting for 2 to 30 minutes, the last one two days before the EEG, he had been afebrile one day. His EEG was normal one week later (right) (from Frantzen *et al.*, 1968)

ted to hospital for their first febrile convulsion and most of them followed closely, both clinically and by EEG, for 5 to 7 years (Frantzen *et al.*, 1968, 1970; Lennox-Buchthal, 1973).

1. A slow or extremely slow EEG tracing was recorded in about one third of the children within a few to six days after the convulsion. The slowing (Fig. 3.6) was most marked in the occipital regions, and was usually asymmetrical even after generalised seizures. When there were lateralising signs, slowing was most marked over the affected hemisphere (with one exception). The slowing was always less and had usually disappeared a week to 10 days later. Since marked slowing did not necessarily recur when the same child had a new febrile convulsion, it was probably related to factors in each acute illness. Though it occurred more often when the convulsion was long (30 minutes) or focal, the difference was not significant. Marked slowing was more frequent when the temperature had been over than when it had been under 39° (P <0.01), and it was more frequent when the illness had lasted more than 36 hours or was accompanied by vomiting or diarrhoea (P < 0.01). This acute abnormality had no clinical prognostic implication. It did occur more often when the child later developed a spike focus, and the spikes were then localised to the area of maximum slowing, but the spike focus did not either predict afebrile convulsions or epilepsy.

2. About a third of the children developed paroxysmal abnormalities at a later age, 2 to 5 years (range 1.5–8.3 years). Since the age when paroxysmal abnormalities appeared was usually later than the initial febrile convulsion, the children who had their initial convulsion after the third birthday were those most apt to have paroxysmal abnormalities on the first EEG. But they were precisely those children whose risk of developing a recurrence was lowest, and there seems therefore to be no sensible cause to select them for prophylactic treatment, as has often been advocated.

The paroxysmal abnormalities were most commonly 3/second spike and wave, either spontaneously (Fig. 3.7) or during photic stimulation or sleep. The spike foci (example in Fig. 3.8) often occupied the region previously affected by acute slowing. The paroxysmal abnormalities did not,

however, predict epilepsy. All three children who developed epilepsy showed paroxysmal abnormalities, but these developed after the onset of the epilepsy and not before it. Of the 67 children who showed paroxysmal abnormalities, 64 were free of seizures (without medication) when they were last seen at the age of 5 to 7 years.

I hope I have convinced the reader that electroencephalography is misleading in the individual child with febrile convulsions. It may be useful for research purposes. For example is there evidence (by CT scan) of cerebral oedema in those children with EEG slowing in the first week, and not in those without?

PHYSIOLOGICAL CONCOMITANTS AND PATHOLOGICAL SEQUELAE OF FEBRILE CONVULSIONS

What happens to the child who has a febrile convulsion? If the convulsion is, as it usually is, brief, very little disruption of normal physiological functions occurs. It is true that any convulsion, with its accompanying paroxysmal discharge in the central nervous system, greatly increases the brain's consumption of oxygen. The motor activity also increases muscular utilisation of oxygen, and it is presumably the increased motor activity that causes the (transient) hyperglycemia (Spirer *et al.*, 1974; Rutter & Smales, 1976).

Concomitant with increased neuronal activity, the level of carbon dioxide in cerebral venous blood increases, and this causes an enormous increase in blood flow through the brain, which partly or completely supplies the increased oxygen demand. These events during a convulsion are well established. The exacerbating features in febrile convulsions are (1) the young age of most of the children, and (2) the additional oxygen demand imposed by the fever.

1. In the adult about 15 per cent of the total circulation goes to the brain. In children of three years, it is about 65 per cent, and may be more at younger ages (Prichard & McGreal, 1958).

2. A rise in temperature of 1°C raises the basal metabolic rate about 15 per cent (Prichard & McGreal, 1958).

To repeat, when the convulsion is brief, the

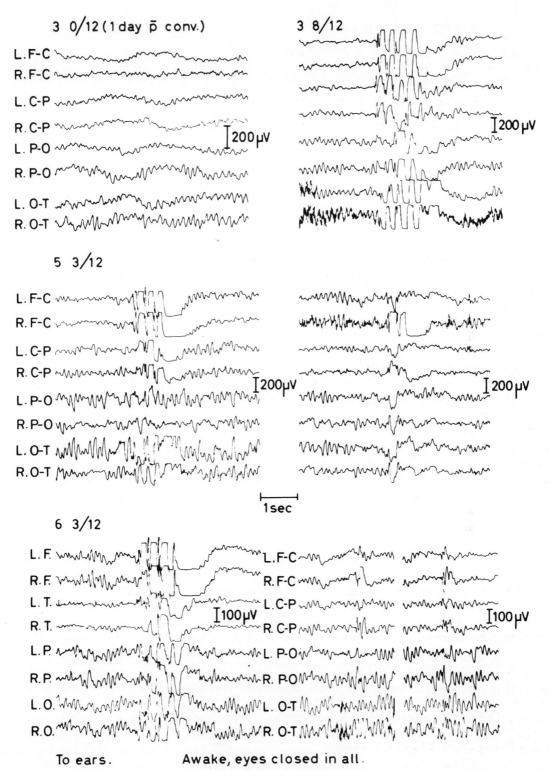

Fig. 3.7 Examples of 3/sec spike-and-wave paroxysms in the waking record of a girl who had a 20-min convulsion with T. 39°C at the age of three years. Two siblings had febrile convulsions. The first EEG (upper left) was normal, as it was three months later (not shown). All subsequent EEGs have showed subclinical spike-and-wave discharges (upper right and middle and lower left), the last when she was six years and three months old. Two EEGs also showed a right frontal spike focus (middle and lower right). No subsequent convulsions (from Frantzen *et al.*, 1968)

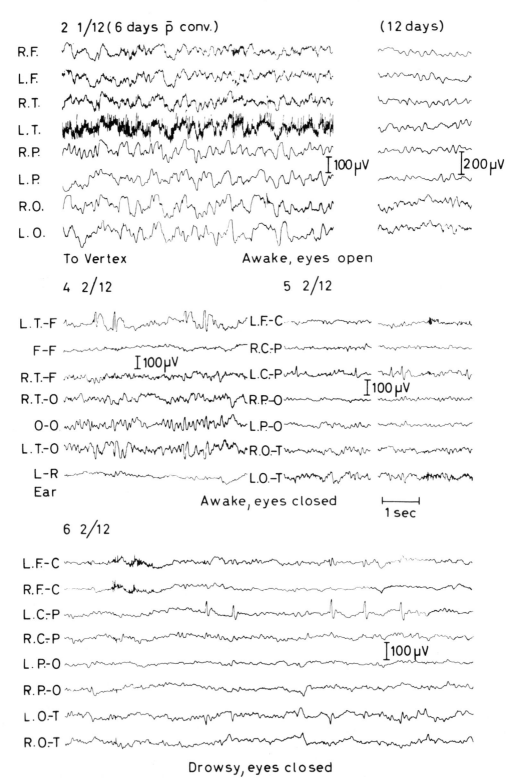

Fig. 3.8 Above, left: the first very slow EEG six days after a brief convulsion with T. 40.1°C of a boy two years and one month old; right, normal six days later. Middle and below: to show the spike focus in the same child in the left temporal region at the age of four years, in the left central region at five and six years of age. No further convulsions. The maternal great grandfather and a maternal cousin had epilepsy (from Frantzen *et al.*, 1968)

increased energy demand of the brain is met, and there is neither clinical evidence of deficit, nor evidence of hypoxia as judged from the lactate/pyruvate ratio in the cerebrospinal fluid (Blennow & Svenningsen, 1974) nor, generally, EEG evidence of abnormality.

There are few studies of changes in cerebral metabolism with febrile convulsions. Salter and Saunders (1970) showed a marked elevation in serum creatine phosphokinase following febrile convulsions in 84 per cent of the children, the number of 'positives' being increased when the determination was obtained on admission and was repeated at 48 hours. Although elevation of serum creatine phosphokinase has been reported in some types of cerebral damage (ref. in Salter & Saunders, 1970), determination of the isoenzyme pattern in a few infants showed that the enzyme was largely derived from skeletal muscle. There was no elevation over control values in infants with fever without convulsions nor in infants with convulsions without fever. Although it is difficult to interpret the findings, the study is an example of the stimulating search for biochemical concomitants of febrile convulsions.

Another example is the study of Siemes, Siegert & Hanefeld (1978) on the blood-cerebrospinal barrier in infants with febrile convulsions. The authors included as controls children with extracerebral infections, and compared them with patients with meningitis or encephalitis. They determined three proteins in the spinal fluid with different molecular weight: albumin, a small molecule; immunoglobulin as moderately large; and α_2-macroglobin as a large molecule. They reasoned that if the brain-cerebrospinal barrier were damaged, this would be reflected in an increased content in the spinal fluid of progressively larger molecules. Their expectation was only partially fulfiled in that 10 of 61 patients (15–90 minutes after a febrile convulsion) had a high content of albumin, none had a high content of immunoglobulin, but five had a high content of α_2-macroglobulin. They did not confirm previous reports that the total protein content in the cerebrospinal fluid tended to be low. The authors pointed out that their findings could hardly be interpreted as indicating a damage in the brain-CSF barrier, but more probably indicated some degree of brain oedema. This probability was supported by the linear relation between the content of albumin in the spinal fluid and the duration of the convulsion.

The situation is quite different when the convulsion lasts from 30 minutes to many hours or is lateralised. Let us consider the concomitants of these extremely severe convulsions, and extrapolate all degrees of involvement for the less severe ones.

The only evidence in human infants who have suffered prolonged or unilateral febrile seizures is that obtained by arteriography, pneumography, electroencephalography and by autopsy or clinical follow-up. X-ray findings indicate severe brain oedema on the side of maximal seizure discharge, i.e. the side opposite the unilateral convulsion (Isler, 1969; Aicardi & Baraton, 1971). The oedema, though mainly due to the hyperaemic response to increased neuronal activity, is increased by the apnoea and increased intrathoracic pressure during the convulsion, and may be due in part to the fever alone (Yannet & Darrow, 1938). Whether the massive unilateral or bilateral oedema is a prerequisite for neuronal degeneration is a matter of dispute but it is indisputable that when massive oedema occurs, cerebral atrophy is apt to follow (Isler, 1969; Aicardi & Baraton, 1971) and to be accompanied by transient or permanent neurological deficit (Gastaut et al., 1960). It is not necessary to take an EEG soon after such a long unilateral convulsion, for it invariably shows extreme slowing on both sides, but mainly over the affected hemisphere.

That a frequent chronic lesion after such severe febrile convulsions is mesial temporal sclerosis with main involvement (ischemic changes and gliosis) of the Sommer or h1 sector of the hippocampus has been amply documented. When the pathology is so gross that the child is left with hemiparesis, and when the history indicates that the febrile convulsion was the traumatic incident (Gastaut et al., 1960), there can be no doubt. Ounsted's evidence, too, seems irrefutable. He and his colleagues studied 100 children with temporal lobe epilepsy; 32 of them had no evidence of cerebral insult aside from a long febrile convulsion that occurred before the third birthday in all but 4 (Ounsted, Lindsay & Norman, 1966; Ounsted, 1967). But perhaps the most convincing evidence is that of Falconer and his colleagues, which he reviewed in 1971. He and his colleagues performed unilateral anterior temporal lobectomy in about 200 patients and followed them for 2 to 10 years. About half the patients had mesial temporal sclerosis, in 35 per cent of the patients attributable to a long febrile convulsion. The episode of status occurred between the ages of six months and four years. That the lesion caused the seizures (and the often accompanying behaviour disorder) is attested by the results of operative removal: two thirds of the patients were rendered free of seizures or nearly so. In all, 96 per cent were benefitted.

The lesion was indistinguishable from the lesions described in chronic epileptics (Sano & Malamud, 1953; Margerison & Corsellis, 1966), and resembled that in children who died in status epilepticus (Norman, 1964; Ounsted et al., 1966): ischaemic nerve cell change and loss of cells and gliosis, especially of the h1 sector of the hippocampus. In autopsied children, more diffuse cell loss involved the cortex, especially the occipital lobes, and the cerebellum (Zimmerman, 1938; Fowler, 1957; Ounsted et al., 1966). The damage to the occipital lobes is undoubtedly related to the mainly posterior slowing on the EEG. In addition there was neuronal loss in the thalamus and, less commonly, in the corpus striatum and inferior olives.

In children who died during a febrile status, cerebral venous congestion and hyperaemia were nearly always mentioned specifically (Herlitz, 1941; Zellweger, 1948; Bamberger & Matthes, 1959). Zimmerman (1938) considered venous congestion, and Gastaut et al. (1960) massive oedema, to be the most important cause of the ischaemic cellular changes.

The experimental studies concern the effect of prolonged convulsions on the brain, they are numerous, but only three of them consider fever as a parameter.

The early experimental studies concerned kittens (reviewed by Lennox-Buchthal, 1973). More recently, Meldrum and his colleagues, in a beautiful series of experiments (reviewed in Meldrum, Horton & Brierly, 1974), showed that prolonged seizures in adolescent baboons produced the histological lesions that have been described in humans: neuronal loss and gliosis in the hippocampus, the h1 or Sommer sector being characteristically damaged, often asymmetrically (Meldrum et al., 1974). The onset of status epilepticus was followed within minutes by a decline in mean arterial pressure, and death during status was due to cardiovascular collapse.

Similar findings were described when the prolonged seizures were induced by bicucullin (Meldrum & Brierly, 1973), only here the lesions involved as well the neocortex diffusely with some accentuation occipitally, and the Purkinje cells of the cerebellum, as has been described in humans and in kittens with febrile convulsions. The brain damage seemed to be due not only to the cerebral epileptic activity, but also to hyperpyrexia, arterial hypotension, mild systemic anoxia and acidosis, occasionally severe hypoglycemia as well. Cerebellar damage was related to hyperpyrexia and arterial hypotension. In a later study on rats, the metabolic stress exerted by hyperthermia exaggerated the neuronal lesions (Blennow et al., 1978). The implications of these well documented studies for the treatment of children with febrile convulsions are discussed on page 83.

The second recent experimental study concerns rats at the age of five and 15 days (Nealis et al., 1978). The animals were used as controls, or were subjected to pyrexia but not allowed to convulse, or were subjected to pyrexia with a convulsion. The rats were then tested for the acquisition of developmental reflexes and for maze-solving ability. There was no difference between the groups in the development of reflexes. The animals that convulsed did, however, make significantly more errors, at the 0.01 level, in maze-solving, the deviation from controls being more marked in animals that had a convulsion with hyperpyrexia at five days than at 15 days (Nealis et al., 1978). Thus, the rat can be used as a model of the neurological sequelae of febrile convulsions.

The experimental findings cited hitherto define the effects of convulsions with fever on the young brain. There has been no clinical study of factors that might account for febrile convulsions. The isolated example was the report of Careddu, Apollonio and Giovannini (1962) that there was evidence of disordered tryptophan metabolism in children at the time of a febrile convulsion, and that the metabolic disorder had returned to normal when the children were free of fever. The finding is still apparently held valid in Italy, and a recent report describes the efficacy of treating the metabolic disorder (Riva *et al.*, 1977). McKiernan *et al.* (1979), on the other hand, found an elevated hydrokynurenine/hydroxyanthranilic acid ratio not only in the children with febrile convulsions but also in children who were febrile without a fit. The authors suggest that the elevated ratio does not indicate vitamin B_6 deficiency but may represent a non-specific response of tryptophan metabolism to stress. In a controlled trial, prophylaxis with vitamin B_6 did not protect against recurrences.

To explain the age-dependent genetically determined susceptibility to febrile convulsions, one suspects that there may be a developmental deficit in some cerebral enzyme system. One such deficit was described by Abood and Gerard (1955): a reduction in ATPase activity in the brains of mice during the period of susceptibility to audiogenic seizures (in a susceptible strain) but not before or after, with a corresponding deficit in oxidative phosphorylation. We therefore tested a susceptible strain and found that they were also susceptible to convulsions with fever, whereas a control strain was not. At the age of peak susceptibility to convulsions, but not before or after, the susceptible mice had a marked diminution in Na, K-activated ATPase, diminished concentration of K^+, diminished K^+-stimulated release of GABA, and diminished oxygen uptake (Hertz *et al.*, 1974). Such a mechanism, if it were found, could explain febrile convulsions in infants.

PROGNOSIS

The risk of recurrence

The size of the risk of recurrences depends on the age of the child. When he is 13 months or

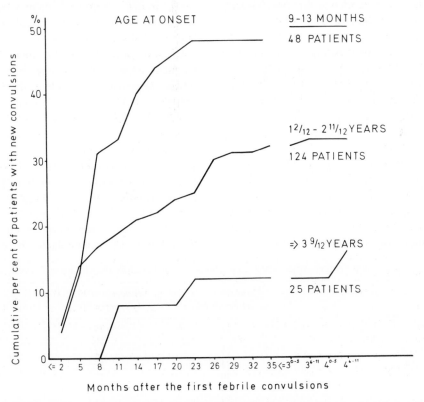

Fig. 3.9 Age at onset and the rate of recurrence. The cumulative rate of recurrence (ordinate) at quarterly intervals after the first febrile convulsion (abscissa). The rate is significantly higher in the youngest patients (p < 0.02 and 0.01)(from Frantzen *et al.*, 1970)

younger, about 50 per cent of the children will have a new febrile convulsion (Fig. 3.9). When he is 14 months to three years old, about 30 per cent, and over the age of three, 10 per cent will suffer a new convulsion. The new convulsions occurred within 20 to 30 months after the first episode. These figures are taken from the 'Gentofte series' (Lennox-Buchthal, 1973). The precise age division may differ somewhat in other series, but agreement is general that recurrences are most apt to occur when the child is under the age of three years, and that nearly all new convulsions have occurred within two years.

In the 'Gentofte series', girl infants were twice as apt to have recurrences as boys, and the children with a positive family history were twice as liable to recurrences as those without.

One might expect that the child with pre-, peri- or postnatal abnormalities would be more apt to develop recurrences than the child without this history, yet there is no unanimity on the subject. There was no such tendency in the 'Gentofte series' (Lennox-Buchthal, 1973).

The risk of afebrile convulsions

As many as 10 per cent (range about 4–20 per cent) of the children have a single or a few subsequent afebrile convulsions. Of the 218 children in the 'Gentofte series', two even had repeated afebrile convulsions, which ceased spontaneously and did not recur during the time of observation, though medication was withdrawn. Ounsted calls this 'remittent epilepsy'.

The risk of epilepsy

Table 3.9 shows the results of a large series of

patients when the findings in benign febrile convulsions and in patients who suffered subsequent epilepsy are compared. Serious prognostic features are, in addition to severe convulsions (long, lateralised or repeated), onset in the first year of life. This susceptibility of the very young brain to damage has not been adequately explained, but it seems to exist. Rasmussen (1979) reviewed the histories and findings of the 1572 patients who underwent cortical resection for medically refractory focal epilepsy at the Montreal Neurological Institute in the years 1928–1977. Of them, 206 patients (13 per cent) had an antecedent history of isolated infantile convulsions, which were febrile convulsions in 29 per cent of the 206. Some of these had a history of birth injury or other factor which could have contributed to the brain lesion, but in nearly half (41 per cent) the convulsion was apparently the sole cause for the later development of recurring seizures.

Other poor prognostic signs are antecedent brain injury (including mental retardation), as described by Nelson and Ellenberg (1976, 1978) and by Wallace (1977), in recent studies. Female sex was mentioned in three reports as being more frequent when the child developed epilepsy after febrile convulsions, and a family history of epilepsy in three studies (Table 37A in Lennox-Buchthal, 1973). Taylor and Ounsted (1971) accounted for the female preponderance in groups with a poor outcome by the fact that girls were younger at the onset. Wallace (1977) saw 12 per cent with continuous recurrent grand mal seizures, usually lower class children, often with a history of perinatal abnormality and long term neurological disorder. Temporal lobe seizures, on the other hand, were related to repeated or pro-

Table 3.9 Clinical features more frequent when febrile convulsions preceded epilepsy than in 'benign' febrile convulsions (FC)

	Incidence of benign FC	Incidence of FC followed by epilepsy %	P
Long convulsions	17	45	< 0.001
Hemiconvulsions	7	30	< 0.001
Repeated convulsions	19	54	< 0.001
Onset in the 1st year	25	39	< 0.001
Antecedent brain injury	10	37	< 0.001
Mental retardation	2	21	< 0.001
Female sex	39	54	< 0.01
Family history epilepsy	8	21	< 0.02

Details in Table 37A from Lennox-Buchthal, 1973.

longed initial convulsions with unilateral features. She believes, therefore, that subsequent grand mal and temporal lobe seizures develop by different mechanisms.

The relation of temporal lobe seizures to severe febrile convulsions was depicted especially clearly by Ounsted and his colleagues (1966), and the relation was established by the beneficial effect of anterior temporal lobectomy and by the histological findings in the resected specimens (reviewed by Falconer, 1971). The lesion has also been produced experimentally.

The risk of epilepsy was exceptionally low in a large series, the Collaborative Perinatal Project of the National Institute of Health of the United States Public Health Service. Although only two per cent of the children developed recurrent afebrile seizures by seven years (and how many of them will turn out to be 'remittent' is not known), the large number – 1706 with febrile convulsions – allowed quantitative estimates of the probability that epilepsy would occur (Nelson & Ellenberg, 1976). The items that increased the risk to 10 per cent were: (1) neurological or developmental abnormalities, whether certain or suspected, before any seizure; (2) an initial convulsion lasting longer than 15 minutes, or multiple or focal. The risk of epilepsy in the rest of the children was one per cent, about the same risk as in the 'Gentofte series' (Lennox-Buchthal, 1973).

Later, Nelson and Ellenberg (1978) added a family history of a febrile seizure as a third risk factor, and found the incidence of subsequent epilepsy to be one per cent when there was one risk factor, two per cent when there were two, and 10 per cent when there were three. The low risk of epilepsy and the absence of any demonstrable evidence of intellectual deficit over that present before the seizure (Ellenberg & Nelson, 1978) lead the authors to the opinion that continuous prophylactic medication is not indicated, unless possibly in the high risk group. To the objection that one cannot foresee whether or not the infant with an initial brief febrile convulsion will subsequently have a severe one, the authors point to their large numbers, which show that after a single brief initial convulsion, 1.4 per cent of the children had a subsequent convulsion lasting over 30 minutes,

and in no instance did the child then develop epilepsy.

These recent American figures are certainly reassuring. Does more prompt and better medical care account for the difference from earlier American series and some contemporary European ones? One can hope that it does. The only criticism one can level against such a massive project is that the children were examined and followed by many persons, not all of equal training. And one wonders how the follow-up could have been so reliable despite the mobility of the American population.

Meantime, those of us in Europe and Canada (and more, I suppose, in the less developed countries) still have the problems of epilepsy and brain damage due to a severe febrile convulsion. The fairly recent data on severe febrile convulsions with subsequent mental and neurological impairment from such countries as Switzerland (Isler, 1969), France (Gastaut et al., 1960; Aicardi & Chevrie, 1970), and England (Ounsted et al., 1966; Wallace & Zealley, 1970) give us no cause for complacency. It makes no difference to the parents or to the affected child whether the percentages are high or low – they know only that the tragedy, which might have been averted, has befallen him, and the physician cannot fail to be equally concerned.

Wallace (1976) found an increase of 'factors associated with suboptimal neurological development' to such a degree that she suggests that 'a convulsion in a febrile child is drawing attention to a development defect'. This agrees poorly with the study of Rasmussen (1979) and with (of recent studies alone) the findings in a large prospective study of consecutive newborn children. Rossiter et al. (1977) compared the 346 children with convulsions (210 with febrile convulsions) with the 4922 newborns without convulsions and found no statistical differences between the children with convulsions and the controls.

TREATMENT

Since the introduction of diazepam for the treatment of status epilepticus (Naquet et al., 1965), treatment of the acute attack has been assured in a way that is, perhaps, as revolutionary as the introduction of phenobarbitone and then of phenytoin for the treatment of epilepsy. It is true that paraldehyde was used effectively by some (0.2 ml/kg intramuscularly, Prichard, 1974), but its use was not widespread, and phenobarbitone and phenytoin were notoriously ineffective because of the long time required to build up adequate blood levels. The use of diazepam to control febrile status was aided by the results of Smith and Masotti (1977), who titrated the dose by giving the drug slowly by the intravenous route. The seizures stopped promptly after a dose of 0.08 to 4 mg/kg: 38 per cent of the infants needed 0.4 mg/kg or less, 53 per cent 0.5 to 1 mg/kg, and only two (of 21 babies) needed 2 to 4 mg/kg. In addition to anticonvulsant medication, clinical experience and experimental evidence indicate the importance of keeping an open airway and giving oxygen. The temperature should be lowered by tepid sponging. When the child is not dehydrated, the use of agents to prevent or reduce brain oedema has been advocated: 1 to 2 mg of dexamethasone, followed by 1 to 2 mg every 4 to 6 hours; and 0.5 g of mannitol per kg body weight as a 20 per cent solution in water intravenously over a period of 10 to 15 minutes (Eiben, 1967). Rutter and O'Callaghan (1978) treat mild hyponatremia by restricting fluids (when the children are not dehydrated).

A further aid to the control of status was the introduction of methods to determine the level of the drug in the blood. Although the plasma level reaches its maximum within minutes after intravenous administration, it falls rapidly and is at an effective level for only 1 to 2 hours (Viala et al., 1971). After intramuscular administration, the peak is reached as late as 30 minutes (Ferngren, 1974), making this route unsatisfactory to control febrile status epilepticus. Whatever the route, a convulsion may recur in several hours, and continuous intravenous infusion is then advocated unless a repeated dose stops the convulsion promptly. Another possibility is offered by the recent report that phenobarbitone 15 mg/kg by mouth or intramuscular injection achieves a blood level over 43 μmol/litre (10 μg/ml) within 45 minutes. The treated patients were not more drowsy than the controls (Pearce, Sharman & Forster, 1977). This would of course be useful only to prevent recurrences in the same illness, not to arrest long convulsions.

Since intravenous administration can be difficult in the young infant in a convulsion, the report was welcomed that the rectal route gives therapeutic levels nearly as fast as the intravenous (Agurell et al., 1975), and one might expect that the rare complication of respiratory arrest would be less. However, when given by the rectal route, the solution supplied for intravenous administration must always be used; the suppository supplied by the drug house gives high levels in the blood too late and too irregularly to be at all useful (Knudsen, 1977). The method is so easy that it can be used in the home, even by the parents, if they are carefully instructed and if they call a physician so he can assure that there is no cause other than fever for the convulsion.

Since I no longer follow children with febrile convulsions, I am grateful to clinicians occupied daily with the treatment of these children (Brown, 1979; Lee & Melchior, 1981, Perret, 1979; Roger, 1979; Wallace, 1979).

How to treat the child with his first febrile convulsion? Agreement seems to be general that brief convulsions pose no threat, but that long convulsions should at all costs be prevented. Some define long as over 15 minutes, some as over 30, some as over an hour. I have described our finding that a brief initial convulsion may well be followed after one or more recurrences, by a severe one. In other words, the child should receive immediate medical attention, and be admitted to hospital for observation (Brown, 1979) or for lumbar puncture if he is under 18 months of age (Rutter & Smales, 1977). After the first febrile convulsion, a second should be prevented if the child has not yet passed his third birthday. To give intermittent medication, i.e. to give phenobarbitone or diazepam at the first sign of fever, is strikingly inadequate, since the convulsion is often the first sign that the child is sick. But if a subsequent convulsion can be stopped immediately at home, while the doctor is on the way, then effective continuous prophylaxis is not necessary. If the mother is intelligent enough and sufficiently thoroughly instructed, rectal diazepam can be given in the home. This is advised routinely in Edinburgh, and the method seems so to cover every contingency that any continuous prophylaxis seems superfluous. I am taking the liberty of quoting Brown (1979) on this point.

'We use rectal diazepam at home as a routine. Our technique is that we use a 1 ml Mantoux syringe. We break off the ampoule top. We do not use the needle at all but the top of the syringe is pushed into the ampoule and the dose sucked up. Then a blob of KY jelly is placed over the anus and the whole syringe is inserted into the rectum about half way. We start off with a dosage of age in years + one, i.e. a three-year-old would be given 4 mg, and this is always given by the mother in hospital under supervision, being shown how to give it before discharge. In this way we know that the mother can give the drug, that there is no danger of her leaving the needle on, there is no need for any aseptic technique if she is worried and nervous at the time that the child is having the fit and it also gives us a chance to see how the child reacts to that dose of drug. We have had one small neonate who went apnoeic with rectal diazepam but we have not had this as a problem in older children. If the dose does not control the attacks we are willing to put up the rectal dosage to 0.5 mg/kg but we usually start on the empirical basis in the first instance. The Pharmacy provides a small kit of syringe, ampoule and Valium® (diazepam) and a small sachet of KY jelly which we give to the patients.'

Diazepam is prescribed to stop convulsions in the home in Stockholm as well (Ferngren, 1977) (0.3–0.4 mg/kg) with good effect and with no toxic symptoms of note. The dose is repeated if the convulsion is still present 20 minutes later.

Continuous prophylactic treatment is the alternative. Many treat only those children with a higher risk for developing epilepsy (i.e. a 'complicated' convulsion or when there is antecedent neurological abnormality) and not the child who has had only a brief febrile convulsion. It seems to me that this therapeutic reasoning is fallacious. The children with an increased risk for epilepsy *have* already suffered brain damage, or an episode that can produce brain damage. In such cases, I agree with Nelson and Ellenberg (1976) that there is no proof that these children benefit by prophylactic anticonvulsant treatment, just as there is no proof that persons with severe head injuries are better off if epilepsy is prevented than they would be if their epilepsy were treated adequately after it has developed. My own experience (1973) has lead me to advocate continuous prophylactic medication for the children who will probably suffer a recurrence, i.e. up to the age of

three years. If one wishes to be absolutely certain that a severe convulsion be prevented, treatment should be up to the age of four years. I stress again that the age is the only reliable guideline; *treatment is not indicated when the EEG is paroxysmal.*

Prophylactic medication with phenobarbitone (3–4 mg/kg if given twice a day, 5 mg/kg if given in a single evening does) has been nearly universally effective in reducing the incidence of subsequent convulsions drastically, from as much as 50 per cent in controls to 10 per cent in treated children, or in preventing them altogether (Faerø et al., 1972; Fois, Malandrini & Beradi, 1974; Thorn, 1975; Wallace, 1975; Wolf, 1977; Wolf et al., 1977). However, even proponents of phenobarbitone seem to agree that it is extremely difficult to convince the mothers to continue with phenobarbitone, sometimes because the child becomes hyperactive, or sleeps irregularly (see especially Thorn, 1975; Wolf & Forsythe, 1978), or because she or the physician fear that it may have an adverse effect on the growing brain. For these reasons sodium valproate is now preferred in many centres in Italy (Cavazzutti, 1975; Galli et al., 1977), France, England and Copenhagen to my knowledge. Because most of the studies are still in the trial stage, there are not yet many final reports, but so far there have been few recurrences in adequately treated children on sodium valproate, 20–30 mg/kg with a blood level of 40–50 μg/ml (Lee & Melchior, 1981). The children take it gladly twice a day, since they enjoy the rasberry syrup it is prepared in (Lee & Melchoir, 1981), and there have been no toxic symptoms of note. Painless prophylactic treatment of the child with a high risk of suffering recurrences seems therefore to be possible. Indeed, Ounsted (1970b) told of a child, a sibling of a child with febrile convulsions, who had a severe febrile convulsion with tragic consequences, though the father had asked the physician for a means of stopping a convulsion because they (the father and children) were to be on vacation, and had been refused. So it may be that siblings, too, should be considered for the possibility of treatment of the acute attack at home, while the parents are waiting for the physician.

REFERENCES

Abood, L.G. & Gerard, R.W. (1955) A phosphorylation defect in the brains of mice susceptible to audiogenic seizure. In Waelsch, H. (ed.) *Biochemistry of the Developing Nervous System*. New York: Academic Press.

Agurell, S., Berlin, A., Ferngren, H. & Hellström, B. (1975) Plasma levels of diazepam after parenteral and rectal administration in children. *Epilepsia*, 16, 277.

Aicardi, J. & Baraton, J.A. (1971) A pneumoencephalographic demonstration of brain atrophy following status epilepticus. *Developmental Medicine and Child Neurology*, 13, 660.

Aicardi, J. & Chevrie, J.J. (1970) Convulsive status epilepticus in infants and children. A study of 239 cases. *Epilepsia* (Amsterdam), 11, 187.

Bamberger, P. & Matthes, A. (1959) *Anfälle im Kindesalter*. Basel: Karger.

Berman, W. & Johnson, B.A. (1977) The value (?) of routine skull radiography in clinical evaluation of children with recurrent convulsions. *Journal of Pediatrics*, 90, 598.

Bird, A.V., Heinz, H.J. & Klintworth, G. (1962) Convulsive disorders in Bantu mine-workers. *Epilepsia* (Amsterdam), 3, 175.

Blennow, G., Brierley, J.B., Meldrum, B.S. & Siesjö, B.K. (1978) Epileptic brain damage. The role of systemic factors that modify cerebral energy metabolism. *Brain*, 101, 687.

Blennow, G. & Svenningsen, N.W. (1974) Cererospinal fluid lactate/pyruvate ratio in children with febrile convulsions. *Neuropädiatrie*, 5, 157.

Broberger, O. (1958) Exanthema subitum och feberkramper. *Nordisk Medicin*, 59, 523.

Brocklebank, J.T., Court, S.D.M., McGuillin, J. & Gardner, P.S. (1972) Influenza-A infection in children. *Lancet*, 2, 497.

Brown, J.K. (1979) Personal communication.

Careddu, P., Apollonio, T. & Giovannini, M. (1962) Troubles du métabolisme du tryptophane dans le mécanisme pathogénique des convulsions hyperpyrétiques. *Pédiatrie*, 17, 359.

Cavazzuti, G.B. (1975) Prevention of febrile convulsions with dipropylacetate (depakine). *Epilepsia*, 16, 647.

Chhaparawal, B.C., Kohli, G., Pohowalla, J.N. & Singh, S.D. (1971) Magnesium levels in serum and in C.S.F. in febrile convulsions in infants and children. *Indian Journal of Pediatrics*, 38, 241.

Collins, A.L. & Lennox, W.G. (1947) The intelligence of 300 private epileptic patients. *Association for Research in Nervous and Mental Disease Proceedings*, 26, 586.

Downham, M.A.P.S., McQuillin, J. & Gardner, P.S. (1974) Diagnosis and clinical significance of para-influenza virus infections in children. *Archives of Disease in Childhood*, 49, 8.

Eiben, R.M. (1967) Acute brain swelling (toxic encephalopathy). *Pediatric Clinics of North America*, 14, 797.

Ellenberg, J.H. & Nelson, K.B. (1978) Febrile seizures and later intellectual performance. *Archives of Neurology* (Chicago), 35, 17.

Faerø, O., Kastrup, K.W., Lykkegaard Nielsen, E., Melchior, J.C. & Thorn, I. (1972) Successful prophylaxis of febrile convulsions with phenobarbital. *Epilepsia* (Amsterdam), 13, 279.

Falconer, M.A. (1971) Genetic and related aetiological factors in temporal lobe epilepsy. A review. Epilepsia (Amsterdam), 12, 13.

Familusi, J.B., Moore, D.L., Fomufod, A.K. & Causey, O.R. (1972) Virus isolates from children with febrile convulsions in Nigeria. *Clinica pediatrica*, 11, 272.

Ferngren, H.G. (1974) Diazepam treatment for acute convulsions in children. A report of 41 patients, three with plasma levels. *Epilepsia*, 15, 27.

Ferngren, H. (1977) Febrile convulsions in children. Acute treatment with diazepam. *Läkartidningen*, 74, 1033.

Fois, A., Malandrini, F. & Berardi, R. (1974) Le convulsioni con febbre. *Clinica pediatrica*, 56, 359.

Fowler, M. (1957) Brain damage after febrile convulsions. *Archives of Disease in Childhood*, 32, 67.

Frantzen, E., Lennox-Buchthal, M. & Nygaard, A. (1968) Longitudinal EEG and clinical study of children with febrile convulsions. *Electroencephalography and Clinical Neurophysiology*, 24, 197.

Frantzen, E., Lennox-Buchthal, M., Nygaard, A. & Stene, J. (1970) A genetic study of febrile convulsions. *Neurology* (Minneapolis), 20, 909.

Galli, V., Gatti, G., Massolo, F., & Modena, I.T.A. (1977) Dipropilacetato di sodio nella profilassi delle convulsioni febbrili dell'infanzia. *Acta neurologica*, 32, 884.

Gastaut, H., Poirier, F., Payan, H., Salamon, G., Toga, M., & Vigouroux, M. (1960) H.H.E. syndrome. Hemiconvulsions, hemiplegia, epilepsy. *Epilepsia* (Amsterdam), 1, 418.

Harker, P. (1977) Primary immunization and febrile convulsions in Oxford 1972–5. *British Medical Journal*, 2, 480.

Herlitz, G. (1941) Studien über die sogenannten initialen Fieberkrämpfe bei Kindern. *Acta paediatrica scandinavica*, 29, Supplement 1, 142.

Hertz, L., Schousboe, A., Formby, B. & Lennox-Buchthal, M. (1974) Some age-dependent biochemical changes in mice susceptible to seizures. *Epilepsia*, 15, 619.

Hippocrates (F. Adams transl.) (1849) *The Genuine Works of Hippocrates*, vol. 1, p. 466. London: The Sydenham Society.

Isler, W. (1969) *Akute Hemiplegien und Hemisyndrome im Kindesalter*. Stuttgart: Thieme.

Kastrup, K.W. (1971) Febrile convulsions and pyurea. *Epilepsia* (Amsterdam), 12, 192.

Knudsen, F.U. (1977) Plasma-diazepam in infants after rectal administration in solution and by suppository. *Acta paediatrica scandinavica*, 66, 563.

Lee, K. & Melchior, J.C. (1981) Personal communication.

Lennox, W.G. (1947) President's address. *Association for Research in Nervous and Mental Diseases. Proceedings*, 26, xv–xix.

Lennox, W.G. (1960) *Epilepsy and Related Disorders*, p. 1168. Boston: Little, Brown.

Lennox, W.G. & Jolly, D.H. (1954) Seizures, brain waves and intelligence tests of epileptic twins. *Association for Research in Nervous and Mental Diseases Proceedings*, 33, 325.

Lennox-Buchthal, M. (1971) Febrile and nocturnal convulsions in monozygotic twins. *Epilepsia* (Amsterdam), 12, 147.

Lennox-Buchthal, M. (1972) Neutropenia and all-boy sibships in children with febrile convulsions. *Developmental Medicine and Child Neurology*, 14, 21.

Lennox-Buchthal, M.A. (1973) *Febrile Convulsions. A Reappraisal*. Amsterdam: Elsevier.

Margerison, J.H. & Corsellis, J.A.N. (1966) Epilepsy and the temporal lobes: A clinical, electroencephalographic and neuropathological study of the brain in epilepsy, with particular reference to the temporal lobes. *Brain*, 87, 499.

McKiernan, J., Mellor, D., Court, S. & Lacey, K. (1980) Hydroxykynurenine/hydroxyanthranilic acid ratios and febrile convulsions. *Archives of Disease in Childhood*, 55, 873.

Meldrum, B.S. & Brierley, J.B. (1973) Prolonged epileptic

seizures in primates. Ischaemic cell change and its relations ictal physiological events. *Archives of Neurology* (Chicago), **28**, 10.

Meldrum, B.S. & Horton, R.W. (1973) Physiology of status epilepticus in primates. *Archives of Neurology* (Chicago), **28**, 1.

Meldrum, B.S., Horton, R.W. & Brierly, J.B. (1974) Epileptic brain damage in adolescent baboons following seizures induced by allylglycine. *Brain*, **97**, 407.

Miller, F.J.W., Court, S.D.M., Walton, W.S. & Knox, E.J. (1960) *Growing up in Newcastle upon Tyne, A Continuing Study of Health and Illness in Young Children within their Families*. London: Oxford University Press.

Millichap, J.G. (1968) *Febrile Convulsions*, p. 222. New York: Macmillan.

Möller, K.L. (1956) Exanthema subitum and febrile convulsions. *Acta paediatrica scandinavica*, **45**, 534.

Naquet, R., Soulayrol, R., Dolce, G., Tassinari, C.A., Broughton, R. & Loer H. (1965) First attempt at treatment of experimental status epilepticus in animals and spontaneous status epilepticus in man with diazepam (Valium). *Electroencephalography and Clinical Neurophysiology*, **18**, 427.

Nealis, J.G.T., Rosman, N.P., De Piero Theslee, J. & Ouellette, E.M. (1978) Neurologic sequelae of experimental febrile convulsions. *Neurology*, **28**, 246.

Nelson, K.B. & Ellenberg, J.H. (1976) Predictors of epilepsy in children who have experienced febrile seizures. *New England Journal of Medicine*, **295**, 1029.

Nelson, K.B. & Ellenberg, J.H. (1978) Prognosis in children with febrile seizures. *Pediatrics*, **61**, 720.

Norman, R.M. (1964) The neuropathology of status epilepticus. *Medicine, Science and the Law*, **4**, 46.

Osuntokun, B.A. & Odeku, E.L. (1970) Epilepsy in Ibadan, Nigeria. A study of 522 cases. *African Journal of Medical Sciences*, **1**, 185.

Ounsted, C. (1951) Significance of convulsions with purulent meningitis. *Lancet*, **1**, 1245.

Ounsted, C. (1952) The factor of inheritance in convulsive disorders in childhood. *Proceedings of the Royal Society of Medicine*, **45**, 865.

Ounsted, C. (1953) The sex ratio in convulsive disorders with a note on single-sex sibships. *Journal of Neurology, Neurosurgery and Psychiatry*, **16**, 267.

Ounsted, C. (1967) Temporal lobe epilepsy: the problem of aetiology and prophylaxis. *Journal of the Royal College of Physicians, London*, **1**, 273.

Ounsted, C. (1970a) Some aspects of seizure disorders. In Hull, D. & Gairdner, D. (eds.) *Recent Advances in Ounsted, C. (1970b) Personal communication.

Ounsted, C., Lindsay, J. & Norman, R. (1966) *Biological Factors in Temporal Lobe Epilepsy*. London: William Heinemann Medical Books.

Patel, C.C. (1971) Acute febrile encephalopathy in Ugandan children. *African Journal of Medical Sciences*, **2**, 127.

Pearce, J.L., Sharman, J.L. & Forster, R.M. (1977) Phenobarbital in the acute management of febrile convulsions. *Pediatrics*, **60**, 569.

Perret (1979) Personal communication.

Prichard, J.S (1974) Convulsive disorders in children. Some notes on the diagnosis and treatment. *Pediatric Clinics of North America*, **21**, 981.

Prichard, J.S. & McGreal, D.A. (1958) Febrile convulsions. *Medical Clinics of North America*, pp. 379–387. Philadelphia & London: W.B. Saunders.

Rasmussen, T. (1979) Relative significance of isolated infantile convulsions as a primary cause of focal epilepsy. *Epilepsia* **20**, 395.

Regnard, J., Huraux, J-M., Bricout, F., Begue, P., Bouillie, J., Grunberg, J., Tournier, G. & Vaudour, G. (1972) Résultats d'une enquête sur la fréquence d'une infection virale contemporaire de convulsions hyperpyrétiques de l'enfant. *Archives francaises de pédiatrie*, **29**, 745.

Riva, E., Borzani, M., Motta, G. & Giovannini, M. (1977) A double-blind trial of pyridoxin pyrrholidoncarboxylate in the treatment of feverish convulsions in children. *Minerva Pediatrica*, **29**, 2001.

Roger, J. (1979) Personal communication.

Rossiter, E.J.R., Luckin, J., Vile, A., Ganly, N., Hallowes, R. & Pearson, R.D. (1977) Convulsions in the first three years of life. *Medical Journal of Australia*, **2**, 735.

Rutter, N. & O'Callaghan, M.J. (1978) Hyponatremia in children with febrile convulsions. *Archives of Disease in Childhood*, **53**, 85.

Rutter, N. & Smales, O.R.C. (1976) Calcium, magnesium and glucose levels in blood and C.S.F. of children with febrile convulsions. *Archives of Disease in Childhood*, **51**, 141.

Salter, D.G. & Saunders, R.A. (1970) Serum creatine phosphokinase elevation following febrile convulsions in infants. *Annals of Clinical Biochemistry*, **7**, 152.

Samson, J.H., Apthorp, J. & Finley A. (1969) Febrile seizures and purulent meningitis. *Journal of the American Medical Association*, **210**, 1918.

Sano, K. & Malamud, N. (1953) Clinical significance of sclerosis of the cornu Ammonis: Ictal psychic phenomena. *Archives of Neurology and Psychiatry* (Chicago), **70**, 40.

Schiøttz-Christensen, E. (1972) Genetic factors in febrile convulsions. An investigation of 64 same-sexed twin pairs. *Acta Neurologica Scandinavica*, **48**, 538.

Schiøttz-Christensen, E. & Hammerberg, P.E. (1975) EEG in twins with febrile convulsions. Follow-up on 59 pairs of the same sex. *Neuropädiatrie*, **6**, 142.

Siemes, H., Siegert, M. & Hanefeld, F. (1978) Febrile convulsions and blood-cerebrospinal barrier. *Epilepsia* **19**, 57.

Smith, B.T. & Masotti, R.E. (1971) Intravenous diazepam in the treatment of prolonged seizure activity in neonates and infants. *Developmental Medicine and Child Neurology*, **13**, 630.

Spirer, Z., Weisman, J., Yurman, S. & Bogair, N. (1974) Hyperglycemia and convulsions in children. *Archives of Disease in Childhood*, **49**, 811.

Stokes, M.J., Downham, M.A.P.S., Webb, J.K.G., McQuillin, J. & Gardner, P.S. (1977) Viruses and febrile convulsions. *Archives of Disease in Childhood*, **52**, 129.

Sørensen, P.N. (1977) Value of routine ophthalmic examination in children with febrile convulsions. *Ugeskrift for Læger*, **139**, 2118.

Taylor, D.C. & Ounsted, C. (1971) Biological mechanisms influencing the outcome of seizures in response to fever. *Epilepsia* (Amsterdam), **12**, 33.

Taylor, D. & Ounsted, C. (1972) *Gender Differences*. Edinburgh: Churchill Livingstone.

Thorn, I. (1975) A controlled study of prophylactic long-term treatment of febrile convulsions with phenobarbital. *Acta Neurologica Scandinavica*, Supplement 60, 67.

Viala, A., Cano, J.P., Dravet, C., Tassinari, C. & Roger, J. (1971) Blood levels of diazepam (Valium) and *N*-desmethyl diazepam in the epileptic child. *Psychiatria, Neurologia, Neurochirurgia*, **74**, 153.

Wallace, S.J. (1975) Continuous prophylactic anticonvulsants in selected children with febrile convulsions. *Acta Neurologica Scandinavica*, Supplement 60, 62.

Wallace, S.J. (1976) Febrile convulsions: neurological sequelae and mental retardation. Neurological and intellectual deficits: convulsions with fever viewed as acute indications of life-long developmental defects. In Brazier, M.A.B. & Coceani, F. (eds) *Brain Dysfunction in Infantile Febrile Convulsions, IBRO Monograph Series*. New York: Raven.

Wallace, S.J. (1977) Spontaneous fits after convulsions with fever. *Archives of Disease in Childhood*, 52, 192.

Wallace, S.J. (1979) Personal communication.

Wallace, S.J. & Zealley, H. (1970) Neurological, electroencephalographic and virological findings in febrile children. *Archives of Disease in Childhood*, 45, 611.

Willis, I. (1685) *The London practise of physick or the whole practical part of physick*. London: George and Crooke.

Wolf, S.M. (1977) The effectiveness of phenobarbital in the prevention of recurrent febrile convulsions in children with and without a history of pre-, peri- and postnatal abnormalities. *Acta paediatrica scandinavica*, 66, 585.

Wolf, S.M., Carr, A., Davis, D.C., Davidson, S., Dale, E.P., Forsythe, A., Goldenberg, E.D., Hanson, R., Lulejian, G.A., Nelson, M.A., Treitman, P. & Weinstein, A. (1977) The value of phenobarbital in the child who has had a single febrile seizure: a controlled prospective study. *Pediatrics*, 59, 378.

Wolf, S.M. & Forsythe, A. (1978) Behavior disturbance, phenobarbital and febrile seizures. *Pediatrics*, 61, 728.

Yannet, H. & Darrow, D.C. (1938) Effect of hyperthermia on the distribution of water and electrolytes in brain, muscle and liver. *Journal of Clinical Investigation*, 17, 87.

Zahorsky, J. (1947) Roseola infantum. A critical survey of recent literature. *Archives of Pediatrics*, 64, 579.

Zellweger, H. (1948) Krämpfe im Kindesalter. 1. Teil. *Helvetica paediatrica acta*, Supplement 5, 3, 1.

Zimmerman, H.M. (1938) The histopathology of convulsive disorders in children. *Journal of Pediatrics*, 13, 859.

PART THREE
CHILDHOOD EPILEPSIES WITH BRIEF MYOCLONIC, ATONIC OR TONIC SEIZURES

J. Aicardi

The epilepsies predominantly characterised by brief myoclonic, atonic or tonic seizures are considered as a separate group because they share several common characteristics: very frequent recurrence of seizures of little clinical significance, some of which may be easily mistaken for minor phenomena such as colics or stumblings; resistance to conventional anticonvulsants; frequent association with mental retardation. The seizures which constitute these epilepsies can be categorised on clinical and EEG grounds as generalised ones according to the International Classification (p. xviii) under the headings of infantile spasms, massive, bilateral myoclonus, tonic and atonic seizures. Although only one type of fit may be observed in some cases, e.g. infantile spasms, more commonly several types are associated in the same patient and it is often impossible to recognise the exact type without simultaneous EEG recording. Falls and head nods which are a hallmark of these epilepsies may be the result of a massive myoclonia, a brief tonic fit or an atonic one, in a standing or sitting child. It is thus justified from a clinical standpoint to consider them jointly. Moreover, two mechanisms are not uncommonly at play in a single fit, e.g. a massive myoclonia may precede immediately loss of postural tone. Other seizure types (absences, partial or grand mal) are often associated and partial or erratic myoclonus is not uncommon, especially during bouts of frequent spells.

Approximately two thirds of the myoclonic and related seizures occur during the first five years. They do not constitute a single syndrome but belong to a number of unrelated disorders. A general classification is presented in Table 3.10 where myoclonic seizures are divided into two groups: (1) Those which are only a symptom of degenerative brain disorders (progressive myoclonic epilepsies); (2) Those which constitute the major component of several epileptic syndromes not due to known underlying progressive diseases. Proper allocation of a particular case to one or the other group may be difficult since apparent progression of the troubles is not infrequent in patients of the second group. This distinction, however, has important practical implications since the progressive disorders of the first group are very severe ones and are genetically determined. These disorders will not be further considered and this chapter will deal only with: (1) infantile spasms; (2)

Table 3.10 Classification of the myoclonic epilepsies and encephalopathies of childhood

Progressive myoclonic encephalopathies
a) Due to known or probable metabolic disturbances
    Tay-Sachs disease
    Juvenile Gaucher disease
    Sialidosis (mucolipidosis I, 'Cherry-red spot myoclonus syndrome')
    Ceroid-lipofuscinosis ('Batten's' disease)
    Lafora body disease
    Non-ketotic hyperglycinaemia
b) Genetic syndromes without known metabolic basis
    Progressive myoclonic epilepsy, 'degenerative' types
    Ramsay-Hunt syndrome
    Juvenile neuroaxonal dystrophy
    Infantile progressive poliodystrophies (Alpers)
    Hallervorden-Spatz disease
    Huntington chorea
    Dominant myoclonus, ataxia and hearing loss
    Myoclonus associated with spinocerebellar degerations
c) Subacute sclerosing panencephalitis
Non progressive myoclonic epilepsies
    Infantile spasms (West syndrome)
    Lennox-Gastaut syndrome
    Cryptogenic myoclonic epilepsy
    Transitional and unclassified types
    Myoclonic absences
    Myoclonic epilepsy of adolescence

Lennox-Gastaut syndrome; (3) cryptogenic myoclonic epilepsy and the borderlands of the Lennox-Gastaut syndrome.

INFANTILE SPASMS (WEST SYNDROME)

Infantile spasms, first described in 1841 by West in his own child, are a form of epilepsy which always occurs in infants before one year, most commonly between three and nine months. Although the term refers only to a particular type of seizures, it has come to designate a syndrome which comprises, in addition to the fits, mental retardation or deterioration and severe electroencephalographic abnormalities known as hypsarrhythmia. In spite of the extensive literature on infantile spasms which has been reviewed in several monographs (Gastaut *et al.*, 1964; Jeavons & Bower, 1964; Lacy & Penry, 1976), the physiopathology of the disorder is still obscure. The reasons for the strict age-dependency and the peculiar clinical and electrical expression are not understood. Huttenlocher (1974) has proposed that abnormalities of dendritic spines could be

important but their significance and specificity are dubious. A brain stem origin for the spasms is suggested by their observation in a hydranencephalic infant (Neville, 1972). However, it has long been recognised that infantile spasms are most commonly associated with diffuse hemispheric lesions of diverse nature. The syndrome may occur in an infant with previous neurological anomalies or retarded development (symptomatic type) or develop in a previously well baby without gross évidence of brain damage (cryptogenic type). This separation is of great prognostic significance but may be more apparent than real since minor – or even gross – pathological changes can be easily missed and since many patients are not submitted to neuroradiological examination. Evidence from CT scan (Gastaut *et al.*, 1978) has demonstrated the frequency of atrophic changes. Such changes, however, should not be the sole basis for classifying cases as symptomatic, especially since recent reports (Lagenstein, Willig & Kühne, 1979; Lyen, Holland & Lyen, 1979) suggest that similar changes may be associated with ACTH or corticosteroid therapy.

The incidence of infantile spasms is about 0.25 to 0.35/1000 live births (Gastaut *et al.*, 1964; Nelson, 1972; Riikonen & Donner, 1979). Boys are affected more often than girls (60 per cent). A family history of epilepsy is uncommon and the occurrence of several cases of West syndrome in a sibship is rare. Two thirds of the patients belong to the symptomatic group but the exact cause remains unknown in half of these. Symptomatic spasms can be due to perinatal brain damage. Anoxic or ischaemic brain lesions (ulegyrias, porencephaly) have been demonstrated in a few cases but the relation between an abnormal birth and infantile spasms is difficult to prove.

Prenatal causes are probably more common. Several brain malformations have been reported including polymicrogyrias, heterotopias, trisomy 21, hydranencephaly, holoprosencephaly (Jellinger, 1970). Pachygyria and callosal agenesis are often associated with infantile spasms. The latter is part of a specific, non-familial syndrome, seen only in girls and which also comprises choroidal lacunae, intraventricular heterotopias and vertebro-costal anomalies (Aicardi, Chevrie & Rousselie, 1969). Tuberous sclerosis is the cause of West syndrome in up to 25 per cent of the cases and can be suspected early when achromic naevi are associated with the spasms. The diagnosis can be confirmed in many cases by the demonstration of subependymal calcifications on CT scan, even during the first year of life (Gastaut & al., 1978). Most cases result from new mutations and the recurrence risk is very low if both parents have no signs of the disorder. Other neurocutaneous syndromes (incontinentia pigmenti, naevus sebaceus, neurofibromatosis) are much less common. Prenatal infections, especially with cytomegalovirus, are probably responsible for some cases (Riikonen, 1978). Prenatal factors are probably important even in the absence of a recognisable disorder, as shown by the abnormally high incidence of a low birth weight for dates among infants with West syndrome (Crichton, 1968; Riikonen & Donner, 1979). Neonatal hypoglycaemia may be an aetiologic factor in some of these infants. While several metabolic abnormalities have been reported in patients with infantile spasms (Lacy & Penry, 1976), only phenylketonuria and nonketotic hyperglycinaemia seem to play a causative rôle.

Postnatal encephalopathies of any cause (traumatic, infectious, or anoxic) can produce infantile spasms. Exceptional cases of tumour are on record (Gastaut et al., 1978). The suggested association between infantile spasms and whooping-cough immunisation seems to be coincidental as the modification of the immunisation schedule in Denmark was not associated with any change in incidence (Melchior, 1977).

The clinical and electrical features of West syndrome are quite distinctive. The onset is between four and seven months in half the cases but it may be after nine months or before three months, especially in symptomatic spasms. The spasms consist of a sudden flexion of the head forwards with bending of the knees and flexion and abduction of the arms. The spasm may last less than one second (lightning spasm) or persist for a few seconds in a brief tonic seizure. In all cases the contraction is slower and more sustained than in true myoclonias. Usually, the spasms recur in series of several dozens, several seconds apart. As the series proceeds, the spasms decrease in intensity and the intervals between the jerks increase. A cry often accompanies each spasm and a smile is not uncommonly seen at the end of a cluster. The spasms are not always generalised and violent. They may be limited to a head nod, at times barely visible. Occasionally the spasms are in extension, resembling a Moro response. They may be asymmetrical in symptomatic cases. There is a tendency for the seizures to be less typical in infants under three months. In all atypical manifestations, the repetitive character is of critical diagnostic importance. In a few patients, however, the spasms fail to recur in series and this is not infrequent at the onset of the syndrome.

Other seizure types (partial motor, adversive) may be associated with the spasms or may precede their onset. They occur almost exclusively in symptomatic forms.

Mental retardation may be obvious before the onset of the spasms in symptomatic cases. In previously well infants a definite behavioural regression is often observed. Social smile disappears, the infant becomes apathetic and hypotonic and is no longer interested in its surroundings. Occasionally these behavioural changes appear before the spasms: West syndrome is the most common cause of mental deterioration in the first year of life and should always be suspected in such a case.

The classical interictal electroencephalographic pattern of West syndrome is known as hypsarrhythmia (Gibbs & Gibbs, 1952). During wakefulness, the record is devoid of background activity and consists entirely of chaotic, high amplitude, asynchronous slow waves haphazardly intermingled with sharp waves or spikes of multifocal origin. During sleep, bursts of synchronous, irregular polyspikes and waves appear on a low-amplitude, poorly organised tracing. The typical hypsarrhythmia may be absent in as many as 40 per cent of the patients (Jeavons & Bower, 1964), especially at onset. A modified pattern with variable admixture of slow waves and spikes, occasionally asymmetrical, is then observed. Especially in infants less than three months, a pattern of complex paroxystic bursts separated by intervals of almost completely inactive EEG (so-called suppression-burst pattern) may be recorded in wakefulness (Maheshwary & Jeavons, 1975). The EEG expression of the spasms is usually a sudden flattening of the tracing sometimes associated with a low amplitude fast activity, rarely with a spike-wave complex. At times, the record remains unchanged. A normal EEG while awake is not sufficient to exclude the diagnosis of West syndrome. Consistently normal records in sleep and wakefulness, however, should raise considerable doubt as to the diagnosis. Normal tracings are more often observed in early true myoclonic epilepsy to which the cases of 'benign myoclonus of early infancy' described by Lombroso & Fejerman (1977) are perhaps related.

Infantile spasms and the hypsarrhythmic EEG pattern both tend to disappear spontaneously before three years of age. The spasms are replaced, in more than half of the cases, by other types of seizures, while the EEG becomes normal or shows focal or diffuse paroxysms (Gastaut *et al.*, 1964; Jeavons & Bower, 1974). Mental retardation, however, persists in approximately 90 per cent of the patients and represents the main disability in this syndrome. Psychiatric disturbances are distressingly common (Thornton & Pampiglione, 1979) and cerebral palsy is an additional handicap in one third of the children. The death rate is between 10 and 20 per cent.

Conventional antiepileptic drugs have very little effect on infantile spasms. Since Sorel's original paper (Sorel & Dusaucy-Bauloye, 1958), ACTH or corticosteroids have been used widely. Doses of 20 to 60 units per day of ACTH, of 10 to 20 mg/kg/d of hydrocortisone or equivalent dosages of prednisolone or dexamethasone are administered for periods of from three weeks to several months in various combinations, with or without associated antiepileptic drugs. No comparative study between the numerous therapeutic schemes is available so that treatment is governed by empirical rules. Our group uses hydrocortisone 15 mg/kg/d for one month without additional antiepileptic drugs.

Hormonal treatment is undoubtedly effective in stopping the fits in 70 per cent of the cases and reverting the EEG to normal in 40 to 50 per cent (Jeavons & Bower, 1974). Recurrences occur in at least 50 per cent of the cases, generally within weeks of stopping therapy. Long-term effects of treatment on mental development are unfortunately much less impressive. The proportion of mentally normal children is around 15 to 20 per cent and in those affected the degree of retardation is usually profound. The best results are achieved in cryptogenic cases with about 35 per cent of normal children, while the results are uniformly poor in symptomatic cases. In the absence of any controlled series it is not known whether mental improvement is due to therapy or results from selection of the best cases for hormonal treatment. Currently, it would seem logical to try to stop the fits and to produce a normal EEG as soon as possible in cryptogenic cases, since the epileptic activity or the unknown process underlying it might play a rôle in the intellectual deterioration. Hormonal therapy however has hazards. Arterial hypertension, electrolytic disturbances and sepsis are quite common and the latter may be fatal. The possible long-term effects of massive and prolonged hormonal therapy on somatic and brain development and other biological functions are not known. In symptomatic cases the risks associated with hormonal treatment are probably not warranted. In such patients, the benzodiazepines (nitrazepam or clonazepam) may control the fits, although they have little effect on the EEG abnormalities (Lacy & Penry, 1976). These drugs are also used by some workers in cryptogenic spasms either as a first choice (Vassella *et al.*, 1973) or in association with hormonal treatment. Their effect, if any, on mental development has not been evaluated.

There is a need for a better assessment of therapy in West syndrome, taking into account several factors which are known to influence strongly the long-term prognosis. These include, in addition to the symptomatic or cryptogenic character of the syndrome, the age of onset and the existence of other fits before the spasms, both of which carry very unfavourable implications. The possible importance of the delay in initiating therapy and of the mental status at onset of the syndrome also needs to be evaluated (Jeavons, Bower & Dimitrakoudi, 1973; Chevrie & Aicardi, 1971). Pending such an evaluation, it is probably wise to use hormonal therapy in all patients whose spasms are not obviously symptomatic.

THE LENNOX-GASTAUT SYNDROME

The term Lennox-Gastaut syndrome was proposed by Gastaut et al (1966) to designate a form of severe epilepsy of childhood with frequently repeated fits of several types and an interictal EEG pattern of diffuse spike-waves at a rhythm of approximately 2 Hz, previously described as 'petit mal variant' (Gibbs & Gibbs, 1952). The term is surrounded by an enormous confusion, due to the fact that the criteria used by various authors to define it are quite different. Some workers select the EEG pattern as the main criterion (Blume, David & Gomez, 1973; Niedermeyer, 1969; Markand, 1977) and include all the clinical correlates of the diffuse slow spike-wave pattern. Others base their description mainly on a clinical picture dominated by falls and massive myoclonias (Kruse, 1968; Doose et al., 1970) and use the clinically descriptive term of 'myoclonic-astatic petit mal' which has often and wrongly been considered synonymous with that of the Lennox-Gastaut syndrome. The EEG correlates in such cases, however, are not always of the 2 Hz spike-wave type and may consist of faster (3 Hz) spike-wave paroxysms. Still others (Aicardi, 1973; Gastaut, 1973; Jeavons, 1977) use combined electroencephalographic and clinical criteria. Much confusion could be avoided by realising that there exists a large group of severe epilepsies of early childhood which share certain common features such as age-dependency, frequent mental retardation, combination of several types of seizures, especially brief atypical ones, and poor response to therapy. These epilepsies are frequently but not always associated with a slow spike-wave pattern. This group, which is not sufficiently homogeneous to be considered a single syndrome, may be variously subdivided, into several overlapping but not identical syndromes according to the criteria selected. In this section the term Lennox-Gastaut syndrome will be restricted to those cases characterised clinically by brief atonic, myoclonic and tonic seizures and electrically by at least some 2 Hz spike-wave activity. Related cases which do not fulfill these criteria will be dealt with briefly in the next section.

The Lennox-Gastaut syndrome is strongly age-dependent. Typical fits rarely appear before two years, only uncommonly develop after seven or eight and tend to be replaced at about ten by uncharacteristic generalised or partial fits. The syndrome is often preceded by other seizure types, especially by infantile spasms. It may thus be considered, like West syndrome, as an age-related response to a variety of non-specific brain insults. The same insults that produce infantile spasms may be responsible for the Lennox-Gastaut syndrome. It may result, in addition, from a number of acquired diffuse brain lesions such as trauma, infections and prolonged seizures. Rare cases of the syndrome in association with localised brain lesions are on record (Bancaud et al., 1973). The rôle played by genetic factors is controversial. The incidence of a family history of convulsive disorders is low (2.5 per cent) in some series (Chevrie & Aicardi, 1972) intermediate in others (Gastaut, 1973) and very high (50 per cent) in some (Doose et al., 1970). These discrepancies may result from the diverse definitions of the syndrome. No cause is found in 20 to 35 per cent of the patients (primary cases). Cases clinically expressed as the Lennox-Gastaut syndrome but due to specific degenerative disorders (e.g. lipidosis) should be excluded since their course and clinical significance are entirely different.

The incidence is difficult to evaluate as a result of the nosological difficulties. It has been estimated at 5 per cent of all the epilepsies and 10.3 per cent (Gastaut, 1973) of the epilepsies of childhood. The typical child is three to five years of age and experiences multiple daily fits resulting in numerous falls during which injuries to the teeth, nose, forehead or occiput may be incurred, such that wearing a protective helmet is necessary. In milder fits the head may nod and the knees sag although the child does not fall. The falls result from different seizure types: brief tonic seizures throwing the patient out of balance; massive myoclonic jerks projecting the child to the ground; atonic or astatic fits which are also responsible for most of the head-nods. The latter two types are often combined in a single seizure, a brief atonia immediately following a myoclonic jerk of the arms and neck (Doose et al., 1970). Periods of brief immobility with a stare, palpebral jerks or slow dropping forward of the head and trunk with occasional simple automatisms (atypical absences) often alternate with the falls. Tonic fits are quite common, especially while the child is asleep and are easily missed. Seizures may be more frequent on awakening. Often, they occur in close succession with clouding of consciousness, interspersed with atonic head nods, brief massive myoclonus, fluttering of eyelids or slight erratic myoclonias of the face, fingers or toes. These periods (petit mal status) last from minutes to hours or days and even weeks, at times in a very mild, almost unrecognisable form. Ataxia is at times noticed during these episodes and may suggest the diagnosis of a progressive disorder. Petit mal status has been reported in 14 to 50 per cent of the patients. In virtually all cases good periods alternate with bad ones with simultaneous fluctuations in intellectual performance.

Other types of seizures are often associated with the tonic, atonic and myoclonic fits which constitute the central ictal pattern of the Lennox-Gastaut syndrome.

The typical interictal EEG features consist of bilateral synchronous slow spike-wave complexes at 1 to 2.5 Hz (Fig. 3.10). These complexes occur in bursts lasting from a few seconds to several minutes. The shape of the complexes is often irregular as are their rate of repetition and topographic distribution. A unilateral predominance is often noted in some records or parts of records but may shift from one side to the other. The paroxysms are little sensitive to hyperventilation or photic stimulation but are strongly activated by sleep during which discharges of 10 Hz rhythms are apt to occur (Gastaut et al., 1966; Niedermeyer, 1969). These discharges are also observed during tonic fits, while other seizures are unaccompanied by any change in the EEG or correspond with a reinforcement of the spikes or a greater synchronisation of the paroxysms. The background activity is usually slow and at times asymmetrical. Other EEG abnormalities are often associated (multifocal or focal spikes, and spike-waves at rhythms faster than 2.5 Hz).

Mental retardation is present from the onset in 20 to 60 per cent of the patients, and in half of the

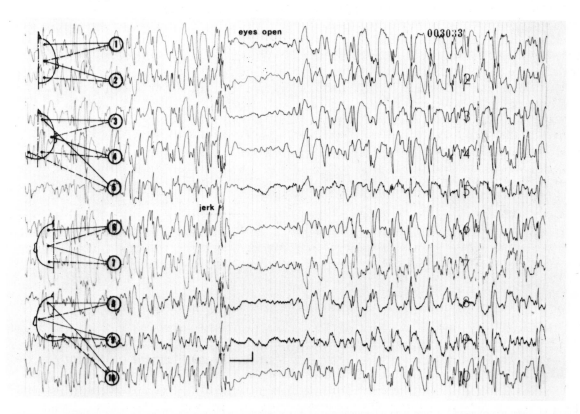

Fig. 3.10 EEG of a patient with the Lennox-Gastaut syndrome. Bilateral spike-wave complexes at 1.5 Hz are interrupted during three seconds following a massive myoclonic jerk. Amplitude and time marker: 50 μ V;I second

cases is severe. After a few years it is found in up to 75 to 95 per cent of the cases. However, there is usually no regression with loss of previously acquired skills, except during episodes of status, and this helps to distinguish the syndrome from degenerative disorders that may mimic it.

The prognosis of the Lennox-Gastaut syndrome is poor. Only a very few patients are able to live independent lives, due to mental retardation or neurological deficits or both. According to Gastaut (1973), 80 per cent will continue to have seizures. Therapy is very disappointing. Conventional anti-epileptic drugs are of little help as are anti-petit mal drugs. The benzodiazepines (Vassella *et al.*, 1973) and sodium valproate (Jeavons, Clark & Maheswary, 1977) are at times effective but often temporarily. Good results have been reported with ketogenic diets (Huttenlocher, 1976; Nellhaus, 1971). ACTH or steroids may be useful to tide some patients over an episode of status but should not be used for long periods. Overtreat-

ment is a major danger in such resistant epilepsies. Evidence has been adduced that limitation of the number of drugs used, may improve the state of consciousness without increasing the frequency of fits (Viani *et al.*, 1977).

CRYPTOGENIC MYOCLONIC EPILEPSY OF CHILDHOOD AND THE BORDERLANDS OF THE LENNOX-GASTAUT SYNDROME.

The borderlands of the Lennox-Gastaut syndrome encompass those cases which belong to the group of severe childhood epilepsies but which do not satisfy the criteria required for inclusion in the syndrome. The size of the group will depend on the comprehensiveness of these criteria. If the sole criterion required is the presence of a slow spike-wave pattern, the borderlands will be limited to cases exhibiting typical myo-atonic seizures with only fast (2.5 Hz or more) spike-wave paroxysms,

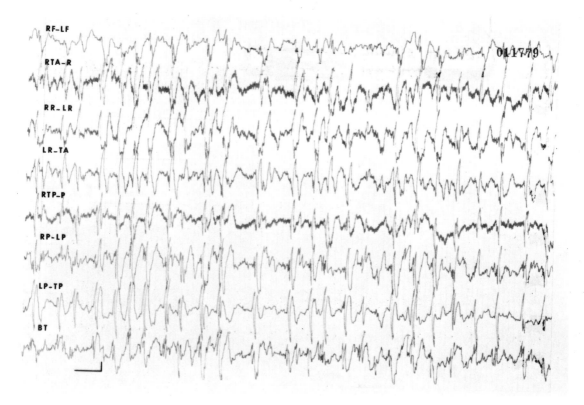

Fig. 3.11 Sleep recording of a patient with infrequent partial motor seizures and atonic fits. Note continuous diffuse slow spike and spike-wave activity. During wakefulness, EEG showed only a left rolandic spike focus. Amplitude and time marker 50 μ V;I second

e.g. cryptogenic myoclonic epilepsy of childhood (Aicardi & Chevrie, 1971; Jeavons, 1975; Aicardi, 1980). With the more restrictive electroclinical criteria we have set forth, the borderlands of the Lennox syndrome will also include cases with a slow spike-wave pattern but without the characteristic seizures.

Cryptogenic myoclonic epilepsy is characterised by the exclusive or predominant occurrence of massive myoclonic or myoclonic-atonic seizures; by the presence of ictal and interictal polyspike-wave bursts at 2.5 Hz or more, without slow spike-waves; by the absence of tonic fits. The onset may be as early as the second semester of life – when it should be distinguished from infantile spasms – or at any time during the first five years. The course is less unfavourable than that of the Lennox-Gastaut syndrome, half the patients being fit-free within five years of onset. One third of the patients remain mentally normal and severe retardation is rare. Transitional forms with some admixture of tonic fits or of slow spike-waves exist and it is currently impossible to decide whether myoclonic epilepsy is an entity in its own right or represents the 'myoclonic' extremity of a spectrum, the more frequent atonic-tonic forms of which constitute the classical Lennox-Gastaut syndrome. In practice, however, the predominance of myoclonic seizures and of paroxysms at 3 Hz has a favourable prognostic significance (Aicardi, 1980).

Epilepsies with diffuse slow spike-wave paroxysms in which tonic, myoclonic or atonic seizures are absent or inconspicuous are difficult to classify. We believe, however, that the slow spike-wave is not in itself sufficient to label them as the Lennox-gastaut syndrome and that, like other epilepsies, they are best classified according to the predominant seizure types.

Most petit mal statuses belong in the Lennox-Gastaut syndrome (Gastaut, 1973) and this probably applies to the cases of 'minor epileptic status' described by Brett (1966). Some however are part of true petit mal and their prognosis is accordingly better.

Recently, cases have been described of children between two and six years of age with almost continuous diffuse slow spike-wave activity during sleep or drowsiness but with only rolandic or frontal spike foci during wakefulness (Tassinari *et al.*, 1977; Dalla Bernardina *et al.*, 1978). Some of these children have only nocturnal or early morning partial motor fits. Others have more or less typical absences and occasional drop-attacks. Such cases should be carefully separated from the Lennox-Gastaut syndrome since their course is a benign one and since they probably represent an atypical form of partial epilepsy with extensive diffusion of the EEG paroxysm during sleep, possibly related to benign epilepsy with rolandic spikes.

REFERENCES

Aicardi, J. (1973) The problem of the Lennox syndrome. *Developmental Medicine and Child Neurology*, **15**, 77.

Aicardi, J. (1980) Course and prognosis of certain childhood epilepsies with predominantly myoclonic seizures. In Wada, J.A. & Perry, J.K. (eds) *Epilepsy, 10th International Symposium, Advances in Epileptology*, 159.

Aicardi, J. & Chevrie, J.J. (1971) Myoclonic epilepsies of childhood. *Neuropädiatrie*, **3**, 177.

Aicardi, J., Chevrie, J.J. & Rousselie, F. (1969) Le syndrome spasmes en flexion, agénésie calleuse, anomalies choriorétiniennes. *Archives Françaises de Pédiatrie*, **26**, 1103.

Bancaud, J., Talairach, J., Geier, S., & Scarabin J.M. (1973) *EEG et SEEG dans les tumeurs cérébrales et l'épilepsie*, p. 266. Paris: Edifor.

Blume W.T., David R.B. and Gomez M.R. (1973) Generalized sharp and slow wave complexes-Associated clinical features and long-term follow-up *Brain*, **96**, 289.

Brett E.M. (1966) Minor epileptic status. *Journal of the Neurological Sciences*, **3**, 52.

Chevrie J.J. & Aicardi J. (1971) Le pronostic psychique des spasmes infantiles traités par l'ACTH ou les corticoïdes.

Analyse statistique de 78 cas suivis plus d'un an. *Journal of the Neurological Sciences*, **12**, 351.

Chevrie J.J. & Aicardi J. (1972) Childhood epileptic encephalopathy with slow spike-wave. A statistical study of 80 cases. *Epilepsia*, **13**, 259.

Crichton J.V (1968) Infantile spasms in children of low birthweight, *Developmental Medicine and Child Neurology*, **10**, 36.

Dalla Bernardina B., Tassinari C.A., Dravet C., Bureau M., Beghini G. & Roger J. (1978) Epilepsie partielle bénigne et état de mal électroencéphalographique pendant le sommeil. *Revue d'EEG et de Neurophysiologie*, **8**, 350.

Doose H., Gerken H., Leonhardt R., Völzke E. & Völz C. (1970) Centrencephalic myoclonic-astatic petit mal. Clinical and genetic investigations. *Neuropädiatrie*, **2**; 59.

Gastaut H. (1973) Evolution clinique et pronostic du syndrome de Lennox-Gastaut. In Lugaresi E, Pazzaglia P. & Tassinari C.A. (eds) *Evolution and Prognosis of Epilepsies*, Bologna: p. 133, Aulo Gaggi.

Gastaut H., Roger J., Soulayrol R. & Pinsard N. (1964) *L'encéphalopathie myoclonique infantile avec hypsarythmie.*

(syndrome de West). Paris: Masson.

Gastaut H., Gastaut J.L., Regis H., Bernard R., Pinsard N., Saint-Jean M., Roger J. & Dravet C. (1978) Computerized tomography in the study of West's syndrome. *Developmental Medicine and Child Neurology*, **20**, 21.

Gastaut H., Roger J., Soulayrol R., Tassinari C.A., Regis H. & Dravet C. (1966) Childhood epileptic encephalopathy with diffuse spike-waves (otherwise known as 'petit mal variant') or Lennox syndrome. *Epilepsia*, **7**, 139.

Gibbs F.A. & Gibbs E.L. (1952) *Atlas of Electroencephalography. Vol. II, Epilepsy.* 2nd edn. Reading: Addison-Wesley.

Huttenlocher P.R. (1974) Dendritic development in neocortex of children with mental defect and infantile spasms. *Neurology* (Minneapolis), **24**, 203.

Huttenlocher P.R. (1976) Ketonemia and seizures: metabolic and anticonvulsant effects of two ketogenic diets in childhood epilepsy. *Pediatric Research*, **10**, 536.

Jeavons P.M. (1977) Nosological problems of myoclonic epilepsies in childhood and adolescence. *Developmental Medicine and Child Neurology*, **19**, 3.

Jeavons P.M. & Bower B.D. (1964) *Infantile spasms. A Review of the literature and a study of 112 cases.* London: Heinemann.

Jeavons P.M. & Bower B.D. (1974) Infantile spasms. In *Handbook of clinical Neurology*, ed. Vinken P.J. and Bruyn G.W., vol. 15, p. 219, Amsterdam: North-Holland.

Jeavons P.M., Bower B.D. & Dimitrakoudi M. (1973) Long-term prognosis of 150 cases of 'West syndrome'. *Epilepsia*, **14**, 153.

Jeavons P.M., Clark J.E. & Maheshwary M.C. (1977) Treatment of generalized epilepsies of childhood and adolescence with sodium valproate ('Epilim'). *Developmental Medicine and Child Neurology*, **19**, 9.

Jellinger K. (1970) Neuropathological aspects of hypsarrhythmia. *Neuropädiatrie*, **1**, 277.

Kruse R. (1968) *Das myoklonisch-astatische Petit Mal*, Berlin, Springer.

Lacy J.R. & Penry J.K. (1976) *Infantile spasms*, New York: Raven Press.

Lagenstein I, Willig R.P. & Kühne D. (1979) Reversible cerebral atrophy caused by corticotrophin. *Lancet*, **1**, 1246.

Lombroso C.T. & Fejerman N. (1977) Benign myoclonus of early infancy. *Annals of Neurology*, **1**, 138.

Lyen K. R., Holland I.M. & Lyen Y.C. (1979) Reversible cerebral atrophy in infantile spasms caused by corticotrophin. *Lancet*, **2**, 37.

Maheshwari M.C. & Jeavons P.M. (1975) Prognosis of

suppression-burst activity in infancy. *Epilepsia*, **16**, 127.

Markand O.N. (1977) Slow spike-wave activity in EEG and associated clinical features: often called 'Lennox' or 'Lennox-Gastaut' syndrome. *Neurology* (Minneapolis), **27**, 746.

Melchior J.C. (1977) Infantile spasms and early immunization against whooping cough. *Archives of Diseases in childhood*, **52**, 134.

Nelhaus G. (1971) The ketogenic diet reconsidered: correlation with EEG. *Neurology* (Minneapolis) **21**, 424.

Nelson K.B. (1972) Discussion. In *The Epidemiology of Epilepsy: A Workshop*, ed. Alter M. and Hauser W.A., NINDS Monograph No 14, p. 78, Washington: US Government Printing Office.

Neville B.G.R. (1972) The origin of infantile spasms: evidence from a case of hydranencephaly. *Developmental Medicine and Child Neurology*, **14**, 644.

Niedermeyer E. (1969) The Lennox-Gastaut syndrome: a severe type of childhood epilepsy. *Deutsche Zeitschrifte für Nervenheilkunde*, **195**, 263.

Riikonen R. (1978) Cytomegalovirus and infantile spasms. *Developmental Medicine and Child Neurology*, **20**, 570.

Riikonen R. & Donner M. (1979) Incidence and aetiology of infantile spasms from 1960 to 1976: a population study in Finland. *Developmental Medicine and Child Neurology*, **21**, 333.

Sorel L. & Dusaucy-Bauloye A. (1958) A propos de 21 cas d'hypsarthmie de Gibbs. Son traitement spectaculaire par l'ACTH. *Acta Neurologica Belgica*, **58**, 130.

Tassinari C.A., Terzano G., Capocchi G., Dalla Bernardina B., Vigevano F., Daniele O., Valladier C., Dravet C. & Roger J. (1977) Epileptic seizures during sleep in children. In Penry, J.K. (ed.) *Epilepsy. The Eighth International Symposium.* New York: Raven Press.

Thornton E.M. & Pampiglione G. (1979) Psychiatric disorders following infantile spasms. *Lancet*, **2**, 1297.

Vassella F., Pavlincova E., Schneider H.J., Rudin H.J. & Karbowski K. (1973) Treatment of infantile spasms and the Lennox-Gastaut syndrome with clonazepam (Rivotril). *Epilepsia*, **14**, 165.

Viani F., Avanzini G., Baruzzi A., Bordo B., Bossi L., Canger R. Porro G., Riboldi A., Sofficutini M.E., Zagnogi P. & Morselli P.L. (1977) Long-term monitoring of antiepileptic drugs in patients with the Lennox-Gastaut syndrome. In Penry, J.K. (ed.) *Epilepsy, The Eighth International Symposium*, p. 131. New York: Raven Press.

West W.J. (1841). On a peculiar form of infantile convulsions. *Lancet*, **1**, 724.

4

Neurology

PART ONE

C.D. Marsden
E.H. Reynolds

INTRODUCTION

'An occasional, an excessive and a disorderly discharge of nerve tissue' (Hughlings Jackson) expresses the concept of seizures (fits). The fits are paroxysms and recurrent, and the symptoms of the fit are the result of excessive and disordered cerebral activity, but the illness epilepsy is more than just the fit (Fig. 4.1).

The word epilepsy does not have a single meaning, and hence it defies definition. One can define a fit, a disease causing fits, a precipitating cause of fits, and the consequences of fits, all of which contribute to the over-all picture of epilepsy. A physiologist can define the parameters of abnormal electrical discharge underlying seizures. The

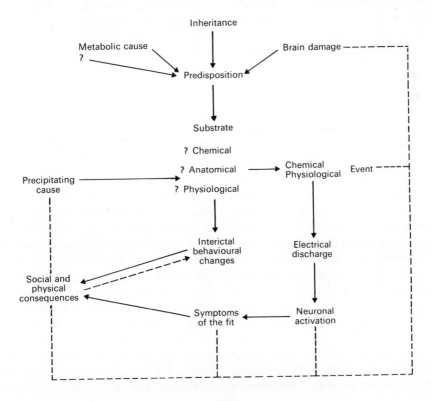

Fig. 4.1

biochemist may, in the future, define a local change responsible for generating that electrical discharge. Such events are also part of epilepsy. But epilepsy is also a social distinction; those diagnosed as having epilepsy are to a greater or lesser extent penalized both economically and socially. For this reason alone, epilepsy remains a medical diagnosis with social consequences that demand restricted use.

It is generally agreed that a cardinal feature of epilepsy is a tendency to *recurrent* seizures. A single seizure, therefore, is not epilepsy. Some seizures have obvious transient causes which do not imply a tendency to recurrence. Thus the patient with renal failure who has a fit, the girl who faints on the stairs and has a fit, the elderly man who has a Stokes-Adams attack and has a fit or any of us who take a drug that precipitates a fit, certainly has had a seizure, but does not have epilepsy as the medical diagnosis. Some have argued (Williams, 1968) that epilepsy is present when recurrent seizures are primarily of cerebral origin. This would exclude all attacks which are caused by disease elsewhere in the body. On the other hand, some recurrent attacks, e.g. hypocalcaemia or cardiac arrhythmia, may be clinically indistinguishable from cerebral disorders and such patients are widely diagnosed as having epilepsy. Furthermore, whether seizure threshold is set primarily by cerebral or extra-cerebral (e.g. hormonal) mechanisms is unknown, and in our present state of ignorance of such fundamental questions it may be premature to restrict the use of epilepsy to apparently cerebral events.

Epilepsy comprises a series of phenomena, each of which poses a different question. The epileptic has a predisposition to recurrent fits, determined by a variety of causes, some identifiable, many unknown. Given a predisposition to fits, the individual attack is triggered by a precipitating cause, which can be identified in some cases but is not apparent in many. Biochemical and electrical events then occur in the brain during the attack, to cause the symptoms of the fit. Both the cerebral substrate and the fits themselves contribute to inter-ictal physical, behavioural and social changes in a proportion of patients, changes that are at least as important as the seizures. This chapter will be concerned with the aetiology, precipitating causes and symptoms of fits, and with the problems of differential diagnosis, investigation and prognosis.

Discussion of each of these topics depends on the sort of seizure the patient suffers. For example, while absence seizures and complex partial seizures are both due to 'an occasional, an excessive and a disorderly discharge of nerve tissue', they have different aetiological backgrounds, different precipitating causes and different symptoms, and raise different problems of differential diagnosis, investigation, treatment and prognosis. In practice we think of the problem of fits, while recognising that we are dealing with a heterogenous group of diseases that may present with this sign of abnormal function of the brain.

To the clinician it is the differences between the various types of fits that is important, although their similarities are crucial to the research worker hunting for the elusive chemical/physiological event responsible for a fit. The latter's aim is to discover how a variety of insults may produce the same sign, and to identify the proximate cause of the fit in order to improve preventive therapy. The clinician, however, is committed to dividing seizures into subgroups in order to provide the best advice for the individual patient. A cornerstone of the clinician's management of the epilepsies is their classification.

THE CLASSIFICATION OF SEIZURES

The terminology and classification of seizures has evolved over many years, creating a variety of interchangeable and confused descriptive terms. The problem has been, and is, to create a single code to cover three basically incompatible systems of classification, namely: that according to clinical symptoms and signs of the fit; that relating to the anatomical and electrophysiological evidence as to the source of the fit; and that defining the aetiology of the fits. An example illustrates the conflict. The symptom complex of a seizure in which there is an abdominal and gustatory aura followed by an impairment of consciousness is often referred to as a *temporal lobe seizure* (Symonds, 1954; Williams, 1966), for usually it indicates temporal lobe pathology and electrophysiological evidence of temporal lobe discharges. However, a similar fit occurs on occasion in patients with a frontal lobe abnormality, and to describe such a fit as a temporal lobe seizure is not entirely accurate. Early descriptions of such fits as *psychomotor attacks* (Gibbs, Gibbs & Lennox, 1937) paid attention primarily to the clinical features of the fit, without prejudice to the anatomical source; further experience led to the realisation that psychomotor seizures usually implicated a temporal lobe origin. An alternative term, again describing the clinical features of the attack rather than the source, is *complex partial seizures*; this is now accepted internationally.

It seems necessary to retain a tripartite system of classification, and it is not always profitable to force clinical symptomatology, anatomical source and aetiology into a single framework, although all three are obviously complementary.

The International League against Epilepsy, under the chairmanship of Henri Gastaut (1969) have attempted the Herculean task of formulating a comprehensive classification of seizures to include the clinical seizure type, EEG seizure type, EEG interictal expression, anatomical substrate, aetiology and age (see p. xviii). Subsequently, further criteria were added by Gastaut, including the presence or absence of interictal neuropsychiatric changes, the response to therapy, and pathophysiology. Others did not accept the original or its modifications and provided alternatives; as Gastaut himself declared, 'Perhaps its

chief advantage is that it can serve as an anvil on which critics can hammer out a classification of higher value'. Indeed, the International League's Commission on classification is attempting to do just this at the present time.

The crucial problem, for any classification, is who is going to use it. As Whitty (1965) has stated, 'Two broad groups of demand for information arise in epilepsy – the practical or clinical, and the more theoretical or pathophysiological. The two cannot be rigidly separated, but they are likely to give rise to differing approaches to classification. On the clinical side, information is required especially about prognosis with or without treatment... From the pathophysiological side, the demand is for information on how the brain works and which parts of it are concerned with which functions... Such multiplicity of aims is scarcely compatible with a unitary classification'.

Our aim in this Chapter is to provide a simple, practical classification which is summarised in Table 4.1. This necessarily oversimplifies a very complex topic, but it does highlight some fundamental concepts, based on the clinical features of fits and differences in their pathophysiology. Thus some fits start with electrical discharges in both cerebral hemispheres simultaneously – *generalised* fits. Others start with a focal discharge in one part of a cerebral hemisphere – *focal* or *partial* fits. If that part of the brain is eloquent, the patient experiences an aura, a consciously remembered

Table 4.1 Classification of seizures

---

1. *Generalised*
    a. Tonic-clonic (grand mal)
    b. Tonic
    c. Atonic
    d. Absence (petit mal)
    e. Atypical absence
    f. Myoclonic
2. *Partial (focal)*
    A. Without impairment of consciousness (simple partial seizures)
    B. With impairment of consciousness (complex partial seizures)
    a. With motor signs (e.g. Jacksonian, versive)
    b. With somato- or special sensory symptoms (e.g. olfactory, visual)
    c. With autonomic features (e.g. epigastric sensations)
    d. With psychic symptoms (e.g. fear, déjà vu)
    e. With automatisms (complex partial seizures only).
3. *Partial seizures secondarily generalised*
    i.e. clinical or electrical evidence of focal discharge before, during or after the generalised seizure
4. *Unclassifiable*

---

experience that may be a motor, sensory, visceral or psychical event. This aura points to the part of the brain where the fit begins. If the site of origin of the fit is silent, the patient may notice nothing until the electrical discharge spreads to an eloquent area, or becomes generalised to involve both hemispheres – *partial fits with secondary generalisation*.

Inevitably such a classification is not comprehensive. Many patients have seizures which do not fit comfortably into any of the categories. Fits with origin in the temporal lobe may manifest many of the categories of focal symptoms. Some syndromes characterised primarily by fits, such as infantile spasms and progressive myoclonic epilepsy, have generalised seizure discharge with atypical absence attacks, atypical myoclonic seizures, and tonic-clonic attacks, and cannot be neatly classified. Many infants and children have partial fits which may or may not be associated with a focal abnormality in the EEG; the latter itself may be erratic and change its position. However, this simple scheme serves most of the clinician's needs.

Some indication of the frequency of different types of fits, generalised and partial, in a series of representative patients, referred with a diagnosis of epilepsy to one centre, is given in Table 4.2.

Table 4.2 Frequency of fits arising from different sources

Temporal lobe	244
Frontal lobe	35
Parietal lobe	11
Occipital lobe	9
Primary generalised	106
Unlocalised	370
Total number of cases	775

Based on a series of cases referred for EEG examination at Leeds, 1951–1961 (Parsonage, 1973)

THE CLINICAL SYMPTOMS OF THE SEIZURE

It is not the purpose of this chapter to describe in detail the clinical phenomena of typical fits. Rather, we will concentrate on certain aspects of fits of practical clinical significance.

Generalised seizures

Tonic-clonic (grand mal) seizures

Clinical features. A typical major motor seizure or *tonic-clonic* fit is unmistakable, consisting of a tonic phase, followed by a clonic phase, the whole lasting for up to two minutes, and followed by a further period of five minutes or so unrousable coma. After this the patient can be awoken, but is confused and disorientated, and usually prefers to sleep for a few hours, to awake often with a headache and sore muscles, but a clear mind. An epileptic cry at the start, cyanosis, frothing at the mouth, emptying the bladder, biting the tongue, or other injury are common but not universal. During the fit the pupils dilate, the pulse may slow initially, then accelerate, the patient sweats profusely, the plantar responses are extensor and the tendon jerks and corneal reflexes are lost. Inevitably the patient loses consciousness and falls in a grand mal attack.

Grand mal seizures do not always conform to this classical sequence, but always involve loss of consciousness and convulsion. On some occasions the seizure may cease after the tonic phase, while sometimes only a clonic seizure occurs. Such limited grand mal fits are especially common in children and infants. Grand mal seizures without muscular contractions probably do not occur. True atonic seizures with collapse of muscle tone are closely associated with absences and myoclonus, and with spike and wave discharge in the EEG.

Prodromal symptoms. Many patients with grand mal fits are aware of an impending fit or flurry of fits days or hours before the event. Such prodromal symptoms are to be distinguished from the aura to a grand mal fit, which precedes it by seconds or a few minutes. The aura is in itself a partial (focal) fit, reflecting an abnormal focal electrical discharge in the brain, while the prodromata are not necessarily signs of seizure activity. Individual patients may complain of prodromal headache, insomnia, irritability, mood change, lethargy, unusual appetite and a variety of other such symptoms. The longer the patient has had fits the more likely he is to be able to recognise such signs. Some of them are due to physiological changes known to precipitate fits, for instance, the water retention preceding menstruation. Others may represent the effects of increasing subclinical seizure discharges, but there is no hard evidence for this. In other patients it is possible that the prodromata are no more than those changes which precipitate their fits; thus anxiety whatever its cause may precipitate seizures, and the patient may come to associate fits with a prodroma of anxiety. The incidence, and significance of these prodromal changes have not been studied much, but might be a profitable field of investigation.

One form of prodroma that is reasonably common and distinctive is myoclonic jerking. Typically such patients develop muscle twitching, particularly of arms and trunk, days or hours before a grand mal fit. Such prodromal myoclonus is said to occur in between 10 and 50 per cent of patients with grand mal fits. In our experience the incidence approximates to the lower figure, but when it occurs it is very distinctive and some patients can accurately predict the day of fit by the onset of jerks on awakening that morning. The subsequent seizure is not inevitable and a few patients may discover means of preventing it, as by rest or extra doses of medication. Whether such premonitory myoclonic jerks represent seizure discharge or not is unclear, but the techniques of continuous EEG monitoring should help to decide.

Focal onset to grand mal. Grand mal fits, either (1) start with bilateral synchronous EEG discharge and abrupt loss of consciousness without aura, (2) may follow an aura indicating a focal origin to the fit, with secondary spread and generalisation, or (3) may follow a focal electrical discharge in a silent area of the cerebral cortex unbeknown to the patient but detectable in the EEG. Grand mal with focal onset, be it evident to the patient as an aura, or to the doctor as an EEG abnormality prefacing a fit, indicates a high likelihood of a focal structural lesion in the cerebral cortex as the cause of the epilepsy. Other phenomena have a similar, predictive value. Thus while a patient may lose consciousness abruptly without warning, an observer may witness head turning or unilateral muscular contraction prefacing the tonic-clonic phase of a grand mal seizure. Similarly, a focal post-ictal paralysis (Todd's paralysis) or post-ictal speech disturbance indicates the focal origin of some grand mal fits. In all these cases the fit begins with a local electrical discharge in some part of the cerebral cortex (the partial fit), then the discharge spreads to involve both hemispheres (secondary generalisation causing the grand mal seizure). The pathophysiology of this march of events during seizures is discussed at length in Chapter 11. Suffice to say that in some way a focal cortical electrical discharge spreads to involve some central structures in the diencephalon and upper brainstem, which then relay bilateral synchronous electrical discharges into both hemispheres to cause the generalised grand mal fit. A partial fit (with local colour and sign) is followed by a generalised seizure.

The nature and location of the neurophysiological events underlying the generalised seizure, be it generalised from onset, or focal in origin with secondary generalisation, is unknown. Penfield (1952) introduced the concept of a centrencephalic integrating system to explain the origin of generalised seizures. Abnormal electrical discharge in this centrencephalic system in diencephalon and upper brainstem causes loss of consciousness and a generalised seizure (of either grand mal or absence type). Grand mal fits of focal origin occur when the abnormal focal cortical discharge spreads to invade this subcortical centrencephalic system. (Partial fits, whatever their cause, may be followed by grand mal fits, but never by absences.) But what happens in patients with generalised epilepsy with no focal origin?

Primary generalised grand mal seizures. Here the patient has grand mal seizures, without aura, without focal EEG onset, and without focal clinical events either during or after the attack. It has been suggested that such patients, who may be said to have primary (or cryptogenic or idiopathic) generalised epilepsy, have a disorder of function of this hypothetical centrencephalic system. This is an attractive, simple, but unproven, hypothesis. Williams (1965) has marshalled clinical evidence against a centrencephalic origin for primary epilepsy. In particular, he argues that cerebral tumours and other pathological processes which are strongly epileptogenic in cerebral cortex rarely cause fits when located in the thalamus or other subcortical areas, or brainstem. This argument may not be decisive, for recent work implicates the cerebellum in seizure control, yet, by and large, cerebellar disease is not marked by seizures. However, the centrencephalic origin of primary seizures remains a concept and an act of faith.

The alternative proposition is described by Elkington (1950) with particular reference to grand mal:

> There is some reason for believing that every major attack has a local commencement in some region of the brain, and that it is in reality a local fit which rapidly becomes general. When such an attack commences with a local aura there is proof positive of local commencement.... When the spread of the disturbance is so rapid as to cause instant loss of consciousness there is no memory to retain the initial event of the attack.

This belief that all grand mal is of focal origin is compatible with the centrencephalic concept if it is assumed that primary generalised epilepsy originates in a focal discharge in the centrencephalic system, but there is no certain evidence that this is the case. A more restricted view is that all grand mal is of focal cortical origin. This view is currently expanding along with the belief that structural lesions, such as Ammon's horn sclerosis, hitherto dismissed as the consequence, not the cause of fits, may, in fact, be the focal origin for fits in many cases (see Ch. 11). Again, this is a hypothesis, attractive for its simplicity and practical consequences, but unproven.

The debate remains whether primary grand mal seizures are due to focal cortical lesions undetectable by the patient, the observer or the EEG, or whether they are due to an abnormality of centrencephalic subcortical structures, an abnormality that so far has escaped recognition.

A concept which is relevant to the debate as to the pathophysiological basis of primary generalised, or indeed secondary generalised, seizures is that of seizure threshold. Seizure activity can occur in all vertebrate nervous systems and the propensity for seizures increases in parallel with the phylogenetic scale, culminating in the highest incidence in man who has the most complex nervous system. Furthermore, it is apparent that all human beings are capable of having a generalised seizure if sufficiently stimulated, as exemplified by convulsive therapy in the treatment of depression. Patients vary, however, in their susceptibility to an induced seizure, perhaps due to variation in seizure threshold, which is presumably set by unknown genetic, neuro-chemical and other

metabolic processes. An unusually low seizure threshold may explain why some patients have spontaneous primary generalised seizures. In others, with a higher threshold, the addition of some insult to the brain, such as a tumour or head injury, may be enough to precipitate seizures, even though the nervous system is compromised by some physical disease or metabolic disturbance. Thus the concept of seizure threshold may explain why patients with identical cerebral pathology do not all have seizures. Furthermore it implies that genetic factors play a role in partial seizures as well as in primary generalised attacks.

Absence (petit mal) seizures

The typical brief staring spells of childhood were earlier called *pyknolepsy*. One of the most significant contributions of EEG investigation to epilepsy was the delineation by Gibbs, Davis and Lennox (1935) of a characteristic paroxysm of three per second bilateral, synchronous, spike and wave discharge accompanying the true petit mal attack. *Petit mal* is now defined as brief absence attacks occurring almost always in childhood, associated with this classical EEG abnormality. Such attacks, and the associated EEG paroxysm, may be provoked by overbreathing.

For some five to ten seconds the child loses consciousness, his eyes stare, and he may show minor movements such as blinking or twitching of the face and arms, but he does not fall. Suddenly consciousness is regained, but there is total amnesia for the brief period of the attack. The patient looks around for a moment, but then resumes his previous occupation. If engaged in conversation before the attack, he will have missed a sentence or so. Such classical petit mal attacks (or *simple absences*) may occur very frequently, even as often as a hundred or more times daily (Lennox, 1945; Gibberd, 1966a; Dalby, 1969).

Not all absence attacks are as simple as this. More complex phenomena, akin to those seen in temporal lobe epilepsy, may occur associated with an otherwise typical EEG paroxysm (Penry & Dreifuss, 1969). Thus the blank spell may last longer and may be accompanied by lip smacking, chewing or mouthing movements. These are sometimes referred to as *complex absences* or *absences with automatisms*. It may be impossible on clinical grounds to distinguish such episodes from temporal lobe 'absences', indeed such a distinction may not be valid, for some patients with temporal lobe epilepsy may show atypical three per second spike and wave discharge in the EEG. The differential diagnosis of true petit mal from other types of 'absence' attack may, on occasions, be impossible either clinically or electrically. One may sometimes be forced to a therapeutic trial of drugs effective against petit mal absences in such circumstances.

Associated with classical absences in some cases are episodes of myoclonic jerking (myoclonic absences) and drop attacks due to sudden collapse of muscle tone. In the former the arms jerk up; the head nods and the trunk flexes as in an exaggerated startle response. The force of this lightning movement may be sufficient to throw the patient to the ground, with injury. On occasion, such myoclonic jerks may be asymmetrical or even unilateral. In drop attacks the patient drops, not slumps, to the ground but can get up immediately.

The association of petit mal, myoclonic jerks and drop attacks was christened the *petit mal triad* by Lennox (1945), but this concept has been distorted by confusion between classical absences with an excellent prognosis, and progressive myoclonic epilepsy, which is a disastrous illness due to a number of causes. In the latter, atypical absence attacks, grand mal seizures, myoclonus and drop attacks all become increasingly severe and are often associated with a progressive dementia or cerebellar syndrome. Such an illness is most commonly seen in childhood and the many known pathological causes are discussed in more detail in Chapter 3. Confusion with simple absences arose because many of such patients show atypical spike-wave discharge in addition to other widespread EEG abnormality. This atypical spike-wave discharge, otherwise known as *petit mal variant* discharge, slow wave and spike, or the two per second spike and wave discharge is associated with a variety of cerebral pathologies and types of seizure, and a very high incidence of progressive mental deterioration (Blume, David & Gomez, 1973) (Table 4.3). To avoid confusion it is perhaps best to distinguish clearly true absences (which may on

Table 4.3 Slow spike and wave abnormality in 84 patients

Age at onset of fits*	5 or less	59	
	6–10	16	
	11–20	5	
	No fits	2	
Outcome* (in 68 cases)	Dead or in custodial care	46%	
	Normal intelligence	30%	
	Retarded	24%	
Aetiology*	Birth injury	14	
	Immunization	3	27%
	Head injury	4	
	Encephalitis	2	
	Family history of fits	22	26%
	Nil	42	50%

* Information was not available for every patient.
(After Blume, David & Gomez, 1973)

occasion be accompanied by myoclonus and drop attacks) with a typical EEG abnormality and excellent prognosis, from the progressive myoclonic epilepsy seen predominantly in childhood due to a variety of cerebral insults which cause progressive brain damage. In practice this is not a difficult distinction, but the delineation of absence attacks plus myoclonus plus drop attacks as a single syndrome has led to conflict in the literature.

Simple absences are uncommon, and are said to occur only in about 3 per cent of epileptic patients (Livingston *et al.*, 1965). Absences start before the age of 15 in nearly all cases, and cease by the age of about 20 in 80 per cent or more of cases (Livingston *et al.*, 1965; Gibberd, 1966b; Dalby, 1969). About 50 per cent of those with absences will develop grand mal seizures (Livingston *et al.*, 1965; Dalby, 1969), and there is some evidence that prophylactic anticonvulsant therapy to prevent grand mal attacks will reduce the number of those who continue to have fits in adult life. Intelligence and development is normal in all but a small minority, who are usually those with additional severe grand mal attacks.

Partial (focal) seizures

Motor fits

Jacksonian seizures. The typical partial motor fit recognised by Hughlings Jackson consists of onset of tonic spasm followed soon by repetitive twitching, usually in the angle of the mouth, thumb and index finger, or great toe, which then spreads in an orderly manner. The fit is due to a discharge in the opposite motor cortex, and the spread or march of the seizure reflects the topography of body representation in the motor strip. Thus the repetitive movements may begin in a hand, spread to arm and face and then down to leg and foot, or may commence in the foot to spread up the leg then down the arm and into the face. The convulsive movements may remain confined to their site of onset, or may spread to involve one-half of the body, and may terminate in a typical grand mal fit with loss of consciousness. If the left hemisphere is the source, speech may be lost during the attack, and additional sensory symptoms are common whichever hemisphere is involved. Whether consciousness is lost during such a partial motor seizure seems to depend on the extent of brain involved. Consciousness is usually preserved if the fit remains confined to its site of origin, but is often lost if half the body is affected. The full-blown typical motor seizure is not seen frequently; more often one encounters fragments of the motor fit, such as tonic spasm alone or clonic spasm alone, with or without spread. Very rarely true inhibition of movement has been described as an epileptic event (Efron, 1961). We have never recognised the inhibitory seizure which must be difficult to distinguish from a post-ictal paralysis or transient ischaemic episode. Partial motor fits may be followed by a prolonged period of paralysis of the affected limbs as described by Todd. In some such cases, particularly in adult life, the fits and the hemiplegia are due to stroke, but not all Todd's paralysis can be so explained. In other patients, again adults by and large, a prolonged Todd's paralysis may be due to the tumour causing the fit, and in such cases if it persists for more than 48 hours full investigation is required. In children, however, Todd's paralysis often occurs without any structural lesion and need not be investigated so aggressively.

Adversive seizures. Another not uncommon form of motor seizure is the adversive attack due to discharge arising in pre-motor areas of the frontal lobe (Penfield & Welch, 1951). Typically the head and eyes are forced away from the affected hemisphere, usually with preservation of consciousness. Sometimes the head turning is accompanied by abduction of the contralateral arm, external rotation of the shoulder and flexion of the elbow. The patient turns his head and eyes to look at his raised arm, thus adopting the posture of a fencer. The force of turning may be so great as to generate circling movements. Such seizures are sometimes accompanied by an epigastric rising aura and other symptoms that might be confused with epileptic discharge arising in the temporal lobe.

Speech in fits. Further mention must be made about speech and fits. Loss of speech (speech arrest) or frank dysphasia if the subject retains consciousness is almost always associated with fits arising in the dominant hemisphere and involving the anterior speech area of Broca, or the parieto-temporal speech area.

Brief stereotyped utterances (speech automatisms) may occur with fits arising in the temporal lobes of either side, most commonly that of the non-dominant hemisphere. The latter must be distinguished from the confused speech that occurs during recovery from fits (Serafetinides & Falconer, 1963).

Sensory fits

Somatic sensory seizures. As with Jacksonian seizures, somatic sensory seizures characteristically commence in one of the preferred sites, such as thumb or mouth, and show a spread or march. The complaint is usually of numbness or pins and needles. Such fits arise from the contralateral sensory strip which is so close to the motor area that they usually occur with motor phenomena. Very rarely pain or burning has been described, but this may be of subcortical origin.

Visual seizures. Two types of visual fits are recognised. Those due to discharge in an occipital pole usually consist of unformed simple visual phenomena such as spots, flashes of light, balls of fire, and revolving objects often throughout the field of vision, but sometimes confined to the appropriate homonymous half field.

Seizures arising in the temporal lobe may uncommonly cause formed and often vivid coloured visual recall of a particular scenario or event, a visual hallucination that is peculiar to the individual patient and is reported in attack after attack.

Auditory events. True epileptic vertigo is uncommon, but rotational or other dysequilibrium may be part of a complex partial seizure (Behrman & Wyke, 1958; Smith, 1960). By contrast, many patients with a variety of fits complain of non-specific dizziness as part of their aura. Complex partial seizures may also include auditory hallucinations, such as sensation of buzzing, hissing, whistling, ringing, sea noises, or the sound of machinery. All these auditory events suggest involvement of the superior temporal gyrus and adjacent cortex.

Olfactory and gustatory sensations. Olfactory hallucinations are frequent in complex partial seizures, as are the closely related hallucinations of taste. Smells and tastes are characteristically unpleasant, such as burnt onions, excreta, burning rubber, or indescribable, but horrible (Daly, 1958a; see also p. 133).

Visceral sensations. Visceral sensations are also a common part of the complex partial seizure, consisting usually of a feeling in the pit of the stomach, often described as a constriction or discomfort, as in fear, which rises into the throat and head. Such an aura may be accompanied by autonomic phenomena, such as tachycardia, sweating, pupillary dilatation and a fall in blood pressure (Van Buren & Ajmone-Marsan, 1960). Whether such a sequence of autonomic events occurring briefly and repeatedly, but without any other evidence of epilepsy, is a form of restricted autonomic epilepsy, is debatable, but has been described with response to anti-epileptic drugs (Fox *et al.*, 1973).

Involuntary micturition, and much more rarely defaecation, is common in tonic-clonic and complex partial seizures. It can, however, occur in isolation as possible evidence of seizure discharge in the frontal lobe, often with loss of awareness such that the patient suddenly finds himself wet without any prior knowledge of impending or completed micturition (Maurice-Williams, 1974).

Psychic fits (see also p. 245)

Many of the symptoms of focal seizures described so far may occur together with other complex phenomena in temporal lobe epilepsy (Tables 4.4 and 4.5). Thus a fit arising in the temporal lobe may be associated with an aura comprising one or all of the following: an epigastric rising sensation,

Table 4.4 Types of fit in 666 patients with temporal lobe epilepsy

Grand mal	57%
Psychomotor attacks*	51%
Minor attacks†	23%
Auras	49%

* Defined as episodes of confusion or amnesia with or without automatism
† Defined as brief attacks in which there was no profound alteration in consciousness
(After Currie *et al.*, 1971)

Table 4.5 Components of temporal lobe fits in 666 patients

Visceral	40%
Motor	14%
Adversive	0.5%
Masticatory	10%
Sensory	
Visual	18%
Auditory	16%
Vertigo	19%
Olfactory	12%
Gustatory	3%
Somatic	2%
Thought disorder	27%
Déjà vu	14%
Other	3%
Speech disorder	22%
Dysphasia	16%
Speech automatism	3%
Emotional disorder	19%
Unpleasant	14%
Panic	1%
Rage	2.5%
Violence	0.75%

(After Currie *et al.*, 1971)

a foul taste and smell, vertigo and auditory hallucinations, formed visual hallucinations, speech disturbance and autonomic phenomena. In addition, the patient may experience profound and disturbing disorders of thought, perception and emotion during the fit (Williams, 1956; Bingley, 1958; Mullan & Penfield, 1959; Penfield & Peroto, 1963).

Thought disturbance. The classical feeling of déjà vu that may be experienced during a complex partial seizure is often indescribable (Cole & Zangwill, 1963). The feeling is an overwhelming sense of familiarity, of it having happened before. Sometimes the experience is linked with a visual and/or auditory hallucination that adds a pictorial image to the familiar scene 'like a re-run of a film'. Sometimes the patient cannot recall the faces, scene, noise, phrase or voice at all, but knows it as familiar. The characteristic feature of such brief ictal events is that the same sequence usually is played each time, that it is repetitively stereotyped, and that like most focal epileptic events it lasts for a brief period only, usually less than a minute or so, and nearly always less than five minutes.

Less common are the phenomena of unreality (jamais vu), in which the patient perceives familiar surroundings as totally unreal, 'as if I'd never seen this room before, yet I've lived in it for 20 years', and that of forced thinking in which a recurrent idea intrudes in each aura.

Perceptual disturbance. Auditory and visual hallucinations, as well as olfactory and gustatory experiences, as epileptic events have already been commented upon. Other perceptual disturbances may also occur, such as illusions of changes in body size, distortions of time ('my heart and the clock suddenly beat at half pace'), or sound receding into the distance.

Emotional experiences. These are frequent in complex partial seizures. Commonest is intense fear (Macrae, 1954; Williams, 1956), which may drive a man to run in terror (cursive epilepsy) (Chen & Forster, 1973), or cower under the bed. Such fear is usually accompanied by an epigastric sensation and often by choking in the throat, such that the patient may fear imminent death. Intense pleasure, or ecstasy, is much rarer. Sometimes the latter may have sexual connotation and one such patient refused to accept any treatment for his fits which were so pleasurable. Laughter may also occur during a seizure (gelastic epilepsy) (Daly & Mulder, 1957; Druckman & Chao, 1957; Gumpert, Hanisota & Upton, 1970), usually of temporal lobe origin. Depression and weeping are uncommon and rage during a fit, as against during the post-ictal automatism that may follow, is scarcely if ever reported.

The complexity of the remembered experience in a temporal lobe seizure can only be illustrated by examples:

A thought comes into my mind, which I know I've thought before; then the smell comes, but I black out too quickly to remember what thought it is. I know it's important, and I've tried to catch it, but no...

I suddenly see a vivid scene of cowboys and indians in colour rushing towards me. I'm terrified and try to run away, but I pass out too quickly. Nobody believes me when I tell this story, they just laugh.

Suddenly I'm standing in a church, but I'm so small that I can't see above the pew, only the ceiling miles up in the sky; the organ is playing a piece of music very slowly; I know it, but I can't remember its name or even sing it now.

Such examples abound and one can only marvel at the range and complexity of the experiences as one listens to each individual's peculiar and often unique form of the fit.

The frequency of the components of complex partial seizures has recently been studied in 666 patients in whom the clinical features suggested temporal lobe epilepsy and/or the EEG showed a definite temporal lobe focal abnormality (in 92 per cent), either slow waves, or sharp waves and spikes (Currie *et al.*, 1971) (Table 4.5). In the 666 cases, epilepsy began under the age of 10 in 12 per cent, between 10 and 15 in 14 per cent, between 15 and 25 in 23 per cent, between 25 and 45 in 32 per cent, and over the age of 45 in 19 per cent. Some 50 per cent of patients did not have their first attack until after the age of 25. Those patients with complex partial seizures represented 25 per cent of those suffering from epilepsy seen in that department between 1949 and 1967.

Automatisms. Periods of automatic, often complex, behaviour may occur during the fit, but usually take place during the post-ictal phase (Liddell, 1953). The only certain way of distinguishing ictal from post-ictal automatism would be to record EEGs during such events, which is rarely achieved.

Automatisms may be defined as 'A state of clouding of consciousness which occurs during or immediately after a seizure and during which the individual retains control of posture and muscle tone but performs simple or complex movements and actions without being aware of what is happening' (Fenton, 1972). Simple automatisms include lip-smacking, chewing, swallowing and fiddling or fumbling with the hands. Complex automatisms consist of semi-purposive action, such as undressing, drinking, washing, searching, wandering, running, speech, or continuation of prior activity. Such complex stereotyped behaviour is well coordinated but inappropriate. Thus a patient during an automatism may make a journey to a pointless destination, may attempt to cook a meal when none is required, may undress in public, urinate, or go to bed. Such complicated behaviour patterns are often repeated from attack to attack in stereotyped form.

Automatisms are of brief duration and last less than five minutes in more than 80 per cent of cases (Knox, 1968). Uncommonly they may be of longer duration, but for practical purposes never longer than an hour. Amnesia for the period of the automatism is usually complete. Aggression during automatism is very rare, apart from a tendency to resist physical interference, and even then dangerous behaviour is almost unknown (Knox, 1968). Despite the increased prevalence of epilepsy amongst prisoners, the fits or what may follow them are rarely the cause of offence (Gunn & Fenton, 1971).

Most automatisms are associated with epilepsy arising in the temporal lobe and it is estimated that about some 75 per cent of those with complex partial seizures will have periods of automatism (Feindel & Penfield, 1954). Such patients will often be able to recall the aura to their attack prior to the period of automatism. Automatism may arise with other forms of epilepsy, but is uncommon. Automatism as the only manifestation of epilepsy is rare, but can occur.

Special types of fits

Status epilepticus

By definition status epilepticus consists of recurrent fits without recovery of consciousness between attacks, in contrast to serial fits where recurrent attacks occur frequently, but consciousness is regained between episodes. True status epilepticus is a medical emergency, and requires urgent intensive treatment. Serial fits occurring very frequently may herald status, but do not carry the still serious consequences of status. Nevertheless, serial fits must be controlled rapidly.

Grand mal status. Repeated grand mal seizures without recovery of consciousness causes increasing pyrexia, anoxia, hypoglycaemia and other metabolic disturbance, tachycardia and hypotension, which combine to produce brain damage and death unless stopped quickly. Of considerable practical importance is the observation that in experimental epilepsy, brain damage may occur even if the systemic manifestations are prevented by curarization (see Ch. 11). This indicates that repeated seizure discharge itself may damage the brain, perhaps by local metabolic change, so that even if the patient in status is maintained in good general condition, the continuing cerebral discharges may lead to cerebral necrosis and must be stopped. Even today grand mal status epilepticus carries an appreciable mortality (10 per cent or so), and an immeasurable morbidity (Table 4.6). Its management is detailed in Chapter 8.

Grand mal status may occur in about 3 per cent of epileptic patients (Oxbury & Whitty, 1971). It may be the first epileptic event in some patients, or may be precipitated in a known epileptic by events such as suddenly stopping antiepileptic

Table 4.6 Causes and consequences of major status epilepticus in 86 adult patients

Cause	Number of patients	Number in whom status was initial event	Death in status	Death within follow up
Tumour	19	10	4	15
Vascular	13	4	0	8
Infection	9	5	1	1
Post-traumatic*	4	1	0	0
Birth injury	4	0	0	3
Other	5	3	1	4
	54	23(43%)	6(11%)	31(57%)
No obvious cause				
Previous epilepsy	28	0	1	6
Indefinite	4	1	0	0
	32	1	1(3%)	6(19%)

* Ten other cases of status after severe head trauma were excluded
(After Oxbury & Whitty, 1971)

drug therapy, intercurrent illness, other drugs, or alcoholic indulgence (Oxbury & Whitty, 1971). Often, however, it occurs without apparent provocation. When grand mal status occurs as the initial episode, it is likely that a recognisable cause will be found. In children this may be an inflammatory disease such as meningitis or encephalitis, hypoglycaemia, hypocalcaemia or other metabolic change, lead poisoning, or the liver disease with encephalopathy known as Reye's syndrome (see Ch. 3 for further details). Most such causes may operate in adult life, but grand mal status as the initial event in an adult is often due to brain tumour, particularly one affecting the frontal lobe, and warrants full investigation (Oxbury & Whitty, 1971). Other causes include hypertensive encephalopathy, cortical venous thrombosis or intracranial abscess formation.

Absence status. Repeated absence attacks causing prolonged periods of confused uncooperative behaviour in children is commoner than is generally appreciated (Bornstein, Coddon & Song, 1956; Niedermeyer & Khalifeh, 1965; Brett, 1966). The physical appearance of such children often does not arouse a suspicion of epilepsy, and the child may be accused of day-dreaming or educational backwardness. However, disorientation, repetitive blinking, myoclonus and drooling are frequently seen, and EEG recording will show continuous or repetitive spike-wave activity. Such events which may last for hours or days, or even weeks, may be terminated by intravenous diazepam.

Complex partial status. Repetitive complex partial seizures rarely may produce a prolonged period of automatic behaviour and amnesia, rather similar to petit mal status, and are associated with repetitive atypical spike-wave activity (Schwartz & Scott, 1971; Escueta *et al.*, 1974). Such events may occur in adults as well as children, but are not common. Their distinction from postepileptic automatisms and other causes of the fugue or twilight state (see below) can only be made with confidence by EEG recording during the attack.

Partial motor status. Repetitive continuous partial motor seizures may occur, usually in adults, particularly with acute structural damage due to trauma or vascular disease, less commonly with tumour. A particular form of repetitive partial motor fit is epilepsia partialis continua, which consists of focal repetitive muscle contractions, usually of the fingers and corner of the mouth, persisting for many days or weeks without loss of consciousness.

Reflex epilepsies

Reflex epilepsy describes fits, most commonly grand mal or partial, which are precipitated by a fixed and clearly recognised sensory stimulus. Although uncommon, reflex epilepsy is of considerable interest, for it gives one of the few clues as to what may trigger fits. A variety of sensory stimuli are recognised to cause reflex epilepsy.

Photosensitive epilepsy (see also Ch. 5). Fits provoked by repetitive flashing lights is the commonest form of reflex epilepsy. Nowadays the flickering television set is the usual stimulus (Charlton & Hoefer, 1964; Binnie, Darby & Hindley, 1973), but in a past era driving down continental highways, with their spaced trees lining the route filtering the sun, was a recognised hazard. Children may even learn to provoke their own fits by shaking their hand in front of their eyes while gazing at a light source (Ames, 1971). Electroencephalography has harnessed photostimulation as a means of exposing abnormality in the EEG of susceptible subjects.

Auditory epilepsy. Sudden noise may be a provocative factor in some patients, while certain music may repeatedly provoke an attack in others (musicogenic epilepsy) (Critchley, 1937). We know of one patient whose grand mal seizures were initially provoked by certain types of classical orchestral and church music, and who could be induced to have a fit by Beethoven's Fifth Symphony. Interestingly, with time the stimulus became less specific, and over the years fits could be provoked simply by entering a church, and now by thinking of a church scene. Such information suggests that the effective stimulus is not the music itself, at least in this patient, but the atmosphere and emotion it engenders (see later).

Reading epilepsy. A very few patients may learn that reading silently or aloud may provoke their fits (Bickford *et al.*, 1957). (We know of no case of writing epilepsy.) In this case it may not be the content of the text that provokes the fit, for reading nonsense may produce the attack, and other stimuli such as playing chess or reading a music score have also been reported as effective. It may be that the passage of vision across the page causes a pattern-evoked visual response, which in susceptible subjects is sufficient to generate epileptic discharges, or that mental decoding of visual information may be responsible. Specific mental effort may be capable of provoking a fit, as in the case of arithmetic epilepsy (Ingvar & Nyman, 1962).

Tactile epilepsy. Touch or muscle stretch may provoke seizure discharge in some patients, usually partial motor epilepsy, or a peculiar form of myoclonus in which a tap to the hand or foot may cause a spike discharge in the cortex followed by a myoclonic jerk of the stimulated limb, or of half the body, or the whole body. Whether this is considered a true epileptic event or not can be argued, but such patients commonly have other forms of fits.

Paroxysmal dystonic seizures. An even more debatable epileptic phenomenon is that of paroxysmal involuntary movements. A number of entities have been described, including paroxysmal choreoathetosis, in which tonic spasm, with on occasion, superimposed dystonic movements, suddenly affect the limbs of one side, or sometimes both, without loss of consciousness, and continues for minutes on end (Lance, 1963; Stevens, 1966). Such attacks may occur daily without known provocation, and the illness may be clearly inherited as an autosomal dominant trait.

In other patients such dystonic seizures may be provoked by movement (Lishman *et al.*, 1962). Sudden action such as rising from a chair, running, or stepping off a kerb may cause the explosive onset of focal or generalised dystonic writhing movements of limbs or trunk such as are seen in torsion dystonia. Consciousness is not lost, but the patient may fall to the ground. Recovery occurs abruptly within a few minutes. Such seizures may be associated with a sensory aura, but are not usually inherited.

In both conditions, consciousness is preserved, the EEG is not abnormal, and other types of fits are most unusual. In these respects such dystonic seizures differ from conventional views of epilepsy due to cerebral cortical discharge, but there seems no reason why they should not be examples of striatal or basal ganglia epilepsy, particularly as they frequently respond to antiepileptic medication.

Other precipitants of seizures

One of the outstanding problems in epilepsy is what triggers a seizure. Mention has already been made of the rare reflex epilepsies, and we are aware of many other precipitating factors. However, by far the majority of fits occur without apparent cause, and what triggers them is a mystery. It is always useful to inquire closely for any precipitatory cause of fits, for such a discovery may enable the patient to avoid specific dangerous circumstances and learn to control his own seizure pattern to some extent. In addition, some patients may only have fits under certain circumstances, and in this case there is room for latitude in applying the label epilepsy with its consequent social and financial restrictions.

Fever. That a pyrexia may trigger fits in childhood is commonplace and poses a particular problem (see Ch. 3). Fever may also trigger fits in patients who have spontaneous seizures, and the differentiation of banal febrile fits in early life, from true epilepsy sometimes triggered by fever is important for prognosis and management.

Nocturnal seizures. Many patients have grand mal seizures only at night, or during daytime sleep or drowsiness (Gibberd & Bateson, 1974). Sleep enhances epileptic discharges in the EEG and may produce abnormality when daytime recordings while alert are quite normal. Sleep induced by barbiturates is thus used as a provocative test in EEG evaluation of epilepsy, particularly in suspected complex partial seizures where the resting EEG may be normal.

Menstrual epilepsy and pregnancy. The incidence of catamenial exacerbation of fits has varied considerably in different series but has been reported in up to 63 per cent of women (Ansell & Clarke, 1956). Cyclical seizures in women unrelated to menstruation have also been documented (Bandler *et al.*, 1957). Although it has long been suspected that premenstrual water retention may be a factor, there is no firm evidence for this. There is, however, experimental evidence that oestrogens may reduce seizure threshold. It is of interest, therefore, that Backström (1976), who studied seven women in detail, found increased tonic-clonic seizures associated with higher oestrogen levels, and that Laidlaw (1956) reported a decrease in seizure frequency during the luteal phase.

The effect of pregnancy (and the contraceptive pill) on seizure frequency is unpredictable. Fits may increase, especially in the puerperium, and the risk of toxaemic fits is greater in epileptic women. Indeed, fits appearing during mild toxaemia may be the first indication of recurrent seizures in later life. However, in some patients, fits decrease during pregnancy, particularly in the first trimester. Epilepsy by itself is neither an indication for advice against procreation, nor for termination of pregnancy. Such decisions are based more on genetic risks and the ability to discharge the responsibility of parenthood, and are the patient's to make after medical counselling.

The risk of increasing fits by concurrent use of the contraceptive pill does not seem to be great, indeed, some patients' epilepsy may be improved. One can only discover by trial, and we would usually not advise against this form of contraception if it is best suited. However, there is evidence that the contraceptive effect of the pill may fail in the drug-treated epileptic patient (see Ch. 8).

While on the subject of pregnancy, mention must be made of the fact that epileptic mothers appear to have a greater than normal risk of bearing a deformed child (Lowe, 1973). The risk is not excessive, perhaps 7 per cent against 3 per cent in the normal population. Although fits themselves, by such means as causing anoxia or trauma, may be responsible in part, the major antiepileptic drugs are known to be teratogenic in some animal species (see Ch. 8).

Stress-induced fits and emotional factors. A variety of stress factors are known to provoke fits in susceptible individuals (Friis & Lund, 1974). Lack of sleep is a common precipitant, often associated with alcohol (see below). Some patients quote physical or mental over-exertion, without emotional background or sleep loss. Intense fear, pain or rage may also be apparent precipitants, and even minor medical manipulations, such as bloodletting, dental treatment, or ear syringing, may provoke a fit in a susceptible subject. In many patients with established recurrent seizures, the frequency of fits clearly waxes and wanes with the individual's life circumstances and emotional responses. Emotional stress precipitated fits in 21 per cent of patients with complex partial seizures (Currie *et al.*, 1971). While it is difficult if not impossible to separate the various potential triggers during a period of misfortune, there is no doubt that such patients' fit frequency is dictated by these events and their consequent effects on mood, happiness and stability. Such a situation may be self-generating, for more fits add to the problems. Some patients will clearly link their fits to their moods, but in such circumstances it is difficult to decide whether the emotional change causes the fits, or is due to the same factor that provokes the fits (i.e. menstrual tension and menstrual epilepsy), or whether the emotional change is a prodromal symptom of the fits (i.e. due to increasing but at that time still sub-clinical seizure discharge).

Some patients may even be able to trigger (or to control) their own fits by thought or will. How they achieve this is usually unclear, but as a phenomenon it is of great interest for it may provide a clue as to how patients can be taught to prevent their own disability. Recent experiments with bio-feedback of epileptic electrical discharge from the EEG to the patient has been overdramatised as a practical solution, but holds promise as a concept and is worth pursuing for what it tells us about epilepsy (see Ch. 6). Patients who can trigger their own fits, be it by use of a recognised reflex stimulus, or by an effort of will, pose particular problems of management for they may learn to use their attacks to manipulate their circumstances. Other patients may feign seizures (hystero-epilepsy is a description not entirely discredited) for the same reasons, often without conscious appreciation of what they are doing. Such patients, often young women, frequently occupy much time and heart-searching in both neurologists and psychiatrists (see Ch. 6 and later).

Drug-induced fits. Many drugs are known to provoke fits in susceptible individuals (Dallos & Heathfield, 1969; Lancet, 1972), including phenothiazines, tricyclic antidepressants, monoamine oxidase inhibitors and isoniazid. Particularly common in this regard is alcohol, often inextricably combined with fatigue, lack of food, and physical and emotional exertion (the hang-over fit).

Fits on withdrawal of drugs are well-known. Alcohol- and barbiturate-withdrawal fits are common. The risks of status epilepticus developing on sudden withdrawal of antiepileptic drugs has already been commented upon. It is important to emphasise at this point that perhaps the commonest cause of recurrence of seizures in epileptic patients is poor compliance with drug therapy, with ensuing withdrawal seizures. Failure to recognise this fact commonly leads to unnecessary polytherapy (Shorvon et al., 1978) (see Ch. 8).

In this context the effect of other drugs on antiepileptic drug metabolism should be mentioned. Many drugs are now known to interact with anticonvulsants, either to increase or decrease their metabolism (see Ch. 8) and fits may be provoked by administration of a drug that lowers serum antiepileptic drug levels.

A practical problem arises when an epileptic patient develops an intercurrent illness requiring treatment with a drug known either to provoke fits itself, or to interfere with antiepileptic drug activity. Such a situation commonly occurs in epileptic patients who develop psychotic illness, either schizophreniform or depressive. Both neuroleptics and antidepressants may cause fits in susceptible individuals, but, in practice, if they are required to treat the psychotic illness they generally have to be used. Extra seizures may be prevented by attention to antiepileptic drug levels and by adjustment of medication. In fact, the use of such drugs only infrequently causes major problems in management.

SYMPTOMS BETWEEN FITS

A fit is a signal of a cerebral epileptic discharge, but between attacks such discharges may continue to be recorded in the EEG without apparent clinical phenomena. An unanswered question in epilepsy is how far do such subclinical seizure discharges cause interictal behavioural phenomena? Undoubtedly there is a high incidence of psychiatric disability amongst patients with epilepsy, including those with temporal lobe fits

Table 4.7 Incidence of psychiatric disability in 666 patients with temporal lobe epilepsy

Nil	56%	
Anxious	19%	
Depressed	11%	
Aggressive	7%	
Obsessive	6%	
Florid-psychiatric disturbance		
Hysteria		3%
Schizophreniform psychosis		2%
Anxiety neurosis		0.5%
Severe depressive illness		0.5%

(After Currie et al., 1971)

Table 4.8 Causes of temporal lobe epilepsy in 666 patients

Tumour		9.5%
Glioma	7%	
Meningioma	1%	
Others	1.5%	
Trauma		7%
Vascular disease*		2%
Angioma		2%
Abscess		1%
Meningitis		0.5%
Others		3%
		25%

* In another 9% there was a history of cerebrovascular diseases which could have been relevant
(After Currie et al., 1971)

(Table 4.7). About a quarter of those with complex partial seizures in this series had a history of psychiatric disorder or aggression. (Of interest is the observation that a definite cause could be found in only about 25 per cent of these 666 patients – Table 4.8.)

Community surveys in unselected populations have confirmed an increased incidence of psychological disturbance in epileptic patients (Pond & Bidwell, 1960; Gudmundsson, 1966; Rutter et al., 1960). The latter study showed that children with epilepsy had two to three times more psychopathology than children with other chronic physical disorders not involving the brain. Some studies have suggested a particular association between personality and psychiatric disorders and complex partial seizures (Rodin et al., 1976) but the evidence is by no means conclusive (Currie et al., 1971). Schizophrenia-like psychoses are rare but have aroused great interest, together with a number of conflicting theories, because of their possible implications for the study of schizophrenia (Slater & Beard, 1963; Reynolds, 1968; Davison & Bagley, 1970; see also Ch. 6). Understandably much more common are depression and anxiety, but these have been little studied. The association of epilepsy and decline in intellectual function has been commented on for centuries (Temkin, 1945), and Lennox (1942) showed that the longer the history of epilepsy the higher the incidence of impaired intellectual skills. The mechanisms involved in this, as in the other inter-ictal personality disorders referred to above, and discussed in detail in Chapter 6 have received little investigation and are poorly understood (Trimble & Reynolds, 1976). Possible factors are illustrated in Fig. 4.1 and Table 4.9. Until now it has proved

Table 4.9 Possible causes of inter-ictal intellectual, personality and psychiatric disturbances

Seizure activity
Brain damage (causing or resulting from seizures)
Genetic
Psychological
Social
Chronic antiepileptic drug therapy

difficult, if not impossible to separate the relative influence of seizure activity, brain damage, genetic factors, psycho-social influences and chronic drug therapy. However, with the recent development of more sophisticated techniques for monitoring these different factors, this should prove to be a fruitful area for future research.

The management and rehabilitation of such problems require expertise from many disciplines, time and care, and provides one of the strongest reasons for special centres for those who suffer from epilepsy.

THE DIFFERENTIAL DIAGNOSIS OF SEIZURES

The wide spectrum of clinical phenomena occurring in fits leads to a variety of diagnostic problems (Parsonage, 1973; Gibberd, 1973). The most important diagnostic features of seizures are their abrupt onset, brief duration and rapid recovery, and stereotyped symptoms which recur time and time again. The best insurance policy against error is a careful complete history and a full interview with a witness to the attacks.

Episodes of unconsciousness

Syncope (Gilliatt, 1974)

A simple faint due to a transient drop in blood pressure accompanied by vagal-mediated slowing of the pulse, pallor and sweating nearly always occurs while standing (reflex syncope). Loss of consciousness is gradual with a premonitory sinking feeling and dizziness, falling is less abrupt than in fits with rare risk of injury, and incontinence is very uncommon. Recovery with nausea and sweating is usually rapid after the horizontal position is achieved. Such simple syncopal episodes are sometimes called vaso-vagal attacks, but Gowers originally used this term to describe a much more prolonged and complex syndrome. Syncope occurs in adolescents and young adults of either sex, under typically provocative circumstances, such as rapidly rising from a chair, prolonged periods of standing in uncomfortable circumstances, as a result of pain or emotional shock, and in hot, stuffy surroundings. Similar postural syncopal attacks also occur in the elderly with some degree of loss of healthy vascular activity, and in patients with autonomic neuropathy such as may occur in diabetes (Sharpey-Schafer & Taylor, 1960) and many other neurological conditions (Johnson et al., 1966; Bannister, 1971). Such postural syncope is the result of a failure of baroreceptor reflexes to adjust heart rate and vascular resistance to abrupt changes in posture (areflexic syncope) (Brigden, Howarth & Sharpey-Schafer, 1950; Barraclough & Sharpey-Schafer, 1963).

Syncope can also be provoked by prolonged coughing (cough syncope) (Sharpey-Schafer, 1953) where a sustained Valsalva's manoeuvre prevents venous return to the heart, during micturition in middle-aged or elderly prostatic men who strain to pass water (micturition syncope) (Proudfit & Forteza, 1959), and in pregnant women in whom syncope can occur lying flat perhaps by an effect of the gravid uterus on the inferior vena cava (Brigden et al., 1950).

A complication that may arise as a consequence of a syncopal attack is that if the patient's head cannot fall below his heart, he may go on to have a typical grand mal fit due to cerebral anoxia. Circumstances in which this may occur include a faint on the stairs or in the lavatory, when the head gets caught on the pan. Careful history-taking will usually indicate that such fits were provoked by syncope, and that the patient is not suffering from epilepsy.

Cardiac dysrhythmias

Abrupt cessation of heart beat or change in rhythm may provoke a faint due to a critical drop in cerebral perfusion. Such Stokes-Adams attacks may be particularly difficult to diagnose unless one has the good fortune to be present at the time. They should be suspected in elderly people with vascular disease, those with known heart disease, and those with heart block. The diagnosis is critical in view of the need for cardiac pacemaking to prevent sudden death in selected cases. Clinical clues are an abrupt onset with pallor followed by flushing, but as with simple syncope a Stokes-Adams attack may cause a fit and the diagnosis can be very difficult. Indeed, some such patients may go on to develop typical spontaneous fits, often temporal lobe in character, perhaps as a result of cerebral ischaemic damage. Whenever such a cardiac dysrhythmia is suspected, a prolonged ECG must be done although it may be normal between attacks.

Another cardiovascular cause for loss of consciousness is the carotid-sinus syndrome (Hutchinson & Stock, 1960), in which elderly patients develop abrupt loss of consciousness on head movement or neck pressure, which may provoke alarming, but transient, cardiac standstill. Patients with aortic stenosis are also prone to sudden episodes of loss of consciousness.

These cardiac causes for syncope are common, especially in the elderly, and are often difficult to separate from epilepsy, so that neurologists hold them in great respect.

Other vascular causes

Loss of awareness, amnesia and even unconsciousness may occur in basilar artery migraine in younger patients (Bickerstaff, 1961a & b) and vertebrobasilar ischaemic episodes in the more elderly. Similar episodes also occur in the rare situations of rheumatoid arthritis or traumatic damage to the cervical spine. In all these situations loss of consciousness is due to brainstem ischaemia and is therefore usually prefaced by other distinctive symptoms such as diplopia, dysarthria, ataxia and perioral paraesthesiae, while visual symptoms may arise from posterior cerebral ischaemia, and headache with or after the attack is common.

Brief loss of consciousness probably does not occur in simple transient ischaemic episodes in carotid territory, but rarely such patients are apparently amnesic for a portion of such an attack, particularly if it involves the dominant hemisphere.

The narcoleptic syndrome

The tetrad of day-time sleep attacks, cataplexy or collapse with emotion, sleep paralysis and hypnagogic hallucinations (Parkes & Marsden, 1974) is not usually confused with epilepsy, but has been regarded as a form of seizure disorder. However, other types of fits do not occur, the EEG shows no epileptic activity, and antiepileptic drugs are of no therapeutic value. Confusion may arise on occasion, as when a child falls asleep in class or at table, or when an adult drops off while at the wheel of a car. Cataplexy may be confused with epileptic drop attacks (as may the relatively common but banal drop attacks that occur in middle-aged women for no known reason). However, consciousness is preserved in such events.

Others

Breath-holding attacks in childhood (and masturbation episodes) may be confused with fits.

Mention must be made of the occasional patient with Menière's disease who loses consciousness during an episode of vertigo.

Nocturnal fits (Gibberd & Bateson, 1974) may be confused with nightmares or night-terrors. The latter are most common in childhood but can occur in adults. A scream calls the parent who finds the child sitting with staring eyes. Recovery is rapid when the child is woken. In fact nocturnal attacks are usually fits, and attacks occurring on waking are nearly always epileptic.

Hypoglycaemia may cause diagnostic confusion, for it may present with states of altered consciousness, and may itself provoke fits. However, clouding of consciousness in hypoglycaemia is gradual and is prefaced by symptoms of sympathetic over-activity, such as faintness, hunger, dryness of the mouth, sweating, fullness of the throat, palpitations and tremor. Such symptoms develop over many minutes, often under characteristic circumstances, such as after a heavy meal in those prone to reactive hypoglycaemia, or in those with one of the varieties of dumping syndromes that may follow gastric surgery.

Transient focal cerebral events

Partial fits may be confused with episodes of transient cerebral ischaemia, which in early life may be due to migraine and in later life to embolic or more rarely flow disturbance in carotid territory. In such cases, short-lived episodes of paraesthesiae or motor weakness may resemble focal sensory or motor fits, but can usually be distinguished by their longer duration (usually ten minutes or more), lack of march of events, and in the case of motor phenomena paralysis rather than tonic or clonic movements. Similarly the visual symptoms of migraine may be confused with focal fits arising in the occipital lobe, but again last five to 30 minutes or so.

A complication arises when, as sometimes happens, a stroke generates focal epilepsy at the onset, but the clinical sequence of events and focal neurological aftermath usually point to the correct diagnosis.

Psychiatric events mimicking epilepsy

While the topic is dealt with at length in Chapter 6, it poses such difficult problems that we will spend some time on it here.

A number of psychiatric syndromes may mimic fits, particularly those of temporal lobe origin. This is not surprising, for many of the symptoms of a temporal lobe attack are those of panic or emotional change, both of which occur as primary events in psychiatrically disturbed patients.

Panic attacks

The panic attack of a phobic anxiety may closely resemble a complex partial seizure (Harper & Roth, 1962), with abdominal discomfort often rising into the throat with a choking feeling, fear, autonomic symptoms, sometimes syncope and even micturition in terror. Often, however, the story of the attack is not quite right, consciousness is not disturbed, the event is clearly precipitated by circumstances, and is unduly prolonged. There usually is evidence of the underlying phobic anxiety state between attacks on formal psychiatric examination. However, it is often extraordinarily difficult to decide between panic attacks and complex partial seizures. In these circumstances an EEG may be requested, and may show abnormality, but in our experience this is best ignored as far as treatment is concerned. Personal error has been towards calling such attacks epilepsy rather than the other way round. If a therapeutic trial is instigated, a sequence of events follows over many months, during which increasing doses of a variety of antiepileptic drugs prove totally ineffective. There is little to be lost by admitting ignorance and deliberately avoiding a diagnosis of epilepsy and antiepileptic drug therapy. If you are wrong, sooner or later true fits will occur and clinch the matter.

Psychopathic rage outbursts

Outbursts of rage and violence are sometimes suspected of being epileptic, particularly by the law and courts. This question arises when some degree of amnesia is claimed and/or when an EEG is carried out and reveals some minor abnormality. There is less difficulty in distinguishing such events from true epilepsy than is the case with panic attacks. The outburst is usually provoked by external circumstances, and a prior motive may be apparent; events during the attack are directed towards an identifiable aim, amnesia is often patchy, and no obvious epileptic phenomenon is reported or seen. In such cases an abnormal EEG is best ignored, for true structured violent attack is almost unknown in epilepsy, apart from the tendency to resent and react vigorously to interference during periods of automatic behaviour (see below). Even in these latter circumstances, violence or aggression is poorly directed towards a goal or carried out in a purposeless fashion. However, on occasion an apparently motiveless crime or attack may be committed, for which amnesia is claimed, and in these cases it can be impossible to say with complete conviction that such an event could not be epileptic in origin, although the balance of evidence suggests that this is unlikely to be the case (Walker, 1961; Fenton & Udin, 1965).

Feigned seizures

Sometimes attacks are seen which clinically resemble epileptic fits, but which are not accompanied by an electrical disturbance in the brain. Whether the patient knowingly feigns such an attack or does so subconsciously is often impossible to discern, and often is immaterial. Such attacks may be a signal of psychiatric illness requiring help (see Ch. 6).

Difficulty arises, firstly, because when one has no more than a second-hand account of such events, it can be well-nigh impossible to distinguish them from true epilepsy; secondly, because many patients with such attacks also suffer from true fits. In such a situation, to observe a feigned fit on one occasion, or to establish a normal EEG during such an episode, does not necessarily mean that all attacks are feigned. It is only by careful and prolonged observation that a balance of evidence may point to such a conclusion, but often with some doubt.

Attacks which are not epileptic can usually be distinguished from true convulsions if witnessed, and often are suspected on history. The event occurs to attract attention, in front of an audience; attacks at night, or alone, or in dangerous circumstances are rarely 'hysterical'. The movements in a 'hysterical' convulsion are spectacular and purposeful, without the typical tonic-clonic sequences of a grand mal fit. They are intensified by restraint and mollified by inattention. Consciousness is often preserved and amnesia is frequently patchy. A subject who speaks is not having a major fit. The tendon jerks, blink, corneal and eyelash reflexes are preserved, and the plantar responses remain flexor. Incontinence, tongue biting and trauma rarely occur.

Many such patients feign fits because they have epilepsy and know about it, others because they have organic neurological disease and have seen fits. 'Hysterical seizures' occur more commonly than not in patients with organic disease. Again a 'therapeutic trial' of anticonvulsant drugs is often doomed to failure in such patients and may itself cause added difficulty by causing drug-toxicity or drug-withdrawal fits. When such a diagnosis is suspected it is often best to admit such patients into units specialised in the management of the problem, where prolonged observation, group therapy, psychiatric treatment and rehabilitation may break what may become a vicious and intractable problem.

Twilight or fugue states

Prolonged periods of altered behaviour with clouding of consciousness or amnesia may be suspected of being epileptic in origin, for a variety of seizure phenomena may induce such a state (see above). Ictal automatisms are brief, lasting a few minutes, but post-ictal automatisms, when frank electrical discharge has ceased in the brain, may last longer. Usually awareness returns and behaviour reverts to normal within minutes, but uncommonly it persists for up to an hour. During such periods of automatic behaviour the patient may undertake complex semi-purposive acts, for which he is subsequently totally amnesic. An initial aura of a temporal lobe fit may be recalled, but often is not. Similar prolonged periods of semi-purposive behaviour with subsequent amnesia may occur during absence status or complex partial status, in which case an EEG during the episode will reveal the ongoing seizure discharges.

Other cases of prolonged fugue are hypoglycaemia, alcoholic intoxication, and drugs (Fenton, 1972). Stroke and cerebral tumour may cause a prolonged amnesia syndrome, and the syndrome of transient global amnesia (Fisher & Adams, 1964) is well established.

However, despite the large number of known organic causes for a fugue, many are of psychiatric origin in the form of prolonged loss of memory commonly described in fiction or the press. Provoking circumstances, psychiatric illness and gain can often be identified in such patients. If doubt exists it is usually best to avoid a label of epilepsy in these circumstances.

Table 4.10 shows the diagnosis established in 31

Table 4.10 Causes of transient loss of memory in 31 patients

Transient global amnesia		19
With associated cerebrovascular disease	9	
With no cerebrovascular disease	10	
Epilepsy		6
Migraine		1
Temporal lobe encephalitis		2
Psychogenic		3

(After Heathfield, Croft & Swash, 1973)

cases of transient amnesia referred to a group of neurologists over a five year period (Heathfield, Croft & Swash, 1973).

THE AETIOLOGY OF SEIZURES

The purpose (and validity) of separating primary or idiopathic epilepsy from symptomatic epilepsy is therapeutic. In the latter we can determine an accepted cause, in the former we cannot. It is likely that many so-called idiopathic epilepsies will become symptomatic as our knowledge advances. The practical aim of this division is to dissect out possible known causes of fits that may be amenable to treatment.

The known causes of fits vary with the age at which they start (Table 4.11). The range of genetic, metabolic, structural and inflammatory causes in infancy and childhood is discussed in detail in Chapter 3. Suffice it to point out that infancy is the time when birth injury, congenital defects, metabolic aberration and infection commonly occur. Between the ages of about three and eight months the syndrome of infantile spasms presents, while from about six months to five years is the time of febrile fits. Primary epilepsy usually starts after the age of three and is then the commonest form of epilepsy. Throughout adult life structural brain damage dominates the list, particularly brain tumours in early and middle adult life, and vascular disease in later years. Head trauma causes fits throughout life.

In this section we propose to discuss in more detail the commonest causes of fits in adult life, namely head injury, brain tumour, cerebral abscess and vascular disease, and to finish with a brief comment on the significance of Ammon's horn sclerosis as a cause of fits. Many other neurological

Table 4.11 Causes of epilepsy presenting at different ages

Neonatal (first month)
  Birth injury – anoxia or haemorrhage
  Congenital abnormalities
  Metabolic disorders – hypoglycaemia, hypocalcaemia, etc
  Meningitis and other infection
Infancy (1–6 months)
  As above
  Infantile spasms
Early childhood (6 months to 3 years)
  Febrile fits
  Birth injury
  Infection
  Trauma
  Poisons and metabolic defects
  Cerebral degenerations
Childhood and adolescence
  Idiopathic or primary epilepsy
  Birth injury
  Trauma
  Infection
  Cerebral degenerations
Early adult life
  Trauma
  Tumour
  Idiopathic or primary epilepsy
  Birth injury
  Infection
  Cerebral degenerations
Late adult life
  Vascular disease
  Trauma
  Tumour
  Cerebral degenerations

and systemic diseases may be associated with fits (Table 4.12), but are beyond the scope of this chapter. In passing it is of practical importance to note that multiple sclerosis may cause fits, particularly partial fits (Matthews, 1962).

Table 4.12 Rarer causes of seizures

Neurological diseases	Systemic diseases
Lipid storage diseases	Pulmonary insufficiency
Leucodystrophies	Anoxia
Demyelinating diseases	Hypocalcaemia
Spinocerebellar degenerations	Hypoglycaemia
Tuberous sclerosis	Pyridoxine deficiency
Sturge-Weber syndrome	Aminoacid abnormalities
Cysticercosis	Water intoxication
Arteriovenous malformation	Renal failure
Subdural haematoma	Liver failure
Syphilis	Reye's syndrome
	Addison's disease
	Acute intermittent porphyria
	Drug withdrawal
	Drug intoxication
	Lead and other poisoning

Post-traumatic epilepsy (see also Ch. 4, part three)

Head injury is now one of the commonest causes of fits. They may develop soon after the injury or months later. The risks of epilepsy are related to whether the dura is penetrated or not. Thus in missile wounds of the head the incidence of fits may be as high as 40 per cent (Caveness, Walker & Ashcroft, 1962), while only about 5 per cent of those with non-missile injuries develop seizures (Jennett, 1962; 1965). Trauma is more likely to cause partial epilepsy, than generalised, but may be responsible for fits in about 5–15 per cent of all cases of epilepsy (Gibbs & Gibbs, 1952).

Fits may occur any time after a severe head injury, but the prognosis varies as to when they first appear. Fits are most common in the first week after a non-missile head injury, and only about 20 per cent of cases will develop their first fits later than this. Of those who develop fits in the first week after injury, some 27 per cent will continue to have persistent recurrent seizures, but in those whose fits develop after two weeks or later the risk is of the order of 70 per cent (Jennett, 1969). Similar trends are evident in patients with missile head wounds. Thus fits developing in the first week after a head injury are of less significance with regard to recurrent long-term epilepsy than fits appearing later on. Even so, about a quarter to a third of those with early fits may develop late epilepsy.

Jennett, Teather and Bennie (1973) have been able to identify factors likely to be associated with persistent post-traumatic epilepsy after non-missile head injuries. In a series of 800 such cases, about 55 per cent had developed epilepsy within a year of injury and 70 per cent within two years. Some 40 per cent of those with a post-traumatic amnesia of 24 hours or longer, some 27 per cent of those with early epilepsy in the first week, and some 25 per cent of those with dural tears had developed late epilepsy.

It is of interest that early epilepsy is commonly partial motor fits, related to the site of trauma, while complex partial seizures are rare. By contrast, late epilepsy is more often of the generalised type or temporal lobe in origin, suggesting some change or difference in the responsible pathological process.

There is some evidence that prophylactic anti-epileptic drugs will reduce the incidence of post-traumatic fits, but careful studies on this critical point are awaited (Rapport & Penry, 1972).

Brain tumour and epilepsy

Brain tumour has gained a notorious reputation as a cause of late-onset epilepsy, because it may be treatable (Parker, 1930; Penfield, Erickson & Tarlov, 1940). In fact, brain tumours are responsible for late onset epilepsy in only about 10 per cent or so of all cases (Sheehan, 1958; Raynor, Paine & Carmichael, 1959; Hyllested & Pakkenberg, 1963; Juul-Jensen, 1964a). The incidence of tumour rises steeply in the case of partial fits, where a figure of 30–40 per cent is more appropriate (Raynor, Paine & Carmichael, 1959; Sumi & Teasdall, 1963). However, the incidence in complex partial seizures is not that high, about 15 per cent or so (Currie et al., 1971). (Table 4.8). In general, these figures are supported by recent studies with the CT scanner in epilepsy (vide infra).

Tumours most likely to cause fits are those affecting the cerebral cortex, and there seems to be an inverse relationship between the malignancy of the tumour and its propensity to cause fits. Meningiomas and benign gliomas characteristically cause seizures, while malignant gliomas do so less frequently. The incidence of fits with different sorts of tumours is in the order of 67 per cent in meningiomas, 70 per cent in astrocytomas and 37 per cent in malignant gliomas (Penfield et al., 1940) (Table 4.13). Secondary deposits usually

Table 4.13 Incidence of seizures due to different tumours

Number of cases	Tumour types	Presenting with fits
64	Astrocytoma	70%
13	Oligodendroglioma	92%
103	Malignant glioma	37%
63	Meningioma	67%
19	Metastasis	47%
32	Pituitary adenoma	9%
(54)	(Abscess)	(50%)
(71)	(Subdural haematoma)	(25%)

(After Penfield & Jasper, 1954)

Table 4.14 Incidence of seizures due to tumours at different sites

Number of cases	Site	Percentage with fits
115	Frontal	53%
74	Parietal	68%
94	Temporal	48%
28	Occipital	32%
20	Third ventricle	32%
12	Thalamic	8%
49	Pituitary region	8%
	Average incidence approximately 37%	

(After Penfield & Japser, 1954)

from lung or breast, are also a relatively common cause of symptomatic fits.

Fits are commonest with tumours of the fronto-parietal region and very rare with lesions in thalamus, basal ganglia or parapituitary area (Williams, 1965) (Table 4.14).

Tumour as a cause of fits in childhood is uncommon, partly because most childhood tumours arise in non-epileptogenic areas, such as the cerebellum, brainstem and diencephalon, also because so many other types of epilepsy appear in childhood.

In general in about 40 per cent of those with fits due to tumour, the fits are the presenting symptom (Penfield & Jasper, 1954). The interval between the onset of fits due to tumour and other symptoms varies considerably. At one extreme is the occurrence of fits almost simultaneously with a rapidly progressive focal deficit due to a malignant glioma. At the other extreme, it may be 20 or more years after the onset of epilepsy before the responsible benign tumour becomes apparent (Douglas, 1971). It is partly for this reason that neurological clinics review regularly those with late-onset epilepsy in whom tumour may be the cause in about 1 in 10 of such cases.

The question as to why some patients with brain tumours develop fits and some do not is not fully answered. It is established that successful removal of tumour often does not stop the fits it causes. The presumption must be that it is the remaining damaged cerebral cortex that is the source of the fits, but the nature of the structural, functional or biochemical lesion responsible is not known.

Brain abscess

Epilepsy is a common complication of supratentorial brain abscess. In a recent study (Legg, Gupta & Scott, 1973), 72 per cent of 70 survivors of supratentorial abscess developed fits in the next month to fifteen years, most commonly in the first year after treatment. Grand mal fits occurred in about 50 per cent of patients, who could have more than one sort of attack. Complex partial seizures developed in a third, and other partial fits in another third of cases. Prophylactic antiepileptic drugs are recommended.

Vascular disease and seizures

Cerebrovascular disease is an even more common cause of adult-onset fits than tumour (Dodge, Richardson & Victor, 1954). It may be responsible for about 10 to 20 per cent of cases of adult-onset epilepsy, but after the age of 50 the figure 50 per cent or more (Juul-Jensen, 1964a; White, Bailey & Bickford, 1953; Woodcock & Cosgrove, 1964). It is estimated that as many as 25 per cent of those with cortical infarcts will have fits (Richardson & Dodge, 1954), although the incidence of fits in non-embolic cerebral infarcts in general is about 8 per cent (Louis & McDowell, 1967). About half of such patients develop their fits within a week of the stroke, and early post-stroke epilepsy seems more prone to spontaneous remission than that developing later.

Mention must also be made of arteriovenous malformations, which cause fits, usually focal in nature in about 40 per cent of cases (Paterson & McKissock, 1956). The combination of fits, migraine-like headache, and subarachnoid haemorrhage is diagnostic, as is the tell-tale cranial bruit.

Fits are said to be rare in subdural haematoma, but certainly occur.

Ammon's horn sclerosis

This theme is discussed and developed in detail elsewhere (Chs 3 and 11) but its practical importance and potential significance are such as to merit further mention.

Stated simply, the facts are that this pathological lesion, Ammon's horn sclerosis, is found commonly in the brain of patients with epilepsy of no apparent cause (Sano & Malamud, 1953; Corsellis, 1957; Margerison & Corsellis, 1966), and also in temporal lobes removed for successful surgical treatment of temporal lobe epilepsy (Falconer, Serafetinides & Corsellis, 1964). It is commonly unilateral (Margerison & Corsellis, 1966). The question arises as to whether this lesion is therefore the source of such epilepsy (Falconer, 1974). Some of these patients give a history of a prior episode of prolonged seizures in childhood, often febrile status epilepticus. Experimental status epilepticus in primates can produce a histological mimic of Ammon's horn sclerosis, often unilaterally (see Ch. 11). The question arises as to whether Ammon's horn sclerosis is caused by severe febrile fits in childhood, and then itself ripens into an epileptogenic scar producing recurrent seizures in adult life. The hypothesis can be and is under experimental test. If established, the consequences are profound. The genetic background to idiopathic epilepsy may be that of febrile fits, which may cause Ammon's horn sclerosis and thereby generate recurrent seizures in a proportion of cases. Aggressive treatment of febrile fits may have the greatest prophylactic impact on epilepsy (along with measures to prevent head injury). Methods will have to be devised to detect the lesion in those with idiopathic epilepsy during life, in order to assess its contribution to the incidence of unexplained fits and to assess a wider range of cases for possible surgical treatment. These and many other notions stem from the development of the hypothesis that Ammon's horn sclerosis, itself a product of epilepsy, may be a frequent cause of fits, a cause both open to prevention and to treatment.

In assessing the possible role of Ammon's horn sclerosis as a cause of temporal lobe epilepsy, the series of Currie et al. (1971) is of interest. A definite cause for the temporal lobe epilepsy was found in 25 per cent of the 666 patients they studied (Table 4.8). An additional 5 per cent of cases gave a history of seizures in infancy, and another 7 per cent had had an isolated fit in childhood; 7 per cent gave a history of an abnormal birth and 11 per cent had a family history of fits. These data do not suggest that fits in childhood are a common cause of temporal lobe epilepsy in

later life, but the information was obtained retrospectively.

THE INVESTIGATION OF SEIZURES

Having recognised epilepsy, the next step in management is to decide how far to press investigation for a cause. This will depend initially on the age of the patient. Epilepsy in infants under the age of six months is of sinister import, and it may well be in those aged under a year. By this time, however, febrile fits are beginning to appear and require less intensive investigation. The management of children with epilepsy is described in detail in Chapter 3, and we will confine ourselves in this section to epilepsy in late childhood, adolescence and adult life.

Needless to say, the initial step in investigating a case of epilepsy is a full history, from both the patient and a witness, and clinical examination. A number of causes of epilepsy may be recognised in the clinic. A history of birth trauma or anoxia, combined with body asymmetry, such as a small thumb or toe, will point to cerebral damage in early life. Tuberous sclerosis and Sturge–Weber syndrome will be indicated by the appropriate skin lesions, and congenital or genetically-determined syndromes may be suggested by a characteristic facial appearance or other signs, as for example in mongolism. General medical examination may point to an extracerebral cause of the fits.

Usually, however, no such clues are apparent. In such cases examination is directly concerned with detecting signs of focal brain damage or raised intracranial pressure. Particularly important are the optic discs and visual fields. The only sign of a temporal lobe lesion may be an upper quadrantanopia. Mild facial weakness, a hemiparesis and extensor plantar response point to a unilateral hemisphere lesion.

Initial outpatient investigation

At this stage simple tests will be required. In older children and adolescents these should include a plain X-ray of the skull and an EEG. Now that multiple haematological and biochemical investigation is automated, we arrange routinely for a full blood count, WR or TPHA test for syphilis, and SMA 12 biochemical screen, which includes a blood sugar and calcium. We have rarely detected a cause for fits by such blood tests, but do them to provide baselines for subsequent monitoring of chronic effects of drug treatment (see Ch. 8). In adults presenting with epilepsy for the first time, an X-ray of the chest is also necessary, and may reveal a bronchogenic carcinoma. In those who have spent time abroad, an X-ray of the thighs may show the calcified cysts of cysticercosis, but this illness is very rare today in this country.

The value of routine X-rays of the skull and EEGs require further comment.

Skull X-ray

Although a routine skull X-ray is usually normal in patients with fits, it can establish the diagnosis of the cause. Thus evidence of raised intracranial pressure, intracranial calcifications in tumour or other lesions, and the bony changes of meningiomas may be detected. Pineal shift may indicate a mass lesion. Asymmetry, particularly of the middle cranial fossae may point to a long-standing atrophic lesion. Such information is crucial in a few cases and a skull X-ray should be undertaken in every epileptic patient (but see also Ch. 9).

EEG (see also Ch. 5)

Much has been written about the EEG in epilepsy. While it provides much interesting information to the doctor, it is not always helpful to the patient. During political unrest or staff shortage it is possible to practise the neurology of epilepsy without EEG data. However, there are certain circumstances in which it is invaluable, provided it is realised that:

a. An abnormal EEG does not indicate epilepsy, which is a clinical diagnosis
b. A number of normal people have abnormal EEGs
c. That a normal EEG does not exclude epilepsy (or brain tumour).

The situations in which an EEG may be expected to help are:

a. In the definitive diagnosis of absence seizures, in particular to separate absences and complex partial seizures
b. To detect a focal as against a generalised abnormality
c. To examine certain regions of the brain that are clinically silent, for example, the frontal lobes.

An initial EEG may also prove of value later in the course of the illness, as for example in assessing the possibility of drug toxicity, or progression of the underlying disease, or in deciding when to stop treatment in those rendered free of fits. In these situations comparison of a recent EEG with the initial record may provide helpful information. The same is true when surgery for epilepsy is contemplated. Since one cannot be sure of the future of any individual with epilepsy, we regard an initial EEG examination as essential in each case of epilepsy.

CT scan (see also Ch. 9)

Two other harmless means of detecting intracranial structural abnormality have become available in recent years, radio-isotope brain scanning and now computerised axial tomography (the CT scan). Both can be undertaken as an outpatient and neither involve more than an intravenous injection. Of the two, the CT scan is the most powerful, for it detects not only tumours, but also atrophy, ventricular dilatation, infarct and haemorrhage.

Gastaut (1976) has summarised the CT scan findings in 1702 epileptic patients of all ages combined from seven research groups. Overall the proportion of abnormalities varied from 34–51 per cent, with a mean of 46 per cent. Amongst these lesions, 56 per cent were atrophic in character. Tumours were found in 8–11 per cent of patients, but this figure rose to 16 per cent in patients over the age of 20, and to 22 per cent when only partial seizures were considered.

The relationship of CT abnormalities to various seizure types is well illustrated by the study of Gastaut and Gastaut (1976) in 401 patients (Table 4.15). A clear difference emerges between the relatively low incidence (11 per cent) associated with primary generalised seizures and the much higher proportion (60–80 per cent) in relation to other

Table 4.15 Abnormalities on CT scan in relation to seizure type

Seizure type	Abnormal CT
Primary generalised	11%
Secondary generalised	61%
Partial	63%
Lennox-Gastaut syndrome	60%
Post-traumatic	80%

(After Gastaut & Gastaut, 1976)

seizure types. These authors also estimate that CT scan detects 20 per cent more cerebral lesions than the combination of long established techniques (skull X-ray, EEG, angiography etc).

These observations have been extended by Yang et al. (1979) who scanned 256 children between the ages of a few days and 17 years (mean 4 years). Abnormalities of the type classified in Table 4.16 were seen overall in 33 per cent. They were able to distinguish a low yield group (2.5–8 per cent) with idiopathic generalised seizures or normal

Table 4.16 Classification of CT findings

1. Normal
2. Bilateral atrophy
   Central atrophy: dilation of lateral ventricles only
   Cortical atrophy: dilation of sulci, lateral ventricles normal
   Generalised atrophy: dilation of sulci and lateral ventricles
3. Focal findings
   Atrophy
   Hemiatrophy
   Porencephalic cysts
   Tumours
4. Other findings
   Pathological calcifications
   Congenital abnormalities of brain
   Evidence of intracranial bleeding

(After Yang et al., 1979)

neurological examination or focal slowing (but not focal spiking) on the EEG (Table 4.17). The highest incidence was seen in neo-natal seizures or a history of seizures beginning in the neo-natal period. Amongst children with mental retardation 45 per cent had abnormal scans. Only 2 per cent of the series had tumours. If the initial scan was normal, contrast enhancement added no new information, but if it initially was abnormal, enhancement gave more information in 10 per cent.

It is possible that the above studies over-

Table 4.17 CT scan findings in children with epilepsy

Low Yield Groups	Abnormal CT
1. Idiopathic generalised seizure	8%
2. Neurological examination and EEG normal (neonates not included)	5%
3. Generalised seizure (idiopathic or known aetiology with normal neurological examination and normal EEG)	2.5%

High Yield Groups	Abnormal CT
1. Partial seizures with elementary symptomatology	52%
2. Partial seizures with complex symptomatology	30%
3. Generalised seizures (known aetiology)	40%
4. Neonates with seizures	68%
5. Children whose seizures began as neonates	100%
6. Focal slowing on EEG	63%
7. Abnormal neurological examination	64%

(After Yang et al., 1979)

estimate the prevalence of CT scan abnormalities as they are mostly based on retrospective analyses from specialised centres. Prospective studies in less selected or community based populations are needed.

Although Gastaut and Gastaut argue that all epileptic patients should have a CT scan, economics in this country would preclude such a course. It is clear, in any case, that patients with primary generalised seizures and with no focal signs on clinical or EEG examination would yield few abnormalities. Although the remote possibility of a tumour may exist in a few such patients it is questionable whether early detection is a great advantage when the only symptoms are seizures. This view would be reversed if it was clear that early surgery for brain tumours carried little risk and was necessary. At present there is little to be lost in observing the low yield group regularly in outpatients. If, however, the seizures fail to respond to optimum therapy with one or two drugs there is an increased likelihood of a detectable brain lesion on the scan (Dellaportas et al., 1980).

Psychometry

Standard psychometric techniques may be useful in documenting the more gross evidence of intellectual decline and/or focal brain lesions, in children or adults with mental retardation, dementia or apparent focal cognitive abnormality. They have proved disappointing in assessing the more subtle but undoubted adverse effects of seizure activity and chronic drug therapy. Attention is now being directed at developing more suitable techniques for the latter problems.

Inpatient investigation

From what has been said already, it is apparent that only those with symptoms or signs (clinical or EEG) of a focal cerebral lesion require further investigation. Even this simple summary requires amplification.

Focal epilepsy in childhood is unlikely to be due to tumour, for reasons stated earlier. Partial fits in children are therefore not in themselves an indication to submit the child to full neuro-radiological study. However, it is here that the simple CT scan may be expected to help, and may delineate the common atrophic lesion causing the partial fits.

Complex partial seizures in adults are also much less likely to be due to tumour than simple partial fits. Unless they are accompanied by signs, or EEG evidence, suggesting tumour, they are not an indication for full neuroradiological study. Again, CT scanning or radio-isotope scanning will help in this problem.

Partial fits in the elderly are just as likely to be due to vascular disease as tumour, and again, the decision as to whether to carry out the more dangerous neuroradiological studies may be resolved by CT scanning or radio-isotope scanning.

If, however, there is strong indication from clinical, EEG, and brain scan information that a tumour may be present, CT scanning, and sometimes carotid angiography and air encephalography will be required. Angiography also is necessary to delineate fully arteriovenous malformations (although epilepsy alone is not always an indication for surgery). However, such full neuroradiological investigation is now only occasionally required in those presenting with epilepsy, and the type and timing of the tests required is usually fairly obvious from the clinical and EEG picture. In passing, it must also be mentioned that lumbar puncture gives no useful information in a case of epilepsy alone. Lumbar puncture is only required when it is suspected that the epilepsy may be due to infection or encephalitis, or to stroke or other intracranial vascular disaster.

Special problems

The solitary seizure

A single fit does not warrant a diagnosis of epilepsy, and if the patient is otherwise healthy, it requires no further investigation or treatment. Only time will tell if this is the first of a series requiring further action.

Provoked seizures

Some patients may only have an occasional seizure under specific circumstances, as for example while watching television, or while taking a provocative drug. Such people are best not labelled as epileptic, and if the provoking factor can be avoided, further investigation and therapy may not be required. In these cases judgement has to be exercised on each individual case as to what course to pursue.

Status epilepticus

Status in a known epileptic requires no further investigation other than that required to manage the problem, or unless otherwise indicated.

Patients whose epilepsy presents as status epilepticus require full investigation, directed in children particularly towards infection or metabolic error as the cause, and in adults towards tumour.

Twilight states

An EEG is the only way to distinguish absence or complex partial status, and may help to point to metabolic or structural causes. Blood sugar estimation is mandatory and other metabolic tests may be required if the situation still exists when the patient is seen. If, however, the patient has fully recovered by the time he reaches medical care, only simple outpatient tests are warranted.

Todd's paralysis

A post-ictal paralysis lasting more than 48 hours justifies full investigation, the extent of which will depend on the age of the patient and the likely cause.

Assessment for surgery

This topic is discussed fully in Chapter 10. Extensive clinical, psychometric, EEG and neuro-radiological investigation is required to establish suitability for surgery.

PROGNOSIS OF SEIZURES

The outcome of epilepsy depends on many factors, including the type of fit, the underlying cause, and probably the quality of treatment.

When epilepsy is symptomatic of some progressive underlying structural or metabolic disorder, the prognosis is that of the cause of the fits. What follows concerns mainly epilepsy of unknown cause or due to static pathology.

Prognosis for tonic-clonic seizures

Considering the frequency of epilepsy, it is surprising how little detailed information is available as to its prognosis. Rodin (1968), in an invaluable review of the literature, questions the widely quoted aphorism 'With current medical therapy approximately 80–85 per cent of all cases can be controlled' (Forster, 1960). Rodin traces this optimistic view to an article by Yahr *et al.* (1952) in which it is concluded that, 'The use of diphenylhydantoin (Dilantin) sodium and pheno-barbitone in this group of 319 patients resulted in 79 per cent control or improvement of seizures regardless of causation. The addition of other anticonvulsants added 6 per cent, giving an overall rate of 85 per cent improvement or control'. However, Rodin points out that only 48 per cent of the patients of Yahr *et al.* were completely controlled, while 37 per cent were improved, and that the duration of complete control varied from less than six months to five and one-half years. Rodin points out that in most studies the incidence of cessation of fits is inversely proportional

Table 4.18 Prognosis for seizures

		Number of patients	Maximum duration of remission	Per cent remitted
Juul-Jensen	1963	969	2 years	32
Alstroem	1950	897	5 years	22
Grosz	1930	91	10 years	11
Bridge*	1949	264	1 month	56
		187	1 year	40
		161	2 years	34
		134	3 years	28
		101	4 years	21
		81	5 years	17

* Data based on 472 epileptic children
(Based on data reviewed by Rodin, 1968)

to the duration of follow-up (Table 4.18). Thus while fits may cease for a year in about 40 per cent of patients with epilepsy, only about 30 per cent are free of fits for two years, about 20 per cent are free of fits for five years, and about 10 per cent are free of fits for ten years. Complementary data on the risk of recurrence of fits after their cessation for a period of two years is provided by Juul-Jensen (1964b), in a study of 200 such patients. Fits recurred in the two years after antiepileptic drugs were withdrawn in 35 per cent. Rodin concludes from his careful study of the literature that '80 per cent of all patients with epilepsy are likely to have a chronic seizure disorder. This does not rule out short-term remissions or changes in seizure patterns, it merely re-emphasises that epilepsy should be regarded as a chronic condition with remissions and exacerbations.'

So far, the data on prognosis has been reviewed for fits in general, irrespective of their age of onset, type, frequency or treatment. Rodin goes on to try and assess from the literature whether there are good criteria to differentiate those patients who will recover from their epilepsy from those who will continue to have recurrent fits. It is worth quoting his conclusions in full.

Reviewing this material the reader will probably be left with a sense of bewilderment. There is agreement in the literature on some points and considerable disagreement on others. It may be best, therefore, to summarise those findings on which the majority of authors agree:
1. Approximately one-third of all epileptic patients were likely to achieve a terminal remission of at least two years.
2. The percentage rises to between 50 and 60 if one considers only those patients who have grand mal seizures without associated minor attacks.

3. It drops to approximately 20 to 30 per cent if one deals with patients who have psychomotor seizures.
4. The percentages of patients who are regarded in terminal remission stand in marked indirect relationship to the length of follow-up.
5. The longer the illness has lasted, the less likely will control be achieved.
6. The more seizures the patient has experienced prior to his first visit to the physician, the less likely will be complete control.
7. The more different seizure types a given patient has experienced, the less likely control.
8. The more abnormal the neurological examination, mental status examination, and the lower the IQ, the more difficult will it be to control the patient.
9. The younger the patient at the time of onset of the illness, the less likely will complete control be achieved; but there are some authors who feel that age at time of onset is not a good prognostic indicator.
10. The initial EEG is of limited value for prognosis, but a persistently abnormal EEG during treatment tends to be associated with poor seizure control.

Opinions are more divided between authors on the importance of heredity, other aetiological factors, nocturnal versus diurnal seizures, and sex.

To summarise, those with a structural cause for their epilepsy, neurological or mental abnormality, partial fits (particularly complex partial seizures), more than one type of fit, and many fits have a bad outlook. Of potential importance is the suggestion that delay in treatment affects prognosis adversely.

Against this general background it is important to examine a number of specific problems. The prognosis for epilepsy in childhood, febrile seizures and absences is discussed in more detail in Chapter 3, but will be mentioned briefly here for completeness.

Prognosis for seizures in childhood

Febrile convulsions

Most patients with epilepsy have their first fit in childhood, and there is a general belief that they will 'grow out of their fits'. This belief is based primarily on the excellent prognosis for uncomplicated febrile fits. The incidence of febrile fits is accepted as about 5 per cent in the general population, but only about 5 per cent of those with febrile fits will develop spontaneous epilepsy. (The exact figure varies between 2 and 14 per cent (Rodin, 1968).) The prognosis for febrile fits is therefore good, although the small proportion who

do go on to have recurrent seizures is of crucial significance (see p. 81).

By contrast with febrile fits, children who develop spontaneous epilepsy do not fare nearly so well. The prognosis for such children depends on the type of fits they suffer.

Absence (petit mal) seizures

The prognosis of those with classical absences is generally believed to be favourable. Livingston et al. (1965), for example, in a follow-up study of 117 cases for five years or more, found that some 79 per cent were controlled of their absences. Dalby (1969), in a similar study of 161 patients with clinical absence attacks and three per second spike-wave paroxysms found that absences ceased in 79 per cent of those with no other type of seizure after a period of observation of five years or more (Table 4.19). In most patients absences

Table 4.19 Prognosis for absences in 161 patients

	Attacks ceased in
All cases	93 (58%)
Absences alone	69 (79%)
Absences and grand mal	24 (33%)
Age at cessation of absences	
0–4 years	1
5–9 years	42
10–14 years	26
15–19 years	16
19 years	8

(After Dalby, 1969)

stopped between the ages of 5 and 14 years. However, grand mal developed in 46 per cent of patients with absences, and attacks ceased in only 33 per cent of these cases. Thus the prognosis of absence seizures depends on whether grand mal occurs as well. Both Dalby (1969) and Livingston et al. (1965) present some evidence to suggest that routine therapy with major antiepileptic drugs, as well as specific drugs to control absence attacks, will decrease the risk of developing grand mal. Thus in Dalby's series only 6 per cent of those given prophylactic major anticonvulsants developed grand mal, as against 22 per cent of those given only anti-absence therapy; corresponding figures from the series of Livingston et al. were 36 per cent and 81 per cent respectively.

In summary, approximately 80 per cent of those with typical absences are likely to lose their fits by the time they reach adult life, provided they do not develop concurrent grand mal attacks, when the prognosis is that of the latter (see above).

The prognosis for those with akinetic or myoclonic attacks is less favourable than in those with isolated typical absences. Thus of 44 such patients in the series of Dalby (1969), only eight (18 per cent) had ceased to have fits. The bad prognosis for those with atypical spikewave paroxysms has already been commented upon (see p. 103) and the appalling outlook for those with infantile spasms is dealt with elsewhere (Ch. 3).

Grand mal and partial seizures

In general, Rodin (1968) concludes that the available data indicates that the prognosis for grand mal and partial fits in childhood is little different for that in adult life. Thus the incidence of remission is inversely related to the duration of follow-up, varying from a figure of about 30 per cent being free of fits for one year to 17 per cent being free of fits for five years. As in adults, those with grand mal seizures alone do best, while those with complex partial seizures and multiple fits do worst.

Prognosis for a single seizure

The management of the solitary fit has already been discussed (see p. 122) and it was concluded that one fit does not in general merit a diagnosis of epilepsy or treatment. This view is based on the belief, and hope, that many patients with a solitary fit will have no further attacks, but evidence to support this view is sparse. Johnson et al. (1972) recently followed the fate of 77 enlisted young naval men who were referred after a single fit, 49 developed a second seizure in the next three years.

Prognosis for seizures during sleep

Present driving laws allow those who only suffer nocturnal epilepsy to drive. Gibberd and Bateson (1974) have recently studied the prognosis of 76 patients with nocturnal seizures alone. One year later, four had developed day-time attacks and fits had ceased in six. Of 61 patients followed for two years, ten had developed day-time fits, and fits had stopped in eight. Of 33 patients followed for five years, ten had developed day-time attacks, and fits had stopped in none. Thus some 30 per cent of those with nocturnal epilepsy may be expected to develop fits during the day in the next five years.

Prognosis for stress-induced seizures

Comment has already been made on the role of physical or mental stress as a precipitant of fits (see p. 114), and in some patients fits may only occur under such provocative circumstances. In a series of 36 such patients followed for 1–12 years (Friis & Lund, 1974), 24 remained free of attacks, ten had further stress convulsions, and two had unprovoked fits. Although only a small series, these data add weight to the view that when a fit is clearly provoked by some adequate external stress stimulus, the risks of such a patient subsequently developing spontaneous epilepsy is relatively low.

Prognosis for complex partial seizures

The prognosis for temporal lobe epilepsy is of particular interest, for it is the commonest type of partial epilepsy (Table 4.2), and the type of epilepsy to which surgical treatment is most commonly applied. Although it is generally held that temporal lobe epilepsy has a poorer prognosis than unlocalised grand mal (see above) the evidence on this matter is far from complete. There have been few studies in which an unselected population of patients with a clinical and EEG diagnosis of temporal lobe epilepsy have been followed for a sufficient length of time to establish firm prognostic guidance. One such study is that of Currie et al. (1971), whose results are summarised in Table 4.20. Only 40 per cent of the 666 patients were free of fits for one year or more, and longer remissions were even less frequent. However, 73 per cent were classified as improved with treatment. Gibbs and Gibbs (1960) studied 739 patients with mid-temporal EEG spike foci, but no other seizure activity. Such an abnormality was increasingly common up to the age of eight years, decreased in incidence between 8 and 15 years, and thereafter

Table 4.20 Prognosis for fits in 666 patients with temporal lobe epilepsy (average follow-up for seven years)

Improved	73%
Free of fits for one year or more	40%
Unchanged	22%
Worse	5%
Working	88%
Deaths*	8%

* Mostly due to cerebral cause of fits, or unassociated with epilepsy

(After Currie et al., 1971)

was rare. Follow-up of 120 children with seizures starting after the age of five and a mid-temporal spike focus, to the age of 18 years revealed that 85 per cent were free of epilepsy and in 55 per cent the EEG had returned to normal. By contrast, patients with temporal lobe epilepsy and an anterior temporal lobe focus on EEG are believed by the Gibbses to have a worse prognosis. In reviewing the available data, Rodin (1968) concludes that the reported remission rate for all patients with temporal lobe epilepsy (irrespective of the duration of remission) is between 20 and 35 per cent, in contrast to a remission rate of between 55 and 63 per cent in patients with pure grand mal.

In general, it appears that remission of temporal lobe epilepsy is less likely than for pure grand mal, but the detailed prognosis for temporal lobe fits with differing ages of onset and EEG abnormality is unclear.

Prognosis for recurrence of seizures on withdrawal of medication

A practical problem of great importance is when to withdraw antiepileptic drugs in those patients whose fits cease. Juul-Jensen (1964b) studied the recurrence of fits in 200 patients who had been free of attacks for two years or more. Fits recurred in the next two years in 35 per cent (in half of these patients the recurrence occurred soon after drug withdrawal). No decisive prognostic features were discovered, although an abnormal EEG increased the risk of recurrence. Zenker et al. (1957) studied 117 children whose drugs were withdrawn after seizure-free periods of one-half to nine years. Fits recurred in 21 per cent and in 36 per cent of those with a persistently abnormal

EEG despite treatment. Studies such as these – and more data are required – form the factual background to the common practice of continuing antiepileptic drugs until the patient has been free of fits for a period of three years. Drugs may then be gradually withdrawn, but fits are likely to recur in some 25 per cent of cases. Common sense suggests that it is unwise to discontinue medication in those with an obvious structural cause for their fits, or a persistently abnormal EEG, the more so as such patients free of fits for three years on drugs are allowed to drive.

Prognosis for intellect and behaviour

In evaluating the prognosis of those with epilepsy in respect of intellect and behaviour, it is necessary to separate those with epilepsy only from those with epilepsy and brain damage. In the latter, the prognosis for intellect and behaviour is that of the underlying cerebral damage and pathology, to which epilepsy is an added complication.

In the case of epilepsy alone there is a long history of attempts to define a mental defect or typical personality in those with the misfortune to suffer fits. Such an erroneous belief stemmed from the frequent association of mental backwardness or behaviour disturbance in brain-damaged epileptics, and similar conclusions were assumed in the case of those with epilepsy alone, by physicians, historians and moralists. Such beliefs were reinforced by the effects of treatments such as bromides, and those of repeated injury, and anoxia. In more recent times many studies of intellectual function in unselected epileptics have suggested that those who suffer epilepsy are, by and large, of lesser intellect than those who do not. For example, Juul-Jensen (1964a) recorded that of 967 patients with epilepsy, 66 per cent were mentally normal, while 13 per cent showed 'severe mental deviation'. Many other studies on intellectual function in those with epilepsy, using a variety of psychological measures, have shown a tendency towards the lower range of normal for averaged data. Such studies are of little relevance to the individual patient, for they ignore the many factors that may compromise the intellectual and behavioural development of a patient with epilepsy. The cause of the fits, the damage caused by the fits, and the drugs and other means of treatment may all contribute to producing some degree of intellectual and behavioural impairment in some epileptic patients. The important point is that in the majority of those with epilepsy alone and who are not intoxicated by medication, intellect and behaviour are normal. Serial studies of intellect in patients with epilepsy alone have not shown evidence of progressive decline (see Rodin, 1968, for review). Intellect may improve in some and decline in others, probably reflecting at least in part the effects of changes in fit frequency and medication. Thus fits themselves are not necessarily associated with either intellectual impairment or behavioural disturbance. This fact is well-known to those who look after such patients and to historians, who point to individuals with epilepsy excelling in all walks of life, but not the public at large who still attach a stigma and doubt to those with fits.

Mortality

Fits themselves rarely cause death, but tragic examples of drowning and other accidental death occur. As with all aspects of prognosis for those with epilepsy, it is difficult to disentangle the effects of fits from those of the disease causing the fits. Henriksen, Juul-Jensen and Lund (1966) have published figures for mortality in a large representative group of non-institutionalised epileptics (excluding those with obvious structural causes) in comparison with life data for the normal population from an insurance company. Mortality in the epileptic population was 2.9 times greater than expected. Death was recorded as due to epilepsy (status or death after a fit) in 26 per cent; suicide in 20 per cent; accidents in 11 per cent, unsuspected brain tumour in 8 per cent; intercurrent unrelated causes in 36 per cent. Risk of death was least in those with normal mentality, idiopathic epilepsy, pure grand mal, and infrequent fits. Such patients usually can be expected to live through a normal life span, while those with brain damage and frequent fits may die prematurely, usually between the ages of 30 and 45 years. Sudden, unexpected and accidental death can rarely be prevented, but status epilepticus

can, and the high incidence of suicide as a cause of death in those with fits is notable.

Prognosis for institutionalisation

The reasons why some patients with fits cannot lead a life within the community obviously depend on the facilities available and the attitudes of doctors, social workers, the family and the population at large. Rodin (1968) compared in detail the significant differences between 57 institutionalised patients and 162 patients living in the community served by hospitals in Michigan. Key factors leading to institutionalisation were, not surprisingly, a very severe seizure disorder resistant to medication, brain damage with severe intellectual impairment rendering life impossible in the community, and behavioural disturbance which could not be tolerated by the community. All the criteria obviously depend on the tolerance and capability of the community and particularly of the family unit, but they represent fairly the reasons for referral for chronic care in this country.

CONCLUSION

The information discussed in this chapter forms the background essential to the neurologist, or other physician, responsible for evaluating a new patient presenting with a history suggestive of epilepsy. Such initial evaluation, diagnosis and investigation, and therapeutic decision usually occupies no more than the first few months or so of a patient's epileptic life. It seems curious that the chapter stops here, for over the next 20 or more years that patient and his doctor may have to engage in continual combat against his fits and their consequences. The success or failure of that battle is one of the major tasks and pleasures of neurology. The additional knowledge and experience required to help such patients deserves a chapter equally long, if not longer, than that already written. Such matters are dealt with elsewhere in this volume, but it is worth asking who should look after epileptic patients. There is no easy answer, for each section of the medical and social community has different fields of expertise to offer the patient. The general practitioner has the considerable benefit of knowing the patient as an individual, his family and his life circumstances. Yet he must nearly always suffer from relative inexperience in the medical vagaries of the illness. With an incidence of about 1 in 200 of the population, the practitioner with an average list may have some 20 epileptic patients in his care at any one time. Many of these may not require the expertise of those with greater experience, but some undoubtedly do. The neurologist may see as many as 200 or more new epileptic patients a year, and may have many hundreds of established epileptic patients attending the clinic. His experience becomes great, but his time is limited. Unless he has a special interest in epilepsy it is almost inevitable that such patients after initial evaluation will fall into the routine of a brief visit on increasingly rare occasions, often to be seen by a member of the junior staff. The neurologist, with his clinical neurophysiological and neuroradiological colleagues is best equipped to undertake the initial evaluation of patients suspected of epilepsy, and from his experience can offer useful advice on specific topics in later years, particularly on treatment. But there are those who also require the help of psychiatrists, and other personnel such as social workers, industrial rehabilitation officers, and lay organisations. For those requiring such help, the concept of centres for epilepsy has been advanced and in certain places instituted. Such centres should provide the full range of expertise required to help those patients with epilepsy whose problems exceed the capacity of their local services. This may not be a large proportion of all those with fits, but patients in this category undoubtedly benefit from such concentrated exposure to all possible therapeutic disciplines. The establishment and adequate continuing finance of such centres must improve the lot of those with the misfortune to suffer from epilepsy.

REFERENCES

Ames, F.R. (1971) 'Self-induction' in photosensitive epilepsy. *Brain*, **94**, 781.

Ansell, B. & Clarke, J. (1956) The role of water retention in menstruating epileptics. *Lancet*, **2**, 7232.

Backstrom, T. (1976) Epileptic seizures in women related to plasma oestrogen and progesterone during the menstrual cycle. *Acta Neurologica Scandinavica*, **54**, 321.

Bandler, B., Kaufmann, I.C., Dyken, J.W., Schleifer, N. & Shapiro, L.N. (1957) Seizures and the menstrual cycle. *American Journal of Psychiatry*, **133**, 704.

Bannister, R.G. (1971) Degeneration of the autonomic nervous system. *Lancet*, **2**, 175.

Barraclough, M.A. & Sharpey-Schafer, E.P. (1963) Hypotension from absent circulatory reflexes: Effect of alcohol, barbiturates, psychotherapeutic drugs, and other mechanisms. *Lancet*, **1**, 1121.

Behrman, S. & Wyke, B.D. (1958) Vestibular seizures. *Brain*, **81**, 529.

Bickerstaff, E.R. (1961a) Basilar artery migraine. *Lancet*, **1**, 15.

Bickerstaff, E.R. (1961b) Impairment of consciousness in migraine. *Lancet*, **2**, 1057.

Bickford, R.G., Whelan, J.L., Klass, D.W. & Corbin, K.B. (1957) Reading epilepsy. *Transactions of the American Neurological Association*, **81**, 100.

Bingley, T. (1958) Mental symptoms in temporal lobe epilepsy and temporal lobe gliomas. *Acta Psychiatrica et Neurologica Scandinavica*, **33**. Supplement **120**, 1–151.

Binnie, C.D., Darby, C.E. & Hindley, A.T. (1973) Electroencephalographic changes in epileptics while viewing television. *British Medical Journal*, **4**, 378.

Blume, W.T., David, R.B. & Gomez, M.R. (1973) Generalised sharp and slow wave complexes. Association clinical features and long-term follow up. *Brain*, **96**, 289.

Bornstein, M., Codden, D. & Song, S. (1956) Prolonged alterations in behaviour associated with a continuous electroencephalographic (spike and dome) abnormality. *Neurology* (Minneapolis) **6**, 444.

Brett, E.M. (1966) Minor epileptic status. *Journal of Neurological Sciences*, **3**, 52.

Brigden, W., Howarth, S. & Sharpey-Schafer, E.P. (1950) Postural changes in the peripheral blood-flow of normal subjects with observations on vasovagal fainting reactions as a result of tilting, the lordotic posture, pregnancy and spinal anaesthesia. *Clinical Science*, **9**, 79.

Caveness, W.F., Walker, A.E. & Ashcroft, P.B. (1962) Incidence of post-traumatic epilepsy in Korean veterans as compared with those from World War I and World War II. *Journal of Neurosurgery*, **19**, 122.

Charlton, M.H. & Hoefer, P.F.A. (1964) Television and epilepsy. *Archives of Neurology* (Chicago) **11**, 239.

Chen, R.C. & Forster, F.M. (1973) Cursive epilepsy and gelastic epilepsy. *Neurology* (Minneapolis) **23**, 1019.

Cole, M. & Zangwill, O.L. (1963) Déjà vu in temporal lobe epilepsy. *Journal of Neurology, Neurosurgery and Psychiatry*, **26**, 37.

Corsellis, J.A.N. (1957) The incidence of Ammon's horn sclerosis. *Brain*, **80**, 193.

Critchley, M. (1937) Musicogenic epilepsy. *Brain*, **60**, 13.

Currie, S., Heathfield, K.W.G., Henson, R.A. & Scott, D.F. (1971) Clinical course and prognosis of temporal lobe epilepsy. A survey of 666 patients. *Brain*, **94**, 173.

Dalby, M.A. (1969) Epilepsy and 3 per second spike and wave rhythms. *Acta Neurologica Scandinavica*, **45**. Supplement **40**, 1–183.

Dallos, V. & Heathfield, K. (1969) Iatrogenic epilepsy due to antidepressant drugs. *British Medical Journal*, **4**, 80.

Daly, D.D. (1958a) Uncinate fits. *Neurology* (Minneapolis) **8**, 250.

Daly, D.D. (1958b) Ictal affect. *American Journal of Psychiatry*, **115**, 97.

Daly, D.D. & Mulder, D.W. (1957) Gelastic epilepsy. *Neurology* (Minneapolis) **7**, 189.

Davison, K. & Bagley, C. (1969) Schizophrenia-like psychoses associated with organic disorders of the nervous system. In: Current Problems in Psychiatry. *British Journal of Psychiatry. Special Publication No. 4*.

Dellaportas, C.I., Galbraith, A.W., Reynolds, E.H., Dawson, J. & Hoare, R.D. (1981) In preparation.

Dodge, P.R., Richardson, E.P. Jr & Victor, M. (1954) Recurrent convulsive seizures as a sequel to cerebral infarction: a clinical and pathological study. *Brain*, **77**, 610.

Douglas, D.B. (1971) Interval between first seizure and diagnosis of brain tumour. *Diseases of the Nervous System*, **32**, 255.

Druckman, R. & Chao, D. (1957) Laughter in epilepsy. *Neurology* (Minneapolis) **7**, 26.

Efron, R. (1961) Post-epileptic paralysis: Theoretical critique and report of a case. *Brain*, **84**, 381.

Escueta, A.V., Boxley, J., Stubbs, N., Waddell, G. & Wilson, W.A. (1974) Prolonged twilight state and automatisms. *Neurology* (Minneapolis) **24**, 331.

Falconer, M.A. (1974) Mesial temporal sclerosis (Ammon's horn sclerosis) as a common cause of epilepsy. *Lancet*, **2**, 767.

Falconer, M.A., Serafetinides, E.A. & Corsellis, J.A.N. (1964) Etiology and pathogenesis of temporal lobe epilepsy. *Archives of Neurology* (Chicago) **10**, 233.

Feindel, W. & Penfield, W. (1954) Localisation of discharge in temporal lobe automatism. *Archives of Neurology and Psychiatry* (Chicago) **72**, 605.

Fenton, G.W. (1972) Epilepsy and automatisms. *British Journal of Hospital Medicine*, **7**, 57.

Fenton, G.W. & Udwin, E.L. (1965) Homocide, temporal lobe epilepsy and depression: A case report. *British Journal of Psychiatry*, **111**, 304.

Fischer, C.M. & Adams, R.D. (1964) Transient global amnesia. *Acta Neurologica Scandinavica*, **40**. Supplement 9, 1–83.

Forster, F.M. (1960) Epilepsy. *Traumatic Medicine and Surgery for the Attorney*, **4**, 481.

Fox, R.H., Wilkins, D.C., Bell, J.A., Bradley, R.D., Browse, N.L., Cranston W.I., Foley, T.H., Gilby, E.D., Hebden, A., Jenkins, B.S. & Rawlins, M.D. (1973) Spontaneous periodic hypothermia: Diencephalic epilepsy. *British Medical Journal*, **2**, 693.

Friis, M.L. & Lund, M. (1974) Stress convulsions. *Archives of Neurology* (Chicago) **31**, 155.

Gastaut, H. (1969) Clinical and electroencephalographical classification of epileptic seizures. *Epilepsia* (Amsterdam) **10**. Supplement 1–28.

Gastaut, H. (1976) Conclusions: Computerised transverse axial tomography in epilepsy. *Epilepsia*, **17**, 337.

Gastaut, H. & Gastaut, J.L. (1976) Computerised transverse axial tomography in epilepsy. *Epilepsia*, **17**, 325.

Gibberd, F. (1966a) The clinical features of petit mal. *Acta Neurologica Scandinavica*, **42**, 176.

Gibberd, F. (1966b) The prognosis of petit mal. *Brain*, **89**, 531.

Gibberd, F. (1973) The diagnosis and investigation of epilepsy. *British Journal of Hospital Medicine*, **9**, 152.

Gibberd, F.B. & Bateson, M.C. (1974) Sleep epilepsy: Its pattern and prognosis. *British Medical Journal*, **2**, 403.

Gibbs, F.A. & Gibbs, E.L. (1952) 'Atlas of Electroencephalography', 2. Reading, Massachusetts: Addison-Wesley Publishing Co.

Gibbs, E.L. & Gibbs, F.A. (1960) Good prognosis of mid-temporal epilepsy. *Epilepsia* (Amsterdam) **1**, 448.

Gibbs, F.A., Davies, H. & Lennox, W.G. (1935) The electroencephalogram in epilepsy and in conditions of impaired consciousness. *Archives of Neurology and Psychiatry* (Chicago) **34**, 1133.

Gibbs, F.A., Gibbs, E.L. & Lennox, W. (1937) Epilepsy: A paroxysmal cerebral dysthythmia. *Brain*, **60**, 377.

Gilliatt, R.W. (1974) Syncope. *Medicine*, **31**, 1823.

Gudmundsson, G. (1966) Epilepsy in Iceland. *Acta Neurologica Scandinavica*. Supplement 25.

Gumpert, J., Hanisota, P. & Upton, A. (1970) Gelastic epilepsy. *Journal of Neurology, Neurosurgery and Psychiatry*, **33**, 479.

Gunn, T. & Fenton, G. (1971) Epilepsy, automatism and crime. *Lancet*, **1**, 1173.

Harper, M. & Roth, M. (1962) Temporal lobe epilepsy and the phobic anxiety-depersonalisation syndrome. Part 1. A comparative study. *Comprehensive Psychiatry*, **3**, 129.

Heathfield, K.W.G., Croft, P.B. & Swash, M. (1973) The syndrome of transient global amnesia. *Brain*, **96**, 729.

Henriksen, P.B., Juul-Jensen, P. & Lund, M. (1966) The mortality of epileptics: A Preliminary Report. *Social Studies in Epilepsy*, No. 5. London: International Bureau of Epilepsy.

Hutchinson, E.C. & Stock, J.P.P. (1960) The carotid-sinus syndrome. *Lancet*, **2**, 445.

Hyllested, K. & Pakkenberg, H. (1963) Prognosis in epilepsy of late onset. *Neurology* (Minneapolis) **13**, 641.

Ingvar, D.H. & Nyman, G.E. (1962) Epilepsia arithmetices. A new psychologic trigger mechanism in a case of epilepsy. *Neurology* (Minneapolis) **12**, 282.

Jennett, W.B. (1962) 'Epilepsy after blunt head injuries'. London: William Heinemann.

Jennett, W.B. (1965) Predicting epilepsy after blunt head injury. *British Medical Journal*, **4**, 1215.

Jennett, W.B. (1969) Early traumatic epilepsy. Definition and identity. *Lancet*, **1**, 1023.

Jennett, B., Teather, D. & Bennie, S. (1973) Epilepsy after head injury. Residual risk after varying fit-free intervals since injury. *Lancet*, **2**, 652.

Johnson, L.C., DeBolt, W.L., Long, M.T., Ross, J.J., Sassin, J.F., Arthur, R.J. & Walter, R.D. (1972) Diagnostic factors in adult males following initial seizures. *Archives of Neurology* (Chicago) **27**, 193.

Johnson, R.H., Lee, G. de J., Oppenheimer, D.R. & Spalding, J.M.K. (1966) Autonomic failure with orthostatic hypotension due to intermediolateral column degeneration. *Quarterly Journal of Medicine*, **35**, 276.

Juul-Jensen, P. (1964a) Epilepsy. A clinical and social analysis of 1020 adult patients with epileptic seizures. *Acta Neurologica Scandinavica*, **40**. Supplement 5, 1–285.

Juul-Jensen, P. (1964b) Frequency of recurrence after discontinuance of anticonvulsant therapy in patients with epileptic seizures. *Epilepsia* (Amsterdam) **5**, 352.

Knox, S.J. (1968) Epileptic automatism and violence. *Medical Science and Law*, **8**, 96.

Laidlaw, J. (1956) Catamenial epilepsy. *Lancet*, ii, **71**, 1235.

Lance, J.W. (1963) Sporadic and familial varieties of tonic seizures. *Journal of Neurology, Neurosurgery and Psychiatry*, **26**, 51.

Lancet (1972). Report from Boston Collaborative Drug Surveillance Programme. Drug-induced convulsions. *Lancet*, **2**, 677.

Legg, N.J., Gupta, P.C. & Scott, D.F. (1973) Epilepsy following cerebral abscess. A clinical and EEG study of 70 patients. *Brain*, **96**, 259.

Lennox, W.G. (1945) The petit mal epilepsies. Their treatment with tridione. *Journal of the American Medical Association*, **129**, 1069.

Liddell, D.W. (1953) Observations on epileptic automatism in a mental hospital population. *Journal of Mental Science*, **99**, 732.

Lishman, W.A., Symonds, C.P., Whitty, C.W.M. & Willison, R.G. (1962) Seizures induced by movement. *Brain*, **85**, 93.

Livingston, S., Torres, I., Pauli, L.L. & Rider, R.V (1965) Petit mal epilepsy. Results of a prolonged follow-up study of 117 patients. *Journal of the American Medical Association*, **194**, 227.

Louis, S. & McDowell, F. (1967) Epileptic seizures in non-embolic cerebral infarction. *Archives of Neurology* (Chicago) **17**, 414.

Lowe, C.R. (1973) Congenital malformations among infants born to epileptic women. *Lancet*, **1**, 9.

Macrae, D. (1954) Isolated fear: A temporal lobe aura. *Neurology* (Minneapolis), **4**, 497.

Margerison, J.H. & Corsellis, J.A.N. (1966) Epilepsy and the temporal lobes: A clinical electroencephalographic and neuropathological study of the brain in epilepsy, with particular reference to the temporal lobes. *Brain*, **89**, 499.

Matthews, W.B. (1962) Epilepsy and disseminated sclerosis. *Quarterly Journal of Medicine*, **31**, 141.

Maurice-Williams, R.M. (1974) Micturition symptoms in frontal tumours. *Journal of Neurology, Neurosurgery and Psychiatry*, **37**, 431.

Mullan, S. & Penfield, W. (1959) Illusions of comparative interpretation and emotion; production by epileptic discharge and by electrical stimulation in the temporal cortex. *Archives of Neurology and Psychiatry* (Chicago) **81**, 269.

Neidermeyer, E. & Khalifeh, R. (1965) Petit mal status (spike-wave stupor). *Epilepsia* (Amsterdam) **6**, 250.

Oxbury, J.M. & Whitty, C.W.M. (1971) Causes and consequences of status epilepticus in adults. A survey of 86 cases. *Brain*, **94**, 733.

Parker, H.L. (1930) Epileptiform convulsions. The incidence of attacks in cases of intracranial tumour. *Archives of Neurology and Psychiatry* (Chicago) **23**, 1032.

Parkes, J.D. & Marsden, C.D. (1974) Narcolepsy. *British Journal of Hospital Medicine*, **12**, 325.

Parsonage, M. (1973) The differential diagnosis of seizures. *Journal of the Royal College of Physicians*, **7**, 213.

Paterson, J.H. & McKissock, W. (1956) A clinical survey of intracranial angiomas with special reference to their mode of prognosis and surgical treatment: a report of 110 cases. *Brain*, **79**, 233.

Penfield, W. (1952) Epileptic automatism and the centrencephalic integrating system. *Research Publications of the Association for Research into Nervous and Mental Diseases*, **30**, 513.

Penfield, W. & Jasper, H. (1954) Epilepsy and the Functional Anatomy of the Human Brain. Boston: Little, Brown & Co.

Penfield, W. & Perot, P. (1963) The brain's record of auditory and visual experience. *Brain*, **86**, 595.

Penfield, W. & Welch, K. (1951) The supplementary motor area of the cerebral cortex. *Archives of Neurology and Psychiatry* (Chicago) **66**, 289.

Penfield, W., Erickson, T.C. & Tarlov, I. (1940) Relation of intracranial tumours and symptomatic epilepsy. *Archives of*

Neurology and Psychiatry (Chicago) **44**, 300.

Penry, J.K. & Dreifuss, F.E. (1969) Automatisms associated with absence of petit mal epilepsy. *Archives of Neurology* (Chicago) **21**, 142.

Pond, D. & Bidwell, D. (1960) A survey of epilepsy in fourteen general practices. *Epilepsia*, **1**, 285.

Proudfit, W.L. & Forteza, M.E. (1959) Micturition syncope. *New England Journal of Medicine*, **260**, 328.

Rapport, R.L. & Penry, J.K. (1972) Pharmacologic prophylaxis of post-traumatic epilepsy. *Epilepsia* (Amsterdam) **13**, 295.

Raynor, R.B., Paine, R.S. & Carmichael, E.A. (1959) Epilepsy of late onset. *Neurology* (Minneapolis) **9**, 111.

Reynolds, E.H. (1968) Epilepsy and schizophrenia: relationship and biochemistry, *Lancet*, **1**, 398.

Richardson, E.P. & Dodge, P.R. (1954) Epilepsy in cerebral vascular disease. *Epilepsia* (Boston) **3**, 49.

Rodin, E.A. (1968) The Prognosis of Patients with Epilepsy. Springfield, Illinois: C.C. Thomas.

Rodin, E.A., Katz, M. & Lennox, K. (1976) Differences between patients with temporal lobe seizures and those with other forms of epileptic attacks. *Epilepsia*, **17**, 313.

Rutter, M., Graham, P. & Yule, W. (1960) A Neuropsychiatric Study in Childhood. In Clinics in Developmental Medicine, No. 35. Spastics International Press, London: Heinemann.

Sano, K. & Malamud, N. (1953) Clinical significance of sclerosis of the cornu ammonis. *Archives of Neurology and Psychiatry* (Chicago) **70**, 40.

Schwartz, M.S. & Scott, D.F. (1971) Isolated petit mal status presenting de novo in middle age. *Lancet*, **2**, 1399.

Serafetinides, E.A. & Falconer, M.A. (1963) Speech disturbances in temporal lobe seizures: A study in 100 epileptic patients submitted to anterior temporal lobectomy. *Brain*, **86**, 333.

Sharpey-Schafer, E.P. (1953) The mechanism of syncope after coughing. *British Medical Journal*, **2**, 860.

Sharpey-Schafer, E.P. & Taylor, P.J. (1960) Absent circulatory reflexes in diabetic neuritis. *Lancet*, **1**, 559.

Sheehan, S. (1958) One thousand cases of late onset epilepsy. *Irish Journal of Medical Science*, **6**, 261.

Shorvon, S.D., Chadwick, D., Galbraith, A.W. & Reynolds, E.H. (1978) One drug for epilepsy. *British Medical Journal*, **1**, 474.

Slater, E. & Beard, A.W. (1963) The schizophrenia-like psychoses of epilepsy. *British Journal of Psychiatry*, **109**, 95.

Smith, B.H. (1960) Vestibular disturbance in epilepsy. *Neurology* (Minneapolis) **10**, 475.

Stevens, H. (1966) Paroxysmal choreo-athetosis. A form of reflex epilepsy. *Archives of Neurology* (Chicago) **14**, 415.

Sumi, S.M. & Teasdall, R.D. (1963) Focal seizures. A review of 150 cases. *Neurology* (Minneapolis) **13**, 582.

Symonds, C.P. (1954) Classification of the epilepsies with particular reference to psychomotor seizures. *Archives of Neurology and Psychiatry* (Chicago) **72**, 631.

Temkin, O. (1945) The falling sickness. Baltimore: The Johns Hopkins Press.

Trimble, M.R. & Reynolds, E.H. (1976) Anticonvulsant drugs and mental symptoms: a review. *Psychological Medicine*, **6**, 169.

Van Buren, J.M. & Ajmone-Marsen, C. (1960) Correlation of autonomic and EEG components in temporal lobe epilepsy. *Archives of Neurology* (Chicago) **3**, 683.

Walker, A. (1961) Murder or epilepsy. *Journal of Nervous and Mental Disease*, **133**, 430.

White, P.J., Bailey, A.A. & Bickford, R.G. (1953) Epileptic disorders in the aged. *Neurology* (Minneapolis) **3**, 674.

Whitty, C.W.M. (1965) A note on the classification of epilepsy. *Lancet*, **1**, 99.

Williams, D. (1956) The structure of emotions reflected in epileptic experiences. *Brain*, **79**, 29.

Williams, D. (1965) The thalamus and epilepsy. *Brain*, **88**, 539.

Williams, D. (1966) Temporal lobe epilepsy. *British Medical Journal*, **1**, 1439.

Williams, D. (1968) The management of epilepsy. *British Journal of Hospital Medicine*, **2**, 702.

Woodcock, S. & Cosgrove, J.B.R. (1964) Epilepsy after the age of 50. A five-year follow-up study. *Neurology* (Minneapolis) **14**, 34.

Yahr, M., Sciarra, D., Carter, S. & Merritt, H.H. (1952) Evaluation of standard anticonvulsant therapy in 319 patients. *Journal of the American Medical Association*, **150**, 663.

Yang, P.J., Berger, P.E., Cohen, M.E. & Duffner, P.K. (1979) Computed tomography and childhood seizure disorders. *Neurology*, **29**, 1084.

Zenker, C., Groh, C. & Roth, G. (1957) Probleme und Erfahrungen beim Absetzen antikonvulsive therapie. *Zeitschrift für Kinderheilkungen*, **2**, 152.

PART TWO
COMPLEX PARTIAL SEIZURES

D.D. Daly

In 1879 John Hughlings Jackson delivered before the Harveian Society three lectures on the diagnosis of epilepsy. In these he described accurately, extensively and completely behaviour which characterises those seizures currently termed complex partial seizures (CPS) (see p. xiii for discussion of terminology). With typical modesty he acknowledged observations and conclusions of a host of predecessors and contemporaries: Bravais, Charcot, Falret, Ferrier, Gowers, Herpin, Reynolds, Todd, Trousseau. However, Jackson himself provided the first systematic description of sequence of events and the first explanation of behaviour in terms of ictal pathophysiology. In the ensuing 100 years, numerous, and often voluminous, descriptions of these seizures have not substantially amended Jackson's concepts although some writers have neglected or adumbrated his contributions. Indeed, during recent decades results of electrical stimulation of exposed cortex (Penfield & Rasmussen, 1950; Penfield & Jasper, 1954) or of stereotactically implanted electrodes (Bancaud *et al.*, 1973; Halgren *et al.*, 1978), careful monitoring of behaviour (Ajmone-Marsan & Ralston, 1957), and simultaneous video and electrographic recordings of spontaneous and induced seizures (Delgado-Escueta, 1979) have illuminated the anatomic substrates and pathophysiology of these seizures while substantiating Jackson's judgements. Among other things such studies have made clear that:

1. Automatisms can occur without ictal invasion of temporal lobes (Ludwig, Ajmone-Marsan & Van Buren, 1975; Geier *et al.*, 1976).
2. Motor arrest, unresponsiveness, mastication and other automatic actions occur indistinguishably in absences (petit mal) and CPS reflecting, in all likelihood, ictal activity in common anatomic systems (Browne *et al.*, 1974; Penry, Porter & Dreifuss, 1975; Escueta *et al.*, 1977).
3. Complex partial status occurs more frequently than previously recognised and in many ways resembles absence status (Andermann & Robb, 1972; Markand, Wheeler & Pollack, 1978; Engel, Ludwig & Fetell 1978).

In the Harveian lectures (Taylor, 1931) Jackson began by distinguishing between *epileptiform seizures* and those of *epilepsy proper* on the grounds that in the former 'consciousness is lost . . . late or not at all . . .' and that the convulsion 'begins very locally on one side . . . and *becomes* universal more gradually . . .' (p. 279)★.

★Jackson defined his concepts precisely and rigorously. However, as Sir Henry Head (1915) bluffly commented about the 'bristling difficulties' of Jackson's papers, 'the style in which they are written makes them peculiarly difficult to read. He was so anxious not to overstate his case that almost every page is peppered with explanatory phrases or footnotes, so that the generalisation can scarcely be distinguished from its qualifications'. To provide ready access to Jackson's extended comments, I have appended paginal references for each quotation.

In discussing those epileptiform seizures now termed CPS, Jackson said (p. 300):

> There are in each case three stages:
> 1. The double state of (1) defect of consciousness along with (2) the positive, the dreamy state.
> 2. A further state, one of loss of consciousness.
> 3. A stage of actions.

The current classification of epileptic seizures adopted by the International League Against Epilepsy (ILAE) (Gastaut, 1970) recognises six categories of CPS (see Introduction):

1. With impaired consciousness only
2. With cognitive symptomatology
3. With affective symptomatology
4. With psychosensory symptomatology
5. With 'psychomotor' symptomatology (automatism)
6. Compound forms

As will become apparent, semantic frameworks underlying the classifications of Jackson and ILAE are essentially identical. Jackson used the phrase 'dreamy state' as a rubric, explaining in a footnote 'the term covers states which are doubtless dissimilar; Voluminous Mental State would be a better name to include them all' (p. 296).

Stage I: THE DOUBLE STATE

Voluminous mental state (cognitive symptomatology)

Jackson defined Voluminous Mental State by direct quotations from his patients:

> One patient would fancy he saw the same things under the same combination of circumstances as he had once before seen them. To illustrate this the patient said pointing to it: 'If I were to see that fender, I should say: "Dear me! I saw that fender before."' (pp. 296–297).
>
> Another patient said: 'I feel as if I was lost – as if I were in some strange country.' (p. 297). Many of his patients spoke in terms of memories or reminiscence: 'It seems as if I went back to all that occurred in my childhood, as if I see everything, but so quick and soon gone that I cannot describe it' (p. 297). Another said: 'It begins . . . by a sort of referring to old things, things that have happened . . .' (p. 296). One patient spoke of 'a peculiar train of ideas as of reminiscence of a former life, or rather, perhaps, a former psychologic state.' (p. 298).

In these experiences patients describe altered interpretations of ongoing events. New experiences seem familiar as if experienced before (déjà vu) or a familiar scene becomes strange or unidentifiable. One of my patients, while driving to her mother-in-law's house, suddenly realised that she did not know where she was or where she was going although she was able to continue driving. Another patient described sitting in her car waiting for her son to finish athletic practice. She experienced her usual aura of 'remoteness' and then realised that she had no idea where she was or why she was sitting in the car. She knew that she was parked near an athletic field, but the place itself seemed completely unfamiliar. She was unsure how long this lasted; the scene regained its familiarity before her son came to the car a few minutes later. She described her feeling of remoteness 'as though a sheet of plate glass was put between me and everything else'; at times an hallucinatory fragrance of lemon blossoms occurred simultaneously. Mullan and Penfield (1959) have classified such instances of altered recognition among 'illusions of comparative interpretation'. In addition to feelings of familiarity or strangeness, they described one patient with prescient sensations, of knowing what people were going to do or say. Gloor (1975) has argued 'that the temporal neocortex and the amygdala act in concert and constitute the functional substrate which enables the animal to relate environmental cues . . . to past experience and to internalised states of drive and motivation'. Halgren et al. (1978) have reported that the two sites at which stimulation was most likely to evoke déjà vu were amygdala and anterior hippocampus.

Some patients have reported altered perception of time. One patient (Mullan and Penfield 1959) said that everything seemed like 'a movie going slow motion'. Other patients experience the reverse – a feeling that all actions 'speed up'.

Many patients describe a thought or idea which comes unbidden to mind. After each seizure they cannot recall, or even characterise, the thought although each insists that in every seizure his 'thought' remains the same. Each remarks that the 'thought' consumes consciousness while ongoing events become dim and remote. At the moment, the idea often seems of overwhelming significance or vast importance. I have described one man with a glioma of the left temporal lobe who regularly experienced a thought which seemed to contain the core of all human understanding of the universe (Daly, 1975). An automatism invariably intervened before he could speak, and afterwards he could never recall the content of his thought. Determined to say something that might contain a clue, he succeeded once. His wife reported that he blurted out 'chicken feathers'!

Affective symptomatology

In discussing 'paroxysms beginning by an epigastric sensation,' Jackson noted (p. 301):

> This is often accompanied or quickly followed by an emotion of fear; the patient may look frightened... Patients have used the following expressions: 'I feel frightened,' 'dread,' 'horror,' 'perfect anguish and despair'... It may of course be suggested that the fear is a normal fear, that the patient is naturally frightened because experience tells him that a fit is coming on. Patients usually repudiate this interpretation.

This was the first assertion of ictal emotion. Twenty years later Jackson returned to this theme (p. 464):

> We have to take heed of all departures from the patient's 'ordinary state of feeling'. And it must be well borne in mind that the departure in uncinate paroxysms is in some cases towards a more pleasurable, although more often towards a more disagreeable, state. Further, what is obviously equally significant, early in the course of a case of epilepsy the feeling in the slight paroxysms may be pleasurable, and, later, disagreeable...

In this same discussion Jackson has paid lengthy tribute to Herpin for early (1867) description of a similar case of ictal fear. Subsequently, almost all identifiable emotions have been reported as ictal experiences (Williams, 1956; Daly, 1958a). In a large series of patients, Currie et al. (1971) have reported 'emotional components' in 20 per cent of CPS; of these, 80 per cent were said to be 'unpleasant'. Their study does not distinguish between subjective experiences of emotion and emotionally tinged behaviour during automatisms An incidence of 5 per cent (Williams, 1956) or 6.7 per cent (Lennox & Cobb, 1933) seems more probable. Nevertheless, all studies report fear or anxiety as the most common emotion.

The intensity of fear ranges from mild anxiety to an engulfing panic. One patient who was literally paralysed with fright said: 'I can't even speak; the terror won't let me' (Daly, 1958a). Some patients fear that they may die: Jackson's patient A.B., a physician, in some attacks experienced

'fear and a sense of impending death...' (p. 468). Children seem particularly prone to characterise their ictal fear in this way.

> Case 1, an 11-year-old girl, began coming to her mother pale and frightened, saying that she had a feeling 'like being dead'. Initially, such episodes were infrequent but later occurred several times per week. Her mother observed that the child gripped objects tightly, stared and did not respond even to a pinch on the cheek. The child pressed her lips firmly together but made no chewing or swallowing movements. An electroencephalogram showed a focus of spikes in left mid-temporal region. Since she began taking carbamazepine five years ago, the child has had no further attacks.

Pleasurable ictal emotions have received relatively less attention. Jackson remarked of one patient with déjà vu 'the sensation is to him pleasing...' (p. 297). In the Morison Lectures, Wilson (1930) commented on one patient who described her seizures as a 'dream of delight' and another who said 'I felt that I had been away somewhere in a pleasant dream, which I was enjoying to the full'. Williams (1956) noted that pleasurable emotions were frequently associated with visual hallucinations or perceptual changes. A previously reported case (Case 5, Daly, 1958a), illustrates both this and transition from an initially pleasant to unpleasant emotion.

> Case 2, a 36-year-old man, eventually proved to have an infiltrating astrocytoma of right mesial temporal lobe. In his initial attack 'suddenly the sunlight appeared to be more intense', and he felt that his perceptions were unusually acute. It seemed to him at the moment that he had viewed the same scene before, although in some strange way it was in a different place and in different circumstances. Sounds became distant. He was nauseated, sweated and had an urge to defaecate. At the same time he felt that he somehow was dissociated from his body and was looking down on the scene. During this episode he experienced a pleasurable emotion which he said was like that 'you have on a sunny day when your friends are all around you'. Several months later the emotion changed, and of it he said: 'It's like being in an old empty house on a dark rainy day, or like being in a deserted office building. It's a feeling of being alone.'

This latter emotion is best characterised as sadness or depression. Feelings described as sadness, loneliness, futility, shame or guilt have been reported by Williams (1956), Daly (1958a), Mullan and Penfield (1959) and Weil (1959). One of Williams' patients (Case 23) became depressed about an hour before her convulsions. She said the depression was 'always with the thought, half-remembered, about "Death and the World" and a compulsive urge to suicide...' Depression tends to be a more enduring emotion than fear or anxiety; in some patients depression lingers even after an automatism or convulsion.

Erotic emotions are rare ictal events. Paraesthesiae of the genitalia may result from focal seizures in somatosensory cortex (Case E.C., Penfield and Rasmussen, 1950; Case R.A., Penfield and Jasper, 1954; Daly, 1958a). Gastaut and Collomb (1954) have emphasised the important difference between subjective erotic experiences and objective sexual behaviour during automatisms. Ictal orgasmic experiences have been documented by Erickson (1945), Mulder, Daly and Bailey (1954), Freemon and Nevis (1969) and Currier *et al.* (1971). Behaviour during an automatism can clearly relate to antecedent, subjective, erotic ictal emotions (Freemon and Nevis, 1969).

Combative or resistive behaviour commonly occurs during confusional stages of automatisms. In contrast, anger as a subjective ictal emotion is extraordinarily rare – if it occurs at all. Mulder and Daly (1952) observed only one patient who characterised his emotion as 'anger.' A single patient of Williams (1956), described as 'a man with pathological tempers,' reported his feelings as follows: 'I feel most uncomfortable. I want to get away. I feel furious and have an unpleasant abdominal sensation, then a sense of terrific release, of elation.'

Ictal emotions usually intrude upon a patient's consciousness without altering perception of ongoing events. Occasionally, affect becomes integrated into perception. Williams (1956) has described a patient who said that during seizures 'his hands would seem too big, they were unnatural, he could not understand why they were there. This was accompanied by intense fear of his hands'. Two patients have said that at onset of seizures any object at which they were looking, for example, a telephone or a chair, suddenly assumed a threatening or malevolent quality totally inappropriate to its character (Daly, 1975). Shifting gaze to another object did not transfer affect; indeed, fear diminished. Returning gaze to the original object led to increasing fear, culminating in loss of consciousness and automatism. Three other patients experienced fear of external attack (Daly, 1958a). A ten-year-old boy said he felt 'as if some men were after me'; a young girl said that she had a sense of fear and a feeling that 'a man is going to grab me'. Another patient felt fear and a conviction that someone was standing behind him although he knew that this was not so. Outside in darkness, 'bushes and shadows change their appearance; they seem to be menacing figures about to attack him. Any noise, such as the rustling of leaves, was interpreted as the sounds of attackers approaching him'.

Psychosensory symptomatology

Jackson recognised a hierarchy of ictal hallucinatory experiences (p. 301): 'coloured vision – a crude sensation warning at the onset of some epileptic paroxysms – is sometimes quickly followed by "seeing faces". The mere statement declares the immense difference in elaborateness... But such elaborate phenomena as spectral faces are... less elaborate than those psychical states we have called "dreamy states," and sometimes spoken of as being voluminous'.

The ILAE classification preserves Jackson's distinctions. 'Crude sensations,' whether of sight, sound or smell, are included among elementary partial seizures. Complex, *i.e.* formed, hallucinations such as 'spectral faces' are classified as CPS under the subheading 'psychosensory symptomatology'. Also included in this category are illusions – distorted perceptions of stimuli.

A. Hallucinations

In the large series reported by Currie *et al.* (1971), sensory components occurred with about equal frequency in each modality: visual 18 per cent, auditory 16 per cent, olfactory 12 per cent, vertiginous 19 per cent and gustatory 3 per cent. However, in my experience, complex hallucinations resembling identifiable perceptions or experiences usually involve vision or hearing.

Russell and Whitty (1955) have observed: 'there is scarcely any aspect of normal vision which is not represented in one or the other of these fits'. Visual hallucinations may be of people or places. For example, one of my patients with right temporal glioma reported seeing the face of an unfamiliar woman; the face was colourless and motionless. Other patients have described landscapes in black and white or natural colours. Cushing and Eisenhardt (1938) have reported a patient with meningioma of the sphenoid ridge who during his seizures saw 'a man and a woman dressed in Louis XIV costumes slowly pass across the field from left to right, or again, a man carrying a cane accompanied by a white dog'. Jackson's description of coloured vision quickly followed by 'seeing faces' parallels Case R.W. of Penfield and Jasper (1954). 'He describes seeing coloured triangles placed irregularly over each other. The triangles flickered. This might be followed by seeing a "robber coming after him with a gun." ... During seizures, the man moved toward him ...'. One of my patients has reported that his seizures begin with coloured squares 'like a checkerboard' which rapidly change into 'stuffed animals, like children play with'. Russell and Whitty (1955) have described a patient who saw numerous small balls of light each of which transformed into a tiny man. These gradually enlarged, and the patient recognised each as an image of himself from the waist up.

In an extensive review of auditory and visual hallucinations, Penfield and Perot (1963) have reported instances of voices, sometimes familiar, calling 'incomprehensible words or phrases'. Occasionally, patients have reported comprehensible words or an entire sentence. Patients have also described hearing music or songs.

Case 3, a ten-year-old boy, had developed seizures at age six years. His first seizures had occurred during hymn singing in church; his parents observed him to stare, pale, gulp and not respond. Subsequently such seizures occurred spontaneously; these were often preceeded by buzzing, humming, or repetitive sounds which he said sounded 'like drums'. Later he reported other sounds 'like voices': sometimes only a single voice, at other times voices of two or more persons. He said that at different times he had heard voices of men, women and children. At times the voices seemed to mumble incomprehensibly, but at other times he had heard intelligible words, such as, 'boy, boy, boy' or 'don't; don't'. Initially music precipitated seizures; later sounds with semi-rhythmic features, for example, a pennant fluttering or tyres thumping on the pavement. Electroencephalograms showed a focus of spikes in the left temporal region; neuroradiological studies gave normal findings.

This patient's seizures typify most ictal auditory experiences. Seizures precipitated by complex sounds or music are relatively rare (Daly & Barry, 1957).

In summing up the character of these auditory and visual experiences, Penfield and Perot (1963) have remarked that without exception the patient passively observes, but does not participate in, these events. If the patient hears voices, he is not involved in a conversation nor does he respond.

The nature of complex hallucinatory experiences remains puzzling. Some patients insist that their experiences are memories of actual events (Mulder & Daly, 1952, Penfield & Perot, 1963, Halgren *et al.*, 1978); however, documentation often proves difficult. Occasionally a patient has reported a scene of extraordinary vividness and complexity which, despite its unchanging vividness, is clearly not a memory (Case 3, Daly, 1975). The element of 'reminiscence' can make an unfamiliar ongoing scene appear familiar; by the same token, an hallucinatory experience could be interpreted as a memory. Jackson, too, apparently doubted that seizures activated neuronal mechanisms in a normal fashion to reproduce memories (p. 295):

I believe all elaborate positive states occur from ... removal of control of higher centres. In the case mentioned [with déjà vu] ... we note that there was a double mental state: the patient had defect of object consciousness (negative) and (positive) increase of subject consciousness; in another way of stating it, he had loss of function of the now-organising nervous arrangements and increased function of the earlier organised.

B. Illusions

Most illusions involve vision or hearing. Objects may appear larger or smaller, closer or more distant. One patient said that a person's face seemed to fill her whole visual field. Light can seem brighter or colours intensify (Case 2); some patients report increased acuity of vision. To others, straight lines appear to curve or the walls of a room to bend in. One woman reported that the checked pattern on her husband's shirt appeared to 'jump about'.

As with vision, sounds may become louder or fainter, closer or more distant. At times voices appear to change pitch or take on an echoing quality.

Occasionally, somaesthetic illusions occur. A limb seems larger or smaller than normal, or occasionally a patient feels a limb is detached from his body. One patient reported that the room looked too large or too small and at the same time his teeth felt 'too large, like marbles' (Daly, 1958b). Ionasescu (1960) has described one patient who felt that his tongue and head were swelling at the same time that objects in the environment were becoming larger or smaller. Other patients reported that the nose or the right ear seemed larger than normal.

STAGE II: LOSS OF CONSCIOUSNESS (PSYCHOMOTOR SYMPTOMATOLOGY)

Abrupt but evanescent changes in behaviour signal loss of consciousness. Failure to respond (unconsciousness) was evident to Jackson and his contemporaries; however, the very brevity of these events has retarded precise and objective description. Cinematography has provided helpful but expensive, and simultaneous display of EEG was technically difficult (Ajmone-Marsan & Ralston, 1957). Television technology has resolved many problems. Multiple video cameras, split-screen display and magnetic-tape recordings allow simultaneous viewing of patient and EEG with chronographic synchronisation (Penry & Dreifuss, 1969). Because absences (ABS) occur frequently or can be readily induced by hyperventilation, they have been more extensively studied (Penry, Porter & Dreifuss, 1975). Prolonged (12 or more hours) monitoring of patients with CPS has led to a gradually enlarging 'library' of spontaneous CPS (Delgado-Escueta, 1979). Such studies have made clear that during CPS and ABS, patients show many identical elements of behaviour and similar ictal sequences suggesting that, despite divergent ictal initiation, CPS and ABS utilise common anatomic systems.

In an early study of pentylenetetrazol-induced CPS, Ajmone-Marsan and Ralston (1957) observed that 'if careful and continuous interrogation of the patient is carried out, then at least 50 per cent of automatisms... begin with a failure to respond before anything else is noted'. Unresponsiveness to all new stimuli, including superficial and deep pain, has been observed within the first two or three seconds by Escueta et al. (1977) (cf. also Case 1 who was unresponsive to a pinch on the cheek). Browne et al. (1974) have studied responsivity during ABS by measuring reaction-time to a loud tone. A threshold detector monitored the EEG permitting delivery of auditory stimuli at preselected intervals from a few to 500 ms after onset of spike-wave discharges. Reaction-times were also measured between seizures. Normal reaction-times occurred at intervals as short as 0.1 s before an ABS. If spike-wave complexes were generalised over the head, within 0.5 s patients failed to respond to 95 per cent of stimuli and remained unresponsive for the initial 2.0 s of ABS. If ABS lasted longer, responsivity returned: at 3.0 s responses occurred to 20 per cent, at 4.0 s to 33 per cent and after 4.1 s to 50 per cent of stimuli.

Arrest of ongoing motor acts, producing momentary immobility, accompanies failure to respond. Frequently patients open their eyes, and tonic contractions of the levators widen the palpebral fissures, giving an impression of staring. Commonly the pupils dilate. A similar sequence occurs at onset of ABS (Orren and Mirsky, 1975; Penry et al., 1975). This behaviour resembles the 'orienting reaction' following stimulation of the amygdala in unanesthetised animals: 'The initial phase consists of an almost immediate arrest of all spontaneous ongoing activities... the animal then exhibits signs of arousal' (Kaada 1972).

Failure to respond does not result solely from an abrupt global inability to initiate movement; on the contrary, arrest of movements follows a brief but stereotyped sequence. Failure to initiate a motor response to a new stimulus appears within one second, followed by disruption of ongoing motor acts. Orren and Mirsky (1975) observed disruption of the tracking phase of opticokinetic nystagmus after 0.5–1.2 s. Using a manual rotor-pursuit test, Goode, Penry and Dreifuss (1970) found motor errors in 70 per cent of ABS lasting less than 2.0 s and 87 per cent of ABS exceeding 3.0 s duration. Disruption of repetitive key-pressing also occurs after about 3.0 s (Mirsky & Van Buren, 1965). On the other hand, predominantly involuntary actions persist longer: respiration is arrested, invariably in expiration, or slowed after 5–10 s (Fischgold & Arfel-Capdeville, 1955; Van Buren & Ajmone-Marsan, 1960; Mirsky & Van Buren, 1965). Table 4.21 summarises the sequence of events in automatisms.

In about one-half of patients, tonic contractions

Table 4.21 Sequence and duration of events in automatisms

Time (seconds)	0	10	30	60	90+
Conscious state	Amnesic		Amnesic	Usually amnesic	Post ictal
Behaviour	Unresponsive eyes open 'stare'		Unresponsive stereotyped chewing blinking, fumbling	Responsive confused perseverative or de novo actions	± global amnesia ± Aphasia
Motor activity	Arrest		Tonic or clonic (80%) rarely: decreased		
Visceral activity					
Cardiac rate	Increased or decreased			Normal	
Vasomotor tone	Pallor or flushing			Normal	
Respiration			Slowed or arrested in expiration	Normal	

produce flexion or extension of an extremity; lateral deviation of head or eyes occurs slightly more frequently (King & Ajmone-Marsan, 1977). At times muscle tone decreases, and occasionally marked hypotonia causes a patient to fall. This seems to occur more frequently with CPS which arise in frontal lobe (Geier et al., 1977). In contrast, during ABS decreased postural tone occurs commonly (22.5 per cent) but increased tone, rarely (4.5 per cent) (Penry et al., 1975). During CPS one-third of patients show clonic contractions; only rarely (13 per cent) are these bilateral, in contrast with clonic contractions of ABS which are invariably bilateral. Unilateral contractions, whether tonic or clonic, are usually contralateral to side of origin; however, deviation of head or eyes is not reliable for lateralisation (King & Ajmone-Marsan, 1977).

Immobility and unresponsiveness to new stimuli are succeeded by a second phase with certain stereotyped actions. In speaking of the 'Uncinate Group of Fits', Jackson remarked: 'at the onset of the paroxysms... there are movements of chewing, smacking of the lips, etc. (sometimes there is spitting)' (p. 467). Repeated opening and closing of the jaws gives an impression of chewing; if accompanied by pursing of lips, the movements are usually described as 'smacking'. Some patients protrude the tongue and lick their lips, or gulp and swallow. Despite such 'alimentary automatisms', patients do not salivate. However, Hecker, Andermann and Rodin (1972) have described five patients who spat during automatisms. In my experience, spitting is not so much rare as disre-

garded by observers. King and Ajmone-Marsan (1977) have observed 'alimentary automatisms' in two thirds of patients with seizures of presumed temporal lobe origin. Penry et al. (1975) observed automatic motor acts involving face or head in 67 per cent of ABS; 'lip-smacking' and chewing accounted for 42 per cent. Repetitive blinking occurs in both CPS and ABS; in the latter, blinking results from clonic twitches synchronous with spikes of the spike-wave complex. Occasionally patients yawn or grimace.

A second type of stereotyped actions involves upper extremities. Patients may rub the face, scratch the head, pluck at clothes or fumble with a button. If a patient is holding an object, he may manipulate it purposelessly; for example, a patient may repeatedly twirl a pencil. Some patients make stereotyped rhythmic movements such as rubbing or patting their thighs. Throughout these two phases, patients are not only unresponsive to new stimuli but amnesic for all events.

In ABS, it is clear that duration of seizures determines occurrence of automatisms. Penry et al. (1975) have observed automatic actions in only 23 per cent of ABS lasting 3 s or less, in 70 per cent lasting 7–10 s but in 95 per cent of ABS lasting 15 s or more. Table 4.22 compares CPS and ABS.

A plethora of autonomic changes initiate or accompany CPS and ABS: pallor, flushing, tachycardia, bradycardia, sweating, piloerection, borborygmi, vomiting and rarely urination or defaecation (Mulder et al., 1954; Van Buren & Ajmone-Marsan, 1960; Mirsky & Van Buren,

Table 4.22 Comparison of ictal behaviour in complex partial seizures (CPS) and absences (ABS)

CPS		ABS
Yes	Aura	No
Yes	Motor arrest	Yes
Yes	Unresponsive	Yes
60–95%	Stereotyped actions	60%
Unilateral	Clonic motor activity	Bilateral
Yes	Perseverative or de novo actions	Yes
Yes	Post-ictal amnesia	No
Yes	Post-ictal aphasia	No
101 ± 47 s	Duration	mean 10.5 s
(Ajmone-Marsan & Ralston, 1957)		(Penry et al., 1975)

1965). In Jackson's time conspicuous bradycardia or pallor occasionally made difficult differentiating between seizures and cardiac syncope.

STAGE III: A STATE OF ACTIONS (AUTOMATISMS)

After 20–60 s, the second phase of stereotyped actions changes rapidly but imperceptibly into a third phase in which the patient responds but in a confused and disorganised way (Escueta et al., 1977). Jackson believed that these 'actions' were post-ictal, initiating a debate that has continued to this day (Jasper 1964). Many terms have been used for these actions: fugues, twilight states, psychic variants, psychomotor seizures (De Jong, 1957). Jackson held: 'they have one common character – they are automatic; they are done unconsciously, and the agent is irresponsible. Hence, I use the term *mental automatism*' (p. 122).

Escueta et al. (1977) believe that these three phases occur in the majority (Type I) of automatisms with CPS. However, they also have observed a small number of seizures which appeared to consist solely of 'reactive automatisms during impaired consciousness' (Type II). Both types may be observed in the same patient. A previously reported patient (Case 3, Daly, 1975) illustrates this:

Case 4, a 43-year-old petroleum geologist, had suffered brief attacks for eight years and two convulsions one year before being seen. In some of his attacks he will suddenly begin talking about topics totally irrelevant to the situation. Usually he speaks of events which have occurred long before. When his wife fails to comprehend, he seems somewhat irritated with her. On one occasion, while discussing oil wells with his business partner, he suddenly began talking about weather conditions which were not only irrelevant but inappropriate for the time of year. His wife observed a slight flushing of the face during these times. On other occasions he will stop what he is doing, stare blankly, bend his head forward and hold it in one hand although he does not seem to be in pain. He then makes one or two grunting sounds, masticatory movements, and rubs his hands on his thighs. On other occasions she has observed that he continues whatever he is doing, for example, eating, working at his drawing board, or petting their dog, but does so in a slow fashion. The episodes last 30–90 s, after which he has difficulty in finding words for another few minutes. After some attacks he dimly recalls his irrelevant remarks, but cannot remember why he made them.

Attempts to classify behaviour during automatisms have provoked extensive but largely inconclusive discussions. Jackson felt that classification was impossible; however, he offered an 'empirical grouping' of five types (p. 299):

a. The patient acts near normally; often the actions are a continuance, although in an imperfect and perhaps grotesque way, of what he was doing...before the fit.
b. The patient walks quietly on the wrong road and finds himself in some strange place; or he runs away from the place...as if terrified; or he appears to be acting as if he wanted to go home, when really he is at home.
c. We have the so-called coordinated convulsion. The patient directly after his fit...lies on the floor, sprawling about, kicking with his heels, etc.
d. She rolls about, struggling and kicking, shouting laughing, and often tries to bite. This condition in a woman is often taken for hysteria, and the mistake is easy, as the prior fit may be slight and transient. It is only for this reason that I state the condition separately from c.
e. The patient is up and about, and violently maniacal.

A conceptually similar classification has been proposed by Penry and Dreifuss (1969). They classify automatisms as:

1. *Perseverative* automatisms in which the patient continues to carry out an action initiated prior to the seizure.
2. *De novo* automatisms in which a new action is 'initiated . . . and occurs only during an ictus'. De novo automatisms further sub-divide into 'reactive', either to external or internal environmental stimuli, and 'released' in which the individual carries out actions which are normally socially inhibited.

At present, this classification seems as useful as any although it does not account for global post-ictal amnesia, an aspect to be discussed shortly. Some seizures of Case 4 can be classed as perseverative automatisms, for example, those in which he continued eating but more slowly, or continued petting their dog. Jackson has described similar actions: 'for example, a patient seized with a slight fit when about to wash himself, twirls his hands about the basin . . .' (p. 298). Jackson also suggested that ictal experiences prior to loss of consciousness might influence behaviour in automatisms: 'to discriminate betwixt the dreamy states is important for another reason. It is possible that when they are followed by loss of consciousness . . . and then by actions, some kinship may be discovered betwixt the particular *dreamy state* and what is done after a paroxysm' (p. 304). Chen and Forster (1973) have described a patient who ran during his automatisms ('cursive' epilepsy). The patient experienced an hallucinatory smell of gasoline at the onset of seizures; this recalled unhappy memories from his childhood, related to a gasoline pump on his father's farm. The patient believed that he ran during his seizures because of these memories. Forster and Liske (1963) have described even more complex actions during automatisms: an organist experienced an automatism while playing hymns during Christmas services. During the automatism, he suddenly began playing jazz but after the automatism returned to the hymn.

In *de novo* automatisms, it is not always clear what determines their content. Thus, Case 4 had no explanation for his talking about weather conditions, a topic not only irrelevant but inappropriate. Jackson has described a patient, one of whose seizures had occurred 'in a place of worship, while sitting in his pew; when his assistant spoke

to him, the patient said: "Do you want to see me on business?"'' (p. 299).

In almost one-half of 200 patients with automatisms, King and Ajmone-Marsan (1977) have observed intelligible speech regardless of hemisphere of origin, but they did not comment on its content. Sometimes the causes of *de novo* automatisms are obvious. Patients who have an automatism during an EEG will scratch their head near an electrode or tug at the wires, obviously trying to alleviate an irritating sensation.

Which actions are classified as 'released' automatisms may rest more upon cultural attitudes of witnesses than the patient. Various kinds of emotional behaviour occur during automatisms. Laughing occurred in 11 of 85 patients with automatisms of non-temporal, largely frontal, origin (Ajmone-Marsan & Goldhammer, 1973) but in only 12 of 199 patients with automatisms of temporal origin (King & Ajmone-Marsan, 1977). Weeping rarely occurs, (3 per cent in automatisms of temporal origin). Laughing and crying can occur in the same patient (Offen *et al.*, 1976; Sethi & Surya Rao, 1976). Combative behaviour occasionally occurs if patients are restrained while confused. Only rarely is combative behaviour organised and directed (Saint-Hilaire *et al.*, 1980).

Jackson recognised that patients can disrobe during automatisms. Usually, patients remove single articles of clothing, for example, a woman may remove her hat, or a man may remove his shoes or necktie. Complete disrobing is almost unknown (Rodin, 1973) and represents an extreme form of 'released' automatism. In the cases reported by Hooshmand and Brawley (1969), disrobing was interpreted as exhibitionism and lead to legal complications.

Jackson observed that, at times, after a 'slight fit' the patient could behave normally but be amnesic for considerable periods. He described an instance of this in the Harveian Lectures (p. 299); however, far more striking was the patient, himself a physician, who described in careful detail four amnesic episodes. The patient's vivid description justifies quoting fully one episode (pp. 403–4):

In October 1887, I was travelling along the Metropolitan Railway, meaning to get out at the fourth station and walk to a house half a mile off. I remember reaching the second station, and I then recollect indistinctly the onset of an 'aura', in which the conversation of two strangers in the same carriage seemed to be the repetition of something I had previously known – a recollection, in fact. The next thing of which I have any memory was that I was walking up the steps of the house (about half a mile from the fourth station) feeling in my pocket for a latch-key. I remembered almost at once that I had a *petit mal* coming on at the second station and was surprised to find myself where I was. I recollected that I had meant to reach the house not later than 12.45, and had been rather doubtful in the train whether I should be in time. I looked at my watch and found it within a minute or two of 12.45. I searched my pocket for the ticket, which was to the fourth station, found it gone and concluded that I must have passed the third station, got out at the fourth, given up my ticket and walked on as I had previously intended, though I had no memory of anything since the second station some 10 or 12 minutes previously.

On another occasion, this physician had an attack while examining a child. During this time, he examined the child, correctly made a diagnosis of 'pneumonia of the left base' and advised the mother to put the child to bed at once. He had no recollection of any of these actions.

Jackson's physician-patient precisely described his symptoms: reminiscence, 'mental diplopia', 'fear and a sense of impending death', global amnesia. Jackson meticulously reported these observations while preserving his patient's anonymity. David Taylor has sought, compassionately, to identify this tragically afflicted man (Taylor & Marsh, 1980).

Such behaviour has been clarified by the finding that bilateral hippocampal ablation in man produces a permanent amnestic syndrome (Milner, Corkin & Teuber, 1968). Walter (1973) has reported on eight patients in whom stimulation of stereotactically implanted electrodes produced unilateral afterdischarge in the hippocampus; this was followed by 'transient confusion and an amnestic state for several minutes to 2 hours...'. He postulated that 'one hippocampus is sclerotic and is the area responsible for the seizure disorder; the other hippocampus is ordinarily intact but, when subjected to the after-discharge, becomes temporarily non-functional'. A crucial study by Penfield and Mathieson (1974) has substantiated this hypothesis. Their patient had CPS some of which terminated in amnesic episodes: 'at home, he might have gone out on the porch, made an observation of the thermometer and barometer located there, and returned to the house to record his observations in the appropriate book, but he would have no recollection of these actions'. The

patient underwent left temporal lobectomy which included the hippocampus; postoperatively, the patient developed an amnestic syndrome which persisted for 13 years until his death. Autopsy showed the right hippocampus to have severe gliosis, rendering it non-functional, and the left hippocampus to have been entirely removed surgically. The behaviour of patients during such seizures resembles the syndrome of 'transient global amnesia', postulated to result from transient ischemia in 'deep temporal structures' (Rowan & Protass, 1979).

COMPLEX PARTIAL STATUS EPILEPTICUS (CPSE)

Since the early 19th century, prolonged tonic-clonic convulsions or convulsions occurring repeatedly without recovery of consciousness in the intervals have been termed status epilepticus or *état de mal*. Recognition of prolonged confusional states as non-convulsive status epilepticus became possible only with the advent of EEG. Absence status or so-called 'spike-wave stupor' was first described in 1945 by Lennox (Andermann & Robb, 1972). Originally considered rare, absence status has been described with increasing frequency; more than 400 cases have been reported since 1966 (Celesia, 1976). CPSE has been regarded as even more uncommon; Celesia was able to document only ten cases prior to his review. In reviewing 60 cases of status epilepticus seen between 1970 and 1974, he found 13 cases of absence status but only two of CPSE. Subsequently a flurry of case reports suggests that CPSE occurs more commonly than previously suspected (Belafsky et al., 1978; Engel et al., 1978; Markand et al., 1978; Mayeux & Lueders, 1978).

Altered consciousness characterises all patients during CPSE. Intervals of staring and total unresponsiveness alternate with stereotyped automatisms with masticatory movements, lip smacking and fumbling or partial responsiveness with confusion and incoherent mumbling of stereotyped but inappropriate phrases. Patients are amnesic for these episodes; in some instances, a patient can have slowly resolving retrograde and anterograde amnesia (Engel et al., 1978).

Comparable alterations of consciousness appear in absence status (Andermann & Robb, 1972). Confusion and mutism occur frequently, but occasionally patients exhibit mutism and unresponsiveness so profound as to suggest catatonic stupor. Amnesia of varying severity also occurs in absence status although instances of anterograde or retrograde amnesia have not been described. In less severe episodes, patients carry out various complex activities but with errors and patchy amnesia. Andermann and Robb (1972) have described one patient who 'decided to keep a luncheon date downtown in a department store restaurant. She went to the wrong department store, wandered about all afternoon and managed to get on the right bus home in the evening.' One of my patients on a 'bad day' drove his car to the hospital for an EEG to confirm the diagnosis! Mastication, rhythmic blinking or clonic twitching of facial muscles occur in absence status as well as CPSE. Absence status can terminate with a tonic/clonic convulsion but comparable termination of CPSE has not been reported. Some authors (Lugaresi, Pazzaglia & Tassinari, 1971; Belafsky et al., 1978) have suggested that absence status consists of a single prolonged attack rather than a series of repeated seizures; however, Andermann and Robb (1972) have commented that 'some patients have a tendency to develop frequent absence attacks interrupted by intervals of only one or few seconds. . . . Awareness is abolished during the absence and returns briefly during the intervals.' Durations of both types of status vary widely, lasting from one hour to several days or, rarely, up to two weeks. A few instances of somewhat different prolonged seizures, perhaps analogous to elementary partial status, have been described. Lugaresi et al. (1971) have described a young woman who 'for several years had seizures localised in the left side of her body. One of these seizures was followed by a prolonged confusional status with visual hallucinations restricted to the left visual field.' Henrickson (1973) has described a patient who, since childhood, had suffered CPS initiated by rising epigastric sensations and fear. At age 39 years, she complained for three months of 'an almost continuous state of anxiety which frequently rose to bouts of maximum fear without impairment of consciousness'. Fluctuations in intensity of fear paralleled changes in discharge frequency of a mesial temporal spike focus in the EEG.

Recent reports have described other forms of status epilepticus with subtly different confusional states and EEG changes (Tharp, 1972; Ellis & Lee, 1978). It seems probable that, as more instances of 'non-convulsive confusional' status are reported, our understanding and ability to differentiate various types of status will also improve. Prolonged behavioural and EEG monitoring may contribute to distinguishing them. Nevertheless, as with CPS and ABS, it appears that many behavioural elements are common to CPSE and absence status.

INTERICTAL BEHAVIOURAL CHANGE

A wide variety of undesirable behaviour has been attributed to persons with epilepsy. Stevens (1975) has compiled a list of 59 derogatory terms ranging, alphabetically, from 'adhesive' to 'wilful', including on the way, 'compulsive', 'emotional', 'impulsive' and 'stubborn'. Initially applied to all persons with epilepsy, the concept of 'epileptic personality' later came to be restricted to persons with so-called 'temporal lobe epilepsy', the majority of whom suffer automatisms. Recently, studies using carefully defined epidemiologic criteria have begun to shed light on this complicated problem. Some studies have attempted to define behavioural aberrations in standard psychiatric terms such as neurosis, psychosis and character disorder (Taylor, 1972; Rodin, 1975; Stevens, 1975). Such studies have also attempted to match patients for age, sex, duration of epilepsy, effectiveness in control of seizures and extent of brain damage as reflected, for example, by psychometric tests. Because of biases, difficult to delineate, which influence referrals of epileptic patients to specialised centres, characterising 'representative' populations becomes difficult. For example, an eightfold variation in prevalence of psychosis is found in two studies from London. In a study of 666 patients from the London Hospital, Currie et al. (1971) found psychosis in 2 per cent; in a study of 100 patients who underwent temporal lobectomy at Guy's-Maudsley, Taylor (1972) found a preoperative prevalence of 16 per cent. An explanation may lie in the fact that Guy's-Maudsley is associated with the Institute of Psychiatry and many of the patients were referred because of severe behavioural disorders as well as seizures.

The continuing studies of Rodin and Stevens have considerably illuminated the question of non-psychotic behavioural disorders. A recent study (Rodin, Katz & Lennox, 1976) has made clear that CPS *per se* are not associated with an increased incidence of behavioural disorders. This study has compared patients with 'temporal lobe seizures' to a control population of epileptic patients with other types of seizures. Epileptic patients with only CPS were not significantly different from a population of epileptic patients with only one other type of seizure. In contrast, epileptic patients with more than CPS, e.g. CPS and convulsions, had significantly greater problems in personality, work and social adjustment; in this regard, they more closely resembled those patients in the control population who had more than one type of seizure. Not surprisingly, patients with more than one 'seizure-type' took more types of antiepileptic drugs in attempting to control seizures and still had more frequent seizures. Thus, studies of Mignone, Donnelly and Sadowsky (1970), Stevens (1975) and Rodin *et al*. (1976) indicate that factors such as frequency of seizures, amount of medication, severity of brain damage (particularly if manifested by mental retardation) and impaired educational and employment background account for behavioural disorders more than epilepsy *per se*.

The question of whether psychosis, CPS and disease of the temporal lobe are related and, if so in what way, has raised extended and often confusing debates. Generally, the debate has now settled on prevalence and nature of permanent psychosis or psychotic episodes characterised by paranoid ideation, hallucinations or both which occur in settings of clear consciousness. This latter qualification excludes instances of CPSE. Certain areas of agreement exist although they cannot as yet be assembled into a parsimonious explanation. Psychosis occurs more frequently in patients with 'alien tissue' (hamartoma), particularly if they are left-handed (Taylor, 1977; Kristensen & Sindrup, 1978) and have their lesions in the left hemisphere

(Flor-Henry, 1972; Taylor, 1977). The psychosis is not a 'non-specific' organic psychosis but an 'epileptic' psychosis (Flor-Henry, 1972; Kristensen & Sindrup, 1979) which is not ameliorated by temporal lobectomy (Taylor, 1972; Jensen & Larsen, 1979). Gender may be important; if so, are females at greater risk (Taylor, 1977; Kristensen & Sindrup, 1978)? In some patients, there seems to be an inverse correlation between frequency of CPS and psychosis (Flor-Henry, 1972; Kristensen & Sindrup, 1978), recalling Landolt's concept of 'forced normalisation' of the EEG.

Ancillary to psychosis is the imputation that patients with CPS or diseased temporal lobes are singularly prone to aggression or attacks of rage and may commit crimes of violence or murder during automatisms. Although such derogations are rarely accompanied by substantiating evidence, data refuting these views have only slowly emerged. Probably this reflects little more than the reluctance of clinicians to report, and editors to publish, 'negative studies'. Kaada (1972) has commented that in animals stimulation of the amygdala never results in directed aggression even in animals normally predatory. Indeed, in man little evidence links lesions in the 'limbic system' to violent behaviour (Goldstein, 1974). Rodin (1973) has found no evidence of ictal or post-ictal aggression in photographically recorded seizures of 150 patients of whom 57 had automatisms. Further, in analysing data on 700 patients from the Epilepsy Centre of Michigan, Rodin found 4.8 per cent whose behaviour was characterised as 'destructive-assaultive'. No evidence suggested a preponderance of CPS in these patients. Gunn and Fenton (1971) have reported results of a survey of prisons and borstals in England and Wales; they identified 158 epileptic prisoners. Of these prisoners, only ten reportedly had had a seizure within 12 hours before or after the offence leading to imprisonment. Gunn and Fenton have concluded that in none was there a clear association between seizure and crime. They also studied 32 patients confined to Broadmoor Hospital because of violent crimes or behaviour; only two violent acts had occurred during post-ictal confusional states. Subsequently, Gunn (1977) has studied 158 epileptic prisoners, 180 non-epileptic prisoners and 67 epileptic patients without criminal records. No evidence suggested that violent crimes occurred more frequently in patients with CPS than in patients with other types of seizure. These various studies indicate that patients with CPS are not prone to outbursts of rage, not prone to commit violent crimes during automatisms, and that no causal association exists between epilepsy in general and criminal behaviour.

DIAGNOSTIC PROCEDURES

Today, for the large majority of patients with CPS, only two diagnostic procedures need be considered: electroencephalography (EEG) and computerised axial tomography (CT). For reasons of cost, an EEG should be done first. When properly used, EEG can provide valuable information about the underlying disorder in patients with CPS; unfortunately, too often clinicians obtain a single EEG with the idea that it will confirm or refute a suspected clinical diagnosis of epilepsy. A single EEG examination in an inter-ictal interval often shows no abnormality (Daly 1979). In a study of 308 epileptic patients, Ajmone-Marsan and Zivin (1970) found that a single EEG, including both waking and sleeping states and activation by hyperventilation and photic stimulation, yielded evidence of epileptiform activity in only 56 per cent. In a second recording made at any time subsequently, an additional 26 per cent of patients had a 'positive recording'. In a more intensively studied sub-group of 79 patients with repeated EEGs over an interval of more than one year, they found a 'positive recording' in 92 per cent of patients. These EEG findings are strikingly similar to those of Currie et al. (1971): of 666 patients diagnosed clinically as 'temporal lobe epilepsy', 92 per cent had 'definite' temporal foci in the EEG. Of these, foci of sharp waves or spikes occurred in 30 per cent, of 'slow waves' in 40 per cent and a mixture of both in 30 per cent.

It is commonly argued that a normal inter-ictal EEG results from 'suppressive' effects of anti-epileptic drugs. The study of Ajmone-Marsan and Zivin (1970) does not substantiate this conclusion. Subsequently, Ludwig and Ajmone-Marsan (1975) have reviewed the effects on EEG of withdrawing antiepileptic drugs in 55 patients with intractable partial seizures. The most common effect was 'non-specific' activation, found in 63 per cent, consisting of generalised spike-and-slow-wave or sharp-and-slow-wave complexes. 'Focal' activation of the EEG was found in only 25 per cent. These studies suggest that repeating an EEG is far more likely to provide useful information than withdrawing medication and avoids the danger of precipitating a burst of seizures or even status epilepticus.

If the waking EEG is within normal limits, sleep as an activating procedure is not particularly effective, eliciting epileptiform discharge in less than 10 per cent of patients (Currie et al., 1971; Klass, 1975). Similarly hyperventilation induces abnormalities or seizures in only 10 per cent of patients with a normal resting EEG (Miley & Forster, 1977). Klass (1975), without giving figures, is more sanguine, observing 'activation of focal temporal abnormalities...occurs often enough to warrant use of hyperventilation routinely for these patients'.

The characteristics of epileptiform discharges can provide useful clues as to aetiology. In summarising a large number of studies, Klass (1975) has reported that bilateral abnormality in the temporal regions was reported in 25–30 per cent of patients; Currie et al. (1971) report 19 per cent. No patient with independent bitemporal discharges has been found to harbour a neoplasm. In a study of patients who underwent temporal lobectomy, Engel, Driver and Falconer (1975) have reported that the EEGs of all patients with hamartomas, or 'alien tissue', had primary medial temporal foci ('medial' being defined as maximum voltage of the generator occurring at a sphenoidal electrode) but that none showed secondary contralateral extra-temporal foci. All patients with mesial temporal sclerosis also showed primary medial temporal foci but occasionally showed secondary contralateral extra-temporal foci. In contrast, no patient with an atrophic lesion on the convexity of the temporal lobe showed a primary medial focus. Klass (1975) offers appropriate cautions about the approximately 25 per cent of patients who will show non-specific paroxysmal discharges such as 'small sharp spikes' or 14 and 6 Hz positive spikes.

CT has dramatically improved the ability to visualise intracranial structures. It is too soon for definitive evaluation, but clearly selected categories of patients with epilepsy have 'high yields' on CT. Gastaut and Gastaut (1976) have reported CT findings in 401 of 500 consecutive epileptic patients seen in a six month period. Of 84 patients with CPS, 60 per cent had abnormal CTs, the abnormality being focal in 36 per cent and diffuse in 24 per cent. Surprisingly, tumours were found in 11 per cent of all patients and in 16 per cent of patients over 20 years of age. In summarising the findings in 1700 patients from seven centres, Gastaut (1976) has noted that in 'partial epilepsies', tumours were found in 22 per cent. The comparable figure from the study of Currie *et al.* (1971), prior to the introduction of CT, was 9.5 per cent. This suggests that use of CT in patients with CPS has strikingly improved our ability to identify causes of these epilepsies.

EEG can help in selecting patients for CT study. Yang *et al.* (1979) have reported studies on 256 infants and children with seizures. In children with CPS, EEG was abnormal in 82 per cent and CT was abnormal in 30 per cent. If the EEG showed focal slowing, abnormal CTs were found in 63 per cent. In contrast, if neurologic examination and EEG were within normal limits, 95 per cent of CTs gave normal findings. In children,

CTs have been particularly helpful in identifying previously unrecognised cases of tuberous sclerosis.

In summary, EEG and CT studies provide safe, non-invasive and repeatable evaluations of the brain. Their use will permit determination of the cause of seizures in a much higher percentage of patients with CPS and early identification of patients with surgically remediable lesions. In passing, it should be noted that the results of surgical excision of low-grade gliomas which present with intractable seizures are as good as resections of atrophic lesions (Rasmussen, 1975).

EPILOGUE

Jackson was one of the major figures of nineteenth century neurology. However, today, as in the day of Sir Henry Head, too few neurologists know at first-hand Jackson's writings. His precise observations and extraordinary powers of analysis enabled him to describe fully and to explain the ictal phenomena we now call complex partial seizures. In this review I have attempted to illuminate his contributions and to pay tribute to this remarkable man. I hope that readers will be encouraged to meet him directly, in his writings.

REFERENCES

Ajmone-Marsan, C. & Goldhammer, L. (1971) Clinical ictal patterns and electrographic data in cases of partial seizures of frontal-central-parietal origin. In Brazier, M.A.B. (ed.) *Epilepsy: Its Phenomena in Man*, p. 236. New York: Academic Press.

Ajmone-Marsan, C. & Ralston, B.L. (1957) *The Epileptic Seizure: Its Functional Morphology and Diagnostic Significance.* Springfield, Illinois: Charles C. Thomas.

Ajmone-Marsan, C. & Zivin, L.S. (1970) Factors related to the occurrence of typical paroxysmal abnormalities in the EEG records of epileptic patients. *Epilepsia*, 11:361.

Andermann, F. & Robb, J.P. (1972) Absence Status – A reappraisal following review of thirty-eight patients. *Epilepsia*, **13**, 17.

Bancaud, J., Talairach, J., Geier, S. & Scarabin, J.N. (1973) *EEG et STEEG dans les Tumeurs Cerebrales et l'Epilepsie.* Paris: Edifor.

Belafsky, M.A., Carwille, S., Miller, P., Waddell, G., Boxley-Johnson, J. & Delgado-Escueta, A.V. (1978) Prolonged epileptic twilight states: continuous recordings with nasopharyngeal electrodes and video-taped analysis. *Neurology*, **28**, 239.

Browne, T.R., Penry, J.K., Porter, R.J. & Dreifuss, F.E. (1974) Responsiveness before, during and after spike-wave paroxysms. *Neurology*, **24**, 659.

Celesia, G.G. (1976) EEG Monitoring in Status Epilepticus. In Janz, D. (ed.) *Epileptology: Proceedings of the 7th International Symposium on Epilepsy*, p. 328. Struttgart: Thieme Publishers.

Chen, R.C. & Forster, F.M. (1973) Cursive epilepsy and gelastic epilepsy. *Neurology*, **23**, 1019.

Currie, S., Heathfield, K.W.G., Henson, R.A. & Scott, D.F. (1971) Clinical course and prognosis of temporal lobe epilepsy: A survey of 666 patients. *Brain* **94**, 173.

Currier, R.D., Little, S.C., Suess, J.F. & Andy, O.J. (1971) Sexual seizures. *Archives of Neurology*, **25**, 260.

Cushing, H. & Eisenhardt, L. (1938) *Meningiomas.* Springfield, Illinois: Charles C. Thomas.

Daly, D. (1958a) Ictal affect. *American Journal of Psychiatry*, **115**, 97.

Daly, D. (1958b) Uncinate fits. *Neurology*, **8**, 250.

Daly, D.D. (1975) Ictal clinical manifestations of complex partial seizures. In Penry J.K. & Daly, D.D. (eds) *Complex Partial Seizures and their Treatment*, p. 57. New York: Raven Press.

Daly, D.D. (1979) Use of the EEG for Diagnosis and Evaluation of Epileptic Seizures and Nonepileptic Episodic Disorders. In Klass, D.W. & Daly D.D. (eds) *Current*

Practice of Clinical Electroencephalography, p. 221. New York: Raven Press.

Daly, D. & Barry, M.J. (1957) Musicogenic Epilepsy: Report of three cases. *Psychosomatic Medicine*, **19**, 399.

DeJong, R.N. (1957) Psychomotor or temporal lobe epilepsy. *Neurology*, **7**, 1.

Delgado-Escueta, A.V. (1979) Epileptogenic paroxysms: Modern approaches and clinical correlations. *Neurology*, **29**, 1014.

Ellis, J.M. & Lee, S.I. (1978) Acute prolonged confusion in later life as an ictal state. *Epilepsia*, **19**, 119.

Engel, J., Driver, M.V. & Falconer, M. (1975) Electrophysiological correlates of pathology and surgical results in temporal lobe epilepsy. *Brain*, **98**, 129.

Engel, J., Ludwig, B.I. & Fetell, M. (1978) Prolonged partial complex status epilepticus: EEG and behavioural observations. *Neurology*, **28**, 863.

Erickson, T.C. (1945) Erotomania (nymphomania) as an expression of cortical epileptiform discharge. *Archives of Neurology and Psychiatry*, **53**, 226.

Escueta, A.V., Kunze, U., Waddel, G., Boxley, J. & Nadel, A. (1977) Lapse of consciousness and automatisms in temporal lobe epilepsy: A video-tape analysis. *Neurology*, **27**, 144.

Fischgold, H. & Arfel-Capdeville, M. (1955) Modifications respiratoires dans les paroxysmes épileptiques. *Electroencephalography and Clinical Neurophysiology*, **7**, 165.

Flor-Henry, P. (1972) Ictal and interictal psychiatric manifestations in epilepsy: specific or non-specific? *Epilepsia*, **13**, 773.

Forster, F.M. & Liske, E. (1962) Role of environmental clues in temporal lobe epilepsy. *Neurology*, **13**, 301.

Freemon, F.R. & Nevis, A.H. (1969) Temporal lobe sexual seizures. *Neurology*, **19**, 87.

Gastaut, H. (1970) Clinical and electroencephalographical classification of epileptic seizures. *Epilepsia*, **11**, 102.

Gastaut, H. (1976) Conclusions: Computerised transverse axial tomography in epilepsy. *Epilepsia*, **17**, 377.

Gastaut, H. & Collomb, H. (1954) Etude du comportement sexuel chez les epileptiques psychomoteurs. *Annales Medico-Psychologiques*, **112**, 696.

Gastaut, H. & Gastaut J.L. (1976) Computerised transverse axial tomography in epilepsy. *Epilepsia*, **17**, 325.

Geier, S., Bancaud, J., Talairach, J., Bonis, A., Enjelvin, M. & Hossard-Bouchaud, H. (1976) Automatisms during frontal lobe epileptic seizures. *Brain*, **99**, 447.

Geier, S., Bancaud, J., Talairach, J., Bonis, A., Szikla, G. & Enjelvin, M. (1977) The seizures of frontal lobe epilepsy: A study of clinical manifestations. *Neurology*, **27**, 951.

Gloor, P. (1975) Physiology of the limbic system. In Penry, J.K. & Daly, D.D. (eds) *Complex Partial Seizures and Their Treatment*, p. 27. New York: Raven Press.

Goldstein, M. (1974) Brain research and violent behaviour. *Archives of Neurology*, **30**, 1.

Goode, D.J., Penry, J.K. & Dreifuss, F.E. (1970) Effects of paroxysmal spike-wave on continuous visual-motor performance. *Epilepsia*, **11**, 241.

Gunn, J. (1977) *Epileptics in Prison*, p. 6. London: Academic Press.

Gunn, J. & Fenton, G. (1971) Epilepsy, automatism, and crime. *Lancet* **1**, 1173.

Halgren, E., Walter, R.D., Cherlow, D.G. & Crandall, P. (1978) Mental phenomena evoked by electrical stimulation of the human hippocampal formation and amygdala. *Brain*, **101**, 83.

Head, H.H. (1915) Hughlings Jackson on aphasia and kindred affections of speech. *Brain*, **38**, 1.

Hecker, A., Andermann, F. & Rodin, E.A. (1972) Spitting automatisms in temporal lobe seizures with a brief review of ethological and phylogenetic aspects of spitting. *Epilepsia*, **13**, 767.

Henriksen, G.F. (1973) Status epilepticus partialis with fear as clinical expression. *Epilepsia*, **14**, 39.

Hooshmand, H. & Brawley, B.W. (1969) Temporal lobe seizures and exhibitionism. *Neurology*, **19**, 1119.

Ionasescu, V. (1960) Paroxysmal disorders of the body image in temporal lobe epilepsy. *Acta Psychiatrica Scandinavia*, **35**, 171.

Jasper, H.H. (1964) Some physiological mechanisms involved in epileptic automatisms. *Epilepsia*, **5**, 1.

Jensen, I., & Larsen, J.K. Mental aspects of temporal lobe epilepsy: (1979) Follow-up of 74 patients after resection of a temporal lobe. *Journal of Neurology, Neurosurgery and Psychiatry*, **42**, 256.

Kaada, B.R. (1972) Stimulation and regional ablation of the amygdaloid complex with reference to functional representations. In Eleftheriou, B.E. (ed.) *The Neurobiology of the Amygdala*, p. 205. New York: Plenum Press.

King, D.W. & Ajmone-Marsan, C. (1977) Clinical features and ictal patterns in epileptic patients with EEG temporal lobe foci. *Annals Neurology*, **2**, 138.

Klass, D.W. (1975) Electroencephalographic manifestations of complex partial seizures. In Penry J.K. and Daly D.D. (eds) *Complex Partial Seizures and their Treatment*, p. 113. New York: Raven Press.

Kristensen, O & Sindrup, E.H. (1978) Psychomotor epilepsy psychosis. *Acta Neurologica Scandinavica*, **57**, 361.

Kristensen, O. & Sindrup E.H. (1979) Psychomotor epilepsy and psychosis. III. Social and Psychological Correlates. *Acta Neurologica Scandinavica*, **59**, 1.

Lennox, W.G. & Cobb, S. (1933) Epilepsy: XIII. Aura in epilepsy: A statistical review of 1,359 cases. *Archives of Neurology and Psychiatry*, **30**, 374.

Ludwig, B., Ajmone-Marsan, C. & Van Buren, J. (1975) Cerebral seizures of probable orbitofrontal origin. *Epilepsia*,

Ludwig, B.I. & Ajmone-Marsan, C. (1975) EEG changes after withdrawal of medication in epileptic patients. *Electroencephalography and Clinical Neurophysiology*, **39**, 173.

Lugaresi, E., Pazzaglia, P. & Tassinari, C.A. (1971) Differentiation of 'absence status' and 'temporal lobe status'. *Epilepsia*, **12**, 77.

Markand, O.N., Wheeler, G.L. & Pollack, S.L. (1978) Complex partial status epilepticus (psychomotor status). *Neurology*, **28**, 189.

Mayeux, R. & Leuders, H. (1978) Complex partial status epilepticus: Case report and proposal for diagnostic criteria. *Neurology*, **28**, 957.

Mignone, R.J., Donnelly, E.F. & Sadowsky, D. (1970) Psychological and neurological comparisons of psychomotor and non-psychomotor epileptic patients. *Epilepsia*, **11**, 345.

Miley, C.E. & Forster, F.M. (1977) Activation of partial complex seizures by hyperventilation. *Neurology*, **34**, 371.

Milner, B., Corkin, S. & Teuber, H.L. (1968) Further analysis of the hippocampal amnesic syndrome: 14 year follow-up study of H.M. *Neuropsychologia*, **6**, 215.

Mirsky, A.F. & Van Buren, J.M. (1965) On the nature of the 'absence' in centrencephalic epilepsy: A study of some behavioural, EEG and autonomic factors. *Electroencephalography and Clinical Neurophysiology*, **18**, 334.

Mulder, D.W. & Daly, D. (1952) Psychiatric symptoms

associated with lesions of temporal lobe. *Journal of the American Medical Association*, **150**, 173.

Mulder, D.W., Daly, D. & Bailey, A.A. (1954) Visceral epilepsy. *Archives of Internal Medicine*, **93**, 481.

Mullan, S. & Penfield, W. (1959) Illusions of comparative interpretation and emotion. *Archives of Neurology and Psychiatry*, **81**, 269.

Offen, M.L., Davidoff, R.A., Troost, B.T. & Richey, E.T. (1976) Dacrystic epilepsy. *Journal of Neurology, Neurosurgery and Psychiatry*, **39**, 829.

Orren, M.M. & Mirsky, A.F. (1975) Relations between ocular manifestations and onset of spike-and-wave discharges in petit mal epilepsy. *Epilepsia*, **16**, 771.

Penfield, W. & Jasper, H. (1954) *Epilepsy and the Functional Anatomy of the Human Brain*. Boston: Little, Brown and Co

Penfield, W. & Mathieson, G. (1974) Memory. *Archives of Neurology* (Chicago), **31**, 145.

Penfield, W. & Perot, P. (1963) The brain's record of auditory and visual experience – a final summary and discussion. *Brain*, **86**, 595.

Penfield, W. & Rasmussen, T. (1950) *The Cerebral Cortex of Man*. New York: Macmillan.

Penry, J.K. & Dreifuss, F.E. (1969): Automatisms associated with the absence of petit mal epilepsy. *Archives of Neurology*, **21**, 142.

Penry, J.K., Porter, R.J. & Dreifuss, F.E. (1975) Simultaneous recording of absence seizures with videotape and electroencephalography: A study of 374 seizures in 48 patients. *Brain*, **98**, 427.

Rasmussen T. (1975) Surgical Treatment of Patients with Complex Partial Seizures. In Penry J.K. & Daly, D.D. (eds) *Complex Partial Seizures and Their Treatment*, p. 415. New York: Raven Press.

Rodin, E.A. (1973) Psychomotor epilepsy and aggressive behaviour. *Archives of General Psychiatry*, **28**, 210.

Rodin E.A. (1975) Psychosocial Management of Patients with Complex Partial Seizures. In Penry J.K. & Daly, D.D. (eds) *Complex Partial Seizures and their Treatment*, p. 383. New York: Raven Press.

Rodin, E.A., Katz, M., and Lennox, K. (1976) Differences between patients with temporal lobe seizures and those with other forms of epileptic attacks. *Epilepsia*, **17**, 313.

Rowan, A.J. & Protass, L.M. (1979) Transient global amnesia: Clinical and electroencephalographic findings in 10 cases. *Neurology*, **29**, 869.

Russell, W.R. & Whitty, C.W.M. (1955) Studies in traumatic epilepsy: 3. Visual fits. *Journal of Neurology, Neurosurgery and Psychiatry*, **18**, 79–96.

Saint-Hilaire, J.M., Gilbert, M., Bouvier, G. & Barbeau, A. (1980) *Epilepsy and aggression*. In press.

Sethi, P.K. & Surya Rao, T. (1976) Gelastic, quiritarian, and cursive epilepsy: A clinicopathological appraisal. *Journal of Neurology, Neurosurgery and Psychiatry*, **39**, 823.

Stevens, J.R. (1975) Interictal Clinical Manifestations of Complex Partial Seizures. In: Penry J.K. & Daly D.D. (eds) *Complex Partial Seizures and their Treatment*. New York: Raven Press.

Taylor, D.C. (1972) Mental state in temporal lobe epilepsy: A correlative account of 100 patients treated surgically. *Epilepsia*, **13**, 727.

Taylor, D.C. (1977) Epileptic experience, schizophrenia and the temporal lobe. *McLean Hospital Journal*, Special Issue, 22.

Taylor, D.C. & Marsh, S.M. (1980) Hughlings Jackson's Dr Z: the paradigm of temporal lobe epilepsy revealed. *Journal of Neurology, Neurosurgery and Psychiatry*, **43**, 758.

Taylor, J. (ed.) (1931) Lectures on the diagnosis of epilepsy (Harveian Society) In *Selected Writings of John Hughlings Jackson*, Vol. 1, p. 276. London: Hodder & Stoughton.

Tharp, B.R. (1972) Orbital frontal seizures: An unique electroencephalographic and clinical syndrome. *Epilepsia*, **13**, 627.

Van Buren, J.M., and Ajmone-Marsan, C. (1960) A correlation of autonomic and EEG components in temporal lobe epilepsy. *Archives of Neurology*, **3**, 683.

Walter, R.D. (1973) Tactical considerations leading to surgical treatment of limbic epilepsy. In Brazier M.A.B. (ed.) *Epilepsy: Its Phenomena in Man*, p. 99. New York: Academic Press.

Weil, A.A. (1959) Ictal emotions occurring in temporal lobe dysfunction. *Archives of Neurology*, **1**, 101.

Williams, D. (1956) The structure of emotions reflected in epileptic experiences. *Brain*, **79**, 29.

Wilson, S.A.K. (1930) Morison Lectures: On nervous semeiology with special references to epilepsy. *British Medical Journal*, **2**, 50.

Yang, P.J., Berger, P.E., Cohen, M.E. & Duffner, P.K. (1979) Computed tomography and childhood seizure disorders. *Neurology*, **29**, 1084.

PART THREE
POST-TRAUMATIC EPILEPSY

B. Jennett

Only a small proportion of head injured patients suffer from fits once they have recovered from the acute stage of the injury. However, head injuries are so common an occurrence that this comprises a size-able number of patients. Most patients are young and in many their susceptibility to fits persists, so that the prevalence of post-traumatic epilepsy is considerable. The significance of even occasional fits to the individual in modern westernised societies has been enhanced by the dependence on car driving as part of many people's lives and livelihoods. For many patients with traumatic epilepsy this is the only serious sequel to their accident, and this likewise emphasises its importance.

With only a fraction of the population at risk of

developing epilepsy, and then often only after a delay of a year or more, there is a premium on the ability of doctors to predict which patients will be affected. Identification of such patients soon after injury makes it possible to give practical advice about the future, in respect of both work and of leisure activities; and to attempt to prevent this complication by giving prophylactic anticonvulsants. A survey of the practice of American neurosurgeons revealed that many failed to protect their head injured patients with antiepileptic drugs, usually because they were uncertain about which patients were at risk, or believed that the risk overall was too low to justify medication (Rapport & Penry, 1972). However, reliable statistics are now available about epilepsy after civilian injuries, to match those published about military injuries after successive wars. The most comprehensive civilian series is that of Jennett (1962,

1975), many of whose findings have subsequently been confirmed by others. This chapter will review the phenomenology of traumatic epilepsy after non-missile injury, making some comparisons with missile injuries; it will outline the prediction rules which have now emerged and which make it possible to assess the risk for an individual patient soon after injury; and will conclude with comments about the strategy of prophylaxis.

EARLY TRAUMATIC EPILEPSY

Fits in the early stages after injury are often considered as a separate category, usually with the implication that fits at this time are of little importance. But how early is early? And do these early fits really not matter?

After both non-missile and missile head injuries fits very much more often begin in the first week

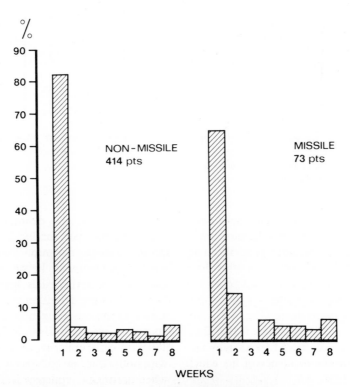

WEEK OF FIRST FIT
(as % of all epilepsy
beginning within 8 weeks)

Fig. 4.2 Week of first fit, as a percentage of all epilepsy beginning within eight weeks

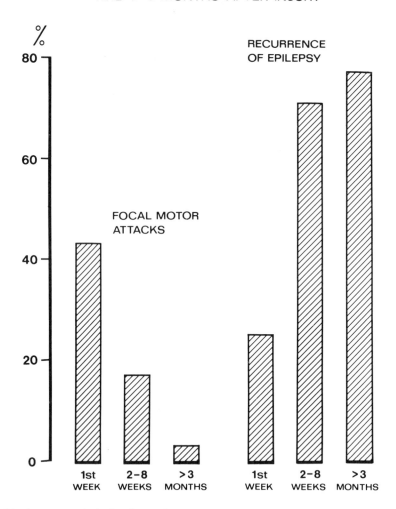

EPILEPSY IN FIRST FEW WEEKS
AND > 3 MONTHS AFTER INJURY

Fig. 4.3 Incidence of focal motor attacks in first few weeks or greater than three months after injury; and the incidence of subsequent epilepsy according to the time of the first fit

than in any of the subsequent seven weeks (Fig. 4.2). These first week fits are much more often limited to focal twitching (without generalisation) than are fits in the next seven weeks, or after three months (Fig. 4.3). Subsequent recurrence of epilepsy is much less common after fits in the first week than when fits occur later (Fig. 4.3). Yet another feature of fits in the first week is that their incidence is differently influenced by various factors, as compared with the incidence of fits which occur later (Table 4.23).

For these various reasons it was proposed by Jen-

nett (1962) that the definition of early epilepsy should be reserved for fits in the first week after injury. Prior to that publication there was considerable disagreement between different authors, but since then there has been acceptance of the first week as the definition for early epilepsy (Table 4.24). In our investigation of 800 patients with epilepsy after non-missile injuries there were over 400 with early epilepsy, over 400 with late and 90 with both. It is late epilepsy which is usually meant when traumatic epilepsy is discussed – because it is this which constitutes persisting disability.

Table 4.23 Influence of various factors on the incidence of early and late epilepsy following non-missile head injury from Jennett, 1975

	Early	Late
Age		
< 5 years	9%	16%
> 5 years	4%	19%
	< 0.05	NS
PTA < 24 hours		
No depressed fracture	2%	6%
Depressed fracture	9%	9%
	<0.001	NS
PTA > 24 hours		
No depressed fracture	10%	9%
Depressed fracture	12%	32%
	NS	< 0.001
Non-missile depressed fracture		
Dura intact	8%	7%
Dura torn	11%	24%
	NS	< 0.001
Missile depressed fracture		
Dura intact	12%	13%
Dura torn	8%	40%
	NS	< 0.001
No depressed fracture/haematoma		
PTA < 24 hours	2%	1%
PTA > 24 hours	9%	5%
	<0.001	< 0.05

Table 4.24 Definitions of early epilepsy in reported series (from Jennett, 1975)

Author	Year	Interval
Ascroft	1941	1 week
Whitty	1947	10 days
Russell & Whitty	1952	1 month
Phillips	1954	14 days
Caveness	1963	14 days
Evans	1963	18 days
Hendrick & Harris	1968	1 week
Courjon	1969	1 week
Stowsand & Bues	1970	1 week
Adeloye & Odeku	1971	1 week
Rish & Caveness	1972	1 week
Braakman	1972	1 week
Jamieson & Yelland	1972	1 week

In half the patients with early epilepsy, the first fit occurs within 24 hours of injury, and in half of these

it is in the first hour. More than half the affected patients have some fits which are focal, at least at onset; and three-quarters of these are limited focal motor attacks. About a third of patients have only a single fit in the first week, but 10 per cent have status, which is commoner under five years of age.

Early epilepsy occurs in about 5 per cent of patients admitted with a head injury to hospital, according to a number of reports from neurosurgeons (Table 4.25). Although these series did

Table 4.25 Incidence of early epilepsy following head injury

Type of patient	n	% with epilepsy	Author
Conservative admission (non-missile)	1000	4.6%	Jennett (1975)
Vietnam military	1030	4.5%	Caveness *et al* (1979)
Admissions	1000	4%	Courjon (1969)
Adult admissions	2354	2%	Stowsand & Bues (1970)
Admissions			
aged < 15 years	814	7%	
> 15 years	4195	5%	Hendrick & Harris (1968)
< 5 years	75	9%	
< 5 years	911	4%	Jennett (1975)

include many mild injuries it seems certain that some degree of selection operated (if only by the inclusion of a proportion of patients transferred from other hospitals because their injuries were more severe). Early epilepsy is more common in patients with intracranial haematoma, with depressed skull fracture, with prolonged post-traumatic amnesia (PTA), and in young children. The epilepsy rate is therefore higher in neurosurgical units which operate a selective admission policy. In Scottish neurosurgical units, which accept less than 5 per cent of all head injured patients admitted to hospital, the early epilepsy rate is 13 per cent (Jennett *et al.*, 1979). By the same token the epilepsy rate is lower (*c*. 1 per cent) in the primary surgical wards to which the vast majority of head injured patients are admitted (in Britain).

Early epilepsy has significance both immediately and for the future. It may confuse the clinical picture in the acute stage, by causing temporary deepening of the conscious state and the appearance of focal signs. When status occurs in children there may be secondary brain damage due to hypoxia or ischaemia. But the most important implication of a fit in the first week is the increased risk of late epilepsy – overall about four times as great as when a fit has not occurred in the first week.

LATE TRAUMATIC EPILEPSY

The incidence of late epilepsy varies greatly according to the nature of the injury – that is what makes it possible to calculate different risk rates for individual patients. The overall incidence therefore depends crucially on the composition of the population; it is about 3 per cent for all hospital admissions in Britain, where many mildly injured patients are taken in for 24– 48 hours; but for a neurosurgical unit with a selective admission policy about 16 per cent of patients will likely develop epilepsy after the first week. For certain patients with depressed fracture, and for those who have had an intracranial haematoma evacuated within 14 days of injury, the rate is much higher. It may be therefore that the risk of epilepsy after civilian injuries is less different from that of military injuries than was previously supposed – if care is taken to compare like with like. Indeed, Caveness *et al*. (1979) has drawn attention to the close parallel between the epilepsy rate in the Vietnam series (93 per cent of which were missile injuries) and the non-missile depressed fractures and haematomas previously reported by Jennett (1975) (Table 4.26). The incidence of early epilepsy was also very similar (Table 4.25; Fig. 4.2).

Features of late epilepsy

More than half the patients who develop this complication have their first fit within a year of injury. However, more than a quarter do not begin until more than four years after injury, and there is always a small continuing risk. Obviously the incidence rate, and the proportion occurring in the first year, depend on the duration of follow-up; variations in this account for some of the discrepancies between different reports.

Focal features occur, at least at the onset of seizures, in about 40 per cent of patients, and a fifth of patients have temporal lobe attacks. It is sometimes asserted that epilepsy reflects a temporary event at a certain stage of the recovery process. Assessment of the tendency of fits to continue will vary according to the duration of follow-up after the first seizure. If the severity is expressed as the number of first fits during a certain interval since injury (say two or four years) this will underestimate the disability in a patient whose first fit occurs late in this period, but who then continues to have frequent epilepsy. Not uncommonly there is a two year remission which is followed by a recurrence of epilepsy. In our study of patients who were followed for two to five years after their first late fit, 80 per cent were found to continue to have some fits; more than a third had frequent fits (Jennett, 1975).

Prediction of late epilepsy

The risk that late epilepsy will develop varies greatly

Table 4.26 Incidence of late epilepsy in first five years after military and civilian injuries (from Caveness *et al*., 1979)

	Vietnam Cases 1030		*Jennett's Cases* 1005 depressed fracture 420 intracranial haematomas	
	n	*cumulative incidence*	*n*	*cumulative incidence*
< 1 year	192	67%	268	66%
1–2 years	62	89%	62	81%
2–3 years	19	95%	40	91%
3–4 years	7	98%	20	96%
4–5 years	7	100%	18	100%
		overall incidence		*overall incidence*
	287	(28%)	408	(29%)

Table 4.27 Risk of late epilepsy after certain injuries

	n	
*Acute intracranial haematoma	128	35%
No haematoma	854	3%
After early epilepsy	238	25%
No early epilepsy	868	3%
Depressed fracture	447	17%
No depressed fracture	832	4%
In patients with neither haematoma nor depressed fracture		
After early epilepsy	124	19%
No early epilepsy	168	1%

*Evacuated within 14 days of injury
All differences significant (P < 0.001)

according to the nature of the injury and early complications (Table 4.27). Three factors dominate: the presence of a depressed fracture, the development of early epilepsy, and the need to evacuate an intracranial haematoma within two weeks of injury (70 per cent of which operations are done in the first week). In most cases therefore a prediction can be made within a week of injury. Patients with haematoma or with early epilepsy have an approximately similar likelihood of developing epilepsy whatever the other features of their injury are. This is not so for patients with depressed fracture – whose risk ranges from less than 3 per cent to over 60 per cent according to various combinations of other features (Fig. 4.4). Depressed fractures associated with a high risk occur relatively seldom (Fig. 4.4); it is therefore possible to reassure some 40 per cent of patients with depressed fracture that there is very little chance that they will develop epilepsy.

The risk of late epilepsy in patients without depressed fracture or intracranial haematoma is less than 2 per cent, even when PTA exceeds 24 hours,

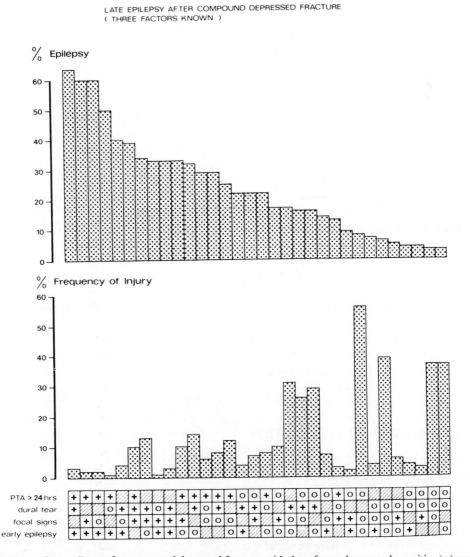

Fig. 4.4 Incidence of late epilepsy after compound depressed fracture, with three factors known to be positive (+) or negative (0).

unless there has been an early fit. It is no more valid to claim that 'severe injuries' have a high probability of epilepsy than it is to claim this for depressed fractures as a whole. There is now enough evidence to make an accurate prediction of the risk in an individual patient a week after injury.

Effect of early management on late epilepsy

The treatment of recently injured patients has improved over the years and this is particularly evident in the statistics from successive wars. Infection of open cranio-cerebral injuries has become much less common, and in the Korean and Vietnam campaigns was eventually as low as 1 per cent. In spite of this there has been no change in the frequency of late epilepsy (Table 4.28), which is pre-

Table 4.28 Incidence of epilepsy after missile injuries in three wars (from Jennett, 1975)

	World War I Ascroft (316)	World War II Walker (295)	World War II Russell (820)	Korea Caveness (211)
All cases	35%	34%	—	35%
Dura torn	41%	—	43%	42%

sumably related to the degree of brain damage and the constitutional susceptibility of the patient. Similarly, in civilian series, the epilepsy rate is similar in those whose depressed fractures had not been elevated and in those subjected to surgery; in those which had been debrided, epilepsy was equally frequent whether or not the bone fragments were replaced or removed (Jennett, 1975). Again the assumption is that epilepsy relates to the brain damage sustained at impact, not to the continued presence of depressed bone.

CONTRIBUTION OF EEG TO PREDICTION

In the early stages after head injury of significant degree many patients have an abnormal EEG, which reflects the brain damage sustained. As time passes the abnormalities become less marked, and in many patients they disappear. Most of the patients who develop late epilepsy continue to have an abnormal EEG – but the difference between this proportion

and that in patients without epilepsy becomes statistically significant only after the first year (since injury). Although patients who have already developed post-traumatic (late) epilepsy more often have an abnormal EEG, this is not of predictive value. About a fifth of patients with late epilepsy have had a normal EEG within a few weeks of injury, whilst many patients with abnormal records in the first year (or even later) never develop epilepsy. Several other authors have expressed the view that EEG is of little use in predicting the likelihood of late traumatic epilepsy developing in the future (Walton, 1963; Courjon, 1969; Terespolsky, 1972).

CHILDREN

Early epilepsy is more common in children (less than 16 years) but on closer examination it is evident that this is due mostly to the more frequent occurrence of fits after mild injuries in young children (less than five years). This finding of Jennett (1975) has been confirmed in two other large studies of children (Stowsand, 1971; Hendrick & Harris, 1968). The only adults encountered with epilepsy after a trivial injury are those with 'immediate' epilepsy – when a fit occurs at the moment the head sustains an impact, a rare event.

Late epilepsy occurs less frequently in patients who were under 16 years at the time of injury; however, the occurrence of an early fit still increases the risk of late epilepsy significantly (Table 4.29). Late epilepsy is a risk even in children under five

Table 4.29 Incidence of late epilepsy (from Jennett, 1975)

	Jennett > 16 years		Jennett < 16 years		Stowsand < 15 years	
No early epilepsy	21/638	3%	8/230	4%	8/230	4%
After early epilepsy	39/120	33%	20/118	17%	8/40	20%
p	< 0.001		< 0.001		< 0.001	

Table 4.30 Incidence of late epilepsy in children (from Jennett, 1975)

	Age < 5 years		Age > 5 years	
Non trivial	5/25	20%	46/180	26%
Trivial	3/17	18%	5/16	31%
All	8/42	19%	51/196	26%

years who have had a trivial injury associated with an early fit (Table 4.30).

PROPHYLAXIS

Two questions call for answers. What level of risk justifies the administration of antiepileptic drugs to a patient who has not yet had a late fit? And what regimen is effective – which drug and dose, when to begin, and how long to continue? Until recently the rationale of prophylaxis was suppression of the tendency to have fits, and the usual recommendation was that drugs should be continued for one or two years. However, there is now some evidence that if medication is begun within hours of injury and maintained for only three months, there may be long-lasting protection (Young *et al.*, 1975; 1979). The assumption is that the development of an epileptic focus is thereby prevented, and that by preventing the first (even the early) fit there will be lasting benefit.

The problem with the practical application of this method, which involves such early treatment, is that it would need to be given even to patients not yet known to be in a high risk category; it could presumably be discontinued after one to two weeks if by then it was clear that the risk was low. It is not clear how this might affect early epilepsy as an indicator of risk. However, two-thirds of early fits occur in the first 24 hours, and half of these in the first hour, so that only a proportion of these early fits would in practice be prevented.

In accordance with modern practice, only one drug should be used. The American trials of early prophylaxis are based on phenytoin but its relative toxicity has led some British workers to recommend sodium valproate.

Epilepsy after intracranial surgery for non-traumatic conditions

It has long been acknowledged that intracranial

surgery may in itself cause epilepsy, but the degree of risk associated with different circumstances has not been established. There has often been epilepsy before operation, during the evolution of the condition requiring surgery (e.g. intracranial tumour or abscess); it is then not possible to know whether any subsequent epilepsy should be ascribed to operative brain damage or to the residual primary pathology. However, a comparison has been made of the post-operative epilepsy rate after removal of acoustic neurinoma by the posterior fossa route and by a combined approach from above and below the tentorium (Cabral *et al.*, 1976a): and after treatment of ruptured aneurysm by carotid ligation and by direct intracranial surgery (Cabral *et al.*, 1976b). In each instance epilepsy more frequently developed when there had been open surgery involving the cerebrum; the risk was between 20 and 25 per cent. More data is needed to determine the level of risk associated with different operations and conditions – in patients who have not had epilepsy pre-operatively. The significance of a fit during the first week after surgery needs to be established – it seems likely that it would be evidence of an increased risk of epilepsy in the future, as it is after accidental traumatic brain damage.

Only when this information is available will it be possible to give soundly based advice about prophylactic antiepileptic drug therapy after surgery, and about when such patients can safely drive again after operation. These matters are of considerable importance since the Ministry of Transport began to recommend suspension of driving licences for a probationary period after certain intracranial procedures, on the basis of the reported frequency of fits in the series referred to above (Lancet, 1980). It seems probable that the approach to prophylaxis being used for traumatic epilepsy (early medication, continued for only a few months) may be appropriate also for post-operative patients.

REFERENCES

Cabral, R., King, T.T. & Scott, D.F. (1976a) Incidence of post-operative epilepsy after a transtentorial approach to acoustic nerve tumours. *Journal of Neurology, Neurosurgery and Psychiatry*, **39**, 663.

Cabral, R., King, T.T. & Scott, D.F. (1976b) Epilepsy after

two different neurosurgical approaches to the treatment of ruptured intracranial aneurysm. *Journal of Neurology, Neurosurgery and Psychiatry*, **39**, 1052.

Caveness, W.F., Meirowsky, A.M., Rish, B.L., Mohr, J.P., Kistler, J.P., Dillon, J.D. & Weiss, G.H. (1979) The nature of post-traumatic epilepsy. *Journal of Neurosurgery*, **50**, 545.

Courjon, J.A. (1969) Post-traumatic epilepsy in electro-clinical practice. In Walker, A.E., Caveness, W.F. & Critchley, M. (eds) *Late Effects of Head Injury*, p. 215. Springfield: Thomas.

Hendrick, E.B. & Harris, L. (1968) Post-traumatic epilepsy in children. *Journal of Trauma*, **8**, 547.

Jennett, B. (1962) *Epilepsy after Blunt Head Injuries*. London: Heinemann.

Jennett, B. (1975) *Epilepsy after Non-Missile Head Injuries*. London: Heinemann.

Jennett, B., Murray, A., Carlin, J., McKean, M., MacMillan, R. & Strang, I. (1979) Head injuries in three Scottish neurosurgical units. *British Medical Journal*, **2**, 955.

Lancet (1980) Epilepsy after head trauma and fitness to drive. *Lancet*, **1**, 401.

Rapport, R.L. & Penry, J.K. (1972) Pharmacologic prophylaxis of post-traumatic epilepsy. *Epilepsia*, **13**, 295.

Stowsand, D. (1971) *Parensen und epileptische Reaktionen im initial-stadium des hirntraumas*. Stuttgart: G.T. Verlag.

Terespolsky, P.S. (1972) Post-traumatic epilepsy. *Forensic Science*, **1**, 147.

Walton, J.N. (1963) Some observations on the value of EEG in medicolegal practice. *Medicolegal Journal*, **31**, 15.

Williams, B. (1979) Craniotomy and fitness to drive. *Lancet*, **2**, 300.

Young, B., Rapp, R., Perrier, D., Kostenbauder, H., Hackman, J. & Blacker, M. (1975) Early post-traumatic epilepsy prophylaxis. *Surgical Neurology*, **4**, 339.

Young, B., Rapp, R., Brooks, W.H. and Madauss, W. (1979) Post-traumatic epilepsy prophylaxis. *Epilepsia*, **20**, 671.

Electroencephalography

PART ONE
M.V. Driver
B.B. McGillivray

INTRODUCTION

As the ECG is to the heart, so in general terms is the EEG to the brain. Both are the electrical concomitants of physiological and pathological events in the corresponding organs occurring at the time the record is being taken. Where the generators of the ECG, atrial and ventricular muscle, are relatively homogeneous and can be treated in a fairly straightforward and understandable way, the generators of the EEG, essentially the neurones of the cerebral cortex, are exceedingly complex and ill understood. Deductions from the EEG thus rely heavily on empirical correlations rather than on a theoretical foundation, which is as yet poorly developed. Recent investigations have gone some way to providing adequate models of the EEG and the basis for rational deductions as will be outlined below. Indeed, these developments presage a much more exciting future for the EEG than most of us had dared hope for even in the last decade.

The first human EEG recording was published by Hans Berger in 1929 although animal recordings had been made long before by Caton (1875) and independently by Beck (1890). Historical accounts are given in Brazier (1961 & 1973a) and Gloor (1969 & 1974). Berger's observations were little noticed until the confirming paper of Adrian and Matthews (1934) brought the EEG to the attention of a wide audience. The first recording of human epileptic activity was published by Gibbs, Davis and Lennox in 1935 and shortly after Grey Walter described the location of cerebral tumours (1936) later proved by surgical removal. It should be recalled that at this time arteriography (Moniz, 1927) was still being developed and air encephalography (Dandy, 1919) was the main, and an unpleasant, investigatory tool.

Early and excessive enthusiasm for the EEG waned in the post-war years as the difficulties in its interpretation came to be appreciated and its potential seemed to be unfulfilled. Now we are able better to fit the EEG into its correct place in the planned investigations of the central nervous system.

The key to its value is that it measures the functional state of the brain. In this it parallels the clinical anamnesis and examination, and psychometry, which also test functional attributes, albeit in different ways. For epilepsy, an essentially functional disorder and one not manifest except with an ictus, it is obvious that the EEG showing inter-ictal abnormalities provides insights which can be obtained in no other way.

It is the purpose of this chapter to explain and evaluate the role of the EEG in the investigation of epilepsy. To this end it is necessary to consider the nature and limitations of EEG recording and the pathophysiology underlying its disturbances.

THE PHYSIOLOGICAL BASIS OF THE EEG

Recent reviews may be found in Creutzfeldt (1974), Andersen and Andersson (1974), Scherrer and Calvet (1972). As a starting-point, we conceive of the nervous system as a processor of information which is its primary if not sole function (there are endocrine and neurotrophic functions). The elementary unit is the neurone which has a cell body or soma, with dendrites which receive information (afferents) and an axon which transmits information (efferent). Information is transmitted along the axon in the form of the axon spike or depolarisation, as an all-or-none phenomenon. The spike duration is about 0.5–1.0 msec. That is, transmission is *digital* or *unitary* in character. The information transmitted may be excitatory or inhibitory on the next cell depending on its synaptic termination.

On arrival at its synaptic terminals, the axon spike produces graded electrical changes in the post-synaptic membrane of the target cell. Such synaptic inputs may produce changes lasting from a few, to several tens or even hundreds of milliseconds in duration. The sum of these post-synaptic graded or analogue events, both inhibitory and excitatory from numerous neuronal inputs, determines the state of the recipient neurone and whether information will be transmitted along its axon. Information passing through the nervous system is repeatedly transformed from digital spikes to analogue waves and back again. From this elementary description it is clear that simple analogies between the brain and digital computers are quite false: not least because although the brain transmits information in a digital way from one place to another, it processes the information by analogue means. As will be shown, there is convincing evidence now that the EEG is comprised of these analogue events, the processing part of the transaction. There is effectively no contribution from the axon spikes or transmission activity except possibly in exceptional circumstances of a massive synchronous input along many parallel axons directly below a recording electrode and oriented perpendicular to it. It should be noted that the spikes referred to are neurone spikes and should not be confused with EEG *spikes* – a descriptive term which refers to the sharp appearance of EEG waves and which are generated by analogue events in the neurones.

In the 1930s at the beginning of electro-encephalography, only neurone spikes were known and it was natural to surmise that the EEG represented the envelopes of such spikes generated in the cells under the electrode and slightly out of synchrony with each other. In fact the correlation between the EEG and the spikes in the subjacent neurone population is extremely poor (Li & Jasper, 1953) in normal circumstances. The introduction of the glass micropipette electrode in the late 1940s enabled the post-synaptic slow potentials (PSPs) already alluded to above to be seen for the first time and several authors suggested they may be the true generators of the EEG (Bishop & Clare, 1952; Bremer, 1949; Calvet, Calvet & Scherrer, 1964; Chang, 1950; Eccles, 1951; Kandel & Spencer, 1961; Li & Chou, 1962; Purpura, 1959). The evidence is now quite convincing (Creutzfeldt, 1974; Scherrer & Calvet, 1972) and is summarised in the diagram of Figure 5.1. The reader should bear in mind that the views expressed here are a rather terse summary of present opinion. The generation of the EEG is likely to be more complex than is indicated.

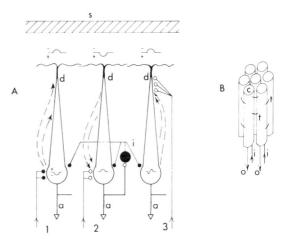

Fig. 5.1 Genesis of the EEG. **A.** Three schematic cortical pyramidal neurones are shown with axons, a, dendrites, d. Input to 1 is inhibitory, indicated by solid black synapses, which produce increased negativity inside the cell. The potential acts as a current source with current flow upwards along the apical dendrite producing a negative potential on the surface. (Note that the EEG convention is negative upwards.) In 2, the input is excitatory (open circle synapses) and current flows away from the apical dendrite into the sink generated by depolarisation with corresponding positive recording on the surface. i, is an inhibitory neurone activated by a recurrent axon. In 3, the input is excitatory at the apical dendrite causing a current sink and surface negativity. s, is a large surface electrode which would record the sum of 1, 2, 3, etc. **B.** Schematic cortical columns, c, with white matter inputs, i, and outputs, o, and loose interactions, t, t.

In the figure, it should be noted that reference is made to the pyramidal cell elements of the cortex only. The detailed structure of the cortex had been very adequately elucidated by Cajal (1909) using silver techniques and he had remarked on the peculiarities of the pyramidal neurones (Golgi type I) which are characterised by a large apical dendrite extending vertically to the cortical surface plexiform layer. This particular orientation and structure ensures that post-synaptic potentials generated in the soma and apical dendrite are electrically conducted to the surface thus giving rise to the potentials recorded there. Potentials arising in horizontally disposed structures or in cell elements not reaching the surface will have little or no effect on the surface potentials.

From the time of Cajal and through many generations of neuroanatomists, it has been the custom to divide the cortex into horizontal layers, usually six, on the basis of the fairly obvious cell laminations, the details of which led to the parcellation of the cortex into numerous sub-types as exemplified in the cortical cytoarchitectonic maps of Brodmann (1909). Many of these cortical areas are known to subserve specific functions and Petsche (personal communication) has found particular EEG patterns related to cytoarchitectonic areas in the rabbit. From the point of view of the generation of the EEG and the detailed functional behaviour of the cortex, however, it is the vertical organisation of the cortex which is of primary interest.

The classical studies of Mountcastle (1957) and Hubel and Wiesel (1962) have revealed the sensory cortex, at least, to be organised in a mosaic of vertical columns each of which appears to be a functional unit for information processing. Szentagothai (1969) has found confirmatory anatomical evidence in support. We come to the view then that the primary EEG generators are the vertically oriented pyramidal (Golgi type I) neurones of the cortex organised in a columnar mosaic.

Returning to Figure 5.1, it is apparent that under any electrode larger than a few millimetres in diameter there will be hundreds of thousands of neurones from which that electrode will pick up post-synaptic potentials. The electrode will show the resultant sum. If one assumes a random pattern in time of the positive and negative potentials in the generating cells then the sum will tend to zero at the surface. There will be no EEG. However, an EEG *is* recorded and often a very large potential. It is evident, therefore, that there must be some degree of correlation or synchronisation of post-synaptic potentials in the cortical generators. The immediate question is, 'How many neurones must be synchronised to produce a detectable EEG?' or better, 'What might be the contribution of a single neurone to the surface potential?' The answer is not known and depends clearly on a number of factors such as the size of the neurone and its apical dendrite and the depth below the surface. These are evaluated by Pollen (1969) and Elul (1972) from a theoretical point of view (it is extremely difficult to devise a practical test) and conclude that somewhere in the order of 0.1 per cent to 1.0 per cent of the relevant neurone population might be required to be synchronised to produce a 100 μV wave on the surface. The figure is surprisingly small but errs if anything on the side of an overestimate.

Since all that we observe on the EEG is a product of synchronisation in the generators, clearly the nature and mechanisms of synchronisation become of paramount importance. A recent symposium (Petsche & Brazier, 1972) contributes to our understanding of the phenomenon, and further reviews may be found in Volume 2 part C of the *Handbook of EEG and Clinical Neurophysiology* (1974) and Petsche (1976).

The mechanisms of synchronisation are multiple and in different circumstances different mechanisms are likely to be involved. For example, the mechanism underlying the generation of the normal 10 cycles per second (Hz) alpha rhythm is quite different from that producing the hypersynchrony associated with an epileptic discharge, and both are different from that which occurs in slowing of the EEG seen with metabolic disturbances and drug intoxication or in association with primary brain disease. This point may be stressed: the EEG is rarely specific to a disease entity or pathology and although we tend to believe that particular wave shapes seen in the EEG reflect a particular mechanism, it is quite possible that the identical waves could be produced in several quite different ways.

For the dominant rhythm in the normal EEG,

the 8–13 Hz alpha rhythm of the posterior quadrants of the brain, a convincing and generally acceptable explanation has been set out by Andersen & Andersson (1974). This is expounded diagrammatically in Figure 5.2. Briefly, the general principle of a negative (inhibitory) feedback (recurrent inhibition) illustrated in the thalamic circuits, appears to be a characteristic of most groups of neurones from spinal cord to cortex, and in all species except those with the most elementary neuraxes. The notion is one which is crucial to the understanding of epileptic phenomena and must be a major factor in preventing runaway excitation (i.e. epilepsy) in the CNS.

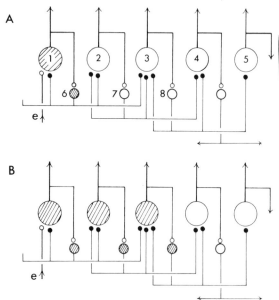

Fig. 5.2 Generation of synchronous activity. The diagram shows five thalamic neurones 1–5, with four inhibitory cells (6–8). **A.** Random excitation, e, fires cells 1 and 6 causing synchronous inhibition of 1, 2, and 3. **B.** These subsequently fire together, having been brought into the same excitatory state, causing synchronous inhibition through the inhibitory neurones of all five thalamic transmission neurones. Firing cells indicated by cross hatching. (Diagram after Andersen & Andersson, 1974.)

The cellular elements and connections in Figure 5.2 have been well worked out for the thalamus, and the cortex is not necessary for the generation of appropriate rhythms. In this theory, the thalamus is the pacemaker for the cortical oscillations which essentially are slaved to the thalamic drive in the normal state. Isolated cortex is quite capable of generating its own rhythms

(Burns, 1950) although these are different from the patterns seen when all the connections are intact. There are known cortico-thalamic connections (Scheibel & Scheibel, 1970) which may modulate thalamic activity even if they are not essential to the generation of normal rhythmical activity.

In the preceding discussion we have been considering synchronisation as a rather passive phenomenon. In epilepsy, a quite different mechanism occurs: active hypersynchronisation of some cell groups, which may recruit large populations to the same activity, i.e. an epileptic discharge.

In the clinical EEG, the signature of this epileptic hypersynchrony is the EEG spike: an event generated in the post-synaptic membranes of cortical cells and characterised by a wave of sharp aspect less than 70 msec in duration, normally electro-negative at the surface and commonly associated with slower waves. The determination of whether a particular sharp wave is a spike of epileptic character, or not, is a matter of experience but also influenced by the EEG context in which it occurs. Thus the sharp waves normally seen with barbiturate activity are not spikes as can be determined from the associated electrical activity. The use of computers to detect spikes requires a more precise definition based on the measurement of *sharpness*, taking into account the rate of change of the potentials forming the ascending and descending limbs of the spike (see discussion in MacGillivray, 1977). In practice, the rule of thumb 'if it's sharp enough to prick it's a spike' works very well.

It must be emphasised that whilst the presence of a spike signifies epileptic activity it does not necessarily indicate that the subject has clinical epilepsy (see further discussion below).

Disruptions of the input to the cortex, hyperexcitability of some neurones, depression of others, will have effects on the EEG recorded from the scalp. Inspection of the record will often allow deductions to be made about the nature of these changes and so it might be, for example, that whilst the patient presents with epilepsy, his EEG shows the features of a tumour. It should be noted too, that the EEG is a short sample in time of brain activity: if the behaviour of the brain is normal at that time, so will be the EEG.

The interconnections between cells, as seen in the histology of the cortex particularly, are so numerous and complex as to lend plausibility to the notion that any one neurone is connected in some way or another to any other neurone in the cortex through intermediaries. The validity of such an idea is not of great consequence since in practice certain preferred functional pathways can be demonstrated which appear to be pre-emptive (cf. the columnar mosaic already referred to for sensory cortex). However, when these normal pathways are damaged with loss of cortical inputs by structural (and probably biochemical) lesions, the residual connections may now exert a dominating influence thus giving rise to different (abnormal) wave forms in the EEG. In these circumstances synchronisation can take place by intra-cortical, cortico-cortical (both U, long association and callosal connections) and reticular influences, or some combination of these. These mechanisms must be frankly speculative at the present time but at least there is evidence for some of them (see discussion on synchronisation in spike and wave epilepsy, Gloor, 1972).

Petsche (1976) has made the point, and it is worth emphasising, that epileptic activity appearing in different parts of the brain during an epileptic seizure is highly organised and has neither the randomness nor the apparent synchrony which inspection of clinical EEG records might suggest. Using computer techniques, he has demonstrated complex but none the less systematic spread of epileptic activity through the cortex, which he relates to intra-cortical U fibres. He has also shown that, in experimental epileptic discharges initiated by electrical stimulation elsewhere, the EEG spike generators are less than 250 microns in width (comprising the *columns* referred to earlier), and are sequentially excited despite the superficial appearance of synchrony. By contrast, the slow wave which accompanies the spike has a much larger generating field, measured in millimetres. In relating these experimental studies to the clinical EEG it must be borne in mind that, even with relatively small electrodes placed directly on the cortex, the EEG pattern is very much that of a low pass filtered version of the intra-cortical activity. With standard EEG electrodes on the scalp, nearly two centimetres away from the generators, the

additional filtering and topographic averaging effects blur time relationships and waveforms very considerably. Although this chapter is not the place to review mechanisms of epilepsy, some mention must be made of slow *depolarising shifts* which are assuming greater importance in epileptogenesis. They reflect substantial ionic shift in glia and dendrites in epileptic foci and very likely provide a mechanism for sustaining the spread of epileptic activity by non-synaptic processes (Prince & Schwartzkroin, 1978). They probably do not directly contribute to routine EEG recordings, which are measured with AC coupled amplifiers, but are likely to underly post-ictal 'silence'.

Fleischauer, Petsche and Wittkowski (1972) and Peters and Walsh (1972) have recently demonstrated another intriguing aspect of synchronisation, namely the organisation of the apical dendrites of cortical pyramidal cells in vertical bundles in intimate contact over quite long lengths. That activity in any one of these dendrites would affect the status of its neighbours seems almost certain (Petsche & Rappelsberger, 1973) and would be an obvious and powerful synchronising mechanism. If validated, this observation carries interesting implications: in the discussion up to this point the EEG generated by post-synaptic potentials has been implied to be entirely an epiphenomenon, like the noise of an engine, and of no immediate consequence in itself for the brain. If Petsche and Rappelsberger are right, however, the EEG may be rather more than this, becoming a part of the electrical environment which itself actually influences the behaviour of the cortex. Such a notion may seem far fetched at this juncture but cannot be dismissed. In a new review, Korn and Faber (1980) bring together evidence of the effect of field potentials on the excitability of neurones at the micro level: it seems as if our Sherringtonian model of the nervous system may have to be substantially modified in a very complex way.

LIMITATIONS OF THE EEG

Because the EEG measures potentials in millionths of volts (μV) and requires sensitive and fairly sophisticated electronic equipment working near theoretical and practical limits (2 μV), it is often thoughtlessly assumed that the recordings themselves must be supersensitive reflections of brain activity. This they are not, as the briefest discussion with any academic neurophysiologist will reveal. Most neurophysiologists are preoccupied with microneurophysiology, the function of the neurone element and its interconnections, about which so much is still to be known. Less attention has been paid to the grosser organisational patterns which are reflected in the EEG and are the routine work of clinical electroencephalography. The EEG is in fact a gross and coarse measure of the behaviour of the neurones of the brain, reflecting as it does the summated properties of large populations of cells. In a peculiar way, therein also is its power: in cerebral function there is a high degree of redundancy in respect of individual neurones; even in the most highly and specifically organised cortex of the primary sensory and motor areas, it requires the loss of several hundreds of thousands of neurones before any behavioural defect is detected either internally by the patient or externally by an observer.

From a theoretical and practical point of view there are a number of factors which can be seen to place obvious limits on the ability of the EEG recording, as currently undertaken, to reveal abnormalities of cerebral function. Essentially these are problems of sampling, in space (topography), in time, and in function.

1. Spatial sampling

The routine EEG recording utilises about 22 electrodes which number is appropriate for conventional 8 or 16 channel machines, and convenient to apply. This gives an average electrode spacing of 5–6 cm. Since heads differ in shape and size, electrodes on the scalp, carefully applied according to agreed measurements from fixed anatomical points, nonetheless bear an inconstant and essentially unknown relationship to gross cortical anatomy, the Sylvian fissure for example (MacGillivray, 1974). Scalp electrodes as little as 2 cm apart can show quite different EEG activity and it is clear that large areas of the brain are inadequately sampled by present techniques. Further,

about a third of the cortex is effectively inaccessible from the scalp, e.g. inferior temporal, occipital and frontal lobes, the insula and the cortex of the median aspect of the hemisphere. Of the accessible cortex, about two-thirds is buried within the sulci and probably non-contributory to the scalp EEG. In short, the cortex actually sampled represents about 20–25 per cent of the whole.

The variable distance of a scalp electrode from the underlying brain, in the parietal as compared with temporal regions for example, adds further difficulties. One begins to doubt, on theoretical grounds, how any useful information is ever obtained from the EEG. In practice things are rather better: extra electrodes can always be placed for particular purposes and although electrodes a few centimetres apart record different EEG patterns, they also record much in common, as indeed do electrodes 5 or even 10 cm apart, i.e. the EEG is reflecting the activity of synchronising systems operating over large areas of brain. It is fortunate that these systems are commonly involved in both epileptic and other pathological circumstances, which is the underlying reason why the EEG is rather more helpful than might be expected.

2. Temporal sampling

This is an obvious limitation; a brain which is behaving normally will produce a normal EEG; five minutes later it could generate an epileptic attack which goes unrecorded. It is this problem that has created increased interest in continuous recording and telemetry.

3. Functional sampling

The routine EEG records the activity of the brain in an *idling* state for the most part. This is clearly an inadequate test of any system and a number of provocative techniques, such as hyperventilation, photic stimulation, drug effects, sleep and evoked potential recording, have been developed as will be described below. These techniques add important information, but many are far removed from the *routine* procedure, besides which they may be difficult to standardise or replicate precisely on another occasion.

The relation of EEG signs to clinical signs will be alluded to later in the text of this chapter, but it may be appropriate to mention that the two are separate phenomena in certain respects. Thus clinical signs are only manifest when specific cortical areas, sensory and motor cortex for example, are malfunctioning, or larger areas of association cortex, parietal lobes for example, or the reticular system (change in consciousness) are involved. Malfunction of small areas of cortex and quite large areas of frontal and temporal lobes can be clinically *silent* whilst electrically very abnormal. The clinician will find all this obvious, but it is remarkable how often it is forgotten and EEG findings written off because there are no supporting clinical signs. There is a fault in the other direction of course, which may be more dangerous from the patient's point of view, namely over- or mis-interpretation of EEG signs, the attribution of pathology for example to a functional abnormality. Experience, as always, strikes a balance between over-enthusiasm and disillusionment.

THE CLINICAL EEG

The EEG is a recording of changes in voltage as they occur at the scalp, selectively presented in order to maximise certain changes of cerebral origin and to minimise changes related to structures and influences from outside the brain. Voltage is a relative concept, and changes of voltage at a point of the scalp can be expressed or displayed only as changes in relation to the voltage of some other point whether on or off the scalp. As is obvious from the facts of electrocardiography, no point on the body surface can be regarded as unchanging in electrical potential and no neutral point can be found to provide a steady and reliable datum from which to measure electrical changes at the scalp. It is found in practice that most of the potential changes of non-cerebral origin, including those due to the action of the heart and to various external electrical fields, affect all areas of the scalp to much the same extent, indicating that differences in potential between points on the scalp and therefore between electrodes attached to the scalp should largely consist of changes due to the function of the underlying brain. *Bipolar* and

common reference (unipolar) recording methods display essentially similar information though in different ways. With bipolar recording each channel of amplification and write-out reflects voltage changes at two electrodes which are considered equally active and important in terms of EEG. These voltage changes are presented separately to the two input terminals of the channel amplifier, the characteristics of each input being identical except that relative negativity at one (the 'first' or 'black' input terminal) results in an upward movement of the recording pen, and vice versa. Bipolar recordings resulting from a first input electrode changing potential towards negativity, and from a second input electrode changing potential by a similar amount towards positivity will therefore be indistinguishable. The method of identifying the electrode showing the maximum change (change at a single electrode in scalp EEG being very rare) and the polarity of that change is described in Appendix 5.1. With common reference recording the 'reference electrode' (usually attached to the nose or ears, or possibly derived in the recorder itself) is considered to be 'inactive' in comparison with the 'active' electrode on the scalp or otherwise favourably placed to respond to cerebral potential changes. Since the reference electrode is conventionally connected to the second or 'white' input terminal, upward pen movements can be interpreted as negative going changes of measurable magnitude at the active electrode. That this apparently attractive method of recording EEG is the less often used reflects both the complexity of the potential changes occurring at the 'active' electrodes and the great difficulty in providing a reference electrode which is truly 'inactive'. However, advances in amplifier technology are undoubtedly improving the value of 'unipolar' recording. Provided a reliable recording has been obtained, appropriate interpretation will give the same information whether a 'bipolar' or 'unipolar' technique has been used.

Differences in electrical potential between one electrode on the scalp and another can be detected when the interelectrode distance is only a centimetre or so, but in practice the common technique is to place the electrodes about 5 cm apart in a grid pattern with symmetrical distribution about the anteroposterior midline. This allows coverage of the convexity of the four lobes of the cerebrum on each side and therefore enables localisation of maximum voltage change to be made with reference to these surfaces of the cerebral hemispheres. It is apparent, as noted earlier, that the scalp EEG can give only a very restricted, indirect and often indefinite view of the voltage changes occurring in the greater part of the brain. The apparatus in common clinical use is capable of providing an accurate representation of between about 0.5 and 100 Hz provided the voltage is above noise level of the amplifier, which is about 2 microvolts (μV). The sensitivity of the apparatus can be adjusted to allow display of any EEG voltages likely to be met with (commonly in the range of 10–100 μV, more in children). Some 8–16 channels, that is, separate representations of voltage change from different electrodes, are commonly recorded, usually by means of an ink-writer system through which paper passes at speeds ranging from 1.5 to 6 cm per second. Additional pens provide a time scale, indications of stimuli and so on, or in more complex apparatus (polygraphs) data related to the heart rate, blood pressure, skin resistance, limb movement or other physiological variables of interest.

Other displays of cerebral electrical activity than that described above are possible, but none is currently in wide clinical use. Rémond's techniques of *spatio-temporal mapping* of potentials and gradients are perhaps best known, a recent develop-ment being the accurate plotting of *isopotential maps of EEG fields* (Ragot & Remond, 1978). While this could well, as is claimed, become the physiological complement of the modern X-ray scanning technique, the need for about 200 scalp electrodes and elaborate data acquisition and processing systems indicates that it is unlikely to be used extensively for some time.

The main determinants of the EEG in health are age and the level of alertness. The record of the alert adult not uncommonly shows very little except for alpha rhythm, the important features of which are its voltage and distribution (mainly parietal/posterior temporal) and frequency (8–13 Hz). The rhythm is broadly symmetrical in the former respects and extremely so in the latter, a 1 Hz difference between right and left being a very significant abnormality. Beta (fast) activity at about 16–30 Hz is described as a normal bilateral fronto-central phenomenon, but is often seen only with difficulty in subjects not on medication (e.g. barbiturates, benzodiazepines). Other apparently spontaneous phenomena may be seen, though these are not of common diagnostic value, and slow waveforms may appear in frontal and posterior temporal areas as a response to hyperventilation being, like the alpha and beta activity, bilaterally symmetrical.

Marked changes occur with the onset of sleep, the new phenomena appearing in sequence being characteristic enough to allow EEG assessment of

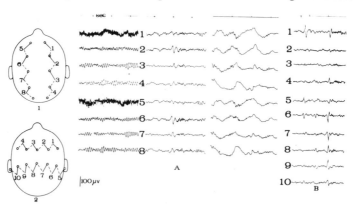

Fig. 5.3 EEG changes in sleep. **A.** Bipolar recordings (electrode pattern 1) showing typical EEGs of a healthy adult awake (alpha rhythm), in light natural sleep, V (Vertex) waves (channels 2, 3, and 6, 7) and sleep spindles (channels 2 and 6, etc.), and in deep barbiturate assisted sleep (very slow waves, with spindles). **B.** Bipolar recording (electrode pattern 2) from a patient with temporal lobe epilepsy, in light sleep. A V wave (channels 1, 4, 5–10 inclusive) shows a phase reversal (i.e. focus) between channels 7 and 8, at the vertex (hence the name), and an abnormal inter-ictal epileptic spike of not dissimilar waveform appears in the right fronto-temporal region (channels 1, 5, 6).

depth of sleep to be achieved. As with the phenomena of the EEG record of the alert state, those of sleep in the normal adult subject are essentially symmetrical (Fig. 5.3). Some of them, however, particularly the 'vertex waves' may be indistinguishable in shape from some of the 'spikes' seen in certain varieties of epilepsy. This and other difficulties in EEG assessment are discussed below.

The adult EEG, as described above, represents the final outcome of a series of changes which have taken place more or less continuously since infancy. These changes are complex and difficult to describe briefly and adequately but essentially they consist, in the awake state, of a reduction in overall voltage and an increase in frequency of the dominant rhythms, together with a progressive loss of prominent rhythmic activity from the anterior half of the head. Bilateral symmetry is broadly maintained throughout, though some features, particularly posterior temporal slow waves of the alert state and the arousal phenomena of sleep (vertex waves, K complexes, spindles) frequently show a degree of asymmetry which is never seen in the healthy adult (Fig. 5.4). Rhythmic positive spikes, frequently seen in parietal and posterior temporal regions of the

child's EEG during drowsiness and light sleep, are probably a normal phenomenon, though when first described were considered evidence of a variety of epilepsy. There is a very wide range of what has to be accepted as *normal* for any given age in childhood and adolescence, and assessment of slight degrees of cerebral dysfunction may be impossible.

THE ABNORMAL EEG

The objective of strict quantitative assessment of the EEG and the establishment of normal limits has been pursued for many years. It will ultimately be attained when adequate computer assisted studies of the healthy have been carried out, but at present the clinical assessment of the EEG depends as it has done heretofore, largely on the visual impression of the electroencephalographer. He scans the record and assesses whether the ongoing continuous or *background* activity seen is appropriate to the patient's age and state of alertness, whether it shows any unusual asymmetry and whether any waveforms not seen in health in the given circumstances, or possibly never seen at all in health, are present. Because of this, the ter-

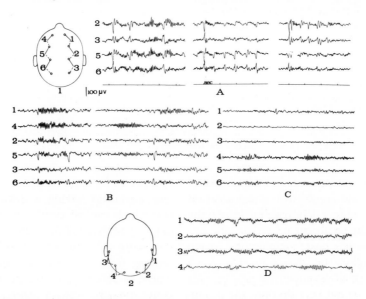

Fig. 5.4 Asymmetrical EEG phenomena in children. Electrode pattern 1: **A**. V wave asymmetries in sleep in a normal child. **B**. Another normal child: spindle symmetry and asymmetry during sleep. **C**. Child with left hemiplegia of infantile type: sleep spindles appear on the left side, none on the atrophic right side. Electrode pattern 2: **D**. Alpha and posterior temporal slow wave distribution asymmetries in an alert normal child.

minology used in descriptions of the clinical EEG tends to be imprecise and the inferences to be drawn from the descriptions possibly not entirely accurate. Thus an EEG which appears normal in all respects except that the background rhythm is unusually slow (say 7 Hz in an adult) may be described as showing a generalised abnormality. This may be true in the sense that the slow alpha rhythm can be recorded over all areas of the scalp but it cannot be true in a physiological sense unless the alpha rhythm is a property of all those parts of the brain function which influences the EEG, which is not so.

In a sense, as indicated above, alpha rhythm, sleep spindles and various other bilateral EEG waveforms can be regarded as having a *local* significance, e.g. in relation to thalamic function. However, the term *local* as used in EEG commonly signifies a unilateral area of cerebral hemispheric dysfunction which manifests itself in one of two ways (Fig. 5.5). The first of these is through

The second manifestation of local cerebral hemispheric dysfunction is the appearance of irregular slow or other morphologically abnormal activity over a similarly limited area of the scalp. The location of the abnormality is made on the principles illustrated in the appendix. In all cases a clear distinction must be made between local brain dysfunction and local brain pathology. The area of cortex which is presumably the immediate seat of the dysfunction manifest by the EEG abnormality is not necessarily, or possibly even commonly, the site of the structural lesion responsible for that dysfunction. This is of great importance in the study of epilepsy where, for example, spikes may be recorded from an area of cortex, subsequent histological examination of which shows no definite structural abnormality and where a posterior temporal deficit of alpha rhythm may be present for a short time after a seizure of anterior temporal origin.

The EEG sign most commonly associated with

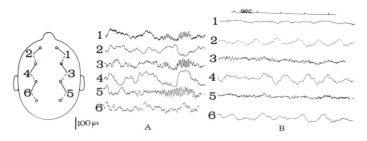

Fig. 5.5 Abnormal EEG features. **A**. An adult patient with a left temporal abscess, asleep: spindle activity, a symmetrical sleep phenomenon in health, is grossly deficient on the left side. Very irregular slow waveforms, inappropriate in health, appear in the left frontal area (note the phase reversal of the slow wave in channels 2 and 4). **B**. An adult with a left temporal abscess, awake: alpha rhythm is deficient on the left side (compare channels 3 and 5 with 4 and 6) and very slow waves of a type not seen in health in the alert state appear on the left (note the phase reversal in channels 2 and 4: this demonstrates that the second electrode in the row was undergoing larger potential changes than the remainder. A recording from other electrodes lower on the scalp would be necessary in order to establish whether this was in fact the most affected electrode).

the localised absence on one side of a phenomenon which in health would appear over equal areas on both sides. Thus with a left parietal lesion the alpha rhythm might be absent over that lobe but recordable over the left posterior temporal region and over both regions on the right side. Such asymmetries of normally symmetrical activity may also be seen with natural beta rhythm, the prominent fast activity induced pharmacologically (e.g. by barbiturate medication) and some phenomena of sleep.

epilepsy in its many varieties is the *spike*, a transient waveform having a distinctly pointed peak and which can be clearly differentiated from the ongoing *background* (e.g. alpha or beta) activity of the record. The duration of spikes is very variable, ranging from 20 ms or so, up to about 200 ms. Those of longer duration (more than 70 ms) are conventionally termed *sharp waves* rather than *spikes* (see reference, Glossary, 1974) but as the distinction is essentially arbitrary it will not be made in this chapter: all sharp transients of supposed significance in the EEG study of epilepsy will be referred to as *spikes*.

It is important to bear in mind that some sharp transients which fit this description of a spike occur in the normal EEG. Amongst these are various sharp waveforms seen in the posterior temporal regions of children and adolescents, also *lambda waves, vertex* or *V waves* and *positive occipital sharp transients of sleep*. These are usually fairly easily differentiated from the spikes of epilepsy by their location, unique appearance in relation to a particular physiological state and bilateral synchrony (Fig. 5.3).

However, difficulties can arise when the epileptic symptoms indicate the possible location of a lesion in the upper central or occipital regions, and in childhood when bilateral synchrony of vertex waves may be incomplete. In addition, the mixed alpha, beta and mu activity of the central areas may, particularly when of high voltage and reinforced by drug-induced fast waveforms, include sharp transients which are morphologically indistinguishable from the spikes of epilepsy. What is possibly a variant of this phenomenon was reported by Negrin and De Marco (1977) who found that focal contralateral parietal spikes appeared following tactile stimulation of the foot in 3–10 year old children (though some of these had a history of febrile convulsions). Note can also be made here of the *14 and 6 per second positive spike phenomenon* first described by Gibbs and Gibbs (1952) and said to be the EEG concomitant of *thalamic or hypothalamic epilepsy*. A very considerable literature on this topic exists, particularly in relation to the significance of the phenomenon in patients with abnormal behaviour, and also in relation to whether, being found so commonly in children and young adults, it can be truly classed as an abnormality (Driver, 1970). Though this particular phenomenon will not be considered further, it is of interest to note here that the predominant phase of the EEG spike of epilepsy is usually electrically negative relative to surrounding areas of scalp (or cortex). This negativity can be interpreted as current flow towards the cortical surface (Fig. 5.1) and therefore, when recorded in the EEG, as towards the overlying scalp. The circumstances in which the relatively rare *positive focal spikes* might be recorded are discussed by

Matsuo and Knott (1977), to whose four categories could be added a fifth, viz. in which a fairly gross cortical defect (e.g. from trauma or an abscess) is present, when the local scalp electrode is quite possibly responding to activity of the deep layers of adjacent active cortex.

The spikes of epilepsy may appear bilaterally synchronously and symmetrically, unilaterally or bilaterally asynchronously and so on, and in each case may occur rhythmically or at irregular intervals, and with or without constant or near constant relationship with another waveform, for example a regular or irregular slow wave to give a *spike–slow* or *spike and wave* complex. Certain combinations of these characteristics tend to be found with particular epileptic symptoms and have been used in various classifications of epilepsy. Thus bilateral synchronous runs of regularly formed spike and wave complexes occurring in approximate three per second rhythmic form, are characteristic of true petit mal or *absence epilepsy*.

Other EEG phenomena are frequently recorded in patients with epilepsy, for example, rhythmic slow waves not associated with spikes. These may have an obvious relation to the seizure itself, as in a psychomotor seizure of temporal lobe origin, or may relate to some presumed non-epileptic dysfunction brought about by a lesion, as possibly with a frontal tumour. In addition, there may be localising features as described above, i.e. the irregular slow waves caused by the presence of a structural lesion, or the local deficits of fast or alpha activity referable either to the lesion itself or to local cortical dysfunction in the immediate post-ictal period.

Where a patient suffers from substantial intracranial pathology, a tumour or infarct for example, and the disorder is manifest at the time of recording, the EEG will usually be abnormal and helpful in location and often as a guide to likely pathology. In the case of a paroxysmal disturbance such as epilepsy, there may be no EEG abnormality unless some form of epileptic activity, not necessarily with any clinical accompaniments, is occurring at the time of the recording. These aspects of the EEG will be discussed below. In general terms, about one-quarter to one-third of routine records taken without activation procedures from

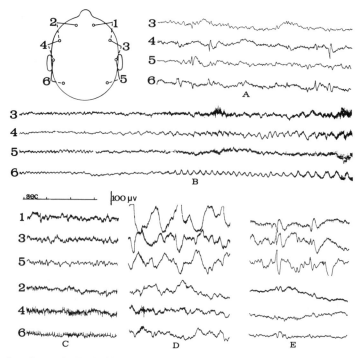

Fig. 5.6 EEG variability in epilepsy. **A.** Typical inter-ictal spikes in an adult patient with temporal lobe epilepsy. Independent spike foci can be seen in the right (channels 3, 5) and left (channels 4, 6) temporal regions (sleep record). **B.** EEG recorded at the start of a temporal lobe seizure (same patient as **A** but on another occasion and now awake). The earliest change is towards loss of alpha rhythm on the left (channels 4 and 6), followed by development of a lateralised rhythm of decreasing frequency on the left side. No spikes of inter-ictal character occurred in the pre-ictal record nor during the subsequent development of the seizure. **CDE** Records from a 12-year-old child with epilepsy due to a right temporal lesion: **C**, inter-ictal; **D**, 1–2 minutes after a seizure (automatism) lasting about half a minute; **E**, about one hour after the seizure.

subjects known to have clinical epilepsy may show no definite abnormality.

PHASES OF THE EPILEPTIC STATE

It is often possible to distinguish several phases in the life experience of a patient with epilepsy. Two are invariable: the seizure or ictus itself and the period between seizures, the inter-ictal state. In addition patients may have phases in which various prodromal symptoms appear, or there may be states dominated by definite aura phenomena. Post-ictal periods of confusion, localised paresis, dysphasia and so on may also occur. What is seen in the EEG may depend very critically on which of these phases was current at the time of the recording (Fig. 5.6). For example, a patient with temporal lobe epilepsy may show a clear left temporal spike focus in the inter-ictal phase, a midtemporal deficit of background rhythm at the time of the aura, prominent left fronto-temporal rhythmic slow waves during the seizure itself, and a posterior temporal irregularity and alpha deficit during the post-ictal period of confusion and dysphasia. A patient with occasional generalised convulsive seizures may show no definite EEG abnormality at all in the inter-ictal phase, but may develop bilateral spikes during the period leading up to the convulsion, and very prominent continuous spike or complex activity during the seizure itself. The post-ictal record may show only grossly irregular slow wave activity bilaterally in all areas.

Fortunately, many patients with epilepsy do show an abnormality during the inter-ictal period when, by necessity, most EEG recording is carried out. Various *activating* techniques can be practised, as will be discussed later, and by their use the great majority of undoubtedly epileptic patients can be induced to present some EEG evidence referable to that state. The most refractory patients in this respect are those of middle and later age who have recently developed infrequent generalised convulsive seizures: numerous recordings in such cases may well show no abnormality of a character definitely suggestive of epilepsy.

It is important to stress at this point that the precise meaning of inter-ictal spikes in the actual symptomatology of epilepsy is more often than not obscure. Focal seizures, particularly those of temporal lobe origin, do not commonly develop in association with an increase in focal spiking. Indeed, those spikes may disappear altogether before the actual clinical seizure phenomena are apparent to the patient or to an observer, to be replaced by a phenomenon of different morphology and possibly different location and distribution over the scalp. It is as though EEG spikes of the inter-ictal period and the various phenomena of the clinical seizure are to a great extent different and not very closely related manifestations of an underlying epileptic dysfunction. If this were so the apparent paradox of the efficacy of barbiturates both in the treatment of epilepsy and in the *activation* of spike foci in the EEG would be resolved. The demonstration of one or more inter-ictal spike foci is therefore not necessarily a complete demonstration of the *focus* of the epilepsy itself, and in some cases it may be necessary to record the EEG immediately before, during and for some time after an actual seizure. This is discussed more fully in a later section.

In children with frequent petit mal absences it may be that clearly *ictal* and *inter-ictal* phases cannot be distinguished in the EEG. The spike and wave bursts accompanying the absences may occur in what seems identical form though possibly of briefer duration, at times when no definite absence is observed. However, experimental procedures have shown that the performance of a task may be adversely affected at the time of these apparently non-ictal bursts which suggests that they do in fact signal an actual ictal event. It may also be true that *inter-ictal* spikes of the type noted earlier also signal an actual epileptic deficit, which sufficiently refined clinical techniques could detect. Such have not yet been developed, and for present purposes the inter-ictal spike is in most cases best regarded as a phenomenon only distantly related in a functional sense to the patient's symptoms.

The point may be made that in order for the patient to experience the effects of a localised epileptic discharge, or an observer to witness such effects, the epileptic activity must occur in at least one of that restricted number of sites in the brain which directly subserve the function experienced or observed. For example, sensorimotor, visual, auditory or olfactory phenomena are only experienced as a result of epileptic activity in particular sites, psychomotor phenomena from the frontal or temporal lobe, dysphasic speech disturbances from the dominant hemisphere and so on. In the case of psychomotor disturbances particularly, and probably most focal epilepsies, it is very likely that quite large areas of the brain have to be involved by the discharge before subjective or objective behavioural features occur. There are many parts of the brain, frontal, parietal and temporal, where these conditions are less frequently met and neither the patient nor the clinician is aware of the quite substantial epileptic discharges revealed by the EEG.

Broadly, one can say that in generalised forms of epilepsy which do not depend on demonstrable or likely brain damage the inter-ictal EEG, bearing in mind the previous paragraphs, shows no specific abnormality whereas the ictal EEG is bilaterally abnormal. In forms of *focal* epilepsy, however, both the ictal and the inter-ictal EEG records are likely to be abnormal. Put another way: the epilepsies most likely to be reflected positively in the effectively random EEG of the *routine* variety are those manifest by frequent *generalised* attacks, particularly petit mal, or by focal symptoms.

CLASSIFICATION OF EPILEPSY AND THE EEG

EEG can contribute to a classification of epilepsy through its ability to demonstrate some evidence of disturbed cerebral electrophysiology. Such a demonstration does not invariably, or possibly even often, enable unequivocal conclusions related to seizure pattern or the underlying pathological basis to be drawn. For example, the 'grand mal EEG pattern' of Gibbs, Gibbs and Lennox (1943) is only rarely found in inter-ictal recordings of patients whose seizures are typically of 'primary grand mal' character. It is more often observed in EEGs of subjects with a variety of generalised seizure types, especially when *akinetic attacks* are the main problem (Rodin, Smid & Mason, 1976). A classification based entirely on EEG features is therefore not satisfactory; clinical, anatomical, etiological and other factors must be considered in addition, and the first of these must provide the basic framework. The role of the EEG is to confirm, amplify, modify or possibly to refute classifications based on clinical observation, to suggest how the results of experimental work may be brought into a classification, and to indicate lines of research which, may clarify doubtful points. A classification of epileptic seizures recommended by a number of international bodies has been published (Gastaut, 1969), together with some additional comments (Masland, 1969). The former is discussed elsewhere (p. xiii). Some aspects only of particular relevance to EEG will be discussed here.

Broadly, the majority of seizures presenting primarily as chronic epileptic problems can be divided into two classes, those with an initial loss or at least modification of consciousness and those without. The EEG features of seizures of the first class are bilateral, symmetrical and synchronous, and they commonly take the form of rhythmically repeating spikes often associated with slow waves. In so far as spike or complex abnormalities are present in the EEG between the seizures, they show approximately constant characteristics though possibly modified in waveform during sleep. The background of such records, that is the alpha or beta rhythms and the activity to be expected in sleep, is commonly normal or, if not, is abnormal in a similar way, for example slow, on both sides. Such records suggest that one of the disturbances present is of mechanisms by which the rhythmic electrical activity of the cerebral cortex is controlled by reticulo-thalamic function. The *centrencephalic* hypothesis of Penfield and Jasper (1954) is based to an important extent on this consideration as is the justification for a subdivision of *centrencephalic epilepsies* in those classifications which use that term. It has been demonstrated by several investigators including Pollen, Perot and Reid (1963) and Weir (1964) that bilaterally symmetrical and synchronous spike

and wave complexes can be induced to appear in the EEG of laboratory animals by simple rhythmical electrical stimulation of parts of the thalamus and reticular formation. In some cases other features of human petit mal, for example eye movements, have also resulted from the same techniques. In addition, the demonstration of a relatively increased alpha frequency stability in periods immediately preceding and following the appearance of a generalised subclinical seizure pattern in the EEG (Simon, Müllner & Heinemann, 1976) does suggest that the origin of the latter is closely related to that of the alpha phenomenon, i.e. to the thalamic nuclei. However, there has been as yet no unequivocal demonstration that petit mal and other varieties of immediately generalised epilepsy are in fact based on an upper brain stem dysfunction, because of which the term *centrencephalic epilepsy* has not met with universal acceptance. Of the several alternative terminologies proposed *primary generalised epilepsy* and *primary subcortical epilepsy* are most commonly met with, though Masland (1969) would prefer *combined generalised epilepsy*. Evidence to be noted later in this chapter, that the cerebral cortex is also significantly involved in the initiation of generalised epileptic seizures, has resulted in the introduction of a further term: *cortico-reticular epilepsy* (Gloor, 1968). This concept also gets support from the reported development of self-sustained 3–4 per second spike-wave complexes in thalamic nuclei following 10 per second stimulation of the cat cortex (Steriade, Oakson & Diallo, 1976).

Epilepsy which is characterised not by an initial loss of consciousness but by some other phenomenon, for example a sudden localised somatic sensation or a series of involuntary movements of a limb, presumably relates to dysfunction of a limited part of the brain. This *focal epileptic seizure* may be the sole manifestation of the fit but it may, after a number of seconds or possibly a minute or two, extend to involve other parts of the body and ultimately a generalised convulsive seizure may develop. These features relate to the increasing extent of involvement of the brain and are reflected in the EEG; the initial changes show as a localised *focus* and this moves, spreads, and possibly changes in waveform as the new clinical phenomena appear. The EEG concomitant of a sensorimotor seizure involving the left hand may therefore be a spike focus recorded over the right central scalp. The inter-ictal EEG may also show focal spikes of similar location but of less frequent and more irregular occurrence in time, and it is in the demonstration of these that the value of the EEG lies. Focal spikes may relate to areas of cortex of very specific function and therefore to focal epilepsy of relatively elementary character. Such would be spikes in the central or occipital regions, associated with epilepsy of somatic sensorimotor or crude visual symptomatology respectively. The logic of such correspondence can be extended to the association of focal spikes with a much more complicated and varied symptomatology of seizure, for example anterior temporal spikes with the various affective, cognitive and psychomotor phenomena comprising the *temporal lobe* seizure. If the next step is taken, any epileptic seizure, however brief, indefinite or apparently inconsis-

tent, or even if apparently generalised from the onset can be regarded as fundamentally *focal* in origin if a clear and unequivocal spike focus can be demonstrated in the EEG.

Broadly speaking, then, a clinical classification consisting of the two main classes of primary generalised and focal onset epilepsy will correspond with an EEG classification based on bilaterally synchronous rhythmic spikes or complexes on the one hand and unilateral focal cortical spikes on the other. However, in practice the EEG may not show just a simple bilateral spike rhythm or a single spike focus: irregularities of spike shape, rhythmicity and synchrony are frequent, as is a multiplicity of spike foci (Figs 5.7, 5.8). The phenomena recorded in many EEG records may therefore raise doubts as to the fundamental basis of the epilepsy, and two questions very commonly arise:

1. Even though the epileptic attacks appear to

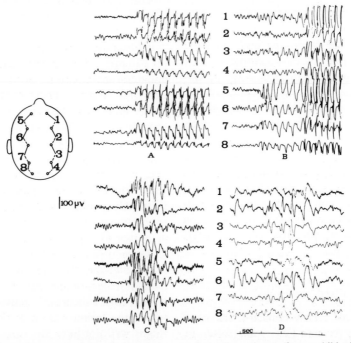

Fig. 5.7 Variation in spike and wave complexes. **A.** Regularly repeating spike and wave from a child with typical petit mal absences and no clinical, EEG or other features to suggest organic brain disease. The complexes showed a high degree of bilateral distribution symmetry and synchrony at all stages of the burst. **B.** Regularly repeating spike and wave of bilateral distribution but preceded by a period of left hemisphere involvement in less well developed complex activity. On other occasions the reverse picture (i.e. earlier involvement of the right hemisphere) or bilateral synchrony of onset were seen. The seizures were of absence type but associated with facial myoclonus which was often more prominent on one side. **C.** Complexes showing greater prominence, particularly of the spike phases, on the left side. These were recorded from a young woman with post concussion symptoms (street accident) but no reported seizures. **D.** Slow and irregular complexes from a youth with a long history of non-convulsive, including psychomotor, and convulsive seizures.

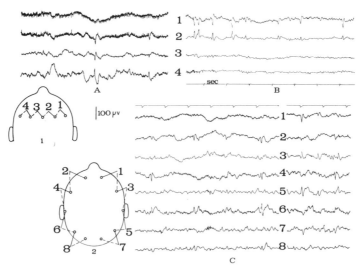

Fig. 5.8 Unilateral and bilateral spike foci. Electrode pattern 1: **A**. Left frontal spike focus with slow waves in a woman of 39 with seizures, often including dysphasia, following left frontal head injury at the age of 8. **B**. Right frontal spike focus in a child of 11 who had recently had two generalised convulsive seizures and otherwise appeared healthy. Records seven years later (no seizures for five years) showed no spikes. Electrode pattern 2: **C**. Bilateral independent spike foci in a young adult with a long history of temporal lobe epilepsy. The first spike shows as a left midtemporal focus (channels 4, 6), the second as a left anterior-middle temporal focus (channels 2, 6), the third has a different distribution over the scalp (channels 2, 4, 6, 8) and the fourth (to the right of the channel numbers) shows as a right anterior temporal focus (channels 1, 3, 5).

be generalised from the beginning and the EEG shows bilateral rhythmic spikes or complexes, is it possible that some localised form of cerebral disease is responsible?

2. Can multiple, possibly bilateral, spike foci be caused by a single localised cerebral lesion which is also directly responsible for the genesis of the seizures?

These questions imply that secondary varieties of generalised epilepsy and also clinically insignificant spike foci may exist. These possibilities, which have received considerable attention in human and animal studies, especially the latter, will be discussed in turn.

1. Secondary generalised epilepsy

Generalised seizures of clearly clinical focal onset or associated initially with an EEG spike focus, in either case probably with focal spikes in the interictal EEG, certainly fall into this category and as one or other *focal* aspect is obvious they can readily be classified as focal in nature. The work of Tükel and Jasper (1952) and Penfield and Jasper (1954) showed that it was possible for bilaterally

synchronous abnormalities to appear in the EEGs of patients with epilepsy apparently caused by unilateral parasagittal, orbital-frontal or anterior temporal lesions. These bilateral abnormalities, which included spike and wave complexes, were thought to reflect an initial cortical dysfunction, related to the presence of the lesion, leading by way of corticofugal pathways to abnormal activation of a centrally placed *subcortical* neuronal system. This in turn led to an abnormal activation of bilaterally projecting pathways and therefore to synchronous epileptic dysfunction of a wide area of cortex of both cerebral hemispheres. Such an EEG picture was called *secondary bilateral synchrony* and the clinical result of the abnormal projection *secondary subcortical epilepsy*. In cases in which this subcortical activation was rapid, or where the lesion was in a *silent* area, the patient might well not have any initial symptoms and the descriptive aspects of the resulting generalised convulsive or minor absence seizure might be indistinguishable from those of an initially generalised or *primary subcortical* seizure. Similarly, if the lesion was deeply situated relative to the scalp, or for some other reason not detectable by common

EEG techniques, the EEG characteristics of the seizure might be similar to those of primary subcortical seizures.

As Jasper and others since have noted, in cases where the presence of a lateralised cerebral hemispheric lesion can be demonstrated, for example by radiography or by a subsequent craniotomy, spike and wave complexes, if present, commonly show a lesser degree of regularity of form, frequency, distribution and symmetry than is the rule with those complexes found in a presumed primary subcortical epilepsy, for example petit mal.

It is not uncommon for patients with what are clinically slightly *impure* forms of generalised seizures to show these *impure* forms of spike and wave in their EEGs, even though other investigations fail to demonstrate a cerebral hemispheric lesion (Fig. 5.7). Only rarely have craniotomies or autopsies been performed in such cases and as a result the true value of the EEG observation by itself is unknown. The observation of Bancaud *et al.* (1974) that electrical stimulation of the medial frontal cortex in patients with epilepsy of presumed organic causation led to spike-wave complexes of typical bilaterally synchronous or centrencephalic character, indicated that there is probably no simple relationship between details of pathology, clinical fit pattern and EEG in generalised epilepsy.

Experimental work in animals with lateralised lesions causing bilateral spikes (for example by Guerrero-Figueroa, 1964) has indicated that appropriate inactivation of the responsible lesion can lead to a bilateral disappearance of the EEG abnormalities. One way of achieving this inactivation is by injection of a soluble barbiturate into the cerebral circulation of the side with the lesion. The intracarotid amylobarbitone test introduced by Wada (Wada & Rasmussen, 1960) for the determination of cerebral hemispheric dominance for speech can be used for a similar purpose in the study of human epilepsy. Practical aspects of the test are noted later, but here it can be said that if the bilateral synchrony is primary the left and right intracarotid injections, given within a 30 minute interval between the two sides, would be expected to have similar (and in practice slight) effects. If the synchrony was secondary, then injection on the side of the lesion would abolish the complexes bilaterally whereas contralateral injection would have only a limited unilateral effect.

The increasing effect in an experimental animal on behavioural and electrographic seizure activity following repeated brief local electrical stimulation of the brain – the *kindling* phenomenon – has been the subject of considerable research in the past decade. Goddard and Douglas (1975) give a good summary of technique and observations, and Pinel and van Oot (1975) discuss clinical implications. The development of spontaneous inter-ictal spikes in the *kindled* animal has also been studied (see references in Fitz & McNamara, 1979) and quantitative aspects of the phenomenon are discussed by Lange, Tanaka and Naquet (1977). Kindling can also be produced by local chemical application and is said to be a possible mechanism for experimental seizures produced by repeated inhalation of industrial solvents (Contreras *et al.*, 1979). The extent to which the kindling process is a valid model of relevance to the development of generalised and other varieties of epilepsy in human beings is not clear, and it is not surprising that study of the electrographic features of clinical epilepsy has been little influenced up to the present. However, kindling and the 'mirror focus' phenomenon noted below offer hypotheses which can be tested, provided EEG observations are made immediately following a potentially 'epileptogenic' insult and frequently repeated during a sufficiently long follow up.

2. Multiple EEG foci from a single lesion

This is a much commoner problem than that of the possibility of secondary spike and wave: probably the majority of patients with forms of focal epilepsy will show more than one spike focus if the EEG studies are pursued vigorously. Experiments involving several species of laboratory animals, including primates, and a great number of techniques inducing epileptic phenomena, have demonstrated that spikes will readily appear in cortical recordings at some distance from the site of the initiating agent and often contralaterally. Also, experience in the operating theatre has demonstrated that areas of cerebral cortex from which spikes of presumed epileptic significance were recorded may prove to be structurally quite normal when examined histologically, and the patient's seizures may continue following their removal.

These observations are important in the consideration of any individual case of focal epilepsy whether or not more than one spike focus is present in the EEG, and some means of distinguishing those spikes which might have localising significance from those which presumably merely reflect intracortical or interhemispheric connections would be extremely useful. Two types of experimental work have offered suggestions as to how this problem might be solved in some circumstances. The first (Ralston, 1958) was to the effect that spikes recorded from the immediate vicinity of an acute artificial epileptogenic lesion tended to be associated with numerous lower voltage fast spiky waves (afterdischarges), whereas those recorded at some distance did not. Unfortunately such a phenomenon appears to be extremely rare in clinical EEG, perhaps because most focal epilepsy encountered in practice is of a chronic type. It could, however, be sought in more acute situations, for example after head trauma. Furthermore, similar afterdischarges have been recorded from the exposed cerebral cortex during surgical operations without consistent establishment of local pathology (Ralston & Papatheodorou, 1960; Engel, Driver & Falconer, 1975). A variant of this concept has been put forward by Babb and Crandall (1976) whose microelectrode recordings, in epileptic patients being investigated for neurosurgery, indicated that there might be significant differences in inter-ictal firing patterns of individual neurones in the vicinity of an epileptogenic lesion and those at a distance. As validation of such experimental work is difficult in the absence of neuropathological studies and a long post-operative follow-up, the technique must be regarded as showing future rather than current promise.

The second type of experimental work of relevance to the multifocal spike problem is that involving study of the *mirror focus*. This was investigated by Morrell (1960) and has since become of widespread interest, particularly in relation to the effects of ablation and commissure section procedures (Lowrie, Maccabe & Ettlinger, 1978). Briefly, the main observations are as follows:

1. An artificial epileptogenic lesion in one cerebral hemisphere of an experimental animal leads to the development of an EEG spike focus in the immediate vicinity of the lesion and also to objective contralateral seizure phenomena.

2. After a period of time, related partly to the location and character of the lesion and partly to the age and species of animal, a second spike focus appears in the homologous area of the contralateral cortex. This is the mirror focus, which is initially time related to the original focal spiking, each contralateral spike appearing after a short interval presumably related to interhemispheric conduction.

3. Eventually the time relationship between the primary and mirror foci disappears and the two foci continue apparently independently of each other.

4. The mirror focus will only develop if at least some of the interhemispheric connections are intact (e.g. corpus callosum or upper brain stem).

5. Removal or other inactivation (e.g. intracarotid barbiturate) of the primary lesion is followed by disappearance of both primary and mirror foci if the spikes are time related, but by persistence of the mirror focus if they are not.

6. Biochemical, radioisotope, microelectrode and other studies have demonstrated changes in the cortex in the vicinity of the mirror focus which show some resemblance to changes produced by the epileptogenic agent on the primary side.

7. Observations concerning objective independent epileptic phenomena on the side of the animal contralateral to the mirror focus are extremely scanty.

The question has to be asked concerning the possible importance of this mirror phenomenon in human studies: is there a class of epilepsies in which the responsible pathological process is clearly lateralised and localised but which gives bilateral spike abnormalities in the EEG? If so, techniques with significant effects in the experimental situation might well enable a clear differentiation to be made between those patients with bilateral spikes related to bilateral structural pathology and those with bilateral spikes and a

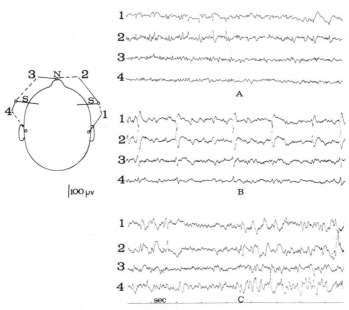

Fig. 5.9 Unilateral and bilateral temporal lobe spike foci. In the electrode pattern **S** indicates a sphenoidal needle electrode and **N** an electrode on the tip of the nose. **A**. Unilateral spike focus in a young woman with a history of temporal lobe epilepsy from childhood. No spikes were recorded at any time from the left side. There are relative excesses of slow activity and deficiencies of fast activity on the right side (compare channels 1 and 4) which support the diagnosis of a right temporal lesion. **B**. Frequent spikes as a focus at the right sphenoidal electrode, often followed after a brief interval by lesser magnitude spikes at the left. It is impossible to say whether the phenomenon on the left represents a mirror focus secondary to that on the right or only indicates current flow from one half of the head to the other (the negative spike on the left appears to be in time with the positive phase of the spike on the right). In subsequent thiopentone-induced sleep the spikes on the left disappeared but a modification in form of those on the right prevented definite conclusions. The patient (aged 26) had a slight left hemiparesis and had generalised convulsive seizures from 3 to 12 years of age and temporal lobe seizures from 14. **C**. Bilateral and independent spike foci in an adult who had had temporal lobe epilepsy since childhood.

lateralised pathology. As it happens, bilateral time-related spikes are not common in the EEGs of patients with focal epilepsy. Bilateral spikes apparently independent in time are far more frequent, particularly in temporal lobe epilepsy, in which variety the clinical seizure pattern may include few or no phenomena of definite lateralising significance (Fig. 5.9). One possible reason for this could be that most cases of temporal lobe epilepsy with bilateral spikes have passed the stage in which the mirror focus is dependent on the primary lesion.

If this were so the chance of distinguishing between the primary and mirror foci, for example by an intracarotid amylobarbitone test, would appear to be small. However, certain observations do point to the distinct possibility that some patients with bilateral spikes have epileptic seizures related to dysfunction of one side only. These are, firstly, that a surgical operation is almost as likely to be effective in cases of temporal lobe epilepsy with bilateral spikes as in those with unilateral (Engel, Driver & Falconer, 1975), and secondly that some patients show a remarkable consistency of fit pattern, including possibly lateralising features, even though bilaterally independent spikes are present in the EEG. It does appear possible, then, that even if a mirror focus is established it may well have no independent truly epileptogenic properties, and its identification therefore becomes worthwhile. Though intracarotid amylobarbitone might not demonstrate the primary nature of a spike on one side and the secondary nature of the contralateral spike, an assessment of seizure *threshold* on the two sides might clearly demonstrate a marked difference: such a procedure, the intracarotid injection of a convulsant drug, has been advocated by Gloor *et al*. (1964) and Garretson, Gloor and Rasmussen (1966), and will be noted later in this chapter.

Classification of epilepsy on purely EEG grounds does therefore present problems, most of them related to the fact that therapeutic surgical procedures are not commonly possible in a way that leads to confirmatory evidence, and necropsy studies in patients who have had extensive EEG examination are very rare. Even at the level of simple sensorimotor epilepsy with a single spike focus localised to the contralateral central region it cannot be stated with absolute confidence that a structural cortical lesion will be demonstrable at operation. If *focal* spikes can transmit from one area of cortex to another and from hemisphere to hemisphere, and if the normal alpha rhythm represents thalamic projection to the cortex, is it not possible for *focal* cortical spikes to be secondary to lesions in deep structures, for example the thalamus? Just as the manifestations of generalised epilepsy, clinically and in the EEG, reflect a widespread bilateral dysfunction of both deep and cortical systems, cannot the manifestations of more restricted forms of epilepsy reflect dysfunction of a limited part of these systems? If it is accepted that cortical spikes can be secondary in this sense then perhaps *focal* is an inappropriate word to describe this variety of epilepsy; a view taken by Gastaut and others which has led to substitution by the word *partial* in the International Classification. It may be, though, that EEG features other than spikes, for example very irregular slow waves or a persistent local deficiency of fast activity, will give an indication that the responsible lesion is cortical rather than subcortical.

Another experimental observation, by Marcus and Watson (1966) must be noted at this point: discrete bilateral cerebral hemispheric lesions can lead to the development of bilaterally synchronous spike and wave complexes even though the midline subcortical grey matter is removed. The precise mechanism of this phenomenon is uncertain, but presumably it depends on a form of interhemispheric recruitment which leads rapidly to generalised bilateral seizure activity. Possibly at least some of the generalised epilepsy and the EEG spike and wave found in children with congenital brain disease, or in children and adults with severe brain damage following trauma or infection, depends on such a process. Spike and wave in the EEG, and presumably generalised forms of epilepsy too, can therefore reflect some at present unknown, but possibly biochemical, defect of function of deep subcortical grey matter, or the presence of a single organic lesion suitably situated in one cerebral hemisphere or bilateral cerebral hemispheric disease. In addition, factors related to white matter function may also be of importance.

The observation (Prince & Farrell, 1969) that intramuscular injection of penicillin in the cat can result both in generalised epileptic seizures apparently resembling petit mal, and to the simultaneous appearance of bilateral spike-wave in the EEG, has provided a model for petit mal which does not depend on localised cerebral manipulation (e.g. by electrical stimulation or lesion induction). Subsequent investigations using this model have shown that

1. the spike-wave first appears in the cortex and only later in subcortical structures, no consistent pacemaker being apparent (Fisher & Prince, 1977)

2. a similar effect is produced by extensive cortical though not by sub-cortical direct application of penicillin (Gloor, Quesney & Zumstein, 1977; also Fisher & Prince 1977)

3. the initiation of spike-wave bursts is closely related to that of the 'spindle' formations of the intact animal's EEG (Quesney *et al.*, 1977)

4. an experimental reduction of cortical excitability causes replacement of the spike-wave by spindles (Gloor, Pellegrini & Kostopoulos, 1979). These findings, together with those obtained from a different experimental model (Steriade, 1974; Steriade & Yossif, 1974) add support to Gloor's (1968) suggestion that the 'centrencephalic' or 'subcortical' concepts of generalised epilepsy be replaced by a 'cortico-reticular' concept. This would recognise both the presumed cortical epileptogenic state and the importance of the triggering propensities of the deeper structures. That the concept is essentially derived from studies of experimental spike-wave rather than directly of petit mal does not detract from its value as a definite move away from a view of generalised epilepsy which, though never accepted by many experienced in clinical epilepsy, had become almost a dogma.

The upshot of these and other experimental findings, as well as experience in the neurosurgical treatment of epilepsy, is that the demonstration of focal spikes or bilateral spike and wave complexes in the EEG may well be but the start of a diagnostic procedure rather than its completion. Further progress in classification may result from the demonstration of other EEG abnormalities, possibly brought out by *activating* techniques, but the greatest progress is likely to be made only if these procedures are invoked in a logical way to provide answers to definite questions which have been based on clinical considerations.

EEG IN THE EPILEPSIES OF CHILDHOOD

A description of the EEG features related to epilepsy in childhood is complicated by the fact that in many cases the disease process responsible for the development of the seizures is still in an acute or at least progressive stage. In such instances the epileptic seizures may be but part of a picture which includes other evidence of gross

cerebral dysfunction, and a final state dominated by chronic epilepsy may not develop owing to death of the child (e.g. Tay Sach's disease and subacute sclerosing panencephalitis) or the development of a *burnt out* non-epileptic state (e.g. following infantile spasms). In these syndromes as in the epilepsies related to severe congenital brain disease (e.g. microcephaly) the EEG tends to show a gross degree of bilateral and often asymmetrical disorganisation with little or no normal activity, and large amounts of mixed spikes and slow waves. The latter may appear more or less continuously or in short periodic or aperiodic bursts. Though none of the electrical features which have been described in relation to some of these syndromes, for example *hypsarrhythmia* with infantile spasms, is pathognomonic, an EEG can be extremely useful when the diagnosis is in doubt. Figure 5.10 gives examples of the gross abnormalities mentioned above, mainly for comparison with the features more commonly met with in the

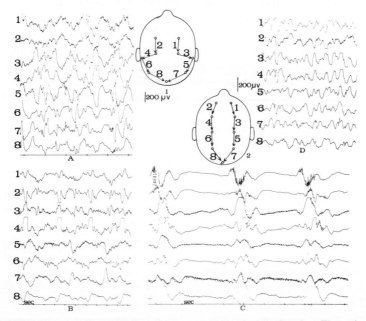

Fig. 5.10 Gross bilateral EEG abnormalities in children with very severe cerebral dysfunction. Electrode pattern 1: **A**. Shows the disorganised mixture of high voltage spikes and irregular slow waves often given the name 'hypsarrhythmia' and commonly found, as here, in association with infantile spasms. **B**. Shows a fairly regular recurrence of high voltage slow waves (channels 2, 4) seen against a disorganised background. The slow waves are predominantly left sided and repeat at about three-second intervals (note the slow paper speed). Their square tops (especially channel 4) are due to limitation of pen movement. The record is from a child with subacute sclerosing panencephalitis, from whom the EEG illustrated in **C** was obtained as the disease progressed. This shows the typical almost regular occurrence of bilaterally distributed mixed slow and spiky waveforms with intervening periods in which little or no EEG activity is recorded. Electrode pattern 2: **D**. Shows a less disorganised but grossly slow EEG from a child with cerebral lipidosis. Spike components occur independently on the two sides. Myoclonic jerking was present, more often so on the right, but not clearly referable to the spikes.

types of childhood epilepsy to be described later. It is suggested that the reader who wishes to pursue the topic of EEG investigation of these most serious diseases of childhood consult Jeavons and Bower (1964) and Harris (1972).

Febrile convulsions in childhood have been the subject of considerable recent attention, both in themselves and in relation to their possible role in the genesis of the sclerotic lesion responsible for a high proportion of chronic temporal lobe epilepsy. EEGs taken within a day or so of such seizures commonly show a grossly and often very irregularly slowed pattern, particularly after more prolonged convulsions. The slow activity gradually subsides over the following week or so but traces can be very persistent. Subsequently, *epileptic* activity is noted in the EEGs of a third or more of these children, commonly taking the form of approximately three per second bilateral rhythmical spike and wave complexes resembling those seen in typical petit mal. Some children, possibly those with the more severe degrees of local brain damage, show focal spikes. Neither of these forms of *epileptic* EEG activity is necessarily associated with a history of epilepsy after the initial febrile convulsions, i.e. they cannot be regarded as of definite prognostic value. A recent monograph (Lennox-Buchthal, 1973) is recommended as further reading (see also Ch. 3).

The remainder of this section will be concerned with the EEG features of syndromes in which, though epileptic seizures may not always be the most constant or more disabling feature, the child is considered possibly to need antiepileptic medication or is stigmatised as being *epileptic*.

1. Petit mal

Almost all children with typical petit mal *absence* attacks will show bursts of bilateral spike and wave activity in the EEG if the recording is carried out appropriately. The spike and wave complexes (Fig. 5.7) commonly repeat rhythmically at about three per second, they show a high (but not absolute) degree of bilateral voltage symmetry, spatial distribution and synchrony as well at the beginning and end of the burst as during its progress. They are usually of maximum voltage (possibly up to about 1000 μV) in the midfrontal regions and

minimum in the posterior temporal regions, though occasionally the reverse is seen. The longer bursts (10 s or so) of such activity appear almost invariably to be associated with some objective diminution of level of consciousness (absence) and, not uncommonly, a deficit in performance can be demonstrated in bursts lasting only one or two seconds (Mirsky & Van Buren, 1965; Tizard & Margerison, 1963). The absences and deficits are not, however, exactly co-extensive in time with the spike and wave: the majority observation has been that the EEG features begin before and outlast the psychological changes, though the reverse has been reported (Mirsky & Van Buren, 1965). Whether this is so or not, a very large part of the daily life of a child with petit mal must be in a state of less than perfect cerebral function (Fig. 5.11). That this affects school performance is also a matter of dispute (Stores, 1978). Goldie and Green (1961) noted that some children with undoubted spike and wave associated petit mal attacks also had periods of inattention during which no spike and wave complexes appeared in the EEG, suggesting on the one hand the possibility that not all such periods in children with petit mal are *epileptic* or on the other that *epileptic* phenomena in petit mal may occasionally not be accessible to EEG techniques. A replication of this study using additional procedures such as 'background' EEG sampling and computer analysis (on the lines of Simon, Müllner & Heinemann, 1976) would be of interest.

As noted in the previous section, irregularities and asymmetries of spike and wave complexes may in some cases indicate that the complexes are

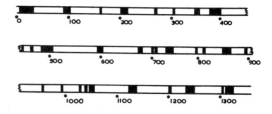

Fig. 5.11 Incidence and duration of spike and wave bursts in a patient with petit mal. Thirty such bursts occurred during a 25-minute EEG recording, indicated by the black bars (figures are seconds elapsed). The 12 longest bursts were associated with obvious absence attacks. Episodes of spike and wave activity occupied 16 per cent of the total recording time, those with associated absences 13 per cent.

secondary to a lateralised cortical lesion or to bilateral organic cerebral hemispheric disease. In the current state of knowledge it is not possible to lay down definite descriptive criteria which will enable a complete separation of primary and secondary generalised epilepsies to be made, though the more extreme departures from three per second and from regularity of form, repetition and bilateral synchrony of onset, almost certainly mean that some form of organic cerebral disease is present. Thus the *petit mal variant* EEG described by Gibbs and Gibbs (1952), essentially a slow (two per second) repetition of rather coarse spike and wave complexes, was shown both by Gibbs on the basis of the patient's history and by Lennox (1953) on the basis of twin studies to be related to brain damage. Incomplete bilateral synchrony of the spike and wave is perhaps the commonest reason why petit mal, and also generalised convulsive seizures in children (since the EEG in such may also show spike and wave complexes), are thought

possibly to be secondary to a cerebral hemispheric lesion. This is rarely borne out by further investigation, for example by air encephalography, in cases where symmetry and synchrony are otherwise typical of true petit mal and where there are no neurological or other features which might suggest brain damage. It has to be borne in mind, as noted above, that the degree of bilateral symmetry of the child's EEG in health is less than the adult's and asymmetries of many phenomena have to be accepted as normal in children which would be very unusual or definitely abnormal in adults. Characteristic examples, including asymmetries of the vertex waves and spindles of sleep, are illustrated in Figure 5.4.

The EEG of children with petit mal commonly changes in sleep, the regular sequences of complexes each consisting of one or more spikes followed by a slow wave giving way to bursts, often lasting several seconds, of multiple spikes with few or no slow waves (Fig. 5.12).

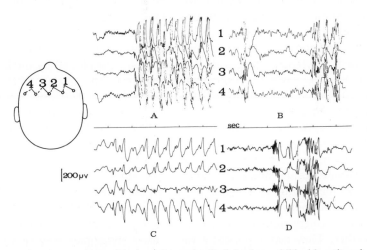

Fig. 5.12 Changes in spike and wave complexes with sleep. **A**, awake, **B**, light sleep: child with petit mal. The asymmetry of some of the complexes (e.g. first in **A**, to the left, and first in **B**, to the right) was thought not to be significant. **C, D**, both light sleep: adolescent boy with petit mal and generalised convulsive attacks since infancy but with recent behaviour disturbance (aggression), occasional automatisms and possibly dysphasic attacks. No definite evidence of localised (e.g. temporal lobe) brain disease was found.

2. Myoclonic and generalised convulsive seizures

Convulsions occurring in children who also have petit mal attacks probably represent only a spread or intensification of the basic *discharge* responsible for the absence. The EEG in such cases commonly

shows spike and wave complexes similar to those seen in simple petit mal, but not infrequently the spike components are multiple and the make-up of the complexes shows an irregularity from one to another, though bilateral synchrony is usually maintained. This variety of complex is seen in the various atonic and akinetic seizures of the International Classification. It is not infrequently difficult during the development and progression of generalised convulsive and myoclonic seizures to distinguish the true cortical spike potentials of the EEG from artefacts related to the electrical activity (EMG) of the face, neck and scalp musculature and to the violent movements of those structures. Simultaneous EMG and movement recording (accelerometer or similar device) is of value in making this distinction, as are specialised computer programmes (e.g. one devised for CNV studies by Shibasaki & Kuroiwa, 1975) and intracerebral recording (Wieser et al., 1978).

Generalised convulsive seizures are very commonly features of those conditions of childhood in which one cerebral hemisphere is extensively damaged with resulting hemiparesis and sometimes mental subnormality also. Simple cerebral hemiatrophy, gross porencephaly and the Sturge-Weber syndrome are examples. The EEG in such cases shows both *lesion* and *epilepsy* features, the former including a unilateral defect of alpha, beta, sleep spindle, and K complex activity, reflecting the non-functioning cortex of one hemisphere, and the latter various spike and complex waveforms as may be met with in other varieties of epilepsy. Not uncommonly epileptic EEG abnormalities appear bilaterally, but not symmetrically. Typically, focal spike and slow and irregular spike-slow complexes of limited or widespread distribution are recorded over the damaged hemisphere, while more regular spike and wave complexes appear on the healthy side. Quite possibly, in some cases, the more regular spike and wave complexes arise through similar processes to those discussed earlier. They may represent a variety of generalised *cortico-reticular epilepsy* which has become modified, at least in its EEG appearance, by the deficiency of normal function in the grossly damaged cortex and other structures on the atrophic side. A hemispherectomy may result not only in a relief from the seizures but also in a disappearance of the contralateral wave and spike complexes.

3. Focal and partial seizures

EEG considerations form only a part of what can

be said about such seizures in childhood, but even so the information available is far too extensive to be dealt with adequately in this chapter. Note will be made here only of temporal lobe epilepsy and the various lines of thought which arise from its consideration. In adults such epilepsy of proven temporal lobe origin is almost invariably associated with an antero-mesial temporal spike focus, which may be unilateral or independently bilateral, and with or without extratemporal secondary spikes. It is usually without inter-ictal diffuse or basal midline spikes or spike and wave complexes even though generalised convulsive seizures may occur at times (Engel, Driver & Falconer, 1975). In children however, with similar *temporal lobe* symptomatology, bursts of bilateral spike and wave complexes similar to those seen in petit mal may be frequent (Fig. 5.13), and demonstration of a clear anteromesial temporal spike focus can be difficult. Follow-up to adult life of some children has demonstrated that the spike and wave bursts become less frequent with the passage of time. One can hypothesise that in many cases of adult temporal lobe epilepsy there has been a progression from a general cerebral tendency to epilepsy (at least as indicated by the EEG) to a purely focal form, though possibly with occasional secondary generalisation. The question then arises as to the meaning of the spike and wave found in the child with temporal lobe epilepsy. Several possibilities present themselves. Firstly, it can represent the same inborn tendency to epilepsy as does the spike and wave found in children with petit mal, but without, for some unknown reason, the associated tendency to absence attacks. In this respect it could be analogous to the spike and wave complexes sometimes seen in the asymptomatic siblings of children with petit mal. Secondly, it could represent an actual tendency to true petit mal attacks which may not be noted or mentioned because of the more severe temporal lobe seizures. In both these possibilities the temporal lobe seizures could perhaps represent the seizure-producing effect of an acquired lesion (e.g. birth trauma, post-natal injury, ear infection and so on) which in hereditarily less susceptible children would not so frequently lead to epilepsy. With either possibility too, the spike and wave complexes could themselves provide a mechanism

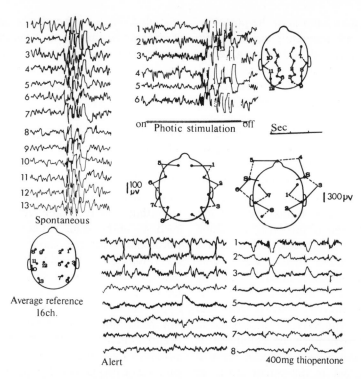

Fig. 5.13 Temporal lobe epilepsy in childhood. Spike and wave bursts occurring spontaneously (top left) and with photic stimulation (top right) in a child with temporal lobe epilepsy who also showed right temporal spikes when awake (bottom left) and asleep (bottom right).

whereby, analogous to the production of a mirror focus or a cortical spike focus secondary to a thalamic spike, a secondary spike focus and possibly later an actual epileptogenic process, could be induced to appear in a susceptible structure, in this case the hippocampus. Thirdly, the spike and wave represents an inborn tendency to epileptic seizures, which, following an intense or prolonged stimulus, as might occur in a *febrile* illness, is expressed as a series of generalised convulsions. During these, susceptible areas of the brain, especially the hippocampus, are damaged in a way which, after a *ripening* period, produces an actual epileptogenic lesion. Fourthly, the spike and wave could itself be secondary to the temporal lobe epilepsy, through the process described in the earlier section in classification. There is no definite EEG evidence at present to decide between these possibilities in individual cases, nor do considerations of family history assist unequivocally. Penfield's hypothesis of *incisural sclerosis* due to birth trauma (Penfield & Jasper, 1954) cannot altogether be excluded as a possibility in some

cases and the findings of Gastaut *et al.* (1959) related to head injury and infection are of relevance.

In cases where there is a definite history of prolonged febrile convulsions or status epilepticus for whatever reason in early childhood the third possibility, that is a secondary hippocampal or mesial temporal sclerosis, appears to be a very likely cause, particularly in view of the experimental evidence given elsewhere in this volume and the clinical studies reviewed by Falconer (1971) and Lennox-Buchthal (1973). Insufficient evidence is at present available regarding the incidence of spike and wave complexes in the EEGs of children with temporal lobe epilepsy due to the hamartomas which account for a large proportion of adult cases. As noted above, demonstration of a clear anterior temporal spike focus may be difficult in children with temporal lobe epilepsy, which could possibly be explained by the *migrating focus* phenomenon described by Gibbs and Gibbs (1960). This represents an hypothesis derived from the observation that in young children the commonly observed spike focus is in the posterior temporal region and with increasing age foci may be seen in the midtemporal and later anterior temporal regions. By no means all posterior foci become anterior foci; the majority remain in the midtemporal regions and carry, according to Gibbs, a good prognosis. Whether a true migration of foci actually occurs or not is undecided, but the observation is an important one and possibly the first signs of a damaged antero-mesial temporal lobe, for example following a period of status epilepticus in infancy, should be sought in the posterior temporal EEG. It may be that the unusual appearance noted involves an alpha irregularity, or a slow wave focus, rather than a definite spike but these may have equal significance in relation to some possibly epileptic behaviour disturbance in childhood. It must be stressed that assessment of what is truly an abnormal degree of asymmetry in the matter of posterior temporal phenomena in childhood is extremely difficult, and warrants special study if the problems of epilepsy in the young are to be dealt with effectively.

The *midtemporal focus* as described by Gibbs was found by Lombroso (1967) in about 1½ per cent of 15 000 records of children aged between 3 and 18 years (all recorded in a hospital and therefore probably *clinical* records). In about 60 per cent of cases showing midtemporal spikes there were features which formed part of a syndrome which Lombroso called *Sylvian seizures*, the main one being somatosensory involvement of the tongue, lips, cheeks, etc. Features suggestive of temporal lobe epilepsy were conspicuously rare. The prognosis of Sylvian seizures, as with the midtemporal spike of Gibbs and Gibbs (1960), was good, 75 per cent of affected children becoming seizure free after five years.

The use of computerised axial tomography has led to the realisation that small temporal lobe lesions of *hamartoma* character may lead to multiple unilateral or possibly bilateral spike or complex abnormalities in the EEG of young children with epilepsy. The possibility of relief by neurosurgery may therefore be contemplated more hopefully than in the past. Only experience will indicate whether adequate criteria for interpreting the EEG in such cases can be devised. Finally, in relation to both temporal lobe and other varieties of epilepsy in childhood, it is important to bear in mind that a very much more useful assessment of the EEG can be made at any stage if previous records are available for comparison.

PRACTICAL PROCEDURES IN THE EEG STUDY OF PATIENTS WITH EPILEPSY

Most laboratories carry out a standard procedure which involves a total of about 20 minutes actual recording. The recording circumstances should be such as to promote patient relaxation, and not uncommonly during about three-quarters of the recording he is undisturbed except for brief periods when he is asked to open and later close his eyes. A period of about 3 minutes' strenuous hyperventilation and another of 2–3 minutes during which photic stimulation or *flicker* is given occupy the remainder of the recording. The details of these procedures are not important here, but one or two points of particular relevance to the study of epilepsy can be made. Firstly, 20 minutes is only a very short time in the daily life of a patient, and since phenomena of relevance to epilepsy may occur at long intervals chance plays an important part in their detection. Secondly, a first EEG recording is a novelty to the patient, and the long preparation time needed might well be conducive to anxiety and excessive muscle and movement artefact in the EEG. Thirdly, a standardised recording procedure will not invariably supply the conditions under which the abnormalities appear in a particular patient. These defects can only be minimised if the EEG is recognised as by far the most important investigation likely to be carried out on a patient with epilepsy; if the recording is carried out in a laboratory with adequate specialist medical and technological staff; and if all details available to the referring physician or surgeon as a result of his interview with the patient are communicated to the laboratory before the recording. An EEG recording carried out merely as a matter of course before the specialist clinician has examined the patient is more often than not of little value.

The number and variety of *activating* techniques in the EEG study of epilepsy is large and no hard and fast rules can be laid down as to which should be employed in given circumstances nor as to how energetically they should be pursued. Enough should be done to answer as far as possible the problems of the particular case, and very good reasons are necessary if any of the possibly unpleasant techniques are to be employed. The more common procedures are listed below, with a few details concerning rationale and technique. Notes concerning their use in particular clinical problems are also given.

1. *Hyperventilation*: the patient is asked to breathe much more deeply than usual and at a faster rate, about 20–25 breaths per minute. Effectively done this leads to a reflex cerebral vasoconstriction and hypoxia, under the influence of which the EEG in health develops increased slow components in the alpha rhythm and bilateral, mainly frontal, slow rhythms appear. Pre-existing abnormalities such as localised slow waves and alpha asymmetries may become more readily assessable when exaggerated by this technique, and occasionally a previously normal EEG becomes abnormal in these respects. The recognition of focal epileptic phenomena is rarely made easier by this procedure, but the spike and wave and multiple spikes of generalised epilepsy are quite commonly more prominent and of far more frequent occurrence after a minute or so of hyperventilation than they were before. This is particularly so in children, in whom an absence or myoclonic attack is often induced. The effects of this procedure, whether of normal or abnormal character, are usually far more prominent in children than in adults. In the latter it can be worthless unless the hyperventilation is sustained for about three minutes and very vigorously pursued.

2. *Photic stimulation*: this is considered in a special section of this chapter.

3. *Sleep*: the frequency of occurrence of experimentally induced EEG spikes can be reduced by electrical stimulation of those parts of the brain concerned with behavioural arousal, for example the *reticular-diencephalic* systems. A similar observation following cerebellar stimulation (Cooke & Snider, 1953 & 1955) suggested a possible therapeutic use of the latter (Cooper *et al.*, 1974). Such observations provide an experimental background to that of Gibbs and Gibbs (1952): the EEG of an epileptic subject is more likely to show spikes or other epileptic features when he is drowsy or asleep than when he is awake and mentally aroused. This 'activating' effect of sleep is particularly noticeable in temporal lobe epilepsy, where the likelihood of recording focal temporal spikes is increased about threefold. Not infrequently, a 'drowsy' or 'sleep' section can be included in the standard EEG recording procedure if disturbance of the patient is minimised by omitting alerting techniques, such as overbreathing and photic stimulation, which are less likely than drowsiness and sleep to lead to the appearance of phenomena of significance. In these circumstances many patients will drift off into light sleep.

In the event that this procedure fails, a second recording is necessary, for which it is advisable to give a sedative drug. A barbiturate (e.g. 200 mg quinalbarbitone for an adult) is most useful, as the induced fast activity provides an additional pointer to cerebral function. However, a sufficient dose of any soporific drug the patient will tolerate is satisfactory.

With this procedure 80–90 per cent of patients with temporal lobe epilepsy will show one or more temporal lobe spike foci and possibly other abnormalities of both epileptic and non-epileptic significance but if not, and the clinical impression of temporal lobe epilepsy is strong, further steps are necessary. With each repeat of a simple sleep EEG the success rate will advance by 1 or 2 per cent, and further advances can be made by repetition after staged withdrawals of antiepileptic medication (see below), by recording during the much deeper sleep induced by intravenous thiopentone or methohexital sodium, and by the use of electrodes which can record from areas unfavourably placed for scalp recording. The *sphenoidal* electrode is the commonest of this type and may occasionally lead to the demonstration of a spike focus which is otherwise invisible. Various types of sphenoidal electrode have been described, that in most common use being a fine insulated wire inserted with the assistance of a rigid needle which is withdrawn after satisfactory placement. Ives and Gloor (1977) describe a recent modification of this method, and Feng and Guo (1979) recommend the use of *acupuncture* needles as electrodes.

It is appropriate to note here that many other drugs, which are not mainly soporific in their properties and may therefore act in a different way to barbiturates, have been utilised with success in the *activation* of temporal lobe spike foci. These include chlorpromazine, hyoscine and procyclidine.

The results of this method of *activation*, whatever drugs and electrodes are used, are such that there are probably few false negatives if three or so recordings are made. It is very difficult to be sure of the exact percentage failure since EEG itself is the main confirmatory technique for the diagnosis, but it is in fact rare for a patient with a strong presumptive diagnosis of temporal lobe epilepsy not to show focal spikes with this technique. That those in this category are not all false negatives is suggested by the series of 59 temporal lobectomies described by Engel, Driver and Falconer (1975) where of the two patients without definite EEG spike foci one had a mesial temporal lesion and did well following lobectomy, the other had no specific temporal lesion and did not improve.

4. *Reduction of antiepileptic medication*: If the patient is already having anticonvulsant medication the possibility must be considered that this is responsible for a failure to demonstrate significant EEG phenomena. However, since withdrawal of barbiturates and other drugs may induce EEG abnormalities with or without actual epileptic seizures in apparently non-epileptic subjects, care must be taken in interpreting the effects of diagnostic withdrawal. It would appear reasonable to assume (as with the use of convulsant drugs noted below) that the appearance in these circumstances of a clearly localised spike or other EEG phenomenon is of significance in relation to a diagnosis of 'focal' epilepsy. On the other hand, a 'generalised' or 'non-specific' activation (for example, a spike-wave burst) need not clearly relate to the patient's habitual attack. This topic is discussed more fully by Ludwig and Ajmone Marsan (1975).

Whether or not EEG investigations are pursued beyond this point depends on the circumstances, but in the authors' view the techniques to be described below have little place in the investigation of temporal lobe epilepsy unless the possibility of neurosurgery is being considered. Even then, they are more useful when the diagnosis has been established and lateralisation is in doubt, rather than as means to determine whether the symptoms are truly epileptic.

5. *Convulsant drugs*: It was noted in the early days of drug-induced convulsant therapy in psychiatry that non-epileptic patients responded with a simple generalised convulsive seizure whereas patients who were also epileptic tended to show some of the characteristics of their spontaneous seizures. This has been confirmed many times since then, and it can be accepted as a working rule that a patient who habitually has only convulsive seizures which are generalised from the beginning will have such a seizure when he is given a sufficient dose of a suitable convulsant drug, whether intravenously or by another route (e.g. by inhalation). Patients who habitually have purely focal attacks will have seizures of similar symptomatology in the same circumstances, and these may later develop into generalised convulsive seizures, particularly if this is also true of the patient's habitual seizures or if there is a history of generalised convulsions in early life. An induced seizure therefore offers a means of investigating the subjective and objective phenomena of the epileptic attacks themselves, and also of the electrical events as recorded in the EEG. It is necessary to stress that this is only so if the patient is known definitely to have epileptic attacks: a normal subject will have a generalised attack if given sufficient convulsive drug, and a patient without known epilepsy but with some localised intracranial disease, for example vascular, may have a focal seizure, apparently as a result of the disturbed cerebral function in the vicinity of the lesion.

In practice, the slow intravenous injection of such drugs (5 per cent leptazol is probably the best) is of greatest value in the study of those focal epilepsies which do not show the high degree of sleep activation of psychomotor epilepsy. This includes the majority of the simple sensorimotor epilepsies and in particular those in which the origin of the seizure is assumed to be in the Rolandic region of either side. It may be that a small amount of leptazol, 100–200 mg or so, will lead to the demonstration of an essentially interictal spike focus, though possibly sufficient (up to a

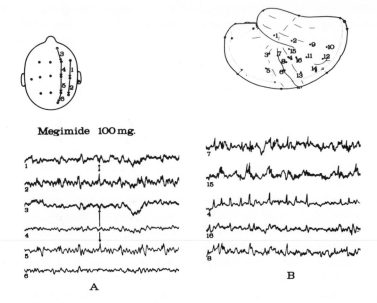

Megimide 100 mg.

A

B

Fig. 5.14 Spikes in focal epilepsy. Records from a young adult with sensorimotor seizures involving the tongue. Standard and sleep records (including use of thiopentone) showed no definite abnormality. Slow intravenous injection of both leptazol (not illustrated) and bemegride led to the appearance of frequent spikes in the right sylvian central area (phase reversals in channels 1, 2 and 3, 5, electrode pattern A, extracted from a 16-channel record). **B**. Electrocorticogram showing several distinct spike foci in a single area in the low right central region. The activity recorded from the other electrodes (not illustrated here) did not include spikes or other abnormal waveforms. The patient was fully conscious at the time of this recording and no convulsive drug injection was necessary.

gram or so) to lead to an actual focal seizure may be necessary before significant localised EEG changes occur (Fig. 5.14).

The technique can also be used in the study of temporal lobe epilepsy, but, as suggested above, in connection with problems of lateralisation rather than primary diagnosis or localisation. For example, if a left-handed patient with invariable ictal dysphasia but bilateral EEG spikes showed a left temporal ictal phenomenon during a drug-induced dysphasic attack it could be concluded that speech representation and seizure initiation were in the left cerebral hemisphere. It may be that because of excess muscle artefact caused by the various ictal movements of the patient, the seizure discharge cannot be discerned in the EEG. In this case a clearly lateralised post-ictal appearance of irregular slow waves, or a lateralised deficit of the fast activity induced by a subsequent intravenous injection of thiopentone will provide equally reliable evidence of lateralisation of the seizure.

6. *Intra-arterial injections*: the use of the intracarotid amylobarbitone and convulsant injec-

tions has been noted in the section on classification and the theoretical basis needs no elaboration. However, a number of points need stressing as these techniques do not in practice tend commonly to give the clear answers expected of them. Possibly the reason for most failures is that the brain disease and associated epilepsy or other disorder of function is not as simple as in the laboratory preparation.

Patients reaching this stage of the investigations without a reasonably logical explanation for their seizures being demonstrated tend to show several different abnormalities in the EEG, and would appear certainly to include a large percentage who have in fact some diffuse, widespread or at least bilateral brain disease. In such it is not to be expected that spikes will disappear bilaterally with an injection on one side and only unilaterally with an injection on the other, or that spike and wave complexes will no longer appear after one injection but will be unaffected by the contralateral procedure. It is also possible to misinterpret a disappearance of focal spikes or spike and wave: they can respond to stimuli unrelated to the pharmacological properties of the injected drug.

Another reason for failure is related to this last point: spike and wave and focal spikes tend to be prominent only when the patient is relaxed or drowsy, whereas the conditions of the intracarotid procedure are of an alerting rather than relaxing nature. It may be necessary to anaesthetise the patient lightly in order to get a state conducive to the appearance of the required EEG phenomena, in which circumstances it is difficult to ensure that the general state of the patient is exactly comparable with the two injections.

Having said this, it must be stated that the intracarotid technique can be a useful procedure in cases where the seizure pattern is such as to suggest an origin invariably in one localised part of the brain, when radiographic and other procedures fail to identify this part, and where the EEG studies have led to equivocal results.

The comparable process of injection of a convulsant drug into the internal carotids in turn and estimating the *seizure threshold* (Gloor *et al.*, 1964) might also, on the basis of animal experiments, be of value in deciding which is the more important side in seizure initiation. However, the possibility that a side for side comparison on that particular occasion does not demonstrate an invariable difference which can be related to the clinical seizures has to be borne in mind.

Additional procedures

Three other procedures which relate to apparatus rather than activation procedures, but which can be used in conjunction with the latter, need also be noted. These are chronically implanted electrodes, telemetry and electrocorticography.

1. *Chronically implanted electrodes,* that is some form of insulated wire or needle electrode stereotactically implanted into cortex or subcortical nuclei through drill or burr holes in the skull, have been used in the study of clinical epilepsy for many years. The main problems associated with such electrodes are that it is often not too clear into what structures they should be inserted, and that the activity recorded from one electrode may not be meaningful in the required sense unless it is compared with that of another electrode in the homologous contralateral area. Such implantations

therefore have tended to involve many electrode insertions through the cerebral cortex on both sides. Even with bilateral recording the results tend to be extremely difficult to evaluate, and in some centres the procedure has been discontinued altogether. In consideration of temporal lobe epilepsy, however, the problems noted above are not so difficult: the amygdala-hippocampal region provides an obvious site and one insertion of a multipolar electrode on each side may be sufficient. Recordings can be taken of the spontaneous ongoing activity, of phenomena occurring in natural and drug-induced sleep, and during spontaneous and induced seizures (Crandall, Walter & Rand, 1963). The procedure also lends itself to telemetering, which is noted below, and to computer assessment (Lieb *et al.*, 1978, which also gives a comprehensive review of the topic).

Implanted electrodes of this type probably offer a definite advantage over the more widely used sphenoidal electrodes in determining the side of onset of a temporal lobe seizure, for which reason they might be considered as the last line of investigation in determination of suitability for a neurosurgical operation for the relief of such epilepsy. Their value in the investigation of clonic muscular twitching has also been demonstrated (Wieser *et al.*, 1978).

2. *Telemetry* is essentially the provision of a radio or similar (e.g. *infra-red*) link between the electrodes, amplifiers and so on attached to the patient and the recording apparatus. Its main justification as a procedure in the study of epilepsy is that is allows the patient to continue with his various activities in the appropriate and habitual environment. The technique would appear to have great potential in the study of seizure frequency and of the factors responsible for the precipitation of the actual seizure, particularly when combined with photographic or television recording of the patient. However, miniature tape recorders which can be concealed in the patient's clothing offer a more simple way of achieving the objective of adequate EEG recording without loss of mobility, and for certain purposes a conventional, though rather long, cable is adequate (Ives, Thompson & Gloor, 1976). Ives and Gloor (1978) describe a complete system for recording EEG and patient activity 'done on a modest budget with no increase

in staff'. Telemetry is considered further in a special section of this chapter.

3. *Electrocorticography*, which includes all recordings of electrical activity of the exposed brain, both superficially and from deep structures, has a history almost as long as that of the scalp EEG. It received a considerable amount of attention in Penfield's work (Penfield & Jasper, 1954) and as a result has been used almost invariably since in surgical operations for the relief of epilepsy. The only aspect of electrocorticography that can be discussed here is to what extent it can be used to guide the surgeon in the operative procedure. Probably more operations have been carried out for the relief of temporal lobe epilepsy than for that of any other single variety, and a start can be made by noting that in such cases both the nature of the epilepsy and the side of the presumed lesion have been determined beforehand. The preoperative EEG has almost invariably shown an anterior temporal spike focus, possibly with an associated irregular slow wave focus and local deficit of fast activity. No EEG evidence to suggest a diffuse or widespread pathology has been recorded. In these circumstances it is not surprising that the surface electrocorticogram, though it increases the detail, rarely provides new information which alters the conclusion drawn from adequate preoperative EEG studies. On rare occasions a clinical impression of temporal lobe epilepsy but without definite EEG support has been confirmed by the demonstration of a temporal lobe spike focus at operation, though possibly even in these cases further EEG recording would have disclosed the spikes. Recordings from deeply inserted electrodes (e.g. in the hippocampus) during the operative procedure commonly yield no further information of value, although the detection of injury potentials may indicate that no gross degree of sclerosis is present. Electrical stimulation may on occasion precipitate what seems to be the patient's habitual seizure but this occurrence does not appear to increase the likelihood that the temporal lobectomy will lead to relief from seizures (Engel, Driver & Falconer, 1975).

The conclusion to be drawn is that where the full capabilities of EEG have been utilised preoperatively, and positive evidence has been obtained of an anterior temporal spike focus, electrocorticography is unlikely to give further information which will influence the operative procedure to be carried out.

The other variety of focal epilepsy for the relief of which a large number of surgical operations have been performed is that involving a sensorimotor symptomatology, suggestive of a lesion of the Rolandic area. The EEG is generally less successful in demonstrating a corresponding abnormality in these cases than with psychomotor epilepsy and a craniotomy may therefore occasionally be carried out on the basis of other information alone. If no cortical lesion is apparent to visual inspection when the brain is exposed, electrocorticography is the only means of localisation of epileptic abnormality. In this respect the technique is almost invariably successful, that is, a clearly delimited spike focus can be demonstrated in a region which could reasonably appear to be involved in the clinical seizure phenomena of the particular case (Fig. 5.14). If recording this spike focus leads to close visual examination of the locality and the detection of some previously unnoticed difference in cortical pattern or colour, and if subsequent incision or needling leads to the demonstration of abnormal tissue, the further course of the operation is clear. Not uncommonly, however, no difference in cortical appearance can be detected in the region of the spike focus, in which case further progress is problematical. Local electrical stimulation may give rise, as it may in normal cortex, to a local electrical after-discharge and to subjective and objective sensorimotor phenomena.

It may be difficult to distinguish between these effects as a possible reproduction of the patient's seizure and a normal response to the stimulus. A conclusion that the actual seizure has been induced is more acceptable if an habitual *march* pattern develops clinically and if ultimately a much wider area of the cortex is involved in the rhythmic spiking. Alternatively a small amount of a convulsant drug may be injected slowly intravenously in order to induce a focal seizure and to record its electrical associates. If no further information can be obtained by these means any local excision that is carried out must be on the basis that cortex in the immediate vicinity of the spike focus is most likely to contain or be adjacent to the responsible lesion. Subsequent histological examination and follow-up studies confirm that this is so in some, but not unfortunately in all cases.

The problem presenting when several separate and apparently independent spike foci can be recorded from what appears to be normal cortex is more difficult. Solution can be attempted on the lines given above but a clear demonstration of the unique epileptogenic properties of the cortex in the vicinity of one electrode is rare.

What is needed in electrical recordings from the exposed brain in the surgery of epilepsy is a reliable differentiation between spikes, or other phenomena, which are topographically related to the epileptogenic lesion and those which are projected to areas of cortex at some distance. Possibly progress towards this will be made when more studies have been carried out on such problems as spike morphology, temporal relationship to other spikes, and spike-background characteristics, and also with the increasing use of microelectrodes. Some work in this direction has been noted earlier in this chapter, including that of Babb and Crandall (1976). The problem of the possible thalamic or other *deep* origin of the focal or *partial* seizure with a projected cortical spike focus might be solved by the same means.

Electrical recordings are also commonly carried out during stereotactic operations for the relief of epilepsy. They are concerned with essentially the same problem as the more widely used neurosurgical procedures, that is the identification of the responsible *focus*, though they have a different purpose in relation to those operations designed to limit the spread of epileptic activity rather than extirpation of its basis. The principles of recording and interpretation are similar to those already discussed here.

This is an appropriate point at which to note that some of the abnormality found in the EEG of patients with focal epilepsy may not be directly related to the 'focus' itself, but to the fact that a form of derived or dependent bilateral or diffuse dysfunction is also present. For example, Brazier *et al*. (1975) demonstrated a global improvement in the EEG following successful surgery, an improvement highly correlated with that observed clinically. Such changes may also be seen following successful drug therapy.

CONTRIBUTION OF THE EEG TO SOME DIAGNOSTIC PROBLEMS

1. The primary diagnosis of epilepsy

The question 'Are the patient's symptoms epileptic?' can rarely, possibly never, be answered from the EEG with an unequivocal negative since, on the one hand, patients with definite epilepsy have been known to have perfectly normal EEG records and, on the other, there are no definite EEG correlates of the various other non-epileptic conditions which could be responsible for the symptoms. The question 'Are there any EEG features in this case which would support a diagnosis of epilepsy?' more readily admits a negative answer. The problem arises quite frequently in relation to episodic aggression or other behaviour disturbance in adolescents and adults, and in relation to absences and faints in children. The former symptoms, if derived from epilepsy, would have a focal and probably temporal lobe EEG correlate, the latter some generalised phenomenon such as spike and wave. A decision has to be made concerning the lengths to which the investigation is to proceed and fortunately in these two common problems it need not be far: with two records, one of them incorporating a 40-minute sleep section, the chances of a false negative would be less than one in ten. If the clinical impression of epilepsy is rather strong and EEG confirmation is sought, a further sleep record could be carried out. The possibility of a *cardiovascular* origin to the symptoms can be investigated by simultaneous EEG and ECG recording (Selby & Driver, 1977).

Where other types of epilepsy are possible different types of investigation may be required. For example with sensory provoked seizures the appropriate stimulus should be sought and used during the EEG investigation. (Poskanzer, Brown and Miller (1962) give a good example of this technique). Possible seizures following excessive fluid ingestion may be similarly investigated.

In respect of the patient with occasional possibly epileptic seizures of late onset in life the EEG is rather unlikely to show any epileptic features at all. Here the problem is better expressed in relation to the possibility of organic brain disease, to which the EEG techniques can be directed. Binnie *et al*. (1979) concluded from a computer assisted

EEG assessment of late onset epilepsy that 90 per cent of patients with cerebral pathology could be detected, and that automatic analysis achieved a four fold reduction in false positive results without increasing the incidence of false negatives.

It has to be remembered in relation to the diagnosis of epilepsy in general, that false positives are possible, for example spike wave complexes in an apparently healthy adolescent. This indicates that the EEG is likely to be most useful when there is a distinct probability rather than a remote chance that the symptoms are epileptic.

2. Relation between EEG abnormality and seizure frequency

In this context, *EEG abnormality* refers to any *epileptic* activity occurring at a time when the patient is not obviously having an epileptic attack. In children with petit mal and patients with generalised convulsive seizures it therefore may include short bursts of spikes or spike and wave complexes which in other respects are best classed as ictal events. The frequency of occurrence of these bursts is very definitely related to the frequency of actual attacks, and the complexes can provide a good index of possible future therapeutic benefit of a particular drug (administered during the recording procedure) as well as benefit derived from a course of therapy already begun.

The relationship between the frequency of extracerebally recorded interictal epileptic phenomena and clinical seizure frequency is much less clear-cut in varieties of focal epilepsy. Though successfully treated cases may show an overall reduction in EEG abnormality in those who continue to have seizures, spikes may be extremely frequent on one occasion and relatively rare on another, both occasions being equally related in time to the previous and the next seizure. This is particularly true in relation to temporal lobe epilepsy where the possibility of different states of mental arousal at the times in question is relevant. In respect of phenomena other than spikes the record may reflect seizure frequency: irregular slow waves and localised alpha and beta deficits tending to be much more prominent at times of frequent seizures. These observations reinforce conclusions drawn from recordings of actual temporal lobe seizures, that the extra-cerebral EEG spike and the epileptic seizure, while both related in some way to the *epileptic* properties of the cerebral lesion, are not very closely related to each other. If this were so, EEG spikes would be unlikely accurately to reflect the therapeutic powers of a particular drug, or the likelihood that a certain cerebral lesion, for example a meningioma or the result of trauma, could provoke epileptic seizures. Though this is borne out in practice it does not follow that EEG recording is of no value at all in these circumstances: *baseline* recordings from the early history of a disease process are very valuable when the need arises to assess the reason for a sudden aggravation of symptoms.

Whether the recording of inter-ictal spikes from appropriate sites within the brain itself could have predictive value in relation to clinical seizure initiation is a matter of controversy. Certainly, observations on penicillin-induced spike foci in cats can provide some evidence relating to impending transition to the ictal state, and such observations might well be applicable to the chronic form of human epilepsy (Sherwin, 1978). Though this was not confirmed by Lieb *et al.* (1978), they supported the possibility that, given observations from within both temporal lobes, the side showing the greater rate of spike activity, and the lesser variation of interspike intervals, was likely to be of the greater significance in the patient's epilepsy. These authors concluded that, though EEG spikes at any particular site did reflect the relative threshold of that site for seizure initiation, they did not provide a prediction of the appearance of the seizure itself. This was possibly because of the importance of other factors such as the chance occurrence of synchrony between several sites. Sherwin (1978) also found that the 'after-discharge' of Ralston (1958), which was referred to earlier in this chapter, was of limited value in providing advance warning of a transition from the inter-ictal to the ictal state, though its claimed status as a pointer to an area of ictal as well as inter-ictal significance was not questioned.

3. Psychiatric aspects

The very extensive literature related to psychiatric aspects of epilepsy, and in particular temporal lobe epilepsy, deals mainly with clinical rather than EEG features, although the latter have been concerned in establishing the nature of the epilepsy and the possible importance of involvement of the dominant as opposed to the non-dominant hemisphere (Slater & Beard, 1963; Flor-Henry, 1976).

Here one is concerned only with diagnostic problems met with when the symptoms could be *psychiatric* or *epileptic*, and a decision has to be made in order to allow appropriate treatment to be given. If the group of organic-based psychoses is eliminated, and these really fall into a different category, the problems become limited to the diagnosis of recurrent episodes of such phenomena as dreamy states, amnesias, illusions, hallucinations, automatisms and so on – all components of what might be a typical psychomotor epileptic attack – and violent, aggressive or other behaviour of a type which could possibly relate to disturbed temporal lobe function of epileptic or non-epileptic character. Patients with such symptoms as part of a clearly *epileptic* picture present no difficulty, but a problem of a different order appears when just one or two of these possibly epileptic symptoms exist in what is otherwise a non-epileptic setting. Very few of these patients will show, even during sleep, the anterior temporal spike so prominent in temporal lobe epilepsy, whereas almost certainly some will show mid temporal or posterior temporal spikes or the '14 and 6 per second positive spike' phenomenon, all of which have been reported as having epileptic significance in psychiatric states, often on very slight grounds (Driver, 1970). Some of these patients, particularly the violent and aggressive, may present very serious management problems and it may well be felt that EEG investigations should be continued beyond the limit suggested above in the consideration of primary diagnosis. This has never led, in the authors' experience, to a definite diagnosis of epilepsy, even when an habitual attack of violent behaviour has been induced by convulsant drug injection.

4. Medicolegal aspects

Several such aspects can be considered, including firstly the primary diagnosis of epilepsy or the possibility of development of epilepsy in post-traumatic cases, particularly where there is actual or impending litigation. These problems have been discussed earlier, but it can be added here that the EEG is a very good indicator of cerebral *dysfunction*, whether epileptic in character or not, and of the location and extent of organic disease responsible for the dysfunction. It therefore has a value beyond the epileptic aspect.

Secondly, in relation to criminal charges: the common experience is that, in the absence of a previous epileptic history, a possible defence that the act was committed during an *epileptic* state is rarely supported by EEG findings. A very large literature has accumulated on this subject, reference to some of which is made in Williams (1969) and Driver, West and Faulk (1974). The latter authors found comparable epileptic abnormalities in groups of prisoners charged with murder and normal controls.

Thirdly, over the question of epilepsy and driving licences: the important information is whether the applicant has seizures or not in circumstances that are likely to occur whilst he is in charge of the vehicle. As noted above, an EEG showing runs of spike and wave or bilateral multiple spikes is a pointer to the likelihood that actual epileptic seizures do in fact occur in present circumstances. On the other hand, a patient who has shown frequent spike and wave complexes invariably in the past but who, possibly because of a change in treatment, has shown none for some time, is probably far less likely to have present attacks. In these circumstances the EEG can be regarded not as definite evidence in itself that the applicant no longer has seizures, but as a support to other evidence to that effect.

In *focal* epilepsy the EEG is unlikely to be of value unless actual ictal rather than inter-ictal activity appears during the recording, or unless phenomena are seen which, on the basis of previous recordings, can be regarded as post-ictal.

TECHNICAL ADVANCES AND THE FUTURE OF THE EEG

Looked at simply in terms of the amount of information, a standard EEG record of 20 minutes' duration represents about 2 million numbers. This forbidding mass of data is at once the challenge for a *number crunching* computer and one reason for the relatively poor success so far of systems designed to resolve the data processing problem. Data compression means data loss and the essential problem is how to extract from the record the information containing elements whilst discarding the rest. Such is the pace of change in computing hardware and costs however, that yesterday's cruncher is today's mini, and the data mass is consequently a lesser problem, but still far from negligible. MacGillivray (1977) and Gotman, Ives and Gloor (1979) discuss the application of automated EEG to the diagnosis of epilepsy, and Barlow (1979) reviews computerised clinical EEG in general.

Several partial systems have been developed although none quite so comprehensive as that of John (1977), who uses a massive array of tests, including multi-system *evoked responses*. The clinical usefulness of such an approach has not, so far, been validated. With all these systems, and there are a dozen or so which are fairly comprehensive in their aspirations, a major problem is still that of *artefacts*: it is unfortunately the case that almost any EEG phenomenon can be simulated by an artefact which fools the human eye, let alone the computer which does only that which human beings tell it to do. With increasing sophistication one can see ways where even this problem can be resolved, but it will need a lot more time yet.

The real value of tools of this sort lies in the objective quantification of the data. Only in this way can we hope to test, validate, or reject the subjective interpretations of clinical practice, form normative and pathological libraries, and define precisely the areas of confusion and misinterpretation which exist currently. At the moment it is an act of faith which some of us, at any rate, believe is not misplaced.

A major future development which might be expected to arise from the use of computers in the clinical environment is the generation of testable heuristic models. Difficulties in the interpretation of the EEG are legion, yet the data are reliable and reproducible. We do not, however, have any useful theoretical infrastructure to help us to know what to do with them.

Aside from the clinical diagnostic aspects, computers have been put to effective use in two areas dealing with rather more limited problems. Rossi has applied a technique developed by Rosadine and co-workers (Rossi, 1973) whereby, given an epileptic spike in any one channel of an EEG recording, the anterior temporal region for example, spikes in all the other channels can be related to this reference precisely in time. Thus it can be determined whether a particular spike leads the others or lags, and by how much, and the statistical relations between spikes can be determined. In this way he has been able to make more appropriate selections of patients for surgery.

The second area is related to the first; Brazier (1973b) has used correlation procedures to trace the path and timing of epileptic activity in the temporal lobe from indwelling depth electrodes. The technique adds new insights into the way epileptic activity moves from one part of the brain to another and has revealed, for example, unexpected tortuous and inconsistent transmission particularly in the temporal lobe. These developments are in their infancy but will undoubtedly add a fund of information of practical value to our knowledge of epilepsy.

Radio-telemetry and portable small pack tape recording, combined with video-recording, provide new insights into the nature and course of epileptic attacks and correlations between behaviour and EEG findings. These techniques have been noted briefly above and are the subject of further discussion in this chapter.

The techniques of evoked responses also hold promise as a diagnostic tool for the detection of some organic brain disturbances (Halliday, McDonald & Mushin, 1973). Variations across subjects are very high and it may be that the topographic distribution of these responses, using the subject as his own control, will offer greater diagnostic finesse. Their value relates obviously to the establishment of lesions which may be causative of epilepsy, and in the proper assessment of the neurologically deprived child who may also be epileptic.

A development outside the specific field of electroencephalography and one which amounts to a revolution in neurodiagnosis and the use of X-rays generally, is computerised axial tomography

(Hounsfield, 1973). This technique is unsurpassed for the detection of structural abnormalities in the brain. It will replace the gamma scan, contrast studies and the majority of arteriograms, and is bound to lead to a reduction in the use of the EEG as a screening procedure for structural lesions. However, as has been emphasised, the EEG looks at the functional state of the brain irrespective of the presence or nature of lesions: as its interpretation and use becomes more sophisticated with development of knowledge about the brain and with developments in computer techniques, the prospects are for an increase rather than a decrease in its use and value.

EDITORIAL COMMENT
John Laidlaw

Almost since its introduction the EEG has played a highly significant part in the study and understanding of epilepsy and, as the authors of this chapter have suggested, properly appreciated, it is likely to prove one of the most valuable methods of elucidating the many unresolved enigmas. Unfortunately, the true value of the EEG has been confounded by the apparent complexities of its technology. All too often a dichotomy has developed between the sophisticated scientist reporting on the EEG and the practising physician trying to relate the reports which he did not understand fully to the management of the patient whom he was trying to help. This dichotomy resulted in, on the one hand, exaggerated ideas of the value of electroneurophysiology, and, on the other, a natural scepticism of a method of investigation which was obscure and too often appeared at variance with clinical judgement.

Our present authors give an excellent critical analysis of the present usefulness of the EEG, firstly, as a method of detecting structural lesions responsible for fits – soon to be overtaken by the equally harmless investigation of computerised axial tomography – and secondly, as an index of the severity of epilepsy by demonstrating the concordance and lack of concordance between *epilep-*

tic discharges in the EEG and clinical fits. However, there are two further ways in which the EEG may be useful in epilepsy which would seem to merit an editorial comment.

The demonstration during the latter half of the nineteenth century of cerebral lesions, appropriately placed and presumably responsible for focal fits, was of immense importance in relieving epilepsy of some of the shrouds of mysticism and demonology. Some half a century later records began to be made on paper of the electrical events in the brain coincident with a fit observed clinically. The medical and scientific importance of the demonstration of the *EEG fit* to the diagnosis and understanding of epilepsy has already been considered in this chapter. Furthermore, it played an essential part in removing finally any lingering doubts and superstitions which doctors may have had about the physical basis of epilepsy. However, I feel that altogether insufficient use has been made of the EEG in helping to allay the fears and prejudices of epilepsy still present among patients and those who are concerned with them. There are quite a number of partial, minor, or modified fits, which are accompanied by EEG events which are dramatically and obviously different from the rest of the record. In some cases such fits are appreciated in part by the patient and are associated with intense fear and indescribable feelings as of obscenity. I had a patient recently, who was so overwhelmed with the horror of what was happening to her and so convinced that she was going mad, that she made several quite determined suicidal attempts. When I showed her the EEG recording during one of her attacks, her sense of relief was pathetic. Some patients with severe epilepsy have EEGs which are grossly abnormal – and it is not necessary to be a clinical neurophysiologist to notice that their records are very different from the normal pattern. The same patients may be difficult to teach or to manage. I have found on many occasions that both nursing staff and instructors find it much easier to understand and sympathise with these *difficult* patients with whom they have to cope, if they can *see something on paper*.

Throughout this book, and particularly in Chapter 8, emphasis has been placed on the deleterious side effects of antiepileptic drugs and of the dangers of overt intoxication. Doubts may even be raised of the efficacy of present antiepileptic drugs in controlling certain types of epilepsy and of the even greater likelihood of overdosage when increasing amounts of many different drugs are used in an attempt to do so. The effect of clinically apparent and sub-clinical *mini* fits on intellectual function has been considered (Ch. 6, 7) but little work has been done on the obtunding effect of antiepileptic drugs, whether in toxic or therapeutic doses. The EEG, which at best is a poor substitute for recent sophisticated methods (Ch. 9) of demonstrating structural cerebral lesions, is the only ancillary method of investigation which attempts to measure disorders of cerebral function. Slowing of the dominant frequency of the background rhythmic activity may provide a sensitive index of the development of toxic or metabolic disorders. It is hardly appropriate in an editorial comment to develop this theme but I would suggest that in the future the EEG, like psychometry and clinical pharmacology, is likely to provide a most useful adjuvant to clinical observation and judgement in avoiding both overt intoxication and latent impairment of intellectual function, which many people feel are a greater disability to the person with epilepsy than the occasional fit.

REFERENCES

Adrian, E.D. & Matthews, B.H.C. (1934) The Berger rhythm. Potential changes from the occipital lobes in man. *Brain*, 57, 355.

Andersen, P. & Andersson, S.A. (1974) Thalamic origin of cortical rhythmical activity. In *Handbook of Electroencephalography and Clinical Neurophysiology*, 2C, p. 90. Amsterdam: Elsevier.

Babb, T.L. & Crandall, P.H. (1976) Epileptogenesis of human limbic neurons in psychomotor epileptics. *Electroencephalography and Clinical Neurophysiology*, 40, 225.

Bancaud, J., Talairach, J., Morel, P., Bresson, M., Bonis, A., Geier, S., Hemon, E. & Buser, P. (1974) 'Generalised' Epileptic seizures elicited by electrical stimulation of the frontal lobe in man. *Electroencephalography and Clinical Neurophysiology*, 37, 275.

Barlow, J.S. (1979) Computerised clinical electroencephalography in perspective. *IEE transactions of biomedical engineering*, 26, 377.

Beck, A. (1890) Thesis (Krakow) quoted by Brazier (1973a).

Berger, H. (1929) Über das Elektrenkephalogramm des Menschen. *Archiv für Psychiatrie und Nervenkrankheiten*, 87, 527.

Binnie C.D., Batchelor, B.G., Gainsborough, A.J., Lloyd, D.S.L., Smith D.M. & Smith, G.F. (1979) Visual and computer assisted assessment of the EEG in epilepsy of late onset. *Electroencephalography and Clinical Neurophysiology*, 47, 102.

Bishop, G.H. & Clare, M.H. (1952) Sites of origin of electrical potentials in striate cortex. *Journal of Neurophysiology*, 15, 201.

Brazier, M.A.B. (1961) *A History of the Electrical Activity of the Brain*. London: Pitman.

Brazier, M.A.B. (1973a) The role of electricity in the exploration and elucidation of the epileptic seizures. In Brazier, M.A.B. (ed.) *Epilepsy, its phenomena in man*, p. 1, New York & London: Academic Press.

Brazier, M.A.B. (1973b) Electrical seizure discharges within the human brain. The problem of spread. In Brazier M.A.B. (ed.) *Epilepsy, its Phenomena in Man*, p. 155. New York & London: Academic Press.

Brazier, M.A.B., Crandall, P.H. & Brown, W.J. (1975) Long term follow-up of EEG changes following therapeutic surgery in epilepsy. *Electroencephalography and Clinical Neurophysiology*, 38, 495.

Bremer, F. (1949) Consideration sur l'origine et la nature des ondes cérébrales. *Electroencephalography and Clinical Neurophysiology*, 1, 177.

Brodmann, K. (1909) *Vergleichende Lokalisationslehre der Grosshirnrinde*. Leipzig: Barth.

Burns, B.D. (1950) Some properties of the cat's isolated cortex. *Journal of Physiology* (London) 111, 50.

Cajal, S. Ramone (1909) *Histologie du Système Nerveux de l'Homme et des Vertébrés*. Paris: Maloine.

Calvet, J., Calvet, M.C. et Scherrer, J. (1964) Etude stratigraphique corticale de l'activaté électroencéphalographique spontanée. *Electroencephalography and Clinical Neurophysiology*, 17, 109.

Caton, R. (1875) The electric currents of the brain. *British Medical Journal*, 2, 278.

Chang, H.T. (1950) The repetitive discharges of corticothalamic reverberating circuit. *Journal of Neurophysiology*, 13, 235.

Contreras, C.M., González-Estrada, T., Zarabozo, D. & Fernández-Guardiola, A. (1979) Petit mal and grand mal seizures produced by toluene or benzene intoxication in the cat. *Electroencephalography and Clinical Neurophysiology*, 46, 290.

Cooke, P.M. & Snider, R.S. (1953) Some cerebellar effects on the electrocorticogram. *Electroencephalography and Clinical Neurophysiology*, 5, 563.

Cooke, P.M. & Snider, R.S. (1955) Some cerebellar influences on electrically–induced cerebral seizures. *Epilepsia* (Boston), 4, 19.

Cooper, I.S., Amin, I., Gilman, S. & Waltz, J.M. (1974) The effect of chronic stimulation of cerebellar cortex on epilepsy in man. In Cooper, I.S. et al (eds) *The Cerebellum Epilepsy and Behavior*. New York: Plenum Press.

Crandall, P.H., Walter, R.D. & Rand, R.W. (1963) Clinical applications of studies of stereotactically implanted electrodes in temporal lobe epilepsy. *Journal of Neurosurgery*, 20, 827.

Creutzfeldt, O. (1974) (Ed) The neuronal generation of the EEG. *Handbook of Electroencephalography and Clinical Neurophysiology*, 2C. Amsterdam: Elsevier.

Dandy, E.W. (1919) Roentgenography of the brain after injection of air into the spinal canal. *Annals of Surgery*, 70, 397.

Driver, M.V. (1970) Electroencephalography and the diagnosis of temporal lobe disease. In Price, J.H. (ed.) *Modern Trends in Psychological Medicine*. London: Butterworths.

Driver, M.V., West, L.R. & Faulk, M. (1974) Clinical and EEG studies of prisoners charged with murder. *British Journal of Psychiatry*, 125, 583.

Eccles, J.C. (1951) Interrelation of action potentials evoked in the cerebral cortex. *Electroencephalography and Clinical Neurophysiology*, 3, 449.

Elul, R. (1972) The genesis of the EEG. *International Review of Neurobiology*, 15, 228.

Engel, J., Driver, M.V. & Falconer, M.A. (1975) Electrophysiological correlates of pathology and surgical results in temporal lobe epilepsy. *Brain*, 98, 129.

Falconer, M.A. (1971) Genetic and related aetiological factors in temporal lobe epilepsy. A review. *Epilepsia* (Amsterdam) 12, 13.

Feng Yingkun & Guo Danhua (1979) The use of acupuncture needles as sphenoidal electrodes in electroencephalography. *Chinese Medical Journal*, 92, 371.

Fisher, R.S. & Prince, D.A. (1977) Spike-wave rhythms in cat cortex induced by parenteral penicillin. 1. Electrographic features. *Electroencephalography and Clinical Neurophysiology*, 42, 608.

Fitz, J.G. & McNamara, J.O. (1979) Spontaneous inter-ictal spiking in the awake kindled rat. *Electroencephalography and Clinical Neurophysiology*, 47, 592.

Fleischauer, K., Petsche, H. & Wittkowski, W. (1972) Vertical bundles of dendrites in the neocortex. *Anat. Entwicklungsgesch.*, 136, 214.

Flor-Henry, P. (1976) Epilepsy and psychopathology. In *Recent Advances in Clinical Psychiatry*. Granville-Grossman, K. (ed.), p. 262. Edinburgh: Churchill Livingstone.

Garretsson, H., Gloor, P. & Rasmussen, T. (1966) Intracarotid amobarbital and metrazol test for the study of epileptiform discharges in man: a note on its technique. *Electroencephalography and Clinical Neurophysiology*, 21 607.

Gastaut, H. (1969) Classification of the epilepsies. Supplement. *Epilepsia* (Amsterdam) 10, S14.

Gastaut, H., Toga, M., Roger, J. & Gibson, W.C. (1959) A correlation of clinical electroencephalographic and anatomical findings in nine autopsied cases of temporal lobe epilepsy. *Epilepsia* (Amsterdam), 1, 56.

Gibbs, F.A. & Gibbs, E.L. (1952) *Atlas of Electroencephalography*, 2. Cambridge, Massachusetts: Addison-Wesley.

Gibbs, F.A. & Gibbs, E.L. (1960) Good prognosis of midtemporal epilepsy. *Epilepsia* (Amsterdam), 1, 448.

Gibbs, F.A., Davis, H. & Lennox, W.G. (1935) The electroencephalogram in epilepsy and in conditions of impaired consciousness. *Archives of Neurology and Psychiatry* (Chicago), 34, 1133.

Gibbs, F.A., Gibbs, E.L. & Lennox, W.G. (1943) Electroencephalographic classification of epileptic patients and control subjects. *Archives of Neurology and Psychiatry* (Chicago), 50, 111.

Gloor, P. (1968) Generalised cortico-reticular epilepsies. *Epilepsia* (Amsterdam), 9, 249.

Gloor, P. (1969) Hans Berger – on the electroencephalogram of man. The 14 original reports on the human electroencephalogram. *Electroencephalography and Clinical Neurophysiology*. Supplement, 28.

Gloor, P. (1972) Generalised spike and wave discharges: a consideration of cortical and subcortical mechanisms of the genesis and synchronisation. In Petsche, H. & Brazier, M.A.B. (eds) *Synchronisation of EEG Activity in Epilepsies*, p. 382. Boston: Little, Brown and Company.

Gloor, P. (1974) Hans Berger – Psychophysiology and the discovery of the human electroencephalogram. In Harris, P. & Maudsley, C. (eds) *Epilepsy: Proceedings of the Hans Berger Centenary Symposium*, p. 353. Edinburgh, Churchill Livingstone.

Gloor, P., Pellegrini, A. & Kostopoulos, G.K. (1979) Effects of changes in cortical excitability upon the epileptic bursts in generalised penicillin epilepsy in the cat. *Electroencephalography and Clinical Neurophysiology*, 46, 274.

Gloor, P., Quesney, L.F. & Zumstein, H. (1977). Pathophysiology of generalised penicillin epilepsy in the cat: The role of cortical and subcortical structures. II. Topical application of penicillin to the cerebral cortex and to subcortical structures. *Electroencephalography and Clinical Neurophysiology*, 43, 79.

Gloor, P., Rasmussen, T., Garretson, H. & Maroun, F. (1964) Fractionated intracarotid Metrazol injection. A new diagnostic method in electroencephalography. *Electroencephalography and Clinical Neurophysiology*, 17, 322.

Glossary of terms most commonly used by clinical electroencephalographers (1974) *Electroencephalography and clinical neurophysiology*, 37, 538.

Goddard, G.V. & Douglas, R.M. (1975). Does the engram of kindling model the engram of normal long term memory? *Canadian Journal of Neurological Sciences*, 2, 385.

Goldie, L. & Green, J.M. (1961) Observations on episodes of bewilderment seen during a study of petit mal. *Epilepsia* (Amsterdam), 2, 306.

Gotman, J., Ives, J.R. & Gloor, P. (1979) Automatic recognition of inter-ictal epileptic activity in prolonged EEG recordings. *Electroencephalography and Clinical Neurophysiology*, 46, 510.

Guerrero-Figueroa, R., Barros, A., Heath, R.G. & Gonzalez, G. (1964) Experimental subcortical epileptiform focus. *Epilepsia* (Amsterdam), 5, 112.

Halliday, A.M., McDonald, W.I. & Mushin, J. (1973) Visual evoked response in diagnosis of multiple sclerosis. *British Medical Journal*, 2, 661.

Harris, R. (1972) EEG aspects of unclassified mental retardation in the brain. In Cavanagh, J.B. (ed.) *Unclassified Mental Retardation*. Edinburgh: Churchill Livingstone.

Hounsfield, G.N. (1973) Computerised axial scanning (tomography) Part I. Description of system. *British Journal of Radiology*, 46, 1016.

Hubel, D.H. & Wiesel, T. (1962) Receptive fields, binocular interaction and functional architecture in the cat's visual cortex. *Journal of Physiology* (London), 160, 106.

Ives, J.R. & Gloor, P. (1977). New sphenoidal electrode assembly to permit long term monitoring of the patient's ictal or inter-ictal EEG. *Electroencephalography and Clinical Neurophysiology*, 42, 575.

Ives, J.R. & Gloor, P. (1978). A long-term time-lapse video system to document the patient's spontaneous clinical seizures synchronised with the EEG. *Electroencephalography and Clinical Neurophysiology*, 45, 412.

Ives, J.R., Thompson, C.J. & Gloor, P. (1976). Seizure monitoring: a new tool in Electroencephalography. *Electroencephalography and Clinical Neurophysiology*, 41, 422.

Jeavons, P.M. & Bower, B.D. (1964) Infantile spasms. *Clinics in Developmental Medicine*, No. 15. London: Heinemann.

John, E.R. (1977) *Neurometrics: Clinical Applications of Quantitative Electrophysiology*. Hillsdale, New Jersey: Erlbaum.

Kandel, E.R. & Spencer, W.A. (1961) The pyramidal cell during hippocampal seizure. *Epilepsia* (Amsterdam), 2, 63.

Korn, H. & Faber, D.S. (1980) Electrical field effect interactions in the vertebrate brain. *Trends in Neurosciences*, 3, 6.

Lange, H., Tanaka, T. & Naquet, R. (1977) Temporo-spatial pattern of subcortical spike activity in kindling epilepsy. A statistical approach. *Electroencephalography and Clinical Neurophysiology*, 42, 564.

Lennox, W.G. (1953) Characteristics and significance of seizure discharges. *Electroencephalography and Clinical Neurophysiology*, Supplement 4, 215.

Lennox-Buchthal, M.A. (1973) Febrile Convulsions. *Electroencephalography and Clinical Neurophysiology*, Supplement 32.

Li, C.L. & Jasper, H. (1953) Microelectrode studies of the electrical activity of the cerebral cortex in the cat. *Journal of Physiology* (London), 121, 117.

Li, C.L. & Chou, S.N. (1962) Cortical intracellular synaptic potentials and direct cortical stimulation. *Journal of Cellular and Comparative Physiology*, 60, 1.

Lieb, J.P., Woods, S.C., Siccardi, A., Crandall, P.H., Walter, D.O. & Leake, B. (1978) Quantitative analysis of depth spiking in relation to seizure foci in patients with temporal lobe epilepsy. *Electroencephalography and Clinical Neurophysiology*, 44, 641.

Lombroso, C.T. (1967) Sylvian seizures and midtemporal spike foci in children. *Archives of Neurology* (Chicago), 17, 52.

Lowrie, M.B., Maccabe, J.J. & Ettlinger, G. (1978) The effects of ablations on primary and secondary epileptic discharges in commissure-sectioned Rhesus monkeys. *Electroencephalography and Clinical Neurophysiology*, 44, 23.

Ludwig, B.I. & Ajmone Marsan, C. (1975) EEG changes after withdrawal of medication in epileptic patients. *Electroencephalography and Clinical Neurophysiology*, 39, 173.

MacGillivray, B.B. (ed.) (1974) Traditional methods of examination in clinical EEG. *Handbook of Electroencephalography and Clinical Neurophysiology*, 3C. Amsterdam: Elsevier.

MacGillivray, B. (1977). The application of automated EEG analysis to the diagnosis of epilepsy. In Rémond, A. (ed.) *EEG Informatics – A didactic review of methods and applications of EEG data processing*. Amsterdam: Elsevier.

Marcus, E.M. & Watson, C.W. (1966) Bilateral synchronous spike and wave electrographic patterns in the cat: interaction of bilateral cortical foci. *Archives of Neurology* (Chicago), 14, 601.

Masland, R.L. (1969) Comments on the classification of epilepsy. Supplement. *Epilepsia* (Amsterdam), 10, S22.

Matsuo, F. & Knott, J.R. (1977) Focal positive spikes in electroencephalography. *Electroencephalography and Clinical Neurophysiology*, 42, 15.

Mirsky, A.F. & Van Buren, J.M. (1965) On the nature of the 'absence' in centrencephalic epilepsy: a study of some behavioural, electroencephalographic and autonomic factors. *Electroencephalography and Clinical Neurophysiology*, 18, 334.

Moniz, E. (1927) L'encéphagraphie artérielle, son importance dans la localisation des tumeurs cérébrales. *Revue Neurologie*, 2, 72.

Morrell, F. (1960) Secondary epileptogenic lesions. *Epilepsia* (Amsterdam), 1, 538.

Mountcastle, V.B. (1957) Modality and topographic properties of single neurons of cat's somatic sensory cortex. *Journal of Neurophysiology*, 20, 408.

Negrin, P. & De Marco, P. (1977) Parietal focal spikes evoked by tactile somato-topic stimulation in sixty non-epileptic children: the nocturnal sleep and clinical EEG evolution. *Electroencephalography and Clinical Neurophysiology*, 43, 312.

Penfield, W. & Jasper, H. (1954) *Epilepsy and the Functional Anatomy of the Human Brain*. London: Churchill.

Peters, A. & Walsh, T.M. (1972) A study of the organisation of apical dendrites in the somatic sensory cortex of the rat. *Journal of Comparative Neurology*, 144, 253.

Petsche, H. (1976) Pathophysiological aspects of epileptic seizures. In Birkmayer, W. (ed.) *Epileptic Seizures – Behaviour – Pain*, p. 11. Bern: Hans Huber.

Petsche, H. & Brazier, M.A.B. (eds) (1972) *Synchronisation of EEG Activity in Epilepsies*. Wein & New York: Springer-Verlag.

Petsche, H. & Rappelsberger, P. (1973) The problem of synchronisation in the spread of epileptic discharges leading to seizures in man. In Brazier, M.A.B. (ed.) *Epilepsy, its Phenomena in Man*, p. 122. New York & London: Academic Press.

Pinel, J.P.J. & Van Oot, P.H. (1975) Generality of the kindling phenomenon: Some clinical implications. *Canadian Journal of Neurological Sciences*, 2, 467–475.

Pollen, D.A., Perot, P. & Reid, K.H. (1963) Experimental bilateral wave and spike from thalamic stimulation in relation to level of arousal. *Electroencephalography and Clinical Neurophysiology*, 15, 1017.

Pollen, D.A. (1969) On the generation of neocortical potentials. In Jasper, H.H., Ward, A.A. & Pope, A. (eds) *Basic Mechanisms of the Epilepsies*, p. 441. Boston: Little, Brown & Company.

Poskanzer, D.C., Brown, A.E. & Miller, H. (1962) Musicogenic epilepsy caused only by a discrete frequency band of church bells. *Brain*, 85, 77.

Prince, D.A. & Farrell, D. (1969) 'Centrencephalic' spike and wave discharges following parenteral penicillin injection in the cat. *Neurology* (Minneapolis), 19, 309–310.

Prince, D.A. & Schwartzkroin, P.A. (1978) Nonsynaptic mechanisms in epileptogenesis. In Chalazonitis, N. & Boisson, M. (eds) *Abnormal Neuronal Discharges*, p. 1. New York: Raven Press.

Purpura, D.P. (1959) Nature of electrocortical potentials and synaptic organisation in cerebral and cerebellar cortex. *International Review of Neurobiology*, 1, 47.

Quesney, L.F. Gloor, P., Kratzenberg, E. & Zumstein, H. (1977) Pathophysiology of generalised penicillin epilepsy in the cat: The role of cortical and subcortical structures. I. Systemic application of penicillin. *Electroencephalography and Clinical Neurophysiology*, 42, 640.

Ragot, R.A. & Rémond, A. (1978) EEG field mapping. *Electroencephalography and Clinical Neurophysiology*, 45, 417.

Ralston, B.L. (1958) The mechanisms of transition of inter-ictal spiking foci into ictal seizure discharges. *Electroencephalography and Clinical Neurophysiology*, 10, 217.

Ralston, B.L. & Papatheodorou, C.A. (1960) The mechanisms of transition of inter-ictal spiking foci into ictal seizure discharges. Part II: Observations in man. *Electroencephalography and Clinical Neurophysiology*, 12, 297.

Rodin, E., Smid, N. & Mason, K. (1976) The grand mal pattern of Gibbs, Gibbs and Lennox. *Electroencephalography and Clinical Neurophysiology*, 40, 401.

Rossi, G.F. (1973) Problems of analysis and interpretation of electrocerebral signals in human epilepsy. A neurosurgeon's view. Brazier, M.A.B. (ed.) *Epilepsy, its Phenomena in Man*, p. 259. New York & London: Academic Press.

Scheibel, M.E. & Scheibel, A.B. (1970) Elementary processes in selected thalamic and cortical subsystems. The structural substrates. In Schmitt, F.O. (ed.) *The Neurosciences*, p. 443. New York: Rockefeller University Press.

Scherrer, J. & Calvet, J. (1972) Normal and epileptic synchronisation at the cortical level in the animal. In Petsche, H. & Brazier, M.A.B. (eds) *Synchronisation of EEG Activity in Epilepsies*, p. 112. Wein & New York: Springer-Verlag.

Selby, P.J. & Driver, M.V. (1977) An unusual cause of apparent epilepsy: ECG and EEG findings in a case of Jervell Lange-Neilson syndrome. *Journal of Neurology, Neurosurgery, and Psychiatry*, **40**, 1102.

Selby, P.J. & Driver, M.V. (1977) An unusual cause of apparent epilepsy: ECG and EEG findings in a case of Jervell-Lange-Neilson syndrome. *Journal of Neurology, Neurosurgery, and Psychiatry*, **40**, 1102.

Sherwin, I. (1978) Inter-ictal – ictal transition in the feline penicillin epileptogenic focus. *Electroencephalography and Clinical Neurophysiology*, **45**, 525.

Shibasaki, H. & Kurojwa, Y. (1975) Electroencephalographic correlates of myoclonus. *Electroencephalography and Clinical Neurophysiology*, **39**, 455.

Simon, O., Müllner, E. & Heinemann, U. (1976) Relation between background activity and subclinical seizure pattern. *Electroencephalography and Clinical Neurophysiology*, **40**, 499.

Slater, E. & Beard, A.W. (1963) The schizophrenia–like psychoses of epilepsy. *British Journal of Psychiatry*, **109**, 95.

Steriade, M. (1974) Interneuronal epileptic discharges related to spike-and-wave cortical seizures in behaving monkeys. *Electroencephalography and Clinical Neurophysiology*, **37**, 247.

Steriade, M. & Yossif, G. (1974) Spike-and-wave after-discharges in cortical somatosensory neurons of cat. *Electroencephalography and Clinical Neurophysiology*, **37**, 633.

Steriade, M., Oakson, G. & Diallo, A. (1976) Cortically elicited spike-wave after-discharges in thalamic neurons. *Electroencephalography and Clinical Neurophysiology*, **41**, 641.

Stores, G. (1978) School children with epilepsy at risk for learning and behaviour problems. *Developmental Medicine Child Neurology*, **20**, 502.

Szentagothai, J. (1969) Architecture of the cerebral cortex. In Jasper, H.H., Ward, A.A. & Pope, A. (eds) *Basic Mechanisms of the Epilepsies*, p. 13. Boston: Little, Brown & Company.

Tizard, B. & Margerison, J.H. (1963) Psychological function during wave-spike discharge. *British Journal of Social and Clinical Psychology*, **3**, 6.

Tükel, K. & Jasper, H. (1952) The electroencephalogram in parasagittal lesions. *Electroencephalography and Clinical Neurophysiology*, **4**, 481.

Wada, J. & Rasmussen, T. (1960) Intracarotid injection of sodium amytal for the lateralisation of cerebral speech dominance. *Journal of Neurosurgery*, **17**, 266.

Walter, W.G. (1936) The location of cerebral tumours by electroencephalography. *Lancet*, **2**, 305.

Weir, B. (1964) Spikes-wave from stimulation of reticular core. *Archives of Neurology* (Chicago), **11**, 209.

Wieser, H.G., Graf, H.P., Bernoulli, C. & Siegfried, J. (1978) Quantitative analysis of intracerebral recordings in epilepsia partialis continua. *Electroencephalography and Clinical Neurophysiology*, **44**, 14.

Williams, D. (1969) Neural factors related to habitual aggression. *Brain*, **92**, 503.

APPENDIX 5.1

Method of localisation of maximum potential change. In the diagram, five electrodes in an antero-posterior row on the scalp are connected in a bipolar fashion in channels 1, 2, 3 and 4 and also sequentially to a common reference electrode on the left ear in channels, 5, 6, 7, 8 and 9. The conventional input arrangement to each channel obliges its pen to move upwards on the paper whenever the electrode connected to its first input (solid black line) goes negative relative to that connected to the second input (broken line), and vice versa with relative positivity. Thus, if the third electrode of the row goes negative, the remainder being unchanged, channel 2 will respond by a downward pen deflection. The *phase reversal* (i.e. opposite pen movement) in two bipolar channels with a common electrode gives the same information as the single deflection in the common reference channel, i.e. it locates the electrode showing the maximum potential change and indicates whether the change was towards negativity or positivity. **A** shows a positive spike in channel 6, seen as an *away going* phase reversal in channels 1 and 2 of **B**, and also a negative slow wave of maximum potential in channel 7, seen as a *toward going* phase reversal in channels 2 and 3 of **B**. The spike therefore affects the second electrode of the row more than the remainder, the slow wave the third electrode. The difference in spike magnitude in channels 1 and 2, and in slow wave magnitude in channels 2 and 3 of **B** indicates that other electrodes are also affected to some extent by these potential changes, i.e., the latter are spread over a *field* rather than confined to a single

point. The calibration mark indicates the sensitivity of the apparatus, i.e. the pen deflection given by a 100 microvolt potential difference between the two inputs to a channel. The difficulty of applying this directly to bipolar recording can be seen in **C** where channel 4 (bipolar) shows a lesser peak to peak alpha amplitude than channels 2 and 3 although, as indicated in the common reference channels 8 and 9, it is in fact over the area of maximum alpha voltage.

PART TWO
PHOTOSENSITIVE EPILEPSY

P.M. Jeavons

INTRODUCTION

The first reference to photosensitive epilepsy was made by Gowers in 1885, not by Apuleius as is so often misquoted. Radovici, Misirliou and Gluckman (1932) first described self-induced epilepsy and Cobb (1947) reported flickering light as a precipitant of fits. The first mention of 'television epilepsy' was made by Livingston in 1952.

Bickford, Daly and Keith (1953) divided their photosensitive patients into three groups, one having fits when exposed to flickering light in everyday life, one having seizures only when exposed to flicker in the EEG laboratory, and one in whom abnormal discharges occurred on intermittent photic stimulation (IPS) without any clinical seizure. Jeavons and Harding (1975) also divided the photosensitive patients into three groups, according to whether fits were only evoked by flicker of everyday life, or were apparently spontaneous as well as being provoked by flicker, or were not apparently evoked by everyday flicker despite having abnormality on IPS. Subsequently analysis of the original patients and other patients seen in the epilepsy clinics suggests that the most useful classification is:

1. Pure photosensitive epilepsy. The fits only occur when the patient is exposed to a flickering light source (or very rarely to a very bright light source which is not flickering). The most common stimulus is television, and the seizures may vary, but are most often tonic-clonic.

2. Epilepsy with photosensitivity. Spontaneous seizures occur as well as those induced by everyday flicker, or there are spontaneous seizures, abnormality is evoked by IPS, but there is no evidence of fits having been provoked by flicker in everyday life.

Pattern-sensitive epilepsy is closely related to photosensitive epilepsy. Pattern-sensitive patients are almost invariably photosensitive and there is increasing evidence that many photosensitive patients are pattern-sensitive, though this may not be suspected unless a correct technique for pattern testing is used.

Seizures due to photosensitivity are probably as common as absence seizures. Of 954 patients seen at my epilepsy clinics, 9 per cent had some form of photosensitive epilepsy. It is important to differentiate photosensitivity from photosensitive epilepsy.

Abnormal response evoked by IPS indicates photosensitivity, but the subject may never have a clinical seizure. Approximately 2–3 per cent of all patients referred for EEG investigation may show spike-wave discharges on IPS (Gastaut, Trevisan & Naquet, 1958; Jeavons, 1966) and brief spike-wave discharges may be found in the clinically normal siblings of patients with photosensitive epilepsy.

The incidence of photosensitive epilepsy in a population aged 5–24 years is probably 1:3970, the figure for males being 1:5441 and for females 1:3087 (G.F.A. Harding, personal communication).

Photosensitive epilepsy usually appears around puberty. Although photosensitivity may be present from as early as three months, the mean age of onset of photosensitive epilepsy is 13.7 years, the mode is 12 years, and the range of age at presentation is 2–58 years. In 76 per cent the onset is between 8 and 19 years.

Females are more likely to be photosensitive than males and the figures in the various subgroups are given in Table 5.1. The figures for myoclonic epilepsy differ slightly from those given by Jeavons and Harding (1975) since the present figures are for those patients primarily diagnosed as myoclonic epilepsy, whilst the previous figures

Table 5.1 Sex ratios in photosensitive epilepsy

	Male	Female
Photosensitive epilepsy	100	169
Self-induced epilepsy	100	233
Impulsive attraction to TV	100	88
Myoclonic epilepsy with photosensitivity	100	260
Myoclonic epilepsy without photosensitivity	100	100
Absences with photosensitivity	100	343
Absences without photosensitivity	100	167

related to any patient with photosensitivity who had myoclonic jerks at any time.

Photosensitive epilepsy is one of the generalised epilepsies and the most common pattern associated with it is spike-wave activity, the slow component being most often at 3 c/s. The peak onset at 12 years is later than absences – the most characteristic of all genetically determined spike-wave epilepsies. Photosensitive epilepsy may be familial (8 per cent) and mothers of photosensitive patients may say that they used to dislike flickering light when they were younger. However, we rarely found abnormality in parents' EEGs, suggesting that photosensitivity had disappeared, presumably after the age of 20 years. This hypothesis cannot be proven for another ten years until we have completed our present follow-up, which started in 1966.

Gerken et al. (1968) and Doose et al. (1969) studied the hereditary aspects of photosensitivity and found that photosensitivity was aged linked, and females predominated. They concluded that the photoconvulsive response (PCR) was a symptom of a very widespread genetically determined susceptibility to convulsions of 'centrencephalic' type. We have confirmed the finding of abnormal responses to IPS in the siblings of probands with photosensitive epilepsy.

Harding, Herrick and Jeavons (1978) reported on the first 12 years of a follow up study of 167 patients untreated with drugs. The mean age at the time of initial investigation was 13.4 years. There was no significant change in the lower sensitivity limit (q.v.) suggesting that photosensitivity does not show any marked improvement over a period of seven years. It is because photosensitivity seems to persist for a longer time than one might expect in epilepsy showing spike-wave discharges that it is important to differentiate photosensitive patients from those with similar seizures but no photosensitivity. Furthermore, spike-wave activity in the basic EEG tends to disappear with a lower dose of sodium valproate than is necessary to abolish photosensitivity in the individual patient.

Although many types of seizure may occur in photosensitive patients they are usually generalised and most commonly are tonic-clonic, myoclonic or absences.

Unlike other types of epilepsy, in which the identification and diagnosis is primarily a clinical matter, an EEG is essential to establish photosensitivity. Increasing awareness of the provocative nature of TV viewing has lead to an increase in a clinical diagnosis of 'television' epilepsy being made before there is laboratory confirmation, but because drowsiness and boredom are powerful precipitants of seizures, and since both are not uncommon with prolonged TV viewing, the diagnosis finally depends on the finding of abnormal paroxysmal discharges evoked by IPS. Since nearly half the patients who have fits provoked by everyday flicker may have a normal basic EEG, it is essential to use an effective method of photic stimulation. Only a correct technique, using a combination of pattern with light stimulation, stimulating the fovea, can guarantee the correct identification of the photosensitive patient (Jeavons & Harding, 1975) and strict criteria and correct technique apply equally to testing for pattern sensitivity (Darby et al., 1980) Details of techniques are given in the appendix, but some explanations follow in the text.

PHOTIC STIMULATION

Photic stimulation is a powerful provocative stimulus and will elicit some EEG response in most subjects. It is a simple and valuable laboratory technique, easily standardised unlike hyperventilation and has been used since 1934 when Adrian and Matthews showed that repetitive flashes of light evoked an EEG response in the occipital regions. In 1946 Walter, Dovey and Shipton first used an electronic stroboscope. Photic stimulation is widely used as a routine procedure in most EEG laboratories and provided that EEG recording is made from anterior as well as posterior regions (a parasaggital montage is preferable) three types of response can be elicited.

1. Responses seen only in the anterior regions (Fig. 5.15), consisting of spikes at the same rate as the flash, and associated with jerking of the muscles round the eye are called *photomyoclonic responses* (Bickford et al., 1953). They are present when the eyes are closed, disappear on eye opening, are a response of muscles to high intensity

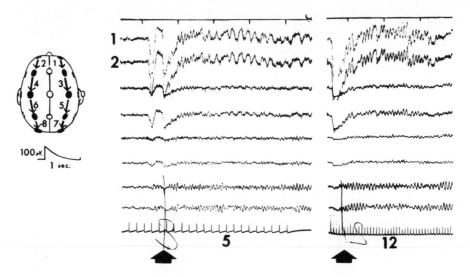

Fig. 5.15 Photomyoclonic response to IPS at 5 and 12 Hz. The activity in channels 1 and 2 is at the same rate as the flash. The black arrows indicate eye closure. (Reproduced from Jeavons, 1969 by kind permission of the editor)

illumination, and have little clinical significance. If the technique described in the appendix is used they will not be elicited, since the lamp has to be placed very close to the eyes and the light must be very bright.

2. Responses seen only in the posterior regions consist of *photic driving*, or *visual evoked potentials*, or *occipital spikes*. Photic driving is a rhythmic response at the same rate or a harmonic or sub-harmonic rate of the flash and although it is said to be symmetrical many patients show a lower amplitude response on the left, and the amplitude

difference may be as much as 50 per cent. An asymmetrical response may be seen in patients who have a unilateral cerebral lesion (Hughes, 1960; Kooi, Thomas & Mortensen, 1960), but such patients usually show asymmetry of alpha rhythm and abnormal slow rhythms and it is rare for asymmetry of photic driving to be the only manifestation of cerebral abnormality. Photic stimulation was found to be of limited value in non-epileptic patients by Coull and Pedley (1978). Photic driving is illustrated in Figure 5.16 which also demonstrates the importance of foveal stimu-

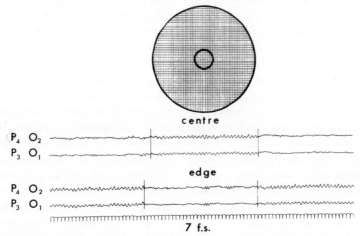

Fig. 5.16 Photic driving response to 7 flashes/second. The vertical lines indicate the patient's change of gaze from the edge of the lamp to the circle in the centre (upper 2 channels) and from the centre to the edge (lower 2 channels). The lamp carries a pattern of small squares

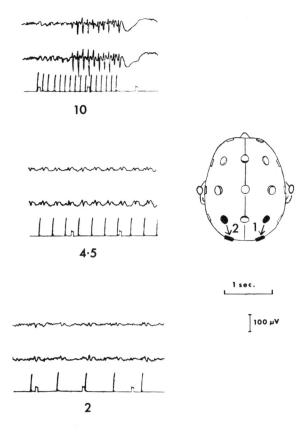

Fig. 5.17 Occipital responses to IPS in one patient. At 2 Hz the visual evoked response has a sharp wave appearance, at 4.5 Hz it appears as a pseudo-spike and wave, and with 10 Hz there are occipital spikes (Reproduced from Jeavons & Harding, 1975, by kind permission of the publishers)

lation – the patient must be looking at the centre of the lamp in order to elicit normal and abnormal responses.

Visual evoked potentials may be seen in the routine EEG if pattern is combined with flash (Fig. 5.17). They occur with slow flash rates or may be seen at the onset of a train of faster flash rates. It is necessary to use an averaging or summation technique to demonstrate the waveform clearly, and the techniques and findings are beyond the scope of this chapter.

Occipital spikes, first described by Hishikawa *et al.* (1967) give a pseudo-spike wave appearance at slower flash rates (below 5 Hz) the spike becoming more apparent at faster rates (Figs. 5.17, 5.18). Occipital spikes are strictly confined to the occipital regions and are rarely seen in routine EEGs unless there is a pattern in front of the lamp of the photostimulator. Their relation to visual

evoked potentials has been described by Panayiotopoulos, Jeavons and Harding (1970, 1972), Dimitakoudi, Harding and Jeavons (1973) and Jeavons and Harding (1975). They are consistently seen in the visual evoked potentials of photosensitive patients and appear on the descending part of the second positive component, provided pattern and light stimulation are combined. Occipital spikes are reduced on monocular stimulation, frequently precede a photoconvulsive response (PCR), and persist when the PCR have been abolished by therapy with sodium valproate (Harding, *et al.*, 1978). Occipital spikes as the sole abnormality evoked by IPS occur in epileptic and non-epileptic patients and must be regarded as a non-specific finding. They certainly do not necessarily indicate photosensitive epilepsy. They may be found at any age from 15 months to 74 years, are not affected by anticonvulsants in any consis-

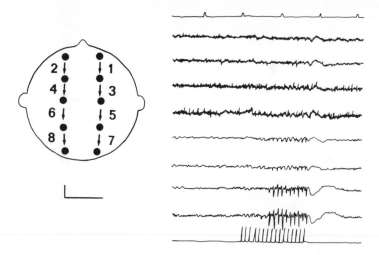

Fig. 5.18 Distribution of occipital spikes evoked by IPS at 10 Hz. Calibration 100 μV and 1 s

tent manner, and nearly half the patients gave no history of epilepsy (Maheshwari & Jeavons, 1975).

3. Responses which are widespread, bilateral, synchronous and involve anterior and posterior regions are known as *photoconvulsive responses* and were clearly differentiated from photomyoclonic responses by Bickford *et al*. (1953). The PCR usually consists of a spike-wave discharge with a 3 c/s component (Fig. 5.19) but there is wide variation in the components (Jeavons, 1969; Jeavons & Harding, 1975). Discharges occur when the eyes are open or closed but are more common with eyes open (Table 5.2). They are rarely found in clinically normal individuals, other than those who are first degree relatives of patients with photosensitive epilepsy. The discharge may be accompanied by a generalised myoclonic jerk.

Photosensitive discharges are found in 2–3 per

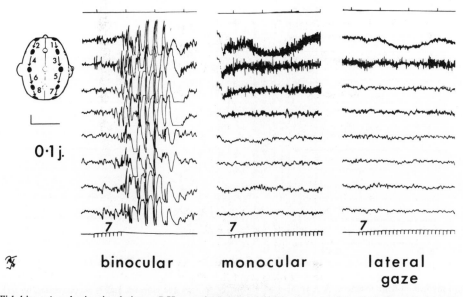

binocular   monocular   lateral gaze

Fig. 5.19 With binocular photic stimulation at 7 Hz a typical photoconvulsive response is evoked after 1 s of exposure. When the patient covers her eye with the palm of the hand a stimulus lasting 3 s evokes no abnormality and none occurs on lateral gaze. Kaiser photostimulator at 0.1 j. Calibration 100 μV and 1 s (Reproduced from Jeavons, 1974, by kind permission of the editor)

Table 5.2 Comparison of IPS with eyes open or closed

Photoconvulsive responses evoked	Number of patients	
Only with eyes open	176	(63%)
More with eyes open than closed	82	(30%)
Only with eyes closed	5	(2%)
More with eyes closed than open	14	(5%)
Total	277	

cent of all patients referred for EEG examination. Their presence indicates a low convulsive threshold, genetically determined, but they do not necessarily indicate either clinical or photosensitive epilepsy since they may occur in patients who have never had a fit induced by flickering light in everyday life. Spike-wave discharges may be evoked by IPS at an early age – our youngest patient was three months old. The finding of such discharges in very young children is not an indication of clinical photosensitivity. Children with febrile convulsions usually show no abnormality in the EEG if it is taken before the age of two years, but after this age spike-wave discharges may be

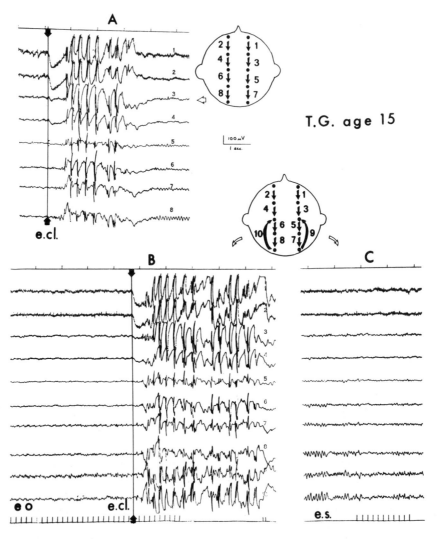

Fig. 5.20 Eyelid myoclonia with absences. **A** A spike-wave discharge follows eye closure, and is accompanied by jerking of eyelids. **B** No abnormality is evoked by IPS at 5 Hz with eyes open but a prolonged discharge occurs on eye closure. **C** No abnormality occurs in response to 5 Hz when the eyes are already closed. (Reproduced from Jeavons, 1978 by kind permission of the publishers)

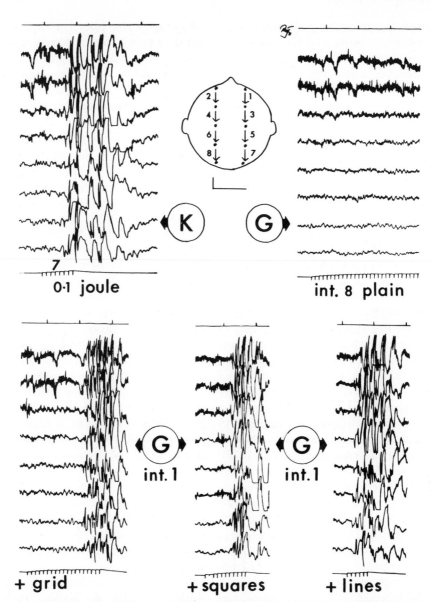

Fig. 5.21 Effect in one patient of pattern combined with IPS. **K** = Kaiser photostimulator with metal protective grid. **G** + Grass photostimulator, with plain glass, or metal grid, or pattern of small squares or vertical line pattern. When no pattern is present no abnormality is evoked. Calibration 100 μV and 1 s (Reproduced from Jeavons *et al.*, 1972, by kind permission of the editor)

present. Since young children will rarely hyper-ventilate properly, photic stimulation is important and may well induce spike-wave, indicating the low convulsive threshold, but not indicating that epileptic attacks will continue into later life.

If photoconvulsive responses are evoked it is more likely that the patient has epilepsy than a non-epileptic condition (provided that no relative had spike-wave in the EEG) but the patient may not show clinical photosensitivity. Most patients with spike-wave on eye closure in the basic record will show a PCR on IPS and will have clinical epilepsy. All patients who have polyspike and wave on IPS have clinical epilepsy, and if a myo-clonic jerk is evoked the patient invariably has clinical epilepsy.

It is important to expose the patient to a wide range of flash rates, starting at 1 Hz and testing up to 60 Hz (see appendix). Each rate is presented separately, with eyes kept open or kept closed throughout. It is essential to distinguish the responses with eyes open, or with eyes closed, from those occurring on eye closure. Cerebral electrical activity is different during the one or two seconds immediately following closure of the eyes – the alpha rhythm may be 2 c/s faster than the basic rate during this brief time and spontaneous spike-wave discharges may occur immediately after eye closure in patients with eyelid myoclonia (Figs 5.20, 5.21).

When testing the effect of IPS in a photosensitive patient it is most important to reduce the risk of inducing a tonic-clonic seizure. If the duration of the stimulus is less than two seconds such a seizure is most unlikely, especially if the lamp is switched off at the first sign of a PCR. It is easy to establish, in any individual, the range of flash rates which will evoke a PCR, and such detailed investigation is important for the individual and also for evaluating the risks of flicker in everyday life. We found that 96 per cent of photosensitive patients were sensitive to flash rates between 15 and 20 Hz, and 98 per cent showed a PCR in response to 16 Hz (Jeavons & Harding, 1975). Television in Europe produces flicker at 50 Hz and 25 Hz, and 49 per cent of patients are sensitive to 50 Hz and 75 per cent to 25 Hz. These two rates should always be tested in the patient who has had fits evoked by TV. Flicker at 8 Hz produced a PCR in 42 per cent of patients, yet this is the fastest rate permitted by the Greater London Council in public discotheques (there is no limit on private discotheques). Adequate protection would only be given if the rate was limited to 5 Hz or less.

By establishing the slowest rate and the fastest rate to elicit a PCR one can quantify the patient's sensitivity range and this measure can be used to assess the efficacy of drugs, and also the prognosis of photosensitive epilepsy. It is, of course, essential to standardise the procedure as described in appendix 5.2.

Photic driving and PCR may only be elicited if the patient looks directly at the centre of the lamp, which must be placed at a distance from the patient's eyes to permit focussing on the glass and the pattern, and if the patient wears spectacles, these should be worn during testing. A pattern of small squares or lines should be placed at the back of the glass (provided this is clear) of the lamp. The effect of such a grid or line pattern is shown in Figure 5.21. The lamp should be placed directly in front of the patient who must stare at its centre. The effect of moving the gaze from the centre is shown in Figures 5.16 and 5.19. Since lateral shift of gaze prevented abnormal discharges we tested the effect of lateral illumination, placing the photostimulator to the side, or using two lamps, one at each side. Provided the patient continued to stare straight ahead abnormal discharges were not evoked, even with very bright bilateral illumination. On the basis of this finding we concluded that seizures were most unlikely to occur in drivers of cars proceeding along tree-lined roads with the sun coming from the side, although passengers may have seizures because they can stare for a long enough time towards the sun.

Monocular stimulation usually inhibits abnormal discharges (Fig. 5.19). The patient is asked to press the palm of the hand firmly in to the side of the nose whilst continuing to stare at the centre of the lamp. It is important to test the effect of monocular occlusion in all photosensitive patients, especially the response to 25 Hz in those with 'television' epilepsy, because of its use in therapy. Both eyes should be tested because in some patients, especially those with different visual acuity in each eye, the procedure may be more effective in one eye.

We have not confirmed the view of earlier workers (Walter & Walter, 1949; Livingston, 1952; Carterette & Symes, 1952; Marshall Walker & Livingston, 1953; Pantelakis, Bower & Jones, 1962; Brausch & Ferguson, 1965; Capron, 1966) that red light is more provocative. If one tests the effect of IPS either immediately on closing the eyes or with eyes closed, the eyelids act as a red filter and under these circumstance red light will be more effective than blue or green. Testing with eyes kept open we found that there was a significant reduction in sensitivity with blue light compared to white light.

CLINICAL ASPECTS OF PHOTOSENSITIVE EPILEPSY

Pure photosensitive epilepsy

Our original study showed that 40 per cent of the photosensitive patients only had fits when exposed to flicker and in 88 per cent the precipitant was television. Other flickering light sources included sunlight reflected from water (swimming baths, rivers whilst fishing), sunlight viewed through the leaves of trees in a breeze, being driven along tree-lined roads with the sun at the side, discotheques, faulty fluorescent lighting, lights in fairgrounds or in amusement arcades. A number of patients experienced unpleasant sensations with patterns, such as the steel steps of escalators, railway sleepers or posts viewed from carriage windows, fluted glass, roof tiles, and striped materials. No patient has so far complained about the diagonal or horizontal white or yellow lines on the roads, although lights in underpasses have evoked sensation. Pattern sensitivity is discussed later.

The provocative effect of television viewing may be due to a number of factors. Viewing distance is one of the most important and nearly half our patients were close to the screen (a distance of 60 cm or less), and were often switching channels or adjusting controls. A faulty picture may itself be a factor, producing slower flicker, but it is probable that it is the approach to the set that is most important. When the picture is viewed from several feet away only the 50 Hz is visible whilst with closer viewing lines are visible and the flicker is at 25 Hz. Pantelakis et al. (1962) found that some patients had fits when the TV set was functioning properly and viewed at a normal distance, whilst others only had fits when close to the set, or when it was faulty. Stefannson et al. (1977) showed that 70 per cent of patients who were photosensitive were also pattern sensitive, more being sensitive to vibrated than static pattern. Jeavons et al. (1972) showed the importance of combining pattern and photic stimulation and Jeavons & Harding (1975) found that only 15 per cent of patients were sensitive to 60 Hz compared to 49 per cent sensitive to 50 Hz, this difference being the main reason why 'television' epilepsy is less common in the U.S.A. where the mains AC frequency is 60 Hz, com-

pared to 50 Hz in Europe. We found that 73 per cent of patients were sensitive to 25 Hz – half the rate of the mains frequency – and this is the rate visible with close viewing. Wilkins et al. (1979) compared the effect of colour and monochrome TV and the epileptogenic properties of patterned and diffuse IPS. There was no significant difference in sensitivity to colour or monochrome TV, although more patients were sensitive to monochrome. Connell et al. (1975) had found colour TV slightly less likely to evoke abnormality. Although statistical proof is lacking there is anecdotal evidence to suggest that colour TV may be less provocative. Wilkins et al. (1979) found that patients who were sensitive to diffuse IPS had a threshold viewing distance greater than 1 m, and in all patients, sensitivity to TV decreased with increase in viewing distance. A small TV screen evoked less abnormality in all patients. For patients who were only sensitive when close to the screen, 25 Hz was a factor. These authors pointed out that whilst conventional visual display units do not present a risk to photosensitive individuals, the increasing use of electronic information retrieval systems and of domestic computers may lead to an increase in 'television' epilepsy.

It is not always possible to obtain an accurate description of fits which occur when watching television, since these often occur when no-one else is in the room, the patient having approached the set to switch or adjust it, and being subsequently found by a member of the family, still unconscious on the floor. In our series, 84 per cent appeared to have had a tonic-clonic seizure, and the predominance of such seizures was found by Gastaut et al. (1960). Absences were rare (6 per cent) and myoclonic jerks even rarer. Partial seizures, usually motor, occurred in 2.5 per cent.

A number of patients with 'television' epilepsy are impulsively attracted to the TV screen. The parents often describe the children as being 'drawn like a magnet to the set'. Such patients show a significantly higher proportion of males (Table 5.1) in comparison to other patients with photosensitive epilepsy, including those with self-induced epilepsy. They are sensitive to a wide range of flash rates, more than half of them are sensitive to everyday flicker, others have spontaneous fits and they are very likely to show spike-wave discharges in the basic EEG. A few appear to use the TV screen for self-induction of seizures, and one of our patients would go close to the set and switch channels in the middle of a programme, for no apparent reason. The attraction to the set may be very strong and with some children it is impossible to leave them alone in the room whilst the TV is on. Children who dislike approaching the set yet are unable to resist the attraction may be treated by some form of monocular occlusion such as eye patching or special spectacles, but most have to be treated with anti-epileptic drugs and the most effective is sodium valproate. This usually prevents the impulsive attraction, although EEG abnormality may still be present on IPS.

Self-induced epilepsy is rare and there have been about 100 reports in the literature since the first case report by Radovici et al. (1932). The patient usually stares at a source of bright light and waves one hand, with fingers outstretched, rapidly across the eyes. There is evidence that the hand movement, in some patients, is part of the ictus rather than the stimulus (Livingston & Torres, 1964; Ames, 1971; 1974; Jeavons & Harding, 1975). Several of the patients in the cine films of Ames appear to have eyelid myoclonia on coming out in to bright sunlight. Many patients who self

induce are said to be mentally retarded (in contrast to our patients with impulsive attraction to TV and to those of Darby et al. described below). Patients are also said to derive satisfaction from self-induction. The use of the TV screen for self-induction has been described by Harley, Baird and Freeman (1967) and Andermann (1971) and blinking as a method was reported by Radovici et al. (1932), Robertson (1954), Andermann et al. (1962) and Green (1966). Self-induced seizures are most commonly absences with spike-wave, though eyelid myoclonia and generalised myoclonic jerks occur. As with other types of photosensitive epilepsy there is a preponderance of females (Table 5.1).

Darby et al. (1980) described a group of patients who induced paroxysmal EEG discharges by eye closure. All patients carried out a slow eye closure movement accompanied by a sustained upwards deviation of the eyes with a characteristic oculographic artefact different from that produced by blinking or voluntary eye closure, and followed by a burst of paroxysmal EEG activity. The incidence of the discharges was reduced by monocular occlusion, or dark glasses and was reduced or disappeared in darkness. There was nothing to suggest that the eye movement was part of a seizure pattern. Three patients derived pleasure from the habit and there was a tendency for it to increase

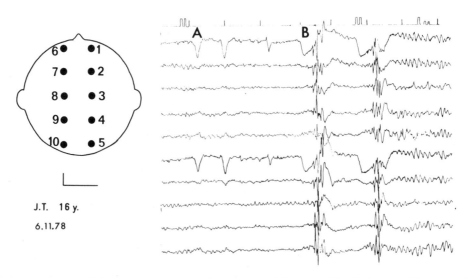

J.T. 16 y.

6.11.78

Fig. 5.22 Paroxysmal discharges follow a slow eye closure. At **A** normal blinks occur. The discharge at **B** is preceded by a slow wave form, repeated in two seconds, after which the eyes remain closed. Calibration 100 μ V and 1 s. Average reference recording

under stress. Only one patient was of subnormal intelligence. In no instance had self-induction been suspected prior to the EEG investigation, and to identify the syndrome it may be necessary to monitor the EEG and oculogram for ten minutes or more. The EEG of one of our patients is shown in Figures 5.22 and 5.23 and the pattern seems to be the same as described by Darby *et al*. (1980) The patient had eyelid myoclonia and her mother noted that she seemed to be attracted by the sun and would blink particularly in bright sunlight. She had myoclonic jerks on spontaneous eye closure.

Patients who show self-induction differ in a number of ways from those who are impulsively attracted to the TV set. The former show a preponderance of females, tend to be mentally retarded, and usually have absences. The latter are predominantly male, are not mentally retarded, and usually have tonic-clonic seizures.

The therapy of self-induction is difficult. Monocular occlusion is rarely successful if the patient is mentally retarded or derives satisfaction from the habit. It is usually necessary to give antiepileptic drugs. Ames and Enderstein (1976) reported some success with clonazepam, and either this drug or nitrazepam or sodium valproate are the most likely to succeed.

Therapy

There are four methods of therapy for photosensitive epilepsy-conditioning, avoidance of the provocative stimulus, protection from the stimulus, and antiepileptic drugs.

Conditioning methods do not seem to be effective (Brabham, 1967; Jeavons & Harding, 1975) although they were used by Forster *et al*. (1964). Protection from the stimulus can be effective and is based on monocular occlusion or the use of special spectacles. Ordinary dark glasses are not effective nor are special tinted or coloured lenses, though if these are to be used blue is probably the best colour. A sophisticated design of spectacles was described by Harding *et al*. (1969) but was not used in practice although it was effective. Wilkins, Darby and Binnie (1977) successfully treated photosensitive patients using a polarising screen in front of the TV set, whilst the patient wore spectacles with one lens polarised in an axis orthogonal to that of the screen, such spectacles being relatively inexpensive.

Protection from the stimulus is often effective, provided that the patient only has fits when exposed to television, though it may be less effective in those who have had fits when viewing from a normal distance and who are sensitive to 50 Hz flicker, or those who have spontaneous spike-wave discharges in the basic EEG. It is more difficult to protect patients from flickering sunlight than from TV. To protect from TV the patient is instructed to view TV from a distance greater than 2.5 m, in a well lit room with a table lamp on top of the set (this reduces relative intensity of light from the screen). A small set is safer than a large one (Wilkins *et al*., 1979) The patient should never

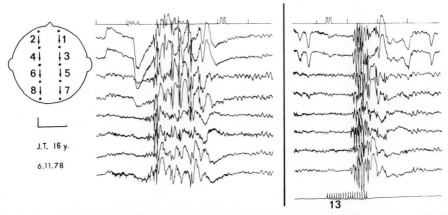

Fig. 5.23 Same patient as Fig. 5.20. A longer irregular spike-wave discharge preceded by a slow eye closure. The photoconvulsive response to 13 Hz consists mainly of polyspikes. Calibration $100\,\mu$V and 1 s.

approach the set to switch channels or adjust controls but if it is necessary to go near to the set the palm of the hand should be firmly pressed in to the side of the nose to ensure monocular stimulation and a similar precaution should be adopted in discotheques if stroboscopic lights are switched on. All patients are shown their EEGs so that they can see the effect of monocular occlusion. In order to reduce the possibility of flickering sunlight provoking seizures polarising spectacles should be worn in sunny weather or when the ground is snow covered, to reduce the flicker from reflections. Ordinary dark glasses or photochromic spectacles are not effective.

Sodium valproate has proved the most effective drug in all forms of photosensitive epilepsy and has the great advantage of lack of sedation, though this may occur with very high dosage. Clonazepam has been reported as abolishing photoconvulsive discharges (Nanda et al., 1977) but it is usually too sedating for children. Ethosuximide may abolish absences induced by IPS, but often has little effect, when given alone, in other types of photosensitive epilepsy and seems to have no effect in pure photosensitive epilepsy.

Because of the infrequency of side effects and especially the lack of sedation, Doose and Gerken (1973) suggested that dipropylacetate might be used in the prophylaxis of symptom free siblings of photosensitive patients. We therefore studied the effect of sodium valproate in photosensitive patients using as a measure the sensitivity range (Jeavons et al., 1976). Spike-wave discharges disappeared first from the basic record, often with a dose of 1 g daily or less, but higher doses were neccessary to abolish the photoconvulsive responses. Occipital spikes were still evoked even when all PCR had disappeared. In pure photosensitive epilepsy control cannot be evaluated on clinical grounds (many patients have only had one or two fits with TV) and assessment is entirely based on the EEG. Complete control means that the EEG no longer shows spike-wave in the basic record nor are there any PCR on photic stimulation, though occipital spikes may still be present. Harding et al. (1978), in a controlled study of sodium valproate, showed that photosensitivity was abolished in 54 per cent and improved by more than 78 per cent in a further 24 per cent. Subsequent withdrawal of sodium valproate lead to a return of photosensitivity, but it is of interest that this return may be delayed for weeks or months after withdrawal, despite a half-life of 6–9 hours.

Rowan et al. (1979), using the sensitivity range as a measure, confirmed the efficacy of sodium valproate in photosensitivity and noted that the maximum effect occurred 1–5 hours after the peak concentration in the blood and lasted up to five days after a single dose of 600 or 900 mg, given to subjects naïve to the drug. In patients already receiving sodium valproate the additional dose had little effect, but all these patients were taking other drugs and in most the daily dose was relatively low (less than 1 g).

We have found that in a number of patients, with various types of epilepsy, a single daily dose is as effective, or more effective, than divided doses (Covanis & Jeavons, 1980).

Epilepsy with photosensitivity

All patients show photoconvulsive responses on IPS, all have seizures not apparently provoked by flicker in everyday life, and some have seizures provoked by such stimuli.

Eyelid myoclonia with absences (Jeavons, 1977)

The characteristic seizure is a brief episode of marked jerking of the eyelids with upward deviation of the eyes, associated with a generalised discharge of spike-wave, and occurring on closure of the eyes (Figs. 5.21, 5.22). The movement of the eyelids is easily visible from a distance, in contrast to the slight flickering of the eyelids with forward staring of the eyes which may occur in simple or complex absences. Patients with eyelid myoclonia also have absences, often complex, and occasional tonic-clonic seizures. All patients are photosensitive and the occurrence in the basic EEG of spike-wave discharges following eye closure is a warning that abnormality will occur on IPS. The discharges on eye closure do not appear in the dark.

The mean age of onset is six years, essentially the same as for absences, but it is important to differentiate this form of epilepsy from absence epilepsy because therapy and prognosis are different. The mean duration in our patients was six years, indicating that therapy is more difficult than in other patients with absences, and this is probably due to the photosensitivity. Eyelid myoclonia is not likely to disappear at puberty. Monotherapy is less successful although sodium valproate alone has controlled all attacks in half our patients. Ethosuximide has not been effective as a sole anticonvulsant, but a combination of this drug with sodium valproate may be needed.

Absences induced by photic stimulation

This is a rare form of photosensitive epilepsy, occurring in 7 per cent. The absences are either simple or complex, can occur spontaneously or in response to flicker in everyday life, though this is rare. The absence induced by IPS is identical to the spontaneous absence, a simple absence lasting 5– 15 seconds, a complex absence lasting up to a min-

ute. Discharges lasting only 1– 3 seconds after the stimulus has ceased are quite common in many patients and are classified as a PCR. Absences induced by IPS are more common in females (Table 5.1), spike-wave discharges are present in the basic EEG in 65 per cent, and half the patients do not have fits with everyday flicker. The spike-wave discharges can often only be induced by a narrow range of flash rates (Fig. 5.24).

This is the only type of photosensitive epilepsy to respond well to ethosuximide, and equally well to sodium valproate.

Myoclonic epilepsy of adolescence (Jeavons, 1977)

The age of onset of myoclonic epilepsy of adolescence is around puberty, rarely earlier than nine years and half our patients are photosensitive. The myoclonic jerks mainly involve the head, arms and

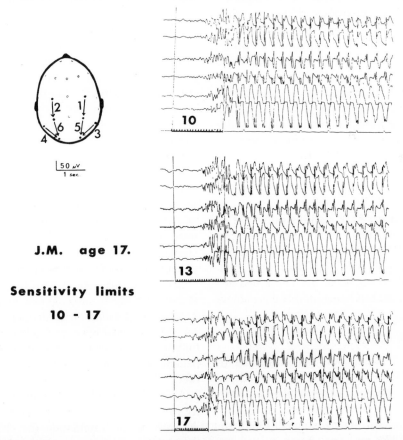

J.M. age 17.

Sensitivity limits 10 - 17

Fig. 5.24 Simple absences induced by IPS over a narrow range of flash rates (10– 17 Hz). The 3 c.s spike-wave discharges start after the cessation of the stimulus. (Reproduced from Jeavons & Harding, 1975 by kind permission of the publishers)

upper trunk, are brief, may be repeated as single jerks over a period of half an hour, occur especially on waking, and in females are more pronounced immediately prior to, or during menstruation, often disappearing during pregnancy. Tonic-clonic seizures are rare, more commonly occurring during sleep, but if diurnal they are often preceded by an exacerbation of jerking. Photic stimulation evokes spike-wave or polyspikewave and a generalised jerk may occur. The basic EEG is often normal, but if a recording is made on waking from sleep, spike-wave or polyspike-wave discharges are commonly seen. The sex ratio differs from that of myoclonic epilepsy without photosensitivity in that females predominate (Table 5.1).

Although the tonic-clonic seizures respond to a variety of antiepileptic drugs the jerks are difficult to control with any drugs other than clonazepam or sodium valproate. Nanda et al. (1977) reported complete control of myoclonic jerks in seven patients and abolition of abnormality on IPS in six of seven photosensitive patients. We prefer sodium valproate because of the lack of sedation and have achieved complete control in eight of nine patients with myoclonic epilepsy of adolescence who are photosensitive, and 18 of 21 who are not photosensitive, the mean duration of the epilepsy in all cases being eight years. Sodium valproate thus seems to be the drug of choice.

Tonic-clonic seizures

Most of these patients have seizures provoked by everyday flicker, but some are identified solely by their response to IPS. Some patients have seizures only during sleep yet consistently show abnormality on IPS. Sodium valproate has controlled seizures in 81 per cent, half being on this drug alone.

Pattern sensitive epilepsy

Pattern sensitive epilepsy was first described by Bickford et al. (1953) and has been reported less frequently than photosensitive epilepsy. Early reports included those of Bickford and Klass (1962, 1969), Gastaut and Tassinari (1966) and Charitan et al. (1970, a,b).

Although there is considerable evidence that sensitivity to pattern is intimately related to photosensitivity, and that pattern plays a significant part in laboratory investigations using IPS, relatively few patients recognise that they are pattern sensitive (Stefannson et al., 1977). We found only 2 per cent who reported symptoms related to viewing patterns (Jeavons & Harding, 1975). The detailed study by Chatrian et al. (1970 a,b) showed that monocular stimulation reduced abnormal discharges evoked by pattern, but they found that patching one eye was not an effective therapy, nor were spectacles blurring vision of one eye. Wilkins, Andermann and Ives (1975) studied a patient who was very sensitive to a wide variety of patterns and confirmed that monocular stimulation was less effective than binocular and that there was a significant reduction in discharges when unfusible binocular patterns were presented. They suggested that the trigger mechanism in pattern sensitivity involved complex cortical cells. Spectacles which blurred the retinal image of one eye were effective in therapy. In a later investigation Wilkins, Darby and Binnie (1979) concluded that paroxysmal EEG activity in pattern sensitive patients depended on the spatial frequency of the pattern (the optimal being between 1 and 4 cycles/degree), the orientation of the pattern, its brightness contrast and its size. They suggested that their findings were compatible with a seizure trigger in the striate cortex.

Stefannson et al. (1977) showed that 70 per cent of patients who were photosensitive were also pattern sensitive in the laboratory, 72 per cent being sensitive to vibrated pattern and 34 per cent to static pattern. All patients who were sensitive to pattern were sensitive to TV. Despite the high laboratory incidence of pattern sensitivity only one patient gave a clinical history of pattern sensitive epilepsy and this suggests that the effect of pattern in everyday life is unrecognised by the patient.

Most EEG laboratories do not specifically test for pattern sensitivity, but in view of the above findings it is obviously important to identify the patient who is at risk from patterns in everyday life.

A simple method for routine testing of sensitivity to pattern is described by Darby et al. (1980). As with photic stimulation the characteristics of the test stimulus are crucial, and for details the original paper should be consulted. The method is summarised in the appendix.

APPENDIX 5.2

Standardised method for photic stimulation (Jeavons & Harding, 1975)
1. The procedure is explained to the patient.
2. The same photostimulator is used in all repeat tests as was used initially.
3. Illumination of the room is standardised by drawing blinds and using artificial light.
4. The lowest intensity light is used initially, increased if there is no abnormality, and standardised in subsequent tests.
5. A pattern of small squares with narrow black lines (0.3 mm), with spacing of 2 mm × 2 mm, or a pattern of parallel lines (1 mm) spaced 1.5 mm apart, is placed behind the glass of the lamp (dry print transfers are cheap and easily available).
6. A circle, of diameter 3 cm, is drawn in the centre of the glass and the patient looks at this circle.
7. The lamp is placed at 30 cm from the eyes.
8. Testing is carried out with eyes kept open or kept closed, and only if no PCR is evoked is the effect of eye closure tested.
9. 16 Hz can be used as an initial test frequency to identify the photosensitive patient. If no PCR is elicited, testing starts at 1 Hz and rates up to 25 Hz are used, followed by 30, 40, 50 Hz.
10. In the photosensitive patient the duration of the stimulus should not usually exceed 2 seconds.

11. In the photosensitive patient testing starts at 1 Hz and increases in steps of 1 Hz until a PCR is evoked. The upper limit is then established by starting at 60 Hz and reducing in steps of 10 Hz.
12. The sensitivity limit is defined as the lowest or highest flash rate which consistently evokes a PCR. The sensitivity range is obtained by subtracting the lower from the upper limit.

Summary of method of testing pattern sensitivity (Darby, Wilkins & Binnie)
1. The black and white stripes should be parallel and of equal size.
2. The optimal width is 2 cs per degree of visual angle (15 minutes of arc) subtending more than 16 degrees.
3. The contrast should be high and brightness above 200 cd/m².
4. The optimal frequency of vibration at right angles is 20 Hz, although vibration by hand cannot exceed 10 Hz.
5. The pattern is circular, diameter 48 cm, with stripes of 2.5 mm.
6. The patient stares at a spot in the centre of the pattern.
7. Viewing is at arms length (57 cm) and the pattern is illuminated by a spot light behind the patient.
8. The pattern is held steady for 30 seconds and is vibrated if no paroxysmal activity is evoked.

REFERENCES

Adrian, E.D. & Matthews, B.H.C. (1934) The Berger rhythm: potential changes from the occipital lobes in man. *Brain*, 57, 355.

Ames, F.R. (1971) 'Self-induction' in photosensitive epilepsy. *Brain*, 94, 781.

Ames, F.R. (1974) Cinefilm and EEG recording during 'hand-waving' attacks of an epileptic, photosensitive child. *Electroencephalography and Clinical Neurophysiology*, 37, 301.

Ames, F.R. & Enderstein, O. (1976) Clinical and EEG response to clonazepam in four patients with self-induced photosensitive epilepsy. *South African Medical Journal*, 50, 1423.

Andermann, F. (1971) Self-induced television epilepsy. *Epilepsia*, 12, 269.

Andermann, K., Berman, S., Cooke, P.M., Dickson, J., Gastaut, H., Kennedy, A., Margerison, J., Pond, D.A. & Tizard, J.P.M. (1962) Self-induced epilepsy. A collection of self-induced epilepsy cases compared with some other photoconvulsive cases. *Archives of Neurology*, 6, 49.

Bickford, R.G. & Klass, D.W. (1962) Stimulus factors in the mechanism of television-induced seizures. *Transactions of the American Neurological Association*, 87, 176.

Bickford, R.G., Daly, D. & Keith, H.M. (1953) Convulsive effects of light stimulation in children. *American Journal of Diseases of Children*, 86, 170.

Bickford, R.G. & Klass D.W. (1969) Sensory precipitation and reflex mechanisms. In Jasper, H.H., Ward, A.A. Pope, A, (eds) *Basic Mechanisms of the Epilepsies*, p. 543. Boston: Little, Brown and Co.

Brabham, J. (1967) An unsuccessful attempt at the extinction of photogenic epilepsy. *Electroencephalography and Clinical Neurophysiology*, 23, 558.

Brausch, C.C. & Ferguson, J.H. (1965) Color as a factor in light-sensitive epilepsy. *Neurology*, 15, 154.

Capron, E. (1966) Etude de divers types de sensibilité électroencéphalographique à la stimulation lumineuse intermittente et leur signification. Thesis, Paris: Foulon.

Carterette, E.C. & Symmes, D. (1952) Color as an experimental variant in photic stimulation. *Electroencephalography and Clinical Neurophysiology*, 4, 289.

Chatrian, G.E., Lettich, E., Miller, L.H. & Green, J.R. (1970) Pattern-sensitive epilepsy, Part 1. An electrographic study of its mechanisms. *Epilepsia*, 11, 125.

Chatrian, G.E., Lettich, E., Miller, L.H., Green, J.R. & Kupfer, C. (1970) Pattern-sensitive epilepsy, Part 2. Clinical changes, tests of responsiveness and motor output, alterations of evoked potentials and therapeutic measures. *Epilepsia*, 11, 151.

Cobb, S. (1947) Photic driving as a cause of clinical seizures in epileptic patients. *Archives of Neurology and Psychiatry*, 58, 70.

Connell, B., Jolley, D.J., Lockwood, P. & Mercer, S. (1975) Activation of photosensitive epileptics whilst watching television: observations on line frequency, colour and picture content. *Journal of Electrophysiological Technology*, 1,

Coull, B.M. & Pedley, T.A. (1978) Intermittent photic stimulation. Clinical usefulness of non-convulsive responses. *Electroencephalography and Clinical Neurophysiology*, 44, 353.

Covanis, A. & Jeavons, P.M. (1980) Once daily administration of sodium valproate in epilepsy. *Developmental Medicine and Child Neurology*, 22, 202.

Darby, C.E., de Korte, R.A., Binnie, C.D. & Wilkins, A.J. (1980) The self-induction of epileptic seizures by eye-closure. *Epilepsia*, 21, 31.

Darby, C.E., Wilkins, A.J., Binnie, C.D. & de Korte, R. (1980) A method for the routine testing for pattern sensitivity. *Journal of Electrophysiological Technology*, 6, 202.

Dimitrakoudi, M., Harding, G.F.A. & Jeavons, P.M. (1973) The inter-relation of the P$_2$ component of the V.E.R. with occipital spikes produced by patterned intermittent photic stimulation. *Electroencephalography and Clinical Neurophysiology*, 35, 416.

Doose, H. & Gerken, H. (1973) Possibilities and limitations of epilepsy prevention in siblings of epileptic children. In Parsonage, M.J. (ed.) *Prevention of Epilepsy and its Consequences*, p. 32. London: International Bureau for Epilepsy.

Doose, H., Gerken, H., Hein-Völpel, K.F. & Völzke, E. (1969) Genetics of photosensitive epilepsy. *Neuropädiatrie*, 1, 56.

Forster, F.M., Ptacek, L.J., Peterson, W.G., Chun, R.W.M., Bengzon, A.R.A. & Campos, G.B. (1964) Stroboscopic induced seizure discharges. Modification by extinction techniques. *Archives of Neurology*, 11, 603.

Gastaut, H. & Tassinari, C.A. (1966) Triggering mechanisms in epilepsy. The electroclinical point of view. *Epilepsia*, 7, 85.

Gastaut, H., Trevisan, C. & Naquet, R. (1958) Diagnostic value of electroencephalographic abnormalities provoked by intermittent photic stimulation. *Electroencephalography and Clinical Neurophysiology*, 10, 194.

Gastaut, H., Regis, H., Bostem, F. & Beaussart, M. (1960) Etude électroencéphalographique de 35 sujets ayant présenté des crises au cours d'un spectacle télévisé. *Revue Neurologique*, 102, 553.

Gerken, H., Doose, H., Völzke, E., Volz, C., & Hien-Völpel, K.F. (1968) Genetics of childhood epilepsy with photic sensitivity. *Lancet*, 1, 1377.

Gowers, W.R. (1885) *Epilepsy and Other Chronic Convulsive Diseases. Their Causes, Symptoms and Treatment*. New York: Wood & Co.

Green, J.B. (1966) Self-induced seizures. *Archives of Neurology*, 15, 579.

Harding, G.F.A., Drasdo, N., Kabrisky, M., & Jeavons, P.M. (1969) A proposed therapeutic device for photosensitive epilepsy. *Proceedings of the Electrophysiological Technology Association*, 16, 19.

Harding, G.F.A., Herrick, C.E. & Jeavons, P.M. (1978) A controlled study of the effect of sodium valproate on photosensitive epilepsy and its prognosis. *Epilepsia*, 19, 555.

Harley, R.D., Baird, H.W. & Freeman, R.D. (1967) Self-induced photogenic epilepsy. Report of four cases. *Archives of Ophthalmology*, 78, 730.

Hishikawa, Y., Yamamoto, J., Furuya, E., Yamada, Y., Miyazaki, K. & Kaneko, Z. (1967) Photosensitive epilepsy: relationships between the visual evoked responses and the epileptiform discharges induced by intermittent photic stimulation. *Electroencephalography and Clinical Neurophysiology*, 23, 320.

Hughes, J.R. (1960) Usefulness of photic stimulation in routine electroencephalography. *Neurology*, 10, 777.

Jeavons, P.M. (1966) Summary of paper on abnormalities during photic stimulation. Proceedings of the *Electrophysiological Technology Association*, 16, 225.

Jeavons, P.M. (1969) The use of photic stimulation in clinical electroencephalography. Proceedings of the *Electrophysiological Technology Association*, 16, 225.

Jeavons, P.M. (1974) The clinical value of the EEG. *Update*, 8, 1077.

Jeavons, P.M. (1977) Nosological problems of myoclonic epilepsies in childhood and adolescence. *Developmental Medicine and Child Neurology*, 19, 3.

Jeavons, P.M. (1978) Electroencephalography. In *Epilepsy Today, Management Guidelines for the Practitioner*. No. 8. Macclesfield: Geigy.

Jeavons, P.M. & Harding, G.F.A. (1975) *Photosensitive Epilepsy*. Clinics in Developmental Medicine No 56. London: Heinemann.

Jeavons, P.M., Harding, G.F.A., Panayiotopoulos, C.P. & Drasdo, N. (1972) The effect of geometric patterns combined with intermittent photic stimulation in photosensitive epilepsy. *Electroencephalography and Clinical Neurophysiology*, 33, 221.

Jeavons, P.M., Maheshwari, M.C., Herrick, C.E. & Harding, G.F.A. (1976). In Legge, N.J. (ed.) *Clinical and Pharmacological Aspects of Sodium Valproate (Epilim) in the Treatment of Epilepsy*, p. 56. Tunbridge Wells: MCS Consultants.

Kooi, K.A., Thomas, M.H. & Mortensen, F.N. (1960) Photoconvulsive and photomyoclonic responses in adults. *Neurology*, 10, 1051.

Livingston, S. (1952) Comments on a study of light-induced epilepsy in children. *American Journal of Diseases of Children*, 83, 409.

Livingston, S. & Torres, I.C. (1964) Photic epilepsy: report of an unusual case and review of the literature. *Clinical Pediatrics*, 3, 304.

Maheshwari, M.C. & Jeavons, P.M. (1975) The clinical significance of occipital spikes as a sole response to intermittent photic stimulation. *Electroencephalography and Clinical Neurophysiology*, 39, 93.

Marshall, C., Walker, A.E. & Livingston, S. (1953) Photogenic epilepsy: parameters of activation. *Archives of Neurology and Psychiatry*, 69, 760.

Nanda, R.N., Johnson, R.H., Keogh, H.J., Lambie, D.G. & Melville, I.D. (1977) Treatment of epilepsy with clonazepam and its effect on other anticonvulsants. *Journal of Neurology, Neurosurgery, and Psychiatry*, 40, 538.

Panayiotopoulos, C.P., Jeavons, P.M. & Harding, G.F.A. (1970) Relation of occipital spikes evoked by intermittent photic stimulation to visual evoked responses in photosensitive epilepsy, *Nature*, 228, 566.

Panayiotopoulos, C.P., Jeavons, P.M. & Harding, G.F.A. (1972) Occipital spikes and their relation to visual evoked responses in epilepsy, with particular reference to photosensitive epilepsy. *Electroencephalography and Clinical Neurophysiology*, 32, 179.

Pantelakis, S.N., Bower, B.D. & Jones, H.D. (1962) Convulsions and television viewing. *British Medical Journal*, 2, 633.

Radovici, A., Misirliou, V. & Gluckman, M. (1932) Epilepsie réflexe provoquée par excitations optiques des rayons solaires. *Revue Neurologique*, 1, 1305.

Robertson, E.G. (1954) Photogenic epilepsy; self-precipitated attacks. *Brain*, 77, 232.

Rowan, A.J., Binnie, C.D., Warfield, C.A., Meinardi, H. & Meijer, J.W.A. (1979) The delayed effect of sodium valproate on the photoconvulsive response in man. *Epilepsia*, 20, 61.

Stefansson, S.B., Darby, C.E., Wilkins, A.J., Binnie, C.D., Marlton, A.P., Smith, A.T. & Stockley, A.V. (1977) Television epilepsy and pattern sensitivity. *British Medical Journal*, 2, 88.

Walter, V.J. & Walter, W.G. (1949) The central effects of rhythmic sensory stimulation. *Electroencephalography and Clinical Neurophysiology*, 1, 57.

Walter, W.G., Dovey, V.J. & Shipton, H. (1946) Analysis of

the electrical response of the human cortex to photic stimulation. *Nature*, **158**, 540.

Wilkins, A.J., Andermann, F. & Ives, J. (1975) Stripes, complex cells and seizures – An attempt to determine the locus and nature of the trigger mechanism in pattern-sensitive epilepsy. *Brain*, **98**, 365.

Wilkins, A.J., Darby, C.E. and Binnie, C.D. (1977) Optical treatment of photosensitive epilepsy. *Electroencephalography and Clinical Neurophysiology*, **43**, 577.

Wilkins, A.J., Darby, C.E. & Binnie, C.D. (1979) Neurophysiological aspects of pattern-sensitive epilepsy. *Brain*, **102**, 1.

Wilkins, A.J., Darby, C.E., Binnie, C.D., Stefannson, S.B., Jeavons, P.M. & Harding, G.F.A. (1979) Television epilepsy – the role of pattern. *Electroencephalography and Clinical Neurophysiology*, **47**, 163.

PART THREE
PROLONGED OBSERVATION AND EEG MONITORING OF EPILEPTIC PATIENTS

R. Cull

R.W. Gilliatt

R.G. Willison

R. Quy

Until a few years ago the admission of an epileptic patient to hospital for observation implied a certain contradiction. The patient would come into the ward and an EEG would be arranged, which might subsequently be repeated with drug-induced sleep or sphenoidal electrodes. During the patient's stay in hospital the total EEG recording time was unlikely to be more than one or two hours. For the rest of his stay the patient was only under observation in the sense that, if he had an attack in the ward, some details of it could be recorded by the nursing staff and shown to the doctor in charge of the case. The chances of the doctor himself being present were small unless the patient was having very frequent attacks. The record made by the nursing staff was often based on details provided by other patients in the ward, particularly in relation to the onset of the attack.

This situation, in which the seizure itself was not usually observed at first-hand, and an EEG was only recorded between seizures, has been greatly improved by the introduction of closed-circuit television (CCTV) for the observation of the patient, combined with long-duration EEG recording carried out in such a way that the patient's mobility is not constrained.

Closed-circuit television can of course be used successfully with conventional EEG recording, provided that mobility of the patient is not important (Penry, Porter & Dreifuss, 1975). For the study of patients during activity, or for the prolonged observation of ambulant patients in hospital, EEG telemetry using radio or cable has obvious advantages, particularly when it is used in conjunction with CCTV. The early development of EEG telemetry was reviewed by Porter, Wolf and Penry (1971); later systems were subsequently reviewed by the same authors (Porter, Wolf & Penry, 1976). Many different systems have been devised, their details varying according to the particular clinical need of the unit concerned. For example, a neurosurgical unit might be particularly interested in the site of origin of EEG spikes immediately preceding a clinical seizure (Ives, Thompson & Gloor, 1976), or in the number of spikes arising in the temporal lobes over a period of observation (Gotman, Ives & Gloor, 1979). To examine the effect of 3-per-second spike-and-wave discharges on a patient's behaviour and performance requires a system providing close-up television coverage of the patient, perhaps with more than one camera, together with a method of quantifying the patient's performance in some standard test (Goode, Penry & Dreifuss, 1970; Porter, Penry & Dreifuss, 1973). Other systems have been reviewed by Stalberg (1976), Kaiser (1976), Mattson (1980) and Rowan et al. (1980).

The use of four-channel portable cassette recorders is a later development, and one which adds a further dimension to EEG monitoring. With this equipment the patient's EEG can be recorded not only in hospital but also at home or at work; in the latter situations, of course, television coverage of the patient cannot be obtained.

This chapter describes three systems which are

in use at the National Hospital, Queen Square, for the monitoring of epileptic patients, and illustrates their application to particular clinical problems.

1. DAY-TIME EEG RECORDING WITH CCTV

The first routine to be introduced was a six-hour session with the patient resting comfortably in a special observation room on the ward floor.

The session usually starts at 10 a.m. and for the first hour the patient may be rather tense and apprehensive of his environment. Although the observation room has been made as comfortable as possible, curtains being used to hide electrophysiological equipment, a patient usually takes some time to settle and relax. While he is free to walk about the room and go across the ward corridor to the bathroom when necessary, he is encouraged to stay as far as possible in a reclining chair in the centre of the room, where he is in full view of the television camera. In the chair he can read, write or watch television programmes. Later his lunch is brought to him. After lunch the patient is encouraged to sleep. For this the room is darkened, the patient being illuminated by an infra-red source so that television monitoring (using a silicon-diode camera with an automatic iris) can be continued. By this time most patients are relaxed and accustomed to the room and few of them have failed to achieve spontaneous sleep. Later in the afternoon the patient is roused and given a cup of tea before the end of the session.

During the session an eight-channel EEG is recorded, using either radio-telemetry or a long cable to pass the signals to the recording system. For radio-telemetry we have used a small eight-channel transmitter, about the size of a cigarette packet, which can be slipped into the breast pocket of a jacket or pinned to a coat or dressing-gown, with a receiving aerial placed in a corner of the room (Bowden *et al.*, 1975). This system has the advantage that the patient is free from any restraint by wires or cables. There are, however, disadvantages compared with the use of a long cable to connect the electrodes to the recording system. For example, a radio-telemetry link is substantially more expensive than cable, it may

need frequent tuning, and it produces more artefacts in the record. Its disadvantages would be justified if recordings were to be continued over the whole area of the ward floor. However, to obtain a television picture we have found it necessary for the patient to stay in one room where he can be viewed by one or, at the most, two cameras. In these circumstances a long cable to carry the multiplexed EEG signals from the patient to an input socket on the wall has proved perfectly satisfactory, provided that the patient has been able to unplug the cable and take it with him if he wishes to go to the bathroom.

After amplification, the EEG signals are stored on eight channels of a 14-channel FM tape-recorder; other channels are used for sound, a coded time signal, and the output of an ultrasonic movement recorder. Four selected EEG channels are displayed on a memory monitor viewed by a second television camera, so that the pictures of the patient from one camera and of four EEG channels from the other can be mixed and displayed on a split screen, together with a digital clock (Fig. 5.25). If two television cameras are used to view the patient, mixing becomes more complex but it is possible to display four channels of EEG and two views of the patient on a single screen. This picture of the patient and his or her EEG is then stored on video-tape.

As little as possible of the recording and data-processing equipment is kept in the room with the patient. Instead, the signals are passed by cable to a laboratory three floors below the ward, where the recordist, doctor and engineer can move about freely, observe the patient on a monitor screen, and change magnetic tape-cassettes as necessary (Bowden *et al.*, 1975).

This system dispenses with the need to keep bulky paper records. When the tapes are reviewed at the end of a session, interesting portions of the primary EEG can be written out on paper from the FM tape but, if the patient and the EEG have remained normal throughout, no paper record need be kept.

The recordist, having put on the electrodes and set up the session, need not be in constant attendance on the patient. The nursing staff on the ward can provide clinical supervision and the recordist is released for other duties, provided that

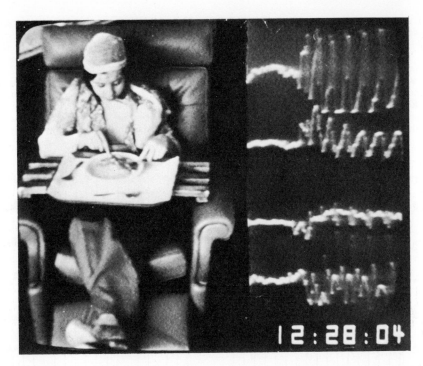

Fig. 5.25 Photograph of TV monitor showing split-screen picture, with patient on the left, and four channels of EEG and digital clock readout on the right. Note the paroxysm of bilateral spike-and-wave activity in EEG record. (From Bowden *et al.*, 1975)

periodic visits are made to the recording laboratory to check the quality of the record and to change tape-cassettes. The recordist is, of course, responsible for darkening the room and settling the patient for sleep after lunch. We have found it helpful to start an eight-channel paper record at this time and to continue it for the hour that the patient is drowsy or sleeping. This may yield evidence of epileptic activity during drowsiness or sleep, even if the patient does not have a clinical attack during the session.

To accelerate review of the material at the end of a session, the television picture of the patient and four EEG channels is recorded not only in real time but also on a separate video-recorder set to run at two or four frames per second instead of 25. By playing this back at the normal speed, a six-hour recording can with practice be reviewed in half or one hour. The times at which clinically relevant phenomena occurred during the session are noted so that these can then be studied in detail.

Six-hour recordings of the type described above are particularly useful in the study of patients with bizarre or unusual attacks which may or may not be epileptic. Results were analysed by Bowden (1976) for the first hundred patients studied by this system during 1974–5. These are reproduced in Table 5.3 and it can be seen that each patient had a routine EEG carried out in the hospital department as well as a long day-time recording by telemetry; the yield of clinical attacks was more than three times greater in the latter. The long sessions with CCTV had the additional advantage that when a clinical attack was recorded, it could be replayed at leisure in the laboratory, and small details could be observed which had not been obvious on first viewing. An illustrative case history is given below.

Case 1

Mrs. C.R. (N.H. No. A83935) was first seen at the age of 59 when she gave a history of infrequent attacks of confusion and altered consciousness for two years. The attacks usually occurred at night; the patient would wake and start to get out of bed. On being asked what was the matter, she would make some reply but might show evidence of confusion (saying perhaps that she wished to put something in a cupboard, or attempting to dress in someone else's clothes). Sometimes she would fall backwards and would be unresponsive with the eyes open for a few minutes before going to sleep again. No stiffening, involuntary movements or incontinence occurred, and in the morning the patient would have no recollection of what had happened. Physical examination revealed no abnormality and investigations were inconclusive. A routine EEG showed a mild excess of slow activity in the right temporal region, and late-onset epilepsy was thought to be the likeliest diagnosis. However, phenobar-

bitone did not prevent infrequent attacks continuing to occur.

The patient was referred back to the clinic at the age of 63, when she was still having episodes of confusion but without actual loss of consciousness. In the attacks, which, as before, were usually nocturnal, the patient might get out of bed and attempt to dress, mumbling in an incoherent fashion. She would get back into bed on her own but might finish up with her head at the wrong end. On another occasion she woke in the morning with bruises and lying on top

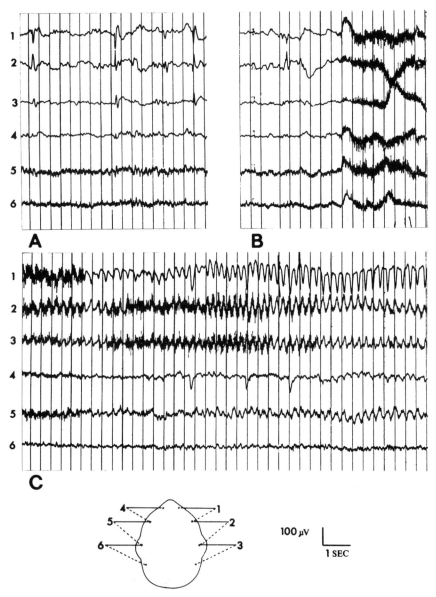

Fig. 5.26 EEG record from Case 1 during post-prandial sleep. **A** shows frequent spike activity arising in the right anterior temporal region. **B** 3 minutes 40 seconds after **A**, a single spike discharge is seen and then the record becomes obscured by muscle artefact. **C** 10 seconds after **B**, the artefact subsides and reveals rhythmical 4 cycles per second activity arising in the right anterior temporal region and spreading to the left side.

of the bed, her eiderdown later being found in the kitchen.

A second routine EEG showed a mild excess of temporal theta activity, more marked on the right side than the left.

At this stage a long EEG recording was carried out using radio-telemetry and CCTV. Recording was started at 11.20 hours and was continued during lunch and the rest period which followed, in which the patient had a natural sleep. The waking record differed little from the previous routine EEGs but as the patient became drowsy high voltage spikes appeared on the right side with a phase reversal in the right fronto-temporal region. At 14.03 hours while the patient was lightly asleep she opened her eyes, lifted her head, moved her jaw and swallowed. There was slight flexion of the neck and trunk and head-turning to the right. During this period which lasted 13 seconds, the EEG was obscured by artefact but the patient then remained quiet with her eyes open and a prolonged paroxysm of rhythmic sharp waves at approximately 4 cycles per second was seen in the right fronto-temporal tracings, which later spread to the left side and which lasted for approximately 30 seconds (Fig. 5.26). After this the patient appeared to wake abruptly and to become aware of her surroundings.

When questioned later in the session the patient denied any unusual occurrence.

Comment

This result illustrates the value of recording a small attack. As is commonly the case, the EEG during the early part of the clinical attack was obscured by movement artefact. However, the record immediately before this showed fairly frequent right temporal spiking; immediately after the movement artefact a prolonged rhythmic discharge in the same region accompanied the later part of the attack.

It can be seen from Table 5.3 that only two thirds of the clinical attacks recorded by Bowden were thought on review to be due to epilepsy. This high proportion of non-epileptic attacks is explained by the selection of patients. Included in this early series was a group of patients who might or might not have had epilepsy in the past but

Table 5.3 Epileptic and non-epileptic clinical attacks obtained during long recordings with telemetry and TV monitoring (average duration 300 minutes) compared with routine EEG recordings in the Hospital EEG Department (average duration 20 minutes) (from Bowden, 1976)

| | Total no. of patients studied | No. of patients in whom clinical attacks recorded | |
		Epileptic	Non-epileptic
Long recording	109	38	19
Routine recording	109	13	4

who were, at the time of the study, thought to be having attacks on a psychological basis. It soon became clear that the prolonged EEG recording with CCTV was particularly valuable in such cases. While epilepsy could never be excluded by the mere absence of a typical discharge pattern in the EEG, there might be clinical details in the television picture which led positively to a diagnosis of hysteria. For example, a well-marked alpha rhythm in an apparently unconscious patient after a violent seizure would be regarded as highly suggestive of a hysterical or simulated attack; blocking of the alpha rhythm by a nurse attempting to rouse the patient would provide clear confirmation of this.

In patients who did not have a clinical seizure during the recording session, the EEG itself often proved helpful in confirming a diagnosis of epilepsy. In his analysis of the 1974–5 patients Bowden found that epileptic activity (paroxysmal activity, random spikes, localised or generalised spike-and-wave bursts) occurred in twice as many patients during long sessions as it did during 20-minute routine recordings (Table 5.4). The fac-

Table 5.4 Number of epileptic patients with epileptic activity in the EEG in long recordings compared with routine recordings (from Bowden, 1976)

	Total no. of epileptic patients studied	No. of patients with epileptic activity in EEG
Long recording	75	66
Routine recording	75	31

tors which result in an increased yield of EEG abnormalities during the longer recordings are of some interest. It has been our impression that the first 30–60 minutes of a recording, while the patient is rather tense and apprehensive, are unlikely to be rewarding. With increased confidence and perhaps boredom on the part of the patient, EEG abnormalities are more likely to appear. Even if absent at this stage, there is a further likelihood of their appearance during post-prandial drowsiness or sleep.

The relation between classical petit mal epilepsy and sleep is a complex one which has been extensively studied by others (Stevens et al., 1971; Sato, Dreifuss & Penry, 1973). Part of the difficulty arises from the fact that the 3 per second spike-and-wave episodes themselves are altered in character during sleep, losing their regularity and consistency of wave form. In deep sleep they may be replaced by single spikes or spike-and-wave complexes which presumably represent inter-seizure rather than seizure activity.

This change is illustrated in Figures 5.27 and 5.28. The patient, a boy of 12, with known petit mal, showed infrequent episodes of generalised 3–4 per second spike-and-wave discharges while awake. The regularity and consistency of wave form is illustrated in Figure 5.27. During post-prandial sleep the number of episodes increased. They tended to become shorter and more irregular in form as sleep deepened (Fig. 5.28).

The use of an automatic system to count spike-and-wave complexes is also illustrated in Figures 5.27 to 5.29. In this system (Jestico et al., 1977) a band pass filter was used to extract the 2–4 Hz component of the spike-and-wave complexes from the EEG signal; when the voltage of activity at this frequency reached a pre-set level (shown in Fig. 5.27), a pulse was generated by the detector, which could be stored and summed, so that the number of spike-and-wave complexes in a 10 or 20-second epoch could be written out by a chart recorder. Also written out on the chart was the filtered and integrated output of slow activity in the EEG, so that the depth of sleep could be assessed.

The full results for the session from which the tracings in Figures 5.27 and 5.28 were taken, are shown in Figure 5.29. The total duration of sleep is signalled by the output of an ultrasonic movement recorder, and it can be seen that body movement virtually ceased between 1300 and 1400 hours. During the first half of this period the content of slow activity in the EEG gradually increased, indicating deepening of sleep. A change can be seen in the middle of the sleep period, after which the patient was only lightly asleep. Isolated episodes of 3 per second spike-and-wave activity had occurred earlier in the session while the subject was awake, individual episodes lasting for 10 seconds or more. Associated with the increasing depth of sleep were more frequent episodes but these were of shorter duration, rarely lasting for more than 5 seconds.

2. OVERNIGHT EEG RECORDING WITH CCTV

Once the daytime system described above had

Figs 5.27–5.29 EEG records and results of automatic analysis from a 12-year-old boy with petit mal epilepsy.

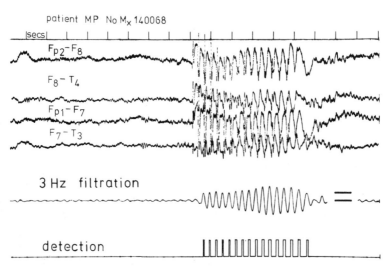

Fig. 5.27 Upper four traces show primary EEG while awake. There is a paroxysm of well-formed 3 per second spike-and-wave activity lasting 5–6 seconds. Fifth trace, EEG from FP_1–F_7, passed through a band-pass filter (3dB points at 4 Hz and 2.2 Hz, attenuation 24 dB per octave). Bottom trace is output of voltage comparator preset to detect amplitude indicated by horizontal bar on right of fifth trace (from Jestico et al., 1977).

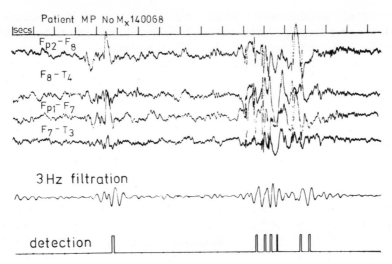

Fig. 5.28 The format is identical with Fig. 5.27. Two briefer and irregular bursts of spike-and-wave activity are seen during slow-wave sleep.

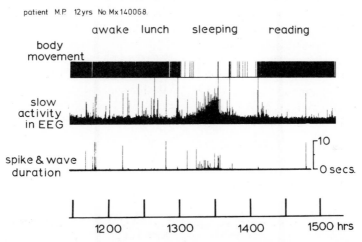

Fig. 5.29 Automatic analysis bar charts showing: upper trace, body movement detected by 41 k Hz ultrasonic system. Second trace, EEG activity from C_3–A_2, amplified, passed through a low-pass filter (–3dB at 5.5 Hz, 24 dB per octave), integrated and plotted as in upper trace. In the third trace, EEG from C_3–A_2 was processed as in Fig. 5.27, but the output of the comparator has been integrated to give time occupied by spike-and-wave discharges during each 10 second epoch. For further explanation see text. (By courtesy of Dr. J. Jestico)

been established, attention could be turned to the special problems of overnight recordings. The same recording room could be used, the reclining chair in the centre of the room being replaced by a bed (Fig. 5.30). The remarkably high quality of the television picture which can be obtained in near-darkness using an infra red light source and a suitable camera is illustrated in Figure 5.31. This makes it possible to obtain a split-screen picture of the patient and the EEG (four channels) through-

out the night, as well as having the full eight-channel EEG recorded separately on FM tape. The television picture is recorded on two video-recorders, one (cassette) recorder running at a normal speed of 25 frames per second and the other (reel-to-reel) recorder slowed to two frames per second. At the former speed the maximal recording time of currently available commercial tape-cassettes is three hours and, in our present system, three of these are used in succession, the recorders being started automatically. When recording at two frames per second a single tape-spool is sufficient for the whole night and the problem of changing tapes or recorders does not arise.

A television monitor with sound is available for the night staff on the ward (Fig. 5.30) and, if a clinical seizure occurs and the time is noted, the relevant portion of the tape can easily be found from the digital clock display on the video-eral impression of the patient's behaviour and EEG during the night to be obtained; the times at which possibly abnormal features occurred can be noted for further study.

Nocturnal observation of this kind is particularly valuable in patients having attacks at night which might be epileptic or which might be nightmares or night terrors. During violent attacks the EEG is likely to be obscured by artefact but the record during the few minutes or

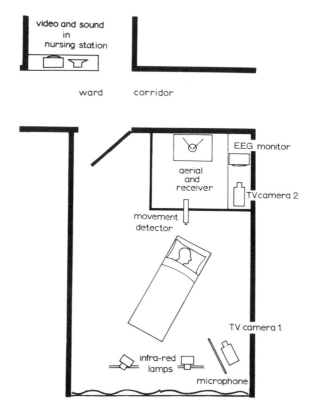

Fig. 5.30 Diagram of recording room and apparatus for overnight recording. The tape recorders are housed in the basement and are linked by cable to the recording room.

recording when the tapes are reviewed in the morning. In such a case it might be unneccessary to search the rest of the tapes as sufficient information would be obtained from the recording of the attack itself. In other circumstances, however, it would be necessary to review the whole of a night's record. For this the time-lapse tape recorder is essential, the tape record at two frames per second being replayed at normal speed (25 f.p.s.). This accelerated review of the tape allows a gen-seconds immediately before the clinical attack may yield valuable information.

As examples of the diagnostic value of night recordings two cases may be cited.

Case 2
A 17-year-old nurse (NH No. 83296) presented with a four-year history of nocturnal attacks in which she would be woken by a choking sensation in the throat with vertigo, vivid visual hallucinations and inability to move her limbs or to speak. From the patient's description, these frightening events were thought to be episodes of sleep paralysis and

hypnagogic hallucination, particularly as they occurred either as she was falling asleep or waking in the morning. However, two members of her family were known to suffer from epilepsy, and the patient's own attacks were clustered around times of menstruation. The patient had been tried with various antiepileptic drugs which had not influenced her nocturnal attacks. Subsequent abrupt withdrawal of the drugs was followed by two diurnal tonic-clonic seizures. Because of the association with drug withdrawal, these were not regarded as definitely epileptic, and no further diurnal attacks had occurred. Previous EEG recordings, including a long daytime telemetry recording with a period of natural sleep, had shown no abnormality. As the diagnosis was uncertain, an overnight recording was made.

Apart from brief waking periods, the recording was un-eventful and showed no abnormality on subsequent video-tape review. A further overnight record was therefore taken a week later. While the first recording had been made with-out acclimatisation to the recording conditions, the patient spent three nights in the recording room before the second session.

During this second recording, two clinical attacks occur-red, each waking the patient from sleep. In both she made a choking sound, turned in bed and sat up abruptly. Figure 5.31 shows the split-screen television picture during the first episode at 01.08 hours. At the onset a burst of somewhat irregular sharp delta activity was seen in the sleep-stage channel, after which she turned her head to the right, and then awoke. Twenty-five seconds later, a 10-second burst of more regular 5 Hz activity was seen in the same distribu-tion, without clinical accompaniment. The patient then sat up, leaned over to the left, cleared her throat, mumbled, and then returned to sleep. This attack was discovered only when the video-tapes were replayed, as the patient had returned to sleep afterwards without calling for nursing assistance. By the following morning she could not recall the attack. A second episode occurred during the same session at 05.30 hours, and was sufficient to wake the patient with characteristic symptoms.

Comment

Although these nocturnal attacks lasted less than two minutes, they were easily detected during the rapid replay of the time-lapse video-tape at six times recording speed. Examination of the corres-ponding real-time video-tapes allowed more detailed study. The stereotyped nature of the attacks and their accompanying rhythmical EEG discharge established the epileptic basis of the patient's symptoms.

Case 3
This 19-year-old clerk (NH No. B02764) had suffered from nocturnal episodes of screaming and abnormal behaviour since the age of three. As a child he would awake several

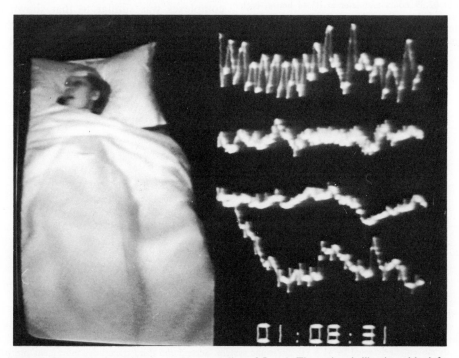

Fig. 5.31 Split-screen TV picture from time-lapse video recording of Case 2. The patient is illuminated by infra-red light. Time 01.08 hours 31 seconds. Telemetered signals on right: Upper trace, EEG channel C_3–A_2 for sleep staging. Second trace, EEG channel F_8–T_4. Third trace, EEG channel F_7–T_5. Lower trace, EOG. signal. A paroxysm of high voltage 5 per second activity is seen in the upper EEG tracing. (By courtesy of Dr. J. Jestico)

nights a week, screaming and seeming frightened; he would sometimes say he had seen little men in his room. These attacks persisted throughout childhood and became more marked after the age of fifteen. They would occur on most nights of the week, sometimes three or four times a night. The screaming became associated with walking round the house in a dazed state, and sometimes by violent behaviour in which he had hit several of his relatives and had broken household fittings. The patient usually had no memory of the nocturnal events, although he could sometimes recall fragments of them. He denied having frequent or frightening dreams.

From the age of three until the age of 18 he had exhibited brief day-time episodes of stiffening and shaking of his arms accompanied by sucking noises. Phenobarbitone treatment had not affected these attacks, and they had ceased six months before his admission. There was no family history of epilepsy. Previous EEGs had shown slight asymmetry of normal rhythms but no other abnormality.

Overnight EEG recording by telemetry was performed after a preceding night had been spent to acclimatise the patient to the recording room. He went to sleep at 23.30 hours, and after brief awakenings, he entered stage 4 sleep soon after 23.50 hours. At 00.26 hours he awoke from stage 4 sleep, screaming. He sat up in bed, held out his hands, and appeared dazed. He then snapped his fingers and left the room to go to the toilet. He returned to sleep soon after getting back to bed, and at 01.08 hours had the first period of REM sleep. At 01.45 hours he awoke from stage 4 sleep, screamed, jumped out of bed and tried to open the door, but stopped and returned to bed. He went back to sleep, but woke again at 02.39 hours and later at 05.44 hours, each time from stage 4 sleep. On each occasion he screamed, sat up and then walked around the room for a few minutes before returning to bed. The EEG record immediately before

each attack showed the changes of stage 4 sleep, and no epileptic activity was seen before, during or after an attack.

Comment

The history of these attacks, their frequency and persistence over many years were against a diagnosis of epilepsy, which had been considered because of a past history of brief attacks of stiffening during the day. The attacks observed on the video-record were typical of night terrors; these characteristically occur during deep slow-wave sleep, in contrast to nightmares which occur during REM sleep (Fisher et al., 1973; Fenton, 1975).

For night studies on patients with petit mal we have again used an automatic system for the registration of spike-and-wave discharges, so that the amount of epileptic activity in the EEG can be related to the patient's level of alertness and to the depth of sleep. An example of the use of our earlier system (Jestico et al., 1977) is shown in Figure 5.32, which is the record of an adult patient with petit mal, taken during the night and early morning. The method of detection of spike-and-wave complexes was similar to that shown in Figures 5.27 to 5.29. For the assessment of the depth of sleep, the integrated output of filtered slow activ-

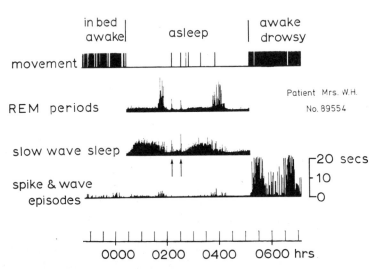

Fig. 5.32 Night study of patient, aged 42, with morning confusion accompanied by 3 cycles per second spike-and-wave in EEG. Upper trace, body movement detected by 41 k Hz ultrasonic system. Second and third traces, eye movement and EEG activity (< 4 cycles per second) recorded as in Fig. 5.29, the vertical height of each line indicating activity integrated and plotted for a 20 second epoch. Fourth trace, EEG from C₃–A₂ processed as in Fig. 5.27, and the output of the comparator integrated to give the time occupied by spike-and-wave discharge during each 20 second epoch. It may be noted that movement artefact sufficient to appear in the EOG and EEG traces (arrowed) did not affect the spike-and-wave analysis (from Jestico et al., 1977).

ity was summed in 20-second epochs, using a sleep channel with the standard electrode placements recommended by Rechtschaffen and Kales (1968). In addition, the output of an eye movement channel was integrated and summed, so that periods of REM sleep could be identified between the slow-wave cycles.

Case 4

The patient (N.H. No. 89554), who was aged 42 at the time of study, was known to have suffered from classical petit mal since the age of seven. Routine EEGs had shown episodes of generalised symmetrical 3–4 per second spike-and-wave activity, and clinical improvement had followed the introduction of ethosuximide ten years previously. Grand mal attacks had started at the age of 18 but were controlled by primidone. At the time of study the patient complained that her petit mal was at its worst in the morning after rising, that she might take more than half an hour to clean her teeth because of the attacks, and that these were sometimes accompanied by incontinence of urine.

In Figure 5.32 it can be seen from the overnight record that several brief spike-and-wave episodes occurred when the patient was lying in bed before going to sleep but none of these lasted more than three seconds. Two complete sleep cycles occurred between midnight and 05.20 hours, each terminated by a REM period. Spike-and-wave activity was reduced or absent during slow-wave sleep, with recurrences during the REM periods. After 05.20 hours the patient was awake but drowsy, and at this time spike-and-wave activity became profuse, many of the discharges lasting for more than 20 seconds. This activity continued until the recording was stopped at 08.15 hours. Between 05.20 and 08.15 hours the patient had 174 episodes of generalised 3 per second spike-and-wave activity, the duration of individual episodes varying from 1.5–109 seconds (mean duration 15 seconds). It was difficult to determine from the television picture of the patient when attacks occurred. On a few occasions small movements of the hands appeared to coincide with the abnormal electrical activity but on others no movement was seen. At the end of the session, when the patient was talking to the nursing staff, interruption of speech was observed in some but not all of the attacks.

Comment

Overnight recording in this patient revealed that much more epileptic activity was occurring in the early morning than had been suspected on clinical grounds. The patient was subsequently helped by altering the timing of her medication to provide better cover in the early morning.

3. EEG MONITORING WITH MINIATURE TAPE RECORDERS

The use of portable cassette-tape recorders for ambulatory ECG monitoring has become an important part of the investigation of patients with cardiac arrhythmias (Camm, Ward & Spurrell, 1978; Brown & Anderson, 1980). This approach is now also being applied to monitoring the EEG of epileptic patients, following the pioneer work of Penry and colleagues (Sato, Penry & Dreifuss, 1976), and of Ives and Wood (1975). It could be argued that such EEG recordings are of little diagnostic value unless the patient's behaviour is also monitored by CCTV. On the other hand, failure to record an attack with the telemetry and CCTV system is likely to occur in patients with infrequent seizures, as this type of monitoring is too demanding of staff to be continued for several days. Furthermore, the patient has to be confined to the area where he is in view of the television camera. There are some circumstances in which EEG monitoring without CCTV is of particular value; for example, in assessing how much epileptic activity is occurring in a patient's EEG at different times, and how this is related to treatment. Classical petit mal epilepsy lends itself particularly to this type of study, since the generalised, high-voltage spike-and-wave episodes in the EEG are relatively easy to detect, whereas the patient's interruption of consciousness and activity may be minimal and therefore difficult to assess clinically. Hence, to supplement the telemetry and CCTV recordings, we set up an EEG ambulatory monitoring system which enables us to obtain long-term EEG recordings from patients whose activity is unrestricted, and who might be in the hospital ward, at a residential centre for epilepsy, or at home.

The EEG data are stored on a four-channel tape recorder (Oxford Medical Systems, *Medilog*) which uses standard audio-cassettes, giving a recording time of up to 24 hours. A major problem in recording the EEG of ambulant patients is the artefact produced by movements of the electrodes and leads, and it has been our experience that conventional EEG records made during seizures are often unreadable because of such artefact. Since, in the absence of a video-picture, a clean recording is essential, we developed a miniature preamplifier that is attached to the scalp with the electrodes (Quy, 1978). This preamplifier has a gain of 1000 and the leads to the electrodes are made very short and flexible; hence artefacts, such as those produced by cable noise, interference from external electromagnetic fields, or movement of the electrodes on the scalp, are greatly reduced. In addition, we developed a type of electrode and an electrolyte paste especially for monitoring active patients over several days (Quy *et al.*, 1980a).

Figure 5.33 shows the system required for recording three channels of EEG and an ECG channel; an event mark can be superimposed onto one of the EEG channels. The electrode montage used with each patient is selected on the basis of previous routine EEG recordings or on the nature of the clinical problem. Any combination of EEG, ECG, eye-movement, body-movement or encoded time signal can be recorded, depending on the purpose of the investigation. The electrodes and preamplifiers can easily be hidden under the hair or by a hat so that recordings can be carried out in the patient's normal environment without causing embarrassment. The tape-recorder is normally carried in a bag at the waist. Using these techniques we are able to obtain high-quality recordings even during tonic-clonic seizures, as demonstrated in Figure 5.34.

A storage-screen system for reviewing the recordings has recently become commercially available (Oxford Medical Systems, PMD-12).

This displays the four data channels in 8 or 16-second pages at 20 or 60 times the recording speed; hence a 24-hour tape can be scanned visually in 30 minutes. Moreover, since each page of data is held stationary on the screen for a brief period we have found it possible to see even short events such as isolated epileptic spikes. The unit also has facilities for generating a time display, automatically detecting an event mark, and producing a paper record by linking to a standard EEG recorder (Stores, Hennion & Quy, 1980). The advantages of using a tape recorder which the patient can wear at home are illustrated by the following case.

Case 5:
This 33-year-old female teacher (N.H. No. B03955) was well until the age of 30 when she began to experience repeated episodes during which she could neither spell words nor write numbers correctly. These attacks lasted 20–30 minutes on some occasions, but she also experienced briefer spells lasting only a few minutes. In addition, she had noticed periods of language difficulty during which she could not talk coherently, would use neologisms, and was unable to understand what was said to her. Such dysphasic episodes might last 3 or 4 hours. A year after the onset of these symptoms, she had a tonic-clonic seizure shortly after waking in the morning. She was 4½ months pregnant at this time.

Clinical examination and investigations, including CT scan, were normal. Routine EEG showed a 2.5 Hz abnormality in the left mid-temporal leads, but no frankly epileptic activity was seen. EEG telemetry with CCTV recording showed runs of high voltage delta activity over the left anterior temporal region, and as the patient became drowsy,

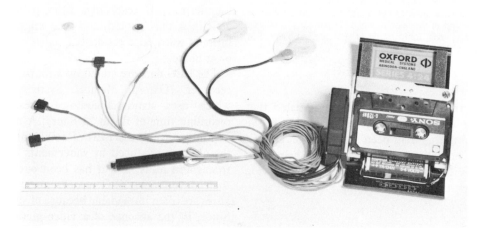

Fig. 5.33 Equipment for ambulatory EEG monitoring. On the right of the photograph is the *Medilog* recorder, unfolded to show the cassette and battery in position. On the left are three 'stick-on' EEG preamplifiers, one with a pair of electrodes attached. Also pictured are a pair of ECG electrodes, a connector pin for a ground electrode, and an event-marker button. The total weight of the recording system is approximately 600 grams.

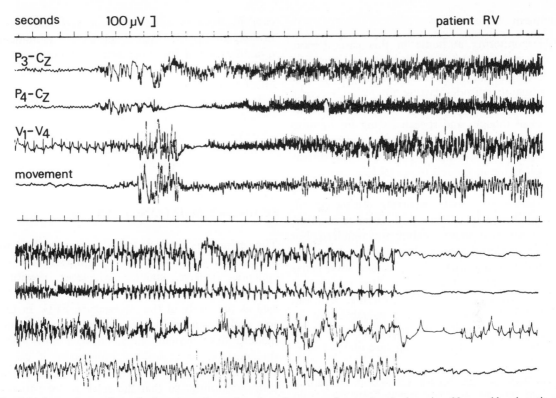

Fig. 5.34 Successive portions of a four-channel record to show the course of a grand mal seizure in a 33 year old male patient while he was at work. Two EEG channels (P_3–C_z and P_4–C_z) and one ECG channel (V_1–V_4) are shown, together with a movement channel obtained from an accelerometer mounted on the head. Approximately 30 seconds have been omitted between the top and bottom portions of the record. The clinical attack commenced with a cry and the patient then fell to his right. Bilateral fast activity can be seen in the EEG before the onset of the clinical seizure, as indicated by the movement recorder. EEG spiking, accompanied by clonic movements, rapidly developed and can be seen to slow in frequency towards the latter part of the record. The patient slept for some 30 minutes after the seizure, during which time the EEG gradually returned to its normal pattern.

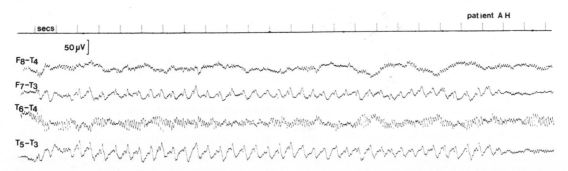

Fig. 5.35 EEG from ambulatory cassette tape record in Case 6. A prolonged run of spikes and sharp slow waves is seen in the left temporal leads, while alpha rhythm continues on the right side.

sharp waves and spikes appeared in this region. However, no clinical attacks were recorded during two 6-hour recording sessions.

Although the patient's symptoms were thought to have an epileptic basis, their very long duration and failure to appear during long EEG telemetry placed the precise diagnosis in doubt. Ambulatory EEG recording was carried out for a

48-hour period while the patient lived her usual life at home. During this time she experienced several typical attacks, lasting a few minutes each. Review of the cassette-tape EEG record showed a striking increase in the paroxysmal left temporal activity during the times of the patient's reported attacks, the EEG discharges lasting up to 30 seconds (Fig. 5.35).

Comment

EEG monitoring at home in this case demonstrated the occurrence of frequent left temporal discharges at the times of her symptoms, these occurring in episodes lasting up to 30 seconds. Although the patient herself had described disturbances of thought and speech lasting for minutes or hours, it was concluded that these were due to the repeated occurrence of brief electrical disturbances arising in the left temporal lobe.

In order to measure the amount of 3 per second spike-and-wave activity occurring during ambulant monitoring in patients with absence seizures, some form of automatic analysis was required. For this we developed a microcomputer-based analyser which detects and quantifies spike-and-wave activity in the EEG at high speed. This system has been described elsewhere (Quy, Fitch & Willison, 1980b). It has proved to be a valuable tool for assessing and adjusting the treatment of patients with petit mal, as the following case illustrates.

Case 6
This 30-year-old man (NH No. A23358) had suffered from epilepsy since the age of nine months. There was a family history of epilepsy. In addition to tonic-clonic seizures, he also had frequent minor attacks of loss of awareness lasting for a few seconds at a time, and known from investigation to be associated with bilaterally synchronous 3 per second spike-and-wave complexes in the EEG. These absence attacks had been poorly controlled during the three years before admission, and he would usually experience several such episodes daily. In addition, he had suffered from less frequent but more prolonged periods lasting up to an hour, during which he would appear dazed and confused and might behave inappropriately.

Ambulatory EEG monitoring with a cassette tape recorder was carried out over a three-day period. Automatic analysis of the EEG tape record revealed frequent bursts of 3–3.5 cycles per second bilateral spike-and-wave activity, some bursts lasting as long as 20 minutes. Some 7915 seconds of this activity occurred in a 24-hour period. The longest periods of spike-and-wave activity occurred in the morning between 08.00 and 09.00 hours and around mid-day (Fig. 5.36).

Sodium valproate was introduced into the patient's drug regime, and ethosuximide and phenobarbitone were gradually withdrawn. This resulted in a considerable improvement in the frequency of his absence attacks, and in a repeat ambulatory EEG recording showed a corresponding reduction in the amount of spike-and-wave activity (down to 2824 seconds in a 24-hour period). This is illustrated in the lower half of Figure 5.36.

Comment

Ambulatory EEG recording was valuable in this case in demonstrating frequent and sometimes prolonged petit mal seizures. Automatic quantification of the 3 per second spike-and-wave activity provided an objective assessment of the effect of altering the drug regime.

It is evident from Figure 5.36 that there was considerable variation in the amount of spike-and-wave activity occurring from hour to hour. This demonstrates how the results of routine EEG recordings can depend very much on the time at which the recording was carried out.

SUMMARY AND CONCLUSIONS

The techniques described in this chapter lead to the general conclusion that the investigation of epileptic patients should, whenever possible, include the observation of a clinical seizure, as well as the study of the interseizure EEG. In the past such a goal might have seemed unrealistic but modern developments in electronics now make this possible in at least a proportion of cases. However, the techniques are both expensive and time-consuming, so that the selection of patients for study requires considerable care.

From our own experience it seems that certain patients are particularly suitable for prolonged observation; for example, those in whom clinical attacks are known to be occurring relatively frequently, although their epileptic nature has been questioned. In contrast, patients with infrequent attacks do not usually justify the commitment of staff time and apparatus to such a study.

Apparatus used for daytime observation and recording can be adapted relatively easily for the study of patients at night; again the most suitable patients are those whose attacks are occurring relatively frequently.

In patients with petit mal epilepsy and 3 per second spike-and-wave discharges, prolonged ambulatory monitoring of the EEG can be carried out by means of a miniature tape-cassette recorder without the need for CCTV, since the epileptic discharges in the EEG are usually a better guide to the activity of the epilepsy than the number of clinical seizures witnessed. Automatic high-speed analysis of the tapes provides a record of the amount of epileptic activity occurring per 15-minute epoch throughout the day and night. Such

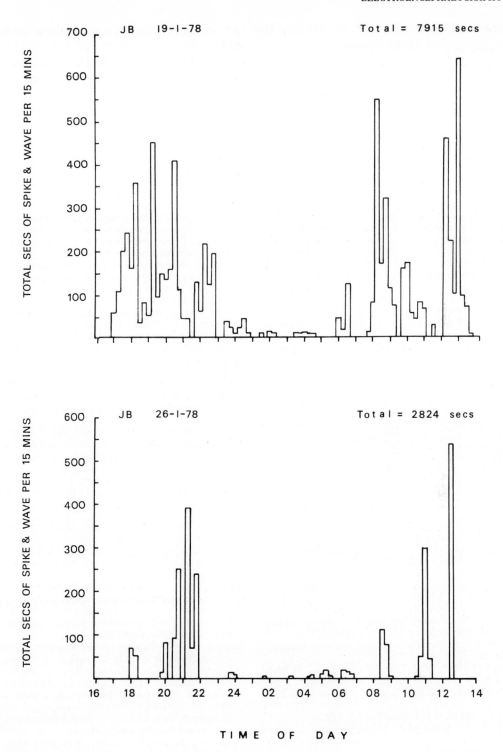

Fig. 5.36 Graphs of the amount of 3 per second spike-and-wave activity per 15-minute interval, based upon automatic analysis of cassette tape recordings from Case 5. Upper record shows frequent spike-and-wave activity during waking hours; lower record was taken one week later, when the patient was taking sodium valproate, and shows marked improvement.

a record is of particular value in checking the efficacy of a patient's drug regime.

Acknowledgements

We are greatly indebted to Mr. P. Fitch, M.Sc., whose engineering skills made these studies possible.

We also wish to thank Dr. J. Jestico for permission to cite unpublished data, and Dr. W.A. Cobb for helpful criticism and advice.

REFERENCES

Bowden, A.N. (1976) The use of EEG telemetry and video-recording in the differential diagnosis of fits. In Nicholson, J.P. (ed.) *Scientific Aids in Hospital Diagnosis*, p. 107. New York: Plenum Press.

Bowden, A.N., Fitch, P., Gilliatt, R.W. & Willison, R.G. (1975) The place of EEG telemetry and closed-circuit television in the diagnosis and management of epileptic patients. *Proceedings of the Royal Society of Medicine*, **68**, 16.

Brown, A.K. & Anderson, V. (1980) The contribution of 24-hour ambulatory ECG monitoring in a general medical unit. *Journal of the Royal College of Physicians of London*, **14**, 7.

Camm, A.J., Ward, D.E. & Spurrell, R.A.J. (1978) Arrhythmias in ambulatory persons: A review and experience of 1,000 consecutive recordings. *Biotelemetry and Patient Monitoring*, **5**, 167.

Fenton, G.W. (1975) The clinical disorders of sleep. *British Journal of Hospital Medicine*, **14**, 120.

Fisher, C., Kahn, E., Edwards, A. & Davis, D. (1973) A psychophysiological study of nightmares and night terrors. *Journal of Nervous and Mental Disease*, **157**, 75.

Goode, D.J., Penry, J.K. & Dreifuss, F.E. (1970) Effects of paroxysmal spike-wave on continuous visual-motor performance. *Epilepsia*, **11**, 241.

Gotman, J., Ives, J.R. & Gloor, P. (1979) Automatic recognition of inter-ictal epileptic activity in prolonged EEG recordings. *Electroencephalography and Clinical Neurophysiology*, **46**, 510.

Ives, J.R. & Woods, J.F. (1975) 4-channel 24-hr cassette recorder for long-term EEG monitoring of ambulatory patients. *Electroencephalography and Clinical Neurophysiology*, **39**, 88.

Ives, J.R., Thompson, C.J. & Gloor, P. (1976) Seizure monitoring: A new tool in electroencephalography. *Electroencephalography and Clinical Neurophysiology*, **41**, 422.

Jestico, J., Fitch, P., Gilliatt, R.W. & Willison, R.G. (1977) Automatic and rapid visual analysis of sleep stages and epileptic activity. A preliminary report. *Electroencephalography and Clinical Neurophysiology*, **43**, 438.

Kaiser, E. (1976) Telemetry and video recording on magnetic tape cassettes in long-term EEG. In Kellaway, P. & Petersen, I. (eds) *Quantitative Analytic Studies in Epilepsy*, p. 279. New York: Raven Press.

Mattson, R.H. (1980) Value of intensive monitoring. In Wada, J.A. & Penry, J.K. (eds) Advances in Epileptology. The Xth Epilepsy International Symposium, p. 43. New York: Raven Press.

Penry, J.K., Porter, R.J. & Dreifuss, F.E. (1975) Simultaneous recording of absence seizures with video tape and electroencephalography. A study of 374 seizures in 48 patients. *Brain*, **98**, 427.

Porter, R.J., Wolf, A.A. & Penry, J.K. (1971) Human electroencephalographic telemetry: A review of systems and their applications and a new receiving system. *American Journal of EEG Technology*, **11**, 145.

Porter, R.J., Penry, J.K. & Dreifuss, F.E. (1973) Responsiveness at the onset of spike-wave bursts. *Electroencephalography and Clinical Neurophysiology*, **34**, 239.

Porter, R.J., Penry, J.K. & Wolf, A.A. (1976) Simultaneous documentation of clinical and electroencephalographic manifestations of epileptic seizures. In Kellaway, P. & Petersen, I. (eds) *Quantitative Analytic Studies in Epilepsy*, p. 253. New York: Raven Press.

Quy, R.J. (1978) A miniature preamplifier for ambulatory monitoring of the electroencephalogram. *Journal of Physiology (London)*, **284**, 23.

Quy, R.J., Willison, R.G., Fitch, P. & Gilliatt, R.W. (1980a) Some developments in ambulatory monitoring of the EEG. In Stott, F.D., Raftery, E.B., Sleight, P. & Goulding, L. (eds) *ISAM 1979: Proceedings of the Third International Symposium on Ambulatory Monitoring*, p. 393. London: Academic Press.

Quy, R.J., Fitch, P. & Willison, R.G. (1980b) High-speed automatic analysis of EEG spike-and-wave activity using an analogue detection and microcomputer plotting system. *Electroencephalography and Clinical Neurophysiology* (in press).

Rechtschaffen, A. & Kales, A. (1968) (eds) A manual of standardized Terminology, Techniques and Scoring System for Sleep Stages in Human Subjects. U.S. Government Printing Office: Public Health Service.

Rowan, A.J., Binnie, C.D., Overweg, J., de Vries, J. & Kamp, A. (1980) The value of prolonged EEG/video monitoring as a routine diagnostic procedure in epilepsy. In Canger, R., Angeleri, F. & Penry, J.K. (eds) Advances in Epileptology, the XIth Epilepsy International Symposium. New York: Raven Press.

Sato, S., Dreifuss, F.E. & Penry, J.K. (1973) The effect of sleep on spike-wave discharges in absence seizures. *Neurology*, **23**, 1335.

Sato, S., Penry, J.K. & Dreifuss, F.E. (1976) Electroencephalographic monitoring of generalised spike and wave paroxysms in the hospital and at home. In Kellaway, P. & Petersen, I. (eds) *Quantitative Analytic Studies in Epilepsy*, p. 237. New York: Raven Press.

Stalberg, E. (1976) Experiences with long-term telemetry in routine diagnostic work. In Kellaway, P. & Petersen, I. (eds) *Quantitative Analytic Studies in Epilepsy*, p. 269. New York: Raven Press.

Stevens, J.R., Kodama, H., Lonsbury, B. & Mills, L. (1971) Ultradian characteristics of spontaneous seizure discharges recorded by radio telemetry in man. *Electroencephalography and Clinical Neurophysiology*, **31**, 313.

Stores, G., Hennion, T.S. & Quy, R.J. (1980) EEG ambulatory monitoring system with visual play-back display. In Wada, J.A. & Penry, J.K. (eds) Advances in Epileptology. The Xth Epilepsy Symposium, p. 89. New York: Raven Press.

6

Psychiatry and epilepsy

PART ONE

T.A. Betts

Epilepsy is important to the psychiatrist, and the psychiatrist is important to epilepsy. Epilepsy lies in the borderland between what is conventionally understood as a province of neurology and what is conventionally understood as a province of psychiatry. Epilepsy and its associated phenomena cannot be understood without a firm grounding in both the neurological and psychiatric sciences.

Epilepsy is unique in terms of the complexity of the relationships that exist between epileptic brain disturbances and behaviour. Epileptic activity in the brain produces changes in behaviour in the person who possesses it and these changes in behaviour produce changes in the behaviour of the people surrounding that person which may well reinforce the behavioural changes that originated as an epileptic phenomenon. It is also becoming increasingly clear that changing the patient's behaviour may actually modify the epileptic experience.

This is a very important concept in the study of epilepsy; hopefully its importance will become clear as the rest of this chapter is read. Clinically as well as theoretically, it is essential to appreciate that the behaviour of people with epilepsy cannot be considered separately in terms of pathophysiology, psychology or sociology, but rather as a result of the interaction of all these influences.

An understanding of epilepsy requires the co-operation of several disciplines. It requires more than that, however, in that each discipline must have some understanding of the role of the others. The treatment of epilepsy is not the prerogative of any one discipline but can be a job for any doctor, whether he be neurologist, psychiatrist, paediatrician or general physician, providing he has a particular interest in epilepsy and is prepared to learn something of the skills and attitudes of other branches of the profession so that he can offer total care to his patient.

This chapter is an attempt to describe the various aspects of epilepsy with which a psychiatrist is particularly concerned, and for which his skills have something to offer.

My two colleagues, Professor Sir Desmond Pond, and Dr Michael Trimble have written their own section which will complement the main body of the chapter. They are writing on aspects of epilepsy which particularly interest them. In addition to covering the other aspects of the psychiatry of epilepsy, I will try to put their section into context. I hope readers will find it stimulating if the three authors do not always agree. Our experience of epilepsy and psychiatry is based on different populations of patients.

THE ROLE OF THE PSYCHIATRIST

There are three main ways in which the psychiatrist has a unique contribution to make to the management of people with epilepsy.

Of people with epilepsy, many are troubled, some are troublesome, and a few are mad. It is probable that psychiatric disturbance of all kinds is commoner in people with epilepsy than in the general population, although this bold statement needs qualification. Most psychiatric disturbance in people with epilepsy can be seen as no more than a reaction to the stress of being epileptic. The skills which psychiatrists and their colleagues in social work and clinical psychology have developed to help people who are stressed are very pertinent here.

Some people with epilepsy, because of concomitant brain damage, or the effect that having epilepsy has had on their emotional development, grow up with persistent disturbances of behaviour in their relationships to other people which classify them as having a personality disorder. This is one of the most contentious areas of the psychiatry of epilepsy. Again the skills that a psychiatrist and his other colleagues possess may have a lot to offer such people. Even more important, perhaps, if we can study these problems carefully enough, we may be in a position eventually to offer some kind of preventative treatment. A few people with epilepsy have such gross disorders of feeling or behaviour or thinking, or in the way they relate to the external world and other people, that they have to be described as actually mad, and here of course the psychiatrist's help is essential.

There are two other ways in which I feel the psychiatrist has a contribution to the management of epilepsy. The first is in helping to diagnose attack disorder. Often the diagnosis of epilepsy is easy but sometimes it is not. With complex partial seizures particularly, it may be difficult to distinguish between a phenomenon relating to epilepsy and a phenomenon relating to psychiatric disturbance. The differential diagnosis of attacks may need psychiatric experience.

Secondly, new and developing methods of treatment in psychiatry, particularly those based on learning theory may have a great deal to offer people with epilepsy in terms of the actual treatment of their seizures. Although still largely experimental, I feel that behavioural treatments will eventually be a powerful adjunct to more conventional forms of therapy.

Since this is a medical textbook I have tended to follow a medical model in describing psychological reactions to epilepsy. There are, however, other equally appropriate models that could have been used, which help to explain why people with epilepsy behave in the way they do. Although it says very little directly about epilepsy, Goffman's book (Goffman, 1963) is well worth reading by those who wish to pursue this idea further. Wing (1974) presents a model of handicap, which although related to schizophrenia, is also extremely applicable to epilepsy and although not formally acknowledged elsewhere, it is really his structure which is being used as the emotional reactions to epilepsy are described. Wing talks of:

a. *Primary handicaps*, which are the result of chronic impairment of physiological or psychological function (e.g. loss of a limb, obsessions, or fits).

b. *Secondary handicaps* – extra handicaps which would not have been present if the primary handicap had not been (e.g. fits leading to hospitalisation which leads to institutionalisation or fits leading to fear which leads to an increased number of fits).

c. *Extrinsic handicaps*, which are pre-existing handicaps which exist independently of the main one but which influence it – like poor social circumstances or a lack of social or cognitive skills which are relevant to treatment planning.

PSYCHOLOGICAL EFFECTS OF HAVING EPILEPSY

To have epilepsy is to be stressed. Stress itself can influence the frequency of fits, and it is possible sometimes for this to become a self-reinforcing phenomenon. If patients can come to terms, or deal with the stress that epilepsy induces, their lives will be made much more comfortable, and their seizure frequency may diminish.

It is therefore important for any doctor who is helping people with epilepsy to know something about the effects of stress, the factors that influence the way an individual reacts to stress and the means available to help people to cope with stress. It is also important for doctors to know when reactions to stress should be classified as abnormal.

The word stress itself of course is ill-defined in the literature: sometimes it is applied to that which causes reactive and unpleasant symptoms in individuals, and sometimes it is applied to the actual symptoms themselves. In this chapter the word stress implies the impact that becoming epileptic has on the patient and also the chronic effects that having epilepsy has on the individual and his relationships with others. In terms of its effects on the individual, help given to him should really be considered under two headings: Firstly, helping him to come to terms with the diagnosis of epilepsy and secondly trying to minimise the effects that epilepsy will have on his life, and on his social life, interpersonal relationships and job.

In looking at how somebody is reacting to a particular stress, it should be remembered that stress reactions in themselves can often be considered as normal, are usually self limiting and are part of the normal biological mechanisms of adaptation to new situations. In considering whether a particular reaction is abnormal or not, one should pay particular attention to whether or not the reaction is helping that person to deal with the situation, or is impeding efforts to deal with it, and also whether or not the reaction is becoming self-reinforcing (i.e. that the person is, for instance, becoming afraid of being afraid).

The term 'normal mental health' certainly does not imply an absence of stress symptoms or emotional conflicts. At any one time, the majority of the population are under some kind of stress and so may be experiencing appropriate feelings or showing evidence of this stress in their behaviour. Indeed, if the criteria are set wide enough, almost every normal person will be classified as having emotional symptoms. For instance, an epidemiological study which used such broad criteria, the Manhatten Midtown Study (Srole *et al.*, 1962) found an estimated eighty seven per cent of the normal population in the survey to have some emotional disturbance. In any population of supposedly ill patients, a careful distinction must therefore be made between normal and abnormal reactions to stress.

The way a particular individual reacts to stress depends on certain factors, some of them independent and some of them interdependent. First, there is the significance of the stress to the individual involved. It has been shown, for instance, that the psychological effects of head injury are partly dependent on the relative meaning of the injury. Dysphasia in a schoolmaster, for instance, is of much more importance in terms of his emotional response to it than dysphasia in a farm labourer.

The support which a person receives from family and friends and society will also affect his ability to cope with a particular stress. Someone recently bereaved, for instance, is much less able to meet the impact of physical illness.

It has also been shown (Slater & Shields, 1969) that the genetic constitution of an individual and the responsiveness of his autonomic nervous system to stress may play an important part in shaping the particular way he presents his stress responses. Lacey, Batemen and Van Lehn (1953) propose the concept of *response specificity* that people respond to stress in a relatively stereotyped way through their autonomic system.

Stress responses are also influenced by a person's educational and cultural background. The West Indian response to stress, for instance, is different from the British, and it is therefore easy to misinterpret the behaviour of immigrants. Stress is not an isolated event and a person's response is influenced by coincident problems and difficulties affecting him at the time. In other words, stress is easier to cope with if one is not already overburdened. Stress reactions are learned as part and parcel of growing up. Children are influenced greatly in terms of the way they learn to respond to stress by the example set by their parents and by the social values of their family.

Various extra influences which fall on people with epilepsy are perhaps particularly pertinent to the way they respond to stress. There is a growing body of evidence to suggest that social learning, particularly in childhood, (which will include learning about how to cope with common stresses and difficulties) is impaired by epilepsy acquired in early childhood, and it is possible that some of the chronic personality difficulties that adults with epilepsy may show are related to mal-learning in childhood.

There is no doubt as well that brain damage, particularly perhaps in the temporal lobes, impairs the ability of a person to respond in a normal way to a stressful situation; minor neurotic symptoms and hysterical reactions are probably commoner in people who are brain damaged.

There is also some evidence to suggest that antiepileptic drugs which are needed by a person with epilepsy may also impair learning and interfere with normal responses to stress. A person with epilepsy then, not only has.to suffer the normal stresses that any chronic illness would impose, but also may be handicapped in terms of responding to those stresses by the illness itself and by its necessary treatment. In some ways, then, epilepsy is a unique illness compared to other chronic handicaps.

COMING TO TERMS WITH EPILEPSY

The first problem for the patient newly diagnosed as having epilepsy is to come to terms with it. It is easy for doctors to believe in the confines of the out-patients (where patients' behaviour is usually subservient and controlled) to believe that this is easy. The patient who nods and smiles when you tell him the diagnosis and says 'Thank you doctor, at least its nothing more serious', is very pleasing, but one should not imagine that he is necessarily going to behave in the same way at home, and even if he does, his friends, parents, spouse or children may not.

It should be remembered by all doctors that there is only a limited amount of information that patients can absorb at any one time in a medical consultation, and even that small amount is drastically reduced if the information given to the patient has emotional import.

Some doctors conceal the truth from their patients about the diagnosis of epilepsy and merely refer in a vague way to blackouts etc. I believe most firmly that all patients with epilepsy should know the diagnosis, but one should remember that in addition to the diagnosis the patient will require a whole range of information about his lifestyle, treatment etc. If one tries to give this information at the same time as giving the patient the diagnosis it will often fall on deaf ears, and the education of the patient with epilepsy about all the implications may take several visits to the out-patients (or visits to the patient's home by a social work colleague), particularly as one is often overcoming the patient's own prejudice and ignorance about the disorder.

In many chronic illnesses, including epilepsy, the use of printed handouts for the patient and his family, (and even the use of videotape material) to further explain the illness is being developed. Many patients as they come to terms with the diagnosis will benefit from the support of fellow sufferers with the disorder. Most countries in the western world are now developing such patient support groups.

As patients come to terms with any emotionally significant or life-threatening physical disability, they commonly show a range of mental mechanisms to deal with the anxieties and stress that the situation has caused. Most of these mental mechanisms are quite normal, and help to maintain emotional equilibrium under stress, and preserve self respect. The work of Bowlby (1960) and Hinton (1967) on children deprived of maternal care, and people facing unpleasant situations such as dying, shows that a very common initial reaction to such unpleasant situations is one of denial, followed by a period of struggle in which the individual consciously tries to assimilate the new knowledge into his self-concept and image. This period of struggle and denial may be particularly painful, and may also of course occur in relatives. It is during this period of denial and struggle that one may see the phenomenon of the patient dragged from one useless consultation to another (often of an esoteric or fringe medicine type) because the devastating truth cannot be accepted. The consultant flattered by being asked to provide a second opinion should remember that the reasons for this may have much more to do with the emotional struggle that the patient is going through than with the consultant's own particular prowess.

The period of denial is often followed by a period of depression as the person begins to assimilate the unpleasant situation into himself. This depression, providing it does not go on for too long and can be worked through, should be regarded as normal. It usually gives way eventually to a period of acceptance and resignation. These reactions need support rather than treatment, except in unusual circumstances. People passing through these emotional reactions may have transient periods of the most profound depression, which unless they become prolonged and therefore pathological, should not be treated since there is evidence that the successful working through of grief is necessary for later emotional stability.

During this struggle to assimilate the diagnosis, in addition to depression, both patients and their relatives may show profound feelings of guilt and also anger. This is particularly likely to happen, of course, if there is some known reason for the epilepsy, like a head injury or a febrile convulsion. It should be remembered that patients often invent their own mythology to explain the cause of their epilepsy and in discussing possible causes for a patient's epilepsy the doctor should be aware of this.

Although not all patients pass through a period of emotional distress on learning of the diagnosis, (some may actually be relieved, have feared far worse, i.e. that they were going mad), it should be assumed that most patients will. It is important as patients go through this period of turmoil that one does not interpret it as anything else than it actually is.

Case 1
This patient was a languages student at University. At the age of nineteen she began to have complex partial seizures. These became frequent, and since they were rather prolonged consisting of absences in which occasionally frightened behaviour would occur, were socially disabling. Despite the concern of her friends, she initially denied there was anything wrong with her and referred to her attacks as her 'little faints'. She developed a blasé flippant attitude to them, so much so that at one time her apparent unconcern made one doctor suspect that she had the *'belle indifférence'* of hysteria (but if one talked to her for long enough, her underlying anxiety became apparent). Later, as she accepted both the diagnosis and its implications (of life-long taking of antiepileptic drugs and restrictions on her future career) she passed through a fairly profound period of depression, but latterly has been able to accept the illness for no more or no less than it actually is, and has found comfort in being able to help others in a worse predicament. Her emotional reaction to her illness was never treated as an illness but merely supported and interpreted, and she was given the opportunity of working through it.

To have epilepsy means to be exposed to the fear of having attacks; it means being somebody who frightens and disturbs others; it means being at a disadvantage in terms of work and personal relationships; it means being open to prejudice (which exists both in the lay public and in the medical and nursing professions) and it means to suffer sometimes disturbing symptoms not always directly connected with epilepsy.

THE SOCIAL EFFECTS OF HAVING EPILEPSY

Among the many problems with which a person with epilepsy has to deal are the unpredictability of his attacks, and the reactions that other people have to his attacks. This description given by one of my patients is typical. 'To awake in a street which for a moment I cannot recognise, lying in a filthy gutter, wet and messy because I soiled myself, my thoughts confused, surrounded by strangers who are half curious, half disgusted, this is the nightmare with which I have to live.' Many people with epilepsy will recognise those feelings. Through most of his life, the person with epilepsy does not appear disabled. He is well. Unpredictably he thrusts his disability unexpectedly on unprepared and uninformed strangers.

There is widespread prejudice against epilepsy in almost all cultures. Among many primitive people, people with epilepsy are regarded with hostility and denied access to whatever medical and social care may be available. Attitudes in Africa in this regard have been particularly well studied. A person with epilepsy may become an outcast from his society, exposed to social and religious taboos, isolated, sometimes denied the right to procreate; seen as different and threatening to the stability of society, and often the victim of cruel and useless medical treatment.

It is easy to be complacent, to say that such things do not happen in our society, and that the primitive reaction to epilepsy is essentially one of rejection. However, we must remember that until very recently similar attitudes and practices occurred in our own societies, and to some extent still exist. In some Western countries laws forbidding people with epilepsy to marry, were repealed only very recently. Officially there is little overt prejudice against people with epilepsy. However, there is still important and significant latent prejudice even amongst those highly educated and with a tradition of liberalism and compassion (the medical, nursing and teaching professions and the churches).

Intensive educational efforts to change public attitudes towards epilepsy have been made particularly in the United States, and as has been shown (Caveness, Merritt & Gallup, 1969) these have had considerable success. As might be expected, the most favourable changes have been found amongst the better educated and younger people living in large towns in the United States. The greatest remaining prejudice against epilepsy was found in the southern states where there seems to be a relationship with racial prejudice. People with epilepsy tend to be viewed with the same hostility as the racial minorities. In western societies, both the coloured man and the person with epilepsy are feared for their supposed primitiveness and violence, and for their unpredictability, (one wonders too whether guilt about how both have been treated enters into the emotional reaction to them).

In Britain ten years ago only 57 per cent of people felt that people with epilepsy should be employed and 32 per cent said that they would object to their child playing with a child with epilepsy (OHE, 1971). It will be interesting to see if these entrenched attitudes can be changed.

That attitudes may be changing in this country is illustrated by a 1979 Gallup Survey (Epilepsy News, 1979) which showed that now 78 per cent of respondents felt that people with epilepsy should be employed and 88 per cent were happy for their children to associate with an epileptic child. Of course, what people say and what they will do are not necessarily the same. How much this poll reflects specific attitude changes to epilepsy or how much it merely reflects a general liberalisation of attitudes in the British people is hard to say. A disquieting feature of the survey was that prejudice is still common in adolescents and young adults reflecting the need for better education about epilepsy in schools.

In purely materialistic terms, money spent on such education in this country would be a way in which preventative medicine might save not only many people much unhappiness but also save an immense amount of time for psychiatrists and their colleagues trying to relieve personality and behavioural reactions to faulty social attitudes.

It is important to emphasise that the medical and related professions themselves are not free from prejudice and may still entertain irrational attitudes about people with epilepsy. The British Medical Association Working Party on Immigration as recently as 1965 recommended that people

with epilepsy should not be allowed to enter this country 'for social and economic reasons'. It is difficult for people even with well controlled epilepsy to enter the medical, nursing or teaching professions. A qualified nurse, for instance, however well controlled her epilepsy, cannot train as a midwife.

Doctors, nurses and some school teachers (and their own teachers in universities and training colleges) are an important source of unbiased education for the public, and removal of prejudice in these groups is therefore very important. The teacher, whether he be medical, nursing or lay has a vital role in educating others about epilepsy. In the classroom the teacher, by his acceptance of the child with epilepsy, his calmness and unconcern if a child has a fit, helps to dispel fear and prejudice by his example in the rest of the class. The British Epilepsy Association provides a valuable information and education service and pays particular attention to organising lectures for teachers.

It is easy for busy doctors immersed in their clinical work to forget the importance that such preventative work may have, and the effect that it may have even on their own practice. As an example of the social consequences of epilepsy, the next case history is presented.

Case 2
This boy began to develop complex partial seizures at the age of 14. Even before treatment began at the age of 15, his attacks had not been very frequent. They consisted of an absence lasting up to five minutes preceded by an abdominal aura. In the absence he would sometimes fall to the ground. For a few minutes after recovering he would be slightly confused and a little querulous but would then recover completely. He usually had an attack on Monday mornings during the first lesson of the day at school. Immediately he would be taken to the school sick room and then transferred in an ambulance to a local hospital from where he would be returned home. The next day his mother would often keep him at home because he had been ill, returning him to school on Wednesday. He might well have an attack on Wednesday or Thursday, and again he would be sent home to start school the following Monday when he would often have another attack.

This pattern of events over a few brief and not very alarming absences per week continued for a year during which time the boy had practically no schooling at all. It was quite clear that he himself was happy with the situation and was probably manipulating people's anxiety levels to maintain it. The situation was only recognised when he was sent up for investigation. It is interesting that when he was seen, this boy was beginning to go through a fairly normal period of adolescent rebellion, particularly with his mother, and occasionally showed some acting-out behaviour. His elder brother had gone through a very similar period about three years before and behaved in very much the same way: this elder brother's rebellion had passed unremarked, but in the patient any minor peccadillo was immediately blamed on his epilepsy. Only careful long term work by a social worker put this problem right and enabled the boy to get a proper schooling. In this case the therapist's work was with the family and school and not with the fits.

A large number of problems with family relationships can be averted by the understanding, sympathy and common sense of the family doctor. Those which are more severe or which have been allowed to develop unnoticed need the special experience of the psychiatrist and his psychologist and social worker colleagues to put right. Reactions of rejection or hostility against the child with epilepsy by parents are common and they are often associated with feeling of guilt as previously mentioned. Some parents, aware of their hostile feelings, will compensate for them with over-concern and over-protection, others will be overtly hostile with equally damaging results although it is a moot point whether overt hostility or kindly over-protection lead to more damage in the long run.

Case 3
At the age of eight, this girl sustained a cerebro-vascular accident of unknown aetiology in the territory of the right middle cerebral artery. After investigation in a neurosurgical unit she recovered quite well although she was left with residual hemiplegia. This, however, did not interfere with her school performance and she eventually obtained a job in the civil service and married. She was the youngest of her family, and particularly after her stroke, was babied by the rest of the family, so that she grew up with a rather histrionic and attention seeking personality. About a year after her marriage she began to develop brief absences accompanied by bilateral twitching in the arms. The attacks worsened rapidly. There had always been a definite startle component to them, but now instead of lasting a few seconds and being followed by instant recovery, they started to last up to half an hour. She would respond to unexpected sounds in her environment by a brief akinetic absence plus a few bilateral jerks of the arms. This was followed by weeping, kicking, screaming and rolling about. She would frequently cry out 'get off' and appeared to be struggling with an imaginary, evil and presumably lecherous assailant. (This change in her attack pattern had followed her visit to hospital for a brain scan which involved an intravenous injection – which she hated – and also a visit to a film called *The Exorcist*).

The family's reaction to these very noisy attacks was interesting in that when she had them, they would rush to her and start rubbing her legs, patting her on the face, and mopping her brow with a damp cloth. At the same time, the mother and the husband would have a bitter quarrel over the struggling body of the girl, the mother accusing the husband

of being the cause of the attacks, saying 'she wasn't like this until she married you', whilst the husband would be hurling similar accusations back at the mother. Eventually the mother took the girl back into her own home to live with her. The frequency of the girl's attacks increased until she was admitted to hospital, having up to half-a-dozen in a single day exhausting both herself and her family. She was rapidly transferred from a general medical ward to a psychiatric unit where the attacks were treated simply by ignoring them and they disappeared fairly rapidly. The startle seizures were controlled with clonazepam. When she went home on weekend leave, the post-ictal elaboration returned and it became apparent that they were the girl's reaction to pre-existing family stresses which had been intensified by the development of her genuine attacks. A family conference was held in which a common policy for dealing with the attacks was thrashed out, and they declined in frequency at home. Over the next few years the elaborated attacks reappeared at times of family stress, and occasionally at such times she also had other brief hysterical symptoms like total aphonia.

She developed a good therapeutic relationship with her social worker who encouraged her to develop independence and self reliance, which was particularly needed after the birth of her child. As she became more mature in her relationships and more self-assertive, her family attitudes to her changed, and eventually her husband left home taking the child with him; she was then rejected by her mother, so that she is now having to make her own way in the world. It seems that neither the family nor the husband were able to accept the girl when she was no longer in a relationship emotionally dependent on them. It is interesting that as she has developed a more mature personality, she has ceased having even her genuine attacks and she has recently been withdrawn from medication.

Over-protection during childhood may well lead to the kind of battle which I have just described, with mother and husband competing to give unnecessary succour to the daughter or wife. It is often as difficult and painful for the victims of such family battles to break away, as it is for the family.

Case 4
This 24 year old girl, born of a prolonged and difficult labour and who later had several febrile convulsions, developed complex partial seizures originating in the left temporal lobe at the age of 11. The seizures consisted of an absence lasting a couple of minutes, during which the girl felt intense jamais vu and had micropsia; occasionally seizures would continue for a great deal longer. They were frequent and showed little response to medication and were most likely to occur in the early morning.

The family's reaction to them was pathological. Mother and father denied themselves the opportunity of having other children and devoted themselves to the care of their child. The mother gave up work, the child was kept in a school near home; due to frequent seizures, school attendance was poor. She was never allowed to play with other children, or to go out on her own, but had to be accompanied everywhere by her mother. She eventually left school and tried to obtain employment. Her mother was so anxious that the girl might possibly have an attack whilst on her own, that her anxieties were communicated to the daughter. She, in turn, became so tense and anxious at the prospect of new employment, that she had many seizures, and she could not keep the job. Consequently she spent a very restricted life at home merely helping her mother with domestic tasks. Occasionally she would go to a youth club, but again was always accompanied by her mother. At the club she met and fell in love with a young man with whom she had a prolonged courtship, marrying six years after they first met. They moved into a house only a few doors away from her parents' house. The girl now finds herself in a very difficult situation. A combination of intensive behavioural treatment and new chemotherapy has made her far more independent and has taught her to deal with her anxieties better, and has significantly reduced the number of her attacks, but she is still trapped in a dependency situation with her mother (who interprets independence as ingratitude) and her husband, who is the kind of man that wanted a dependent domesticated woman to look after him.

Several studies (Pond & Bidwell, 1959; Bagley, 1971) have shown that the earlier the age of the onset of epilepsy, the more likely it is that the child will have behavioural problems during childhood, and also in later life. Pathophysiological factors are obviously important, but it is likely that faulty attitudes at school and in the family contribute to this finding.

I have already referred to the prophylactic value of educating the public about epilepsy and changing their attitudes towards it. The family doctor, the neurologist, the psychiatrist and their associated colleagues such as health visitors, clinical psychologists and social workers have an even greater opportunity within the family effectively to manipulate attitudes and so to prevent the development of the failures to live with epilepsy which are described in Chapter 15.

STRESS DISORDERS

Having looked at general reactions to stress, it is appropriate here to consider whether stress disorders are more common in people with epilepsy and to describe the form that they take.

It has been said previously that many stress responses are normal. Stress responses become abnormal either when they are very severe, so that they interfere significantly with the person's life or with the life of others, or when they become prolonged and continue to exist long after the stress itself has resolved, or when they are maladaptive (in other words they inhibit the persons correct response to a particular stress so that it cannot be solved), or when they become self-reinforcing so that the stress symptoms themselves become the stress.

Reinforcement can also occur because of the effect that the patient's symptoms have on other people, or because the patient's symptoms do, in an unhealthy way, solve the problem. Psychiatrists talk about *'primary gain'* which the patient himself may obtain from his symptoms, and *'secondary gain'* which is the reinforcement or encouragement that other people may unwittingly give to the patient's symptoms. As we have seen, some parents have a need to have a child who is totally dependent on them, and may as the child comes to adolescence encourage his dependency needs. Some patients whose symptoms are cutting them off from a stressful situation (like the development of paraplegia in a teenager who is in conflict about whether or not to leave home) may find that there is a kind of collusion between himself and other people so that his symptoms are reinforced by other people who cheerfully push the paralysed teenager around in a wheelchair and help him to adapt to the life of somebody who is paralysed.

Just as we cannot consider epilepsy in isolation (epilepsy is certainly not just having fits) so we cannot consider psychiatric symptoms in isolation but we have to take into account not only the patient's reaction to them but also the reaction of other people, and the situation in which they are occurring.

The particular stress disorder which occurs in an individual is the sum of many forces and influences acting on him and is partly determined by his constitution and by his previous experience. Stress disorders tend to be fairly consistent although modified by the factors we have already considered and they can also be modified by treatment.

The commonest stress disorder is probably an anxiety state, which may be seen as a 'flight or fight' reaction which has become distorted by the requirements of civilisation. Some people under stress develop disabling depressive symptoms and some may show maladaptive ritualistic or obsessional behaviour. Others, (although this is now rare) 'cut off' from their stress and develop hysterical conditions. Occasionally people under stress may break down into acute psychotic states. Stress is, of course, also a most important causative factor in some physical illnesses and a significant adjunct to many others. The rôle of stress in the precipitation of fits will be considered later on in this chapter. The types of maladaptive responses to stress which have been described are not necessarily exclusive, many people who are anxious, for instance, can also feel depressed and vice versa.

By and large, stress disorders should not be seen as illnesses. There is no doubt that psychiatric illnesses in the true sense occur and these will be considered later on in this chapter. Except perhaps in rare situations, however, it is unhelpful to see anxiety or mild depression or hysteria as an illness particularly as this tends to imply that there is a 'medical' treatment.

Do stress disorders occur more commonly in people with epilepsy than in the general population? The answer is that they probably do, and that, epilepsy in some ways is unique in causing stress disorders. (It should be remembered, however, that life experiences may be *pathogenic* in a disorder, in other words they may actually *cause* the disturbance or they may be *pathoplastic*, in other words, they alter the *form* that the disturbance takes in the particular individual).

Studies of the epidemiology of stress disorders and psychiatric illness in people with epilepsy have been made, but there are many difficulties in carrying out an accurate epidemiological survey of the psychological difficulties of people with a chronic relapsing disorder like epilepsy. It is known for instance that only about half the people with epilepsy in the community treated by their general practitioners will be seen at a hospital clinic. Those that are seen are often referred not because of the severity of their epilepsy as such, but because of other handicaps both physical and mental or because of co-existant personality and stress disorders. Any studies that concentrate on a hospital population of people will therefore be biased by the selected population being studied.

Although general practitioners frequently know a great deal about their patients' social problems, emotional disorders and psychological difficulties, such information may not be recorded

or assessed accurately. It is also true that there are in the general population some people with epilepsy (and certainly many people with mental disorders) who do not seek help from their general practitioners. The sickest people often may be those least likely to seek help. Again, therefore, it is likely that those who do seek help from their general practitioner will be a biased sample. Some people with epilepsy may not themselves realise that they have it, or their families may accept it without asking for help. In one study (Betts, 1974) of people with epilepsy admitted to psychiatric hospitals, it was found that 28 per cent of the sample (who had proven epilepsy) had never consulted their general practitioners about their attack disorder, and were not receiving medication.

To determine accurately the relationship between epilepsy, stress disorders and mental illness, therefore, field studies should be carried out in which a *total* population of a particular town or district is sampled by specially trained personnel who can carry out a formal examination of all the people with a particular disorder. Even such a study will miss those people in the population who have been removed to institutions.

Therefore, the results of the studies carried out in the past few years should be interpreted cautiously. There does seem to be general agreement, however, that stress disorders (neurotic disorders) are commoner in people with epilepsy than in the general population (Pond, Bidwell & Stein, 1960; Gudmundsson, 1966).

A survey of all handicapped children on the Isle of Wight suggested that about one-third of children with epilepsy had significant psychiatric disturbance. This proportion rose in those cases which had associated neurological symptoms, and was particularly high in those who were mentally handicapped as well (Graham & Rutter, 1968). The survey showed that the prevalence of psychiatric disorder was twice as frequent in children with epilepsy compared with children who had other chronic disabilities (e.g. asthma) and was about four times the expected rate in the general child population.

It may be that one other unique factor in the burden that epilepsy imposes on people (apart from the fear of the attacks themselves and the limitations on day to day living) is the fear of *loss of control* which epilepsy engenders. In this regard a comparison can be made between people with epilepsy and sufferers from Menières's Syndrome, some of whom may also be toppled to the ground by their vertigo. Patients with this disease may also feel very keenly the ignominy of their disability, which they are also helpless to control, and it has been shown that they too are particularly liable to develop anxiety and depression (Pratt & Mackenzie, 1958).

ANXIETY

As we have said, anxiety is part of normal experience. It becomes pathological when it becomes reinforcing, or when it prevents the individual from dealing with the problem which is causing the anxiety. Anxiety has a psychological component (a feeling of morbid dread or fear, which is subjectively most unpleasant) and a somatic component which consists of symptoms referrable to stimulation of the sympathetic and the parasympathetic autonomic nervous systems (palpitation, nausea, diarrhoea, muscle aching, shaking etc.) In some patients the psychological component is prominent and in some the somatic component. Since anxiety often presents with somatic symptoms it can easily be mistaken for physical illness, and the corollary is also true. In epilepsy it is particularly important to distinguish between querulousness, irritability and agitation found in organic brain disease and anxiety itself. Likewise, anxiety is often a component of depression, and in somebody who is agitated it is important to look for a possible underlying depressive illness.

Anxiety may be generalised and therefore be with the person all the time (so-called free-floating anxiety) or it may be situational, occurring in response to certain definite identifiable stimuli to which the patient is exposed (so called phobic anxiety, occurring only when the patient is travelling, or going into shops or when he encounters, say, cats or moths). In somebody who has anxiety symptoms, it is important to distinguish if there is a phobic element, as this may alter the management. As will be seen later, patients who become acutely anxious often have so-called panic attacks and these can be sometimes difficult to distinguish

from epilepsy itself. A variety of severe phobic anxiety is called agoraphobia; the patient is crippled by intense anxiety as he steps over the threshold of his home, and may in fact become totally housebound.

In my experience, phobic anxiety and agoraphobia seem particularly common in people with epilepsy, and relate clearly to the patient's fear of having a seizure in a crowded place or in the street. Often, as we shall see later, the patient's anxiety increases the likelihood that he will have seizures so that as the seizure anxiety increases so does the frequency of seizures and the two reinforce each other.

The management of anxiety involves careful investigation of the patient and his symptoms with a physical history and examination followed by detailed analysis of his emotional symptoms and life situation. Some patients with anxiety need counselling to help them to discover the best way of dealing with the situation that is making them anxious. Some, whose anxiety relates to interpersonal conflict, may need formal psychotherapy (in other words, a therapeutic relationship with a professional therapist who uses his interpersonal skills, and the emotional relationship that develops between him and the patient to guide him to an understanding of the emotional or interpersonal conflict which is causing the anxiety). Formal psychotherapy is a skilled undertaking with a large investment in terms of time and resources, and although sometimes extremely useful need not be applied routinely in every patient who is anxious.

Behavioural methods of treatment (that is treatment aimed at helping the patient to overcome his symptoms or to control them without worrying too much about the antecedents of the anxiety) are gaining popularity. They were originally used successfully in patients with phobic anxiety, but are now being used in those with free-floating anxiety. There are various available methods of teaching a patient to control his anxiety, involving types of relaxation training or biofeedback which will be described in the section on the self-control of seizures. The advantages of behavioural methods is that they teach the patient self-reliance and self-control.

In my view, the use of psychotropic medication in those who are anxious should be kept to an absolute minimum. Far too many people in this country are given minor tranquillisers or hypnotic drugs to deal with neurotic symptoms which can be much better dealt with by other methods. Once started, tranquillisers are difficult to stop; they lead to dependence, they are a potent source of overdoses and they teach the patient nothing about self-reliance. These views against the use of psychotropic medication in anxiety may seem severe, but they do apply particularly to patients with epilepsy, as most minor tranquillisers of the benzodiazepine group have antiepileptic properties and it may be even more difficult to take a patient with epilepsy off diazepam or chlordiazepoxide than somebody who is not epileptic. Occasionally other medication may be useful temporarily in treating anxiety, particularly beta-blocking drugs if the anxiety has a large somatic component (Tyrer, 1974). If tranquillisers are used they should be given in short courses of two or three weeks during which time the patient must be encouraged to deal with the situation which is causing his anxiety. Furthermore it should be remembered that the treatment of anxiety is not just the giving of a tranquilliser but that counselling and self-help methods must also be employed.

DEPRESSION

Depression is a term much used but often little defined. As a symptom of a reaction to stress it is probably less common than anxiety, but can be much more disabling.

Depression like anxiety has both psychological and somatic components. It is a feeling of pathological sadness or lowness (which may pass beyond ordinary human understanding), often accompanied by feeling of guilt, unworthiness and self-blame.

In severe depression even delusions and hallucinations of a gloomy nature may occur. These psychological symptoms are accompanied by biological symptoms of a change in sleep pattern, loss of weight, loss of appetite and loss of libido. In milder forms of depression the appetite and sleep changes sometimes go in the reverse direction and there is oversleeping and overeating, with a consequent weight gain.

Classically, two forms of depression are described, reactive and endogenous (or neurotic and psychotic) implying that in some people depressive symptoms are a clear result of life stress or interpersonal difficulty and in other patients no such relationship can be seen, and it is assumed that depression is an illness *sui generis*. This is sometimes a useful concept, although it is probable that in the majority of patients with a depressive illness no clear separation can be made. Endogenous depressive illnesses do seem to be more common in people with epilepsy and will be discussed further in the section on psychotic illness. The management of depression again involves a detailed history and examination of the patient, both physically and mentally, and an enquiry into his life circumstances.

Some depressions can be supported and worked through using techniques of counselling or psychotherapy. In contrast to anxiety however, many patients will need chemical support as well; the indications for using drugs even in reactive depression are much stronger than in anxiety. The tricyclic antidepressants should be considered first, although their convulsant action needs to be remembered. Apart from the drug treatment, patients with depression need the support of somebody who understands how disabling depression can be. As a person's depression starts to improve, so he will need careful rehabilitation, because, like anxiety, there is no doubt that depression can be self-reinforcing. The loss of confidence in one's abilities which depression can engender may eventually be more disabling than the depression itself and can persist long after the depression is over.

In the management of depression the risk of suicide must always be kept in mind. Those with epilepsy have a readily available source of dangerous antiepileptic drugs with which to take an overdose. It is probable that suicide attempts (as well as completed suicide) are more common in people with epilepsy than in the general population (Mackay, 1979). A patient with epilepsy is also more likely to repeat previous overdoses. Part of the explanation for the increased incidence of repeated overdoses in people with epilepsy may of course lie in the chronic nature of the epileptic patient's problems which are not resolved by the overdose attempt.

In a busy general hospital I see many people with epilepsy who have taken overdoses of their antiepileptic drugs. One particular phenomenon which is not well described in the text books is worth reporting, and that is that following recovery of consciousness in patients who have taken large overdoses of such drugs as phenytoin, phenobarbitone, primidone or the benzodiazepines, there may be an interval of several days of unruly acting-out behaviour which may be mistaken for the patient's normal state.

Case 5
A 17-year-old girl with poorly controlled epilepsy (probably because of her reluctance to take antiepileptic drugs) discovered herself to be pregnant, and immediately swallowed a large quantity of phenobarbitone and phenytoin. She was admitted to hospital unconscious, and recovered consciousness 24 hours later. Shortly after regaining consciousness she was found on a window ledge of the general hospital to which she had been admitted, threatening to jump. When taken back to bed and restrained, she bit, fought and scratched the nursing staff, broke two thermometers on her bedside locker and attempted to swallow them, and later broke a cup and attempted to cut her wrists. Unless constantly watched, she would get out of bed and dash round the wards, screaming and shouting and attempting to leave the hospital. She was therefore transferred to a psychiatric unit (where this kind of behaviour after antiepileptic drug overdosage was well known), and therefore her behaviour was contained rather than treated, as it has been found that sedating such disturbed patients merely makes them worse.
An EEG at this time showed changes compatible with drug intoxication, but there was no evidence of sub-ictal epileptic activity (which might have been the cause of her mental state). Three days after her admission to the psychiatric unit her behaviour rapidly settled and a pleasant and co-operative, if somewhat troubled, teenager emerged from underneath it. Her antiepileptic drug was changed to one she found more tolerable: her compliance with treatment improved, and she was counselled about her pregnancy, which she decided to keep.

In patients with epilepsy, threats of suicide should always be taken seriously and carefully assessed. Any patient who is depressed should be asked specifically about whether or not he has had any thoughts or plans of harming himself. (Many patients are relieved to be asked this question). It has been shown that most people who succeed in killing themselves have given clear warning to somebody of their intention beforehand. Patients who are considered likely to make active attempts at suicide (whether their depression is reactive or endogenous) should be admitted to hospital for treatment of their depression, and if necessary they should be compelled to come into hospital.

Even if initial assessment suggests that the patient is not potentially suicidal, it is important to keep in close touch with him until the depression has clearly resolved. It should also be remembered that somebody with intractable epilepsy, which has not responded to treatment, may attempt to take his life, not because he is depressed, but because he feels this is a rational solution to an intolerable situation.

A high seizure frequency may make effective treatment of the depression more difficult and concomittant with the treatment of depression every effort should be made to bring the patients' seizures under as good control as possible, short of intoxication. (It should be remembered that the symptoms of depression can resemble those of drug intoxication and vice versa). It cannot be emphasised too strongly that if a family doctor or neurologist has any doubts about the suicidal intentions of a depressed patient whom he is treating, it is important that the patient is referred urgently for a psychiatric opinion.

Symptomatic alcoholism is common in depression and may also occur in people with epilepsy, although one survey has suggested that drinking problems are less common in people with epilepsy than in the general population (Mackay, 1979). If alcoholism does occur in somebody with epilepsy it complicates considerably the management of the epilepsy. Excessive alcohol intake may cause fits (as may alcohol withdrawal), although it can be debated whether such 'Rum Fits' constitute established epilepsy. However, alcohol affects the metabolism of antiepileptic drugs, and it is difficult to control serum levels if they are liable to be influenced by excessive and erratic alcohol intake. Patients who drink excessively are usually unreliable in the taking of prescribed drugs.

There is no evidence that moderate drinking needs to be forbidden in people with epilepsy (who are already subject to many restrictions), although in view of the potential epileptogenic effects of hydration, an excessive fluid intake should be avoided.

Those patients with anxiety and depression who are faced with a loss of employment or severe social disadvantage (like the break-up of marriages), will need further measures to help them. Antidepressants or a therapeutic relationship will not be enough, and skilled help from a social worker can be of tremendous importance to such patients. Deterioration which has evoked a call for psychiatric help will often be associated with an increased frequency of fits and the psychiatric problems themselves may be exacerbating the difficulties in controlling the epilepsy. In-patient care, with careful observation of fits, medical management, adjustment of antiepileptic drugs with biochemical control, and a controlled programme of work rehabilitation is essential. Even specialised neurological units with a good psychiatric support may not be able to look after patients long enough, or provide adequate work programmes, and specialised psychiatric units, which in many other ways are more suitable, may not have all the necessary facilities. (In this regard the placement of Employment Rehabilitation Units on general hospital sites – as at the Queen Elizabeth Medical Centre in Birmingham – is to be encouraged as it makes liaison a great deal easier). For the patients just described with multiple handicaps the Special Centres for Epilepsy where there are complementary hospital and residential units, may be particularly useful.

Effective treatment and management of the patient depends not on the skills of one particular discipline but rather on the understanding by each specialist discipline of the skills of the others and on their constructive co-operation. A member of any discipline who treats epilepsy must have a good working knowledge of the skills of the other disciplines which are necessary for the total care of a patient with epilepsy, and must know when to call in other specialised help. Any psychiatrist who sets out to treat the psychological complications of epilepsy must also have a very sound knowledge of epilepsy itself.

OTHER STRESS DISORDERS

Some people under stress develop compulsive ritualised behaviours (such as compulsive hand washing, checking, or thinking) which can be seen as a magical attempt to ward off the anxiety induced by the particular stress. Compulsive disorders are particularly likely to become self-reinforcing and are subjectively most unpleasant. There is no evidence that they are more common in people with epilepsy than in the general population, (indeed one wonders why this is so) and they seem to respond best to behavioural methods of treatment. (This should be distinguished from the 'obsessional personality' which is a rigid pedantic personality structure not uncommon in those who are brain damaged.)

Some people under stress, in order to escape an intolerable situation, develop hysterical symptoms. There is no word in psychiatry which has been more abused and misunderstood than hysteria. To a psychiatrist, hysteria means the unconscious adoption of conversion symptoms of an organic nature (often a pseudo-neurological character) which resolve the conflict or stress for the patient often in a symbolic way (e.g. the paralysis of the writing hand which prevents a student from writing his final examination papers). Most psychiatrists would agree that the symptoms or signs presented are adopted unconsciously in hysteria although the borderline between conscious simulation of a disorder and conscious malingering is difficult to define. Hysteria nowadays in Britain is rare, and usually easy to recognise, particularly as it usually results from an acute traumatic situation for the patient.

The problem arises with chronic symptoms which *may* be hysterical. It is certainly true that acute hysterical symptoms, unless rapidly treated, may become chronic, particularly as they are easily reinforced by the reaction of other people to them. However, it cannot be emphasised enough that in a patient with chronic neurological symptoms for which no adequate cause can be found, the diagnosis of hysteria must only be made on positive diagnostic criteria for hysteria and not just be a diagnosis of exclusion. Many patients with a definite organic lesion may over-elaborate their symptoms in order to draw the attention of an often doubting medical profession to them. Cases of firmly diagnosed hysteria often turn out later to have either organic or other psychiatric pathology to account for them (Slater, 1965).

Hysteria has usually been treated by some form of psychotherapy but there is a growing interest in treating hysteria along behavioural lines (Bird, 1979) as will be considered when hysteria is described in the section on the differential diagnosis of attack disorders.

Occasionally, people under stress break down into what appears to be an acute psychotic illness of either an undifferentiated or schizophrenic type. In some patients who break down like this under acute stress, there is no doubt that it is an unconsciously simulated psychotic disorder (like the Ganser Syndrome), which can be seen as a variant of hysteria, often with a clear message from the patient to the outside world 'Look how mad you have made me', but occasionally an acute schizophrenic illness can be precipitated by stress. Such illnesses have a good prognosis if the stress can be removed and in people with epilepsy need to be distinguished from those psychotic illnesses of a schizophrenic type which are found in association with epilepsy itself.

PERSONALITY DISORDERS IN PEOPLE WITH EPILEPSY

There is a long felt belief that people with epilepsy are more prone to disorders of personality than people without epilepsy. This question needs to be considered critically, rather than with the prejudices of those who have preconceived ideas or those who are over-anxious to alleviate the problems that their patients have by refusing to accept that some people with epilepsy may have problems in interpersonal relationships.

A personality disorder is not easy to define. It is true, however, that some people seem to have chronic problems of adjustment to society or with living, or relating to other people which appear to be persistent and long standing (often dating from childhood) which produce stress symptoms either in the person himself or in those who have to live with him. Problems arise in the definition and measurement of such apparent personality disorders as the definition of a personality disorder is very much bound up with the values of the particular society which is defining it. A particular trait may be seen by one society as pathological; in another it may even be the norm. In societies such as ours, which are changing rapidly, definitions become even more difficult.

The diagnosis of a personality disorder must rest on definitive reliable criteria which any psychiatrist can recognise, and not on the personal prejudices either of the psychiatrist or of society. Attempts have been made recently to try to clarify and refine the concept of personality disorder, and even to develop rating scales which can be used to define it accurately. (Walton & Presly, 1973; Tyrer & Alexander, 1979; Tyrer et al., 1979).

Most of the published observations on the relationship between personality disorder and epilepsy, however are not based on reliable criteria which have been scientifically evaluated but are based merely on descriptions of the patient's behaviour. Such descriptions (which classify people as, for example, 'obsessional' or 'hypochondriacal' or 'overdependent') miss 90 per cent of the patient's other behaviours, and it may be better to see patients on a continuum from normality in terms of a particular personality trait, and also to see their personalities as multi-dimensional. As Walton and Presly (1973) point out, any classification of personality disorder should be based on clinical observation of behaviour rather than intuitive hunches. No symptom of neurotic or psychotic illness is required to make the diagnosis, the abnormality is in the personality itself and is based on the clinical history and examination and the observation of behaviour, and as Tyrer et al. (1979) point out, on a history from a relative who has known the patient for some time. Deviation from normal behaviour shows itself primarily in the patient's relationship with other people and is a continuing, not an episodic, phenomenon. Various personality traits have been attributed to people with epilepsy from time to time. The most famous, (or infamous) personality type historically related to epilepsy is of course the 'epileptic personality' itself.

The balance of evidence suggests that a small number of patients with chronic epilepsy living under conditions of institutionalisation or environmental handicap may develop a characteristic pattern of personality change which has attracted many descriptive adjectives in its time; many of them pejorative. Such patients are commonly described as pedantic, circumstantial, meticulous, religiose, egocentric, hypercritical, hypochondriacal, suspicious and quarrelsome and possessing a slowness and stickiness of thought which may suggest subnormality or early dementia. Such patients, even if few in number, in an institution are bound to colour opinion and must also represent a continuing problem in management.

It is surprising how widely this view is still held. Indeed, not so very long ago (Henderson & Gillespie, 1950) it was held that this epileptic personality was an accentuation of a pre-existing epileptic constitution which was responsible for the fits and any mental deterioration that occurred.

The problem in an institution is that if one has ideas about the personality of patients it is extremely easy to find evidence which supports one's hypothesis, and indeed the hypothesis may even become self-filling. If one is expecting a certain form of behaviour from a patient one may well behave towards him in such a way as actually to induce the behaviour.

The other problem about having a fixed belief that certain patients have an abnormal personality characteristic, is that one is then not motivated to change them, (although there is some evidence that even organic personality traits can be treated and changed).

However, there is little doubt that the constellation of personality traits described above does occur and is to be found in people with epilepsy. This apparent association is due to factors of selection in that those with unfavourable personality traits will tend to enter institutions more often than those whose personalities enable them to manage much better in the outside world and, once admitted, tend to stick there. Referral of patients with epilepsy to general hospital out-patients unconnected with psychiatry is still more likely to occur if the patient has psychological problems (Pond et al., 1960).

The epileptic temperament, if it exists, or when it occurs, is the result of multiple handicap – childhood environmental and physical deprivation, brain damage and, perhaps, the chronic effects of antiepileptic drugs. A temperament in many ways similar can be found in patients with other non-epileptic prolonged disabilities. For example, rheumatoid arthritis and chronic pain cause personality change (Merskey & Tonge, 1974). The same is doubtless true of epilepsy especially if it is severe and affects a person predisposed to emotional illness by reason of his earlier life experiences.

Some authors suggest that the 'epileptic personality' may be a brain damage syndrome, (Guerrant et al., 1962) and there is some evidence that a similar clinical picture may occur in those with bitemporal lobe damage but without epilepsy (Slater, Beard & Glitheroe, 1963).

It is certainly true that the epileptic personality has lost its importance in the thinking of those psychiatrists with an interest in epilepsy as indeed has the interest in trying to substantiate the relationship between epilepsy and other types of personality disorder. The methodological drawbacks and difficulties are well described by Tizard (1962).

There remains, however, a generally held view in the literature and elsewhere that people with epilepsy are aggressive. Whether aggressiveness is more common in people with epilepsy than in the general population has never been tested formally except in children where the evidence is conflicting. One study (Mellor, Lowitt & Hall, 1974) suggested that epileptic children are somewhat more miserable than their peers but if anything are less aggressive. Bagley (1971) found an increase in aggressiveness in certain types of epilepsy in children. (It should be remembered that aggression in someone with epilepsy may be the result of severe subnormality or a symptom of associated mental illness.)

Whether or not aggressiveness is more common in adults with epilepsy than in the general population is open to question, but there is no doubt that people with epilepsy are feared for their aggressiveness. In my experience this is an irrational fear which stems from a small group of hospitalised epileptic patients who may show aggressiveness and from the general fear of epilepsy itself.

Some people may, following their epileptic seizure, have outbursts of self-limiting extreme violence – so called 'Epileptic Furore'. Whether this is itself an ictal phenomenon is uncertain. What is true is that it is becoming very rare nowadays. Violence may also occur after temporal lobe attacks which in themselves may pass almost unnoticed. A few patients with epilepsy may have clear-cut episodes of rage in between their epileptic attacks which may be difficult to control, and which colour the views that mental nurses may have of patients with epilepsy. In an institution like a mental hospital, chronic patients are largely in the care of nurses who may have worked on the same ward as the patient for many years. The medical staff may not see the patient for more than perhaps half an hour a year, unless he causes trouble. In addition, the medical staff tend to take on trust what the nurses tell them about particular patients, especially as the junior staff are often little versed in the language and culture of the country. If the nurses' views of the relationship between personality disorder and epilepsy are fixed and archaic, then fixed and archaic descriptions will be given of the patient.

The management of those few patients with epilepsy who do show extreme rage whether it is ictal, peri-ictal or apparently unassociated with ictal events is controversial.

Case 6

I first saw this man in 1967 when he had been in hospital for 11 years having been admitted at the age of 35. He had a history of meningitis as a child and also a history of a forceps delivery. His epilepsy began at the age of 11, and was described as 'grand mal' in type. From the age of 20 he almost invariably suffered a severe epileptic furore after each fit, and was eventually admitted to a mental hospital because of these furores. Following his admission to hospital he continued to have many epileptic fits (up to about 20 a month) and for a long time was the terror of the hospital being confined to a locked room on a locked ward, and there was a record of several homicidal attacks on staff and patients. Most of the homicidal episodes occurred after a major tonic-clonic seizure but occasionally, in between his major seizures he would have sudden short lived outbursts of homicidal violence. They would start without warning or obvious precipitant and last for five to thirty minutes (during which time he was entirely unapproachable). He seemed to have no memory of them afterwards. At the time of his admission he appeared to be suffering also from a paranoid psychosis, in which he was described as having ideas of reference, grandiose delusions and auditory hallucinations. This psychotic state cleared within a few months after his admission without specific treatment.

He had been taking large doses of phenytoin and phenobarbitone since his admission. His epilepsy had not been investigated until 1967 when an EEG showed phase reversal of spike-and-wave activity in the right anterior mid-temporal region. In addition to his regular antiepileptic drugs, chlordiazapoxide, 25 mg three times a day was added in 1967. Subsequently, he had no further fits and there were no further aggressive outbursts. His whole personality seemed to change in that he became pleasant and sociable, and within six months of starting chlordiazapoxide he was allowed out into the grounds for the first time ever. He eventually started work in the occupational therapy unit. He was seen again by me in 1979 (Betts & Skarrott, 1979). He was still in hospital although clearly he would have been quite suitable for hostel accommodation if any had been available. He was a pleasant cheerful man with a wry sense of humour,

and a good grasp of current affairs. There was no evidence of a dementing process. The chlordiazapoxide had been withdrawn in 1974; he had had occasional short-lived aggressive episodes since that time (but none for two years) and he had had no seizures since originally taking chlordiazapoxide, although he remained on heavy doses of phenobarbitone and phenytoin.

Case 7

This man had already been in hospital for 29 years when first seen by me in 1967. He was 19 years old on admission. His epilepsy was known to have begun at the age of 13 and was simply described in his notes as 'grand mal' in type. In 1967 he was still having a couple of fits a month. He was admitted originally 'confused and demented, and elated with auditory hallucinations'. This seems to have been an acute organic psychosis of paranoid type, which disappeared quite rapidly after his admission to hospital without any specific treatment. Subsequently, he suffered from many attacks of epileptic furore following his tonic-clonic seizures and occasionally would suffer from acute aggressive outbursts in between his major seizures. These rages occurred without provocation although it was noted that a specific phrase 'who's got wooden legs' would always precipitate an aggressive outburst.

This, at one time, unfortunately became a source of amusement for some of the nursing staff. In 1967 he was taking 240 mg of phenobarbitone a day in divided doses; this dosage has continued until the present day. His medical notes had continued to describe him as suffering from 'epileptic insanity' although no psychotic features had been observed in his mental state for many years and also he was described as suffering from 'epileptic dementia', although in fact he was correctly orientated in space and time and had a reasonable knowledge of current events. On review in 1979 he was found to be pleasant, and equable in temperament. He was a somewhat simple man of seventy who showed no evidence of a dementing process and no psychotic features. His last seizure occurred in 1974, and since then there had been no further episodes either of furore or of aggressive outbursts.

These patients are representative of the epileptic patients with aggressive outbursts that can be found in mental hospitals. In them there seems to be a relationship, even if not a direct one, between seizures and the aggressive outbursts as both seem to wane at about the same time. They do not resemble at all closely the patients described by Maletzky (1973) with the 'episodic dyscontrol syndrome'. These were men without epilepsy (but many of them had temporal lobe EEG abnormality) who were subject to episodes of senseless unprovoked violence in the setting of severe personality disorder: some improved with phenytoin.

The treatment of such violent aggressive outbursts is difficult and somewhat controversial. Occasionally, patients may respond well to the exhibition of benzodiazepine drugs, whether intravenously or by chronic oral medication; but not all will do so, and it should be remembered that these drugs, like alcohol and the barbiturates may have a disinhibiting action, making the violence worse. I have already mentioned the phenomenon of those patients who, following overdoses of antiepileptic drugs show transient 'acting out' behaviour. This can also happen in patients who have been given large doses of diazepam intravenously to control status epilepticus, indeed it may also produce transient pseudo-seizures. Some patients may be better controlled with parenteral or oral phenothiazines, butyrophenone drugs, or chlormethiazole. A particularly useful drug for calming the acutely disturbed is droperidol which can be given safely intravenously. Patients with acute aggressive outbursts, are often better left alone as the outburst is usually self-limiting.

Some patients, then, do have *episodes* of severe aggression. It is widely reported in the literature, although no controlled studies have been done, that many patients with epilepsy are *chronically* irritable and aggressive. I am not certain that this is necessarily more than one would find in an equivalent population of either institutionalised patients or normal people; but if it is accepted for a moment that perhaps some people with epilepsy do show undue aggressiveness, is it possible to find any correlation between the aggression and their social and epileptic history? There have been several reviews (Taylor, 1969b; Serafetinides, 1965; and an unpublished Birmingham study). All three studies suggested that male epileptics are more likely to be aggressive than women and also showed that the earlier the onset of the epilepsy, the more likely it was that aggression would develop later, which would suggest strongly the importance in the pathogenesis of aggression of early social disadvantage and failures of social learning. Taylor and Serafetinides suggested that there is a connection between aggression and temporal lobe epilepsy, but no such relationship was found in the Birmingham study. Serafetinides indeed suggested that patients with left temporal lobe lesions are more likely to be aggressive.

The populations studied however are not comparable. The first two studies were considering patients with intractable epilepsy selected for surgery because of unilateral temporal lobe lesions whereas the Birmingham study covered a much wider and probably more representative population of patients with epilepsy admitted to mental hospitals (Betts, 1974). Many questions about the relationship between aggression and epilepsy remain unanswered and further work using control populations is clearly necessary.

The evidence to date suggests that although brain mechanisms may be important, the influence of social and learning factors may be paramount in causing aggression in people with epilepsy. This is important because prevention may be possible with better management of children with epilepsy.

One important factor that has come out of studies of aggressiveness in epilepsy (Taylor, 1969) is that in those patients going forward for temporal lobe surgery, aggressiveness is a good prognostic sign in terms of successful rehabilitation after the operation, and cessation of fits. It is interesting that the other psychiatric disorders that may occur in association with temporal lobe epilepsy are seldom improved by temporal lobectomy, and may even be made worse. It has been suggested that some of the depressive illnesses which occur after otherwise successful temporal lobe surgery, (Hill et al., 1957) are the result of the 'turning in' of this aggression onto the patient himself. Post-operative depression is certainly common after temporal lobectomy, or indeed after successful drug treatment of temporal lobe epilepsy, but this may have other causes.

Gunn (1969) in his study of epileptics in prisons, found little evidence of an increased degree of aggressiveness and violence in epileptic prisoners although he recognised that some more difficult patients might have been sent to the special hospitals. He also found that in those people with epilepsy in prisons who were aggressive there was no particular correlation with any type of epilepsy. Others also have found no evidence that aggressiveness is especially common in temporal lobe epilepsy (Guerrant et al., 1962; Small, Hayden & Small, 1966). Lishman (1968) in his study of the psychiatric sequelae of brain injury found that aggressiveness was more common after frontal rather than temporal lobe injuries.

EPILEPSY AND CRIME

If there is uncertainty about a relationship between epilepsy and aggressiveness, what is the relationship between epilepsy and crime itself? It has long been held that there is such a relationship (Lombroso, 1889). In a survey of prison and borstal receptions in England and Wales, followed by a study of a representative sample of male epileptic prisoners (Gunn, 1969) showed that the prevalence of epilepsy in the prison population is well above that to be expected. Many of these epileptic prisoners were also psychiatrically abnormal, but they were not more aggressive than the general population of prisoners. They did however have significantly more depressive symptoms than their fellow prisoners and had attempted suicide more often. There was no relationship between the kind of crime the prisoners had committed and whether or not they had epilepsy, and no relationship between type of crime and type of epilepsy.

No explanation could be found for the apparent increase in criminal acts in people with epilepsy, although it is likely that what relationship there is will be a social one rather than a physiological one.

A further study (Gunn & Fenton, 1971) of epileptic patients in a special hospital to assess the possible connection between criminal acts and epileptic automatism showed that automatism is an extremely rare explanation for crime in people with epilepsy. Many people with epilepsy are socially disadvantaged and deprived, and tend to drift into crime and possibly they are caught more easily. Most people with epilepsy in prison are there for thieving, as is the general prison population, and the increased prevalence of people with epilepsy in prison is almost certainly related to social rather than medical factors.

EPILEPSY AND SEXUALITY

The general public again tends to equate epilepsy with hypersexuality in the same way as they tend to associate it with criminality and violence. How much of this prejudice can be blamed on Lom-broso (1889) is uncertain, but the actual facts about sexuality in epilepsy are very different.

There is a relationship between sexuality and temporal lobe epilepsy (Shukla, Srivastava & Katiyar, 1979). Temporal lobe lesions may produce disturbances of sexual function, usually hyposexuality with lowered sex drive, occasionally total impotence, and, in women, loss of sexual response (Hierons & Saunders, 1966). Social and psychological factors may play at least as important a part as biological ones, although accumulating evidence does suggest that there is a neurophysiological factor present.

There is some evidence that successful treatment of the epilepsy, particularly by surgery, may improve sexual performance (Taylor, 1969a). There has been no evidence presented to show whether conventional sex therapy of a psychotherapeutic or behavioural sort would influence epileptic hyposexuality, which may in part have a neurophysiological basis, although it should not be forgotten that even apparent organic impotence may respond at least in part to behavioural methods of treatment (Betts, 1975), and there is scope here for further research.

There is possibly a slight increase of perverse sexuality in temporal lobe epilepsy although the evidence for this is slight. It has recently been reviewed by Hoenig and Kenna (1979), and again neuro-physiological factors as well as social ones may be playing a part. The temporal lobes, after all, are probably the seat of sexual awareness in man and it is therefore not surprising that aberrations in performance in these areas in the brain may give rise to aberrations in sexual behaviour. There is very little evidence that hypersexuality – except of a primitive kind such as excessive masturbation – occurs in epilepsy, although it may do so in very rare cases. Often, of course, hypersexuality is bound up with mental illness or severe brain damage.

Occasionally sexual functioning may get bound up in the epileptic event itself, as in those patients whose attacks sometimes have a sexual component (Mitchell, Falconer & Hill, 1954), or in those patients whose major seizures are triggered off by a sexual experience as a form of reflex epilepsy (Hoenig & Hamilton, 1960).

THE ROLE OF THE PSYCHIATRIST IN THE DIFFERENTIAL DIAGNOSIS OF ATTACKS

Professor Pond, in Part Two, will be considering the overall differential diagnosis of epilepsy; I want to concentrate on the role of psychiatrist in this exercise, particularly as it is becoming clear from various sources that epilepsy is often misdiagnosed and that psychological factors play quite a large part in this.

Some people with epilepsy are misdiagnosed as suffering from other conditions, and therefore not correctly treated; some patients are diagnosed as having epilepsy when in fact they have other conditions (Betts, 1974). There is also a considerable body of patients with epilepsy who, in addition, have other attack disorders as well. Emotional outbursts may be mistaken for epilepsy. Epilepsy may cause an apparent emotional outburst, and, as will be developed in the next section of this chapter, undoubtedly emotional states influence profoundly the frequency of epileptic seizures themselves, and indeed the emotional management of epilepsy is becoming increasingly important.

The psychiatrist may have an advantage in the diagnosis of certain forms of disturbed behaviour and epilepsy, although before doing so he needs a good knowledge of the varieties of epileptic experiences. Available to him are techniques of observation and behavioural management which are not commonly found on ordinary medical wards, and in addition, a psychiatric ward is a place where disturbed behaviour is probably more tolerated than in an ordinary hospital ward, and, if trained, his nursing staff also are capable of making valuable observations. The following case histories illustrate some of the diagnostic difficulties involved.

Case 8

A man of 36 developed the symptoms of severe depression and was admitted to his local psychiatric hospital where he appeared profoundly depressed with psychomotor retardation, delusions of guilt and unworthiness and definite suicidal intentions. He was accordingly treated with electroconvulsive therapy (ECT); he had previously been in good health and there was no history of a previous attack disorder. A few hours after the second application of ECT, whilst fully recovered from it, he had a witnessed tonic-clonic convulsion. The course of ECT was not continued and following this spontaneous seizure, his depression rapidly improved.

Neurological examination was normal, as were several EEG's; he was not put onto antiepileptic drugs. When followed up a year later he had had no further seizure. However in a discharge summary from the hospital, he was described as 'having epilepsy'. His general practitioner accordingly informed both him and his employing authority of this diagnosis. He was immediately dismissed from his job and a year later was still finding difficulty in gaining employment. Spontaneous convulsions occurring during ECT, although rare, are recognised as a definite phenomenon, perhaps analogous to seizures which occur with amitriptyline and other tricyclic drugs. It was likely that this seizure was an indication of no more than a low convulsive threshold (a view in keeping with my experience of other patients with spontaneous seizures occurring during a course of ECT) and that this man did not have epilepsy.

Case 9

This woman, aged 38, had a long history of psychiatric illness. For some years before admission to a psychiatric hospital she had become agoraphobic, being unable to pass over the threshold of her front door without experiencing symptoms of anxiety. She became particularly anxious when entering shops and shortly before her admission to hospital began to experience peculiar attacks of depersonalisation in this situation, eventually falling to the floor if she entered a supermarket. She was aware of a rising tide of anxiety before these phenomena happened; suddenly, the anxiety would seem to leave her, and was replaced by intense depersonalisation. She became aware of a feeling of lightheadedness, tingling in her hands and feet followed by tetany of the hands and feet, and she would then pass into a brief period of apparent unconsciousness. When one of these attacks was witnessed, she was put into an ambulance and initially taken to a nearby general hospital, but from there transferred to the local psychiatric hospital. During the course of her investigations there, an EEG was performed which showed some dysrhythmia in the right temporal lobe (a not uncommon finding in people with phobic anxiety). On the basis of this abnormal EEG she was diagnosed as having temporal lobe epilepsy and was referred for neuro-surgical advice. She was seen at the request of the neuro-surgeon before surgery was contemplated, admitted to a general hospital psychiatric unit, treated with intensive behaviour therapy, and eventually made a full recovery from the attacks which were clearly not epilepsy, but panic attacks. The phenomena of lightheadedness, tingling, tetany, and then apparent unconsciousness, which were considered as epileptic, are of course symptoms and signs of hyperventilation which, rarely, may even cause a major convulsion.

Case 10

An art student was referred to a psychiatrist with study difficulty. Her general practitioner asked about the advisability of psycho-analysis to ease her guilt feelings. She described increasing difficulty in studying over the previous six months, her concentration had become impaired, and she described both memory difficulty and difficulty in understanding certain words. In addition, she had begun to experience guilt feelings and had spent a long time trying to understand them with the help of her chaplain, as she was deeply religious. She described them as being like an intense feeling of guilt lasting up to a minute at a time, and coming unpredictably sometimes several times a day. When she was asked if other people would be able to recognise when she was having the attacks she said 'Oh yes, because I always make one of my puddles as well', and described how she wet herself during the attacks of guilt. A diagnosis of temporal lobe epilepsy was made and she was admitted to hospital for investigation which revealed an infiltrating tumour of the left hemisphere.

Case 11

This woman believed herself to be a witch as did many of the inhabitants of the small Herefordshire village where she lived. She had been able to predict many natural disasters and had become an object of fear and veneration in her village. She eventually became greatly distressed by her prophecies and by the effect they were having on others and she had several episodes of depression and was referred for further investigation. A careful history showed that she was not predicting natural disasters in a direct way, but would develop sudden brief intense feelings of apprehension of impending disaster. These would repeat themselves at intervals until a natural disaster would occur, and her reputation would then be further enhanced. These forebodings did not occur every time there was a natural disaster, and it was clear that selective forgetting of occasions when she did not predict correctly and retrospective falsification of memory were responsible for her reputation. Careful nursing observation on the ward revealed that she was having a brief attack disorder in which she would suddenly slump forward for a few seconds, breathing stertorously with a vacant glazed expression. During the attack she could not be roused, and would wake up suddenly although she was dazed for a few seconds afterwards; she was quite unaware of having had an attack although she remembered a premonitory feeling before it. The relationship between her attacks and the premonitory experiences became clear, when it was found that there was EEG evidence of a temporal lobe epileptic focus. The association of brief intense ictal emotion and temporal lobe epilepsy has been described in a detailed paper, (Williams, 1956).

Case 12

This woman had had an undiagnosed attack disorder thought to be psychogenic for eight years before she was referred for a second opinion. Her turns started the day after the delivery of her third child; unwanted. Although she had had them for eight years, only her husband had ever witnessed one. She could only describe them vaguely although she knew that in them she was very badly frightened. She described feeling hot and very anxious for no apparent reason and she thought they lasted for about fifteen minutes. At first they might come on at any time, but for some time they had occurred invariably on a particular day of her menstrual cycle. In addition to these symptoms she was undoubtedly prone to depression and anxiety and had a marked obsessional personality. She had had a very unhappy childhood, with a complete disruption of normal family relationships. Over the eight years she had had frequent EEG examinations, all of which revealed no abnormality and had taken a large amount of psychotropic medication including tranquillisers and antidepressants, all of which had failed completely to relieve her symptoms. Most doctors who had seen her over this eight year period thought she was suffering from anxiety attacks. For some reason it was eight years before anyone got

a description from her husband, the only witness of the attacks. What he had observed was very different from his wife's account. He said the attacks were very brief, seldom lasting more than thirty seconds; he appreciated when she was having one since she became vacant and clouded and he was not able to reassure her. After the attacks, she was intensely anxious and frightened. She was admitted to a specialised unit for observation at the phase of her menstrual cycle when an attack might be expected. The attacks began, as anticipated, and were as her husband had described. They began quite suddenly; for twenty to thirty seconds she was dazed and unrousable and was observed to flush violently over the face and upper arms and she chewed and smacked her lips. She came to suddenly, although she appeared somewhat dazed and confused for some seconds afterwards, and was also intensely frightened (it was this part of the attack that she remembered).

During the day of the attacks themselves, but at no other time, her EEG showed evidence of strong epileptic activity in her left temporal lobe. She is an example of how during a temporal lobe attack, time sense may become distorted so that the patient gives an inaccurate estimate of how long the attack lasts.

Case 13

This 40-year-old man was admitted to a psychiatric unit having been diagnosed by physicians as suffering from hysteria. In the preceeding three months having had no previous physical or psychiatric history, his work as a store clerk in a large factory had been difficult because every time he raised his hand above his head to get something from the shelf, his whole arm would stiffen and go rigid and remain in this position for some minutes before slowly relaxing to his side. The process only affected his right arm. It would occasionally happen at other times quite spontaneously. His doctors could find no cause for his symptoms which were therefore deemed to be hysterical, and he was referred for psychiatric treatment. His psychiatrist was reluctant to accept the diagnosis of hysteria in a stable man of 40 with no previous psychiatric history, and with no obvious gain from his symptoms. However, before further investigation could be undertaken, he went into status epilepticus and later died. At the post mortem, the cause of this particular variant of tonic motor epilepsy induced by movement was apparent in an infiltrating secondary deposit from a bronchial carcinoma in the left parietal area.

Case 14

This 72-year-old man was admitted at the request of a consultant physician for treatment of his hysterical seizures which had commenced two weeks after his wife's death from a slow and painful illness. The seizures were occurring up to 30 times a day and consisted largely of incoherent shouting. Epilepsy had been considered but rejected as a diagnosis because his EEG was normal. Observation of his seizures on the psychiatric ward showed that they were indeed occurring 20-30 times a day and would consist of a sudden cessation of movement and speech, accompanied by a glazed expression and unresponsiveness when spoken to; his head and eyes would then turn to the left, and there would follow incoherent vocalisation. Recovery occurred after about 30 seconds although he was a little confused for a few seconds after apparently recovering his senses. He was aware of having shouted, but not of the other components of the attack. During the attack itself, an EEG showed phase reversed spike-wave activity localised to the posterior left temporal area, although investigation showed no underlying structural abnormality in the temporal lobe. He was given 100 mg of carbamazepine twice daily and within four days the attacks had stopped and have not since returned. The serum levels of carbamazepine were within the therapeutic range, even with such a low dose. It was interesting that the physician who had referred him came in to see him on the ward and remarked that he felt that the man's response to medication proved that the attacks were hysterical because he had responded to what the physician regarded as 'a homeopathic dose'.

Case 15
This 45-year-old man was referred for in-patient treatment of his intractable epilepsy by another physician. His attacks had begun suddenly, a month after his wife's unexpected death. In the attacks he would have a premonitory feeling of unsteadiness or dizziness, and would then slump forward lying inert and unrousable for as long as two or three minutes. These attacks could occur several times a day, had prevented the man from working for some months, and had failed to respond to antiepileptic drugs. On admission he was taking a mixture of phenytoin, phenobarbitone, ethosuximide and troxidone; his EEGs had been consistently normal. After one or two of the attacks were witnessed, doubt was felt about whether they were in fact epileptic particularly as during the attack it was noticed that he became very pale, flushed after the attack and that during the attack his pulse rate was extremely slow. 24 hour ECG monitoring showed that he had a marked cardiac dysrhythmia with runs of ventricular abnormalities leading presumably to low cerebral perfusion pressure, and a 'cerebral grey out'. His antiepileptic drugs were withdrawn completely (after which he said that he felt a great deal better in himself) and he was treated by a cardiologist.

In practice, a psychiatrist most often has to distinguish epilepsy from a simple faint or an anxiety or panic attack or from simulated epilepsy, although there are other rarer diagnostic difficulties. The greatest diagnostic confusion can occur in the person who actually has epilepsy, but who also has a very good psychological reason for having attacks. In addition, of course, epilepsy assumes protean forms and in a minority of cases, a diagnosis may be exceedingly difficult or even impossible.

What is particularly important in the differential diagnosis of attacks is that there should be accurate and unprejudiced observation by experienced and trained observers. It is easy for a doctor with some knowledge of psychopathology and little experience of the varieties of epilepsy to prejudge an attack in favour of a psychogenic origin, and so fail to make the observations essential to the correct diagnosis, as in some of the case histories outlined above. This is particularly likely to happen if he takes the unsupported diagnosis of observers without finding out exactly what they saw during the attack, and also particularly likely to happen if the attacks start at a time of stress for the patient. The EEG may be very helpful but as in some of the case histories, it may actually be misleading.

Epileptic attacks are usually repetitive and brief and the majority of fits last seconds or minutes (the rarer attacks which last longer, more often come the psychiatrist's way). Epileptic fits, even the most bizarre, tend to be stereotyped. There are, however, important exceptions to this particularly when the epilepsy is becoming established, or when there is a progressive underlying lesion causing the epilepsy. If attacks occur during sleep, they are more likely to be epilepsy, although Lishman (1978) records an example of a psychogenic attack disorder occurring during sleep.

The incidence of epileptic attacks is erratic; there may be groups of fits with variable periods of freedom. It is important to enquire whether there is an association with precipitating factors such as phases of sleep and the circadian rhythm, emotional stress, the menstrual cycle, or those specific stimuli which may be responsible for the exceptional case. Attacks which are epileptic are very commonly followed by a period of confusion and even very minor attacks may lead to undue sleepiness. The noting of such important diagnostic features may be difficult and underline the value of accurate observation.

Very slight minor attacks may lead to sequelae which easily may be misinterpreted as psychologically induced. It is particularly important to observe any true alteration of effective relations to the external environment during and immediately after such episodes. Although the problem of the attack disorder which is difficult to diagnose may be uncommon it is apparent that particular skills are needed for its assessment and they may often fall within the compass of psychiatric units specialising in the problems of epilepsy.

An analysis of cases observed on such a unit over the last five years and followed up for at least a year afterwards (Betts *et al.*, 1981) is of interest. In this period 133 patients with attack disorders were admitted, of whom 78 were admitted with a diagnosis – made before admission by other authorities – of epilepsy. After observation of their attacks, it was felt that 16 of these patients (20 per cent) did not suffer from epilepsy, but suffered from some other kind of attack disorder, and were therefore withdrawn from antiepileptic drugs.

55 patients were admitted diagnosed by other authorities as having an attack disorder other than epilepsy. Of these 55 patients, it was felt, after observing their attacks in hospital, that 36 (65 per cent) did have epilepsy, whereas 19 did not. However, a completely clean separation between epilepsy and non-epilepsy could not be made in this series. Of those patients *with* epilepsy, 22 had *additional* attacks which were felt to be not epileptic, a group referred to as 'epilepsy plus'.

Of the attacks which were not epilepsy the commonest were hysteria, or simulation, followed by anxiety attacks. Those attacks which were mistaken for epilepsy included some seizures which were alcohol related, and occasional patients with migraine, faints, encephalitis, amitriptyline induced seizures and the basilar artery syndrome. In two patients in this series it could not be decided what the attacks were, although it was felt fairly confidently that they were not epilepsy. It is important with undiagnosable patients like this that one does not treat them as if they have epilepsy, unless one is certain of the diagnosis. Time will often make the diagnosis if nothing else does. In those patients with epilepsy plus other attack followed by simulation, or elaboration of a attacks followed by simulation, or elaboration of a genuine epileptic attack.

It is interesting that out of these 133 patients, 17 were admitted for treatment of severe intractable epilepsy which had failed to respond even to heroic treatment. Of this particular sub-group of patients with 'frequent epilepsy', 24 per cent did not have epilepsy at all, but were being treated heroically for what were primarily anxiety or simulated attacks. 23 per cent did have intractable epilepsy, most of whom responded to drug or behavioural treatment. The remainder had epilepsy 'plus', and it was the 'plus' attacks which were the intractable ones (these again were simulation or panic attacks). It was felt that many patients were also suffering from drug intoxication and when drugs were reduced or withdrawn the frequency of the seizures declined.

It is important to recognise that even rapidly recurring seizures which may resemble near status epilepticus can have a psychogenic origin. This certainly occurred in the Birmingham series (Betts *et al.*, 1981) and has been reported by others (Poulose & Shaw, 1977). As mentioned earlier, pseudo-seizures may occur also as a complication of the treatment of status epilepticus.

Increasing interest in the problem of pseudo-seizures has been shown in recent years, and it has been suggested that there are psychological differences between patients with pseudo-seizures and those that do not have them, which can sometimes be helpful in distinguishing the two. (Finlayson & Lucas, 1979; Roy, 1977). This does not account for the patients who have both genuine seizures and pseudo-seizures, which as will have been seen above was a common combination in the Birmingham series. In this series, however, the epilepsy plus group differed significantly from the other two groups in that they were younger and all but one were female. There were no age or sex differences between the epilepsy and the non-epilepsy groups.

A recent suggestion to help to distinguish between genuine and non-genuine seizures has been made by Trimble (1978), that in patients with generalised epilepsy the serum concentration of prolactin rises to high levels after a seizure, but this does not occur in those patients whose attacks were thought to be hysterical. This observation needs replicating at other centres, but may be very useful. In some centres split screen videotape techniques are used where both the patient's behaviour and his EEG can be recorded at the same time for later analysis. Such apparatus is extremely expensive and can only be used at one or two special centres. In my experience videotape has the advantage that it can be replayed again and again so that an attack sequence can be studied in detail although video replay keeps the viewer at one remove from actuality.

Therefore, the commonest psychological attacks which have to be distinguished from epilepsy are panic or anxiety attacks and simulation. Anxiety attacks may become very stereotyped; they may appear spontaneously without warning or may come in clusters. Typically the patient feels a mounting tide of panic in which both the psychological and physical symptoms of anxiety are prominent and there is a dread either of going mad, or of imminent physical dissolution.

The attack is accompanied by over-breathing of which the patient is often unaware, and this provokes symptoms of lightheadedness and peripheral tingling as described in Case 9. Later, frank tetany in the hands and feet may occur. Eventually if the over-breathing continues the patient may become unconscious and may take some time to recover. If the anxiety attack has been particularly prolonged the patient may feel tired and sleepy afterwards, and may also complain of a headache.

It is easy for a vicious circle to be set up in which the fear of the attacks themselves, of losing control in public places, raises the general anxiety level and so makes attacks more likely to occur. The first stages of the attack may also act as a stimulus for the further development of the attack. When a patient begins to get his first feeling of panic he expects that the rest of the attack is inevitable, becomes more anxious and a full blown attack therefore develops which fulfils his expectations.

Although there is usually an obvious event of emotional significance in a patient's life which brings on an attack, one can be provoked merely by the apprehension of having one.

The distinction from epilepsy has to be made very carefully since it is quite common in some people for epileptic attacks to be brought on by anxiety, and over-breathing, of course, may precipitate fits. Sometimes the situation occurs of the patient whose epilepsy is brought on by anxiety (or by over-breathing) and the epilepsy which results then causes further anxiety. It can be very difficult in these circumstances to decide which came first, and also what is the correct form of management.

Case 16
This man of 36 was referred from another consultant with a diagnosis of intractable temporal lobe epilepsy which large doses of several antiepileptic drugs had failed to control. Two years before, following a road accident, he had begun to develop attacks which were described as starting with 'an aura of fear' and which were accompanied by stereotyped

behaviour, which was described as an automatism. This was sometimes followed by a tonic-clonic seizure. The attacks were occurring many times a week and had totally disrupted his life and the life of his family – he had also been dismissed from a couple of jobs because of his epilepsy.

On admission to hospital he was noted to be intoxicated with the various antiepileptic drugs he was taking and the usual policy of gradually withdrawing them was pursued. He became very apprehensive as they were withdrawn, and warned that he would have many fits as a result. It was interesting that, as so often happens both with people with epilepsy and also those with pseudo-seizures, he did not have an attack for about ten days after his admission to hospital. He had several attacks on his first weekend visit home, however, being returned to hospital in an ambulance accompanied by various worried relatives. He then began to have many attacks whilst in hospital and most of them followed the same curious stereotyped form. Nurses would notice that he had become somewhat distant and vague; he would then suddenly jump to his feet, run to the nearest water tap which he would turn on (it was always the cold tap), and then allow a stream of cold water to flow over his head whilst holding his nose and groaning incoherently. His attacks would usually terminate after this, and he would lie on his bed for about half an hour recovering, declaring himself to have an headache and to feel sleepy. On two or three occasions, however, whilst kneeling with the cold water pouring over his head, he would have an undoubted tonic-clonic seizure.

If he was arrested in his dramatic flight down the ward to find the nearest cold tap, however, it was possible to hold a rational if somewhat fraught conversation with him, and there was no evidence of a diminution in or clouding of consciousness and he would express himself at that time as feeling intensely anxious and frightened and said that the sensation of the cold water, plus the act of holding his nose, seemed to prevent the anxiety from becoming more intense. It was also noted that at these times he was hyperventilating and it seemed that his nose holding was a way of slowing his breathing.

EEG's before and after a seizure failed to reveal any significant abnormality, and, during one of his EEG's, hyperventilation precipitated one of his seizures up to nose holding with no concomitant EEG change. There was no doubt, however, that occasionally, what came to be regarded as acute panic attacks were followed by genuine tonic-clonic seizures. As he came to be better known (when detoxified he became a somewhat amiable rogue) the connection between his anxiety attacks and his road accident became more clear, in that the car he was driving when he had the accident was stolen, he was uninsured, he did not have a driving licence and he was also drunk. He had been terrified ever since that the police might investigate the accident and charge him with the various offences that he had committed. However, in the accident itself he had suffered a head injury with slight concussion afterwards and it was interesting that air encephalography of the brain revealed a discrete area of cortical atrophy in the right parietal area consistent with the previous head injury.

He was treated by an intensive regime of behaviour therapy aimed at anxiety reduction and whilst on the ward he completely stopped having his anxiety attacks and after this no spontaneous tonic-clonic seizures were seen. It was concluded that he was suffering primarily from anxiety attacks which occasionally were severe enough to precipitate a tonic-clonic seizure from hyperventilation, due perhaps to a low convulsive threshold induced by his head injury. He was eventually discharged and attended an employment rehabilitation unit.

Unfortunately, with the stresses of work and family life, he began to have panic attacks again and eventually had another tonic-clonic seizure and persuaded his general practitioner to put him back on to antiepileptic drugs. The reason that he was keen to go back on drugs was to gain respectability in the eyes of his family, who when told that his attacks were primarily anxiety attacks, rejected him and told him to 'pull himself together'. When he had a further tonic-clonic seizure at home following rehabilitation they became very angry with the hospital, insisted he changed consultants and complained to their Member of Parliament who instituted enquiries into the 'gross incompetence' of the hospital. It was difficult to convince the MP that one could have an epileptic attack without necessarily being 'an epileptic'.

The complex nature of this man's attacks illustrates the difficulties that arise in deciding whether attacks are primarily psychogenic or primarily physiogenic, and also the importance, if after prolonged study of a patient, one does decide that the attacks are primarily psychogenic, that one treats not just the patient but also the family and their response to the attacks, and, if necessary, educates other members of the medical profession who may also be involved in the care of the patient. This calls for close contact with the patient after discharge and often intense social work support for the family as well.

The Birmingham figures (Betts *et al.*, 1981) quoted above suggest that many of the patients seen have been like this man, and in any patient with intractable epilepsy which has not responded to a large number of antiepileptic drugs, it is important to ask oneself again whether the attacks really are epilepsy or whether they might not be something else. Many of the patients I have seen who have had either panic attacks or who simulated epilepsy, have carried that pejorative label 'Known Epileptic'. One should never assume that a known epileptic actually suffers from epilepsy.

Occasionally psychiatric symptoms such as depersonalisation or déja vu experiences occurring in people without epilepsy may resemble epileptic phenomena. The question may be raised, for instance, whether a patient with recurrent depersonalisation is actually suffering from a complex partial seizure, a decision made more difficult by the fact that many such patients do have temporal lobe abnormalities on EEG examination. These

psychogenic experiences can usually be distinguished from epilepsy because they are less clear cut, less stereotyped, .of less rapid onset and departure, and tend to be more prolonged. Observation of the patient during the episode will usually clarify the diagnosis. The patient who is experiencing an attack of depersonalisation or an auditory or visual hallucination, but who is quite clearly completely in contact with his surroundings, is in a state of clear consciousness, and who is showing no other ictal behaviour, is probably not suffering from epilepsy.

Careful observation of the patient's behaviour before, during and after the attack is necessary to determine whether the sensorium is intact, whether there is post-ictal confusion or amnesia and whether there are ictal accompaniments such as lip smacking and chewing or autonomic changes such as flushing, pallor or sweating.

Case 17
A girl with known complex partial seizures, consisting of brief absences, began to complain of true auditory hallucinationary experiences. It was felt that these might be ictal but they went on for a long time (two or three hours), and from her description appeared to be occurring in clear consciousness; she was subjectively distressed by her experiences. Observation of her behaviour while she was hallucinated indicated that her sensorium was completely intact and there was no evidence of an element of confusion or clouding of consciousness and she could walk about the ward and perform her usual ward tasks without difficulty. Afterwards, she had a complete recollection of events during the hallucinationary periods and showed no change in behaviour during them. It was concluded that these were not ictal.

It has become my custom in assessing patients with doubtful attack disorders to screen the patient carefully for hypoglycaemia which means taking blood for estimation of glucose and insulin levels, during the attack if possible, estimations of blood glucose over a prolonged period of fasting and occasionally such tests as the tolbutamide tolerance test. In addition many patients may also need several sessions of continuous 24 hour ECG monitoring until one has a record during an attack in order to rule out cardiogenic causes.

One of the main roles of the psychiatrist is in distinguishing simulated epilepsy from genuine epilepsy. In some societies epilepsy has social value and purpose and in some animal populations it has been shown to have protective or survival value, particularly the common reflex epilepsy found in small mammals. Although at first glance it would appear to be without value in man, occasionally it can get bound up in the life of a tribe or society in such a way as to have some reward so that attacks are deliberately induced or simulated. Many voodoo dancers of the West Indies over-breathe themselves into a state of tetany and unconsciousness but the man who over-breathes himself into a tonic-clonic seizure becomes invested with magical properties. There is no doubt too that breath-holding spells in children are a way of indicating distress, seeking attention, or withdrawing from unpleasant situations, and although they are not epileptic they illustrate that attacks can sometimes be used for social purposes.

It is generally held that in Britain simulated epilepsy is now uncommon, and when it does occur it is almost invariably in people who already have epilepsy. The Birmingham figures quoted above, however, do suggest that it can still be found in its own right. It has been my impression that in Birmingham it is particularly common in women of our Asian sub-culture, but very few of these patients that I have seen are willing to come into hospital for further investigation. Language difficulties have also made it impossible to determine completely what is happening in this group.

Epilepsy may be simulated either unconsciously as part of a hysterical illness or consciously as part of the repertoire of the malingerer. It is often difficult to distinguish where the borderline between these two conditions lies (and there has been some argument about whether in fact they should be distinguished), but most psychiatrists in this country would feel that they can be and should be. Merskey (1979) has just produced an excellent review of the whole subject of hysteria.

Simulated epilepsy is usually easy to distinguish from the real thing provided careful observation is made. It cannot be emphasised too much that the diagnosis is made by observation of the attack, and it is important that, if the doctor cannot see the attacks himself, he should get a detailed account from nurses or other witnesses. He must have their *account* rather than their *opinion*. It should be remembered that many unusual forms of behaviour do occur in epilepsy and although lack of corroborating EEG evidence is suspicious in a patient who is having frequent seizures, the

absence of epileptic activity in the EEG does not necessarily mean that the attacks are not genuine.

The simulator tends to fall with a dramatic cry or to pitch himself down and thrash about in a way entirely different from a true epileptic seizure. If the performance fails to obtain the objective desired, then embellishments may well be added. Intervention by other people may modify the course of the attack in a way not usually seen in epilepsy. Although the patient may appear to be unconscious, careful observation will show that there is no true alteration in the level of consciousness. Recovery from the attacks is usually rapid and without the post-ictal confusion often seen in genuine epilepsy; incontinence is rare and injury seldom occurs. What is presented is usually an acted-out version of the layman's view of epilepsy, and since that view is often of coupling epilepsy with aggression, the patient will often shout vigorously and lash out at people who try to restrain him. One should always be suspicious of the patient who proudly tells you 'it takes six people to hold me down'. However, perverse pride in the strength of one's epileptic achievement is not entirely confined to the simulator. Sometimes it can be difficult to distinguish between genuine and simulated epilepsy and occasionally, as found in the Birmingham series, impossible. If it is impossible to tell, I feel it better to treat the patient as though they did not have epilepsy and only treat the attacks as epileptic when one is certain. Even when certain, one should be prepared to revise the diagnosis from time to time, and should certainly never accept uncritically the diagnosis of epilepsy which has been given to the patients by others.

Case 18
This woman was transferred to a psychiatric unit via a medical ward where she had been admitted at the request of her general practitioner with what was described as 'near status epilepticus'. She had begun to have epileptic attacks some ten years before. At first they were infrequent but in the two years before admission she was having three or four major convulsions a day, despite heroic doses of antiepileptic drugs. On admission she was ataxic and dysarthric. This had been ascribed to her uncontrolled epilepsy but in fact was due to taking too many drugs. From the time of her admission to the medical ward she had had numerous seizures in which she would fall, emitting a loud cry and would then thrash about, screaming loudly, banging her head hard on the ground as she did so, often drawing blood, and making a great deal of noise.

Apart from the signs of drug intoxication, no physical abnormalities were discovered. She had a rather unpleasant personality and antagonised most of the nursing staff. After she had been rude to a senior member of the consultant staff during one of her attacks, at the same time attempting to bite his ankle, her removal to the psychiatric ward was requested. When she arrived on the psychiatric unit, the usual policy of discreet observation of the attacks without intervention was followed, and she was noted to have two types of attack. Occasionally she had a brief episode of confusion lasting no more than ten seconds, (usually occurring at the dinner table), in which she would drop whatever she was carrying, stare fixedly at the wall and chew and swallow in a dazed way. The other kind of attack was the major event, already described, which always occurred at times of frustration or anger, or when she was asked to do something that did not suit her (like helping with the ward chores). At these times she would fling herself violently to the ground often throwing herself out of a chair to do so, and kick and scream in a manner reminiscent of a three year old in a tantrum.

It was decided to reduce her antiepileptic drugs steadily and to ignore her attacks in the hope that they would then stop. As might be expected, ignoring her attacks made them rise to a crescendo. She would go off the ward to have her attacks in a neighbouring lift, or in front of visitors, some of whom became quite angry at the 'callous way' she was being treated by the staff on the ward. However, on a psychiatric ward with a common therapeutic plan formulated after discussion with all members of the staff, the anxieties that such patients arouse can be supported and contained. The policy of ignoring the attacks was continued. Suddenly, after about ten days they stopped abruptly and more attention could then be paid to the patient's real problems.

It was decided that she did have genuine epilepsy, and indeed when her antiepileptic drugs had been reduced to a very low level, she had two spontaneous tonic-clonic seizures. It was clear, however, that most of her attacks were not genuine epilepsy but that she was using simulated epilepsy for secondary gain in a battle with her husband. The threat of having these attacks was sufficient to keep him at home in the evenings and to get him to do the various domestic chores around the house, which he had done uncomplainingly for several years. Undoubtedly her behaviour had been made worse by excessive drugs with the resulting intoxication.

Her rehabilitation was largely concerned with preventing her husband from allowing the same pattern of behaviour to develop when she returned home, and encouraging her to talk out her anger, frustration and difficulties rather than resorting to seizure behaviour.

Case 19
A student teacher aged 20 began to have attacks in front of her class, which became so frequent and so unpleasant as to force her removal from teaching. She was subsequently admitted to a gynaecological hospital for investigation as, in addition to these attacks, she had stopped menstruating. It proved impossible to manage her in the gynaecological hospital because when any attempt was made to get her out of bed, she collapsed on the floor. She became bedfast and a nurse had to sit with her at all times (otherwise she would fall out of bed), and some three nurses had to escort her to the toilet. She was transferred to a psychiatric unit, and at this time was having several attacks a day. She said that she had no warning of the attack but would merely find herself

on the floor, obviously having fallen, but with no memory of having done so. She did not feel sleepy or confused afterwards. Careful observation revealed that she would sink gently to the floor without hurting herself and lie as though asleep for several minutes, although it was noticed that her eyelids would be flickering. On several occasions she fell out of bed in an attack. At these times she would edge herself carefully towards the side of the bed for several minutes before she would suddenly fling herself out of bed and drop to the floor. Her attacks were ignored in the usual way and very soon disappeared as her underlying problems were discovered, and she started to talk them out.

I am interested when observing my own children at play, to see that when they wish to 'play dead' they behave in very much the same way as this girl was doing, sinking to the floor, lying flaccid and inert but with a curious eyelid flutter as they take surreptitious peeps at their surroundings. There is a rich field for study here by a sociologist with behavioural interests, or a clinical ethologist.

It has been indicated above, that my usual policy for patients with diagnostically puzzling attacks, is never to interfere with the course of the attacks unless it is life-threatening. Nurses are taught to do nothing but observe and record exactly what happens. This policy is explained to the patients and in itself is therapeutic since it means that *secondary gain* does not accrue to those who are simulating their attacks and that even genuine epileptic fits are not rewarded. After an attack, whether genuine or not, a patient is expected to get up as quickly as possible and continue with ward activities. He is not put to bed and certainly is not excused the ward washing-up or similar chores.

It is difficult sometimes to train new doctors and nurses to do nothing when somebody has a seizure. Nurses may well have come from wards where active intervention in an epileptic attack was mandatory and have been taught to operate mouth gags and even those archaic instruments known as mouth openers. A doctor, particularly if inexperienced, when summoned to a patient who is convulsing, or who has just finished convulsing, feels that he must do something, and the unfortunate patient is often injected with antiepileptic drugs or diazepam which may cloud his mental state or actually induce the condition it was supposed to prevent. Worse still, after a seizure the patient's drug regime may be changed in a haphazard and irrational way. It is easier to control doctors' and nurses' over enthusiasm on a psychiatric ward, where a common policy of management can be thrashed out with staff and patients alike, or, in a special unit where every patient has epilepsy.

The relationship between epilepsy and hysteria is a notoriously difficult one. The term 'hysterical fits' means a state of subjective loss of consciousness, without ictal discharges, perhaps in response to psychological stimuli. Ideally to confirm the diagnosis these fits should be shown to serve the purpose of solving a psychic conflict and the patient should recognise subsequently that he has not suffered an epileptic form of impairment of consciousness.

It is important to distinguish true hysteria from deliberate malingering, as the management is somewhat different, and also to distinguish it from hyperventilation and panic attacks, which may be confused with hysterical attacks, particularly in adolescents.

It should also be remembered that many epileptic discharges, especially in the temporal lobes, are so modified by treatment that they may appear as brief episodes of loss of consciousness, at times resembling generalised absences and at other times even seemingly hysterical behaviour (hysterical in the layman's sense of acute emotional disturbance). Pond (1974) has indicated that a brief epileptic discharge may be followed by a post-ictal state in which consciousness is modified and in which an unruly so-called hysterical state may appear. In such a state the patient may respond with kicking, jerking or screaming if touched, or may respond to commands in a way which suggests that he is aware of his environment and is *putting on an act*. In such cases, careful clinical examination is important as it may demonstrate focal impairment of a cortical function such as dysphasia.

Case 20
A girl of 16 who had been subject to occasional tonic-clonic seizures since the age of ten began to suffer brief lapses of consciousness from which she would not recover completely but she would remain in a somewhat dazed state and if approached by anybody would cry out with fear as she misidentified them as the devil. Her level of consciousness fluctuated markedly so that at times she appeared to be quite psychotic. During this post-ictal state, which might last two days, she would often rise from her bed and attempt to escape from imaginary pursuers; at these times it was noted that she would stagger wildly and clutch onto the wall for support in a dramatic and exaggerated fashion. Physical examination during one of these attacks, however, revealed that she had developed a transient left hemiparesis which disappeared when she suddenly regained her faculties a few hours later. At these times there was persistent spike-wave discharge in the posterior part of the right temporal lobe on EEG examination.

In a series of 666 patients with temporal lobe epilepsy, it was found (Currie *et al.*, 1971) that seventeen suffered from gross hysterical disorders such as paresis and ataxia. Phenytoin intoxication, as well probably as other drug intoxication, may release such gross hysterical behaviour and signs (Niedemeyer *et al.*, 1970). These disorders usually settle with adjustment of dosage and adequate control of serum levels. Patients with brain damage may be especially liable to hysterical symptoms (Slater, 1965) so that it can be seen why patients with epilepsy are amongst those most at risk of hysterical behaviour and symptoms.

In addition to these direct organic provocative factors, psychological problems undoubtedly contribute to the production of hysterical fits. The fact that fits are the favourite hysterical symptoms in those with epilepsy is understandable since the patient models the psychological complaint on the pattern of his pre-existing physical one. As might be expected, hysterical fits can be provoked by a variety of emotional problems such as family dissension, difficulty at work or in love. Nevertheless, apart from excessive use of antiepileptic drugs, failure to control fits or to adjust to epilepsy plays a large part in upsetting the patient and generating extra attacks. It may seem paradoxical that an individual wishing to be rid of an illness should enhance its effects, but it is recognised often enough in clinical practice that patients respond in a way that over-emphasises their disability almost as though by exaggerating the symptoms they may draw attention more forcibly to the failure to control them. Such patients need help which is best given by a degree of sympathetic acceptance, not marred by rejection as fakers or deceivers. Doctors, particularly those concerned with physical symptoms and signs, often find it difficult to appreciate that patients need help whatever may be the cause of their troubles.

The treatment and management of hysterical patients require such acceptance, together with an effort to unravel their individual fears. As with anxiety the psychiatric treatment of hysteria may be highly technical or fairly simple. In patients known to have epilepsy it is best at first to establish that there is no evidence of intoxication. Waiting for a few weeks to allow intoxication to resolve cures a number of cases. At the same time, some may undergo spontaneous remission or improvement from being in a supportive hospital environment.

Psychological treatment thereafter follows the usual lines. Discussion with the patient about his problems; family interviews to obtain background information, and family therapy to alter family attitudes and responses to the patient's attacks. When informing the patient that his attacks are simulated it is often best to approach the matter in a roundabout way, talking to him first about general matters and only rarely relating the symptoms to problems, until the problems become explicit, and allowing the patient himself to make the connection. Emphasis on the upsetting nature of the illness often provides common ground for the patient and the doctor. Occasionally hypnosis provides a face-saving manoeuvre to remove symptoms, although it will not discover a repressed problem unless the patient is ready for the discovery to be made.

Although the differential diagnosis of hysteria and epilepsy and the relationship of hysteria to epilepsy are of great importance to this book, the detailed management of hysteria is beyond its scope and readers are referred to Merskey's monograph (Merskey, 1979).

EMOTIONAL AND PSYCHOLOGICAL CONTROL OF FITS

It has been known for a long time that certain physical and emotional stimuli and certain somatic and mental states can influence either directly or indirectly the number of attacks which a patient is having. Occasionally patients may have a measure of control over their fits. I feel that a great deal more attention should be paid to these phenomena, partly because they may help to

explain one of the fundamental problems of epilepsy – why do fits occur when they do – and partly because they may hold out therapeutic possibilities.

Such states should be of increasing interest to the psychiatrist. Physical stimuli adequate to precipitate attacks may on occasions be replaced by the psychological equivalent of such stimuli and many of the methods of psychological treatment whose aim is a reduction of anxiety or a lowering of arousal, may have some therapeutic benefit in these forms of epilepsy and indeed in epilepsy in general.

Photic epilepsy induced by flickering light, sudden changes in light intensity or complex patterns, is the commonest form of reflex epilepsy. A variation of this is television epilepsy which is particularly common in young adolescents. Rarely, reading may provoke attacks in which initial twitching of the jaw progresses to a generalised convulsion if the subject does not stop reading at once.

Case 21
This 20-year-old student was referred with a study phobia to a psychiatrist. He gave a history that in the previous year at university, whenever he attempted to study hard at night, he had a blackout and was either found by his friends wandering in a dazed state outside his room, or slumped before his open books. He said that when reading he suddenly became aware of a throbbing in his throat, followed by a twitching in his jaw, and then remembered no more for up to an hour. This was clearly reading epilepsy which disappeared when he was given antiepileptic drugs.

Photic stimulation is the commonest way in which subjects, usually children, induce their own seizures physically, although this type of directly self-induced epilepsy is rare. Visual self-inducers are characterised by exceptionally high light sensitivity, frequent seizures and sub-normal intelligence. Most of these visually-induced attacks are of the generalised absence or myoclonic type and the frequency of attacks depends to a certain extent on the available light intensity, for example, they are commoner in Australia than Great Britain.

Most children that do this cannot give an adequate explanation of their behaviour, although it would seem from observation that pleasure and escape from stress or boredom are important aetiological factors. Some seem almost compelled to do it in the same way that some children with television epilepsy seem irresistably drawn towards a television set. Whether this urge is an epileptic phenomenon or related to some other phenomena, like counter-phobic behaviour, is not known. Self-induced visual epilepsy is very difficult to treat, and in many cases it is necessary to help the family rather than the child, and advise them on how the child and his symptoms should be handled.

Hyperventilation is another common form of induced epilepsy in children and adolescents; some people with self-induced epilepsy seem able to produce an attack at will, or on request, but without any realisation of how they do it. Some unconsciously hyperventilate; others do it by an effort of concentration.

Seizures may be precipitated by other sensory stimuli such as loud unexpected sounds; an element of startle is essential since a loud sound that the patient is expecting will not induce an attack (Doube, 1965).

Musicogenic epilepsy, another rare condition, has aroused considerable interest. In most patients with musicogenic epilepsy, an affective associative response to the music is required to bring on a fit. In a few cases, however, there is evidence that the musical sound itself is the epileptogenic stimulus possibly at a subcortical level.

A number of other stimuli effective in inducing fits have been described including voice and language, movement, skin touching or tapping, vibration, eating food or the sight of it, immersion in hot or cold water, taste and sexual stimulation (Gastaut & Tassinari, 1966).

The important emotional and psychological component to most cases of reflex epilepsy is perhaps best illustrated by Goldie and Green's (1959) classic study. They described a man who could produce a reflex fit by rubbing his face. The psychological stimuli of preparing to rub his face, or thinking about rubbing it, were as effective as actually rubbing it in provoking epileptic EEG activity or the actual attack itself.

The reflex epilepsies are difficult to treat; it may be impossible to shield the patient from the provoking stimulus without great difficulty, or it may be that the patient himself does not want to be shielded, either because he likes the stimulus or because it gives him some kind of emotional

pleasure. Antiepileptic drugs are often unsatisfactory. Recently attempts have been made, mainly by Forster (1972) to use conditioning or extinction techniques which may have great possibilities in treating the reflex epilepsies, although they are at present too time-consuming for wide spread use. They may also work by a therapeutic shift of the patient's attention away from the triggering stimulus (Mostofsky & Balaschak, 1977).

Forster presents the particular triggering stimulus to the patient continually until the convulsive and EEG responses to the stimulus have extinguished. He may also train the patient to give himself a different stimulus if he encounters the actual triggering stimulus (as say when reading) which prevents the usual convulsive response. Forster appears to have had a great deal of success with these techniques and is also engaged in developing portable devices which can continue the patient's treatment at home, as much of the treatment at the moment is laboratory based.

SELF CONTROL

The phenomenon of the self-control of seizures has been well known since the days of Hughlings Jackson and Gowers but seems to have been studied curiously little, and in many cases little effort seems to have been made to discover exactly what it is that some patients actually do to stop their attacks. Symonds (1959) reviewed the evidence that voluntary mental and physical activity could inhibit seizures. It is well known that patients with sensory or motor epilepsy can sometimes inhibit their attacks, once they have started, either by vigorous sensory stimulation of the involved area, or by brisk muscular activity.

Patients in my experience who can stop their seizures in this way do not always feel comfortable afterwards and they may feel better if they allow themselves to have an attack at a time and place of their own choosing. Symonds was more concerned with those patients who could inhibit seizures by an effort of concentration or an effort of will. This may involve thinking very hard about not having an attack or the repetition of some phrase which has the property of stopping the attacks, or occasionally the induction of an emotional state in which the attack will not occur. Of Symonds' patients, 5.3 per cent could stop their attacks in this way, although how they did it was not usually obvious. Patients may not volunteer to their doctors that they have these control mechanisms and they may only be discovered by accident.

Although we know little about how these patients actually do stop their seizures, it is known that desynchronising and other control mechanisms do exist in the brain and quite possibly could be better utilised. That certain psychological methods of treatment might be used in potentiating such control mechanisms is illustrated by the example of the woman that Efron (1956) described, where a controlling mechanism which the patient herself had noticed and brought to the attention of her doctor, was shaped and refined, so that it became easier to use. It would be interesting to see whether patients with sensory auras could be treated in the same way.

It has been held for a long time that emotional states can lead to an increase in the number of patients' attacks, and therefore one could suppose that altering emotional states could reduce seizure frequency. Direct induction of seizures by emotional stimuli is probably rare and certainly Gastaut and Tassinari (1966) in their extensive review could find very little evidence that direct induction occurs. However, most doctors experienced in epilepsy are aware that changes in a patient's emotional state often towards higher arousal may lead to an increased number of attacks (Servit et al., 1963). In recent years, a fair amount of laboratory evidence has emerged to support these beliefs.

Mattson et al. (1970) carried out a detailed and important neurophysiological study of the effects of psychic stress on the frequency of seizures, although not as a direct stimulus. In other words, in a patient under stress more seizures than usual are likely to occur but not as a direct result of the stress itself. A search was made for any measure of an increase in arousal or stress that could be related to the increase in seizure frequency.

There was little relationship between any of the usual parameters of arousal (for instance plasma cortisol levels) and seizure frequency, but it was noted that increase in seizure frequency under stress was related to involuntary hyperventilation with a resulting fall in carbon dioxide concentration. The aetiological importance of this finding was supported by the observation that such an increased seizure frequency under stress could be prevented if the patient was made to breathe an increased concentration of carbon dioxide. It is suggested that involuntary overbreathing may be an important psychophysiological precipitant of seizures, as it is in those patients who induce their attacks deliberately by hyperventilation.

Gotze et al. (1967) using telemetered EEG recordings, showed that physical exercise tended to normalise the EEGs of patients with epilepsy. In patients after exercise, who were made to hyperventilate, less EEG abnormality was produced than if they had hyperventilated without previous physical exercise. It would seem therefore that physical exercise raises the seizure threshold and reduces the likelihood of seizures occurring.

It may be that involuntary hyperventilation was also responsible for the effect that Stevens (1959) noticed in her experiment which showed that emotionally stressful interviews had an adverse effect on EEG stability in a large proportion of people with epilepsy. Hyperventilation is often seen in those who are anxious, and of course is amenable to behavioural manipulation.

The telemetered EEG is a powerful tool in the study of the effects of various kinds of stress and emotional states on both EEG and seizure activity. Two studies in this field (Vidart & Geier, 1968; Bureau et al., 1968) are of interest. Vidart was concerned with adults, and measured the occurrence of diffuse episodes of spike-and-wave activity in the EEGs of patients with known epilepsy as they went about a normal life. Intellectual work which did not overtax the capacity of the patient to deal with it, such as mental arithmetic, caused a reduction in EEG abnormalities, and presumably therefore a reduction in seizure frequency. If the intellectual effort required to solve the problem exceeded a level critical for the patient, the number of abnormalities increased again (Bureau et al., 1968). As might be expected, fatigue and tiredness increased the amount of spike-and-wave activity in the EEG. The relationship between a patient's mental state and abnormalities in the EEG was shown to be complex. Changes in mood might either increase or decrease the amount of abnormal epileptic activity.

Stressful events always seemed to increase the amount of abnormal activity occurring, whereas if interest was shown in the patient, the number of abnormalities would decrease. In adults or children, boredom or inactivity led to the most abnormalities per unit time in the EEG, whereas if their attention was engaged and they were interested in their work, then the amount of EEG activity decreased dramatically.

Such states as emotional stress, sleep deprivation, fatigue, boredom and prolonged overtaxing intellectual effort and hyperventilation seem therefore to be important factors in precipitating seizures. Physical exercise and interesting intellectual work seem to decrease seizures. In this field it is clear that psychological methods may have an important part to play in the management of seizures, and that further research is necessary. There is no doubt that psychological methods of treatment along behavioural lines are probably the treatments of choice for people who self-induce their seizures; and it is also a reasonable assumption to make, that those seizures which are associated with an increase in anxiety will also be amenable to psychological methods of treatment aimed at reducing anxiety levels.

Scattered reports occur in the literature (Pinto, 1972; Standage, 1972; Mostofsky & Balaschak, 1977) which suggest that anxiety-reducing treatment using relaxation or desensitisation are effective in treating patients whose anxiety levels are increasing their seizure frequency, and the behavioural treatment results both in a reduction in anxiety and a reduction in the frequency of seizures or even their disappearance.

Case 22
This 28-year-old woman had had occasional tonic-clonic fits between the ages of five and eleven, and had then remained seizure-free until the age of 26 when she suddenly had an attack in a supermarket. At the time this happened, she was under a great deal of marital and personal stress, and had been feeling anxious for some weeks. She was still taking antiepileptic drugs. She was extremely embarassed about the spectacle she had made of herself and although the marital and personal stress later resolved itself, she continued to feel anxious whenever she approached the particular supermarket in which the fit had occurred. On several occasions, her anxiety levels were so high that further seizures occurred there. As a result she became more generally anxious and attacks began to occur in other places, at home or in the street, and she eventually became so frightened of going out that she became totally house-bound. Her antiepileptic drugs were

increased but had no apparent effect on her seizure frequency.

She was admitted to hospital for behavioural treatment of her agoraphobia. This consisted of intensive relaxation training so that she would have some control over her anxiety feelings, followed by gradual exposure to the outside world, with encouragement and verbal reward as she was able to progress outside the hospital. As a result, her anxiety symptoms diminished markedly but she was still afraid of having a seizure in a supermarket or public place. Accordingly, Standage's (1972) method of getting the patient, whilst relaxed, to imagine themselves having a seizure (desensitisation in imagination) was used. As a result she lost her fear of attacks and from that time she has not had another one despite being able now to go anywhere. Her drugs were subsequently withdrawn.

An interesting variant of desensitisation was described by Feldman and Paul (1976), in which video-tape recordings of the patients' seizures were played back to five patients. The authors believed that the videotapes provided a means by which the patients could acquire otherwise unrecognised or forgotten information and thereby identify specific emotional triggers which precipitated their seizures. The videotapes were therefore used as a specific adjunct to classical psychotherapy. Another way of seeing the procedure, however, would be as a desensitisation to the seizures themselves. With the wider availability and use of videotape this method deserves to be explored further.

Certainly in the patients I see where epilepsy is made worse by anxiety, behavioural methods of treatment have now an established place in management. The question arises as to whether behavioural methods of treatment, or indeed psychotherapy itself, has a part to play in the management of epileptic fits when neither self-inducement, anxiety or high arousal appear to be playing a precipitating part. This matter is still controversial and has not been subjected to vigorous experimental proof, but there are indications (Mostofsky & Balaschak, 1977) that even in patients where there does not appear to be an emotional precipitant, behavioural methods aimed at extinguishing seizure behaviour may be beneficial. In their extensive review, Mostofsky and Balaschak discuss the various methods that have been used for seizure control which include operant conditioning (that is, reward of non-seizure behaviour or punishment of seizure behaviour), desensitisation, relaxation, psychotherapy, habituation and extinction programmes (as described by Forster, 1972), and biofeedback.

They point out the difficulties of assessing exactly what it is in a behavioural programme to which the patient is actually responding (i.e. many behavioural programmes involve relaxation and it may be that it is to this that the patient is responding rather than to the specific behavioural changes that the therapist is inducing). They call for a much greater control over experimental variables in the study of the behavioural treatments of epilepsy. Hopefully better experimental design and more careful selection of patients may lead to further information about the usefulness of behavioural techniques in epilepsy. The problems that experimenters have in teasing out the actual technique which is the therapeutic one, resembles, in some ways, those that bedevil people setting up clinical trials for the drug treatment of epilepsy. (In some ways those conducting behavioural experiments are possibly more aware of the confounding experimental variables.) Study of the available literature on the subject of the behavioural treatment of epilepsy does however suggest that sometimes it is impossible to decide whether the patient being treated actually did have epilepsy, or whether it was pseudo-seizures that were being treated and whether the patient was particularly anxious about having attacks, and whether specific triggering mechanisms were being treated rather than the seizures themselves.

What is really needed is a study of behavioural techniques on a *fresh* population of patients with epilepsy (not just patients who fail to respond to conventional medical methods) and if possible a population who have not yet begun to be treated by drugs. I suspect that behavioural methods, evaluated this way, would always remain an adjunct to more conventional methods although they may be valuable in the individual patient. They certainly need an extensive formal trial to prove their worth. There is one point about these methods which so far has been under-emphasised. Review of results to date suggests that often a placebo affect is operating and is responsible for the actual reduction in seizure frequency. This may well be true, but we should be asking ourselves, even if the significant reduction in a patient's seizure frequency is due to a placebo affect, exactly what it is

that the placebo is doing, because the seizure reduction itself is real. Anything that throws light on possible brain mechanisms that appear to extinguish seizures and which we can learn to control, is worth pursuing.

In this regard, the interest that has been shown in biofeedback methods of treatment is certainly justified. Of all the behavioural methods used in the treatment of epilepsy biofeedback has perhaps excited the most interest. Biofeedback is a method of helping patients to alter certain physiological functions of which normally they are unaware. Electronic devices are used to pick up signals from, say, muscles or blood pressure, heart rate or the brain. These electronic signals are then converted to visual or auditory signals which the patient can recognise and begin to learn how to alter. Thus, for instance, muscle tension can be shown to be rising or falling by amplifying muscle potentials and providing noise from them through a microphone. As the noise rises or falls, so the patient can learn to adapt his muscle tension to produce more or less noise, and therefore more or less muscle tension. A good description of biofeedback and its clinical uses is provided by Basmajian (1979). Biofeedback training is now widely used in a variety of ways as an agent of anxiety reduction and this in itself may be useful to the patient with epilepsy, but various techniques of biofeedback directly related to suppressing paroxysmal EEG activity are being developed. Mostofsky and Balaschak (1977) provide a useful review.

Perhaps the greatest proponent of biofeedback in the treatment of epilepsy has been Sterman (1973) who made the original observation that cats taught to enhance the amount of sensorimotor rhythm (SMR) in their EEG (SMR is a 14 to 16 cycles per second rhythm which occurs over the sensorimotor cortex) became seizure-resistant when exposed to noxious chemicals. Therefore he began to experiment with training patients with epilepsy to produce a similar rhythm, and has extended his studies up until the present day (Sterman & MacDonald, 1978). His original work on looking at the sensorimotor rhythm has extended to enhancing other frequencies in the brain, and also the suppression of certain slower frequencies. Sterman has had consistently encouraging results although he has found that in those patients who do respond to biofeedback training, continued practice is needed if satisfactory results are to be maintained.

Other workers in this area have not had quite such satisfactory results and indeed some (Lockard et al., 1977) urge caution and suggest that it may sometimes have deleterious effects. Some limited support of Sterman's work however has come from other workers (Wyler, Robbins & Dodrill, 1979). This latter study is particularly interesting for its suggestion that possibly the more normal the personality of the patient the better their response to biofeedback.

EEG biofeedback on this side of the Atlantic has not received such an enthusiastic reception, and by and large the majority of work that has been carried out in this country has led to inconclusive results (MacDonald & Quy, 1979). This last study suggested strongly that placebo, experimenter and various other effects not specific to biofeedback training, may be largely responsible for the therapeutic benefits achieved.

The place of biofeedback therefore is not clear in the treatment of epilepsy, but it is certainly true that further research must be done in this area. The evidence to date suggests that perhaps some forms of EEG biofeedback do have normalising and desynchronising effects in the EEGs and brains of some patients with epilepsy (Sterman & MacDonald, 1978). Further research must try to elucidate exactly what this effect is and whether or not there are better ways of achieving it. Even if biofeedback turns out largely to be a placebo effect, it once again is important to find out what effect the placebo is actually having. To date the technique has largely been tried on patients with intractable epilepsy in terms of their response to antiepileptic drugs (such patients until recently have also been used to assess new drugs, with sometimes misleading results). Once again biofeedback must at some time be tried in newly diagnosed patients with epilepsy before they have had antiepileptic drugs if its efficiency and validity is ever to be tested fully.

PSYCHOTIC ILLNESS IN EPILEPSY

Dr. Trimble, in Part Three, will be concentrating on the relationship between epilepsy and schizophrenia, which is one of the psychotic illnesses, and I will therefore say little about schizophrenia itself apart from applying some perspective to the relationship between schizophrenia and epilepsy. There are, however, other psychotic illnesses.

The first general point that should be made about psychotic illness and epilepsy is to say that this is an area of controversy and that, unfortunately, the terminology used varies in its meaning from country to country. The term schizophrenia, for instance, has a broader and somewhat looser diagnostic meaning in the United States than it does in Europe (except for Russia). English speaking psychiatrists on both sides of the Atlantic describe specific 'organic brain syndromes' in which there is a characteristic psychiatric disturbance accompanied by evidence of organic brain impairment: these on the continent are often referred to as a psychosis. Descriptions of the relationship between complex partial seizures and psychosis are bedevilled by the term 'psychomotor epilepsy' which to some people means epilepsy originating in the temporal lobe and confirmed by the EEG, and to other authors it is a clinical description of a type of fit, perhaps 20 per cent of which do not originate in the temporal lobe. Such terminological confusion leads to muddle in terms of assessing other authors' work.

The word psychosis itself is open to different interpretations, and the distinction between psychosis and neurosis anyway is becoming blurred. I shall take it to mean a qualitative change from normal behaviour, which is neither understandable in ordinary human terms, nor in terms of the patient's life experience and environmental circumstances (although they may colour the form the psychosis takes), and which appears to have the form of an illness and to follow the illness model. There are three main groups.

1. Schizophrenic illnesses. These are global disruptions of personality in which there is disturbance of thinking, behaviour, emotional relationships, feeling and perception which occur together in a characteristic way.

2. Affective disorders. These are primary disturbances of mood (depression or pathological elation) which are accompanied by secondary symptoms such as depressive hallucinations or delusions.

3. Organic psychosyndromes. These include confusional states, changes in behaviour in the context of epilepsy associated with sub-ictal activity, delirium and dementia, which will be considered in a separate section.

Most British psychiatrists would consider that manic, depressive and schizophrenic illnesses represent such exceptional departures from normal that it is probable that they will be found eventually to be associated with physiochemical disturbances in the brain, and that they are true illnesses.

As will become clear from reading Part Three, contradictory views are held about the aetiology of the various psychotic mental states that occur in epilepsy. In some states there appears to be a direct relationship between the mental condition and an increase in epileptic activity, in others there appears to be a relationship to a decrease in epileptic activity and in yet others it would appear possible that both the psychotic symptoms and the epilepsy are the result of the same basic neuronal disorder. To be diagnosed as schizophrenic or as manic or depressive, these states should not be *directly* associated with epileptic attacks, and must occur in the setting of a normal level of consciousness, although they may be associated with a change in attack frequency.

Schizophrenia and epilepsy

Most studies of the relationship between schizophrenia and epilepsy have been confined to special or post-graduate institutions which probably see a very selected population of patients both with schizophrenia and with epilepsy. The majority of patients with psychiatric illness in this country are treated in mental hospitals and it is perhaps appropriate to draw one or two ideas and lessons from studies of mental hospital populations, which are likely to be less selected, in considering the relationship between epilepsy and schizophrenia.

In a study of psychotic patients in mental hospitals extending over twelve years (Betts & Skarrott, 1979) it is clear that paranoid symptoms are common in institutionalised people with epilepsy and it is probable that they form a continuum. On the one extreme are paranoid changes in personality occurring in a brain damaged patient who res-

ponds poorly to changes in his environment and who is suspicious and hostile and has poorly formulated grandiose, religiose or mystical ideas. On the other extreme is a patient with a fully developed paranoid schizophrenic psychotic illness (with formal persecutory and grandiose delusions).

Many of these psychotic illnesses seem to develop out of a previous paranoid personality. Sensitive paranoid thinking and ideas gradually change into a paranoid delusional system which comes to occupy a larger and larger part of the patient's psychic life and thus alters his behaviour to such an extent as to require treatment. Auditory hallucinatory experiences develop as the condition progresses and may be accompanied either by evidence of organic brain damage, or by other signs or symptoms sufficient to compel the diagnosis of schizophrenia.

Other paranoid illnesses seem to develop suddenly out of an apparently clear blue sky and may occur at a time of increasing attack frequency (usually then accompanied by signs and symptoms that suggest organic brain disease or delirium). Paranoid illnesses may also develop insidiously in patients with a previously normal personality as their attack frequency dies away.

In my experience in the chronic wards of mental hospitals where the more severely disabled psychotic epileptics tend to collect, undifferentiated paranoid psychoses, either organic or developing out of a long-standing paranoid personality, are far more common than true paranoid schizophrenia, although the latter, as will be seen from Part Three of this chapter, has acquired great notoriety. I would personally agree with continental authors who find a full-blown paranoid schizophrenic syndrome in epilepsy relatively rare. In my own series of cases (Betts & Skarrott, 1979) 50 per cent of the chronic epileptic population of two mental hospitals in the Birmingham region had paranoid illnesses (which had usually been responsible for the patients' admission to hospital and their subsequent detention), but only a few of them could be said, using strict diagnostic criteria, to have paranoid schizophrenia. The comparative rareness of this syndrome is also illustrated in a study of people with epilepsy admitted to psychiatric care of Birmingham in one calendar year (Betts, 1974). Of the 72 patients admitted with both epilepsy and psychiatric disorder, only three had paranoid psychotic illnesses. None of these patients satisfied the criteria of a paranoid schizophrenia.

A similar paucity of schizophrenia in epilepsy was found by Stevens (1979), in a study of psychiatric admission in America. Stevens, who has consistently criticised the English and continental view of the special relationship between epilepsy and schizophrenia, indeed believes that there is a biological antagonism between them.

Undoubtedly confusion arises because in the literature different diagnostic criteria for paranoid schizophrenia have been used by different authors. I have adopted the customary British meaning of paranoid schizophrenia as a psychotic illness which includes one or more of the so-called first rank symptoms of schizophrenia (Mellor, 1970). Unfortunately other operational definitions of schizophrenia exist.

It is likely that patients who have both paranoid symptoms and epilepsy may accumulate in the chronic wards of mental hospitals as they may be particularly difficult to rehabilitate. However, a 12 year follow-up of a mental hospital population showed that some *had* been rehabilitated. My experience of such a population also suggests that too much emphasis has been placed on the time relationship between the onset of the epilepsy and the onset of schizophrenia. Indeed, Slater himself has modified his position on this (Slater & Moran, 1969). The recomputing of his original data throws some doubt on the precise significance of the duration of the proceeding epilepsy before the onset of the psychosis. In the chronic mental hospital population (Betts & Skarrott, 1979) as many patients started their schizophrenia *before* their epilepsy, as did those who started their epilepsy before schizophrenia (a proportion started both together). The clinical impression was gained that those patients who did start with schizophrenia first were more aggressive before the epilepsy started than the majority of schizophrenic patients. The schizophrenia-first group also appeared to dement fairly rapidly after the onset of the epilepsy. Follow-up of these patients, however, did not really confirm the original impression of the development of a dementing process, but tended to suggest that there are immense

difficulties in assessing the degree of dementia in a patient who at the time of assessment has a marked thought disorder.

Whether patients begin with epilepsy first, or schizophrenia first, they eventually seem to lose both. The majority have temporal lobe epilepsy and if they do, they lose their tonic-clonic seizures first, and secondly complex partial seizures. The end state is one of institutionalisation, but with little evidence of organic brain impairment in most patients. Often, the epilepsy and the psychosis seem to disappear at about the same time, and study of this particular group of psychotic epileptic patients suggests that there is a close relationship between the epilepsy and the mental disorder, in that they are both an expression of some underlying disorder in the temporal lobe, and whether epilepsy or schizophrenia started first, was fortuitous.

In this regard, there are hints throughout the literature that many patients with classical schizophrenic illnesses have a lower convulsive threshold than the normal population, and therefore have an increased frequency of epilepsy, even at the start of their illness (Hill, 1957): there is also some support in the literature for the view that in psychotic patients with temporal lobe epilepsy, behavioural disturbances and epilepsy increase and decrease in intensity together (Brady, 1964).

No formal trial of treatment of these organic psychotic states of epilepsy has ever been attempted but it is my impression that they are more likely to respond to powerful neuroleptic drugs which are non-sedative (like haloperidol, pimozide or trifluoperazine). Because they are often related to organic brain disease, depot preparations of neuroleptic drugs should be avoided if possible and 'drug holidays' to prevent tardive dyskinesia are probably important. Certainly a large number of these patients seem to end up with tardive dyskinesia eventually. ECT is usually not indicated. The long term prognosis would seem to be reasonable. The following case histories illustrate some of the complex inter-relationships between these psychotic states and epilepsy.

Case 23
This woman of 53 developed epilepsy at the age of 40, following the removal of a left temporal tuberculoma. Her

attacks had usually been generalised without aura although EEG evidence showed clearly their temporal lobe origin. Until recently she had had relatively few attacks and was controlled with a mixture of phenobarbitone and phenytoin. Three years before her first psychiatric admission, she developed status epilepticus and was unconscious for some time after her fits were controlled. She was left with a gross dysmnesic state which slowly cleared over the following year. As this improved, so she began to develop paranoid symptoms, becoming hostile towards her neighbours and entertaining delusional ideas about them. She finally exhibited a complex delusional system involving Jehovah's Witnesses and the Post Office whom she felt were tampering with her mind and had inserted an electronic listening device into her brain, so that her thoughts were broadcast to other people. She began to develop auditory hallucinations and her behaviour became so disturbed at home that she needed admission to hospital. She was treated with small doses of haloperidol and within a fortnight the delusional ideas encapsulated and then disappeared and she was no longer troubled by auditory hallucinations. On a small dose of haloperidol she remained well, but two years after her original psychiatric admission she was readmitted with a further exacerbation of her psychosis following self-withdrawal of the haloperidol. Since then she has been maintained on it and has continued well. She has not had a fit since the onset of her original psychotic illness.

Case 24
This woman of 30 with poorly controlled left temporal lobe epilepsy began to develop religious ideas which gradually became so obtrusive and insistent that she would read her Bible loudly and continually all day long, both at work, on the bus going to and from work, and at home. Her readings became more angry and vociferous and eventually she began to express religious delusions that she had had a visitation from The Almighty and had been sent with a special purpose to clean the world of sin. As her symptoms became more florid she showed by her behaviour that she had developed auditory hallucinations although she always denied them. Her epilepsy continued although there was a clear relationship between the intensity of her psychotic symptoms and the temporary absence of her fits. On several occasions after spontaneous attacks of serial epilepsy, lasting two or three days, her psychotic symptoms would clear temporarily. On admission to hospital she was found to have clear evidence of brain damage and an air encephalogram showed marked atrophy of the left temporal lobe. She was treated with large doses of haloperidol and on this regimen her psychotic symptoms gradually abated and practically disappeared so that she was able to return to sheltered employment. Since her original admission, she has continued without obvious psychotic symptoms and has had the occasional epileptic seizure, although her epilepsy itself now seems to be gradually disappearing of its own accord. She has begun to develop signs of tardive dyskinesia.

Case 25
This woman was admitted to a mental hospital at the age of 27 with a history of the insidious onset of a schizophrenic illness. On admission she displayed delusions of passivity and influence, ideas of reference, somatic illusions, and auditory hallucinations which failed to respond to treatment. At the age of 32 she began to have tonic-clonic seizures,

often at night, not very frequently but described as very severe when they did occur, as she would remain unconscious for several hours afterwards. Both the epilepsy and the psychosis continued. The psychotic symptoms disappeared after she was given haloperidol at the age of 46. For the next ten years of her life, no trace could be found of a psychotic illness on formal mental state examination, although she continued to have two or three major tonic-clonic seizures a year despite treatment with phenobarbitone and phenytoin. About once or twice a year she would have episodes of acute excitement, lasting two or three hours, in which she would become quite aggressive and destructive. These were unpredictable and swiftly resolved and she seemed to have little memory of them. Shortly before her death at the age of 57 she began to have more tonic-clonic seizures than usual, although her mental state remained unchanged and there was no evidence of dementia or organic brain impairment. She was found dead one morning; there was no post mortem examination, (it is not uncommon for epileptic patients in institutions to be found dead). EEG examination at the age of 46 had shown right temporal slow-wave activity but no epileptic discharges.

Primary disturbance of mood

Misery, unhappiness and reactive depression and anxiety have already been considered (p. 234 to p. 240). Brief changes in mood from elation to depression are well recognised in people with epilepsy, particularly by continental authors who call them dysphoric states, and have been described by Landolt (1958) in association with 'forced normalisation' of the EEG or with a decline in attack frequency. They are somewhat similar to the prodromal symptoms, often affective, occasionally seen in patients with epilepsy two or three days before an attack. The patient with prodromal affective symptoms is likely to have more prolonged affective changes if his attack frequency is lessened. It is from this setting of mood instability that the true depressive states of epilepsy probably arise.

There is no doubt that endogenous depressive episodes are common in people with epilepsy and seem to occur when the attack frequency itself is declining (Flor-Henry, 1974; Betts, 1974). Although in clinical terms the depressions of epilepsy are similar to endogenous depression occurring in people without epilepsy, they do seem to have a special characteristic of coming and going with a rapidity which is unusual in ordinary depressive illnesses. Occasionally the rapid switching in and out of depression suggests an ictal experience.

Case 26

This 63-year-old man tumbled off a ladder in a fit whilst painting his house. One of his lumbar vertebrae was shattered. Whilst lying in an orthopaedic ward, alone in the early hours of the morning, he cut his throat with a razor blade, and his life was barely saved. On admission to the psychiatric ward he was in a profound depressive stupor; he had life-long poorly controlled epilepsy, and was still having up to 12 major seizures a week, despite heroic attempts to control them with antiepileptic drugs. He had had several previous psychiatric admissions for depressive illnesses. Because of his precarious physical condition, his depression was not treated for a few days. In that time it was noted that he was passing very rapidly from the depth of profound despair and depression to near normality and back again. In the middle of a sentence he might slump forward into an intense stupor, the picture of unhappiness, responding painfully and slowly to all questions, and full of suicidal ideas, only suddenly, some minutes or an hour or so later, to lift in mood back to an almost normal state. His EEG showed generalised spike and wave discharge. He was treated with clonazepam. A relatively small dose of this drug rendered him attack free and within a few days of starting it his depressive mood changes disappeared and have not returned.

Case 27

This 23-year-old girl developed complex partial seizures at the age of 16. There was a previous history of febrile convulsions as a child. The attacks were initially frequent and responded poorly to antiepileptic drugs. Physical examination showed no abnormality although an EEG showed some right posterior spike and wave activity. A year before her admission to hospital, her seizures appeared spontaneously to decline in frequency, and she had not had one for three months. Shortly after her attacks stopped, she quite suddenly became profoundly depressed with early morning waking, loss of weight and appetite, loss of sexual interest, and marked diurnal variation in mood. She developed profound ideas of guilt related to childhood masturbatory episodes, and was admitted to hospital following a determined attempt at suicide with her antiepileptic drugs. Treatment with amitriptyline in hospital failed to resolve the depression (although there was a concomitant return of her seizures, and in addition she had two tonic-clonic attacks which she had never had before). Amitriptyline was therefore stopped. Because of the severity of her depression and her continuing suicidal feelings, she was treated with a course of electro-convulsive therapy. After six applications of ECT, her depression had largely resolved and she was able to go home. It is interesting that the electrically induced seizures produced a remission in her depression which the spontaneous tonic-clonic seizure had not, (this is not always the case). Over the subsequent year she had two further short-lived episodes of depression which did not require hospitalisation or treatment as they resolved fairly rapidly, and since then she has been both depression and seizure free.

In the epileptic admission study already referred to (Betts, 1974) depression was the commonest formal psychiatric diagnosis made on the patients admitted, and there was a significant relationship between decline in attack frequency and the onset of the depressive symptoms. These depressive states of epilepsy are little described in the literature yet in my experience are the most important psychiatric complication of epilepsy, particularly as they may result from successful treatment of fits and in turn lead to suicide. Successful suicide is of course more common in people with epilepsy than in the general population. (Henriksen, Juul Jensen & Lund, 1970).

The treatment of these depressive states may be difficult and paradoxically the use of electro-convulsive therapy may be necessary to clear the depression. Conventional antidepressant medication may not be helpful particularly as tricyclic antidepressants especially amitriptyline, have epileptogenic properties. They can cause epileptic fits in normal people, and in those with low convulsive thresholds, and must be used cautiously in people with epilepsy (Betts *et al.*, 1968). In practice, if an antidepressant is needed, I tend to use either maprotiline or trimipramine as both appear to be less epileptogenic, and are reasonably effective antidepressants.

Flor-Henry (1974) showed that there is a significant correlation between dominant temporal lobe lesions and schizophrenia, and non-dominant (usually right) temporal lobe lesions and depressive symptoms, a finding confirmed by Lishman in his study of the head injured (Lishman, 1968). Manic-depressive illness itself seems relatively rare in epilepsy, but pure mania has been described as being commoner than would be expected by chance (Dongier, 1959). Whether the manic excitement described by some continental authors is actually psychomotor over-activity occurring in a mild confusional state is uncertain. I have seen a large number of patients with psychotic illnesses related to epilepsy, but have never seen one who was manic.

Organic mental illness and epilepsy

Brain damage and impairment of brain function is often found in epilepsy. It may be responsible for, or a factor in, mental illness occurring in people with epilepsy. The neuropsychology of epilepsy is reviewed by Dr Dodrill in Chapter 7, and I need do no more than review one or two aspects which are relevant to psychiatric practice.

In a person with epilepsy who is of limited or subnormal intelligence, almost invariably both the epilepsy and the subnormality are related to a single aetiological cause. In general terms, epilepsy itself does not cause reduction in intelligence, and studies which have suggested that it does have usually looked at highly selected populations. However there is now good evidence that both ictal activity (Jus & Jus 1962) and sub-ictal activity (Goode, Penry & Dreifuss, 1970) may interfere with registration of information and also occasionally cause a brief retrograde amnesia. Epileptic activity occurring in specific brain areas, particularly the left temporal lobe may also interfere with intellectual functioning and learning in children, and therefore cause behaviour problems (Stores, 1978). There is also growing evidence that antiepileptic drugs may play a part in learning difficulty in children with epilepsy (Stores, 1978) and these effects, occurring at an early age, may partly account for the observation that patients with temporal lobe epilepsy have a lower intelligence the earlier the onset of their epilepsy (Taylor & Falconer, 1968). It has been shown that actual mental retardation in children with epilepsy is restricted to those who have suffered acute cerebral insults in the form of perinatal damage, head injury or infection, or who have had status epilepticus at an early age (Ounsted, Lindsay & Norman, 1966).

Up until recently, discussion about the effects of brain damage and epileptic activity, whether ictal or sub-ictal, and medication on intelligence and learning, was difficult to quantify due to the relative crudity of tests of intelligence, intellect and cortical functioning. However, recent advances in the neuropsychology of epilepsy (Dodrill, 1978), have led to more discriminatory tests of intellectual and cognitive function. Also being developed are reliable tests of vigilance, attention, performance and learning in a laboratory setting (Hutt & Fairweather, 1971; Hutt, 1979). There is little doubt from these studies that specific cognitive, learning and performance deficits do occur in people with epilepsy, and that for children with epilepsy special teaching methods and skills are necessary to obtain optimum learning performance (p. 284).

Epilepsy and dementia

It used to be accepted without much question that people with epilepsy were liable to dement, and the concept of epileptic dementia was a part of older psychiatric teaching. This concept requires critical examination.

Dementia may be described as a syndrome of chronic, irreversible and usual progressive intellectual and memory loss in which both recall and retention of information are affected. Usually recent memory is more affected than distant memory. An important early sign of dementia is an emotional lability with which may go a 'catastrophic reaction' in which the patient over-reacts emotionally to quite trivial changes in his environment.

As the disorder progresses, so there is a deterioration of judgement and critical faculties which may lead to inappropriate behaviour. There may also be a release of previously controlled elements in the patient's personality, revealing themselves for the first time, so that, for instance, anti-social behaviour may be expressed in a previously well-behaved middle-aged man.

Poverty of thought and ideation occurs. Patients show difficulty in shifting from one topic to the next and eventually develop severe perseveration. They lose the ability to think logically or handle symbols and develop 'concrete thinking'. Later they may become disorientated in time and place, but very rarely in person, and they suffer from episodes of confusion; infection and sedatives may make confusion worse. Very often chronic emotional changes occur, usually those of depression and may appear when the patient is aware of his failing powers.

The diagnosis of dementia is largely a clinical diagnosis although assisted by psychological tests and radiological investigation. It should not be a diagnosis that is made lightly and only after the fullest possible investigation. The value of careful investigation of people suspected of having dementia has been shown by Marsden & Harrison (1972), who found that a proportion of patients referred with a diagnosis of dementia did not have the condition at all and that some who were demented had treatable causes of the dementia.

Follow-up studies of patients with dementia (Mann, 1973), show that even in patients diagnosed radiologically as having dementia, some turn out on follow-up not to have the disorder at all. Both clinical, radiological, and also psychological investigations in patients with suspected dementia may therefore give rise to misleading results, particularly in the case of psychological testing which is relatively crude and inaccurate except in advanced cases. However, the recent introduction of more specific and sensitive psychological tests is to be welcomed, particularly the Halstead Reitan Neuropsychological Battery, a version of which has been prepared for patients with epilepsy (Dodrill, 1978). It should lead to improved accuracy of psychological investigation as it becomes more widely used in this country.

The inaccuracies in the diagnosis of dementia should be particularly borne in mind in considering the relationship between epilepsy and dementia. Whether epilepsy itself is associated with progressive dementia is uncertain. The term 'epileptic dementia' occurs quite commonly in the psychiatric literature, but is often mistaken either for the chronic changes that occur in psychotic illnesses, or for the personality changes that occur in epilepsy, or for institutionalisation, or for depression, which so often occurs in epilepsy, or for chronic drug intoxication.

Apart from those children who suffer devastating brain insults as a result of febrile status epilepticus, it is unlikely that even repeated epileptic fits lead to any degree of dementia. In those people who do have epilepsy and have presenile dementia, almost certainly the two syndromes are the result of a single brain disease of a progressive nature (for an example see Betts, Smith & Kelly, 1968). It is occasionally speculated that some people with epilepsy are suffering from chronic viral infections or from the punch-drunk syndrome (Traumatic Encephalopathy). These hypotheses are unproven, apart from occasional case reports, and are still speculative. Interest in the neuropathology of dementia is certainly increasing (Dayan, 1974) and some of these speculative ideas should be investigated further.

It should be expected, however, that people with epilepsy who are brain damaged, even if the brain damage is static, will tend to dement earlier than the general population as they have already lost some of their cortical reserves. It is still generally accepted that considerable neuronal damage may occur without any apparent loss of intellectual function, but that after a critical level of brain tissue has been lost there will be a rapid and obvious loss of function.

In assessing a patient with suspected dementia associated with epilepsy, full investigation should be undertaken both neurological and psychiatric. Psychological testing should be employed by using relevant tests (Dodrill, 1978). Psychiatric illness, drug intoxication, and apathy and inertia due to chronic illness should be rigorously excluded. Computer Assisted Tomography of the brain or air encephalography should also be carried out, although it should be noted that air encephalography is not as predictive of the prognosis of dementia as was thought originally (Mann, 1973). Occasionally cerebral biopsy may be necessary to elucidate the cause of a particular dementing syndrome (Sim, Turner & Smith, 1966) although use of this particular form of investigation is becoming rare.

The confusional states of epilepsy

Various organic mental states occur in people with epilepsy either with a time relationship to a clinical seizure or occurring at the same time as subictal seizure activity in the EEG. They are becoming increasingly recognised and have psychiatric and forensic importance. Their classification has been confused and arbitary and they have gone under a bewildering variety of names. A division of these states into three groups has been made by continental authors (Bruens, 1974).

a. Post-ictal twilight states

These may occur after any type of fit; any attempt to restrain the confused patient may lead to outbursts of aggression. The EEG shows profuse irregular slow activity. Hughlings Jackson thought that such states might be due to the exhaustion of cerebral neurones, but it is possible that they may represent a continuing ictal event. It is also possible that the now very rare epileptic furore is related to these states. Some patients, however, after their seizure are not aggressive but remain in a prolonged confused dream-like state which seems to occur regularly after their attacks.

Case 28

This 30-year-old publican had been in good health and there was no evidence of previous seizure activity. One evening whilst working with his wife in their public house, he went down into the cellar to change a beer cask and failed to return after a few minutes. His wife, who suspected that he was having an affair with one of the barmaids, crept down to the cellar to see what was going on. When she got into the cellar she saw her husband in the throes of a tonic-clonic seizure. Shortly after the attack ended, her husband rose in a dazed fashion from the floor, and kicked in several of the barrels in the cellar. His wife remonstrated with him, and was irritably pushed out of the way by her husband who then ran up the stairs into the bar and began to assault his customers. Although he hurt several of them, his violence did not seem to be directed against any one in particular. If people kept out of the way he failed to pursue them, but if they tried to restrain him, he would respond with violence. The police were summoned and he was eventually taken away with some difficulty to a local hospital where in the casualty department further attempts were made to restrain him. During the struggle, two members of the staff were injured but attempts to inject him with a sedative were fruitless. He was eventually locked in a side room where, left to himself, he quietened down very rapidly and fell asleep. Subsequent investigations revealed a temporal glioma which was ultimately fatal. Similar behaviour occurred following further seizures but without the violence as no further attempts were made to restrain him and he was just confused and irritable. Attempts at conversation with him during such states were fruitless, as although he was clearly awake he rarely made any reply.

b. Absence status

This is a mental state directly related to generalised epileptic discharges. Since its first description by Lennox in 1945, in which it was termed petit mal status, it has been described by several authors under different names. I would personally use a term coined by Roger, Lob and Tassinari (1974) that of *generalised status epilepticus expressed as a confusional state*. This describes a clinical picture and avoids using terms like absence and petit mal because not all patients who develop absence status have either a previous history of convulsions or of absences (Roger, Lob & Tassinari, 1974: Ellis & Lee 1978). Indeed these states do sometimes seem to start *de novo* in middle age without a previous epileptic history. They are characterised by a confusional state which varies in intensity and presentation from patient to patient and also varies

within the same patient from time to time. There may be only a slight degree of confusion, often then accompanied by apparent histrionic or neurotic behaviour, but with clear-cut evidence of an organic deficit on formal psychological testing. There may be episodes of severe confusion, often with a patchy loss of intellectual function (i.e. the patient may remember one thing but forget others during the attack, or may have transient signs of parietal lobe disturbance). There may be the most profound stupor. Those confusional states which are related to previous epilepsy of a generalised nature seem to respond well to intravenous diazepam or clonazepam, but often respond poorly to other antiepileptic drugs, whereas the ictal confusional states of middle-age seem to respond to conventional drugs, once the underlying epileptic diathesis is identified. Occasionally, during the ictal period, in addition to the confusion previously described, frank psychotic symptoms may appear. These can often be seen as the patient's attempt to explain puzzling internal feelings which cannot be understood. This phenomenon is commoner in the acute prolonged confusional states of later life (Ellis & Lee, 1978)

Case 29

This 13-year-old girl, who had had recurrent generalised absences and tonic-clonic seizures since the age of three, poorly controlled with conventional medication, was admitted from a neurological ward to a psychiatric unit with the diagnosis of schizophrenia made by the neurologists. On admission she was fatuous and giggling, appeared to have visual hallucinations, and described herself as married to a well-known pop singer. In addition to this, however, she was vague and distant, appeared to be disorientated and had little memory of recent events. She had been admitted to the neurological unit in this state some days previously. EEG examination on her admission to the psychiatric unit showed generalised three per second spike-wave activity. Oral nitrazepam was given and within a day the EEG abnormally had stopped and a somewhat bewildered but now normal 13 year old girl emerged from underneath the apparent psychotic behaviour. On reviewing her history it would seem that in the preceding few years, she had had many attacks like this lasting up to a day which had greatly interfered with her school work. Under a small dose of nitrazepam these attacks no longer occurred although she continued to have the occasional tonic-clonic seizure. Her school work improved markedly.

c. 'Psychomotor' status

In which a prolonged alteration in mental state results from epileptic discharge in the cortex, usually in the temporal lobes. This has not been described extensively in the British literature, but in my experience it is commoner than is generally thought. The condition is better described in the continental literature and the patients I have seen follow quite closely the descriptions given there. I have appended three case histories to illustrate the clinical features. Some twilight states which resemble 'psychomotor' status but which are chronologically related to seizures, appear to occur in other types of epilepsy. These are the ones particularly described by Landolt (1958) who maintained that such twilight states can result from overdosage of antiepileptic drugs a statement with which I would agree.

Case 30

This 40-year-old man had never sought help before for the brief seizures which he had had for 20 years, and which were of a brief muddled feeling accompanied by a déja vu experience. He had had one of his usual attacks on the bus on his way to work; after the attack he walked away from his regular bus stop in a dazed state, removing his clothing as he did so. Completely naked, he wandered up and down a shopping precinct muttering incoherently. He was arrested, struggling violently, and covered in the regulation blanket, removed to a police station. When questioned he did not make coherent replies except occasionally to mutter 'protest'. He remained in this state for 12 hours and then suddenly recovered his senses, and demanded to know where he was and who had removed his clothing. He has not shown similar behaviour since, but passed through a transient period of depression on knowing what he had done. Subsequent investigation showed a right temporal epileptic focus on EEG.

Case 31

A man of 23 was found wandering in a dazed fashion in the middle of a large city. He had given no coherent reply to questions by the police, and search of his clothing revealed no identifying mark or documents. He was accordingly admitted to a psychiatric hospital where he was observed to spend most of his time in a catatonic-like stupor, crouched in a chair. Occasionally he was thought to be visually hallucinated as he seemed to be watching some insect or bird flying round his room. Rarely he would become violently aggressive when he would dash up out of his chair and fly around the ward overturning tables and chairs, and smashing windows for a few minutes before returning to his previous still posture. He was thought to have catatonic schizophrenia and was treated with psychotropic drugs but with little effect. A week after admission whilst asleep in bed he was observed to have a tonic-clonic fit. On awakening the next morning he was lucid and rational, knew his name and where he came from, and was surprised to find himself in hospital. Over the next few hours, the previous psychotic state returned; an EEG at this time showed continuous spike-wave discharge from the left temporal lobe. He was given intravenous diazepam and his mental state returned to normal, at the same time as the abnormal EEG discharges stopped. He made a complete recovery with regular antiepileptic drugs.

Case 32

A woman with left temporal lobe epilepsy stopped her antiepileptic drugs suddenly. A day later she passed into a peculiar clouded mental state in which she was irritable and tearful and had obvious memory difficulty. Definite organic impairment was confirmed on formal mental state testing. She would not eat, lost weight rapidly and complained of bone pain. She would wander distracted round the house in a confused state and was incapable of looking after her children. An EEG showed continual epileptic activity in the left temporal area, which previously had only been present during her actual attacks. Ten days after this episode started she awoke one morning in a normal frame of mind; on that day the EEG abnormality had disappeared and has not returned.

These cases illustrate the wide variety of phenomena which may be seen in association with continual epileptic activity occurring in one temporal lobe, though if looked for confusion and evidence of organic impairment can always be found. Pseudo-neurotic behaviour may also be prominent. Sometimes, automatisms are the main feature to be seen in the patient's mental state, and occasionally the patient may wander away in the twilight state in a kind of fugue. Twilight states may be prolonged and last for several days.

More profound confusional states can also occur in epilepsy and some people with epilepsy develop a frank delirium although not apparently as an ictal experience. Epileptic delirium was frequently described in the older literature on epilepsy and is, in fact, still encountered. The usual characteristics of delirium are present (psychomotor overactivity, perceptual distortions, hallucinatory experiences usually of a visual nature, confusion, disorientation in time and place and a degree of clouding of consciousness). Delusional ideas may also be present, usually persecutory (although I have seen the occasional patient with a depressive element to their delirium).

Landolt (1958) associates these delirious states with supression of fits and forced normalisation of the EEG. However, I would agree with other continental authors (Bruens, 1974) that forced normalisation does not occur in states in which there is also clouding of consciousness. It has been my experience that these delirious conditions are relatively common, often associated with the patient's admission to hospital, and usually seemed to be associated with a sudden increase in attack frequency and carry a relatively good prognosis (Betts, 1974). It has usually not been possible to do an EEG at the time of the patient's admission but it has been my clinical impression that one is seeing a confusional state related to frequent seizures rather than to ictal activity itself.

Case 33

This man of 60 had had about four tonic-clonic fits a year from the age of 30 which had never been investigated, although he had been taking phenobarbitone for years. Just before his sixtieth birthday he had eight attacks within a week, possibly connected with a reduction in his antiepileptic drugs. During this period he became suspicious, truculent and hostile, and later became physically aggressive and overactive and developed florid paranoid ideas, imagining that he was being spied upon, that his neighbours were pumping gas under his doors: he appeared to have auditory hallucinations and began to see visions of the devil. Finally he attacked his son-in-law with an axe, mistaking him for the devil himself. On removal to hospital he was noted to have the classical symptoms of delirium, and was markedly confused with severe disorientation and a poor retentive memory. His antiepileptic drugs were increased and within a few days the exited delirious state disappeared pari passu with cessation of his seizures, and the mental state has not returned.

This patient seems to have been left with no residual organic deficit although in my mental hospital experience some patients who develop a delirious state related to epilepsy seem afterwards to have a permanent organic defect state, although it can be difficult to say whether or not they had had it before.

Acknowledgements

I am particularly grateful to two friends and colleagues who have assisted in the preparation of this chapter. Dr Pauline Skarrott, a former student, gave much enthusiastic help with a resurvey of a population of people with epilepsy in mental hospitals, a survey which has greatly influenced my view of the fate of people with epilepsy who are mentally ill. Judith Baron, a colleague from social work, read an early draft of this chapter and made several valuable suggestions.

REFERENCES

Bagley, C. (1971) *The Social Psychology of the Child with Epilepsy*. London: Routledge & Kegan Paul.

Basmajian, J.B (1979) *Biofeedback: Principles and Practice for Clinicians*. Baltimore: Williams & Wilkins.

Betts, T.A. (1974) A follow-up study of a cohort of patients with epilepsy admitted to psychiatric care in an English city. In Harris, P. & Mawdsley, C. (eds) *Epilepsy – Proceedings of the Hans Berger Centenary Symposium*, p. 326. Edinburgh: Churchill Livingstone.

Betts, T.A. (1975) Disturbances of sexual behaviour. *Clinics in Endocrinology and Metabolism*, Vol. 4, No. 3, 619.

Betts, T.A. & Skarrott, P.H. (1979) Epilepsy and the mental hospital. Paper presented at International League Against Epilepsy Scientific Meeting, Oxford, November 1979.

Betts, T.A., Smith, W.T. & Kelly, R.E. (1968) Adult metachromatic leucodystrophy (sulphatide lipidosis) simulating acute schizophrenia *Neurology* (Minneap), **18**, 1140.

Betts, T.A., Kalra, P.L., Cooper, R. & Jeavons, P.M. (1968) Epileptic fits as a probable side effect of amitriptyline. *Lancet*, **1**, 390.

Betts, T.A., King, A., Pidd, S.A. & Skarrott, P.H. (1981). 'Queer Turns' – A Study of Patients with Undiagnosed Attack Disorders. To be published.

Bird, J. (1979). The Behavioural Treatment of Hysteria. *British Journal of Psychiatry*. **134**, 129.

Bowlby, J. (1960) Grief and Mourning in Infancy and Early Childhood. *Psychoanalytic Study of the Child*. **15**, 9.

Brady, J.P. (1964). Epilepsy and Disturbed Behaviour. *J. Nerv. Ment. Disease* **138**, 468.

Bruens, J.H. (1974) Psychoses in Epilepsy. In Vinken, P.L. & Bruyn, L.W. (eds) *Handbook of Clinical Neurology*, 15, Ch. 32. Amsterdam: North Holland Publishing Co.

Bureau, M., Guey, J., Dravet, C. & Roger, J. (1968) A Study of Distribution of Petit Mal Absences in the Child in Relation to his Activities. *Electroencephalography and Clinical Neurophysiology*. 25, 513.

Caveness, W., Merritt, H. & Gallup, G. (1969) A survey of public attitudes towards epilepsy in 1969. Washington: U.S. Dept. of Health Education & Welfare, Public Health Service.

Currie, S., Heathfield, K.W.G., Henson, R.A. & Scott, D.F. (1971) Clinical Course and Prognosis of Temporal Lobe Epilepsy: A survey of 666 Patients. *Brain*, **94**, 173.

Dayan, A.D. (1974) The brain ageing and dementia. *Psychological Medicine*. 4, 349.

Dodrill, C. (1978) A neuropsychological battery for epilepsy. *Epilepsia*. **19**, 611.

Dongier, S. (1959) Statistical study of clinical and electroencephalographic manifestations of 536 psychotic episodes occurring in 516 epileptics between clinical seizures. *Epilepsia*. 1, 117.

Doube, R. (1965) Sensory precipitated seizures – a review. *J. Nervous and Mental Disease*. **141**, 524.

Efron, R. (1956) The effect of olfactory stimuli in arresting uncinate fits. *Brain*. **79**, 267.

Ellis, J.M. & Lee, S.I. (1978) Acute prolonged confusion in late life as an ictal state. *Epilepsia*. **19**, 119.

Epilepsy News (1979) **12**.

Feldman, B.G. & Paul, N.G. (1976) Identity of emotional triggers in Epilepsy. *J. Nervous and Mental Disease*. **162**, 345.

Finalyson, E. & Lucas, A.R. (1979) Pseudo-epileptic seizures in children and adolescents. *Mayo Clinic Proceedings*. **54**, 83.

Flor-Henry, P. (1974) Psychosis, neurosis and epilepsy. Developmental and gender related effects and their aetiological contribution. *British Journal of Psychiatry*. **124**, 144.

Forster, F.M. (1972) The classification and conditioning

treatment of the reflex epilepsies. *International Journal of Neurology*. **9**, 73.

Gastaut, H. & Tassinari, C.A. (1966) Triggering mechanisms in epilepsy. *Epilepsia*. **7**, 85.

Goffman, E. (1963) *Stigma. Notes on the management of spoiled identity*. New Jersey: Prentice Hall.

Goldie, L. & Green, J.M. (1959) A study of the psychological factors in a case of sensory reflex epilepsy. *Brain*. **82**, 505.

Goode, D.J., Penry, J.K. & Dreifuss, F.E. (1970) Effects of paroxysmal spike wave on continuous visual motor performance. *Epilepsia*. **11**, 241.

Gotze, W., Kupicki, S.T., Munter, F. & Teichman, J. (1967). Effect of exercise on seizure threshold. *Diseases of the Nervous System*. **28**, 664.

Graham, P., & Rutter, M. (1968). Organic brain dysfunction and child psychiatric disorder. *British Medical Journal*. **3**, 695.

Gudmundsson, D. (1966) Epilepsy in Iceland. *Acta Neurologica Scandinavica*. **43**, Supplement 25. 1.

Guerrant, J., Anderson, W.W., Fisher, A., Weinstein, M.R. Jaros, R.M. & Deskins, A. (1962) *Personality in Epilepsy*. Springfield, Illinois: C.C. Thomas.

Gunn, J.C. (1969) *Epileptics in Prison*. M.D. Thesis. University of Birmingham, England.

Gunn, J.C. & Fenton, G. (1971) Epilepsy, automatism and crime. *Lancet*, **1**, 1173.

Henderson, D. & Gillespie, R.D. (1950) *A Textbook of Psychiatry*, 7th edn. London: Oxford University Press.

Henrikson, B., Juul Jenson, P. & Lund, M. (1970) The mortality of epileptics. In Brackenridge, R.D.C. (ed.) *Life Assurance Medicine: Proceedings of the 10th International Conference of Life Assurance Medicine*. London: Pitman.

Hierons, R. & Saunders, M. (1966) Impotence in patients with temporal lobe lesions. *Lancet*. **2**, 761.

Hill, D. (1957) The electroencephalogram in schizophrenia. In Richter, D. (ed.) *Schizophrenia Somatic Aspects*. London: Pergamon Press.

Hill, D., Pond, D.A., Mitchell, W. & Falconer, M.A. (1957) Personality changes following temporal lobectomy for epilepsy. *Journal of Mental Science*. **103**, 18.

Hinton, J. (1967) *Dying*. Harmondsworth: Penguin.

Hoenig, J. & Hamilton, C.M. (1960) Epilepsy and Sexual Orgasm. *Acta Psychiatrica Scandinavia*. **35**, 448.

Hoenig, J. & Kenna, J.C. (1979) EEG abnormalities and transexualism. *Brit. J. Psychiat*. **134**, 293.

Hutt, S.J. (1979) Cognitive processes and EEG activity in patients with epilepsy. Paper presented at the International Conference on Psychology and Medicine. University College of Swansea, Wales.

Hutt, S.J. & Fairweather, H. (1971) Some effects of performance variables upon generalised spike wave activity. *Brain*. **94**, 321.

Jus, A. & Jus, K. (1962) Retrograde amnesia in petit mal. *Arch. Gen. Psychiat*. **6**, 163.

Lacey, J.T., Bateman, D.E. & Van Lehn, R. (1953). Autonomic response specificity. *Psychosomatic Medicine*. **15**, 8.

Landolt, H. (1958) In Lorentz de Haas (ed.) *Lectures on Epilepsy*, p. 91. Amsterdam: Elsevier.

Lishman, W.A. (1968) Brain damage in relation to psychiatric disability and head injury. *British Journal of Psychiatry*. **114**, 373.

Lishman, W.A. (1978) *Organic Psychiatry*. London: Oxford University Press.

Lockard, J.S., Wyler, A.R., Finch, C.A., & Hurlburt, K.E.

(1977) EEG operant conditioning in a monkey model. 1. Seizure data. *Epilepsia*. **18**, 471.

Lombroso, C. (1889) *L'uomo Delinquente*. Turin Bocca.

MacDonald, L.M. & Quy, R.J. (1979) Biofeedback of the electroencephalogram in the treatment of epilepsy. Paper presented to the International Conference on Psychology and Medicine. University College of Swansea. Wales. July 1979.

Mackay, A. (1979) Self poisoning – a complication of epilepsy. *British Journal of Psychiatry*. **134**, 277.

Maletzky, B.M. (1973) The episodic dyscontrol syndrome. *Diseases of the Nervous System*. **34**, 178.

Mann, A.H. (1973). Cortical atrophy and air encephalography: a clinical and radiological study. *Psychological Medicine*. **3**, 374.

Marsden, C.D. & Harrison M.J. (1972) Outcome of investigation of patients with presenile dementia. *British Medical Journal* **2**, 249.

Mattson, R.H., Heninger, G.R., Gallagher, B.B. & Glaser, G.H. (1970). Psychophysiologic precipitants of seizures in epileptics. *Neurology (Minneapolis)*. **20**, 407.

Mellor, C.S. (1970) The first rank symptoms of schizophrenia. *British Journal of Psychiatry*. **117**, 15.

Mellor, D.H., Lowitt, I. & Hall, D.J. (1974) Are epileptic children behaviourally different from other children? In Harris, P. & Mawdsley, C. (eds) *Epilepsy: Proceedings of the Hans Berger Centenary Symposium*, p. 313. Edinburgh: Churchill Livingstone.

Merskey, H. & Tonge, W.L. (1974) *Psychiatric Illness*, 7th edn. London: Baillière and Tindall.

Merskey, H. (1979) *The Analysis of Hysteria*. London: Baillière and Tindall.

Mitchell, W., Falconer, M.A. & Hill, D. (1954). Epilepsy with fetishism relieved by temporal lobectomy. *Lancet*. **ii**, 626.

Mostofsky, D.I., Balaschak, B.A., (1977) Psychobiological control of seizures. Psychological Bulletin **84**, No. 4, 723.

Niedemeyer, E., Blumer, D., Holscher, E. & Walker, B.A. (1970) Classical hysterical seizures facilitated by anticonvulsant toxicity. *Psychiatric Clinics* (Basle). **3**, 71.

Office of Health Economics (1971) Epilepsy in Society. London.

Ounsted, C., Lindsay, J. & Norman, R. (1966) *Biological factors in temporal lobe epilepsy*. London: Heinemann.

Pinto, R. (1972) A case of movement epilepsy with agoraphobia treated successfully by flooding. *British Journal of Psychiatry*. **121**, 287.

Pond, D.A. (1974) Epilepsy and personality disorders. In Vinken, P.L. & Bruyn, G.W. (eds) *Handbook of Clinical Neurology*, 15, Ch. 31. Amsterdam: North Holland Publishing Co.

Pond, D.A. & Bidwell, B.H. (1959) A survey of epilepsy in 14 general practices II. Social and psychological aspects. *Epilepsia*. **1**, 285.

Pond, D.A., Bidwell, B.H. & Stein, L. (1960) A survey of epilepsy in 14 general practices. I. Demographic and medical data. *Psychiatrica, Neurologica, Neurochirgia* (Amsterdam) **63**, 217. Publishing Co.

Poulose, K.P. & Shaw, A.A. (1977) Rapidly recurring seizures of psychogenic origin. *American Journal of Psychiatry*. **134**, 1145.

Pratt, R.T.C. & Mackenzie, W. (1958) Anxiety states following vestibular disorders. *Lancet*. **2**, 347.

Slater, E. (1965) The diagnosis of hysteria. *British Medical Journal*. **1**, 1395.

Slater, E. & Shields, J. (1969) Genetical aspects of anxiety. In Lader, M.H. (ed.) *Studies in Anxiety*. Ashford: Headley Brothers.

Slater, E. & Moran, E.A. (1969) Schizophrenia like psychoses of epilepsy: relation between ages of onset. *British Journal of Psychiatry*. 115, 599.

Small, J., Hayden, M. & Small, I. (1966) Further psychiatric investigations of patients with temporal and non temporal lobe epilepsy. *American Journal of Psychiatry*. 123, 303.

Srole, L., Langner, T.S., Michael, S.T., Opler, M.K. & Rennie, T.A.C. (1962) *Mental Health in the Metropolis, the Mid-town Manhattan Study*. 1. New York: McGraw Hill.

Standage, K.F. (1972) Treatment of epilepsy by reciprocal inhibition of anxiety. *Guys Hospital Reports*. 121, 217.

Sterman, M.B. (1973) Neurophysiologic and clinical studies of sensorimotor EEG biofeedback training and some effects on epilepsy. *In Biofeedback and Self Control*, p. 363. Chicago: Aldine Publishing Co.

Sterman, M.B. & MacDonald, L.R. (1978) Effects of central cortical EEG training on the incidence of poorly controlled seizures. *Epilepsia*. 19, 207.

Roger, J., Lob, H. & Tassinari, C.A. (1974) Generalised status epilepticus expressed as a confusional state (petit mal status or absence status epilepticus). In Vinken, P.L. & Bruyn, G.W. (eds) *Handbook of Clinical Neurology* 15, p. 167. Amsterdam: North Holland Publishing Co.

Roy, A. (1977) Hysterical fits previously diagnosed as epilepsy. *Psychological Medicine*. 7, 271.

Serafetinides, G. (1965) Aggressiveness in temporal lobe epileptics. *Epilepsia*. 6, 33.

Servit, Z., Machek, J., Stercova, A., Kristof, M., Servenkova, V.A., & Dudas, B. (1963) Reflex influences in the pathogenesis of epilepsy in the light of clinical statistics. In Servit, Z. (ed.) *Reflex Mechanisms in the Genesis of Epilepsy*. Elsevier: Amsterdam.

Shukla, G.D., Srivastava, O.N., & Katiyar, B.C. (1979). Sexual disturbances in temporal lobe epilepsy – a controlled study. *British Journal of Psychiatry*. 134, 288.

Sim, M., Turner, E. & Smith, W.T. (1966) Cerebral biopsy in the investigation of presenile dementia. *British Journal of Psychiatry*. 112, 119.

Slater, E., Beard, A.W. & Glithero, E. (1963) The schizophrenia – like psychoses of epilepsy. *British Journal of Psychiatry*. 109, 95.

Stevens, J.R. (1959) Emotional activation of the electroencephalogram in patients with convulsive disorders. Journal of Nervous and Mental Disease. 128, 339–351.

Stevens, J.R. (1966) Psychiatric implications of psychomotor epilepsy. *Archives of General Psychiatry*. 14, 461.

Stevens, J.R. (1979) The biological background of psychosis in epilepsy. Paper presented at the 11th Epilepsy International Symposium. Florence.

Stores, G. (1978) School children with epilepsy at risk for learning and behaviour problems. *Developmental Medicine and Child Neurology*. 20, 502.

Symonds, C. (1959). Excitation and inhibition in epilepsy. *Brain*. 82, 133.

Taylor, D.C. (1969) Sexual behaviour and temporal lobe epilepsy. *Archives of Neurology*. 21, 510.

Taylor, D.C. (1969) Aggression and epilepsy. *Journal of Psychosomatic Research*. 13, 229.

Taylor, D.C. & Falconer, M.A. (1968) Clinical socio-economic and psychological changes after temporal lobectomy. *British Journal of Psychiatry*. 114, 1247.

Tizard, B. (1962) The personality of epileptics. *Psychological Bulletin*. 59, 196.

Trimble, M.R. (1978) Letter. *British Medical Journal*. 2, 1682.

Tyrer, P. (1974) *The role of bodily feelings in anxiety*. London: Oxford University Press.

Tyrer, P. & Alexander, J. (1979) Classification of personality disorder. *British Journal of Psychiatry*. 135, 163.

Tyrer, P., Alexander, J., Cicchetti, D., Cohen, M. & Remington, M. (1979) Reliability of a schedule for rating personality disorder. *British Journal of Psychiatry*. 135, 168.

Vidart, L. & Geier, S. (1968) Work, fatigue and the psychic state in epileptic patients: a telemetric EEG study. *Electroencephalography and Clinical Neurophysiology*. 25, 511.

Walton, H.J. & Presly, A.S. (1973) Use of category system in the diagnosis of abnormal personality. *British Journal of Psychiatry*. 122, 259.

Williams, D. (1956) The structure of emotions reflected in epileptic experiences. *Brain*. 79, 29.

Wing, J. (1974) Paper 5 in *People with Handicaps Need Better Trained Counsellors*. Central Council for Education and Training of Social Workers.

Wyler, A.R., Robbins, C.A., and Dodrill, C.B. (1979) EEG operant conditioning for control of epilepsy. *Epilepsia* 20, 279.

PART TWO
THE DIFFERENTIAL DIAGNOSIS OF ATTACKS AND THE BORDERLANDS OF EPILEPSY

D.A. Pond

The word 'attack' is meant to cover in the broadest sense episodic disturbances of consciousness and/or behaviour that usually last seconds or minutes rather than hours or days and are often stereotyped in form. Such complaints are among the commonest ever made by patients to their general practitioner who, in turn, refers them to a wide variety of general physicians, neurologists and psychiatrists. As far as this book is concerned, the differential diagnosis of attacks refers essentially to the differentiation of epileptic attacks from non-epileptic attacks. The term, 'the borderlands of epilepsy', first came into general use as a result of Gowers' famous little book of that name. It concerns the slightly different question of what types of attack can be diagnosed as having an epileptic basis.

By far the most important information required for making the correct diagnosis of attacks comes from a minute account of what actually happens in the attacks, preferably from observers as well as the sufferer. An exact description of one particular attack seen from the very beginning is more helpful than an impressionistic summary of many. Words such as 'epileptiform', 'hysterical', and so on, should not be used as they anticipate the diagnosis, often erroneously.

The non-epileptic causes of attacks may be conveniently, if roughly, divided into vascular, biochemical, and psychogenic, but in each group there are a number of different physiological mechanisms at work producing the clinical phenomena of patients' attacks. Because loss of consciousness, however partial and transient, is typical of all forms of epileptic attacks, special attention will be paid to the aetiology and pathogenesis of attacks that involve disturbances of consciousness.

ATTACKS ON A VASCULAR BASIS

Attacks on a vascular basis leading to a disturbance of consciousness may result from cerebro-vascular or extra-cranial, mainly cardiac, causes. By far the commonest form, especially in young people is the simple faint due to a temporary failure of the blood supply to the brain. The phenomenology is well known and scarcely needs detailed description. The sufferer is standing, sometimes sitting, but never lying down unless he or she has already got serious heart disease. There is usually a sensation of 'going off', combined with pallor, slow small pulse, and sweating. As the blood supply to the brain is restored, a few jerks of the body from the cerebral anoxia, or rarely, more definite epileptic phenomena, are occasionally seen. Faints are quite often precipitated by a situation of sudden acute stress or anxiety.

More sinister are impairments of consciousness resulting from heart disease of which the Stokes-Adams attack is the most typical. In such cases there is always other evidence of pre-existing heart disease and the differential diagnosis within the

cardiac causes of attacks need not be further discussed here.

Attacks on a cerebro-vascular basis are nowadays sometimes referred to as transient ischaemic attacks. They are varied in form, depending on which blood vessels of the brain are involved, but the basilar artery territory, which includes the brain stem and mid-brain, is the one most likely to produce transient disturbances of consciousness often associated with focal paralyses and disturbances of speech. These attacks usually last minutes or hours rather than seconds.

It is convenient at this place to mention the common clinical problem in old people of 'drop attacks' or senile falls. In these the patient may suddenly find himself upon the ground, having no warning or just a sensation that his legs are giving way under him. The sudden fall may cause a bang on the head still further complicating the clinical picture with 'concussion', so-called, causing amnesia and confusion of a few seconds' duration. In persons who have had a definite cerebro-vascular accident in the past, probably large enough to leave behind prominent neurological signs, such as hemiplegia, the cerebral scar may become epileptogenic and focal epileptic attacks start, which are sometimes confused with further cerebro-vascular accidents. A particularly interesting clear-cut cause of sudden attacks, especially in older people, results from kinking of the vertebral artery when persons stretch up and hyper-extend their neck to reach something above them. In such persons the carotid circulation around the Circle of Willis may be insufficient to maintain the blood supply to the brain stem, and almost instantaneous unconsciousness can occur.

Under the term 'vascular' heading may be included, for convenience, attacks of labyrinthine origin, usually called Menière's disease. In these a sudden paroxysmal giddiness may be so intense as to cause loss of posture. Some headaches, particularly of the migrainous variety probably also have a basis in vascular spasm. The symptomatology may resemble focal epileptic attacks, but the time course is minutes, not seconds. Very rarely can the cerebral spasm of migrainous origin be so severe as to produce permanent scarring from cerebral anoxia, which may later become epileptogenic. There are, however, other possible mechanisms relating migraine and epilepsy.

BIOCHEMICAL DISORDERS

This term again is a rag-bag of causes not easily classifiable in any other way. Several metabolic diseases can cause unconsciousness but rarely brief enough to constitute an attack as defined above. Hypoglycaemia is commonest, though all too often diagnosed without proper laboratory confirmation. Spontaneous hypoglycaemia from, for example, tumours of the islets is rare; the most common cause is insulin overdose in an unstable diabetic. Definite epileptic atacks, usually of the major variety, are precipitated by many metabolic disorders; for example, hypoparathroidism, hypoglycaemia, hypocalcaemia, but the epileptic attack is rarely the only presenting symptom and extensive endocrine investigations are not routinely warranted as part of the diagnostic work up of a new case of epilepsy.

Under this heading may be included the very important group of drug effects, including stimulants, sedatives and above all, alcohol. Drugs, such as amphetamines and antidepressants in overdose, can cause convulsions, and these may occur with barbiturate withdrawal, especially after overdosage or sudden stopping of medication given chronically. Alcohol is probably one of the commonest causes of single epileptic attacks as they present in the casualty departments of city hospitals dealing with the floating homeless population. As both barbiturates and alcohol are often taken irregularly, various types of attacks can be seen in chronic cases which do not seem to be simply caused by epileptic attacks whether major or minor. Drowsy and amnesic episodes, 'blackouts' (a favourite word used by this type of patient) inexplicable falls, and apparently psychogenic fugue states or furores in middle-aged people, should be an indication for a spot drug check on blood or urine. The EEG in these cases may show a considerable amount of non-specific, usually symmetrically fast and occasionally slow activity. The clinical state and the blood, drug and alcohol levels at the time of the EEG must be known before it can be properly assessed. Epileptic phenomena are, of course, commonly seen during withdrawal states from these drugs. Provided the patient remains off them, such an attack need not necessarily imply a continuing tendency to subsequent attacks, and so indicate the need for regular antiepileptic drug therapy.

Finally, under this heading, may be mentioned functional biochemical changes seen in the breath-holding spells of very young children, and, even more commonly, the tetany, numbness and tingling following hyperventilation that commonly occurs in some neurotic adults.

PSYCHOGENIC ATTACKS

The term, 'psychogenic' is preferable to 'hysterical'. The disturbances of behaviour can occur in a variety of psychiatric conditions. For example, some patients with catatonic schizophrenia may have sudden periods of mutism, immobility or outbursts of violence. The temper tantrums and rage attacks of behaviour problem children are also not hysterical, if this term is to be used with its proper psychiatric meaning. The malingerer who simulates attacks, is also a different psychological problem rarely seen in civilian practice. Nevertheless, the commonest forms of psychogenic attacks are hysterical in the sense that they occur in neurotic personalities with other evidence of emotional disturbance, and show evidences of secondary gain. The forms of seizure are very variable, and no typical patterns can be described. In fact, the protean nature of the attacks is one of the diagnostic features. Another important point is that the attacks usually occur when the subject is not alone, and the attention paid to the seizure by others often results in the increase of the violence of the movements or noises made. This interaction of the patient with his immediate environment may occur even when he is seemingly unconscious and with subsequent amnesia for the attack.

THE BORDERLANDS OF EPILEPSY

Particular difficulties can occur when patients have attacks of more than one kind; for example, both epileptic and hysterical seizures, or epilepsy and some other medical cause of attacks, such as diabetes or asthma. These questions lead naturally to a consideration of the borderlands of epilepsy.

The term, 'borderlands of epilepsy', as already mentioned, came into general use after Gowers' (1907) famous little book of more than 70 years ago. At that time it was generally accepted that there was a disease of genuine or idiopathic epilepsy, distinct from symptomatic epilepsy, so that the concept of the borderland of the former condition had some validity. Gowers' little book is still worth reading for the accurate detail and elegant description of conditions which still cause diagnostic confusion. He discusses mainly faints, vaso-vagal attacks, vertigo, migraine and sleep symptoms. To these mainly medical disorders are often added in the borderlands various psychiatric symptoms, such as childhood temper tantrums and other episodic behaviour disorders, hysterical attacks, fugues, and even sometimes non-paroxysmal psychiatric disorders.

Now that all epilepsy is regarded as symptomatic, the question of borderlands has to be looked at rather differently. The unique diagnostic feature of epilepsy is the clinical attack proved to be related to simultaneous neurophysiological disorders of specifically epileptic type. If this diagnosis could be made every time with certainty, then logically there would be no borderlands. Clinical phenomena would either be due to epilepsy or due to some other pathological disturbance.

Until recently the routine scalp EEG was almost the only method of identifying specific epileptic discharges during clinical seizures, but two significant technical advances have widened the scope of recording. The first is the use of telemetry so that recordings can be taken from freely moving subjects. The second is that recording electrodes can now be accurately placed in various parts of the brain and left in situ for many days. For the most part these technical advances have not demonstrated any epileptic basis to the majority of the medical and psychological symptoms listed above. They have tended rather to confirm the epileptic basis of minor disturbances of behaviour and consciousness that were always suspected to be epileptic, anyway.

It must be stressed that only the specific high voltage hypersynchronous discharge typical of epilepsy should be accepted as evidence of an epileptic basis to any particular symptom. The non-specific abnormalities such as bursts of fast and slow (for example, 14 and 6 cycles per second) activity cannot be regarded as giving evidence of an epileptic basis to even paroxysmal symptoms. Such an extension of the concept of epilepsy was for a while particularly popular in the field of child neuropsychiatry. There may certainly be a place for a concept of a non-epileptic paroxysmal cerebral disturbance as a cause of episodic behaviour disturbances, but this is another matter outside the scope of this chapter.

It follows therefore from the above that a classification of episodic phenomena in terms of their relationship to an ictus is a logical way of considering somatic and psychological symptoms in relationship to epilepsy. Table 6.1 will therefore be briefly discussed.

Table 6.1 Relationships between psychiatric symptoms and epileptic attacks

Pre-ictal
1. Epileptic attacks as cause of psychological symptoms – 'Working up to a fit'?
2. Epileptic attacks as effect of psychological conditions:
   a. Specific triggers, e.g. musicogenic epilepsy; self-induced photic stimulation.
   b. Non-specific; e.g. tension, excitement.

Ictal
Loss of consciousness, total or partial
Elementary (and ? complex) sensory experiences (auras).
? Epileptic equivalent.

Post-ictal
Confusional states
'Furores', fugues.

Non-ictal
Non-episodic behaviour disorders, neurotic symptoms.
(Effects of underlying brain damage).
(Effects of medication).

The pre-ictal phase is unique in that the psychological disorders seen may be part cause of the subsequent epileptic attack or part result of whatever physiological disturbance leads to the fit. It is also the least understood period from the neurophysiological point of view. General 'psychological' stress, even if pleasurable, is so often recorded as precipitating epileptic attacks that it has to be accepted, though the evidence is inevitably anecdotal. More interesting and inexplicable are the specific triggers of which musicogenic epilepsy is the best known, though actually rare. Another rare group is formed by those patients (usually children and often subnormal and emotionally disturbed) who discover for themselves the epileptogenic properties of intermittent photic stimulation. It is not certain how far these patients have a different physiological mechanism (as opposed to psychological disposition or attitude) from the much commoner groups of photo-sensitive epileptics where there is no psychological component to the stimulus and its effect is usually unpleasant and actively avoided.

The possibility of a pre-ictal psychological condition being the effect rather than the cause of the subsequent fit has always been raised by the oft repeated observation that some chronic epileptic patients are 'working up to a fit'. It is usually manifested by increasing irritability and tension but no relevant neuro-physiological observations have ever been made even by telemetry and indwelling electrodes so the question remains open.

As regards ictal disorders, it is a safe generalisation that any complex mental state occurring in an epileptic attack has always some disturbance of consciousness. Only brief focal sensory auras may be an exception and they are so ego-alien an experience that the sufferer can give a clear account, and the patients always have (or have had) other forms of epilepsy, so there are few diagnostic difficulties. The situation is, however, confused by the long tradition of the epileptic equivalent or similar term from which the patient is said to suffer in lieu of his usual definite epileptic attacks. The term is even more unwarrantably extended by some to include episodic disturbances of behaviour in persons never having epilepsy – Marchand and Ajuriaguerra's (1948) old but otherwise excellent book is marred by such extensions. The reasoning is fallacious and much harm can result from the wrong diagnosis which may lead to the overlooking of significant psychological factors.

Grand mal status is too characteristic a condition to be misdiagnosed but minor status, i.e. recurrent attacks of petit mal or absence variety, is a rare cause of an apparent confusional state. Its real nature may not be diagnosed without an EEG at the time, though usually there are small fleeting signs such as flickering of the eyelids which may give a clue to the careful observer.

The post-ictal period is one in which occur most episodic psychiatric disturbances seen in people with epilepsy. They may occur after major seizures but are more perplexing after some minor focal cortical attacks, especially of the psychomotor type (that of course most commonly arise from temporal lobe epileptogenic foci). The very name 'psychomotor' bears witness to the frequency with which disturbances occur that on careful observation can be clearly differentiated from the stereotyped movements such as lip-smacking, fumbling and the autonomic changes of the actual ictus. The irregular slow, often asymmetrical and low voltage EEG is best evidence of the post-ictal disturbance of cerebral activity that causes the lowering of cortical control which in turn predisposes to the acting out of psychological stresses. As in the case of the complex aura the abnormal cerebral activity is a necessary but not sufficient cause of the disordered behaviour which is also affected by past experiences, personality factors and the actual situation of the attack. Clumsy attempts at restraint may, for example, lead to the patient lashing out through misinterpreting the actions as assault. Occasionally the post-ictal period may be prolonged up to hours by serial seizures or recurrent brief minor attacks that are difficult to separate from the general confusional state.

The great majority of psychiatric disturbances in persons with epilepsy cannot be related to actual attacks in any of the above ways. They are varied in form and discussed in detail in other parts of this chapter. All that need be noted here is best summarised in Table 6.2 which lists the factors that have to be considered in every case.

Table 6.2 Factors affecting psychological disorders in persons with epilepsy

1. The general genetic or constitutional endowment.
2. The brain damage or disorder which is causing the epileptic attacks.
3. The effects of the epileptic attacks themselves.
4. Past and present psychosocial factors.

REFERENCES

Gowers, W.R. (1907) *The Borderlands of Epilepsy*. London: Churchill.
Marchand, L. & De Ajuriaguerra, J. (1948) *Epilepsies: Leurs formes cliniques, leurs traitments*. Paris: Desclée de Brouwer.

PART THREE
PSYCHOSIS AND EPILEPSY

M. Trimble

INTRODUCTION

The relationship between psychosis and epilepsy has been commented on since antiquity. Early ideas connected epilepsy, madness, possession, and similar states with the moon, and some defined epilepsy as a 'disease of the moon' (Tempkin, 1971). In the nineteenth century the growth of mental hospitals led to an increasing number of patients with epilepsy coming under the care of neuropsychiatrists, and several provided figures specifically on this relationship. Esquirol (1838) reported that of 385 epileptic females, 12 were monomaniacs, 30 were manic, and 34 were furious. Prichard (1822) used the term 'epileptic delirium' to describe phases of insanity in which 'an appearance of maniacal hallucination displayed itself, but more generally the disorder resembles phrenitic delirium'. Morel (1860) introduced the term 'larval epilepsy' for those cases in which there was automatic activity, without necessarily clear loss of consciousness, in which behaviour disturbances occurred including anger, violence and emotional outbursts. Falret (1860) drew attention to the 'more immediate mental prodromes' of epilepsy, and distinguished them from folie épileptique which usually followed epileptic attacks but in some patients actually substituted for them. The suggestion was that the convulsions and the delirium were both manifestations of the same underlying disease process. Hughlings Jackson (1875) also discussed temporary mental disorders after epileptic fits. Observing patients mainly in the wards of general hospitals he introduced the term 'epileptic insanity', and suggested that the epilepsy was the actual cause of the psychiatric disorder. Echeverria (1873) reported that nocturnal epilepsy was more likely to be complicated by insanity than daytime epilepsy, and that hallucinations occurred in 86 per cent of cases, 62 per cent of which were auditory. He divided the types of psychiatric illness into three, namely intermittent, remittent, and continuous.

A comprehensive account of mental states found in epilepsy was first given by Turner (1907). He commented on paroxysmal psychoses which either precede, succeed, or replace the convulsive episodes and which included hallucinatory, delusional, maniacal, melancholic or psychasthenic states. He also commented that a number of epileptic patients passed 'eventually into a state of continued delusional insanity, requiring asylum treatment...'. Although up to that time a number of other authors had commented on the interparoxysmal mental state, the majority of reports were concerned with mental deterioration and epileptic dementia rather than psychotic states per se (Gowers, 1881). Following this, reports of a chronic schizophrenia-like psychosis associated with epilepsy gradually appeared. Slater and Beard (1963) have reviewed the earlier literature on this syndrome. Giese reported six cases in 1914. Gruhle (1936) quoted 23 authors who described individual cases, and commented particularly on the gradual development of a chronic paranoid psychosis in established epileptic patients. He felt that these cases did not represent combinations of two different diseases, but they were truly symptomatic schizophrenias. Glaus (1931) documented 12 cases in detail in which schizophrenia, with paranoid syndromes predominating, occurred.

The increasing use of the EEG and the identification of temporal lobe lesions in association with epilepsy led to the recognition that psychiatric disorders were much commoner in cases with focal temporal lobe epilepsy than in other forms of epilepsy (Gibbs, 1951). Pond (1957) referred to the chronic paranoid-hallucinatory state in epilepsy as a definitive entity, and noted that all patients with this condition had temporal lobe epilepsy with typical complex auras. The epileptic attacks began some years before the psychotic symptoms and the latter often appeared when the epileptic fits were diminishing in frequency. Hill (1953) also commented on this clinical condition again noting the relationship to temporal lobe seizures. Since these descriptions a number of more comprehensive studies have been carried out including those of Slater and Beard (1963), Flor-Henry (1969), Bruens (1971) and Kristensen and Sindrup (1978). These are discussed further below. Although one conclusion to be drawn from these studies is that a relationship between psychosis and epilepsy exists, it is clear that the early authors in particular concentrated on peri-ictal psychotic disorders, and only more recently have chronic inter-ictal states been the subject of major investigation.

An alternative view has been expressed, namely that epilepsy and psychosis are biologically antagonistic (Marchand & Ajuriaguerra, 1948). Von Meduna (1937) initiated convulsive therapy in psychotic disorders on clinical observations that spontaneous seizures were effective in alleviating psychotic symptoms. This seeming paradox was resolved by Davison and Bagley (1969). They suggested that while there is an affinity between the two disorders, there are some individual cases in which an antagonism can be noted between schizophrenic symptoms and convulsions, whether spontaneous or induced. These relationships will now be discussed further.

THE ANTAGONISM HYPOTHESIS

The relationship between psychotic states and epilepsy can thus be subdivided into peri-ictal conditions in which a clear neurophysiological relationship exists between the epileptic seizure and the mental state, and inter-ictal states which are chronic disorders. The peri-ictal psychotic symptoms include ictal hallucinations and related phenomena, and ictal and post-ictal automatisms during which psychopathology may be seen associated with alteration of consciousness. Paranoid ideas and hallucinations may be observed in these states, and the EEG is always abnormal. Often generalised slow activity is seen, although in some patients petit mal status or complex partial seizure status may be reported. In some of these conditions the abnormal behaviour may persist for hours or even days with prolonged states of confusion, automatic behaviour and psychotic experiences.

A different phenomenon was described by Landolt (1958). He recorded changes in the EEG both during preseizure dysphoric episodes and during limited periods of frank psychosis which sometimes lasted days or weeks. During these episodes he noted improvement of a previously abnormal EEG with, what he termed, 'forced normalisation'. At the end of psychotic episodes the EEGs in his patients returned to abnormality. The majority of his cases had temporal lobe epilepsy. Dongier (1959) collected information on 536 psychotic episodes that occurred in 516 epileptic patients. Consciousness was disturbed in 69 per cent, and delusions occurred in 54 per cent. 40 per cent had 'centrencephalic epilepsy', 44 per cent had psychomotor epilepsy. Patients with clouding of consciousness were more likely to have centrencephalic epilepsy than focal or psychomotor epilepsy. A relationship was observed between disturbance of consciousness and the presence of diffuse delta waves or continuous bisynchronous spike-way discharges on the EEG. In 78 cases EEG abnormalities disappeared during the psychosis. 53 per cent of these did not show clouding of consciousness. Delusions in particular were more frequent in patients in whom a pre-existing focal discharge disappeared, and in these patients the duration of the episode was particularly long, sometimes being several weeks. These observations, in addition to a number of documented clinical cases in the literature (see Davison & Bagley, 1969) indicate that it is possible to define a group of patients in which there is a well-defined antagonism between psychotic symptoms and epileptic activity. Both Landolt and Dongier implied a relationship of this phenomenon to temporal lobe epilepsy, and in some of these cases, in particular those described by Landolt, the schizophreniform nature of the mental state was emphasised.

Several different explanations have been put forward to explain these phenomena. Landolt regarded the EEG changes as causal to the development of the psychosis. Reynolds (1968) drew attention to biochemical explanations noting that antiepileptic drugs could precipitate a psychosis, and that epileptic fits could be induced by antipsychotic drugs in schizophrenic patients. In particular he highlighted the relationship between folic acid and both the mental state and seizures, and the ability of antiepileptic drugs to lower folic acid levels. An alternative hypothesis suggested involves dopamine (Trimble, 1977). The most efficacious antipsychotic drugs block dopamine, and drugs such as amphetamine, which are dopamine agonists, can lead to a psychosis indistinguishable from schizophrenia. A number of clinical observations and laboratory experiments have shown that dopamine agonists raise the seizure threshold, and dopamine antagonism decreases it, often provoking seizures (Meldrum Anlezark & Trimble, 1975). There thus appears to be a relationship between psychosis, epilepsy and dopamine such that dopamine antagonism resolves a psychosis but lowers the seizure threshold, whereas dopamine agonism increases the seizure threshold but may provoke or exacerbate psychosis. Alterations of dopamine activity, that may occur spontaneously or result from the administration of antiepileptic or antipsychotic drugs, could thus underlie these clinical observations of antagonism.

ON THE AFFINITY BETWEEN EPILEPSY AND PSYCHOSIS

Neither schizophrenia nor epilepsy are rare disorders, and the appearance of both conditions in the same person may well result from chance. Slater and Beard (1963) estimated the expectation of this coincidence and statistically predicted the number of new cases expected each year in the Greater London Area. In their studies they easily collected 69 fresh cases which they considered to be far in excess of chance. They criticised some earlier papers which had suggested a low prevalence of epilepsy in schizophrenic populations (Bartlet, 1957) on statistical grounds, and suggested that patients who suffered from epilepsy developed a schizophrenia-like illness with a markedly increased frequency. A number of other authors have reported an increased prevalence of epilepsy amongst schizophrenic patients. Kraepelin suggested that epilepsy occurred as a precursor to dementia praecox, and it was noted in around 16 per cent of his cases (Kraepelin, 1919). Yde, Lohse & Faurbye (1941) in 715 patients with schizophrenia noted epilepsy to be twice as common as in the general population.

The most comprehensive study to-date was that of Slater and Beard (1963). They studied 69 patients who had a combination of epilepsy and schizophrenia. 11 had chronic psychosis that had been preceded by recurrent short-lived confu-

sional states, 46 had a psychosis that was 'highly typical of paranoid schizophrenia', and 12 had hebephrenic schizophrenia. In these patients there was no evidence of abnormal premorbid personality or family history of psychiatric disturbance that suggested a predisposition to develop schizophrenia. The mean age of onset of the psychosis was 29.8 years, and it occurred after the epilepsy had been present for a mean of 14.1 years. Although in most patients it was not possible to relate the onset of the mental illness to any change in the quantity or quality of the fits, in some cases the psychotic symptoms appeared when the fit frequency was falling. Nearly all patients had delusions in a setting of clear consciousness, and mystical delusions were common. In a summary of their clinical findings they state that all the cardinal symptoms of schizophrenia were seen at one time or another. However, catatonic phenomena were unusual, affective responses remained warm, and periodic mood swings were noted in most patients. Depressive episodes, although short-lived, could be severe. They were unable to document any relationship between the antiepileptic drugs that the patients were receiving and the subsequent psychotic illness, but noted that the commonest form of epilepsy was temporal lobe epilepsy. Although clinical neurological findings were usually negative, air encephalography, which was carried out on 56 cases, showed abnormalities in 39, usually that of atrophy. In 19 cases there was dilatation of one or both temporal horns.

Bruens (1971) studied 19 epileptic patients with psychotic states, the duration of which varied from 2.5 months to 29 years. Nine cases had a paranoid syndrome with systematised delusions. Hallucinations and delusions were particularly marked in the symptomatology and religious colouration was common. In 16 of the patients temporal lobe epilepsy was noted. A conspicuous sub-group consisted of five cases that showed a temporal focus and bilaterally synchronous spike-wave complexes. He reaffirmed Slater's suggestion that there was a fairly constant interval between the onset of the epilepsy and the onset of the psychosis, and assumed a causal relationship between the two disorders. In contrast to Slater he commented that none of the psychoses noted filled the strict criteria for a diagnosis of schizophrenia, the quality of phenomenology not being typical.

That these sorts of observations are not confined to western cultures is indicated from the studies of Asunti and Pillutla (1967) who found a schizophrenia-like psychosis in 11 out of 42 epileptic patients in Western Nigeria. These patients had many of the characteristics described by Slater and Beard including the preservation of affect, and a correlation between duration of the epilepsy and the onset of the psychosis.

Slater's results were criticised by Stevens (1966) who suggested that the high proportion of patients with temporal lobe epilepsy in this series was an artefact due to sampling in specialised hospitals that deal with difficult cases, and that the formula used for calculation of the probabilities of occurrence of epilepsy and schizophrenia in the general population would not apply to a specifically referred one. In addition she suggested the relationship between the age of onset of the epilepsy and that of schizophrenia was an artefact due to the different ages of onset of the two disorders.

In spite of Stevens' reservations, a number of studies have emphasised further the relationship between temporal lobe abnormalities and psychosis. Gibbs (1951) in a study of 275 cases noted that 17 per cent of patients with anterior temporal spike activity had features of psychosis. Ervin, Epstein & King (1955) noted that in a group of 42 patients with temporal spikes, 34 had received a clinical diagnosis of schizophrenia. The most severe psychiatric disturbances were noted in those with psychomotor seizures. Rodin *et al.*, (1957) presented six cases in detail in which psychomotor epilepsy was associated with 'schizophrenic' symptomatology. Glaser (1964) evaluated 37 patients with psychomotor temporal lobe seizure states who had psychotic episodes lasting from one to many days. He emphasised the disturbances of thought processes with loss of train of associations and word-finding difficulties that occur in these patients. Flor-Henry (1969) undertook a comprehensive but retrospective study of 50 cases of temporal lobe epilepsy who had at one time been classified as psychotic. A non-psychotic control group was also examined. When compared with the controls the schizophreniform psychotics were found to have fewer

psychomotor seizures, and to have epilepsy lateralised particularly to the dominant hemisphere. No overall difference was noted in the incidence of major seizures between the two groups. Of particular interest was the laterality effect that he noted. Thus patients with non-dominant foci tended to be manic depressive as opposed to schizophrenic. These laterality effects were confirmed by Gregoriadis *et al.*, (1971) in a group of 52 hospitalised psychotic-epileptic patients.

Another controlled investigation has recently been undertaken on 192 patients with complex partial seizures and psychosis by Kristensen and Sindrup (1978). They noted that the fit frequency for complex partial seizures was lower in the psychotic group, and that an interval with a median of 18 years occurred between the onset of the epilepsy and the psychosis. They subdivided their patients depending on whether the seizures were accompanied by automatisms, or epigastric aura, or were 'superficially initiated' (psychical seizures). In the psychotic group there was a significantly greater number of patients with automatisms. Clinical neurological and otoneurological examination showed a greater proportion of psychotic patients to have findings indicative of an organic brain lesion.

Summarising the evidence presented, it would seem that many authors have shown a relationship between complex partial seizures and chronic inter-ictal psychotic illness. In particular a paranoid schizophreniform picture appears to result. The precise relationship of this to process schizophrenia has to be clarified. There seems to be a relationship in some patients between the emergence of the psychosis and the diminishing frequency of seizures, another manifestation of antagonism. Dominant hemisphere lesions are more likely to produce these effects. It should be noted that there are a number of reports which have failed clearly to detect this association (Stevens, 1975; Small & Small, 1967). However, many of these have used rating scales to assess psychopathology which, while useful from the point of view of assessing personality, are not designed as diagnostic tools. In addition, as Flor-Henry (1976) points out, these often have studied epileptic populations, and since the incidence of schizophrenia in partial seizures is small, larger samples would be needed for statistically significant relationships to be detected.

A number of different explanations have been put forward to explain the association between chronic psychosis and epilepsy. The majority of them take as their starting point the now established relationship between temporal lobe-limbic system mechanisms and affective experiences. There are two main contrasting hypotheses. The first is that the schizophrenia-like illnesses are epileptic in origin and should be referred to as 'epileptic psychoses'. The second is that they are a manifestation of organic neurological damage and thus not specific for epilepsy. The former view has been most strongly expressed by Flor-Henry (1969). Criticising the absence of a control population in some of the older studies, noting the constant observation of an inverse relationship between frequency of psychomotor seizures and the onset of the psychosis, and commenting on the laterality effect that he noted, he suggested that it was not structural damage, but the characteristics of the seizures that lead to the clinical picture. Continuing abnormal epileptic neuronal activity was thought to be responsible therefore for the schizophrenic syndrome. Support for this suggestion comes from depth electrode studies in psychotic patients who do not have epilepsy. Abnormal activity in the deep temporal structures is associated with suppression of surface cortical activity, and when patients are psychotic abnormal spike wave activity may be detected in these areas, which is not seen on conventional surface electrodes (Heath, 1977).

The alternative position was taken by Slater and Beard (1963). They noted a significant proportion of the psychotic patients had a defined organic basis for their epilepsy, and that the onset of the psychosis was related to the duration of the epilepsy. Their conclusion stressed the importance of an underlying structural lesion in the temporal lobe. A similar view was taken by Kristensen and Sindrup (1978). Kiloh (1971) made the point that almost any diffuse brain disease may on occasion be associated with a similar clinical picture and epilepsy is often not present. He suggested the psychoses were a reflection of a certain stage of what, in the long run, was a dementing process. Follow-up studies of such patients do not however lend support to this view. Bruens (1971) put forward the idea that both organic and psychodynamic events potentiate each other. The patient is unable to protect himself against the vicissitudes of life except by using pathological defence mechanisms, which result in psychosis. Pond (1962), suggested it was the abnormal experiences associated with temporal lobe epilepsy which gradually became integrated into a person's psychic life that led to the development of the psychosis. However these explanations do not account for the laterality findings, and as Slater and Beard point out, do not take into account the volitional disturbances, thought disorder, and hebephrenic symptoms noted in these patients.

Symonds (1962) pointed to the 'epileptic disorder of function'. He suggested that the loss of balance between excitation and inhibition at synaptic junctions leads not only to the paroxysmal phenomena of epilepsy, but also that the 'continuous disorder of neuronal function' leads to inter-ictal symptoms, the nature of which will be related to the site of the focal activity. It was, he suggested, not the loss of neurones in the temporal lobe that was responsible for the psychosis, but the disorderly activity of those that remain. However if there does exist a number of years between the beginning of the epilepsy and the onset of the psychosis, as some of the studies suggest, modification of this idea may be necessary. The discovery in experimental neurophysiology of kindling may provide an important link here. Thus it is extremely difficult to kindle epileptic seizures in certain parts of the limbic system, particularly those that are catecholaminergic. Kindling of the mesolimbic dopamine system leads not to seizures, but to marked behaviour changes which persist after the kindling has ceased (Stevens and Livermore, 1978). The possibility arises that in man similar mechanisms exist such that chronic subictal activity leads to a kindling process within dopaminergic pathways, overactivity in which leads to the development of abnormal behaviour patterns and psychosis. In that the behaviour changes associated with kindling of the mesolimbic dopamine system are enhanced by the administration of dopamine agonists, it is probable that the kindling itself is associated with altered post-synaptic function of dopamine receptors. As noted, increased dopamine activity tends to increase the seizure threshold. As with the mechanism of antagonism discussed above, these neurophysiological observations may be invoked to explain the clinical findings of an association between persistent abnormal temporal lobe activity and psychosis, and the tendency of its development to be associated with a declining seizure frequency.

TREATMENT AND PROGNOSIS

Psychoses associated with peri-ictal disturbances require that the patient is observed during the episode to make sure that he comes to no harm. The use of psychotropic drugs is often not indicated. Major tranquillisers such as phenothiazines and butyrophenomes are contraindicated in these situations as they may lead to further seizures and aggravation of the behaviour problem. If tranquillisation is required benzodiazepines or chlormethiazole are more appropriate. Aggressive outbursts are rarely ictal, and usually occur as the result of the injudicious use of restraint of patients in a confusional state. In that the mental state returns to normal during the inter-ictal phase, control of the epilepsy and prevention of further episodes needs the most attention. Where anti-epileptic drug therapy is inadequate this must be regulated, but where compliance is a problem rationalisation of therapy such that the patient is taking the minimal number of doses on the minimal number of occasions is imperative.

For the inter-ictal psychoses psychotropic drugs are the treatment of choice. If there appears to be a reciprocal relationship between the onset of the psychosis and diminution of seizure frequency then gradual reduction of the antiepileptic drugs with the addition of psychotropic drugs should be undertaken. Although major tranquillisers, such as chlorpromazine (Largactil) or haloperidol (Haldol), are known to lower the seizure threshold, their therapeutic potential may reside in this process. If it is the patient's mental state which is causing the greatest problems in management, rather than the seizures, then it is more logical to treat that accordingly. It is important to monitor serum antiepileptic levels following the administration of major tranquillisers since they interfere with the metabolism of the antiepileptic drugs, and toxicity, with worsening of the behaviour problem, can readily be provoked. Development of affective symptoms will require the administration of antidepressants and, where clinically indicated, ECT should be administered. In long-term management, especially where the clinical picture is accompanied by dysphoric and recurrent depressive mood changes, the use of carbamazepine (Tegretol) as an anticonvulsant may be helpful. Monotherapy is preferable to polytherapy.

The only series to study outcome of these disorders was that of Slater and Beard (1963). They followed up their patients 2–25 years after the onset of the psychotic illness. 18 of their patients were in hospital, but 30 lived permanently at home. The outcome appeared better than in 'process' schizophrenia and their employment record was surprisingly good. The epilepsy tended to become less troublesome and one-third had obtained a complete remission from their specifically schizophrenia-like symptoms. 11 of the patients had a temporal lobectomy and in eight of them the schizophrenic symptoms receded.

REFERENCES

Asunti, T. & Pillutla, V.S. (1967) Schizophrenia-like psychoses in Nigerian epileptics. *British Journal of Psychiatry*, **113**, 1375.

Bartlet, J.E.A. (1957) Chronic psychosis following epilepsy. *American Journal of Psychiatry*, **114**, 338.

Bruens, J.H. (1971). Psychosis in Epilepsy *Psychiatria Neurologia Neurochiurgia*, **74**, 175.

Davison, K. & Bagley, C.R. (1969) Schizophrenia-like psychoses associated with organic disorders of the central nervous system. In Herrington, R.N. (ed.) *Current Problems in Neuropsychiatry*, p. 113. Kent: Headley Brothers.

Dongier, S. (1959) Statistical study of clinical and electroencephalographic manifestations of 536 psychotic episodes occurring in 516 epileptics between clinical seizures.
Epilepsia, **1**, 117.

Echeverria, M.G. (1873). On epileptic insanity. *American Journal of Insanity*, **30**, 1.

Ervin, F., Epstein, A.W. & King, H.E. (1955). Behaviour of epileptic and non-epileptic patients with temporal spikes. *Archives of Neurology and Psychiatry*, **74**, 488.

Esquirol, E. (1838). *Des maladies mentales*. Paris.

Falret, J. (1860). De L'état mental des épileptiques. *Achives générales de medicine*, **16**, 661.

Flor-Henry, P. (1969). Psychosis and temporal lobe epilepsy. *Epilepsia*, **10**, 363.

Flor-Henry, P. (1976) Epilepsy and psychopathology. In Granville-Grossman, K. (ed.) *Recent Advances in Clinical Psychiatry, Vol. 2*. Edinburgh: Churchill Livingstone.

Gibbs, F.A. (1951). Ictal and non-ictal psychiatric disorders in temporal lobe epilepsy. *Journal of Nervous and Mental Disease*, **113**, 522.

Glaser, G.H. (1964). The problem of psychosis in psychomotor temporal lobe epileptics. *Epilepsia*, **5**, 271.

Gruhle, H.W. (1936) Ueber den Wahn bei Epilepsie Zeitschrift ges Neurol Psychiat., **154**, 395.

Glaus, A. (1931). Ueber Cominationen von Schizophrenie und Epilepsie *Zeitschrift für diegesante neurologie und psychiatrie*, **135**, 450.

Gowers, W.R. (1881). *Epilepsy and other chronic convulsive disease*. London.

Gregoriadis, A., Fragos, E., Kapsalakis, Z. & Mandouralos, B. (1971). A correlation between mental disorders and EEG and AEG findings in temporal lobe epilepsy. *Proceeedings of the Vth World Congress of Psychiatry*, Mexico.

Heath, R.G. (1977) Subcortical Brain Function Correlates of Psychopathology and Epilepsy. In Shagass, C., Gershon, S. & Friedhoff, A.J. *Psychopathology and Brain Dysfunction*, 51. New York: Raven Press.

Hill, D. (1953). Psychiatric disorders of epilepsy. *The Medical Press*, **229**, 473.

Jackson, J.H. (1958). On temporary mental disorders after epileptic paroxysms (1875) Reprinted in Taylor, J. (ed.) *Selected Writings of John Hughlings Jackson*, Vol. 1. London: Staples Press.

Kiloh, L.G. (1971) Psychiatric aspects of epilepsy. In Winton, R.R. (ed.) *Geigy Symposium on Epilepsy*. Australia: Geigy.

Kraepelin, E. (1919). *Dementia Praecox and Paraphrenia* Edinburgh: Livingstone.

Kristensen, O. & Sindrup, E.H. (1978). Psychomotor epilepsy and psychosis. *Acta Neurologica Scandanavica*, **57**, 361.

Landolt, H. (1958). Serial encephalographic investigations during psychotic episodes in epileptic patients and during schizophrenic attacks. In Lorentz de Haas (ed.) *Lectures on Epilepsy*. London: Elsevier.

Marchand, L. & De Ajuriaguerra, J. (1948). *Epilepsies: Leurs formes Cliniques, Leur traitements* Paris: Desclée de Brouwer.

Meldrum, B., Anlezark, A. & Trimble, M. (1975). Drugs modifying dopamine activity and behaviour, the EEG and epilepsy in Papio papio. *European Journal of Pharmacology*, **32**, 203.

Morel, B.A. (1860). D'une forme de délire, suite d'une surexcitation nerveuse se rattachant à une variété non ecore décrite d'épilepsie. *Gazette Hebdoma daire de médecine et de Chirurgie*, **7**, 773.

Pond, D.A. (1957). Psychiatric aspects of epilepsy *Journal of the Indian Medical Profession*, **3**, 1441.

Pond, D. (1962). The schizophrenia-like psychoses of epilepsy – Discussion *Proceedings of the Royal Society of Medicine*, **55**, 311.

Prichard, J.C. (1822). *A Treatise on Diseases of the Nervous System*. London.

Reynolds, E.H. (1968). Epilepsy and schizophrenia. Relationship and biochemistry. *Lancet*, **1**, 398.

Rodin, E.A., De Jong, R.N., Waggoner, R.W. & Bagchi, B.K. (1957). Relationship between certain forms of psychomotor epilepsy and schizophrenia. *Archives of Neurology and Psychiatry*, **77**, 449.

Slater, E. & Beard, A.W. (1963). The schizophrenia-like psychoses of epilepsy. *British Journal of Psychiatry*, **109**, 95.

Small, J.G. & Small, I.F. (1967). A controlled study of mental disorders associated with epilepsy. *Recent Advances in Biological Psychiatry*, **9**, 171.

Stevens, J.R. (1966). Psychiatric implications of psychomotor epilepsy. *Archives of General Psychiatry*, **14**, 461.

Stevens, J.R. (1975). Inter-ictal clinical manifestations of complex partial seizures. In Penry, J.K. & Daly, D.D. (eds) *Advances in Neurology, Vol. II*. New York: Raven Press.

Stevens, J.R. & Livermore, A. (1978). Kindling in the mesolimbic dopamine system: animal model of psychosis. *Neurology*, **28**, 36.

Symonds, C. (1962). The schizophrenia-like psychoses of epilepsy – Discussion *Proceedings of the Royal Society of Medicine*, **55**, 311.

Tempkin, O. (1971) *The falling sickness*. Baltimore: Johns Hopkins Press.

Trimble, M.R. (1977). The relationship between epilepsy and schizophrenia: A biochemical hypothesis. *Biological Psychiatry*, **12**, 299.

Turner, W.A. (1907). *Epilepsy: A Study of the Idiopathic Disease*. New York: Macmillan and Co.

Von Meduna, L. (1937). *Die Konvulsiontherapie der schizophrenie*. Halle Marhold.

Yde, A., Lohse, E. & Faurbye. A. (1941) On the relationship between schizophrenia, epilepsy and induced convulsions. *Acta Psychiatrica Scandanavica*, **16**, 325.

7

Neuropsychology

C.B. Dodrill

INTRODUCTION

As applied to the study of human beings, *neuro-psychology* evaluates ability, personality, and behavioural correlates of brain lesions and other pathological conditions affecting the nervous system. It is a discipline arising from both neurology and psychology. From neurology, information is obtained about the central nervous system. From psychology, the techniques of precision in measurement are borrowed. Neuropsychology rests on the assumptions that the brain is systematically organised, that the behaviour of the organism is related to the condition of the brain, and that an index of the condition of the brain can be inferred by evaluating carefully the behaviour and abilities of the organism. It is also assumed that the neurological status of the brain will determine how far deficits may affect the organism's future activities. The two questions that neuropsychology asks for any patient are, 'What, if any, neurological dysfunction or impairment in brain functions exists?' and 'What impact will such a condition have upon performance in daily life?'

Neuropsychology is of immense importance in the total evaluation of the individual with epilepsy. By definition, an individual with a seizure disorder has a brain which is dysfunctional, at least intermittently. Furthermore it is known that in most cases one can detect the presence of a seizure disorder by means of multiple EEGs, all of which may be recorded interictally. When a patient is referred for an EEG it is not expected that a clinically obvious attack will be recorded, and such is not necessary to confirm the presence of a seizure disorder. This fact is well known to physicians but its significance with respect to neuropsychology is generally overlooked. It means that abnormal brain functioning persists between attacks in individuals with epilepsy. In addition, no one would dispute the contention that the brain is the seat of abilities. It is therefore reasonable to expect alteration in abilities not just during but also between attacks and it is also reasonable to assume that such alterations may affect a person's performance in daily life.

The purposes of this chapter are to describe the basics of neuropsychological assessment and to summarise some of the research which correlates important variables related to epilepsy with impairment in brain functions as identified by neuropsychological tests. The nature of neuropsychological evaluations will first be discussed, and will be followed by a partial review of the literature dealing with neuropsychological testing. Finally, a neuropsychological battery developed specifically for the evaluation of epilepsy will be presented and its use illustrated.

THE NATURE OF NEUROPSYCHOLOGICAL EVALUATION

The brain is an extremely complex organ which has many functions. Therefore it is readily apparent that one cannot evaluate fully the intactness of the brain without also evaluating many of these functions. It was on this basis that many years ago Halstead (1947) perceived that a full battery of tests was needed in order to make even reasonably adequate comments about brain functioning. Although this may seem elementary, it underlines that clinical neuropsychological evaluation can make a major contribution by a careful, detailed, and systematic evaluation of brain functions. There is no way, for example, that a professional can hope to obtain even a semi-adequate assessment of brain functions by having a patient draw a few figures. Furthermore, it is simply not possible to obtain an adequate index of recovery from a brain insult such as a severe head injury by merely talking to a patient and performing the simplest of memory, perceptual, and motor tests. Yet, these judgements are made every day on the basis of obviously inadequate observations. A valid systematic evaluation must be made of a broad range of functions including memory (both verbal and nonverbal), ability to attend to the task, motor skills, perceptual abilities (auditory, visual, tactile), cognition, visuo-spatial functions, and language-related abilities.

Although the evaluation of a broad range of abilities is important, more is required for a thorough neuropsychological evaluation. Such tests should provide information which can be used in complementary ways in order to relate neurological problems to those of adjustment. The majority of tests used by psychologists (such as tests of intelligence) provide only an indication of level of performance. This is important because it gives information about how a person compares with others and it is therefore used in neuropsychological testing. However, a person may perform poorly for a variety of reasons, only one of which may be because of brain injury or impairment in brain functions. One cannot, for example, say that an individual is necessarily brain damaged simply because of low intelligence although brain damage is found more often in those who are mentally deficient.

Because of the limitations in assessing only the level of performance, three other approaches to dealing with neuropsychological test information have been developed in detail by Reitan (1969) and are employed regularly. Briefly, the first of these compares the relative performances of the right and left sides of the body. This approach is borrowed from neurology where it is regularly employed. It has the important advantage of using the patient as his own control and may show up definitely pathological defects of performance. The second additional approach demonstrates specific signs of neurological deficit such as dys-

phasia or constructional dyspraxia which may have diagnostic value. The absence of such specific signs does not mean, of course, that mental function is necessarily normal. Finally, the information provided by a full neuropsychological battery allows for a pattern analysis from which may be inferred the nature, location and extent of the brain damage and the impact which it is likely to have upon functioning in life. The extent to which inferences about neurological problems can be made has been documented by Reitan (1964) who, using these complementary methods of neurological inference, was able to show a striking ability to define extent, location, and type of lesion based solely upon neuropsychological test findings and with no reference whatever to the history. The ability to make such inferences from neuropsychological test results is not widely known. However in my opinion this should not be the major function of neuropsychology, which should focus instead upon the impact of lesions upon performance in life. Nevertheless it is important to appreciate that accurate inferences about the nature of lesions can be made providing that one has sufficiently sensitive tests and that a sufficiently detailed evaluation is carried out.

In 1935, Halstead established the first full-time neuropsychological laboratory for the study of the effects of brain lesions upon human beings. In his work, he soon recognised the validity of the matters just discussed and set out to develop a comprehensive battery of neuropsychological tests, each of which would be sensitive to problems of brain function and which when taken together could provide a basis for making valid inferences about the condition of the brain. The many tests that he used are described in his monumental work, *Brain and Intelligence* (Halstead, 1947). Of these tests, five were finally adopted for use by Reitan and are perhaps among those test measures which are best validated and most widely used by neuropsychologists today.

Category Test. This is a complex test of problem solving ability. It uses a slide projecter which presents figures on the back of a milk-glass screen. In each of seven groups, the patient must determine what principle underlies correct responses and feedback is obtained about whether answers are right or wrong by a bell and a buzzer, respectively. The test evaluates a patient's ability to solve problems, to adapt to new and different situations, and to utilise effectively feedback given about the correctness of responses. The score is the number of items out of 208 which are incorrect.

Tactile Performance Test. This test employs a form of the Seguin-Goddard form board. The patient is blindfolded before the test begins and does not see the board at any time. The task is to put a series of blocks into the proper spaces on the board first using only the preferred hand, then only the non-preferred hand, then both hands taken together. The time required for each trial is recorded as well as the total for all three trials. After the task is over, the blocks and board are removed and the patient is required to draw a picture of the board putting in as many blocks as can be remembered and also trying to put them in the drawing where they were on the board. Both the number of blocks remembered (Memory Component) and the number correctly localised (Localisation Component) are indicators of 'incidental memory' since the patient is not forewarned that a picture of the board will be required at the end of the test. Like the Category Test, this test requires a substantial ability to solve problems and adapt to a novel situation with a strong emphasis upon tactile, kinaesthetic, motor, and visuo-spatial skills.

Seashore Rhythm Test. Thirty pairs of rhythmic beats are presented by a tape recorder and the subject must indicate whether the rhythms within each pair are the same or whether they are different. The test seems to require sustained attention to the task and ability to perceive and deal with non-verbal stimuli.

Speech-sounds Perception Test. Nonsense words are given over a tape recorder and the patient must select from four alternatives the word that is said. The words all have beginning and ending consonants with a central 'ee' vowel sound. This test evaluates auditory discrimination of verbal materials.

Finger Oscillation (Finger Tapping) Test. This test uses a manual tapper and the patient propels a key up and down as rapidly as possible. Several ten-second trials are averaged for the index finger of each hand. This test appears to be rather purely dependent upon motor speed.

In addition to these tests, Reitan added some additional measures and those usually used with adults include the following:

Aphasia Screening Test. This is Reitan's modification of the Halstead-Wepman Aphasia Screening test (Halstead & Wepman, 1949) which provides for the assessment of a number of types of aphasia and apraxia. The test requires the patient to name, spell, read, write, pronounce, calculate, and so on. The results are evaluated for specific signs of neurological deficit.

Trail Making Test. This test consists of two parts. In Part A, a person merely draws lines connecting circles numbered 1 to 25 in order. Part B requires the alternation of numbers and letters in an ordered fashion. This test appears to require the ability to keep more than one aspect of the stimulus situation in mind and to think flexibly in going from one type of stimuli to the next.

Lateral Dominance Examination. This test is used primarily to evaluate preference in handedness but it also includes a measure of grip strength with a hand dynamometer and an indicator of name writing speed. These two last test measures are obtained for both the preferred and non-preferred hands.

In addition to the above test measures, Reitan also included a general measure of intelligence and one of emotional functioning. For adults, these tests are the Wechsler-Bellevue Intelligence Scale (or Wechsler Adult Intelligence Scale) and the Minnesota Multiphasic Personality Inventory (MMPI). These are also regularly used in our evaluation of epileptic patients.

The above series of tests is used in many places around the world and is generally known as the Halstead-Reitan Neuropsychological Battery. Except for instances in which general measures of intelligence are used alone, this battery appears to have been applied more often to the evaluation of those with seizure disorders than any other. Representative studies which have used the battery will now be reviewed.

NEUROPSYCHOLOGICAL CORRELATES OF SEIZURE HISTORY VARIABLES

Most of these investigations reported in the literature have used measures of intelligence alone. However, such tests were never designed to evaluate the adequacy of brain functions and do not do so as well as the more specialised neuropsychological test measures. Since complete reviews of the performances of epileptic patients on tests of intelligence have already been published (Lennox & Lennox, 1960; Tarter, 1972) detailed findings of results already well known will not be given here.

Aetiology

The results of a long series of studies summarised by Tarter (1972) indicate that individuals with seizure disorders of known aetiology average approximately 5–10 fewer IQ points than those whose aetiology is unknown. In a more detailed study using the Halstead-Reitan approach, Kløve and Matthews (1966) found that individuals with epilepsy of known aetiology consistently performed more poorly than persons who had seizures of unknown aetiology but that in most cases the differences did not reach statistical significance. Of the tests described above, only the Trail Making Test, the Tactile Performance Test (Time Component) and the Halstead Impairment Index (a summary measure of performance on the Halstead tests) produced statistically significant differences. This study is perhaps the most carefully controlled one in the literature and it suggests that it is only with respect to motor and psychomotor problem-solving tasks that aetiology makes a consistent and reliable difference. One should recall in fact that the majority of tests of intelligence have a standard error of approximately five points so that this much fluctuation may be expected from one administration to the next without indicating any real differences between patient groups. This finding argues against overgeneralisation and over-interpretation of research findings.

Age at onset and duration of disorder

In general, studies have suggested that the earlier the age at onset and the longer duration, the lower the abilities. The differences demonstrated, however, are usually modest with some suggestion that

they are greatest in cases with generalised tonic-clonic attacks (DeHaas & Magnus, 1958; Lennox & Lennox, 1960). Using the general Halstead-Reitan approach, Dikmen, Matthews, and Harley (1975) considered only individuals with major motor seizures and only the extreme groups of age at onset (age 0–5, age 17–50). Statistically reliable differences on 9 of 14 variables appeared between these groups which always favoured the group with the later age at onset. Even under these rather ideal circumstances for producing statistically significant differences, however, the differences were modest and it is not clear that many would have been found had the full range of individuals been evaluated including those with age at onset 6–16 years. Intellectual and psychomotor problem-solving tasks produced the greatest differences.

The minimal nature of positive findings with these variables is further confirmed by work done in our own epilepsy centre with a diverse group of 305 adult epileptic patients. A statistically significant relationship was demonstrated between the age at onset and the Wechsler Adult Intelligence Scale Full Scale IQ with a correlation of 0.24 ($p < 0.001$) but no relationship was demonstrated with the Halstead Impairment Index (correlation of 0.00). The duration of the disorder was not significantly related to the WAIS Full Scale IQ (correlation of -0.07) but a significant relationship was found with the Halstead Impairment Index (correlation of 0.22 ($p < 0.001$). Although some of these findings are statistically reliable, it is apparent that they account for only a small fraction of the variation in performance scores (about 4 per cent). Thus, *when people with epilepsy are considered as a whole*, these relationships are clearly not potent ones.

Seizure type

Some studies have found no general relationship between seizure type and mental abilities whereas others have demonstrated decreased mental functions in those having primarily tonic-clonic attacks. Rarely has it been possible to show decreased intelligence in association with petit mal absences although difficulties with other types can usually be demonstrated (Lennox & Lennox,

1960). In the most complete neuropsychological evaluation that has been done, Matthews and Kløve (1967) simultaneously considered the question of aetiology and seizure type among adults having primarily complex partial seizures, primarily generalised tonic-clonic seizures, or both. In general, individuals with major attacks did more poorly than those with complex partial seizures, and those with known aetiology did worse than those with unknown aetiology. In this study, seizure type was more potent than aetiology in its correlation with performance but the two factors together showed the greatest differences in scores.

Seizure frequency

Although one might expect that decreased performance might be associated with increasing seizure frequency, the literature shows no such consistent trend. In the one detailed neuropsychological study which considered the question, Dikmen and Matthews (1977) used only patients with major motor attacks and demonstrated a small number of differences favouring persons with fewer attacks. It appears highly likely that had persons other than those with major motor seizures been included, no such relationships would have been demonstrated. In my own laboratory, I was able to determine reliably seizure incidence in 258 heterogeneous adult epileptic patients and found seizure incidence for the last 30 days to be correlated 0.10 ($p > 0.05$) with the Halstead Impairment Index and 0.00 with WAIS Full Scale IQ. Thus, there was no general relationship between seizure frequency and performance.

Research on the above variables is somewhat discouraging to review since only very modest relationships are found in the majority of instances. This underlines the complexity of measuring performance, and the need for caution in interpreting and explaining results.

PERFORMANCE AND ANTIEPILEPTIC DRUGS

Every physician dealing with epilepsy has received reports from patients on antiepileptic drugs which suggest that the medication may have some effect on their ability to think, remember, and perform in daily life. Many efforts have therefore been made to evaluate formally the effects of antiepileptic drugs upon performance. In examining these studies, one should be aware of four limiting factors. Firstly, the use of normals in antiepileptic drug studies produces results of limited general applicability since it is not clear that normals respond to the drugs as do individuals who have taken them chronically. Secondly, changes in drug regimens are often accompanied by changes in seizure frequencies and the net effects may be confounded. Thirdly, the use of a placebo in comparison with an active agent is not an effective technique for evaluating changes in performance even though it may be an effective approach for evaluating changes in seizure frequency. The reason for this is that such studies, by definition, compare an active agent with an inactive one and, since the addition of active agents in general tends to decrease performance, the outcome of the study with respect to tests of performance (not seizure frequency) is predictable to a considerable degree before the study is begun. Finally, the majority of studies that have been done evaluating the effects of antiepileptic drugs have used only one test as a measure of performance and so a pattern of deficits is not shown. This is particularly important since our own studies over a decade have demonstrated patterns of difficulties associated with each drug.

The neuropsychological impacts of phenytoin (Dilantin) are of special interest because of the wide use of this drug. In one study, Matthews and Harley (1975) evaluated the effects of this drug in combination with those of primidone and phenobarbitone and classified patients as toxic or non-toxic based upon serum levels. Differences favouring the non-toxic group appeared on a few measures of attention and concentration, on indicators of motor coordination, and on static tremor. Dodrill (1975a) studied patients who were on phenytoin alone and compared those with high and low serum levels above and below 120 μmol/1 (30 μg/ml) as well as those who were clinically classed as toxic or non-toxic. A series of results from this study pointed to decreased *motor* performance with increased serum levels and toxicity. However, no other functions were affected. This study is remarkable in that no other antiepileptic drugs were involved and also because the high serum level group had a very high average level of 172 μmol/l (43 μg/ml) which should have made it easier to demonstrate other mental deficits.

The other antiepileptic drug which has received the most attention is phenobarbitone. Somerfeld-Ziskind and Ziskind (1940) demonstrated no decreased mental ability when the administration of phenobarbitone was compared with a control epileptic group which essentially was untreated. In fact, mental age as evaluated by the Stanford-Binet Intelligence Scale actually increased in the group given phenobarbitone. However, the number of seizures experienced by that group was substantially less than that by the other. This study illustrates the pervasive finding that despite any adverse effects which may be associated with antiepileptic drugs, it is routinely better to administer these agents and stop the seizures than not to do so. In a well-executed study with normals, Hutt et al. (1968) found that increasing phenobarbitone serum levels was associated with decreased performances on tasks requiring sustained attention, psychomotor performance, and spontaneous speech. These findings are consistent with those of the study by Matthews and Harley (1975) and it is suggested that phenobarbitone has effects maximally evident on tasks requiring sustained attention, but that it may have effects on motor coordination as well.

Carbamazepine is another drug which has received some attention because of its presumed 'psychotropic' effects. Dalby (1975) reviewed approximately 40 studies and found evidence for such an effect in approximately half of these. Most commonly reported was improvement in mood and behaviour as well as reduced aggression and irritability and a possible decrease in depression. However, these conclusions were based on subjective observations rather than objective testing. Rodin, Rim, and Rennick (1974) used a double-blind placebo versus carbamazepine design and demonstrated some loss in ability with carbamazepine. Dodrill and Troupin (1977) used a

battery of neuropsychological tests with a single agent double-blind cross-over design and compared carbamazepine with phenytoin. With seizure control about the same by either drug, some limited improvements in performance with carbamazepine were observed on mental tasks requiring problem solving and sustained attention. Emotional status and personality adjustment as evaluated by the MMPI also showed slight improvement. It was observed that duller persons and those with more extensive psychiatric problems improved the most with carbamazephine. The changes appeared to be due to starting cambamazepine rather than the stopping of phenytoin.

Studies related to other antiepileptic drugs may be mentioned briefly. One study of methoin (mephenytoin) demonstrated that there was slightly better attention to a task with methoin than with phenytoin (Troupin, Ojeman & Dodrill, 1976). Sodium valproate is only now coming under detailed scrutiny in the United States and therefore very little can be said about it at the present time in terms of performance correlates. Although some studies already exist in the current literature none have appeared which have used it as a sole antiepileptic drug, and studies which have contrasted it with a placebo cannot be used to support the contention that it is associated with decreased performance.

Over several years of working specifically with antiepileptic drugs and their effects, I have observed that when antiepileptic drug serum levels fall within therapeutic ranges and when there are no overt signs of toxicity, it is rarely possible to demonstrate performance deficits due to the medication. A review of all of the studies reveals only one (Dodrill, 1975b) in which there were truly striking differences in performance when two different groups of drugs were administered. This agent, sulthiame, is not used in the United States and apparently is used elsewhere only in combination with other drugs. In general, the effect on performance correlates with antiepileptic drugs is less than with the other variables discussed in this chapter. In certain cases, of course, there may be unusual protein binding or metabolic interactions of significance. However, unless there are at least slight clinical signs of toxicity, it is unlikely that drugs can be shown to cause performance difficulties.

THE NEUROPSYCHOLOGICAL BATTERY FOR EPILEPSY

All of the neuropsychological tests discussed previously have been developed and standardised on groups of patients with a variety of neurological disorders and none was designed specifically for work with people with epilepsy. Thus, the effects of medication for seizures, seizures themselves, and the correlates of important EEG variables were not considered in the development of the tests. As a matter of fact, the majority of tests thus far described were developed before it was apparent that such variables would affect performance significantly. Further, no one has developed normal standards for people with epilepsy on even these tests, nor were sex differences taken into account. Existing neuropsychological batteries and even the Halstead-Reitan Neuropsychological Battery covered poorly the difficulties often complained of by patients, such as problems with memory or sustaining attention to a task.

These considerations led me to believe that the development of a Neuropsychological Battery for Epilepsy would be of assistance in dealing with patients having seizure disorders. The full development of this neuropsychological battery has been reported (Dodrill, 1978). Briefly, the deficits noted clinically with this group were catalogued together with the difficulties in performance documented from studies of the effects of seizures upon performance, of drugs, and of the correlates of important EEG variables. In pilot, principal, and cross-validation studies, approximately 100 prospective neuropsychological variables were reduced to 16 which had been tested for their ability to pin-point deficits associated with epilepsy, for a lack of overlap with one another, and for general applicability to normal and patient groups. These 16 test measures, known as discriminative measures because of their ability to differentiate those with, from those without epilepsy, include six from Halstead's Neuropsychological Battery, five from the tests that Reitan added, and the following additional tests.

Stroop Test. This is a test of reading rate and sustained attention to the task. A colour plate is used which has printed on it colour names (red, green, blue, orange) each of which is always printed in an incongruous colour. Thus, 'red' may be printed in green, blue, or orange, and 'green' may be printed in red, blue, or orange. In Part I of this test, the person reads through the words as quickly as possible, ignoring the colours in which they are printed. The time required is one of the discriminative measures. In Part II, the person must give the colour of the print while ignoring the word. This latter task proves to be extremely difficult for most people and for those with brain problems it is exceptionally hard. When the time required for Part I is subtracted from that for Part II, a measure of 'static' or interference is identified which appears to be an indicator of distractibility. This is also a discriminative measure.

Wechsler Memory Scale. The Logical Memory and Visual Reproduction portions of the Wechsler Memory Scale (Form I) are administered, since they have been previously used as indicators of verbal and non-verbal memory (Milner, 1975). In the verbal test, the person repeats as much as possible of two short stories which are given orally and the number of elements recalled is recorded. In the non-verbal (Visual Reproduction) portion, four drawings are reproduced after ten-second exposures and a single score is provided.

Seashore Tonal Memory Test. This test is somewhat like the Seashore Rhythm Test used by Halstead. A series of notes is played twice and in the second playing one note is changed. The patient must identify which note is changed in each of 30 trials. This is a harder test than the Seashore Rhythm Test and appears to evaluate sustained attention to the task.

Using all 16 test measures, norms were established for a highly diverse group of adult epileptic patients. For each of the 16 tests, a point was found in the performances of the control group below which approximately 25 per cent of these individuals scored. This was established as a 'cut-off' point and scores below this point were said to fall outside normal limits. In general, between 60 and 70 per cent of epileptic patients fall in this range. For an individual of average intelligence, the interpretation of the battery rests in some part upon the total number of tests falling outside normal limits and the following standards are used as general guidelines.

Within normal limits. 0–4 tests outside normal limits. Up to four tests may be expected to fall outside normal limits on the basis of chance alone and individuals with scores in this range usually show no impairment in brain functions whatever.

Borderline. 5–6 tests outside normal limits. Individuals here may or may not demonstrate some evidence of impairment in brain functions as for example in different performances of the right and left sides of the body. Even when such is demonstrated it is so minor that it has no detectable impact on ability to adjust to life.

Very mild impairment. 7–8 tests outside normal limits. Individuals falling in this range typically demonstrate convincing evidence of impairment in brain functions but it is so slight that it has only a limited impact on adjustment.

Mild impairment. 9–11 tests outside normal limits. Persons whose performances fall in this range almost always demonstrate both definite evidence of neurological problems and also of at least some impact upon ability to function.

Moderate impairment. 12–14 tests outside normal limits. Patients with performances falling in this range are easily identified as impaired and a portion of this group is able neither to live independently nor to function in normal employment.

Severe impairment. 15–16 tests outside normal limits. Individuals here routinely show striking neurological impairment which has a marked impact on abilities in every or nearly every area. They will need assistance in sheltered or semi-sheltered employment and living conditions.

Case material

D.D. was a 20 year old caucasian male referred for a neuropsychological evaluation as part of his presurgical work-up at our epilepsy centre. He was diagnosed as having complex partial seizures with occasional secondary generalisation and a large number of these partial attacks had occurred in the month prior to the evaluation. There was no family history of seizures. Sudden noises and emotional upsets appeared to precipitate some of the attacks. Repeated EEGs demonstrated focal epileptiform discharges over the right fronto-temporal area as well as moderate diffuse abnormalities. An intra-carotid sodium amytal test ('Wada' test) showed that speech was clearly related to the left cerebral hemisphere. At the time of the evaluation, this 84 kg man was taking 1500

mg of carbamazepine, 1000 mg of primidone, and 38 mg of clorazepate per day.

The results of the neuropsychological evaluation are presented in Table 7.1. The results from the 16 specialised neuropsychological tests are given in the middle of the page and the general indicators of intelligence, personality, and preference in handedness are given at the bottom of the page.

A review of the discriminative measures provides information of interest. First of all, some 9 of 16 (56 per cent) of the specialised neuropsychological tests were performed in a range designated as outside normal limits (mild impairment). Examination of the scores does not point to any one area where the deficiencies are striking but rather shows limited difficulty with a number of tests. Probably the greatest of these pertain to his inability to attend to the task under distracting conditions and it was observed that his performances on both Seashore tests and on the Stroop Test were deficient. Other poor results included a relatively poor visuo-spatial memory (Wechsler Memory Scale), language-related problems (Aphasia Screening Test), decreased motor speed (name writing), and deficient problem solving (Category Test). Thus, difficulties were noted in a variety of tests and although none of these were overwhelming, they would almost certainly make him less able to function in life.

The 16 discriminative measures were also examined for laterality and a series of performances were found which implicated the right cerebral hemisphere. The relatively poor memory for non-verbal materials has already been mentioned and is in some contrast to his good memory for verbal material. On the Tactile Performance Test there was scarcely any improvement at all on the second trial when the left hand was used and because of memory factors, we would have expected an improvement of perhaps 30–35 per cent. In addition, it was observed that his left hand was slow on the Finger Tapping Test and we would expect the left hand to perform about 90 per cent as well as the right hand even in this strongly right-handed person. Finally, it was observed that the left hand was relatively slow on the name writing procedure. In terms of letters per second executed, we would expect the left hand to take approximately three times as long as the right but a considerably longer period was required. Furthermore, there were four perceptual errors made on the left side of the body but only one made on the right. The left cerebral hemisphere was implicated only by seven errors made on the Aphasia Screening Test.

It is concluded from the specialised neuropsychological measures that there is evidence for organic involvement of both cerebral hemispheres but that the right cerebral hemisphere is definitely involved more than the left. Thus, it appeared that the EEG focus and whatever caused that focus had very definite behavioural correlates, which included certain aspects of functioning traditionally related especially to the right temporal lobe but also the posterior inferior frontal lobe and, to some degree, to the parietal lobe as well.

Intelligence was evaluated by means of the Wechsler Adult Intelligence Scale and Table 7.1 demonstrates that he scores in the lower ranges of normal or average performance. In the emotional area, the MMPI suggested that he may be seen as peculiar or odd by others. He may also tend to keep a social distance from people and to have limited social skills. Immaturity, dependency, and passivity were also indicated and the possibility was raised that at least some of his physical complaints may have a functional basis.

Two months after his neuropsychological evaluation, he

Table 7.1 Summary of neuropsychological tests on patient D.D., a 20-year-old male with complex partial seizures and a focus in the right temporal area.

NEUROPSYCHOLOGICAL REPORT -- EPILEPSY CENTRE

Name D.D.   Hospital No.   Date 5/5/77   No. 709
Age 20   Education 12   Handedness R   Race C   Occupation Unemployed

NEUROPSYCHOLOGICAL BATTERY FOR EPILEPSY

Discriminative Measures

Stroop Test	Part I		216(6)★	Category Test		88★
Part II 320(13)	II–I		194★	Tactile Performance Test		
Wechsler Memory Scale (Form I)				Preferred 4.5	Total time	9.9
Verbal (Stories)			21	Nonpreferred 4.2	Memory	8
Visual-Spatial (Drawings)			8★	Both Hands 1.3	Localization	5
				Seashore Rhythm Test		23★
Perceptual Examination	R	L		Seashore Tonal Memory Test		19★
Misperceptions	0	0				
Suppressions	0	0		Finger Tapping		
Finger Agnosia	0	0		Preferred 55	Nonpreferred 46	101
Agraphagnosia	1	4		Trail Making Test		
Astereognosis	0	0		Part A 57	Part B	146★
Total Errors	1	4	5	Aphasia Screening Test		
Astereo. Time	11	9		Expressive 4	Receptive 1	7★

Name Writing (Let/Sec)
  Pref. 1.23   Nonpref. 0.24   0.40★   Constructional Dyspraxia   Ques.
★Performance falls outside normal limits.   Total tests outside normal limits: 9/16(56%)

General Measures

	Wechsler Adult Intelligence Scale			Minnesota Multiphasic Personality Inventory				Lateral Dominance Examination	
								R	L
VIQ 88	Info	8	Dig Sym 7	? 50	Pd 69	Es 31		R	L
PIQ 95	Comp	7	Pic Com 11	L 66	Mf 65	Ep 31	Hand 7	0	
FSIQ 90	Arith	11	Bl Des 11	F 76	Pa 65	A 18	Eye 2	0	
VSS 47	Simil	7	Pic Arr 10	K 46	Pt 69	R 24	Foot 2	0	
PSS 47	Dig Sp 7		Obj Ass 8	Hs 77	Sc 88	Man Anx 22	Dyna. 53.5	49.5	
TSS 94	Vocab	7		D 72	Ma 63	Cr. In. 11			
				Hy 73	Si 67				

---

was taken to surgery and a low grade glioma was excised from the right temporal lobe. Follow-up one year later demonstrated a substantial decrease in seizure frequency although occasional attacks persisted. In general, slight improvement on the neuropsychological tests was demonstrated at that time and this is often seen with individuals for whom the surgical procedure has been substantially or fully effective. Emotional status also showed some improvement although he continued to remain somewhat withdrawn socially.

CONCLUSIONS

We have found that a neuropsychological evaluation complements other forms of neurological assessment and that it provides an objective assessment of epilepsy and its impact upon behaviour. At approximately twice the cost of a standard EEG and six to eight hours of patient time, this entirely non-invasive procedure may be used which approaches the brain from the viewpoint of functioning rather than having the goal of establishing structural or electrical problems. In addition, the procedure provides a good index of what can be expected of a person with respect to performance in daily life and information is thereby provided which is not available through other methods of assessment. Because of these assets, neuropsychological evaluation is very frequently used at our Epilepsy Centre in order to provide a more complete assessment of the problems and prospects for our epileptic patients.

REFERENCES

Dalby, M.A. (1975) Behavioural effects of carbamazepine. In Penry, J.K. & Daly, D.D. (eds) *Advances in neurology*, (Vol. 11). New York: Raven Press.

De Haas, A. & Magnus, O. (1958) In De Haas, A. (ed.) *Lectures on epilepsy*. New York: Elsevier.

Dikmen, S. & Matthews, C.G. (1977) Effect of major motor seizure frequency upon cognitive-intellectual functions in adults. *Epilepsia*, **18**, 21.

Dikmen, S., Matthews, C.G. & Harley, J.P. (1975) The effect of early versus late onset of major motor epilepsy upon cognitive-intellectual performance. *Epilepsia*, **16**, 73.

Dodrill, C.B. (1975a) Diphenylhydantoin serum levels, toxicity, and neuropsychological performance in patients with epilepsy. *Epilepsia*, **16**, 593.

Dodrill, C.B. (1975b) Effects of sulthiame upon intellectual, neuropsychological, and social functioning abilities among adult epileptics: Comparison with diphenylhydantoin. *Epilepsia*, **16**, 593.

Dodrill, C.B. (1978) A neuropsychological battery for epilepsy. *Epilepsia*, **19**, 611.

Dodrill, C.B. & Troupin, A.S. (1977) Psychotropic effects of carbamazepine in epilepsy: A double-blind comparison with phenytoin. *Neurology*, **27**, 1023.

Halstead, W.C. (1947) *Brain and intelligence: A quantitative study of the lobes*. Chicago: University of Chicago Press.

Halstead, W.C. & Wepman, J.M. (1949) The Halstead-Wepman aphasia screening test. *Journal of Speech and Hearing Disorders*, **14**, 9.

Hutt, S.J., Jackson, P.M., Belsham, A. & Higgins, G. (1968) Perceptual-motor behaviour in relation to blood phenobarbitone level: A preliminary report. *Developmental Medicine and Childhood Neurology*, **10**, 626.

Kløve, H. & Matthews, C.G. (1966) Psychometric and adaptive abilities in epilepsy with differential etiology. *Epilepsia*, **7**, 330.

Lennox, W.G. & Lennox, M.A. (1960) *Epilepsy and related disorders* (2 Vols.) Boston: Little, Brown & Company.

Matthews, C.G. & Harley, J.P. (1975) Cognitive and motor-sensory performances in toxic and non-toxic epileptic subjects. *Neurology*, **25**, 184.

Matthews, C.G. & Kløve, H. (1967) Differential psychological performances in major motor, psychomotor, and mixed seizure classifications of known and unknown etiology. *Epilepsia*, **8**, 117.

Milner, B. (1975) Psychological aspects of focal epilepsy and its neurosurgical management. In Purpura, D.P., Penry, J.K. & Walter, R.D. (eds) *Advances in neurology* (Vol. 8). New York: Raven Press.

Reitan, R.M. (1964) Psychological deficits resulting from cerebral lesions in man. In Warren, J.M. & Abert, K.A. (eds) *The frontal granular cortex and behaviour*. New York: McGraw-Hill.

Reitan, R.M. (1969) The neurological model. In L'Abate, L. (ed.) *Models of clinical psychology*. Atlanta: Georgia State College.

Rodin, E.A., Rim, C.S. & Rennick, P.M. (1974) The effects of carbamazepine on patients with psychomotor epilepsy: Results of a double-blind study. *Epilepsia*, **15**, 547.

Somerfeld-Ziskind, E. & Ziskind, E. (1940) Effect of phenobarbital on the mentality of epileptic patients. *Archives of Neurology and Psychiatry*, **40**, 70.

Tarter, R.E. (1972) Intellectual and adaptive functioning in epilepsy: A review of fifty years of research. *Diseases of the Nervous System*, **33**, 763.

Troupin, A.S., Ojemann, L.M. & Dodrill, C.B. (1976) Mephenytoin: A reappraisal. *Epilepsia*, **17**, 403.

8

Clinical pharmacology and medical treatment

PART ONE

A. Richens

INTRODUCTION

The following case history illustrates some of the problems that can occur in the drug treatment of epilepsy. The management of these problems will form the basis of this chapter.

Case 1
Philip had been born with dextrocardia, congenital heart block and mild pulmonary stenosis. Although his heart condition caused him little disability, at the age of seven he began to have attacks of altered consciousness. These attacks, consisting of blankness, confusion and automatisms, appeared epileptic rather than syncopal and an electroencephalogram confirmed this by demonstrating a right posterior temporal lobe focus. At first his attacks were infrequent, but gradually they worsened until they disrupted his schooling to a considerable degree. He failed to reach an average standard and had difficulty in reading. At about 14 years of age it was thought that some of his attacks were syncopal in nature although no evidence was obtained to support this suspicion. His pulse rate was noted to be 30 beats/minute at this time, and he had a systolic murmur in the pulmonary area.

On leaving school Philip worked for a while in a leather works and later in a wool mill, but left because of the danger of injury during fits. At about this time he was assessed for temporal lobe resection but was considered unsuitable as there was no clear neurosurgical target. In late 1972, when aged 22, he was interviewed for possible admission to the National Hospitals – Chalfont Centre for Epilepsy in order that his capability for employment could be assessed. At interview he was noted to be slightly ataxic and slow of speech. He was receiving three Mysoline with phenytoin tablets (each containing 250 mg of primidone and 100 mg of phenytoin), sulthiame 600 mg and diazepam 15 mg daily.

Philip was admitted after Christmas, and continued to receive the same dose of drugs, although primidone and phenytoin were prescribed separately rather than as com-

bined tablets. Two weeks after admission he developed a pyrexia, vomiting and generalised lymphadenopathy. Although the pyrexia settled spontaneously he became confused and severely ataxic, with gross incoordination of all four limbs. His walking was so severely affected that he required elbow crutches to steady himself. A serum phenytoin level was measured at this point and gave a result of 180 μmol/l* (45 μg/ml, which was considerably in excess of the accepted therapeutic range of 40–80 μmol/l (10–20 μg/ml).

As this toxic level fully accounted for his clinical condition it was decided to lower the level not by reducing the dose of phenytoin but by withdrawing sulthiame, a known inhibitor of phenytoin metabolism. A month later his walking was greatly improved although he still had residual nystagmus. As his serum phenytoin level was still slightly above the therapeutic range at 116 μmol/l (29 μg/ml), the dose of phenytoin was reduced to 200 mg daily. This resulted in a marked fall in phenytoin level to 28 μmol/l (7 μg/ml) one month after reduction, but as his fits appeared to be occurring more frequently the dose was increased gradually by 25 mg increments until a level within the therapeutic range was established. The relationship which was found between the dose and the serum concentration of phenytoin is illustrated in Figure 8.1 (PH). A satisfactory dose was found to be 250 mg daily, which he continued to receive together with primidone 750 mg daily until his discharge in September 1974. On leaving the Chalfont Centre, Philip was able to take up a job in an engineering firm and his employer appeared to be entirely satisfied with his work.

Unfortunately, this happy state of affairs was interrupted by an emergency admission to a local hospital because he had developed vertigo, vomiting, confusion and a behaviour disorder. The latter became so difficult to manage, despite heavy sedation with chlorpromazine, that admission to a mental hospital was entertained. Eventually, however, arrangements were made for him to return to the Chalfont Centre. On admission he was grossly confused and hullucinated, had marked tremor, nystagmus and ataxia, and showed some choreoathetoid movements of his arms. The cause of these symptoms was soon discovered; instead of receiving five 50 mg tablets of phenytoin daily, for the previous ten days he had been give the same number of 100 mg tablets as the result of a dispensing error. His serum phenytoin concentration was 152 μmol/l (38 μg/ml). The drug was discontinued for a few days and then started again at the

*Serum drug levels are given throughout this and other chapters in μmol/l and μg/ml. Conversion factors are given in Appendix 8.1

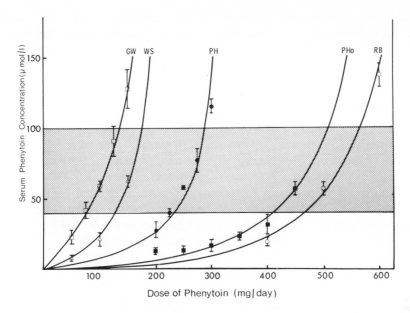

Fig. 8.1 Relationship between phenytoin dose and serum level in five patients in whom steady state concentrations were measured at several different doses. Further details of PH and GW are given in the case histories on p. 292 and p. 298 respectively. Each point represents the mean ± S.D. of 3-8 separate estimations of the serum level. The curves were fitted by computer using the Michaelis-Menten equation. The stippled area indicates the 'therapeutic range' of serum levels but is more generous than the usually quoted 40-80 μmol/l (*note*: 4 μmol/l = 1 μg/ml) (Reproduced from Richens and Dunlop, 1975, by kind permission of the editor)

correct dose. He rapidly improved and was able to leave again three weeks later. Subsequently Philip was fitted with a cardiac pacemaker, but without obvious influence on his fits.

This case report illustrates several of the problems which are encountered in the management of severe epilepsy. The possibility that some of Philip's fits were syncopal, or were genuinely epileptic but provoked by poor perfusion of an existing cerebral lesion due to a low cardiac output, is interesting to speculate upon but is outside the scope of this chapter. However, the difficulties which occurred with his drug therapy pose a number of questions which it is the purpose of this chapter to try to answer.

Philip has a temporal lobe focus which causes characteristic complex partial seizures without secondary generalisation. This type of seizure has a reputation for being difficult to treat, and for this reason patients like Philip often end up receiving a variety of drugs in combination. One drug alone fails to stop the fits so a second is added, then a third, and so on. After several years of increasingly complicated polypharmacy it may

reasonably be asked whether the patient is deriving a useful benefit from drug therapy or whether he is merely being subjected to the inconvenience of unnecessary adverse effects. What is the evidence that two drugs are better than one, and three better than two in patients with difficult fits? What, indeed, is the evidence that treating complex partial seizures with antiepileptic drugs benefits the patient at all?

Apart from the fact that the risk of adverse effects is increased with every new drug added to a patient's therapy, the likelihood of clinically important drug interactions becomes considerable with multiple drug therapy. In Philip's case, inhibition of phenytoin metabolism by sulthiame was largely responsible for the toxicity which he showed after his first admission. How common a problem is this, and what other drugs can precipitate toxicity by interfering with drug metabolism? Can several drugs in combination produce toxicity by an additive effect without the serum concentration of any one drug being in the accepted toxic range?

Other factors may have been involved in producing Philip's phenytoin intoxication. On admission a change was made from a combined preparation to individual preparations of primidone and phenytoin. Although the dose of the two drugs remained the same, is it possible that the 'biological availability' of the individual preparations (i.e. the amount of drug absorbed from each) was increased by the change in tablets? Problems of this nature have been described with different brands of phenytoin as well as with a variety of drugs used in other fields of medicine.

An alternative explanation is that Philip was not taking the full dose of his tablets at home, but began to do so when more closely supervised after admission to the Chalfont Centre. How often is lack of 'patient compliance' a cause of therapeutic failure in epilepsy? Are physicians naïve in believing that most of their patients take the prescribed medicine in the right dose and at the right time?

Undoubtedly, a contributing factor to Philip's intoxication was the fact that he is a relatively slow metaboliser of phenytoin. Whereas most patients require 300 mg or more to achieve a therapeutic serum concentration of the drug, Philip had a toxic level on this dose. He could tolerate at most 275 mg daily although on 200 mg his serum level was subtherapeutic. What is the cause of this difference between patients, and is there any way of predicting whether a person will be a slow or a fast metaboliser? What, also, is the reason for the non-linear relationship between serum phenytoin level and dose which is seen in Figure 8.1, giving rise to a very small dose range within the therapeutic range of serum concentrations?

The aim in adjusting Philip's phenytoin dose was to produce a serum level within the range of 40–80 μmol/1 (10–20 μg/ml) which was considered to be the therapeutic range in the laboratory which performed the estimations. How valid is this range? Are no patients able to tolerate a level above 80 μmol/1 (20 μg/ml)? Is it essential in all patients to achieve a level in excess of 40 μmol/1 (10 μg/ml) before fits become adequately controlled? If a patient is taking phenobarbitone or primidone in addition, is the therapeutic range of serum phenytoin levels the same as if he was receiving phenytoin alone? Coming back to the first question asked, what is the evidence that this range applies to the use of phenytoin in complex partial seizures which are notoriously drug-resistant? Are we simply deluding ourselves into an apparently precise scheme for managing fits when we ought to be examining much more closely the efficacy of the established drugs in the various types of epilepsy? Even worse, will we make the mistake of treating the serum level rather than the patient himself?

The introduction of serum level monitoring has been hailed as a major step forward in the routine management of epilepsy: Before we accept this view with uncritical enthusiasm we should examine carefully the evidence in favour of a management programme which involves regular measurement of drug levels. This will be the main theme of this chapter.

PHARMACOKINETICS IN THE NORMAL ADULT AND CHILD

Phenytoin

Of the various antiepileptic drugs in common use (Appendix 8.2), phenytoin has been studied in greatest depth because it is the most widely used, is relatively easy to measure in serum, and has some interesting pharmacokinetic properties which are responsible for the wide variation in response to the drug. A full account of its pharmacokinetics has been given by Richens (1979) and the important facts are summarised in Table

Table 8.1 Summary of pharmacokinetic data on phenytoin

Range of daily maintenance dosage	Adult: 150–600 mg/day Child: 5–15 mg/kg/day
Minimum dose frequency	Adult: once daily Child: twice daily
Time to peak serum level	4–12 hours (oral) many hours (IM)
Percentage bound to plasma proteins	90% (85% in neonates)
Apparent volume of distribution	0.45 l/kg
Elimination half-life in adults	9–140 hours (saturation kinetics)
Time to steady state after starting therapy	7–21 days
Major inactive metabolite	5-(p-hydroxyphenyl)-5-phenylhydantoin
Other metabolites	Diphenylhydantoic acid 3,4 dihydrodiol Catechol metabolites

8.1. The structural formula is given in Appendix 8.3.

Absorption. Phenytoin is usually administered either as the sodium salt or as the acid. The latter presents bioavailability problems unless it is in a microcrystalline form which presents a large surface area for dissolution. In an amorphous form it is poorly and erratically absorbed. The sodium salt, which is macrocrystalline in form, is reliably absorbed. It is much more soluble than the acid form and although it may reprecipitate as the latter at the acid pH of the stomach, it will do so in a finely divided form. The most important determinant of phenytoin absorption is therefore particle size rather than whether it is in its acid or salt form.

The excipient in a formulation may influence bioavailability by altering the rate of deaggregation of the particles. In Australasia in 1968 an outbreak of phenytoin intoxication occurred when the manufacturers of Dilantin capsules changed the excipient from hydrated calcium sulphate to lactose, which resulted in an unexpected increase in bioavailability (Tyrer *et al.*, 1970). In Scandinavia, inequivalence between the various marketed preparations has been a cause of concern (Lund, 1974a). In particular, one preparation, Difhydan, contains phenytoin acid in an amorphous form with a highly variable particle size, leading to poor bioavailability compared with other preparations. Marked changes in serum concentration have occurred on changing from one brand to another. In the USA and West Germany, less dramatic but nevertheless clinically important generic inequivalence has been reported (Gugler *et al.*, 1976; Rambeck *et al.*, 1977). In the USA and UK, a chewable microcrystalline tablet formulation for paediatric use (Epanutin Infatabs) appears to be better absorbed than standard tablets (Stewart *et al.*, 1975), although only marginally better than capsules (Smith & Kinkel, 1976). In agreement with these observations, British Pharmacopoeia tablets are slightly inferior to capsules (Richens, 1976). The bioavailability of phenytoin and implications for therapeutic use have been reviewed in detail by Neuvonen (1979).

Although parenteral preparations of phenytoin are generally recommended for intramuscular administration, they are very poorly absorbed and it is questionable whether they should ever be used by this route. In order to concentrate the drug in a convenient volume, the solvent is made very alkaline, about pH 12, and when this is buffered to physiological pH in the tissues, crystals of drug precipitate. These have a relatively small surface area for redissolution and up to half of the drug may still be present in the muscle 24 hours after injection (Wilensky & Lowden, 1973). Furthermore, considerable muscle damage may result (Serrano & Wilder, 1974). Serum concentrations produced by intramuscular administration may therefore be inadequate, and a change from oral to intramuscular administration to cover, for instance, an abdominal operation, may cause seizures. On the other hand, rebound intoxication may occur on resumption of oral therapy because considerable quantities of drug remain to be absorbed (Wilder & Ramsay, 1976). Although a scheme has been described for changing from oral to intramuscular administration (Wilder *et al.*, 1974) it is more satisfactory to give the drug by intravenous infusion (into a saline drip) in a single daily dose.

Distribution and plasma protein binding. Phenytoin is approximately 90 per cent bound to plasma proteins in adults (Porter & Layzer, 1975). The binding is mostly to albumin (Odar-Cedarlof & Borga, 1976), but secondary low affinity sites on other proteins bind the drug when it is displaced from albumin by other drugs (Monks *et al.*, 1978). Bilirubin can cause displacement in the neonate (Fredholm *et al.*, 1975).

There has been controversy on the importance of intersubject differences in protein binding, but the most reliable data indicates that variation in the free drug concentration is no greater than two-fold provided the albumin concentration is within the normal range (Yacobi *et al.*, 1977) Hypoalbuminaemia is associated with a reduction in the total quantity of drug bound, and therefore the total serum concentration, but the free drug level will not be greater than normal.

Ideally, it would be better to measure the free drug concentration as a therapeutic guide rather than the total serum concentration. However, methods for separating free and bound drugs are too cumbersome for routine use and this, together with the inaccuracy of measuring low concentrations of the drug, make monitoring of free levels impractical for other than research purposes at the present time.

An alternative approach, which circumvents separation of bound and free drug in serum, is to measure the salivary concentration. It appears that the salivary glands act as a simple dialysis membrane across which the free drug molecules in plasma are able to diffuse and equilibrate (Reynolds *et al.*, 1976; Paxton *et al.*, 1977). Although the ratio of the plasma concentration of free drug to salivary concentration of total drug is close to unity, there is considerable variation in individual values from one subject to another (Reynolds *et al.*, 1976). How much of this is real and how much is due to methodological difficulties is uncertain. Contamination of the mouth by liquid or chewable preparations can cause erroneous results for up to three hours after dosing, and this is a particular problem in children, in whom the use of salivary levels are most desirable.

Phenytoin diffuses rapidly into the tissues. Following intravenous administration, the distribution phase lasts about two hours. The drug binds to brain tissue to about the same extent as it binds to serum proteins, and therefore the brain and

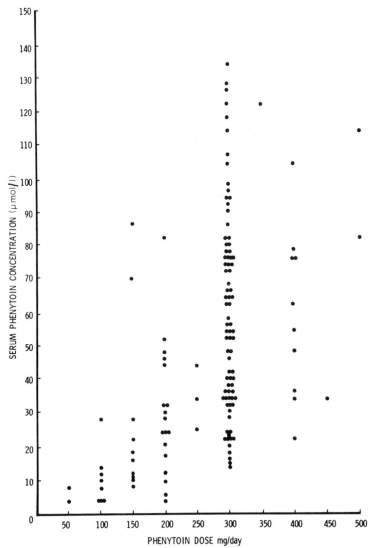

Fig. 8.2 Relationship between phenytoin dose and serum level in 137 patients treated chronically with phenytoin and usually at least one other antiepileptic drug (excluding sulthiame) (*note*: 4μmol/1 = 1μg/ml)

serum concentrations are almost identical (Houghton et al., 1975b). Penetration into brain is rapid and its use in status epilepticus therefore has a sound basis (Wilder et al., 1977). As might be expected, phenytoin penetrates more slowly into cerebrospinal fluid but once it has equilibrated the concentration of phenytoin mirrors that of the free drug concentration in serum (Lund et al., 1972; Houghton et al., 1975b).

Dose–serum concentration relationship. As phenytoin is cleared slowly the serum concentration on repeated dosing is relatively stable even with once daily administration. However, steady state concentrations vary considerably between patients, as they do for most lipid soluble drugs which are cleared by hepatic metabolism (Fig. 8.2) A median dose of phenytoin in adults of 300–350 mg/day may be enough to produce a therapeutic concentration in one patient (e.g. GW in Fig. 8.1) while another may require in excess of 500 mg/day (e.g. RB in Fig. 8.1). Although age, sex and body weight influence the dose — serum level relationship in adults, the relative contribution of each is relatively small (Sherwin et al., 1974; Houghton et al., 1975a). For example, replotting the data in Figure 8.2 to take into account body weight (Fig. 8.3) results in only a marginal improvement in the dose-level relation-

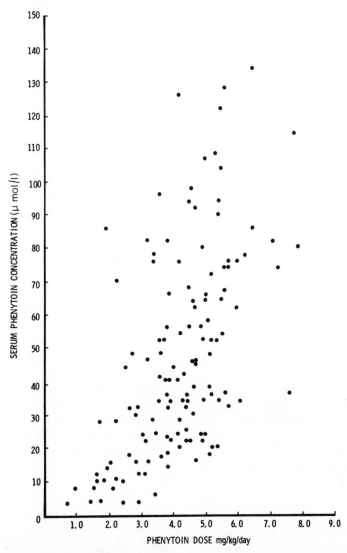

Fig. 8.3 As in Fig. 8.1, but dose has been converted to mg/kg

ship. Barot *et al.* (1978) found that body surface area correlated most strongly with dose requirements in adult patients.

In children, body size becomes a major determinant of dose (Borofsky *et al.*, 1972). The dose/kg of body weight required to produce a given serum concentration increases as body weight falls. Although there is general agreement that calculations based on body surface area provide the most reliable guide to dosage in children (Catzel, 1966), in practice it is usually satisfactory to dose according to bodyweight. A suitable scheme for starting doses is given in Table 8.2. Because there is a

Table 8.2 Starting doses of phenytoin in children and infants. The doses have been chosen to produce an average serum concentration of 40 μmol/l (10 μg/ml)

Body weight kg	Phenytoin dose mg/kg/day	mg/day*
6–10	10.0	100
11–15	9.0	125
16–20	8.0	150
21–25	7.0	175
26–30	6.5	200
31–35	5.5	200
36–40	5.5	225
41–45	5.5	250
46–50	5.0	250
51–60	5.0	300

*Doses rounded off to suit 25 mg dose units

wide inter-individual variation in serum levels produced by a given dose of phenytoin, the doses suggested will give levels that are too low in some, and toxic in a few. They should be regarded as doses which will on average produce therapeutic levels.

Other dosage schemes have been published for phenytoin by Buchthal and Lennox-Buchthal (1972a), but it fails to take into account the saturation kinetics of the drug (see below). If dose increments are made in a patient using this scheme, intoxication is likely to result. Once a serum level of 40 μmol/l (10 μg/ml) has been achieved, the maximum increment permissible is about one-sixth of the dose.

Metabolism. Phenytoin is extensively metabolised in the liver, less than 5 per cent appearing unchanged in the urine. The rate at which it is metabolised is under genetic control which is thought to be polygenic in nature. There is a continuous unimodal distribution of rates of metabolism with very slow and very fast metabolisers at the extreme ends of the distribution. Race may also be important; Arnold and Gerber (1970) found that negroes metabolised phenytoin more slowly than caucasians.

The major metabolite of phenytoin is 5-(p-hydroxyphenyl)-5-phenylhydantoin (p-HPPH), which is pharmacologically inactive. It is conjugated to a glucuronide and excreted in the urine.

The conversion of phenytoin to this metabolite by microsomal enzymes in the liver is saturable within the therapeutic range of serum levels. This means that the liver is unable to increase its rate of metabolism in proportion to the serum concentration (which it is generally able to do, a situation called *first order kinetics*). Instead it moves towards a situation in which a fixed amount of drug is removed regardless of the serum level (a situation called *zero order kinetics*).

The saturable nature of phenytoin metabolism is of considerable practical importance, because it leads to a non-linear relationship between the dose and serum level. The importance of this is highlighted by the case report which opened this chapter; in Figure 8.1 it can be seen that in this patient (PH) an increment of only 55 mg would carry the serum level from the lower limit to the upper limit of the therapeutic range. How many physicians on seeing a patient who had responded inadequately to 200 mg of phenytoin daily would have made an increment of 100 mg, especially if he had known that the serum level was only 28 μmol/l (7 μg/ml)? The dose-serum level relationship for four additional patients is also illustrated. The same pattern is seen in each patient, although the dose range yielding a therapeutic level varies considerably, presumably because of genetic differences in the amount of hydroxylase enzyme available for metabolism. One of these patients (GW) is one of the slowest metabolisers I have encountered and his case history is interesting.

Case 2
Graham was admitted to a school for epileptic children when he was ten years old, having had major fits since the age of 18 months. His IQ on admission was 77 (revised Stanford Binet test), but six years later was recorded as only 57. He showed little aptitude for school work and it was recommended that employment at a simple repetitive task, particu-

larly in farming, might suit him. This proved to be the case, but because he was unable to live independently he was transferred to an adult residential centre when he was 16. His fits had been difficult to control and at the time of transfer he was receiving phenobarbitone 120 mg, primidone 750 mg, phenytoin 100 mg, ethotoin 500 mg and dexamphetamine five mg daily. A number of EEG recordings had shown large slow waves anteriorly and over the temporal lobes, but the cause of his fits remained uncertain. The rare occurrence of a minor fit, in which he slumped to the floor and then remained in a dazed and confused state for 10–20 minutes, suggested a focal origin.

Following his transfer a number of changes in his drug therapy were made in order to achieve better control of his fits. The doses of the drugs he was receiving on admission were adjusted, but any increase, particularly in phenytoin or ethotoin, produced intoxication. Eventually ethotoin and dexamphetamine were discontinued and the dose of phenytoin kept at 100–150 mg/day. Later, pheneturide was tried but had to be stopped again because it produced ataxia. (Pheneturide inhibits phenytoin metabolism – see p. 000). Four years after Graham was admitted to the adult centre, in 1965, a fungal infection of his finger nails was noted which, on culture, proved to be due to Trichophyton rubrum. Over

the next ten years Graham received a number of courses of griseofulvin in doses of 500–1000 mg/day, but entirely without success. (Anticonvulsant drugs modify the absorption and metabolism of griseofulvin – see p. 000).

In 1967, it was decided to try beclamide in order to reduce the frequency of his fits, and this he received for the next two and a half years, in addition to phenytoin, phenobarbitone and primidone. His drug treatment and fit frequency over eight years from the start of beclamide treatment have been plotted out month by month in Figure 8.4. In July 1967 and June 1969 signs of drug intoxication were noted, causing the dose of phenytoin to be temporarily lowered on the first occasion, and a bolder reduction of phenobarbitone and a withdrawal of beclamide on the second. Following this second reduction he became brighter and remained so for the next five years. Although Graham was not able to achieve much in the way of academic success because of his mental handicap, he nevertheless worked slowly but surely in his job on the farm. He had always been a little unsteady on his feet, but this did not seem to worry him unduly.

In March 1974, an increase in his phenytoin dose was made, from 150 mg to 200 mg daily. Shortly afterwards he became slower and more ataxic than usual, and had coarse nystagmus on lateral gaze. A small adjustment was made in

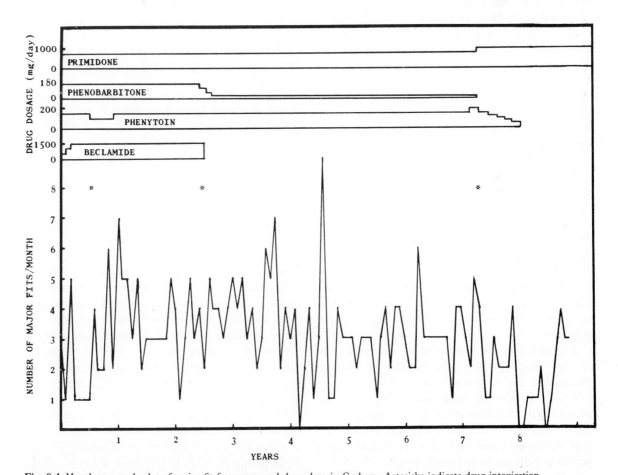

Fig. 8.4 Month to month plot of major fit frequency and drug dose in Graham. Asterisks indicate drug intoxication

the dose of primidone and phenobarbitone, but without effect. His serum phenytoin level was then measured and gave a result of 180 μmol/l (45 μg/ml). An immediate reduction to 150 mg daily was made, and over the following nine months the dose was gradually lowered in 25 mg decrements. The relationship between the dose and serum level is seen in Figure 8.1. It can be seen that a level within the 'therapeutic range' would have been achieved by a dose of 75–125 mg, accounting for his sensitivity to hydantoins which had been commented on in his earlier case records.

The gradual withdrawal of phenytoin, leaving him on only 1000 mg of primidone caused a marked improvement in his general well-being and apparently, in his fits (a point which will be taken up later – see p. 330).

This case report illustrates one of the problems created by wide variability in the rate of metabolism of phenytoin. Although Graham was treated with a smaller-than-average dose of phenytoin it was still too great for his metabolic capacity. Slow metabolisers are more likely than average to receive toxic doses of the drug, just as fast metabolisers are likely to be undertreated, because these patients' dose requirements fall outside the usual prescribing range. It is understandable if a physician feels that a dose of 75 mg of phenytoin daily is unlikely to be having much of a therapeutic effect, or if he is hesitant to increase the dose above 500 mg daily even if a patient is not showing evidence of toxicity. In the absence of serum level monitoring, most choose to adhere to a conventional 300 mg/day (Fig. 8.5).

The steepness of the dose-serum level relationship within the therapeutic range is important in a number of ways:

1. If phenytoin therapy is regulated by monitoring serum levels, increments in dose should be limited to 50 mg or less when the level comes close to the lower end of the therapeutic range.

2. Monitoring serum phenytoin levels is essential if the dose is to be correctly tailored. Finding the correct dose on clinical grounds alone is very difficult.

3. A small increase in the biological availability of the drug (p. 295) will readily increase a therapeutic level to a toxic one.

4. The effects of drug interactions will be exaggerated. Addition of a second drug which either inhibits or induces phenytoin metabolism (See Tables 8.21 and 8.22) will produce a disproportionate change in phenytoin level.

5. It is possible that a temporary disturbance of

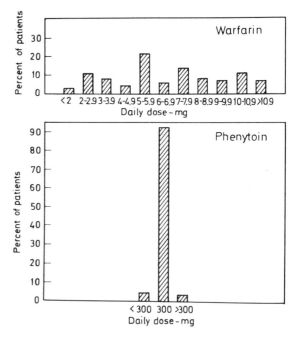

Fig. 8.5 Range of maintenance doses prescribed to 200 outpatients on warfarin and a further 200 receiving phenytoin. Monitoring the prothombin time leads to accurate individualisation of warfarin dose, but the greater difficulty of measuring the response to phenytoin results in the physicians' adhering to standard doses. (Serum phenytoin levels were not monitored in these patients.) (Reproduced with permission from Koch-Weser, 1975)

body function, as might occur during a viral infection, could produce a critical change in enzyme activity. Perhaps even small variations during health may do the same. This might account for some of the episodes of intoxication occurring in an otherwise well-controlled patient.

These practical problems make phenytoin therapy difficult to manage, particularly if the therapeutic range of serum levels suggested by Buchthal, Svensmark and Schiller (1960) is used as an objective. We need to be quite sure that this range is optimum for all patients with epilepsy because if some patients are well controlled at 'subtherapeutic' levels, the control would be expected to be much more stable. This question is fully discussed later (p. 316).

In order to assist the prescriber in achieving serum levels within the therapeutic range various schemes have been devised for adjusting dosage. Each demands at least one measurement of the serum phenytoin level, from which a prediction can be made of the increment in dose necessary to increase the level into the therapeutic range. The simplest method (Fig. 8.6) is the nomogram devised by Richens and Dunlop (1975) and modified by Rambeck *et al*. (1980). It requires only one accurately measured serum level. The direct linear plot method devised by Mullen (1978) is more accurate, but requires measurement of the serum level at two different doses, which considerably detracts from its clinical value.

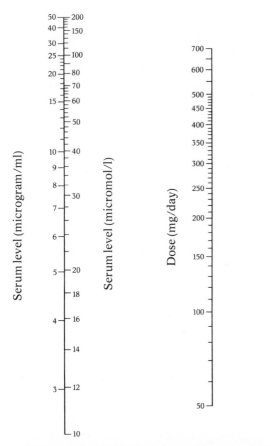

Fig. 8.6 Nomogram for adjusting phenytoin dose. Given a single reliable serum concentration on a known dose of phenytoin, the dose required to achieve a desired level can be predicted. A line is drawn connecting the observed serum concentration (left hand scale) with the dose administered (centre scale) and extended to intersect the right hand vertical line. From the point of intersection, another line is drawn back to the desired serum level (left hand scale). The dose required to produce this level can be read off the centre scale. *Note*: This nomogram will give misleading predictions if the serum concentration measurement is inaccurate, if the patient's compliance is in doubt or if a change in concurrent treatment has been made since measurement of the serum level. (Reproduced with permission from Rambeck *et al*., 1980)

Renal excretion. Less than five per cent of the daily dose is excreted unchanged in the urine (Karlen *et al*., 1975). About 70 to 80 per cent is eliminated as p-HPPH, mainly in the conjugated form. The ratio of metabolite to parent drug is determined both by genetic differences in drug metabolism and by the steady-state serum concentration of the parent drug (Houghton & Richens, 1974a). As the latter rises, the hydroxylation mechanism becomes saturated and p-HPPH production fails to rise in proportion, and therefore relatively more parent drug appears in the urine. p-HPPH appears to be actively excreted by the renal tubules as its clearance exceeds that of the glomerular filtration rate (Bochner *et al*., 1973).

Plasma half-life and dose interval. For drugs which lack an active metabolite, the plasma half-life of the parent compound determines the frequency of administration of doses, the time taken to reach a plateau serum level, the interval that should elapse between changes in dose, and the time taken for complete elimination of the drug following its withdrawal. Thus a knowledge of the half-life is essential if a drug is to be used effectively.

The object of therapy is to maintain an adequate serum level at all times, and it is therefore usual practice to space doses no greater than one half-life apart. If a second dose is given one half-life after the first oral dose, the peak serum concentration due to the second dose will rise to a higher value than after the first. Similarly, subsequent doses will produce progressively higher and higher levels until an equilibrium is reached in which the rate of elimination of the drug equals the rate of absorption. If doses are given at regular intervals this accumulation will, for practical purposes, be complete after five half-lives have elapsed. One of the common misconceptions concerning phenytoin is that steady state is achieved in something like five days in the adult, i.e. five times the half-life of 22 h reported by Arnold and Gerber (1970). In fact, because phenytoin metabolism is saturable, the effective plasma half-life gradually lengthens as the steady-state concentration rises (i.e. the clearance gradually decreases.) On average, the effective half-life at very low serum concentrations is about 13 h, but this lengthens to 46 h when the steady-state concentration reaches the top of the therapeutic range (Houghton & Richens, 1974a). The time to steady state therefore depends upon the dose and the final concentration reached, and may be as long as two weeks or more in a patient given a dose yielding a high therapeutic or toxic concentration. Similarly, the rate of elimination of the drug on discontinuing therapy may be much slower than expected, particularly in a patient who started with a toxic serum concentration.

Also, the fluctuation in serum concentrations may be less than expected. The higher the steady state serum concentration, the smaller (in percentage terms) is the fluctuation in the serum concentration. Figure 8.7 represents a theoretical plot of the fluctuation in serum concentration with once daily dosing at a subtherapeutic, therapeutic and toxic steady state concentration. It can be seen

that the degree of fluctuation is quite acceptable for clinical purposes, and this accords with the finding that once daily dosage in adults (Strandjord & Johannessen, 1974) is compatible with effective control of seizures. In practice, many patients find that twice daily dosing, once after breakfast and again after the evening meal, is most satisfactory. Nevertheless, it is much appreciated if the midday dose can be dropped, because many patients forget it or find it inconvenient to take.

In children, twice daily dosing is preferable because the serum concentration 16–24 hours after a single daily dose may be inadequate. The serum half-life of phenytoin is shorter and the steady state serum level for a given dose/kg is lower in children than in adults, the difference increasing with decreasing age (Borofsky et al., 1972). Phenytoin exhibits saturable metabolism in

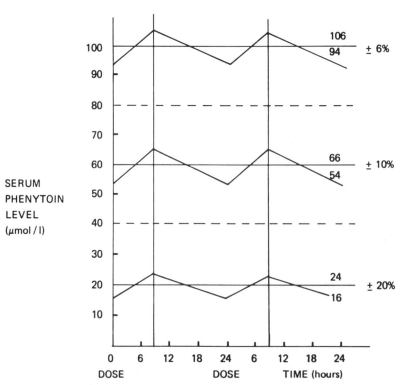

Fig. 8.7 Theoretical plot of the fluctuation in serum phenytoin concentration with once daily dosing. Calculations have been made at three steady-state concentrations, subtherapeutic, therapeutic and toxic. The therapeutic range of serum concentrations 40–80 μmol/l (10–20 μg/ml) is indicated with dotted lines. Half-life data provided by Houghton & Richens (1974) have been used. Peak and trough concentrations, together with the percentage fluctuations have been calculated. The fluctuation decreases as the serum concentration rises because saturation kinetics effectively lengthen the elimination half-life. (Reproduced with permission from Richens, 1980)

children as in adults (Eadie & Tyrer, 1980).

If an immediate therapeutic effect is required, a loading dose can be administered (Wilder *et al.*, 1973) but an unexpectedly high frequency of generalised skin rashes during the second week of treatment developed in children loaded with 6 mg/kg eight-hourly for four doses followed by a daily dose of 6 mg/kg (Wilson *et al.*, 1976).

Methoin (mephenytoin) (Troupin et al., 1976)

This is an hydantoin compound related to phenytoin (Appendix 8.3), and of a similar potency. It is metabolised by N-demethylation to an active metabolite, 5-ethyl-5-phenylhydantoin (Nirvanol), which is more active as an anticonvulsant than the parent compound. Subsequently the metabolite is broken down to an inactive metabolite, 5-ethyl-5(p-hydroxyphenyl)hydantoin, which is excreted in the urine.

Little data is available on the pharmacokinetics of methoin and Nirvanol. In steady-state the serum concentration of the parent drug accounts for only about 8 per cent of the combined concentration of methoin and Nirvanol. The elimination half-life of Nirvanol is longer than that of the unchanged drug, but the values quoted for the former (e.g. 74 and 144 hours in two patients; Troupin *et al.*, 1976) were measured following administration of the parent drugs and were therefore artificially lengthened by continuing production of Nirvanol. In one patient the half-life of methoin was 32 hours.

It is unlikely that extensive pharmacokinetic data will become available on this drug because its bone-marrow toxicity has led to a decline in its use.

Ethotoin (Sjö et al., 1975a)

This hydantoin compound has only one-fifth of the anticonvulsant potency of phenytoin. Like the latter drug it exhibits saturation kinetics, and lacks an active metabolite. It is approximately 90 per cent bound to plasma proteins.

Carbamazepine (Bertilsson, 1978; Pynnönen, 1979) (Table 8.3)

Absorption. Carbamazepine is slowly absorbed

Table 8.3 Summary of pharmacokinetic data on carbamazepine

Range of daily maintenance dosage	Adult: 400–1800 mg/day Child: 10–30 mg/kg/day
Minimum dose frequency	Adult: twice daily Child: twice daily
Time to peak serum level	4–24 hours
Percentage bound to plasma proteins	75%
Apparent volume of distribution	1.2 l/kg
Elimination half-life	Single doses: 20–55 hours After chronic therapy: 10–30 hours (adults) 8–20 hours (children)
Time to steady state after starting therapy	Up to 10 days (but subsequent fall may occur from auto-induction)
Major active metabolite	10,11-epoxide
Other metabolites	Dihydrodiol Hydroxy-metabolites Iminostilbene

because the drug has a low solubility. The extent of absorption has not yet been determined but is probably incomplete because it may be increased by taking the drug with meals (Levy *et al.*, 1975).

Distribution and plasma protein binding. Carbamazepine is readily lipid soluble and therefore distributes to the tissues rapidly. The plasma protein binding of carbamazepine is 70–80 per cent. The salivary concentration closely reflects the free concentration in plasma (Chambers *et al.*, 1977) and can therefore be used in monitoring therapy, but the same reservations apply to salivary carbamazepine levels as to phenytoin (see above). The presence of other antiepileptic drugs does not influence carbamazepine binding. The epoxide metabolite (see below) is about 50 per cent bound.

Metabolism. Carbamazepine is largely metabolised into a stable epoxide metabolite, carbamazepine 10,11-epoxide, which is pharmacologically active (Faigle *et al.*, 1977) and is present in measurable amounts in plasma. It is further metabolised to hydroxy-derivatives which are excreted in the urine. Only about 2 per cent of the drug is excreted unchanged.

Dose-serum concentration relationship. When single blood samples from many different patients are analysed for carbamazepine there is little correlation between the dose and serum concentration. In addition to the usual variation in rate of metabolism between individuals, there are probably two reasons for this: a. the incomplete, and therefore presumably variable, bioavailability of the drug, and b. auto-induction of its own metabolism. It has been shown that predictions of the steady-state serum concentration cannot be made from single dose studies; the actual level always falls short of the predicted level because auto-induction causes the drug to be broken down increasingly rapidly. On the other hand, a linear relationship between dose and serum level can be found within patients (Perucca, Bittencourt & Richens, 1980). The increase in serum level which is produced by a dose increment is usually less than predicted, however, possibly because of increasing enzyme induction.

When carbamazepine is given with other drugs such as phenytoin, phenobarbitone and primidone, it is much more difficult to achieve a therapeutic serum carbamazepine level (see p. 361). An absorption interaction or enzyme induction by the other drugs are two possible explanations for this observation, but on current evidence it is not possible to decide which. In practical terms, however, it means that the dose of carbamazepine when used alone should be much smaller than when used in conjunction with other drugs.

The serum concentration of the 10,11-epoxide metabolite in adults is about 15–55 per cent of the concentration of the unchanged drug (Morselli et al., 1975). In children the range is wider, 5–80 per cent, but is on average higher because of the faster metabolism of the drug. The same is true when carbamazepine is given together with other enzyme-inducing drugs (Rane, Höjer & Wilson, 1976). The antiepileptic potency of the epoxide in man is uncertain, but the metabolite probably contributes to the overall pharmacological effect, particularly when allowance is made for its lower degree of plasma protein binding (one-half of the plasma concentration is free compared with only one-quarter of the parent drug).

Plasma half-life and dose interval. When single doses of carbamazepine are given to volunteers, half-life values of up to 55 hours have been recorded. Following chronic administration the half-life shortens because of auto-induction of its metabolism. A steady state serum concentration will be reached in 5–10 days but a subsequent fall

in the concentration will occur as induction slowly rises to a maximum over the first 3–4 weeks of therapy. With half-life values of 10–30 hours after chronic dosing in the adult, twice daily dosing is appropriate. It should be remembered that carbamazepine is relatively slowly absorbed, and this tends to smooth out fluctuations in the serum concentration. Johannessen et al., (1977) showed that the variation in serum level with twice daily dosing is about 50 per cent of the mean value. However, it is my experience that individual doses greater than 400 mg in the adult often cause adverse effects 2–3 hours after dosing, and it may be necessary to divide the daily dose into more than two administrations when higher doses are being used.

Sodium valproate (Pinder *et al.*, 1977; Gugler *et al.*, 1979) (Table 8.4)

Sodium valproate is the sodium salt of valproic acid, which is also known as dipropylacetic acid, 2-propylpentanoic acid, or 2-propylvaleric acid. In some countries a magnesium salt is available, in others the drug is marketed as the acid or the amide (depamide). There are only minor differences in the pharmacokinetics of these preparations because the common substance present in the plasma is valproic acid.

The structure of sodium valproate differs considerably from traditional antiepileptic drugs

Table 8.4 Summary of pharmacokinetic data on sodium valproate

Range of daily maintenance dosage	Adult: 600–3000 mg/day Child: 20–50 mg/kg/day
Minimum dose frequency	Once daily? (see text)
Time to peak serum level	1–4 hours (uncoated tablets)
Percentage bound to plasma proteins	92% (but see text)
Apparent volume of distribution	0.15 l/kg
Elimination half-life in adults	8–20 hours
Time to steady state after starting therapy	4 days
Major metabolites	Glucuronic acid conjugate 3-keto-2-propylvaleric acid (β-oxidation product) 5-hydroxy-2-propylvaleric acid (Ω-oxidation product)

(Appendix 8.3). Its structure is that of a simple two-chain fatty acid.

Absorption. Sodium valproate is absorbed completely and rapidly, with peak serum levels occurring at 1–4 hours after ingestion of the uncoated tablets or syrup. Absorption is delayed if taken after a meal. Depamide, the amide of valproic acid, is slowly converted to the free acid following absorption; the serum concentration of valproic acid peaks at 3–6 hours after administration of this precursor substance. A common adverse effect produced by sodium valproate, and particularly valproic acid, is nausea. This is dose-related and attempts to give individual doses of 600 mg or more is often not tolerated. This can be largely offset by using enteric-coated tablets and these are especially useful when daily doses of 1500–3000 mg are required. They appear to be reliably absorbed and have the additional advantage of smoothing out the fluctuations in serum level throughout the day (although the importance of this can be questioned – see below).

Distribution and plasma protein binding. The distribution of valproic acid is restricted largely to the extracellular water. Brain concentrations are therefore low relative to plasma. Its plasma protein binding is about 90–95 per cent at low therapeutic concentrations, but as the plasma level rises the extent of binding falls progressively (Gugler *et al*., 1980). This gives rise to a non-linear relationship between dose and serum level such that the total concentration of drug in the serum fails to rise in proportion to the dose (Gram *et al*., 1980). It binds to free fatty acid binding sites and therefore an interaction with these endogenous substances occurs. Valproic acid will cause a clinically significant displacement of phenytoin (see p. 360). Salivary concentrations are low and cannot be used for monitoring free plasma levels (Gugler *et al*., 1980).

Dose-serum concentration relationship. As mentioned above, there is a non-linear relationship between dose and serum level because of changes in plasma protein binding. However, the free concentration of the drug and therefore the therapeutic effect is linearly related to dose because this is what determines the rate of metabolism. Attention must be paid to the time of sampling because valproic acid has a short half-life (see below) and con-

siderable fluctuations in serum level occur throughout a 24 hour period. This is one reason why most studies have shown a poor correlation between serum level and dose in large groups of patients.

Metabolism. Valproic acid is largely metabolised by β - and Ω-oxidation. In addition to the metabolites listed in Table 8.4, various other minor degradation products have been identified (Jakobs & Loscher, 1978). None of the metabolites is known to be pharmacologically active.

Renal elimination. About 20–40 per cent of the administered dose is recovered as conjugated compounds in the urine, mainly conjugated valproic acid and the 3-keto derivative. Only about 1–4 per cent of the parent compound is excreted unchanged.

Plasma half-life and dose interval. When sodium valproate is administered alone the plasma half-life varies from 8–20 hours. In patients receiving other drugs, however, shorter values of 5–10 hours can be measured, and this is presumably the result of induction of the oxidation of valproic acid. These short half-lives suggest that sodium valproate should be administered 2–4 times daily, and this has been general practice. However, there is evidence from monkeys with alumina-gel foci (Lockard & Levy, 1976) and from photosensitive patients (Rowan *et al*., 1979) that the antiepileptic effect of the drug may come on more slowly than would be predicted from the time to peak plasma concentration following a single dose, and that it

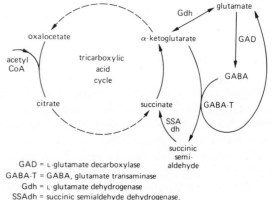

GAD = L-glutamate decarboxylase
GABA-T = GABA, glutamate transaminase
Gdh = L-glutamate dehydrogenase
SSAdh = succinic semialdehyde dehydrogenase.

Fig. 8.8 Metabolism of GABA in nervous tissue. Valproic acid is known to inhibit the enzymes responsible for the breakdown of GABA, particularly succinic semialdehyde dehydrogenase and, to a lesser extent, GABA glutamate transaminase

may long outlast the presence of the drug in the plasma. If valproic acid has its effect by modifying the activity of enzymes responsible for the degradation of the inhibitory neurotransmitter, ϑ-aminobutyric acid (GABA) (Sawaya, Horton & Meldrum, 1975) (Fig. 8.8), a slow onset and offset of action might be expected. Once daily administration therefore appears to be feasible; indeed, Covanis and Jeavons (1980) have reported that seizure control was at least as good with once daily administration as with divided dosage. It is essential to use the enteric-coated formulation if this policy is being adopted, and even then gastrointestinal adverse effects or drowsiness may make a return to divided dosage necessary.

Phenobarbitone (Table 8.5)

Phenobarbitone is a substituted barbituric acid with a phenyl and ethyl group attached in position 5 (Appendix 8.3). It is one of the few barbiturates with useful antiepileptic activity on chronic administration.

Table 8.5 Summary of pharmacokinetic data on phenobarbitone

Range of daily maintenance dosage	Adult: 30–240 mg/day Child: 2–6 mg/kg/day
Minimum dose frequency	Once daily
Time to peak serum level	1–6 hours (oral and intramuscular)
Percentage bound to plasma proteins	45%
Apparent volume of distribution	0.8 l/kg
Elimination half-life	Adult: 50–160 hours Child: 30–70 hours
Time to steady state after starting therapy	Up to 30 days
Major metabolite	p-Hydroxyphenobarbitone

Absorption. The rate of absorption of phenobarbitone is variable. Jalling (1974) found peak serum concentrations 1–6 hours after oral administration, but slower absorption has been described in earlier reports (Sjögren, Solvell & Karlsson, 1965). This may be due to differences in pharmaceutical formulation and relationship to meals. Preparations of phenobarbitone and its sodium salt are available, but there does not appear to be a consistent difference in the absorption of the two compounds. The absorption is virtually complete.

When given intramuscularly, phenobarbitone reaches a peak serum concentration in 0.5–6 hours (Jalling, 1974; Graham, 1978), but this is too slow for the emergency treatment of status epilepticus.

Distribution and plasma protein binding. The distribution of phenobarbitone is sensitive to variations in plasma pH because it has a pKa value of 7.2. Acidosis causes a shift of the drug from plasma to tissues. It is about 45 per cent bound to plasma proteins, mainly to albumin and α-globulins. This relatively low degree of binding means that the drug is less susceptible to alterations in plasma protein concentrations, renal disease and drug interactions in which there is competition for binding sites. CSF concentrations reflect the free level in plasma (Houghton *et al.*, 1975b), but salivary concentrations do not, because they are sensitive to pH changes (Schmidt & Kupferberg, 1975). It is therefore unwise to use saliva for monitoring purposes. Penetration of the drug into the brain is relatively slow, which is another reason why phenobarbitone is not ideal for treating status epilepticus.

Table 8.6 Starting doses of phenobarbitone in children and infants. The doses have been chosen to produce an average serum concentration of 60 μmol/l (14 μg/ml)

Body weight Kg	Phenobarbitone dose	
	mg/kg/day	mg/day*
6–10	4.5	45
11–15	4.0	60
16–20	3.5	60
21–25	3.0	75
26–30	2.5	75
31–35	2.5	90
36–40	2.0	90
41–45	2.0	90
46–50	2.0	100
51–60	2.0	120

*doses rounded off to suit 15, 30, 60 and 100 mg dose units

Dose-serum concentration relationship. Over the therapeutic range of serum concentrations there is a nearly linear relationship between dose and serum level within subjects. For this reason phenobarbitone is a simpler drug to manage clinically than phenytoin. As with other drugs, however, there is considerable variation between subjects in the serum level produced by a given dose. Children metabolise the drug more quickly than

Table 8.7 Summary of pharmacokinetic data on primidone

Range of daily maintenance dosage	Adult 250–1500 mg/day Child 15–30 mg/kg/day
Minimum dose frequency	Twice daily
Time to peak serum level	2–5 hours
Percentage bound to plasma proteins	less than 20%
Apparent volume of distribution	0.6 l/kg
Major active metabolites	Phenobarbitone Phenylethylmalonamide (PEMA)
Elimination half-life in adults	Primidone 4–12 hours Derived phenobarbitone 50–160 hours Derived PEMA 29–36 hours (but see text)
Time to steady state after starting therapy	Up to 30 days for derived phenobarbitone

adults and therefore require a larger mg/kg dose. A suitable scheme for starting doses in children is given in Table 8.6.

Metabolism and renal elimination. Approximately half of the administered dose is metabolised to p-hydroxyphenobarbitone which is rapidly excreted both unchanged and as a glucuronide (Butler, 1978). The metabolite lacks antiepileptic activity. Unchanged phenobarbitone also appears in the urine, accounting for 20–40 per cent of the dose. Alkalinization of the urine increases the excretion of the parent compound and this has been taken advantage of in treating overdosage. The renal clearance can be increased from 4–5 mls/min to 30 mls/min by bicarbonate administration.

Methylphenobarbitone

Methylphenobarbitone differs from phenobarbitone in having a methyl group substituted in position 1 of barbituric acid ring. It is 20 times less soluble than phenobarbitone and there is doubt over the extent of its absorption, which may account for the fact that 2 mg of methylphenobarbitone is equivalent to 1 mg of phenobarbitone when given orally. Its absolute bioavailability has never been determined, however. Following absorption, it is demethylated to phenobarbitone with a half-life of about 20 hours (Eadie *et al.*, 1978). Steady-state serum levels of the parent compound are only about 10–15 per cent of the derived phenobarbitone. Methylphenobarbitone may be active in its own right, but in view of the

low serum levels of this compound, most of the pharmacological effect resides with the metabolite. There seems to be no advantage in giving methylphenobarbitone rather than phenobarbitone.

Primidone (Table 8.7)

This substance is a desoxybarbiturate which was first marketed as an antiepileptic drug in 1952 (Handley & Stewart, 1952). It is partly oxidised to phenobarbitone *in vivo* (Fig. 8.9).

Absorption. Peak serum concentrations are achieved within 2–5 hours after administration of a single dose, but on chronic administration peak levels appear to occur later (Booker *et al.*, 1970; Gallagher & Baumel, 1972).

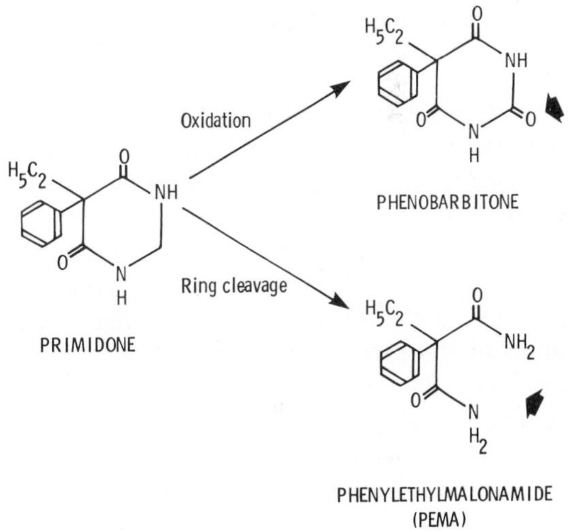

Fig. 8.9 Main metabolic pathways of primidone

Distribution and plasma protein binding. The degree of binding of primidone to plasma proteins is low, and can be ignored for practical purposes. Salivary concentrations are 75–100 per cent of the plasma concentration, the difference presumably being due to the small amount bound to plasma proteins.

Metabolism. Primidone is metabolised in the liver to phenobarbitone and phenylethylmalonamide (PEMA). On average, about 20–25 per cent is converted to the former and therefore a daily dose of 1000 mg of primidone should be regarded as the equivalent of administering 200–250 mg of phenobarbitone. However, there is considerable inter-subject variation in the extent of conversion, and this leads to a wide scatter of serum phenobarbitone : primidone concentration ratios (see below). The metabolism to phenobarbitone is very slow after single dose administration, and measurable serum concentrations of this compound are found only after 24–28 hours (Baumel et al., 1972). However, on chronic administration, and also when given in single doses to patients receiving other enzyme-inducing antiepileptic drugs (p. 361), the conversion occurs more quickly. Metabolism to PEMA is rapid following a single dose of primidone; the metabolite is measurable within 1–2 hours and peaks at 7–8 hours. At the start of therapy, marked central nervous system adverse effects (dizziness and sedation) may occur with quite small doses; this reaction appears to be related to serum concentrations of the parent drug rather than to the metabolites.

Elimination half-life and dose interval. Primidone has a half-life of only 4–12 hours and therefore considerable fluctuation in the serum concentration occurs throughout a 24 hour period. The derived phenobarbitone has a much longer half-life (50–160 hours) and therefore the serum concentration of this metabolite exceeds the concentration of the parent compound despite the fact that only 20–25 per cent is converted to phenobarbitone. PEMA also accumulates because it is eliminated more slowly than primidone. Its true elimination half-life when administered as such is about 15 hours (Richens, unpublished). When derived from primidone, its half-life is overestimated because it is being generated from the parent drug at the same time as it is being eliminated.

The ideal dose interval for primidone administration is uncertain because the rôle played by unchanged primidone and PEMA in the anticonvulsant effect of the drug has not been determined. In animals both these substances have been shown to have a protective effect in experimental seizures (Gallagher, Smith & Mattson, 1970; Baumel, Gallagher & Mattson, 1972), but whether they contribute to the overall effect in the treatment of epilepsy is less certain. However, Oxley et al. (1980) have shown that, in some patients, primidone is a superior antiepileptic drug to phenobarbitone when given in doses which

produce similar serum phenobarbitone concentrations. Whether the parent drug itself or the derived PEMA accounts for this additional activity is not known. In view of these doubts a minimum dose frequency of twice daily would seem to be appropriate.

Dose-serum concentration relationship. An approximately linear relationship exists between primidone dose and the derived serum phenobarbitone concentration. The ratio of serum primidone to serum phenobarbitone concentration at steady state is, on average, about 1 : 2.5, but there is a wide scatter between subjects due to differences in the rate of metabolism. Also, the ratio is affected by the large fluctuation in serum primidone level resulting from its short half-life. The co-administration of other enzyme-inducing antiepileptic drugs, i.e. phenytoin and carbamazepine, increases the ratio by increasing the rate of metabolism (see p. 361).

Urinary excretion. No data are available in adults, but in children it has been shown that up to two-thirds of a dose of primidone may be excreted unchanged (Kaufmann, Habersang & Lansky, 1977).

Sulthiame

Little information is available on the pharmacokinetics of this drug. It is absorbed fairly rapidly and completely (Diamond & Levy, 1963). About two-thirds of the dose is excreted unchanged in the urine, the remainder being eliminated mainly as a hydroxylated derivative. It has an important inhibitory effect on phenytoin metabolism (p. 363), which may partly account for its antiepileptic activity.

Ethosuximide (Sherwin, 1978) (Table 8.8)

Absorption. Ethosuximide is rapidly and completely absorbed from the gastrointestinal tract, peak serum levels occurring after 1–4 hours (Buchanan, Kinkel & Smith, 1973; Goulet, Kinkel & Smith, 1976). Absorption is quicker with syrup preparations.

Distribution and plasma protein binding. Plasma protein binding of the drug is negligible, and therefore the drug is present in saliva and CSF in

Table 8.8 Summary of pharmacokinetic data on ethosuximide

Range of daily maintenance dosage	Adult 500–1500 mg/day Child 10–25 mg/kg/day
Minimum dose frequency	Once daily
Time to peak serum level	1–4 hours
Percentage bound to plasma proteins	Negligible
Apparent volume of distribution	0.7 l/kg
Major inactive metabolites	2-(1-hydroxyethyl)- 2-methylsuccinimide 2-(2-hydroxyethyl)- 2-methylsuccinimide 2-acetyl- 2-methylsuccinimide
Elimination half-life	Adult 40–70 hours Child 20–40 hours
Time to steady-state after starting therapy	Up to 14 days (adults) Up to 7 days (children)

concentrations that approximate to that of plasma (McAuliffe *et al.*, 1977).

Dose-serum concentration relationship. There is evidence that a non-linear relationship exists between dose and serum level such that increments in dose produce disproportionate increases in serum level (Browne *et al.*, 1975). However, the non-linearity over the therapeutic range of serum concentrations is not sufficient to have important practical implications, in contrast to phenytoin (p. 300). A daily dose of 20 mg/kg yields a serum level of about 450 μmol/l (65 μg/ml) on average (Browne *et al.*, 1975).

Metabolism and urinary excretion. Ethosuximide is extensively metabolised to two hydroxylated metabolites and a ketone derivative (Table 8.8). The hydroxylated metabolites are excreted largely as glucuronides. Only 12–20 per cent of the drug is excreted unchanged in the urine.

Elimination half-life and dose interval. The elimination half-life of ethosuximide is long enough for once daily administration to be adopted (Buchanan *et al.*, 1976), although with larger doses gastrointestinal adverse effects may make this impractical.

Phensuximide (Porter et al., 1977)

Phensuximide is N-methyl-2-phenylsuccinimide. It is less potent than ethosuximide and its clinical use is declining. Doses of up to 3000 mg daily are required. It is rapidly absorbed and is metabolised

by N-desmethylation with a half-life of 4.5–12 hours.

Methsuximide (Porter et al., 1977)

Methsuximide is N, 2-dimethyl-2-phenyl-succinimide. Its metabolite, N-desmethyl-methsuximide, is pharmacologically active and accumulates because it has an elimination half-life of about 36 hours compared with 1–2 hours for the parent drug. The antiepileptic activity of the drug rests almost entirely with the metabolite because its concentration in plasma is, on average, several hundred times greater than that of the parent drug (Strong *et al.*, 1974).

Benzodiazepines

All of the 1,4-benzodiazepine drugs have anti-epileptic actions in addition to tranquillising and hypnotic effects. Their clinical usage has been determined more by marketing convenience than by differences in their pharmacology. Indeed, pharmacokinetic studies have subsequently shown that several compounds have been promoted for inappropriate uses. The elimination half-lives of two benzodiazepines which have commonly been used for hypnotic purposes, nitrazepam and flurazepam, are long, and therefore hangover effects are more marked than with some of the other compounds that have traditionally been used as tranquillisers (Table 8.9). Only two of the benzodiazepines, diazepam and clonazepam, will be discussed in detail.

Diazepam (Mandelli, Tognoni & Garattini, 1978) (Table 8.10)

Absorption. When given orally, diazepam is rapidly absorbed (Hillestad *et al.*, 1974; Gamble *et al.*, 1975). Administration after a meal delays the peak serum level but appears to increase the extent of absorption (Greenblatt *et al.*, 1978). Diazepam is very insoluble in water and is prepared for parenteral use in a vehicle which is irritant and often causes local thrombophlebitis on intravenous administration. The drug will come out of solution if diluted with small amounts of saline, but it may be diluted with large amounts

Table 8.9 Elimination half-lives of some commonly used benzodiazepine drugs

Drug	Half-life of parent compound (hours)	Active metabolite	Half-life of active metabolite (hours)
Diazepam	20–60	N-desmethyldiazepam (Nordiazepam)	30–90
Clorazepate	Very short	N-desmethyldiazepam	30–90
Nitrazepam	20–40	none	
Flurazepam	Very short	Desalkylflurazepam	24–48
Oxazepam	5–20	none	
Lorazepam	9–22	none	
Temazepam	6–10	none	
Clonazepam	20–60	none	

Table 8.10 Summary of pharmacokinetic data on diazepam

	Diazepam	N-Desmethyldiazepam
Range of daily adult maintenance dosage	5–60 mg/day	
Minimum dose frequency	Twice daily	
Time to peak serum level (oral)	0.5–2 hours	
Percentage bound to plasma proteins	97%	97%
Apparent volume of distribution	1-2 l/kg	
Major active metabolite	N-desmethyldiazepam Temazepam Oxazepam	Oxazepam
Inactive metabolites	Conjugated derivatives	Conjugated derivatives
Elimination half-life	20–60	30–90
Time to steady state after starting therapy		Up to 20 days

for intravenous infusion (p. 337). However, there is some uncertainty about this practice (Morris, 1978). When given intramuscularly, its absorption is slow and unpredictable (Hillestad et al., 1974; Gamble et al., 1975; Kanto, 1975) and it is therefore inadvisable to administer diazepam by this route for an emergency, e.g. status epilepticus, although it may be acceptable in situations where a slower and more prolonged effect is required. Diazepam solution for parenteral administration is rapidly absorbed when given per rectum using a needle-less syringe inserted into the rectum or by a specially designed applicator (Agurell et al., 1975; Kundsen, 1977; Dulac et al., 1978, Meberg et al., 1978). By this route of administration, peak serum levels occur within 6–10 minutes in many patients, although are seen later in some. Rectal diazepam can be used prophylactically for febrile convulsions (p. 85) but for the acute treatment of convulsions it is less satisfactory than intravenous administration when this is possible (Knudsen, 1979). Suppositories are much more slowly and erratically absorbed than the solution, and produce much lower serum levels.

Distribution and plasma protein binding. Following intravenous injection diazepam distributes very rapidly to body tissues. Peak brain concentrations are seen within 1–5 minutes. It is highly bound to plasma proteins, and CSF and salivary levels correspond to the free fraction (Di Gregorio, Riraino & Ruch, 1978).

Metabolism and urinary excretion. Diazepam is extensively metabolised by demethylation and hydroxylation. Its major metabolite, N-desmethyldiazepam (nordiazepam), is pharmacologically active and accumulates because it has a longer half-life than the parent drug (Bond, Hailey & Lader, 1977). The hydroxylated derivatives of diazepam and N-desmethyldiazepam are temazepam and oxazepam respectively; both are pharmacologically active but have short half-lives. All three metabolites are conjugated with glucuronic acid and excreted in the urine (Mandelli, et al., 1978). Only traces of the parent drug are excreted.

Elimination half-life and dose interval. The long half-life of diazepam, and particularly its N-desmethyl metabolite, allows the drug to be administered once daily. With larger doses, however, the sudden rise in the serum concentration may cause adverse effects and divided dosage may then be preferable. On the other hand a single daily administration last thing at night may have advantages if a hypnotic effect is desirable. The serum concentration of N-desmethyldiazepam is usually higher than that of the parent drug in steady state.

Clonazepam (Pinder et al., 1976) (Table 8.11)

Clonazepam is fairly rapidly absorbed, producing peak serum levels within 1–3 hours although sometimes the peak may occur later (Berlin & Dahlstrom, 1975). It distributes equally rapidly and is about 85 per cent bound to plasma proteins. It is extensively metabolised to 7-aminoclonazepam and 7-acetaminoclonazepam, both of which are inactive (Sjö *et al.*, 1975b). The elimination half-life is usually long enough (20–60 hours) for once daily dosage to be possible in adults, but as with diazepam divided dosage is preferable if adverse effects related to peak levels are to be avoided. The half-life is shorter in children (22–33 hours, Dreifuss *et al.*, 1975). Other enzyme-inducing antiepileptic drugs can lower serum clonazepam levels (Sjö *et al.*, 1975b).

Table 8.11 Summary of pharmacokinetic data on clonazepam

Range of daily adult maintenance dosage	1–10 mg/day
Minimum dose frequency	Once daily
Time to peak serum level (oral)	1–3 hours
Percentage bound to plasma proteins	85%
Apparent volume of distribution	2–5 l/kg
Inactive metabolites	7-aminoclonazepam 7-acetaminoclonazepam
Elimination half-life	20–60 hours
Time to steady state after starting therapy	Up to 14 days

PHARMACOKINETICS IN SPECIAL SITUATIONS

Neonates (Morselli, 1977)

Neonates who have not been exposed to enzyme-inducing drugs *in utero*, metabolise most drugs

slowly at birth. During the first month of life the enzyme systems mature and are capable of metabolising antiepileptic drugs much faster than in the adult. During childhood, the rate of metabolism gradually slows until it reaches adult levels. In neonates who have been exposed to enzyme-inducing drugs *in utero*, the trans-placentally-transferred drugs are metabolised at least as quickly as in the mother. For example, Rane *et al.* (1974) found half-lives of 6.6–34 hours for transplacentally-transferred phenytoin in the neonate.

Phenytoin levels are lower in cord plasma and plasma from neonates than in maternal plasma (Fredholm *et al.*, 1975). The reason for this is that the plasma protein binding of the drug is lower in the neonate because endogenous substances such as steroids, free fatty acids and bilirubin compete for protein binding sites.

With drugs that are excreted unchanged in the urine in substantial amounts, e.g. phenobarbitone, the immature renal excretory function and low mean urinary pH may contribute to the slow elimination of these drugs from the plasma of newborn infants.

Pregnancy

There is general agreement that serum antiepileptic drug levels may fall progressively throughout pregnancy (Eadie, Lander & Tyrer, 1977; Dam *et al.*, 1979). The reason for this is not yet understood, but may involve an increase in the rate of metabolism resulting from an increased metabolic capacity of the maternal liver, the development of drug metabolising activity in the foetal liver, and a reduction in plasma protein binding of drugs. Fit frequency often increases during pregnancy, and may be related to this fall in drug levels (Mygind *et al.*, 1976). Hormonal factors, however, may also play a part.

The excretion of antiepileptic drugs in breast milk has always been a matter of concern and many epileptic women have been advised not to breast feed. In fact, the quantities of drugs excreted are usually small (Table 8.12). A possible exception is ethosuximide which, because of its negligible plasma protein binding, is excreted in sufficient amounts to produce a low therapeutic serum level in the infant when the mother has a

Table 8.12 Approximate drug intake in breast-fed infants nursed by an epileptic mother. (Based on data of Kaneko, Sato and Suzuki, 1979)

Drug	Milk : serum concentration ratio	Infant dose* mg/day(mg/kg/day)
Phenytoin	0.20	1.5 mg (0.5 mg/kg)
Phenobarbitone	0.45	5.5 mg (1.8 mg/kg)
Primidone	0.80	6.0 mg /2.0 mg/kg)
Carbamazepine	0.40	1.5 mg (0.5 mg/kg)
Ethosuximide	0.80	24.0 mg (8.0 mg/kg)

*Infant dose calculated on a milk intake of 500 ml/day for a 3 kg infant and a therapeutic maternal serum drug concentration

high therapeutic serum level, which should be an unusual circumstance. Also, high maternal doses of diazepam might possibly cause hypotonia in the infant (Cole & Hailey, 1975). On the other hand, abrupt withdrawal of some drugs at birth, e.g. phenobarbitone and benzodiazepine drugs, may give rise to withdrawal symptoms, and a slower reduction in dose associated with breast feeding might conceivably have advantages.

Disease

Most of the reported pharmacokinetic studies of antiepileptic drugs have been performed in normal volunteers or in patients who were healthy other than having epilepsy. Sometimes it is necessary to administer these drugs to patients with diseases of other systems, and these diseases may radically change the way in which they are handled.

Gastrointestinal disease

It is likely that the absorption of drugs can be modified in patients who have undergone gastric or small bowel surgery, or who have small bowel conditions such as coeliac disease. This possibility has been little investigated although one study showed good absorption of phenytoin and ethosuximide in a patient with a jejuno-ileal bypass (Peterson & Zweig, 1974).

Hypoalbuminaemia

The importance of changes in plasma albumin concentration on the protein binding of drugs has been mentioned earlier (p. 295). For a given serum drug concentration, the amount of a highly bound drug which remains unbound increases as the plasma albumin falls, and because it is the latter fraction which produces the concentration gradient for drugs to enter the brain, a reduced albumin level may cause drug toxicity at apparently therapeutic serum levels. This possibility should be borne in mind if a patient shows unexpected toxicity at normal serum levels.

Liver disease (Blaschke, 1977)

Antiepileptic drug disposition may be altered in several ways by liver disease:

a. The development of portal-systemic anastamoses in cirrhosis may allow drugs to bypass the liver on absorption, leading to an increased bioavailability.

b. Systemic metabolism may be reduced by hepatocellular disease.

c. Plasma protein binding may be reduced by hypoalbuminaemia and by competition for binding sites by high levels of bilirubin. Drugs which are extensively bound to plasma proteins are likely to be most affected. Thus, there is good evidence that the plasma protein binding of phenytoin is reduced in cirrhosis, resulting in a lower total serum concentration of the drug but a higher free fraction (Hooper et al., 1974). The pharmacological effect of the drug would therefore be greater than predicted by measurement of the serum level. However, if hepatocellular function is significantly impaired, phenytoin toxicity may result (Kutt et al., 1964a). Acute viral hepatitis can also disturb phenytoin binding and metabolism (Blaschke et al., 1975). The disposition of benzodiazepine drugs (Andreasen et al., 1976) and valproic acid (Klotz, Rapp & Mueller, 1978) may be similarly affected. Although carbamazepine binding may be reduced (Hooper et al., 1975) an increased toxicity of this drug in liver disease has not been reported. Phenobarbitone disposition appears to be little affected.

Renal disease (Reidenberg & Drayer, 1978)

Although renal excretion plays a small part in the elimination of most antiepileptic drugs, renal failure can indirectly alter the distribution of drugs by reducing their binding to plasma proteins. The free fraction may be increased at least two-fold for phenytoin (Sherwin et al., 1976) and valproic acid (Gugler & Mueller, 1978). The impaired binding may be partly due to a lowered serum albumin concentration, but a more important factor is probably a change in the molecular configuration of albumin or the presence of endogenous inhibitors of binding (Reidenberg & Drayer, 1978). Serum phenytoin and valproic acid levels are therefore a poor guide of the therapeutic effect of these drugs unless allowance for the reduced binding is made. There is evidence that induction of phenytoin metabolism may also contribute to the lower serum levels in renal disease (Odar-Cederlöf & Borga, 1974).

Phenobarbitone is cleared partly by urinary excretion, and creatinine clearance values below 30 ml/min may be associated with phenobarbitone toxicity (Lous, 1966).

Other diseases.

It is likely that cardiac failure alters the disposition of antiepileptic drugs although this has not been studied. Acute viral infections have been shown to inhibit drug metabolism and therefore drug toxicity may be mistaken for symptoms of the intercurrent infection. Drugs given for concomitant diseases may also influence the pharmacokinetics of antiepileptic drugs (p. 359).

DRUG LEVELS IN THE MANAGEMENT OF EPILEPSY (Richens, 1976; Reynolds, 1980)

Since the development of spectrophotometric techniques for measuring phenobarbitone and phenytoin in the late 1940s and early 1950s, a variety of methods have been described for estimating these compounds. The most widely used is gas chromatography although immunoassay techniques may supplant gas chromatography in the future. Immunoassay offers the advantage of rapid estimation without a preliminary extraction procedure to separate the drug from interfering compounds. Gas chromatography, although specific and accurate, is not well suited to the routine laboratory because it requires special skills on the part of the operator, and the number of specimens that can be handled per day is small, with the result that a restriction on the number of requests for drug estimations has to be made. High performance liquid chromatography is a newer technique which, like gas chromatography, is specific and accurate and is likely to be used increasingly. Details of these techniques can be found in a number of reviews (see Pippenger, Penry & Kutt, 1978).

Concern about the accuracy of estimations is obviously necessary, for there is no point whatsoever in going through the costly exercise of measuring a drug level if the result is as likely to mislead the clinician as to help him. Careful attention to quality control within the laboratory is necessary if the clinician is to have confidence in the results (Ayers et al., 1980). Several interlaboratory quality control schemes have been set up to assist the analyst to achieve accuracy (Pippenger et al., 1978; Griffiths et al., 1980).

Whether the report is helpful to him, however, depends upon the reasons which made the clinician decide to request a drug level. There are a number of sound reasons in clinical practice for measuring the serum level of a drug, whether an antiepileptic drug or any other type of compound. These will be spelled out because they should be borne in mind whenever a decision to monitor a drug is made.

Reasons for monitoring drug levels

1. When there is wide interindividual variation in the rate of metabolism of a drug, producing marked differences in steady state levels between patients.
2. When saturation kinetics occur, causing a steep relationship between dose and serum level within the therapeutic range.
3. When the therapeutic ratio of a drug is low, i.e. when therapeutic doses are close to toxic doses. Most of the available antiepileptic drugs have a low ratio.
4. When signs of toxicity are difficult to recognise clinically, or where signs of over-dosage or under-dosage are indistinguishable.
5. During pregnancy or when gastro-intestinal, hepatic or renal disease is present, which is likely

to disturb drug absorption, metabolism or excretion.

6. When patients are receiving multiple drug therapy with the attendant risk of drug interaction. If a drug is being added which is known to alter the metabolism of an existing drug, it is wise to monitor the level of the latter.

7. Where there is doubt about the patient's reliability in taking his tablets (i.e. his compliance). Up to 50 per cent of epileptic outpatients do not take what is prescribed (Mucklow & Dollery, 1978). Serial samples, particularly on admission to hospital, may identify these patients.

8. During research studies such as controlled therapeutic trials. A correlation between the serum level of a drug and its therapeutic or toxic effect is sound evidence that the effect really is due to the drug.

Obviously, for research studies the decision to measure serum levels will be based on different criteria from routine estimations performed to improve the clinical management of the individual patient. Sufficient evidence from prospective studies relating serum level and effect must be available in order that the results can be interpreted in a way that will lead to improved management. Unfortunately this is not always the case and the 'therapeutic ranges of serum levels' which are widely quoted have sometimes been derived simply from observing the ranges of levels normally encountered in patients whose fits appear to be controlled by standard doses of the drugs in question. For some drugs, therefore, there is little to be gained by measuring levels – indeed the clinician may be deluding himself by using an apparently scientific approach to the control of epilepsy, and succeeding only in treating the serum level rather than the patient. There is little to be gained from having the most precisely controlled serum level of a drug if the patient's epilepsy is in fact resistant to it. Perhaps it would be worthwhile examining each drug in turn to consider the evidence for and against monitoring levels.

Phenytoin

The soundest case can be made out for measuring phenytoin levels. Running through the points

listed above, the rate of metabolism of the drug varies widely from person to person and this is exaggerated by saturation of the enzyme system involved. The therapeutic range of serum levels is close to the toxic range; indeed in some patients they seem to overlap. Sometimes phenytoin intoxication is difficult to recognise when it presents in an unusual way, such as odd neuropsychiatric symptoms, encephalopathy or even as an increase in fit frequency. Sometimes the clinical signs are taken as an indication for more intensive antiepileptic drug therapy (Ahmad et al., 1975). These are very compelling reasons for measuring phenytoin levels routinely. Perhaps it may be worthwhile spelling out the clinical situations in which measuring serum phenytoin levels will be of value.

1. When fits are not controlled by greater-than-average doses of the drug. The important question here is whether an optimum level of the drug has not yet been achieved because the patient is a rapid metaboliser or is failing to take his tablets, or whether his epilepsy is resistant to phenytoin.

2. If a patient shows clinical signs of phenytoin intoxication, namely coarse nystagmus, ataxia and slurred speech, it is useful to confirm that they are drug-induced by estimating the serum level. Sometimes a normal or low level may be found in a patient whose cerebellar signs are caused by cerebellar pathology rather than acute intoxication (see p. 349).

3. If a patient presents with odd neuropsychiatric symptoms or dyskinetic movements. These can result from phenytoin intoxication even in the absence of nystagmus.

4. If a previously well-controlled patient has a sudden increase in fit frequency. This can result from a fall in the serum level (e.g. because he is failing to take his tablets) or from a rise to toxic levels (e.g. from a change in biological availability of a formulation).

5. If another drug which might interfere with phenytoin metabolism is added to the patient's treatment. Sulthiame is important in this respect (Houghton & Richens, 1974b).

6. In the management of status epilepticus in a patient who has been receiving maintenance doses of phenytoin (p. 337).

7. In the management of epilepsy in childhood,

Table 8.13 Number of patients without seizures in various plasma concentration intervals. Patients treated only with phenytoin

Concentration of phenytoin in plasma μ mol/l (μg/ml)	0–39 (0–9.9)	40–79 (10.0–19.9)	above 80 (above 20.0)
Number of patients	95	33	20
Percentage of total material	64.2	22.3	13.5
Number of patients without seizures during the last two months	41	24	19
Percentage seizure-free in each group	43.2	72.5	95.0

(Taken from a retrospective survey by Lund, 1973)

in which dosage adjustment can be more difficult.

8. If the epilepsy is complicated by other diseases which might affect phenytoin handling.

9. During pregnancy.

Buchthal *et al*. (1960) were the first to attempt to define a therapeutic range of serum concentrations for phenytoin. In a prospective study in 12 hospitalised patients with frequent fits they found no clinical response until the serum concentration exceeded 40 μmol/l (10 μg/ml). As clinical signs of toxicity were frequently encountered with levels above 80 μmol/l (20 μg/ml) they considered that a therapeutic range of 40–80 μmol/l (10–20μg/ml) would give optimum control of fits without toxicity. This view has been reiterated by Kutt and McDowell (1968) and this range has been

widely used in the management of phenytoin therapy.

However, Buchthal and his colleagues studied only a small number of patients with severe epilepsy and their conclusions may not be valid for ambulant patients with mild or moderate epilepsy. Although a number of retrospective studies have been performed in patients of this type, the results have been conflicting. Lund (1973) found that higher concentrations were associated with better control of epilepsy, particularly with levels in excess of 40 μmol/1 (10 μg/ml) (Table 8.13), but Triedman, Fishman and Yahr (1960) and Haerer and Grace (1969) had previously found no correlation. In two studies, the relationship was reversed, i.e. a lower serum concentration was found in

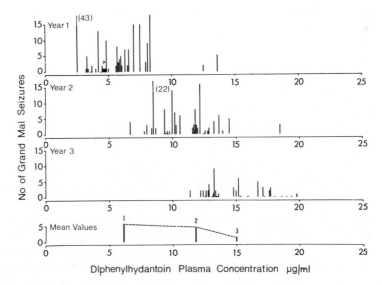

Fig. 8.10 Relationship between the annual number of grand mal seizures and corresponding mean concentration of phenytoin (diphenylhydantoin) for each of 32 patients with epilepsy observed prospectively for three years. Annual mean values for the whole group are given at the bottom. (Reproduced from Lund, 1974b, by kind permission of the editor.) (*note*: 1 μg/ml = 4 μ mol/l)

patients with adequately controlled fits (Stensrud & Palmer, 1964; Travers, Reynolds & Gallagher, 1972).

Obviously, restrospective studies are an unsatisfactory way of examining the problem because too many factors are left uncontrolled. For this reason, Lund (1974b) set up a three year prospective study in 32 patients with grand mal epilepsy (Fig. 8.10). The patients were selected because they had at least one grand mal attack during a two month control period. During the first year, plasma phenytoin levels averaged 24.4 μmol/l (6.1 μg/ml) but during the second and third years the levels were increased to 46.8 μmol/l (11.7 μg/ml) and 60 μmol/l (15.0 μg/ml) respectively by a change in the brand of phenytoin or by increments in dosage. The total number of fits occurring during the three years were 186, 132 and 52 respectively. Although the improvement in control was independent of the type of epilepsy,

the optimal phenytoin level for each patient was dependent upon the severity of the epilepsy (Fig. 8.11).

This latter observation is important because it suggests that many epileptic out-patients with mild epilepsy may be controlled with serum levels that would be termed 'subtherapeutic' using the criteria of Buchthal et al. (1960). The main limitation of both prospective studies is that the selection criteria excluded patients with mild epilepsy. No doubt if patients of this type were included, a dose-response curve would be found to the left of the curves plotted by Lund (Fig. 8.11), and would intersect the plasma concentration axis at a level well below 40 μmol/l (10 μg/ml). On the other hand, there are likely to be patients with severe epilepsy who produce a curve to the right, and whose fit frequency will never fall to zero despite toxic doses of phenytoin alone. An alternative approach to studying serum level response

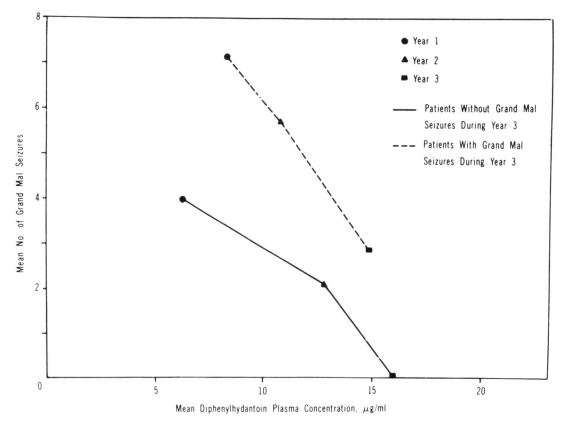

Fig. 8.11 Mean data from Fig. 8.10 plotted according to whether seizures were completely controlled or not during the third year of the study by Lund. (1974b). (Reproduced by kind permission of the editor.) (*note*: 1 μg/ml = 4 μmol/l.)

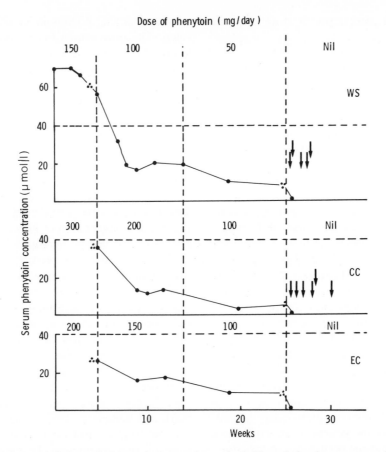

Fig. 8.12 Gradual withdrawal of phenytoin therapy in three patients who had been fit free for many years. The horizontal dashed line represents the lower limit of the usually quoted 'therapeutic range' of serum levels. Each arrow represents a major fit. A further plot of patient CC is illustrated in Fig. 8.13. (Reproduced from Richens, 1976, by kind permission of the publisher) (*note*: $4\,\mu M = 4\,\mu\,mol/l = 1\,\mu g/ml$)

relationships is to make gradual dose reductions in patients who have been receiving long-term maintenance therapy with phenytoin but who have not had a fit for many years. Figure 8.12 illustrates the serum phenytoin levels in three patients over a period of 20–25 weeks in which the phenytoin dose was slowly reduced to zero. Despite the phenytoin levels falling to subtherapeutic values of around 8 μmol/l (2 μg/ml), no fits occurred until the final dose unit was stopped. A few days later, however, two of the three had a number of major fits, their first for at least five years. Perhaps a larger study would reveal many patients like these, who need quite low phenytoin levels to achieve full control of fits. Increasing the level into the 'therapeutic range' would serve only to increase the likelihood of adverse effects in these patients.

Here, then, is the importance of treating the patient and not the serum level. The rigid use of a lower limit of $40\,\mu$ mol/1 ($10\,\mu$g/ml) to the therapeutic range is not in the interest of many patients and may lead to misguided dose changes.

It should be noted that the three patients in Figure 8.12 were receiving phenobarbitone in addition to phenytoin. This raises the important question of whether simultaneous administration of phenobarbitone reduces the phenytoin level necessary to achieve control of fits. If so, does a combination of three or four drugs in low dosage achieve the same control, with fewer adverse effects, than one drug used in high dosage? There is a school of thought that believes this is so. Obviously, if it is, the application of a standard therapeutic range of levels to all patients despite their receiving an assortment of drug combinations is invalid.

There is general agreement that clinical signs of phenytoin intoxication become frequent when the serum level rises to somewhere between 80 and 120 μmol/l (20 and 30 μg/ml) (e.g. see Buchthal et al., 1960; Kutt et al., 1964b; Lascelles, Kocen & Reynolds, 1970; Lund, 1973). The incidence of toxic effects at a particular concentration varies considerably from one report to another, no doubt depending on the clinician's criteria for intoxication. Although Kutt et al. (1964a & b) found a good correlation between the serum level and the clinical signs of toxicity a number of authors report patients with levels greater than 160 μmol/l (40 μg/ml) in the absence of clinical signs (e.g. Triedman et al., 1960; Buchthal et al., 1960; Loeser, 1961). Conversely, some patients may show nystagmus at serum levels below 60 μmol/l (15 μg/ml) (Haerer & Grace, 1969). However, it may be difficult to decide whether nystagmus or ataxia in these patients is due to phenytoin or to underlying brain damage which has perhaps occurred during major fits. Obviously, rigid use of an upper limit to the therapeutic range is not only unnecessary but may deny some patients the benefit of an extra therapeutic effect without the occurrence of toxicity.

In conclusion, therefore, the object in the management of phenytoin therapy should be to increase the serum concentration until complete control of fits is achieved, whether this is at 20 μmol/l in a patient with mild epilepsy, 60 μmol/l in one with moderate epilepsy, or 100 μmol/l in severe disease. A knowledge of the serum level makes it possible to achieve this optimal treatment without risk of over-dosage. The inflexible use of a range of 40–80 μmol/l imposes unnecessary and harmful limits on clinical judgement. Figure 8.16 provides a simple nomogram for making dosage increments, taking into account the saturation kinetics of phenytoin. If adequate control is not possible within this range, it is permissible to increase the level further by small increments in dosage if signs of toxicity are absent. If control is then not achieved without producing intolerable adverse effects, the clinician has one of two choices, either to substitute an alternative drug or to add a second drug while maintaining the phenytoin level at a subtoxic value. The main reason for monitoring phenytoin levels during this period is to give guidance in choosing dosage increments and to assist in recognising drug toxicity.

Phenobarbitone

Although a number of indications listed for phenytoin apply also to phenobarbitone, the clinical value of phenobarbitone estimations is far less. This is probably because the relationship between the serum concentration of phenobarbitone and its actions on the central nervous system may not be as close as has been assumed. It is well recognised that tolerance occurs to the sedative effects (Butler et al., 1954) such that a serum level of 20 μmol/l (4.8 μg/ml) produced acutely may have a greater sedative effect than a level of 200 mol/l (48 μg/ml) which has been maintained chronically. Whether tolerance occurs to the antiepileptic activity is less certain. Although it has been found in mouse (Schmidt et al., 1980) it has not been formally studied in man. Buchthal, Svensmark and Simonsen (1968) found no tendency for 'escape' from control to occur during a follow-up time of two months in 11 patients started on phenobarbitone, but as tolerance would be expected to develop during the 20–30 day period when the serum level was rising to a plateau, it would have been masked.

Buchthal et al. (1968) studied 11 hospitalised patients with grand mal fits occurring from once a week to once a month. They were treated with phenobarbitone alone and were not fully controlled until the serum level exceeded 42 μmol/l (10 μg/ml). No toxic effects were seen in this study, but earlier Buchthal and Svensmark (1959) had found that drowsiness occurred at levels of 105–210 μmol/l (25–50 μg/ml). Plaa and Hine (1960) reported mental slowness and ataxia in four phenobarbitone-treated patients whose serum levels varied from 150–325 μmol/l (36–77 μg/ml), although several other patients had levels above 125 μmol/l (30 μg/ml) without evidence of intoxication. Sunshine (1957) reported levels of up to 250 μmol/l (60 μg/ml) in patients who were free of symptoms.

The difference in the incidence of intoxication in these studies no doubt arises partly because different criteria were used to judge toxicity. Mental slowness and drowsiness are difficult qualities to judge, particularly if the clinician is looking for changes over several months in a patient who is already impaired by brain damage. A slow-witted patient with a low IQ may appear asymptomatic on a large dose of phenobarbitone whereas an intelligent man with a responsible job may feel intellectually impaired by quite small doses. Nevertheless, there may, in addition, be variation between patients in their sensitivity to the drug and their ability to acquire a tolerance to its central effects.

Despite these difficulties, Buchthal and Lennox-Buchthal (1972b) considered that the therapeutic range for phenobarbitone was 40–105 μmol/1 (10–25 μg/ml), although most authorities would consider this range much too low. As some degree of sedation probably occurs within this range, and because there is no clear-cut level at which sedation suddenly becomes prominent, the upper level of the therapeutic range depends upon the tolerance which the patient and his physician have for the sedative effects of the drug.

In conclusion, it is likely that the relationship between the serum level and tissue effect of phenobarbitone is not a constant one but depends on the degree of tolerance that has developed. As one of the fundamental principles behind therapeutic drug monitoring is that this relationship should be constant, it seems that the value of measuring phenobarbitone levels may be less than was previously thought. Perhaps this accounts for the fact that a substantial proportion of patients are found to have 'toxic' levels on routine monitoring without much in the way of obvious toxic signs. Certainly the syndrome of phenobarbitone intoxication is much less clear-cut than for phenytoin.

Primidone

With primidone the situation is more complicated because it is converted into the two active metabolites phenobarbitone and PEMA (p. 307) as well as possibly being active in its own right (Baumel *et*

al., 1972). Indeed, Oxley *et al.* (1980) showed that primidone had advantages over phenobarbitone in some patients, and concluded that the additional benefit was probably due to the unchanged drug and/or PEMA. Thus, for a full assessment it may be that the levels of all three compounds need to be measured. However, for this to be justified, the relative potencies of the three compounds would need to be known so that the overall antiepileptic effect could be assessed. This is not possible on present evidence. The most practical approach is to monitor derived phenobarbitone.

One potential value of measuring unchanged primidone is in detecting non-compliance, for the patient who arrives at the clinic having taken the drug for only a few days beforehand will have a low ratio of phenobarbitone to primidone in his serum. Apart from this, primidone estimations for routine purposes are not helpful. Perhaps the position will be different when further research has clarified the relationship between primidone levels and fit control. Many laboratories report on primidone levels because the drug gives a measurable peak on a chromatogram run for phenytoin or phenobarbitone. The clinician is probably better off concentrating on these latter two drugs and ignoring the primidone value.

Carbamazepine

Serum levels of this drug show considerable variation from patient to patient and are markedly influenced by the presence of other enzyme inducing drugs. A knowledge of the serum level is therefore helpful in dosage tailoring. In general the dose will be much lower in patients receiving monotherapy. In a prospective study in 45 adult institutionalised patients, Cereghino *et al.* (1974a) found serum concentrations ranging from 23–58 μmol/l (5–13.7 μg/ml), with 70 per cent of values between 23 and 46μmol/l (5 and 10 μg/ml). In infants and children Sillanpää *et al.* (1979) found a good therapeutic effect at serum concentrations of only 12–18 μmol/l (2.9–4.3 μg/ml). Adverse effects usually do not occur until serum levels of around 40–50 μmol/l (9.5–12 μg/ml) are reached, but there is considerable variability between patients. Blurring of vision and diplopia are the most common dose-related adverse effects and result from a disturbance of extra-ocular muscle balance. Although these symptoms are often a good indication of a pending toxicity, some patients may become hyponatraemic and show impaired water balance before other signs of toxicity appear (Perucca *et al.*, 1978). This may be the reason why carbamazepine toxicity is associated with an increase in fit frequency. Certainly it justifies routine monitoring.

As carbamazepine has a relatively short half-life on chronic treatment, standardisation of the time of drawing the blood sample is preferable (see below).

The serum concentration of the active epoxide metabolite is too low to be important in adults, although in infants and children it may sometimes be almost as high as the parent drug, and as it is less protein bound it may contribute appreciably to the therapeutic effect (Rane *et al.*, 1976; Sillanpää *et al.*, 1979). Insufficient evidence is available, however, to justify routine monitoring of the epoxide.

Sodium valproate

The position with regards to monitoring valproic acid levels is not clear at present. The drug appears to have a somewhat greater therapeutic ratio than some of the more traditional drugs although the occurrence of hair loss, tremor, CNS adverse effects, platelet deficiency and perhaps hepatotoxicity seem to occur mainly at high serum levels i.e. above 800 μmol/l (Henrikson & Johannessen, 1980). As was pointed out on page 305, sodium valproate appears to have a 'hit-and-run' effect and if this is confirmed it lessens the value of drug level monitoring because the serum level, and fluctuations in it, will not correlate closely with the antiepileptic effect. Nevertheless, Gram *et al.* (1980) have shown that increasing the serum levels within a range of 113–344 μmol/l in a group of 13 patients produced a clear improvement in fit control; the design of their trial, however, allowed time for the effect to plateau following a change in dose. It should be noted that the serum levels in this study were much below the normally quoted therapeutic range of 350–700 μmol/l, despite which a good response was seen.

The short half-life of valproic acid leads to marked fluctuation in the serum level during a 24 hour period, and therefore standardisation of sampling is essential (see below).

Clonazepam

As with phenobarbitone, tolerance occurs to the effect of clonazepam (and other benzodiazepine drugs) and therefore the same limitations apply to the monitoring of this drug. Furthermore, serum levels of clonazepam are much lower than for most of the other antiepileptic drugs and therefore technical difficulties in measurement loom large. In fact, the poor quality of results returned in external quality control checks indicate that they may be more misleading than helpful (Griffiths *et al.*, 1980). There are no satisfactory studies of the relationship between serum levels and clinical effect, although Morselli (1978) reported that plasma levels over 580–640 nmol/l (180–200 ng/ml) were associated with an increase in seizure frequency, improvement occurring on reduction to 130–160 nmol/l (40–50 ng/ml).

Ethosuximide

As it is used mainly in children, routine monitoring may have a place, although the serum level appears to be reasonably predictable for a given dose in mg/kg provided the age of the patient is taken into account (Sherwin & Robb, 1972). Regular monitoring was found to reduce non-compliance and allowed drug requirements to be individualised, resulting in an improvement in control (Sherwin, Robb & Lechter, 1973). Two prospective studies have been carried out to study the relationship between control of absence seizures and plasma levels of ethosuximide. One, involving only 18 patients but with intensive study over a nine-week period (Penry *et al.*, 1972), showed that plasma levels in the completely controlled patients were in the range of 290–500 μmol/l (41–70 μg/ml). However, as only four of the 18 achieved 100 per cent control it is difficult to draw firm conclusions about the therapeutic range. Patients who had absences which were only partly controlled had plasma levels in the range of 230–740 μmol/l (32–104 μg/ml). In a second study involving 117 patients (Sherwin & Robb, 1972), 45 per cent were completely controlled with ethosuximide and most of these patients had plasma levels above 280 μmol/l (40 μg/ml). A number of patients had levels in excess of 700 μmol/l (100 μg/ml) and the authors suggest that the therapeutic level for some may be as high as 850 μmol/l (120 μg/ml). In a follow-up study, the dose of ethosuximide was altered in 27 patients, with control being achieved in some when their levels approached 280 μmol/l (40 μg/ml). Thus, there is good evidence from these studies that control of absence seizures is related to the plasma level of the drug, and that most patients require a level of up to 700–850 μmol/l (100–120 μg/ml) to achieve optimum control. There does not appear to be a clear correlation between serum levels and adverse effects (Sherwin, 1978). The active metabolite of methsuximide, N-desmethylmethsuximide, is responsible for the antiepileptic effect of the drug. A therapeutic range of up to 200 μmol/l (40 μg/ml) for the metabolite has been suggested (Strong et al., 1974) but further work is required to define the precise range.

Troxidone

The active metabolite of troxidone, dimethadione, accumulates so that its concentration in plasma is about 20 times higher than that of the parent compound. Retrospective studies indicate that most patients whose absence seizures are controlled have dimethadione concentrations greater than 5400 μmol/l (700 μg/ml) (Booker, 1972b).

Timing of blood sampling

The shorter a drug's elimination half-life the greater the fluctuation in serum levels throughout a 24 hour period. Although the frequency of dosing is adjusted to compensate for this, it is seldom practical to administer a dose during the night and therefore an early morning trough occurs which, for a drug like sodium valproate may be only about one half of the peak level. With phenobarbitone and phenytoin (Fig. 8.7) this fluctuation can usually be ignored, and a random sample will give a reasonable estimate of the steady state level. With carbamazepine, the fluctuation is greater and

therefore standardisation is preferable. There is no ideal time, but if the conclusions reached by Nicholson, Dobbs and Rogers (1980) on digoxin apply also to carbamazepine, a sample taken 6 hours after dosing, using a twice daily regime, would be the best compromise. For sodium valproate a shorter interval of about 4–5 hours after dosing would be most suitable.

In practice, blood samples will usually coincide with the time of the patient's clinic visit because it is inconvenient to do otherwise. The advantage to be gained from attempting to achieve the pharmacokinetic ideal is usually too small to be justified. In residential institutions or with hospital in-patients, however, it is possible to achieve standardisation without too much inconvenience. In out-patients, a certain degree of standardisation is likely to be reached by a regular clinic always taking place at the same time. If this clinic is an afternoon one, and if twice daily dosing is encouraged, most of the samples will be taken at a time which does not deviate too far from the ideal.

Abuse of drug monitoring

Perhaps a note of warning should be sounded at this point. Too often in modern medicine is the test result treated rather than the patient, and this is particularly so when clinical decisions are not easy to make, such as in treating the patient with severe epilepsy. Booker (1972a) views this problem in the following terms:

Unfortunately, we have seen occasional adverse effects from the availability of serum level determinations. The values have tended to regress over time not to the mean which might be expected but to the published 'therapeutic' levels. Subjects with low levels have had their doses increased, and doses associated with high levels have been decreased. In a few cases, we have seen seizures recur or toxicity develop, so that the treatment of a laboratory value instead of the patient is not always to the benefit of the latter. To say that the fault lies with the physician and not the methodology, while correct, ignores the fact that physicians are human. As such, faced with the increasing complexity and amount of scientific data upon which his practice must be based, the clinician will intuitively turn to simple algorithms that will reduce the complexity of his problems to simple decisions. Unfortunately, these will be increasingly based on laboratory values. Thus, in the application of population values, i.e. therapeutic and toxic levels, to the treatment of an individual subject, we must always continue to treat the patient and not the laboratory value. Nevertheless, knowledge of the serum levels is a valuable resource for the clinician.

Table 8.14 Which drugs should be monitored?

Drug	Therapeutic levels† (μmol/l)	Value rating‡	Comments
Phenytoin	Up to 80	*****	Monitoring essential for good therapy. Accurate dosing difficult without serum levels, because of saturable metabolism. Low therapeutic ratio, disguised toxicity and frequency of drug interactions add weight to the case for routine monitoring.
Carbamazepine	Up to 50	****	Monitoring useful. Clinical symptoms (especially eye symptoms) are often helpful in determining dose limit, but water intoxication and increase in fit frequency may be caused by high serum level. Standardisation of sampling time advisable.
Ethosuximide	Up to 700	***	Monitoring in children is less acceptable, but can be helpful as a guide to correct dose.
Phenobarbitone	Up to 170	**	Therapeutic ranges misleading. Development of receptor tolerance limits value of routine monitoring.
Primidone (unchanged)		*	Phenobarbitone is major metabolite – this should be monitored if indicated.
Sodium valproate	Up to 700	*	Timed specimens essential. Little evidence that management is improved by monitoring. Possibility of 'hit and run' effect.
Clonazepam		*	Sedation is usually dose-limiting; serum levels unhelpful because of development of receptor tolerance.

†The upper limit given is to be interpreted very flexibly. It is permissible to exceed the range if the patient does not show clinical signs of toxicity. Lower limits to the therapeutic ranges are not given, for reasons stated in the text.
‡The more stars, the greater the value of routine monitoring.

Conclusions: which drugs should be monitored?

Table 8.14 summarises the evidence discussed above, and attempts to put a star rating on each of the commonly-used antiepileptic drugs. Top of the list is phenytoin, for which serum level monitoring is essential if the drug is to be used properly. At the bottom is clonazepam, for which the measurement of serum levels may actually worsen drug management.

MODE OF ACTION

The mode of action of antiepileptic drugs is poorly understood and a review of the evidence is outside the scope of this chapter. The reader is referred to Glaser, Penry and Woodbury (1980) for a comprehensive account.

DRUG TREATMENT OF THE EPILEPSIES

In his survey of published papers on the therapeutic efficacy of antiepileptic drugs, Coatsworth (1971) classified studies into two types: clinical trials, i.e. prospective studies in which some sort of formal design was evident, and case reports, i.e. studies in retrospect. Needless to say, the latter were in the majority (140 reports) and usually produced conclusions which were much more favourable to the test drug than more sophisticated clinical trials, presumably because the clinician's enthusiasm for the new compound was more in evidence in the former. However, in only two of the 110 clinical trials reviewed was observer bias completely eliminated by the use of a double-blind design, although a third used a single-blind technique. A further weakness in these studies was the lack of an adequate description of the type of epilepsy being studied. In 11 per cent of clinical trials and 29 per cent of case reports the information was either not recorded or unclear. Because of these weaknesses in design and reporting, few firm conclusions could be drawn. If only the clinical trials were considered, disregarding unsophisticated testimonials of the case report category, the following generalisations were possible (Coatsworth & Penry, 1972):*

*The clinical trials reviewed were of those drugs marketed in the United Sates of America at the time, and therefore excluded carbamazepine, sodium valproate and clonazepam.

1. Ethosuximide consistently showed good results in the treatment of petit mal and should be considered the drug of choice in this seizure type. Phensuximide showed similar results.

2. Trimethadione (troxidone) is somewhat less effective in petit mal and is not effective in generalised convulsive seizures.

3. Diphenylhydantoin (phenytoin), mephenytoin (methoin) and primidone appear to be effective in generalised convulsive seizures. Primidone is not effective in petit mal seizures.

4. Trials using phenacemide gave consistently poor results and it should be a drug of last resort, if used at all.

5. Psychomotor seizures are best treated with diphenylhydantoin, mephenytoin, methsuximide and primidone. The trials in this category are relatively few, however.

6. Clinical trials using phenobarbital (phenobarbitone) and reporting by frequency summary were insufficient to allow any conclusion about its use.

The final conclusion is perhaps the most surprising, for although phenobarbitone has been used since 1912 there is still no satisfactory evidence on which to base its use in epilepsy. Although few would doubt its efficacy in major seizures, it is notable that the lack of controlled trials in the various types of epilepsy is an important hindrance to our rational use of the drug. Obviously, one of our chief objectives following the introduction of a new drug for epilepsy should be to ensure that it receives comprehensive assessment in properly controlled clinical trials as early as possible following its introduction into clinical practice. Only in this way will the quality of antiepileptic therapy improve. Since Coatsworth published his monograph, a number of trials have been reported which have used a double-blind technique to compare a test drug with a placebo or with an established antiepileptic drug. These trials will be reviewed in the remainder of this section and an attempt will be made to indicate drugs of choice in the various types of epilepsy, as well as to provide a practical guide for the clinician who is faced with the day-to-day management of the disease.

Drugs in tonic-clonic and partial seizures

Tonic-clonic seizures can be primary in origin or can result from secondary generalisation of a focal discharge (see Ch. 4). The difference in response depending on the origin of these seizures has been little studied, although Lund (1974b), in a prospective three-year study, demonstrated that both types responded to phenytoin. Those starting focally, however, showed a marginally poorer response than primary seizures (Table 8.15). Booker (1972a) studied retrospectively 107 patients with various types of epilepsy, mostly tonic-clonic and complex partial seizures, finding that those with primary generalised tonic-clonic seizures more often had their fits completely controlled by hydantoin or barbiturate drugs than patients with partial seizures (Table 8.16). This finding, although limited by the retrospective nature of the study, supports the traditional view that complex partial seizures are resistant to drug therapy (Penfield & Erickson, 1941; Gibbs, 1947; Aird & Tsubaki, 1958). Rodin (1968) found a control rate of only 20–30 per cent in patients with temporal lobe epilepsy compared with 50–60 per cent in those with tonic-clonic seizures. The prognosis of the epilepsies are dealt with more extensively in Chapter 4.

Table 8.15 Plasma phenytoin levels and number of grand mal fits in 14 patients with primary tonic-clonic seizures and 18 patients with tonic-clonic seizures starting focally

	Primary tonic-clonic seizures		Tonic-clonic seizures starting focally	
	Plasma phenytoin level μmol/l (μg/ml) $\pm$ SD	Mean number of tonic-clonic seizures	Plasma phenytoin level μmol/l (μg/ml) $\pm$ SD	Mean number of tonic-clonic seizures
Year				
1	28 ± 20 (7.0 ± 4.9)	7.6	30 ± 21 (7.6 ± 5.3)	5.7
2	46 ± 23 (11.5 ± 5.8)	5.9	46 ± 25 (11.5 ± 6.2)	3.5
3	57 ± 20 (14.3 ± 4.9)	1.4	63 ± 24 (15.8 ± 6.0)	1.8

(modified from Lund, 1974b)

Table 8.16 Response to phenytoin, phenobarbitone or primidone treatment in 107 patients with tonic-clonic or partial seizures. Controlled = less than one seizure per year, all patients having had more seizures in the past.

Seizure type	Controlled	Uncontrolled	Significance of difference
Tonic-clonic*	26	15	0.01 (x^2)
Other†	15	51	

* A few also had absences
† Mostly complex partial seizures with or without occasional secondary generalisation
(Modified from Booker, 1972a)

Hydantoins and barbiturates (including primidone)

Most clinicians have a preference for one drug or the other, based on whether they feel that the sedative effects of phenobarbitone are better or worse than the more numerous adverse effects caused by phenytoin. Opinion is swinging away from phenobarbitone, largely because phenytoin is now a much better understood drug particularly from the pharmacokinetic point of view. Primidone is usually not regarded as the drug of first choice because it is tolerated less well than the other two drugs. However, some authorities (e.g. Forster, 1959) regard primidone as the drug of choice for temporal lobe epilepsy, although there is no controlled evidence to support this opinion. Surprisingly, many authorities have stated that phenobarbitone is ineffective in temporal lobe epilepsy although it is the chief active moeity of primidone. Nevertheless, Oxley et al. (1980) have shown that primidone is more effective than phenobarbitone in a proportion of patients with mixed seizure types, presumably because of the additional activity of PEMA and unchanged primidone.

Comparing phenytoin to phenobarbitone and primidone, White, Plott and Norton (1966) found no difference between these three drugs in a carefully-controlled trial in 20 patients with partial seizures. If anything, there was a trend towards phenytoin being the superior drug (Table 8.17). The three test drugs had a significantly greater dose related effect than an identical placebo tablet. Combinations of two of the three drugs were about as effective as twice the amount of either the combined agents used alone.

Table 8.17 Effects of phenytoin, phenobarbitone and primidone, used singly or in combination, on partial seizures, scored by 'demerit points'. The higher the score, the more frequent were the fits.

Drug and dose (mg/day) Phenytoin	Phenobarbitone	Primidone	Mean demerit points per day
—	—	—	0.916
—	150	—	0.590
—	—	750	0.577
300	—	—	0.439
—	300	—	0.295
—	—	1500	0.271
300	150	—	0.213
300	—	750	0.178
—	150	750	0.177
600	—	—	0.105

(Modified from White et al, 1966)

A similar trial design was used by Cereghino et al. (1974b) in their study of albutoin. In this trial, phenytoin was found to be superior to primidone, and both drugs were superior to albutoin. In children, Millichap and Aymat (1968) found that primidone and phenytoin were equally effective in controlling major seizures.

Comparisons of phenobarbitone and phenytoin have produced conflicting results, no doubt because of the differences in dose schedules, drug formulation and type of epilepsy. For example, Ruskin (1950) and Ives (1951) found that phenobarbitone was superior to phenytoin in grand mal epilepsy, whereas Weinberg and Goldstein (1940) and McLendon (1943) had previously concluded that phenytoin gave the most satisfactory results. On the other hand, Gruber et al. (1956) found that the two drugs were, weight for weight, equal in efficacy, but contradicted this in a later publication (Gruber, Brock & Dyken, 1962). In this latter study, in which the patients' usual treatment was discontinued for the purpose of the trial, the authors concluded that the following doses of drugs were equivalent in effect in major epilepsy: phenobarbitone 30 mg, methylphenobarbitone 128 mg, primidone 93 mg, phenytoin 200 mg, and methoin 112 mg. The effect of ethotoin was too weak to derive a comparative dose, although 470 mg of the drug was considered to be equivalent to 70 mg of phenytoin. These results need to be intrepreted cautiously, however, because if the doses are doubled the effect of the hydantoin drugs will increase disproportionately because of their saturation kinetics.

This study indicated that methylphenobarbitone is a much less potent drug than phenobarbitone, weight for weight. Earlier, however, Millman (1937) found that methylphenobarbitone in a dose only 50 per cent higher than that of phenobarbitone produced a much greater reduction in fit frequency. The conclusion that methoin is about twice as potent as phenytoin is in agreement with the uncontrolled findings of Ruskin (1950). Methoin, however, was found to be twice as toxic.

Carbamazepine

Evidence has accumulated that carbamazepine is a highly effective drug in the major epilepsies and that its initial reputation of being toxic to the bone marrow has not been sustained with further experience.

Rodin, Rim and Rennick (1974) treated 37 patients with psychomotor epilepsy with capsules of identical appearance containing either placebo or 200 mg of carbamazepine added to existing phenytoin or phenobarbitone therapy. The dose of carbamazepine was adjusted to give serum concentrations of 21–29 μmol/l (5–7 μg/ml). A highly significant effect in favour of carbamazepine was seen, both for complex partial seizures and for secondarily generalised tonic-clonic seizures.

Comparisons of carbamazepine with conventional drugs in major epilepsy have shown it to be of equal efficacy. Bird et al. (1966) compared its effect with that of phenytoin, phenobarbitone or primidone given singly or in combination in a group of 46 mentally subnormal patients. No difference in fit frequency was found between those patients whose treatment was changed to carbamazepine and those who remained on their conventional therapy. Other controlled studies have reached similar conclusions. Cereghino et al. (1974a) studied 45 patients with mainly partial and secondarily generalised convulsive seizures. Regular medication was replaced by one of three treatments on a double-blind basis: phenytoin 300 mg daily, phenobarbitone 300 mg or carbamazepine 1200 mg daily. Each patient received each test drug for 21 days in a randomised sequence. The

effects of the three drugs were clinically and statistically indistinguishable. Troupin, Green and Levy (1974) found no difference between carbamazepine and phenytoin when used as sole treatment in patients with complex partial and tonic-clonic seizures, and Doose et al. (1970) in an open comparative study found carbamazepine equal in effectiveness to phenytoin and primidone.

In reviewing over 250 papers on carbamazepine, Cereghino et al. (1974a) considered that the following conclusions seemed appropriate:

1. Carbamazepine would appear to be a major antiepileptic drug and not merely a supplemental medication
2. Carbamazepine does not help all patients
3. Results would appear to be best with tonic-clonic (grand mal) and partial seizures with complex symptomatology (temporal lobe seizures)
4. Absence seizures (petit mal) do not appear to be influenced by carbamazepine
5. Patients experiencing several types of seizures have a variable response to therapy
6. A wide variety of side effects are seen, paticularly during initiation of therapy, but usually are not severe enough to discontinue the drug
7. Initial fears about toxicity, particularly bone marrow depression, seem exaggerated in view of subsequent experience with the drug
8. A transient leukopenia, presumably due to initiation of carbamazepine therapy, is a recurring clinical impression
9. A psychotropic effect has been noted but not definitely proven. (Carbamazepine is chemically related to the tricyclic antidepressant drugs)
10. Carbamazepine does not appear to normalise the EEG, and the EEG cannot be relied on to correlate with clinical control of seizures
11. In patients with uncontrolled seizures despite multiple drug therapy, carbamazepine, if effective, appears to exert an independent action and cannot replace the previously administered drugs
12. Determinations of serum carbamazepine levels would appear to be clinically useful, but, despite a number of adequate methodologies, have seldom been reported

These conclusions have been fully supported by subsequent clinical trials. In a double-blind comparison of carbamazepine and phenytoin, Troupin et al. (1977) found that the drugs were of equal efficacy in patients with partial (mainly complex) and major generalised seizures, but carbamazepine produced fewer adverse effects. In a similar group of patients, Rodin et al. (1976) showed that carbamazepine and primidone were equally effective, but more adverse effects were related to carbamazepine than to primidone. In both studies, however, carbamazepine treatment was associated with an improvement in mood, in support of the suggestion that this compound possesses a psychotropic effect (Dalby, 1975).

In children and infants with partial seizures Sillanpää et al. (1979) found that carbamazepine was a highly effective drug even in doses as low as 9–10 mg/kg, which, in patients of this age, produce serum levels well below the accepted therapeutic range (p. 319).

Sodium valproate

Three placebo-controlled studies have been performed in patients with major epilepsy. Meinardi (1971) studied 42 'drug resistant' patients with various types of epilepsy and found that one in three appeared to benefit. Richens and Ahmad (1975) performed a cross-over trial in 20 institutionalised chronic epileptic patients who had frequent fits which had proved difficult to control with standard drugs. Most had partial fits, usually of temporal lobe origin, with or without secondary generalisation. When added to existing therapy, sodium valproate produced a significant effect on both partial and tonic-clonic seizures. In this trial an increase in serum phenobarbitone levels was seen which may, in part, have accounted for the antiepileptic effect of the drug. Furthermore, it may have been responsible for the initial drowsiness which occurred in many patients, an observation which has been made in previous studies (Jeavons & Clark, 1974). A reduction in phenobarbitone or primidone dosage is often necessary. More recent evidence, however, suggests that the sedation, even amounting to coma, which is provoked in some patients on addition of sodium valproate to phenobarbitone therapy may be caused by a pharmacodynamic interaction, i.e. an interaction at the receptor sites in the central nervous system. The nature of these receptor sites is, of course, unknown but it is tempting to suggest that GABA transmission might be involved. An interaction of a similar nature has been reported with clonazepam. Furthermore, central sedative effects and occasional behavioural changes, have been observed in patients on sodium valproate alone.

Gram et al. (1977) were able to improve on the trial design used by Richens and Ahmad (1975) by reducing the dose of phenobarbitone or primidone in order to maintain a constant serum phenobarbitone throughout the trial. A mean dose reduction of 33 per cent was required in order to achieve this. Nevertheless, they were able to show a good effect of sodium valproate in patients with mixed seizure types.

In general, it has been shown that sodium valproate is less effective in partial seizures than in primary generalised tonic-clonic or absence seizures (Simon & Penry, 1975; Pinder et al., 1977). No controlled studies have been performed in which sodium valproate has been compared with other drugs in major epilepsy. It is therefore not possible to give firm recommendations concerning its advantages or disadvantages as a drug of first choice. However, it is likely that it lacks the efficacy of the more traditional drugs in partial epilepsies and should probably be reserved for primary generalised seizures.

Sulthiame

This drug is a sulphonamide derivative with carbonic anhydrase inhibiting properties. Although it has been shown to be active in anticonvulsant screening tests in animals, the case for its efficacy in man rests upon uncontrolled case reports in which it has usually been added to patients' conventional treatment. One controlled trial, however, has been performed in which sulthiame has been compared with phenytoin as sole treatment in 67 patients with focal seizures with or without secondary generalisation (Green et al., 1974). Only 21 patients completed the trial. During sulthiame treatment 17 patients dropped out because of increased seizures compared with seven during phenytoin treatment. A further 16 patients left the trial because of drug toxicity during sulthiame treatment compared with three during phenytoin administration. Only four remained on sulthiame after the trial even though 10 had fewer seizures during sulthiame treatment. In the remaining six, the toxicity of sulthiame was considered to weigh against its continuance. EEG recordings showed that more epileptic activity occurred in the patients' records when they were receiving sulthiame (Wilkus & Green, 1974). The authors concluded that sulthiame has little value as a primary anticonvulsant agent in major epilepsy, although it could not be said it was completely devoid of anti-convulsant activity because it was compared only with phenytoin, not with a placebo.

Undoubtedly, sulthiame is effective when added to established therapy because it is a powerful inhibitor of the metabolism of phenytoin, phenobarbitone and primidone (see p. 363), and an elevation of the serum levels of these drugs would be expected to have a useful effect in patients whose levels were previously sub-therapeutic. However, drug intoxication is a major risk, and, in addition, sulthiame adds characteristic adverse effects of its own, notably hyperventi-lation, parasthesiae of the extremities, anorexia and weight loss. Whether sulthiame has antiep-ileptic activity in its own right is uncertain.

Two controlled trials (Moffatt, Siddiqui & MacKay, 1970; Al-Kaisi & McGuire, 1974) found a significant improvement in the disturbed behaviour of mentally subnormal patients. Aggressiveness and hyperactivity in particular were reduced suggesting a sedative effect of the drug. This is supported by the observations of Green et al. (1974) that patients on sulthiame were less alert and performed less well on tasks in which time was a factor in scoring.

Beclamide

Although claimed to have a central stimulant rather than sedative effect, this drug is not widely used. It is, at best, a weak anticonvulsant in major epilepsy. Wilson, Walton and Newell (1959) found a small, but significant effect in a placebo-controlled trial. The weakness of its action is sup-ported by the observation that substitution of a placebo for the active drug in six patients made no difference to the control of fits (Kaye, Jones & Warrier, 1959). However, a placebo-controlled trial in mentally subnormal patients, some of whom were epileptic, showed an improvement in their severe behaviour disorders (Price & Spencer, 1967).

Benzodiazepines

Although intravenous administration of diazepam and other benzodiazepine drugs has proved invaluable in the management of status epilepticus (p. 337), long term oral treatment has been dis-appointing because the effect on major seizures has been poorly sustained. The use of the ben-zodiazepines in epilepsy has been fully reviewed by Browne and Penry (1973).

Diazepam. Most long-term trials of diazepam have been uncontrolled and consisted of the addi-tion of the benzodiazepine to the usual anticonvul-sant treatment of patients with uncontrolled fits. The optimistic conclusions of these trials have not been substantiated by controlled studies.

The disappointing effect of diazepam given orally may be because the doses have been too small to produce serum levels within the optimum range for their anticonvulsant action. Booker and Celesia (1973) observed that the levels produced by 30–40 mg of oral diazepam did not exceed 0.5 μg/ml, whereas on intravenous injection the level required to suppress inter-ictal spike dis-charges in the EEG usually exceeded this value.

Furthermore, central nervous system tolerance may become important with chronic therapy, accounting for reports of a diminishing effect with time. There is increasing evidence that this is a major disadvantage of diazepam therapy. Although undoubtedly effective as a tranquilliser or antiepileptic drug when first administered there is little evidence that these effects are sustained with chronic therapy. Escalation of the dosage will regain the therapeutic effect but further tolerance develops. Finally, when the drug is discontinued, marked withdrawal effects can occur, including seizures in non-epileptic subjects and a rebound increase in fit frequency in established epilepsy.

Clonazepam. Clonazepam has been better asses-sed, presumably because it was marketed from the outset as an antiepileptic drug. In practice, it is doubtful whether it has advantages over other benzodiazepine drugs for chronic use in epilepsy. In 21 patients with complex partial seizures Birket-Smith et al. (1973) found that clonazepam was significantly more effective than a placebo when added to the patients' existing therapy. In 12 patients clonazepam was the preferred treat-ment, in one placebo was preferred and in eight there was no difference. In another placebo-controlled study Edwards and Eadie (1973) found a reduction in fit frequency in grand mal epilepsy, but partial seizures, especially those originating in the temporal lobe, tended to respond less well than generalised epilepsy. In these two trials, a high incidence of drowsiness, giddiness, aggression, irritability and diplopia was seen. Mikkelsen *et al*. (1975) found that 10 out of 17 patients with partial seizures with or without secondary generalisation became seizure free, whereas only 3 were so on placebo. However, somnolence and incoordination occurred in the majority.

A diminishing effect with chronic therapy appears to occur with clonazepam, as with diazepam.

Other benzodiazepine drugs. All of the available benzodiazepine drugs have antiepileptic properties, although few have been formally studied as long term therapy. Clobazam a 1,5-benzodiazepine, has been assessed in an uncontrolled trial (Gastaut & Low, 1979) but tolerance occurred rapidly. Probably all the benzodiazepines suffer this disadvantage.

Practical management of major generalised and focal seizures

It will be obvious from what has been said above

that a completely rational choice of drug for each type of epilepsy is not possible on the published evidence available. Nevertheless, the clinician needs to make a choice based on the best of current evidence. Table 8.18 represents an attempt to do so.

When to start treatment

It may seem trite to say that before antiepileptic therapy is started a correct diagnosis should be made. Nevertheless, a clear distinction between epileptic and non-epileptic attacks is of major importance because the attachment of the label 'epilepsy' has medical, therapeutic and social implications that will greatly influence the patient's future life. The differential diagnosis of epilepsy is discussed fully in Chapters 4 and 6.

The decision to treat an individual patient should take into account not only the number of attacks, but the circumstances in which they occurred; the presence or absence of precipitating factors, the severity and type of attack, whether or not there is accompanying neurological or

Table 8.18 Drug treatment of the epilepsies based on an abbreviated version of the International Classification of Epileptic Seizures (Gastaut, 1970)

Type of seizure	Drugs of choice

1. Partial seizures (seizures which produce clinical manifestations referable to a part of one hemisphere)
  (i) With elemetry symptomatology (focal motor, sensory and autonomic symptomatology)
  (ii) With complex symptomatology (impaired consciousness and cognitive, affective, psychosensory and psychomotor symptomatology)
  (iii) Becoming secondarily generalised (focal seizure leading to tonic-clonic seizure)
	(Carbamazepine
	(Phenytoin
	(Primidone
	(Phenobarbitone

2. Generalised seizures (seizures which do not produce clinical manifestations referable to part of one hemisphere) (i) Absences (petit mal and atypical petit mal)	(Sodium valproate (Ethosuximide
(ii) Bilateral massive epileptic myoclonus (myoclonic jerks)	(Sodium valproate (Clonazepam
(iii) Infantile spasms	(ACTH (Clonazepam

(iv) Clonic seizures
  (v) Tonic seizures
  (vi) Tonic-clonic seizures
	(Phenytoin
	(Carbamazepine
	(Primidone
	(Phenobarbitone
	(Sodium valproate

(vii) Atonic seizures (viii) Akinetic seizures	(Sodium valproate (Clonazepam
3. Unilateral seizures (tonic, clonic or tonic-clonic seizures which are unilateral)	As for 2 (iv)–(vi) above

psychiatric disability, and the patient's social environment. No hard and fast rules can therefore be made. Most neurologists, however, would agree that anticonvulsant therapy is indicated in a healthy 18 year old presenting with a history of two or three grand mal fits without an obvious provocative cause, or in a child suffering from classical petit mal absences with accompanying three per second spike-and-wave in this EEG record. On the other hand, the indications for prescribing antiepileptic drugs for a patient presenting with a history of occasional complex partial seizures and a marked behavioural disturbance are less compelling.

It is necessary always to balance the harmful effects of antiepileptic therapy, some of which may not be immediately obvious (see p. 348), against the potential benefit. As newer and, hopefully, less toxic drugs become available, the case for early treatment in patients with established epilepsy, or prophylactic therapy in patients in whom there is a high risk of seizures, will be stronger. It is known that the incidence of epilepsy following penetrating head injuries or certain neurosurgical procedures is high (see Ch. 4) and it is the usual practice in many neurosurgical units to prescribe prophylactic anticonvulsant therapy in order to prevent epilepsy developing. In fact, 60 per cent of neurosurgeons in the United States have such a policy (Rapport & Penry, 1973). Whether prophylaxis has any advantage over treating seizures when they occur is unproven, however. While the drugs are being administered there is a lower incidence of seizures (North et al., 1980) but whether any long-term benefit is derived on stopping prophylactic therapy is open to doubt, although a claim has been made that this is so (Young et al., 1979). Regretably, the lack of an appropriate control group in this study leaves the authors' case unproven.

Dose scheme for tonic-clonic and partial seizures

Once a decision has been made to treat major epilepsy, one of the drugs of choice should be selected and started in a low to average dose (see Tables 8.2, 8.6, and 8.19). Sufficient time should then be allowed for the serum drug level to reach steady state and for the patient's response to therapy to be assessed. If the response is inadequate the dose should be increased gradually until full control has been achieved or until signs of drug toxicity occur. If monitoring serum levels is possible, particularly for phenytoin, the dose of drug can be adjusted more skillfully but ultimately the decision that a maximum dose has been reached is largely a clinical one.

If intoxication occurs before an acceptable degree of control has been achieved, a gradual change to an alternative drug should be made, tailing off the first drug slowly while slowly introducing the second drug.

If the second drug fails, it is time to try a combination of two drugs, but if the policy outlined by Shorvon et al. (1978) is adhered to this will not

Table 8.19 Satisfactory starting doses of the commonly-used antiepileptic drugs in adults. These dose frequencies take into account the serum half-life of the drug and the immediate adverse effects to single doses. Phenytoin and phenobarbitone doses for children are given in Tables 8.2 and 8.6

Drug	Dose units available in UK (mg)	Starting dose	Range of maintenance doses (mg/day)
Phenytoin	25, 50, 100	100 mg twice daily	150–600
Methoin	100	100 mg daily	100–600
Carbamazepine	100, 200	100 mg twice daily	400–1800
Phenobarbitone	15, 30, 60, 100	30 mg at night	30–240
Primidone	250	125 mg at night	250–1500
Sodium valproate	200, 500	200 mg twice daily	600–3000
Ethosuximide	250	250 mg twice daily	500–1500
Troxidone	300	300 mg twice daily	900–2100
Diazepam	2, 5, 10	5 mg twice daily	5–60
Nitrazepam	5	2.5 mg twice daily	5–20
Clonazepam	0.5, 2	0.5 mg twice daily	1–10

be necessary in the majority of patients, at least not in the early stages of treatment. Regrettably, however, as the epilepsy becomes more established an increasing proportion of patients require combination therapy, and there is a hard core of patients who remain poorly responsive to drugs, whether given singly or in various combinations of two three or more drugs.

Although monotherapy is preferable, a logical combination of two drugs is often a very effective way of treating mixed seizure types, e.g. absence seizures or myoclonic jerks occurring together with tonic-clonic fits.

Drug-resistant epilepsy

If the response to full doses of two drugs is inadequate, addition of a third may be entertained but probably seldom justified. At this point the patient's response to treatment should be carefully reviewed because it is possible that the seizures are completely unresponsive to drug treatment or, indeed may actually be made worse. Furthermore, with full doses of two or more drugs, adverse effects may become a major problem – the patient may become slow-witted, ataxic, acne-scarred, swollen-gummed and osteomalacic in exchange for little therapeutic benefit. Here a good record of fit frequency over months or years will be of enormous help. This is illustrated by Figure 8.4 in which a month-to-month plot of a patient's major fits and drug therapy over nine years reveals the resistant nature of his attacks. Fit frequency seems independent of treatment in this patient. A combination of four drugs at the beginning of the period of study produced no greater benefit than one drug at the end. Indeed, withdrawal of phenytoin, with only primidone remaining, was followed by two successive months free of major fits, the first time this had been observed during the eight years in which he had been followed.

In reviewing a group of over 200 patients, Booker (1972a) distinguished two groups, those whose epilepsy was well controlled on moderate doses of one or two drugs, and those whose epilepsy was partially controlled but who continued to have large numbers of fits. Whereas the former usually had grand mal epilepsy of relatively late onset and were generally free from other stigmata of neurological disease, the latter group usually had complex partial and/or mixed seizures and showed clinical and psychometric evidence of chronic encephalopathy. A small number of patients showed little or no response to three or four drugs given simultaneously, just like the patient described above, although they had definite signs of drug intoxication.

These patients create a therapeutic dilemma for the clinician because the balance between the benefits and hazards of high dose multiple therapy can be precarious. It is often difficult to assess how much benefit a patient is deriving from drug treatment when several years have elapsed since its start, especially if many drugs have been tried in a variety of permutations. Furthermore, it can be difficult to assess how much a patient's mental slowness and blunted affect is caused by drug therapy, and how much is due to accompanying brain damage. If there is any doubt, a bold reduction in drug therapy is justified and will occasionally produce a dramatic improvement in the patient's mental state while at the same time not affecting, or sometimes even reducing, fit frequency (Shorvon & Reynolds, 1979).

However, a policy of major drug reductions sometimes has its hazards. The author has seen a number of patients who have run into disaster following a well-meaning reduction in drug therapy in an attempt to achieve the ideal of monotherapy. In a substantial proportion of patients on combination therapy, this is not a realistic policy. The patient illustrated in Figure 8.13, for instance, had not had a fit for 15 years while on a combination of phenytoin and phenobarbitone, but following a gradual withdrawal of phenytoin he began to experience tonic-clonic fits once again. A return to his existing therapy failed to regain control of his attacks, and at the time of writing, six years after the drug reduction, his epilepsy is still uncontrolled despite several changes of therapy.

Although, in despair, it is sometimes tempting to withdraw all therapy in an apparently drug-resistant patient, in the author's experience this is rarely successful. It is easy to underestimate the effect that drug treatment is having on secondary generalisation in a partial epilepsy.

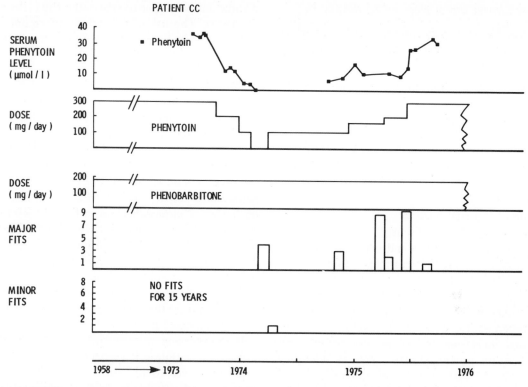

Fig. 8.13 Follow up on patient CC illustrated in Fig. 8.12. Despite returning to the initial therapy (and later increasing the dose further) the patient's fits remained uncontrolled

Hazards of polytherapy

This is not to say that irrational polypharmacy is not highly undesirable. The points against this type of management are several in number:

1. Although it has been argued that several drugs in low dosage will produce additive antiepileptic effects without the toxicity that one drug in high dosage would cause, there is no evidence in support of this contention. There is no reason why central sedative effects should not be additive just as the therapeutic effects are. This is supported by the observation that drug intoxication can occur in a patient on multiple therapy without the serum level of any one drug being within the toxic range.

2. Interactions between antiepileptic drugs occur commonly and can be of considerable practical importance. Some drugs which are used as supplementary therapy, e.g. sulthiame, can pre-cipitate drug intoxication by inhibiting the metabolism of other antiepileptic drugs (p. 000).

3. If an adverse reaction occurs it is difficult to know which drug is responsible if several are being given simultaneously.

4. It is not known how much the administration of a second or third drug alters the therapeutic range of serum levels of the first. It may be that monitoring serum levels is an aimless exercise if several drugs are being given together.

5. Many patients do not comply with polytherapy, because they refuse to take so many tablets, because they are confused about what they should take or because they know better than their doctor how much the drugs upset them.

Enough has been said to make it obvious that polypharmacy is a practice to be avoided. Wherever possible, one drug should be used to its fullest, and if this is done, serum level monitoring will be of great assistance.

Factors carrying a poor prognosis for therapy

It is possible to identify a number of factors which carry a poor prognosis or produce resistance to drug therapy.

1. Seizures dating from birth or developing early in life
2. Seizures of infantile (salaam) spasm or akinetic type
3. Evidence of underlying structural or degenerative cerebral pathology
4. A severe diffuse slow wave abnormality in the EEG
5. Complex partial seizures

Gordon (1974) has discussed many other factors, social, psychological and neurological, which can lead to failure in treatment. Rodin (1968) found that patients who presented early and who had had only a few attacks had the best prognosis. This suggests that early treatment might improve the prognosis for it is known that brain damage, perhaps increasing the propensity to fits, may occur during prolonged major seizures. The prognosis for the various types of epilepsy is considered at length in Chapters 3 and 4.

Value of the EEG in regulating therapy

The EEG is invaluable as an aid to identifying the type of epilepsy from which a patient is suffering, and therefore in enabling a logical choice of drug to be made. As a guide to the regulation of therapy, however, it is less useful. It should be remembered that the clinical EEG records cerebral activity for a period of only 30 minutes or so during a patient's waking day, and on one occasion the recording may coincide with a period of normal electrical activity and on the next day with an episode of disturbed function. Single records may therefore be unhelpful or even misleading. This has been noted in a number of therapeutic trials, but particularly when carbamazepine has been the drug under study (Cereghino *et al.*, 1974a). Even prolonged EEG telemetry has failed to show a correlation between the clinical and EEG response to carbamazepine (Rodin *et al.*, 1974). On the other hand, the improvement in the incidence of absences produced by ethosuximide therapy is accompanied closely by a reduction in the number of spike-and-wave paroxysms in the EEG (Penry *et al.*, 1972). The use of telemetry and ambulatory recording procedures is discussed in Chapter 5.

When to stop treatment

The EEG has often been used as a guide in deciding whether or not drug therapy can be withdrawn in a patient who has been free of attacks for two to four years. Holowack, Thurston and O'Leary (1972), however, found it unhelpful in indicating the prognosis on withdrawal of therapy. Clear-cut paroxysmal activity in the EEG was considered not to be a contra-indication in patients with well controlled seizures, particularly if serial records had shown improvement during the seizure-free period. Bad prognostic features were (a) a long duration of seizures before control had been achieved, (b) the presence of structural brain damage, and (c) the occurrence of partial, particularly Jacksonian, attacks.

If the decision to stop antiepileptic therapy is made, the withdrawal of drugs should be slow, preferably over 6–12 months. The chance of a recurrence of seizures in children who have been fit-free for four years is about one in four (Holowack *et al.*, 1972), and in adults who have been fully controlled for two years the recurrence rate during the first four years following withdrawal of therapy is about one in three (Juul-Jensen, 1964).

Treatment of accompanying psychiatric disorders

The various types of psychiatric disturbance which can accompany chronic epilepsy are discussed in Chapter 6. Two therapeutic problems can be encountered in treating disorders of this nature in the epileptic patient who is receiving one or more drugs for major epilepsy. These drugs induce the activity of liver enzymes and this effect can result in a much more rapid turnover and excretion of drugs such as the tricyclic antidepressants and phenothiazines (p. 366). The epileptic patient who is receiving two or three anticonvulsant drugs in combination, is likely, therefore, to have therapeutically ineffective levels of these psychotropic drugs if standard doses are used. If failure occurs in treating these patients, there should be no hesitation in increasing the dose beyond the usual limits.

The convulsant activity of tricyclics and phenothiazines is now fairly well documented and should be borne in mind when prescribing for an epileptic patient. On no account, however, should severe depression or psychosis go untreated because of this small danger. The importance of tricyclic antidepressants as a cause of fits has been discussed by Betts et al.(1968), Legg and Swash (1974), and Trimble (1978).

Treatment of absence seizures

The conclusion reached by Coatsworth and Penry (1972) on reviewing 79 case reports and clinical trials of drugs in absence seizures was that ethosuximide was the drug of choice. However, the position has now changed with the introduction of sodium valproate, which many would now regard as the drug of first choice.

Sodium valproate

Sodium valproate is particularly effective in absences accompanied by classical 3 per second spike-and-wave in the EEG. Most studies have shown that about two-thirds of patients with simple or complex absences show a good response (75–100 per cent reduction in seizures) with sodium valproate (Simon & Penry, 1975; Pinder et al., 1977).

In an open clinical study which included 42 children with typical (simple) absences or absences with automatisms (complex absences), no fewer than 36 achieved complete control of clinical seizures (Jeavons, Clark & Maheshwari, 1977). Villarreal et al. (1978) recorded spike-and-wave activity by EEG telemetry in 25 patients with absence seizures and found that a reduction occurred in 19. The reduction in absence seizures seen in this study was less encouraging than in the report of Jeavons et al. but the difference is probably accounted for by the fact that the patients monitored by Villarreal et al. were older and usually had other types of seizure in addition.

In a controlled comparative trial of sodium valproate and ethosuximide in 19 patients with absence seizures, Suzuki et al. (1972) showed that

sodium valproate was indistinguishable from ethosuximide. However the latter drug has the disadvantage of not being active against coexisting tonic-clonic fits. Indeed, it has been suggested that it can precipitate major seizures, although this claim has been disputed (Heathfield & Jewesbury, 1964). Whether this is so or not, sodium valproate has the clear advantage of suppressing tonic-clonic fits in addition to the absence seizures (see below).

Succinimides

Phensuximide (1953) was the first of these compounds to be introduced for the treatment of petit mal epilepsy and was followed by methsuximide (1957) and ethosuximide (1960). Methsuximide has been found to be consistently less effective than the other two drugs (Coatsworth, 1971). Ethosuximide is the most widely used.

Since Coatsworth's survey was published, two studies have been reported in which plasma levels of ethosuximide have been related to clinical control of petit mal absences and both confirm the effectiveness of the drug. Penry et al. (1972) studied 18 children who had absence seizures. Some also had major seizures for which they were receiving phenytoin, phenobarbitone or primidone; these drugs were continued throughout the trial. Assessment included EEG telemetry, a battery of neuropsychological tests and intensive observation by trained observers. Four patients had a 100 per cent decrease in seizure frequency and another five had a decrease greater than 95 per cent. At the end of the trial, 10 of the patients had no spike-and-wave discharges in a 12 hour EEG recording, whereas all had had such activity in the control week at the beginning of the trial.

A second study, on a larger scale although less detailed, has been performed by Sherwin and Robb (1972). 53 of 117 patients with absence attacks were completely controlled on ethosuximide therapy. When the dose of ethosuximide was increased in 16 patients with uncontrolled seizures, complete control or marked improvement was seen in ten. On the other hand, a decrease in dose in 12 controlled patients was a decrease in dose in 12 controlled patients was associated with the reappearance of attacks in five. In both of these studies plasma levels over

280 μmol/l (40 μg/ml) appeared to give the best chance of complete control of seizures. A dose of 20 mg/kg was necessary to produce, on average, a level of this order.

Oxazolidinediones

Although the six case reports reviewed by Coatsworth (1971) reported complete control or marked improvement in the majority of patients with petit mal absences treated with troxidone, the results of seven clinical trials gave less favourable results. In four, the degree of improvement was only mild or moderate. The number of case reports and clinical trials of paramethadione were too few for any conclusions to be drawn, although in one trial (Davis & Lennox, 1949) this drug was found to be as effective as troxidone. On the whole, oxazolidinediones appear to give less favourable results than the succinimides or sodium valproate. Their use is now seldom necessary.

Benzodiazepines

There is evidence from animal experiments that benzodiazepine drugs can suppress the type of electrical activity which is associated with petit mal absences in man (Browne & Penry, 1973). This has stimulated a number of clinical trials in which benzodiazepines have been injected intravenously in patients with three per second spike-and-wave abnormalities; diazepam, nitrazepam and clonazepam all suppress spontaneous discharges of this type. Absence status is very sensitive to parenteral benzodiazepines.

The deficiencies of long-term trials of benzodiazepine drugs in petit mal epilepsy have been described by Browne and Penry (1973): 'absence or petit mal seizures are not well defined by most authors and can mean anything from all seizures other than grand mal to the very precise definition of absence seizures (see Gastaut, 1970). Furthermore, most reported clinical trials of benzodiazepines for absence seizures have been performed on patients who have failed to have their absence seizures controlled by other anticonvulsants, who have had a benzodiazepine added to their usual anticonvulsant medications, and who were evaluated in the absence of blind techniques

by a physician relying principally on the mother's history to determine drug efficacy.' Of 28 reports evaluated by these authors, only nine included ten or more patients, of which 22–94 per cent had a 50 per cent or greater reduction in absence seizure frequency when treated with a benzodiazepine drug. Mikkelsen et al. (1976) have shown in a controlled trial that clonazepam is superior to placebo in absence seizures, and Chandra (1973) demonstrated a superior response with this drug than with diazepam. A number of uncontrolled studies also report a good effect of clonazepam in absence seizures.

The major disadvantage, however, of benzodiazepine drugs in treating this type of epilepsy is their sedative effect, which is tolerated particularly poorly in children. As both sodium valproate and ethosuximide are effective drugs in absence seizures, there is seldom a need in practice to use benzodiazepine compounds in the treatment of this type of seizure.

Practical management of absence seizures

Sodium valproate is the drug of first choice. It should be started in a dose of 10 mg/kg and increased as necessary to achieve satisfactory control. The use of enteric coated tablets will reduce the incidence of gastro-intestinal adverse effects and will make it possible to administer the drug once daily. As mentioned earlier there is evidence that once daily administration will produce a steady therapeutic effect despite the short half-life of the compound.

If control is not achieved with sodium valproate alone it is probably sensible to add ethosuximide rather than to change completely to the latter. In the experience of Jeavons et al. (1977), this appeared to be effective, particularly when absences are accompanied by myoclonus. Ethosuximide should be started in a dose of 10 mg/kg and increased until control of seizures is achieved. Serum level monitoring will help to achieve the optimum dose of ethosuximide (Sherwin & Robb, 1972). A plateau serum concentration will be reached in about seven days in children.

If combinations of sodium valproate and ethosuximide are not fully effective (which is unusual), clonazepam or troxidone can be tried. It is probably better to avoid combining large doses of clonazepam and sodium valproate, because a high incidence of drowsiness has been reported (Jeavons *et al.*, 1977).

Coexisting absence and tonic-clonic seizures

One in two or one in three children with absence seizures will ultimately develop tonic-clonic seizures (Rodin, 1968). The broad spectrum activity of sodium valproate is therefore an advantage in treating absence seizures. If coexisting tonic-clonic or other types of seizure remain uncontrolled, carbamazepine or phenytoin can be added. The former drug is preferable for two reasons; first, it causes fewer adverse effects than phenytoin (gum hyperplasia, acne and hirsutes are particularly undesirable in the young), and secondly, phenytoin and valproate compete for plasma protein binding sites and make serum phenytoin levels more difficult to interpret (p. 359). Phenobarbitone and primidone are poorly tolerated in children, causing behaviour disturbances and hyperkinesia, and should be avoided if possible.

Treatment of the myoclonic epilepsies

The myoclonic epilepsies of early childhood represent a heterogeneous group of disorders which are discussed in detail in Chapter 3. In infantile spasms ACTH or corticosteroid therapy has become a conventional form of treatment and there is good evidence that an immediate improvement in the clinical and electroencephalographic abnormalities occurs (Jeavons & Bower, 1974; Hrachovy *et al.*, 1979). There is little difference in the efficacy of ACTH or corticosteroids (Jeavons & Bower, 1974). However, there is general agreement that the long-term prognosis is not influenced by this treatment, and is usually poor (Jeavons & Bower 1974; Pollack, Zion & Kellaway, 1979).

Of the other myoclonic epilepsies, there are those which are notoriously drug resistant, such as the Lennox-Gastaut syndrome, while others are more amenable to therapy, such as *true myoclonic epilepsy* or *myoclonic epilepsy of childhood*. The co-existence of atonic-akinetic seizure in general signify a more resistant epilepsy. Head-nodding

attacks, atypical absences or tonic-clonic fits may occur in addition.

In general myoclonic phenomena respond best to treatment with a benzodiazepine drug, sodium valproate or ethosuximide. Six large studies reviewed by Browne and Penry (1973) reported a 50 per cent or greater reduction in myoclonic seizure frequency in 36–100 per cent of patients treated with chlordiazepoxide, diazepam or nitrazepam. Studies in which the latter two drugs have been compared indicate that nitrazepam is equal in efficacy or perhaps slightly superior to diazepam. The optimum dose of diazepam is twice that of nitrazepam.

A number of uncontrolled reports have been published describing the use of clonazepam in myoclonic epilepsies, and the results have been uniformly favourable (see reviews by Pinder *et al.*, 1976; Browne, 1976). One controlled study showed a clear superiority of clonazepam over placebo (Mikkelsen *el al.*, 1976). Atonic-akinetic seizures appear to benefit to a similar extent (Pinder *et al.*, 1976). Post-anoxic intention myoclonus can be effectively treated with clonazepam (Goldberg & Dorman, 1976).

A satisfactory comparative study of the response of myoclonic epilepsies to clonazepam and to sodium valproate has not been performed. Sodium valproate, however, appears to be of a similar efficacy to benzodiazepine drugs. Jeavons *et al.* (1977) included 56 patients with various types of myoclonic epilepsy in their report and most showed a very good response, in particular those with myoclonic jerks of childhood or adolescence. Patients with myoclonic-astatic epilepsy (Lennox-Gastaut syndrome) did less well, although half derived considerable benefit and for a notoriously drug-resistant condition this is very encouraging.

Other drugs such as phenytoin, phenobarbitone and primidone are used in myoclonic and akinetic epilepsies, particularly when other types of fit co-exist, but no controlled trials of these drugs have been performed. On the whole, the response of myoclonic seizures to these drugs is poor.

Treatment of photosensitive epilepsy

Photosensitive epilepsy is discussed in detail in

Chapter 5. A majority of patients achieve complete control of photosensitivity with sodium valproate and this would appear to be the drug of first choice (Harding, Herrick & Jeavons, 1978). Clonazepam is effective, but is more sedative (Nanda et al., 1977).

Prophylaxis of febrile convulsions

Febrile convulsions are discussed in detail in Chapter 3. A policy of prophylaxis in children who have had a single febrile convulsion has been advised by Ounsted, Lindsay and Norman (1966). The argument in favour of this is that febrile convulsions which are severe and prolonged can cause structural damage in the temporal lobe leading to chronic epilepsy. There is good evidence that phenobarbitone and sodium valproate, given continuously up to the age of three years or so, will reduce the incidence of recurrent convulsions (Faerø et al., 1972; Wolf et al., 1977; Wallace & Aldridge Smith 1980). By inference, the number of children suffering ischaemic brain damage leading to chronic epilepsy should be reduced, but this remains to be demonstrated.

Although prophylactic therapy is in keeping with the general aims of medical practice, i.e. promoting preventive rather than curative medicine, there are two reasons for being hesitant about its general acceptance; (a) the correct drug and dosage to produce effective prophylaxis is uncertain, and (b) there is a natural disquiet about treating a large number of children, of whom only a proportion may have had a seizure, with drugs (e.g. phenobarbitone) which are likely to impair learning ability and cause behaviour disturbances. Furthermore, it needs a highly motivated parent for the approach to be successful, and many are understandably hesitant about giving regular treatment to an apparently well child.

An alternative approach is intermittent treatment, i.e. treatment given at the time of a febrile episode in order to prevent a convulsion occurring or to stop it as soon as it begins. Rectal administration of the parental form of diazepam is particularly promising in this respect (p. 85) because it is rapidly absorbed and can be administered at home by a parent.

Treatment of major status epilepticus

Major status epilepticus is a grave medical emergency in which the mortality can be up to 21 per cent (Rowan & Scott, 1970; Oxbury & Whitty, 1971). Apart from the immediate mortality the incidence of neurological and mental sequelae is high, and it seems likely that damage to the temporal lobes during status epilepticus in childhood can cause Ammon's horn sclerosis leading to chronic temporal lobe epilepsy (see Ch. 3 & 11). Status epilepticus therefore requires immediate and effective treatment if uneventful recovery is to occur because the prognosis is related to the time interval between the onset of status and the start of effective treatment. The following guide should be adhered to:

1. Initial doses of drugs should be given intravenously not intramuscularly. Some drugs, e.g. diazepam and phenytoin (see below), are slowly absorbed from intramuscular sites of injection and it is, therefore, inappropriate to use them in this way in status. Rectal administration is not appropriate unless medical help is unavailable.

2. Adequate doses should be administered from the start (Janz & Kautz, 1964).

3. There should be no hesitation in repeating doses if status returns.

4. If status returns despite two or three single dose administrations, a continuous infusion should be used. Benzodiazepines and thiopentone are not suitable for intravenous infusion (see below). A switch from parenteral to oral treatment should not be made too early.

5. Other measures may need to be taken, such as tepid sponging and administration of aspirin for febrile convulsions in children, and rehydration and correction of acidosis by administration of intravenous fluids (Melekian, Laplane & Debray, 1962). In neonates, rapid detection and treatment of underlying metabolic disorders is essential (Ch. 3). Care should be taken to maintain an unobstructed airway, as is usual with any patient in coma. Intubation and ventilation should be instituted if status and/or drug treatment impairs oxygenation.

6. Once control of seizure activity is achieved, careful consideration should be given to the

patient's maintenance therapy. Measurement of drug levels on a specimen taken immediately on admission will be invaluable, but in the heat of the moment this will often be forgotten. If the facilities are available, it is reasonable to request an urgent result for it may influence the early management. A low level will suggest that the patient has not been taking his drugs regularly, or that the prescribed dose has been too low. Rowan and Scott (1970) found that omission or reduction of anticonvulsant therapy was a common precipitating factor. Early administration of parenteral supplements of phenytoin or phenobarbitone may prevent a recurrence of the status epilepticus, and serial measurement of the levels while the patient remains in hospital will allow an optimum therapeutic level to be achieved.

Although there are many reports testifying to the effectiveness of various drugs in treating status epilepticus, almost no studies have been performed in which two drugs have been compared. Of the drugs available, the consensus of opinion is that an intravenous injection of diazepam or clonazepam is the most effective initial treatment for status. Although intravenous short-acting barbiturates, e.g. thiopentone, are also very effective, the incidence of respiratory depression is much greater. Intravenous injection of phenytoin may also be effective, particularly if the patient has not been receiving this drug chronically or if the episode of status has been precipitated by his failure to take it as prescribed, but intoxication can occur if the patient already has a therapeutic level in his serum. Chlormethiazole given by intravenous infusion is very effective but has not been widely used. Although paraldehyde has unpleasant physical properties it remains an effective drug.

Diazepam

Browne and Penry (1973), in a detailed review of the use of benzodiazepines in epilepsy, have summarised the results of treating various types of status epilepticus with diazepam. It appeared to be very effective in most types of status epilepticus, but particularly absence status. In complex partial, tonic and clonic status epilepticus it was somewhat less effective and in infantile myoclonic

status the drug achieved temporary control only. Focal EEG discharges are usually suppressed less readily than bilateral spike-and-wave activity. Most authors agree that diazepam is a drug of first choice in treating status epilepticus in infants and children (Bailey & Fenichel, 1968; McMorris & McWilliam, 1969; Wojcik & Lombroso, 1971) and in adults (Nicol, Tutton & Smith, 1969). However, the recent introduction of clonazepam may have altered the situation (see below).

Intravenous diazepam is a relatively safe drug (Greenblatt & Koch-Weser, 1973) but in status epilepticus it can cause respiratory depression and hypotension, especially if the injection follows administration of a barbiturate (Prensky et al., 1967; Sawer, Webster & Schut, 1968; Bell, 1969), but the incidence of these adverse effects with diazepam is probably less than with other drugs, such as the barbiturates. Diazepam is supplied as ampoules containing 10 mg in 2 ml. The intravenous administration of one ampoule over two minutes is usually adequate to terminate major status, although larger doses are sometimes necessary. Children will, of course, require smaller doses. After an initial rapid rise, the brain level falls quickly after intravenous administration because the drug redistributes to other tissues, and therapeutic levels are maintained for only one to two hours at most (Ferngren, 1974).

Diazepam is not satisfactory when given by infusion. Apart from the fact that there are solubility problems (p. 000), the parent drug and its active desmethyl metabolite accumulate, and after large doses have been infused coma may last for several days after the status has been controlled.

Clonazepam

This drug has been available for a much shorter time than diazepam, and therefore experience in its administration for status epilepticus is less extensive. It appears to be highly effective in treating both major and absence status epilepticus (Martin & Hirt, 1973; Ketz, 1973; Beck & Tousch, 1973) and two comparative studies have shown it to be at least as effective as diazepam (Bergamini et al., 1970; Gastaut et al., 1971). Whether it should be used in preference to diazepam can only be answered by a properly conducted comparative trial. In one study, clonazepam was found to have a longer duration of action (Congdon & Forsythe, 1980). On a weight-for-weight basis, clonazepam is about ten times more potent than diazepam.

Chlormethiazole

Intravenous infusion of 0.8 per cent solution of chlormethiazole has been shown to be effective in terminating status epilepticus (Laxenaire, Tridon & Poire, 1966; Harvey, Higenbottam & Loh, 1975). Too rapid an infusion may result in hypotension. As has been observed with diazepam, focal EEG discharges are less easily suppressed than bilateral spike-and-wave activity. For this reason, it has been suggested that the infusion should continue until all the paroxysmal electrical activity has been suppressed (Laxenaire et al., 1966). Chlormethiazole has the great advantage of a short duration of action and therefore control over the patient's state is good; the degree of sedation can rapidly be altered by a change in the rate of infusion. Its chief disadvantage is its propensity to produce thrombophlebitis. It is probably under-used; if single doses of a benzodiazepine are not effective, an infusion of chlormethiazole is a good second line treatment.

Phenytoin

Intravenous injection of phenytoin sodium is more effective than phenobarbitone sodium when given in adequate intravenous doses, because it crosses the blood-brain barrier more rapidly. For initial treatment Wallis, Kutt and McDowell (1968) used doses of 1000 mg given slowly into an infusion tube, the rate of infusion not exceeding 100 mg per minute because large doses of the solvent given too rapidly can produce hypotension, apnoea and cardiac asystole. Subsequently 300–500 mg daily was administered orally or intramuscularly. The latter route of administration, however, cannot be recommended because the drug crystallises in the tissues, causing local damage and haemorrhage, and is absorbed very slowly (p. 295). Although a method has been described for managing temporary intramuscular administra-

tion of phenytoin, it is much more satisfactory to give the drug once daily by intravenous infusion until the patient can take the dose orally. Monitoring serum phenytoin concentration will enable the optimum level to be achieved and will minimise the risk of intoxication.

Short-acting barbiturates

Amylobarbitone, hexobarbitone, quinalbarbitone and thiopentone have all been given intravenously in the control of major status epilepticus. Brown and Horton (1967) found that the suppressing dose of thiopentone sodium was much smaller than the sleep dose and had no significant effect on consciousness. No adverse effects or difficulties in management were encountered in any patient. The initial dose was usually 150–250 mg.

Alternatives to thiopentone sodium are pentobarbitone sodium 300–500 mg or amylobarbitone sodium 400–800 mg. There is no evidence indicating whether these are less effective or more effective than thiopentone sodium. Thiopentone should not be given by intravenous infusion. Although the distribution half-life (which determines duration of unconsciousness after an induction dose) is short, the elimination half-life is long (Cloyd, Wright & Perrier, 1979) and coma may last for several days, as occurs after diazepam infusions.

Phenobarbitone

Although often given by intramuscular injection in major status, phenobarbitone sodium is not rapidly absorbed, taking up to six hours to reach a peak serum level (Jalling, 1974). Even when given intravenously, phenobarbitone sodium has a rather delayed onset of action because equilibration between serum and brain occurs slowly. Up to 800 mg may have to be given by slow or intermittent intravenous injection before adequate brain levels are achieved. Although no longer the drug of choice for immediate treatment, phenobarbitone has an important place in the subsequent management because long-term therapy must be continued or started as soon as the acute episode is satisfactorily controlled. If the patient had previously been taking phenobarbitone orally, parenteral administration needs to be continued until oral therapy can be resumed. The suitability of the drug, or its dose, for long-term therapy may need to be reviewed.

Paraldehyde

Before the benzodiazepine drugs were introduced, paraldehyde was considered by many to be the drug of choice for treating major status epilepticus. Whitty and Taylor (1949) recommended giving 8–10 ml intramuscularly as soon as possible, massaging the injection site to promote absorption, although it takes up to 30 minutes to act. If status continues, they suggested giving further injections of 5 ml every 30 minutes until it ceases. Alternatively the drug can be given slowly intravenously in normal saline. Paraldehyde is soluble in water to the extent of one part in eight. Rectal administration of 4–8 g has also been used, but the onset of action is slower. Whitty and Taylor (1949) found that paraldehyde often worked where phenobarbitone sodium had failed. The unpleasant smell of the drug, its irritant nature, occasionally resulting in a cold abscess at the site of the injection or, if badly placed, sciatic nerve palsy, and its ability to dissolve some of the earlier plastic syringes have led to a decline in its use. However, most modern syringes are now stable enough to contain the drug for immediate administration and therefore given intramuscularly it may still have a useful place in the emergency treatment of children in status, when finding a suitable vein for administration of intravenous diazepam may be difficult, especially for the inexperienced.

Althesin

Munari et al. (1979) have reported successful use of Althesin (a mixture of two steroid derivatives, alfaxalone and alfadolone) in status.

General anaesthesia and curarisation

When fits have continued despite administration of full intravenous doses of the above drugs, general anaesthesia and full curarisation can be used with intermittent positive-pressure respiration (James & Whitty, 1961). The rationale of this procedure is to suppress peripherally the motor manifestations of the convulsions, because if they continue they will ultimately prove lethal. Curarisation will, of course, abolish the clinical manifestations of status, and therefore continuous EEG monitoring is required to assess the electrical activity. Continued administration of antiepileptic drugs is necessary in order to suppress the electrical discharge. In this situation chlormethiazole is appropriate.

Treatment of absence status

As mentioned earlier, both diazepam and clonazepam are highly effective in terminating absence status, although, on occasion, tonic status may be precipitated by administration of benzodiazepines (Tassinari et al., 1972; Prior et al., 1972).

Treatment of 'pre-status'

Some patients with severe epilepsy frequently have a series of major or minor fits occurring at close intervals during the course of a day. Although these episodes may not fall within the definition of 'status epilepticus', there is nevertheless reason for concern lest the fits evolve into status. Intravenous diazepam may not be necessary in these patients, although the administration of a drug to avert status is wise. Intramuscular diazepam, although rather slowly absorbed, may be suitable but needs to be given in doses of 20 mg in adults. If the patient is conscious, oral administration is perferable. Rectal administration of diazepam solution or paraldehyde is suitable in this situation, particularly when oral administration is not possible or if 'pre-status' occurs frequently in patients who live at home. Diazepam suppositories, although more slowly absorbed, have a more prolonged action and may be useful in averting recurrent seizures.

APPENDIX 8.1

Throughout this textbook serum anticonvulsant levels have been given in units with which the reader may be unfamiliar, μmol/l. For those who are accustomed to values expressed in μg/ml, these have always been added in parenthesis. The following is a list of factors for converting μg/ml to μmol/l.

Drug	Factor
Phenytoin	4.0
Methoin	4.6
Ethotoin	4.9
Phenobarbitone	4.3
Primidone	4.6
Carbamazepine	4.2
Carbamazepine-10, 11-epoxide	4.0
Ethosuximide	7.1
N desmethylmethsuximide (metabolite of methsuximide)	5.3
Troxidone	7.0
Dimethadione (metabolite of troxidone)	7.7
Diazepam	3.5
Clonazepam	3.2
Valproic acid (from sodium valproate)	6.9

	Britain	USA
Benzodiazepines	Diazepam(Valium) Nitrazepam(Mogadon) Clonazepam(Rivotril)	Diazepam(Valium) * Clonazepam (Clonopin)
Others	Carbamazepine (Tegretol) †	Carbamazepine (Tegretol) Phenacemide (Phenurone)
	Sulthiame(Ospolot) Sodium valproate (Epilim)	* Sodium valproate (Epilim)
	Beclamide(Nydrane) Acetazolamide(Diamox)	* Acetazolamide (Diamox)

* Not available in the USA at the time of writing
† No longer available in Britain
Note: The following compounds are also approved by the Food and Drug Administration in the USA for use as antiepileptic drugs: amobarbital(Amytal Sodium) ampoules, amphetamines, chlordiazepoxide(Librium) and quinacrine(Atabrine).

APPENDIX 8.2

Antiepileptic drugs available in Britain and the United States of America. The names listed are generic (approved), while those in parentheses are brand (trade) names.

	Britain	USA
Hydantoins	Phenytoin(Epanutin)	Phenytoin (Dilantin)
	Ethotoin(Peganone)	Ethotoin (Peganone)
	Methoin(Mesontoin)	Mephenytoin (Mesantoin)
Barbiturates	Phenobarbitone	Phenobarbital
	Methylphenobarbitone (Prominal)	Mephobarbital (Mebaral)
	Primidone(Mysoline)	Primidone (Mysoline)
Succinimides	Ethosuximide (Zarontin)	Ethosuximide (Zarontin)
	Methsuximide (Celontin)	Methsuximide (Celontin)
	Phensuximide (Milontin)	Phensuximide (Milontin)
Oxazolidinediones	Troxidone(Tridione)	Trimethadione (Tridione)
	Paramethadione (Paradione)	Paramethadione (Paradione)

APPENDIX 8.3

Structural formulae of some commonly used antiepileptic drugs.

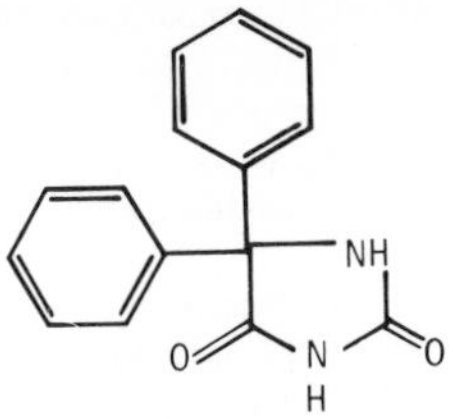

PHENYTOIN

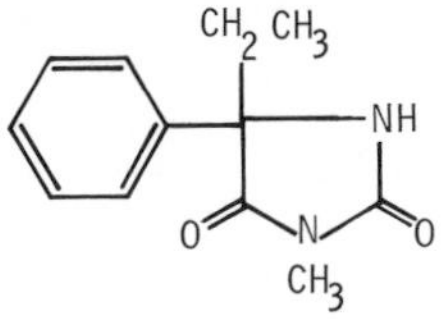

METHOIN

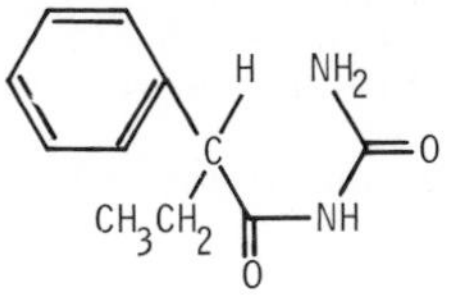

PHENETURIDE

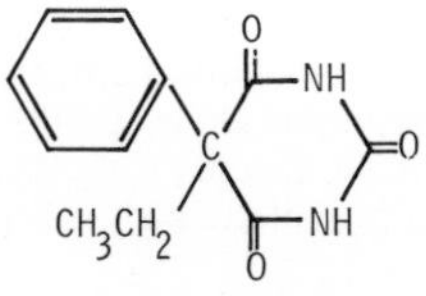

PHENOBARBITONE

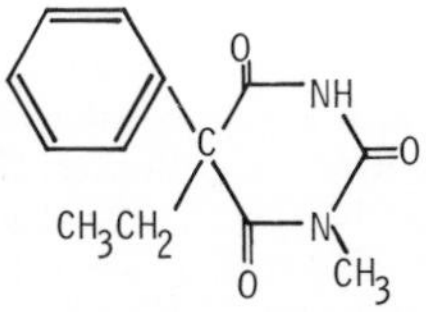

METHYLPHENOBARBITONE

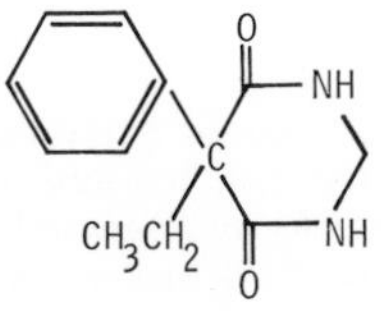

PRIMIDONE

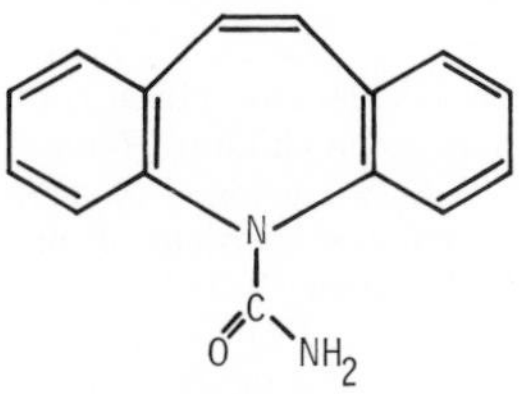

CARBAMAZEPINE

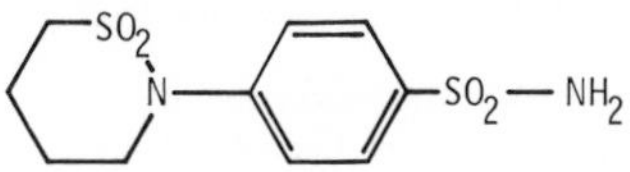

SULTHIAME

8.3(i)

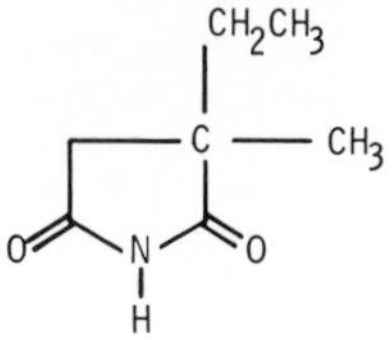

ETHOSUXIMIDE

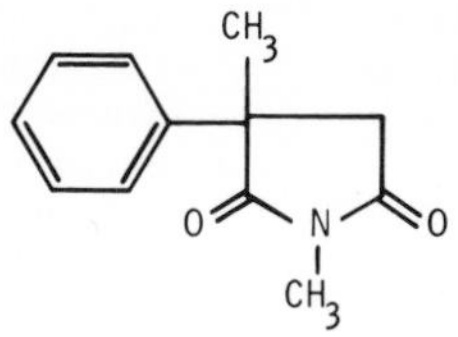

METHSUXIMIDE

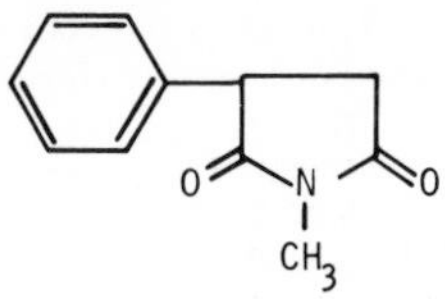

PHENSUXIMIDE

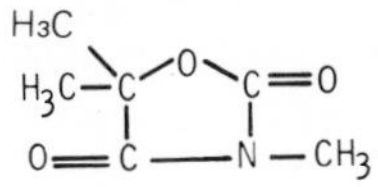

TRIMETHADIONE

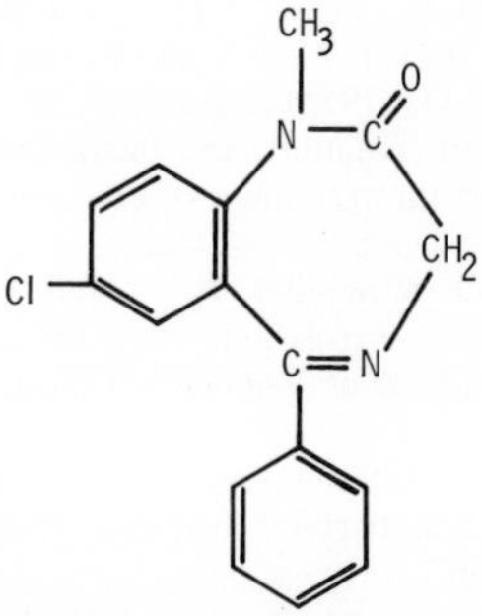

DIAZEPAM

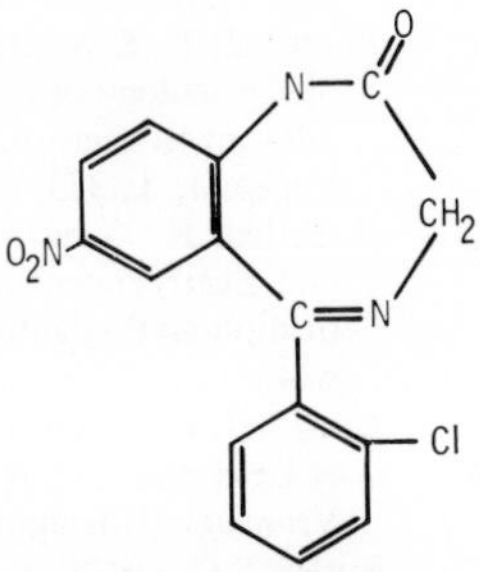

CLONAZEPAM

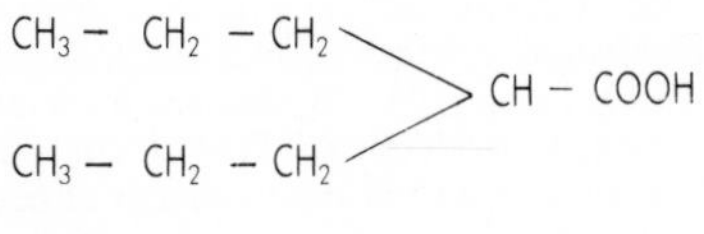

Valproic Acid

8.3(ii)

8.3(iii)

REFERENCES

Agurell, S., Berlin, A., Ferngren, H. & Hellstrom, B. (1975) Plasma levels of diazepam after parenteral and rectal administration in children. *Epilepsia*, **16**, 277.

Ahmad, S., Laidlaw, J., Houghton, G.W. & Richens, A. (1975) Involuntary movements caused by phenytoin intoxication in epileptic patients. *Journal of Neurology, Neurosurgery and Psychiatry*, **38**, 225.

Aird, R.B. & Tsubaki, T. (1958) Common sources of error in the diagnosis and treatment of convulsive disorders: a review of 204 patients with temporal lobe epilepsy. *Journal of Nervous and Mental Diseases*, **127**, 400.

Al-Kaisi, A.H. & McGuire, R.J. (1974) The effect of sulthiame on disturbed behaviour in mentally subnormal patients. *British Journal of Psychiatry*, **124**, 45.

Andreasen, P.B., Hendel, J., Greisen, G. & Hvidberg, E.F. (1976) Pharmacokinetics of diazepam in disordered liver function. *European Journal of Clinical Pharmacology*, **10**,115.

Ayers, G., Burnett, D., Griffiths, A. & Richens, A. (1980) Quality control of drug assays. *Clinical Pharmacokinetics* (in press).

Arnold, K. & Gerber, N. (1970) The rate of decline of diphenylhydantoin in human plasma. *Clinical Pharmacology and Therapeutics*, **11**, 121.

Bailey, D.W. & Fenichel, G.M. (1968) The treatment of prolonged seizure activity with intravenous diazepam. *Journal of Pediatrics*, **73**, 923.

Barot, M.H., Grant, R.H.E., Maheendran, K.K., Mawer, G.E. & Woodcock. B.G. (1978). Individual variation in daily dosage requirements for phenytoin sodium in patients with epilepsy. *British Journal of Clinical Pharmacology*, **6**, 267.

Baumel, I.P., Gallagher, B.B. & Mattson, R.H. (1972) Phenylethylmalonamide (PEMA). An important metabolite of primidone. *Archives of Neurology* (Chicago) **27**, 34.

Beck, H. & Tousch, C. (1973) Traitement des états de mal épileptiques par le clonazépam. *Semaine des Hôpitaux de Paris (Thér)*, **49**. Supplement 21.

Bell, D.S. (1969) Dangers of treatment of *status epilepticus* with diazepam. *British Medical Journal*, **1**, 159.

Bergamini, L., Mutani, L., Fariello, R. & Liboni, W. (1970) Elektroenzenphalographische und klinische Berwertung des neuen Benzodiazepam Ro 5-4023. *Zeitschrift fur EEG-EMG*, **1**, 182.

Berlin, A. & Dahlstrom, H. (1975) Pharmacokinetics of the anticonvulsant drug clonazepam evaluated from single oral and intravenous doses and by repeated oral administration. *European Journal of Clinical Pharmacology*, **9**, 155.

Bertilsson, L. (1978) Clinical pharmacokinetics of carbamazepine. *Clinical Pharmacokinetics*, **3**, 128.

Betts, T.A., Kalra, P.L., Cooper, R. & Jeavons, P.M. (1968) Epileptic fits as a probable side effect of amitriptyline. *Lancet*, **1**, 390.

Bird, C.A.K., Griffin, B.P., Miklaszewka, J.M. & Galbraith, A.W. (1966) Tegretol(carbamazepine): a controlled trial of a new anticonvulsant. *British Journal of Psychiatry*, **112**, 737.

Birket-Smith, E., Lund, M., Mikkelsen, B., Vestermark, S., Zander-Olsen, P. & Holm, P. (1973) A controlled trial on Ro 5-4023 (clonazepam) in the treatment of psychomotor epilepsy. *Acta Neurologica Scandinavica*, **49**. Supplement 53, 18.

Blaschke, T.F. (1977) Protein binding and kinetics of drugs in liver disease. *Clinical Pharmacokinetics*, **2**, 32.

Blaschke, T.F., Meffin, P.J., Melmon, K.L. & Rowland, M. (1975) Influence of acute viral hepatitis on phenytoin kinetics and protein binding. *Clinical Pharmacology and Therapeutics*, **17**, 685.

Bochner, F., Hooper, W.D., Sutherland, J.M., Eadie, M.J. & Tyrer, J.H. (1973) The renal handling of diphenylhydantoin and 5-(p-hydroxyphenyl)-5-phenylhydantoin. *Clinical Pharmacology and Therapeutics*, **14**, 791.

Bond, A.J., Hailey, D.M. & Lader, M.H. (1977) Plasma concentrations of benzodiazepines. *British Journal of Clinical Pharmacology*, **4**, 51.

Booker, H.E. (1972a) Phenobarbital, mephobarbital, and metharbital. Relation of plasma levels to clinical control. In Woodbury, D.M., Penry, J.K. & Schmidt, R.P. (eds) *Antiepileptic Drugs*, p. 329. New York: Raven Press.

Booker, H.E. (1972b) Trimethadione and other oxazolidinediones. Relation of plasma levels to clinical control. In Woodbury, D.M., Penry, J.K. & Schmidt, R.P. (eds) *Antiepileptic Drugs*, p. 403. New York: Raven Press.

Booker, H.E. & Celesia, C.C. (1973) Serum concentrations of diazepam in subjects with epilepsy. *Neurology* (Minneapolis) **29**, 191.

Booker, H.E., Hosokowa, K., Burdette, R.D. & Darcey, B. (1970) A clinical study of serum primidone levels. *Epilepsia*, **11**, 395.

Borofsky, L.G., Louis, S., Kutt, H. & Roginsky, M. (1972) Diphenylhydantoin: efficacy, toxicity and dose-serum level relationship in children. *Journal of Pediatrics*, **81**, 995.

Brown, A.S. & Horton, J.M. (1967) *Status epilepticus* treated by intravenous infusions of thiopentone sodium. *British Medical Journal*, **1**, 27.

Browne, T.R. (1976) Clonazepam. A review of a new anticonvulsant drug. *Archives of Neurology* (Chicago) **33**, 326.

Browne, T.R. & Penry, J.K. (1973) Benzodiazepines in the treatment of epilepsy. A review. *Epilepsia*, **14**, 277.

Browne, T.R., Dreifuss, F.E., Dyken, P.R., Goode, D.J., Penry, J.K., Porter, R.J., White, B.G., & White, P.T. (1975) Ethosuximide in the treatment of absence (petit mal) seizures. *Neurology* (Minneapolis) **25**, 515.

Buchanan, R.A., Kinkel, A.W. & Smith, T.C. (1973). The absorption and excretion of ethosuximide. *International Journal of Clinical Pharmacology and New Drugs*. **7**, 213.

Buchanan, R.A., Kinkel, A.W., Turner, J.L., Heffelfinger, J.C. (1976) Ethosuximide dosage regimens. *Clinical Pharmacology and Therapeutics*, **19**, 143.

Buchthal, F. & Lennox-Buchthal, M.A. (1972a) Diphenylhydantoin. Relation of anticonvulsant effect to concentration in serum. In Woodbury, D.M., Penry J.K. & Schmidt, R.P. (eds) *Antiepileptic Drugs*, p. 193. New York: Raven Press.

Buchthal, F. & Lennox-Buchthal, M.A. (1972b) Phenobarbital. Relation of serum concentration to control of seizures. In Woodbury, D.M., Penry, J.K. & Schmidt, R.P. (eds) *Antiepileptic Drugs*, p. 335. New York: Raven Press.

Buchthal, F. & Svensmark, O. (1959) Aspects of the pharmacology of phenytoin (Dilantin) and phenobarbital relevant to their dosage in the treatment of epilepsy. *Epilepsia*, **1**, 373.

Buchthal, F., Svensmark, O. & Schiller, P.J. (1960) Clinical and electroencephalographic correlations with serum levels of diphenylhydantoin. *Archives of Neurology* (Chicago) **2**, 624.

Buchthal, F., Svensmark, O. & Simonsen, H. (1968) Relation of EEG and seizures to phenobarbital in serum. *Archives of Neurology* (Chicago) **19**, 567.

Butler T.C. (1978) Some quantitative aspects of the pharmacology of phenobarbital. In Pippenger, C.E., Penry,

J.K. & Kutt, H. (eds) *Antiepileptic Drugs: Quantitative Analysis and Interpretation*, p. 261. New York: Raven Press.

Butler, T.C., Mahaffee, C., & Waddell, W.J. (1954) Phenobarbital: Studies of elimination, accumulation, tolerance, and dosage schedules. *Journal of Pharmacology and Experimental Therapeutics*, **111**, 425.

Catzel, P. (1966) *Paediatric Prescriber*. Oxford: Blackwell Scientific Publications.

Cereghino, J.J., Brock, J.T., Van Meter, J.C., Penry, J.K., Smith, L.D. & White, B.G. (1974a) Carbamazepine for epilepsy. A controlled prospective evaluation. *Neurology* (Minneapolis) **24**, 401.

Cereghino, J.J., Brock, J.T., Van Meter, J.C., Penry, J.K., Smith, L.D., Fisher, P. & Ellenberg, J. (1974b) Evaluation of albutoin as an antiepileptic drug. *Clinical Pharmacology and Therapeutics*, **15**, 406.

Chambers, R.E., Homeida, M., Hunter, K.R. & Teague, R.H. (1977) Salivary carbamazepine concentrations. *Lancet* i, 656.

Chandra, B. (1973) Clonazepam in the treatment of petit mal. *Asian Journal of Medicine*, **9**, 433.

Cloyd, J.C., Wright, B.D., and Perrier, D. (1979) Pharmacokinetic properties of thiopental in two patients treated for uncontrollable seizures. *Epilepsia*, **20**, 313.

Coatsworth, J.J. (1971) *Studies on the Clinical Efficacy of Marketed Antiepileptic Drugs. NINDS* Monograph No. 12. Washington: US Government Printing Office.

Coatsworth, J.J. & Penry, J.K. (1972) General principles. Clinical efficacy and use. In Woodbury, D.M., Penry, J.K. & Schmidt, R.P. (eds) *Antiepileptic Drugs*, p. 87. New York: Raven Press.

Cole, A.P. & Hailey, D.M. (1975) Diazepam and active metabolites in breast milk and their transfer to the neonate. *Archives of Diseases in Childhood*. **50**, 741.

Congdon, P.J. & Forsythe, W.I. (1980) Intravenous clonazepam in the treatment of status epilepticus in children. *Epilepsia*, **21**, 97.

Covanis, A. & Jeavons, P.M. (1980) Once-daily sodium valproate in the treatment of epilepsy. *Developmental Medicine and Child Neurology*, **22**, 202.

Dalby, M.A. (1975) Behavioural effects of carbazepine. In Penry, J.K. & Daly, D.D. (eds) *Complex Partial Seizures and their Treatment. Advances in Neurology, Vol. 11*. New York: Raven Press.

Dam, M., Christiansen, J., Munck, O. & Mygind, K.I. (1979) Antiepileptic drugs; metabolism in pregnancy. *Clinical Pharmacokinetics*, **4**, 53.

Davis, J.P. & Lennox, W.G. (1949) A comparison of Paradione and Tridione in the treatment of epilepsy. *Journal of Pediatrics*, **34**, 273.

Di Gregorio, G.J., Piraino, A.J. & Ruch, E. (1978) Diazepam concentrations in parotid saliva, mixed saliva and plasma. *Clinical Pharmacology and Therapeutics*, **24**, 720.

Diamond, S. & Levy, L. (1963) Metabolic studies on a new antiepileptic drug, Riker 594. *Current Therapeutic Research*, **5**, 325.

Doose, H., Helmchen, H., Ketz, E., Künkel, H., Matthes, A., Oberhoffer, G., Penin, H., Rabe, F., Scheffner, D. & Voigt, U. (1970) Modern methods of assessing antiepileptic drugs. (Results with carbamazepine.) *Pharmakopsychiat. Neuropsychopharm.*, **3**, 227.

Dreifuss, F.E., Penry, J.K., Rose, S.W., Kupferberg, H.J., Dyken, P. & Sato, S. (1975) Serum clonazepam concentrations in children with absence seizures. *Neurology* (Minneapolis) **25**, 255.

Dulac, O., Aicardi, J., Rey, E. & Olive, G. (1978) Blood levels of diazepam after single rectal administration in infants and children. *Journal of Pediatrics*, **93**, 1039.

Eadie, M.J. & Tyrer, J.H. (1980) *Anticonvulsant Therapy. Pharmacological Basis and Practice*, 2nd edn. Edinburgh: Churchill Livingstone.

Eadie, M.J., Lander, C.M. & Tyrer, J.H. (1977) Plasma drug level monitoring in pregnancy. *Clinical Pharmacokinetics*, **2**, 427.

Eadie, M.J., Bochner, F., Hooper, W.D. & Tyrer, J.H. (1978) Preliminary observations on the pharmacokinetics of methylphenobarbitone. *Clinical and Experimental Neurology*, **15**, 131.

Edwards, V.E. & Eadie, M.J. (1973) Clonazepam – clinical study of its effectiveness as an anticonvulsant. *Proceedings of the Australian Association of Neurology*, **10**, 61.

Faerø, O., Kastrup, K.W., Lykkegarrd-Nielsen, E., Melchior, J.C. & Thorn, I. (1972) Successful prophylaxis of febrile convulsions with phenobarbital. *Epilepsia*, **13**, 279.

Faigle, J.W., Feldmann, K.F., & Baltzer, V. (1977) Anticonvulsant effect of carbamazepine. An attempt to distinguish between the potency of the parent drug and its epoxide metabolite. In Gardner-Thorpe, C., Janz, D., Meinardi, H. & Pippenger, C.E. (eds) *Antiepileptic Drug Monitoring*, p. 104. Avon: Pitman Press.

Ferngren, H.G. (1974) Diazepam treatment for acute convulsions in children. *Epilepsia*, **15**, 27.

Forster, F.M. (1959) Advances in the medical treatment of epilepsy. *Wisconsin Medical Journal*, **58**, 375.

Fredholm, B.B., Rane, A., & Persson, B. (1975) Diphenylhydantoin binding to proteins in plasma and its dependence on free fatty acid and bilirubin concentration in drugs and newborn infants. *Pediatric Research*, **9**, 26.

Gallagher, B.B., Smith, D.B. & Mattson, R.H. (1970) The relationship of the anticonvulsant properties of primidone to phenobarbital. *Epilepsia* (Amsterdam) **11**, 293.

Gallagher, B.B. & Baumel, J.P. (1972) Primidone. Biotransformation. In Woodbury, D.M., Penry, J.K. & Schmidt, R.P. (eds) *Antiepileptic Drugs*, p. 361. New York: Raven Press.

Gamble, J.A.S., Dundee, J.W. & Assaf, R.A.E. (1975) Plasma diazepam levels after single oral and intramuscular administration. *Anaesthesia*, **30**, 164.

Gastaut, H. (1970) Clinical and electroencephalographical classification of the epileptic seizures. *Epilepsia*, **11**, 102.

Gastaut, H. & Low, M.D. (1979) Antiepileptic properties of clobazam, a 1, 5-benzodiazepine, in man. *Epilepsia*, **20**, 437.

Gastaut, H., Courjon, J., Poiré, R. & Weber, M. (1971) Treatment of *status epilepticus* with a new benzodiazepine more active than diazepam. *Epilepsia*, **12**, 197.

Gibbs, F.A. (1947) New drugs in the treatment of epilepsy. *Annals of Internal Medicine*, **27**, 548.

Glaser, G.H., Penry, J.K., Woodbury, D.H. (eds) (1980) *Antiepileptic Drugs: Mechanisms of Action*. New York: Raven Press.

Goldberg, M.A., & Dorman, J.E. (1976) Intention myoclonus: successful treatment with clonazepam. *Neurology* (Minneapolis) **26**, 24.

Gordon, N. (1974) Why does the medical treatment of epilepsy sometimes fail? In Harris, P. & Mawdsley, C. (eds) *Epilepsy. Proceedings of the Hans Berger Centenary Symposium*, p. 187. Edinburgh: Churchill Livingstone.

Goulet, J.R., Kinkel, A.W. & Smith, T.C. (1976) Metabolism of ethosuximide. *Clinical Pharmacology and Therapeutics*, **20**, 213.

Graham, J. (1978) A comparison of the absorption of phenobarbitone given via the oral and the intramuscular route. *Clinical and Experimental Neurology*, 15, 154.

Gram, L. Flachs, H., Würtz-Jørgensen, A., Parnas, J. & Andersen, B. (1980) Sodium valproate, relationship between serum levels and therapeutic effect: a controlled study. In Johannessen, S.I. et al. (eds) *Antiepileptic Therapy: Advances in Drug Monitoring*, p. 217. New York: Raven Press.

Gram, L., Wulff, K., Rasmussen, K.E., Flachs, H., Würtz-Jorgensen, A., Sommerbeck, K.W. & Løhren, V. (1977) Valproate sodium: a controlled clinical trial including monitoring of drug levels. *Epilepsia*, 18, 141.

Green, J.R., Troupin, A.S., Halpern, L.M., Friel, P. & Kanarek, P. (1974) Sulthiame: evaluation as an anticonvulsant. *Epilepsia*, 15, 329.

Greenblatt, D.J. & Koch Weser, J. (1973) Adverse reactions to intravenous diazepam: a report from the Boston collaborative drug surveillance program. *American Journal of Medicine and Science*, 266, 261.

Greenblatt, D.J., Allen, M.D., McLaughlin, D.S., Harmatz, J.S., & Shader, R.I. (1978) Diazepam absorption: effects of antacids and food. *Clinical Pharmacology and Therapeutics*, 24, 600.

Griffiths, A., Hebdige, S., Perucca, E. & Richens, A. (1980) Quality control in drug measurement. *Therapeutic Drug Monitoring*, 2, 51.

Gruber, C.M., Mosier, J.M., Grant, P. & Glew, R. (1956) Objective comparison of phenobarbital and diphenylhydantoin in epileptic patients. *Neurology* (Minneapolis) 6, 640.

Gruber, C.M., Brock, J.T. & Dyken, M. (1962) Comparison of the effectiveness of phenobarbital, primidone, diphenylhydantoin, ethotoin, metharbital and methylphenylethylhydantoin in motor seizures. *Clinical Pharmacology and Therapeutics*, 3, 23.

Gugler, R. & Mueller, G. (1978) Plasma protein binding of valproic acid in healthy subjects and in patients with renal disease. *British Journal of Clinical Pharmacology*, 5, 441.

Gugler, R. & Von Unruh, G.E. (1980) Clinical pharmacokinetics of valproic acid. *Clinical Pharmacokinetics* 5, 67.

Gugler, R., Manion, C.V. & Azarnoff D.L. (1976)5) Phenytoin: pharmacokinetics and bioavailability. *Clinical Pharmacology and Therapeutics*, 19, 135.

Gugler, R., Eichelbaum, M., Schell, A., Fröscher, W., Kiefer, H., Schulz, H.U. & Müller, G.(1980) The disposition of valproic acid. In Johannessen, S.I. *et al.* (eds) *Antiepileptic Therapy: Advances in Drug Monitoring*, p. 125. New York: Raven Press.

Haerer, A.F. & Grace, J.B. (1969) Studies of anticonvulsant levels in epileptics. 1. Serum diphenylhydantoin concentrations in a group of medically indigent outpatients. *Acta Neurologica Scandinavica*, 45, 18.

Handley, R. & Stewart, A.S.R. (1952) Mysoline: a new drug for the treatment of epilepsy. *Lancet*, i, 742.

Harding, G.F.A., Herrick, C.E. & Jeavons, P.M. (1978) A controlled study on the effect of sodium valproate on photosensitive epilepsy and its prognosis. *Epilepsia*, 19, 555.

Harvey, P.K.P., Higenbottam, T.W. & Loh, L. (1975) Chlormethiazole in treatment of status epilepticus. *British Medical Journal*, 2, 603.

Heathfield, K.W.G., & Jewesbury, E.C.O. (1964) Treatment of petit mal with ethosuximide: follow-up report. *British Medical Journal*, 2, 616.

Henriksen, O. & Johannessen, S.I. (1980) Clinical observations of sodium valproate in children: an evaluation of therapeutic serum levels. In Johannessen, S.I. et al. (eds) *Antiepileptic Therapy: Advances in Drug Monitoring*, p. 253. New York: Raven Press.

Hillestad, L., Hansen, T., Melsom, H. & Driveness, A. (1974) Diazepam metabolism in normal man. 1. Serum concentrations and clinical effects after intravenous, intramuscular, and oral administration. *Clinical Pharmacology and Therapeutics*, 16, 479.

Holowack, J., Thurston, D.L. & O'Leary, J. (1972) Prognosis in childhood epilepsy. *New England Journal of Medicine*, 286, 169.

Hooper, W.D., Bochner, F., Eadie, M.J. & Tyrer, J.H. (1974) Plasma protein binding of diphenylhydantoin. Effects of sex hormones, renal and hepatic disease. *Clinical Pharmacology and Therapeutics*, 15, 276.

Hooper, W.D., Dubetz, D.K., Bochner, F., Cotter, L.M., Smith, G.A., Eadie, M.J., & Tyrer, J.H. (1975) Plasma protein binding of carbamazepine. *Clinical Pharmacology and Therapeutics*, 17, 433.

Houghton, G.W. & Richens, A. (1974a) Rate of elimination of tracer doses of phenytoin at different steady-state serum concentrations in epileptic patients. *British Journal of Clinical Pharmacology*, 1, 155.

Houghton, G.W. & Richens, A. (1974b) Inhibition of phenytoin metabolism by sulthiame in epileptic patients. *British Journal of Clinical Pharmacology*, 1, 59.

Houghton, G.W., Richens, A. & Leighton, M. (1975a) Effect of age, height, weight and sex on serum phenytoin concentration in epileptic patients. *British Journal of Clinical Pharmacology*, 2, 251.

Houghton, G.W., Richens, A., Toseland, P.A., Davidson, S., Falconer, M.A. (1975b) Brain concentrations of phenytoin, phenobarbitone and primidone in epileptic patients. *European Journal of Clinical Pharmacology*, 9, 73.

Hrachovy, R.A., Frost, J.D., Kellaway, P. & Zion, T. (1979) A controlled study of prednisone therapy in infantile spasms. *Epilepsia*, 20, 403.

Ives, E.R. (1951) Comparison of efficacy of various drugs in treatment of epilepsy. *Journal of American Medical Association*, 147, 1332.

Jakobs, C. & Loscher, W. (1978) Identification of metabolites of valproic acid in serum of humans, dog, rat and mouse. *Epilepsia*, 19, 591.

Jalling, B. (1974) Plasma and CSF concentrations of phenobarbital in infants given single doses. *Developmental Medicine and Child Neurology*, 16, 781.

James, J.L. & Whitty, G.W. (1961) The electroencephalogram as a monitor of *status epilepticus* suppressed peripherally by curarization. *Lancet*, 2, 239.

Janz, D. & Kautz, G. (1964) The aetiology and treatment of *status epilepticus*. *German Medical Monthly*, 9, 451.

Jeavons, P.M., & Bower, B.D., (1974) Infantile spasms. In Vinken, P.J. & Bruyn, G.W. (eds) *Handbook of Clinical Neurology Vol. 15: The Epilepsies*, p. 219. New York: American Elsevier.

Jeavons, P.M. & Clark, J.E. (1974) Sodium valproate in the treatment of epilepsy. *British Medical Journal*, 2, 584.

Jeavons, P.M., Clark, J.E., & Maheshwari, M.C. (1977) Treatment of generalised epilepsies of childhood and adolescence with sodium valproate (Epilim). *Developmental Medicine and Child Neurology*, 19, 9.

Johannessen, S.I., Barruzzi, A., Gomeni, R., Strandjord, R.E. & Morselli, P.L. (1977) Further observations on carbamazepine and carbamazepine – 10,11-epoxide kinetics in epileptic patients. In Gardner-Thorpe, C., Janz, D., Meinardi, H. & Pippenger, C.E. (eds) *Antiepileptic Drug Monitoring*, p. 110. Avon: Pitman.

Juul-Jensen, P. (1964) Frequency of recurrence after discontinuance of anticonvulsant therapy in patients with epileptic seizures. *Epilepsia*, 5, 352.

Kaneko, S., Sato, T. & Suzuki, K. (1979) The levels of anticonvulsants in breast milk. *British Journal of Clinical Pharmacology*, 7, 624.

Kanto, J. (1975) Plasma concentrations of diazepam and its metabolites after per oral, intramuscular and rectal administration. *International Journal of Clinical Pharmacy and Biopharmaceutics*, 12, 427.

Karlen, B., Garle, M., Rane, A., Gutova, M. & Lindeborg, B. (1975) Assay of diphenylhydantoin (phenytoin) metabolites in urine by gas chromatography. Metabolite pattern in humans. *European Journal of Clinical Pharmacology*, 8, 359.

Kaufmann, R.F., Habersang, R. & Lansky, L. (1977) Kinetics of primidone metabolism and excretion in children. *Clinical Pharmacology and Therapeutics*, 22, 200.

Kaye, N., Jones, I.H. & Warrier, G.K. (1959) Nydrane as an anticonvulsant. *British Medical Journal*, 1, 627.

Ketz, E. (1973) *Status epilepticus – Behandlung mit Rivotril. Schweizerische medizinische Wochenschrift*, 103, 1134.

Klotz, V., T. & Mueller, W.A. (1978) Disposition of valproic acid in patients with liver disease. *European Journal of Clinical Pharmacology*, 13, 55.

Knudsen, F.U. (1977) Plasma-diazepam in infants after rectal administration in solution and by suppository. *Acta Paediatrica Scandinavica*, 66, 563.

Knudsen, F.U. (1979) Rectal administration of diazepam in solution in the acute treatment of convulsions in infants and children. *Archives of Diseases in Childhood*. 54, 855.

Koch-weser, J. (1975) The serum level approach to individualisation of drug dosage. *European Journal of Clinical Pharmacology*, 9, 1.

Kutt, H., Winters, W., Scherman, R. & McDowell, F. (1964a) Diphenylhydantoin and phenobarbital toxicity. The role of liver disease. *Archives of Neurology* (Chicago)3 11, 649.

Kutt, H., Winters, W., Kokenge, R. & McDowell, F. (1964b) Diphenylhydantoin metabolism, blood levels, and toxicity. *Archives of Neurology* (Chicago) 11, 642.

Kutt, H. & McDowell, F. (1968) Management of epilepsy with diphenylhydantoin sodium. *Journal of the American Medical Association*, 203, 969.

Lascelles, P.T., Kocen, R.S. & Reynolds, E.H. (1970) The distribution of plasma phenytoin levels in epileptic patients. *Journal of Neurology, Neurosurgery and Psychiatry*, 33, 501.

Laxenaire, M., Tridon, P. & Poire, P. (1966) Effect of chlormethiazole in treatment of *dilerium tremens* and *status epilepticus*. *Acta Psychiatrica Scandinavica*, 42. Supplement 192, 87.

Legg, N.J. & Swash, M. (1974) Clinical note: Seizures and EEG activation after trimipramine. *Epilepsia*, 15, 131.

Levy, R.H., Pitlick, W.H., Troupin, A.S., Green, J.R. & Neal, J.M. (1975) Pharmacokinetics of carbamazepine in normal man. *Clinical Pharmacology and Therapeutics*, 17, 657.

Lockard, J.S. & Levy, R.H. (1976) Valproic acid: reversibly acting drug? *Epilepsia*, 17, 477.

Loeser, E.W. (1961) Studies on the metabolism of diphenylhydantoin (Dilantin). *Neurology* (Minneapolis) 11, 424.

Lous, P. (1966) Elimination of barbiturates. In Johansen, S.H.

(ed.) *Barbiturate Poisoning and Tetanus*, p. 341. Boston: Little Brown.

Lund, L. (1973) Effects of phenytoin in patients with epilepsy in relation to its concentration in plasma. In *Biological Effects of Drugs in Relation to their Plasma Concentration*. Edited by D.S. Davies & B.N.C. Prichard, p. 227. London: Macmillan.

Lund, L. (1974a) Clinical significance of generic inequivalence of three different pharmaceutical preparations of phenytoin. *European Journal of Clinical Pharmacology*, 7, 119.

Lund, L. (1974b) Anticonvulsant effect of diphenylhydantoin relative to plasma levels. A prospective three-year study in ambulant patients with generalised epileptic seizures. *Archives of Neurology* (Chicago) 31, 289.

Lund, L., Berlin, A. & Lunde, P.K.M. (1972) Plasma protein binding of diphenylhydantoin in patients with epilepsy. Agreement between the unbound fraction in plasma and the concentration in the cerebrospinal fluid. *Clinical Pharmacology and Therapeutics*, 113, 196.

Mandelli, M., Tognoni, G. & Garattini, S (1978) Clinical pharmacokinetics of diazepam. *Clinical Pharmacokinetics*, 3, 72.

Martin, D. & Hirt, H.R. (1973) Clinical experience with clonazepam (Rivotril) in the treatment of epilepsies in infancy and childhood. *Journal of Neuropaediatric Biology, Neurology and Neurosurgery*, 4, 245.

McAuliffe, J.J., Sherwin, A.L., Leppik, I.E., Fayle, S.E. & Pippenger, C.E. (1977) Salivary levels of anticonvulsants: A practical approach to drug monitoring. *Neurology* (Minneapolis), 27, 409.

McLendon, S.B. (1943) A comparative study of 'Dilantin Sodium' and phenobarbital in Negro epileptics. *Southern Medical Journal*, 36, 303.

McMorris, S. & McWilliam, P.K.A. (1969) *Status epilepticus* in infants and young children treated with parenteral diazepam. *Archives of Disease in Childhood*, 44, 604.

Meberg, A., Langslet, A., Bredesen, J.E., & Lunde, P.K.M. (1978) Plasma concentration of diazepam and n-desmethyldiazepam in children after a single rectal or intramuscular dose of diazepam. *European Journal of Clinical Pharmacology*, 14, 273.

Meinardi, H. (1971) Clinical trials of antiepileptic drugs. *Psychiatry, Neurology and Neurosurgery*, 74, 141.

Melekian, R., Laplane, R. & Debray, P. (1962) Considérations cliniques sur les convulsions du course des déshydrations aigrés. *Annales de Pédiatrie*, 9, 290.

Mikkelsen, B., Birket-Smith, E., Brandt, S., Holm, P., Lund, M., Thorm, I., Vestermark, S. & Zander-Olsen, P. (1976) Clonazepam in the treatment of epilepsy. A controlled clinical trial in simple absences, bilateral massive epileptic myoconus, and atonic seizures. *Archives of Neurology* (Chicago) 33, 322.

Mikkelsen, B., Birket-Smith, E., Holm, P., Lund, M., Vestermarks, S. & Zander – Olsen, P. (1975) A controlled trial on clonazepam (Ro 5 – 4023, Rivotril) in the treatment of focal epilepsy and secondary generalised grand mal epilepsy. *Acta Neurologica Scandinavica*, 51, (Suppl. 60) 55.

Millichap, J.G. & Aymat, F. (1968) Controlled evaluation of primidone and diphenylhydantoin sodium. Comparative anticonvulsant efficacy and toxicity in children. *Journal of the American Medical Association*, 204, 738..

Millman, C.G. (1937) Luminal and Prominal in epilepsy. A comparative study. *British Medical Journal*, 2, 61.

Moffatt, W.R., Siddiqui, A.R. & MacKay, D.M. (1970) The

use of sulthiame with disturbed mentally subnormal patients. *British Journal of Psychiatry*, **117**, 673.

Monks, A., Boobis, S., Wadsworth, J. & Richens, A. (1978) Plasma protein binding interaction between phenytoin and valproic acid *in vitro*. *British Journal of Clinical Pharmacology*, **6**, 487.

Morris, M.E. (1978) Compatibility of diazepam injection following dilution with intravenous fluids. *American Journal of Hospital Pharmacy*, **35**, 669.

Morselli, P.L. (1977) Antiepileptic drugs. In Morselli, P.L. (ed.) *Drug Disposition during Development*, p. 311. New York: Spectrum Publications.

Morselli, P.L. (1978) Clinical significance of monitoring plasma levels of benzodiazepine tranquillisers and antiepileptic drugs. In Deniker, P., Radouco-Thomas, C., & Villeneuve, A. (eds) *Neuropsychopharmacology*, p. 877. Oxford: Pergamon Press.

Morselli, P.L., Gerna, M., de Maio, D., Zanda, G., Viani, F. & Garattini, S. (1975) Pharmacokinetic studies on carbamazepine in volunteers and in epileptic patients. In Schneider, H., Janz, D., Gardner-Thorpe, C., Meinardi, H. & Sherwin, A. (eds) *Clinical Pharmacology of Antiepileptic Drugs*, p. 166. Berlin: Springer-Verlag.

Mucklow, J.C., & Dollery, C.T. (1978) Compliance with anticonvulsant therapy in a hospital clinic and in the community. *British Journal of Clinical Pharmacology*, **6**, 75.

Mullen, P.W. (1978) Optimal phenytoin therapy: a new technique for individualising dosage. *Clinical Pharmacology and Therapeutics*, **23**, 228.

Munari, C., Casarou, D., Matteuzzi, G. & Pacifico, L. (1979) The case of Althesen a drug-resistant status epilepticus. *Epilepsia*, **20**, 475.

Mygind, K.E., Dam, M. & Christiansen, J. (1976) Phenytoin and phenobarbitone plasma clearance during pregnancy. *Acta Neurologica Scandinavica*, **54**, 160.

Nanda, R.N., Johnson, R.H., Keogh, H.J., Lambie, D.G. & Melville, I.D. (1977) Treatment of epilepsy with clonazepam and its effects on other anticonvulsants. *Journal of Neurology, Neurosurgery and Psychiatry*, **40**, 538.

Neuvonen, P.J. (1979) Bioavailability of phenytoin: Clinical, pharmacokinetic and therapeutic implications. *Clinical Pharmacokinetics*, **4**, 91.

Nicol, C.F., Tutton, J.C. & Smith, B.H. (1969) Parenteral diazepam in *status epilepticus*. *Neurology* (Minneapolis) **19**, 332.

Nicholson, P.W., Dobbs, S.M. & Rodgers, E.M. (1980) Ideal sampling time for drugs assays. *British Journal of Clinical Pharmacology*, **9**, 467.

North, J.B., Penhall, R.K., Hanieh, A., Hann, C.S., Challen, R.G., Prewin, D.B. (1980) Post-operative epilepsy: a double-blind trial of phenytoin after craniotomy. *Lancet*, **1**, 384.

Odar-Cederlöf, I. & Borga, O. (1974) Kinetics of diphenylhydantoin in uraemic patients: consequences of decreased plasma protein binding. *European Journal of Clinical Pharmacology*, **7**, 31.

Odar-Caderlöf, I. & Borga, O. (1976) Impaired protein binding of phenytoin in uremia and displacement effects of salicylic acid. *Clinical Pharmacology and Therapeutics*, **20**, 36.

Ounsted, C., Lindsay, J. & Norman, R. (1966) *Biological Factors in Temporal Lobe Epilepsy*. London: William Heinemann Medical Books.

Oxbury, J.M. & Whitty, C.W.M. (1971) Causes and consequences of *status epilepticus* in adults. A study of 86 cases. *Brain*, **94**, 733.

Oxley, J., Hebdige, S., Laidlaw, J., Wadsworth, J. & Richens, A. (1980) A comparative study of phenobarbitone and primidone in the treatment of epilepsy. In Johanessen, S.I. et al. (eds) *Antiepileptic Therapy: Advances in Drug Monitoring*, p. 237. New York: Raven Press.

Paxton, J.W., Whiting, B. & Stephen, K.W. (1977) Phenytoin concentrations in mixed parotid and submandibular saliva and serum measured by radioimmunoassay. *British Journal of Clinical Pharmacology*, **4**, 185.

Penfield, W. & Erickson, T.C. (1941) *Epilepsy and Cerebral Localisation*. London: Baillière.

Penry, J.K., Porter, R.J. & Dreifuss, F.E. (1972) Ethosuximide. Relation of plasma levels to clinical control. In Woodbury, D.M., Penry, J.K. & Schmidt, R.P. (eds) *Antiepileptic Drugs*, p. 431. New York: Raven Press.

Perucca, E., Bittencourt, P. & Richens, A. (1978) Effect of dose increments on serum carbamazepine concentration in epileptic patients. *Clinical Pharmacokinetics*, (in press).

Perucca, E., Garratt, S., Hebdige, S. & Richens, A. (1978) Water intoxication in epileptic patients receiving carbamazepine. *Journal of Neurology, Neurosurgery and Psychiatry*, **41**, 713.

Peterson, D.I. & Zweig, R.W. (1974) Absorption of anticonvulsants after jejunoileal bypass. *Bulletin. Los Angeles Neurological Society*, **39**, 51.

Pinder, R.M., Brogden, R.N., Speight, T.M. & Avery, G.S. (1976) Clonazepam: a review of its pharmacological properties and therapeutic efficacy in epilepsy. *Drugs*, **12**, 321.

Pinder, R.M., Brogden, R.N., Speight, T.M. & Avery, G.S. (1977) Sodium valproate: a review of its pharmacological properties and therapeutic efficacy in epilepsy. *Drugs*, **13**, 81.

Pippenger, C.E., Penry, J.K. & Kutt, H. (Eds) (1978) *Antiepileptic Drugs: Quantitative Analysis and Interpretation*. New York: Raven Press.

Plaa, G.L. & Hine, C.H. (1960) Hydantoin and barbiturate blood levels observed in epileptics. *Archives internationales de pharmacodynamie (et de thérapie)*, **128**, 375.

Pollack, M.A., Zion, T.E., & Kellaway, P. (1979) Long-term prognosis of patients with infantile spasms following ACTH therapy. *Epilepsia*, **20**, 255.

Porter, R.J. & Layzer, R.B. (1975) Plasma albumin concentration and diphenylhydantoin binding in man. *Archives of Neurology* (Chicago) **32**, 298.

Porter, R.J., Penry, J.K., Lacy, J.R., Newmark, M.E., & Kupferberg, H.J. (1977) The clinical efficacy and pharmacokinetics of phensuximide and methsuximide. *Neurology* (Minneapolis) **27**, 375.

Prensky, A.I., Raff, M.C., Moore, M.J. & Schwab, R.S. (1967) Intravenous diazepam in the treatment of prolonged seizure activity. *New England Journal of Medicine*, **276**, 779.

Price, S.A. & Spencer, D.A. (1967) A trial of beclamide (Nydrane) in mentally subnormal patients with disorders of behaviour. *Journal of Mental Subnormality*, **13**, 75.

Prior, P.F., Maclaine, G.N., Scott, D.F. & Laurance, B.M. (1972) Tonic *status epilepticus* precipitated by intravenous diazepam in a child with petit mal status. *Epilepsia*, **13**, 467.

Pynnönen, S. (1979) Pharmacokinetics of carbamazepine in man: a review. *Therapeutic Drug Monitoring*, **1**, 409.

Rambeck, B., Boenigk, H.E. & Stenzel, E. (1977) Bioavailability of three phenytoin preparations in healthy subjects and in epileptics. *European Journal of Clinical Pharmacology*, **12**, 285.

Rambeck, B., Boenigk, H.E., Dunlop, A., Mullen, P.W.,

Wadsworth, J. & Richens, A. (1979) Predicting phenytoin dose: a revised nomogram. *Therapeutic Drug Monitoring*, 1, 325.

Rane, A., Höjer, B. & Wilson, J.T. (1976) Kinetics of carbamazepine and its 10,11-epoxide metabolite in children. *Clinical Pharmacology and Therapeutics*, 19, 276.

Rane, A., Garle, M., Borga, O. & Sjöqvist, F. (1974) Plasma disappearance of transplacentally transferred phenytoin in the newborn studied with mass fragmentography. *Clinical Pharmacology and Therapeutics*, 15, 13.

Rapport, R.L. II, & Penry, J.K. (1973) A survey of attitudes towards the pharmacological prophylaxis of post-traumatic epilepsy. *Journal of Neurosurgery*, 38, 159.

Reidenberg, M.M. & Drayer, D.E. (1978) Effects of renal disease upon drug disposition. *Drug Metabolism Reviews*, 8, 293.

Reynolds, E.H. (1980) Serum levels of anticonvulsant drugs. Interpretation and clinical value. *Pharmacology and Therapeutics*, 8, 217.

Reynolds, F., Ziroyanis, P., Jones, N. & Smith, S.E. (1976) Salivary phenytoin concentrations in epilepsy and in chronic renal failure. *Lancet*, 2, 384.

Richens, A. (1976) *Drug treatment of epilepsy.* London: Henry Kimpton.

Richens, A. (1979) Clinical pharmacokinetics of phenytoin, *Clinical Pharmacokinetics*, 4, 153.

Richens, A. & Ahmad, S. (1975) Controlled trial of sodium valproate in severe epilepsy. *British Medical Journal*, 4, 255.

Richens, A. and Dunlop, A. (1975) Serum phenytoin levels in the management of epilepsy. *Lancet*, 2, 247.

Rodin, E.A. (1968) *The prognosis of patients with epilepsy.* Springfield, Illinois: C.C. Thomas.

Rodin, E.A., Rim, C.S. & Rennick, P.M. (1974) The effects of carbamazepine on patients with psychomotor epilepsy: results of a double-blind study. *Epilepsia*, 15, 547.

Rodin, E.A., Rim, C.S., Kitano, H., Lewis, R. & Rennick, P.M. (1976) A comparison of the effectiveness of primidone versus carbamazepine in epileptic outpatients. *Journal of Nervous and Mental Disease*, 163, 41.

Rowan, A.J. & Scott, D.F. (1970) Major *status epilepticus.* A series of 42 patients. *Acta Neurologica Scandinavica*, 46, 573.

Rowan, A.J., Binnie, C.D., Warfield, L.A., & Meijer, J.W.A. (1979) *Epilepsia*, 20, 61.

Ruskin, D.B. (1950) Comparative results in seizure control using phenobarbital, Dilantin and Mesantoin. *American Journal of Psychiatry*, 107, 415.

Sawaya, M.C.B., Horton, R.W. & Meldrum, B.S. (1975) Effects of anticonvulsant drugs on the cerebral enzymes metabolizing GABA. *Epilepsia*, 16, 649.

Sawyer, G.T., Webster, D.D. & Schut, L.J. (1968) Treatment of uncontrolled seizure activity with diazepam. *Journal of the American Medical Association*, 203, 913.

Schmidt, D. & Kupferberg, H.J. (1975) Diphenylhydantoin, phenobarbital and primidone in saliva, plasma and cerebrospinal fluid. *Epilepsia*, 16, 735.

Schmidt, D., Kupferberg, H.J., Yonekawa, W. & Penry, J.K. (1980) The development of tolerance to the anticonvulsant effect of phenobarbital in mice. *Epilepsia*, 21, 141.

Serrano, E.E. & Wilder, B.J. (1974) Intramuscular administration of diphenylhydantoin. Histologic follow-up. *Archives of Neurology* (Chicago) 31, 276.

Sherwin, A.L. (1978) Clinical pharmacology of ethosuximide. In Pippenger, C.E., Penry, J.K., & Kutt, H.P. (eds) *Antiepileptic Drugs: Quantitative Analysis and Interpretation*, p. 283. New York: Raven Press.

Sherwin, A.L., & Robb, J.P. (1972) Ethosuximide. Relation of plasma levels to clinical control. In Woodbury, D.M., Penry, J.K. & Schmidt, R.P. (eds) *Antiepileptic Drugs*, p. 443. New York: Raven Press.

Sherwin, A.L., Robb, J.P. & Lechter, M. (1973) Improved control of epilepsy by monitoring plasma ethosuximide. *Archives of Neurology* (Chicago) 28, 178.

Sherwin, A.L., Harvey, C.D., Leppik, I.E., & Gonda, A. (1976) Correlation between red cell and free plasma phenytoin levels in renal disease. *Neurology* (Minneapolis) 26, 874.

Shorvon, S.D., & Reynolds, E.H. (1979) Reduction of polypharmacy for epilepsy. *British Medical Journal*, 2, 1023.

Shorvon, S.D., Chadwick, D., Galbraith, A.W. & Reynolds, E.H. (1978) One drug for epilepsy. *British Medical Journal*, 1, 474.

Sillanpää, M., Pynnönen, S., Laippala, P. & Säkö, E. (1979) Carbamazepine in the treatment of partial epileptic seizures in infants and young children: a preliminary study. *Epilepsia*, 20, 563.

Simon, D. & Penry, J.K. (1975) Sodium di-n- propylacetate (DPA) in the treatment of epilepsy. A review. *Epilepsia*, 16, 549.

Sjö, O., Hvidberg, E.F., Larsen, N.E., Lund, M. & Naestoft, J. (1975a) Dose dependent kinetics of ethotoin in man. *Clinical and Experimental Pharmacology and Physiology*, 2, 185.

Sjö, Ö., Hvidberg, E.F., Naestoft, J. & Lund, M. (1975b) Pharmacokinetics and side effects of clonazepam and its 7-amino-metabolite in man. *European Journal of Clinical Pharmacology*, 8, 249.

Sjögren, J., Solvell, L. & Karlsson, I. (1965) Studies on the absorption rate of barbiturates in man. *Acta Medica Scandinavica*, 178, 553.

Smith, T.C. & Kinkel, A. (1976) Absorption and metabolism of phenytoin from tablets and capsules. *Clinical Pharmacology and Therapeutics*, 20, 738.

Stensrud, P.A. & Palmer, H. (1964) Serum phenytoin determinations in epileptics. *Epilepsia* (Amsterdam) 5, 364.

Stewart, M.J., Ballinger, B.R., Devlin, E., Miller, A. & Ramsay, A.C. (1975) Bioavailability of phenytoin – a comparison of two preparations. *European Journal of Clinical Pharmacology*, 9, 209.

Strandjord, R.E. & Johannessen, S.I. (1974) One daily dose of diphenylhydantoin for patients with epilepsy. *Epilepsia*, 15, 317.

Strong, J.M., Abe, T., Gibbs, E.L. & Atkinson, A.J. (1974) Plasma levels of methsuximide and N-desmethylmethsuximide during methsuximide therapy. *Neurology* (Minneapolis) 24, 250.

Sunshine, I. (1957) Chemical evidence of tolerance to phenobarbital. *Journal of Laboratory and Clinical Medicine*, 50, 127.

Suzuki, M., Maruyama, H., Ishibashi, Y., Ogawa, S., Seki, T., Hoshino, M., Maekawa, K., Yo, T. & Sato, Y. (1972) A double-blind comparative trial of sodium dipropylacetate and ethosuximide in epilepsy in children, with special emphasis on pure petit mal seizures. *Medical Progress*, (Japan) 82, 470.

Tassinari, C.A., Dravet, C., Roger, J., Cano, J.P. & Gastaut, H. (1972) Tonic *status epilepticus* precipitated by intravenous benzodiazepines in five patients with Lennox-Gastaut syndrome. *Epilepsia*, 13, 421.

Travers, R.D., Reynolds, E.H. & Gallagher, B.B. (1972) Variation in response to anticonvulsants in a group of epileptic patients. *Archives of Neurology* (Chicago) 27, 29.

Triedman, H.M., Fishman, R.A. & Yahr, M.D. (1960) Determination of plasma and cerebrospinal fluid levels of Dilantin in the human. *Transactions of the American Neurological Association*, **85**, 166.

Trimble, M. (1978) Non-monoamine oxidase inhibitor antidepressants and epilepsy: A review. *Epilepsia*, **19**, 241.

Troupin, A.S., Green, J.R. & Levy, R.H. (1974) Carbamazepine as an anticonvulsant: a pilot study. *Neurology* (Minneapolis) **24**, 863.

Troupin, A.S., Ojemann, LM. & Dodrill, C.B. (1976) Mephenytoin: a reappraisal. *Epilepsia*, **17**, 403.

Troupin, A., Ojemann, L.M., Halpern, L., Dodrill, C., Wilkus, R., Friel, P. & Feigl, P. (1977) Carbamazepine – a double-blind comparison with phenytoin. *Neurology* (Minneapolis) **27**, 511.

Tyrer, J.H., Eadie, M.J., Sutherland, J.M. & Hooper, W.D. (1970) Outbreak of anticonvulsant intoxication in an Australian city. *British Medical Journal*, **4**, 271.

Villarreal, H.J., Wilder, B.J., Willmore, L.J., Bauman, A.W., Hammond, E.J., & Bruni, J. (1978) Effect of valproic acid on spike and wave discharges in patients with absence seizures. *Neurology* (Minneapolis) **28**, 886.

Wallace, S.J. & Aldridge Smith, J. (1980) Successful prophylaxis against febrile convulsions with valproic acid or phenobarbitone. *British Medical Journal*, **280**, 353.

Wallis, W., Kutt, H. & McDowell, F. (1968) Intravenous diphenylhydantoin in treatment of acute repetitive seizures. *Neurology* (Minneapolis) **18**, 513.

Weinberg, J. & Goldstein, H.H. (1940) Comparative study of effectiveness of Dilantin sodium and phenobarbital in a group of epileptics. *American Journal of Psychiatry*, **96**, 1029.

White, P.T., Plott, D. & Norton, J. (1966) Relative anticonvulsant potency of primidone. A double blind comparison. *Archives of Neurology* (Chicago) **14**, 31.

Whitty, C.W.M. & Taylor, M. (1949) Treatment of *status epilepticus*. *Lancet*, **2**, 591.

Wilder, B.J. & Ramsey, R.E. (1976) Oral and intramuscular phenytoin. *Clinical Pharmacology and Therapeutics*, **19**, 360.

Wilder, B.J., Serrano, E.E. & Ramsay, E. (1973) Plasma diphenylhydantoin levels after loading and maintenance doses. *Clinical Pharmacology and Therapeutics*, **14**, 797.

Wilder, B.J., Serrano, E.E., Ramsey, E. & R.A. (1974) A method for shifting from oral to intramuscular diphenylhydantoin administration. *Clinical Pharmacology and Therapeutics*, **16**, 507.

Wilder, B.J., Ramsay, E., Willmore, L.J., Feussner, G.F., Perchalski, R.J. & Shumate, J.B. (1977) Efficacy of intravenous phenytoin in the treatment of status epilepticus; kinetics of central nervous system penetration. *Annals of Neurology*, **1**, 511.

Wilensky, A.J. & Lowden, J.A. (1973) Inadequate serum levels after intramuscular administration of diphenylhydantoin. *Neurology* (Minneapolis) **23**, 318.

Wilkus, R.J. & Green, J.R. (1974) Electroencephalographic investigations during evaluation of the antiepileptic agent sulthiame. *Epilepsia*, **15**, 13.

Wilson, J., Walton, J.N. & Newell, D.L. (1959) Beclamide in intractable epilepsy: a controlled trial. *British Medical Journal*, **1**, 1275.

Wilson, J.T., Hojer, B. & Rane, A. (1976) Loading and conventional dose therapy with phenytoin in children; kinetic profile of parent drug and main metabolite in plasma. *Clinical Pharmacology and Therapeutics*, **20**, 48.

Wojcik, J.S. & Lombroso, C.T. (1971) Neonatal seizure states. Electroencephalography and diazepam. *Paediatrics*, **47**, 957.

Wolf, S.M., Carr, A., Davis, D.C., Davidson, S., Dale, E.P., Forsythe, A., Goldenberg, E.D. Hanson, R., Lulejian, G.A., Nelson, M.A., Treitman, P., & Weinstein, A. (1977) The value of phenobarbital in the child who has had a single febrile seizure: a controlled prospective study. *Paediatrics*, **59**, 378.

Yacobi, A., Lampman, J. & Levy, G. (1977) Frequency distribution of free warfarin and free phenytoin fraction values in serum of healthy human adults. *Clinical Pharmacology and Therapeutics*, **21**, 283.

Young, B., Rapp, R., Brooks, W.H., Madauss, W. & Norton J.A. (1979) Post traumatic epilepsy prophylaxis. *Epilepsia*, **20**, 671.

PART TWO
ADVERSE REACTIONS TO ANTIEPILEPTIC DRUGS

M. Dam

In this context adverse reactions to antiepileptic drugs refer to unwanted effects of drugs, often occurring delayed and insidiously. The symptoms and signs are often related to increased serum levels or to the duration of the treatment. Other predisposing factors typical for the individual patient may certainly also contribute, however.

It is only in the last few years that attention has been paid to the more chronic toxic effects of antiepileptic therapy. Many physicians are still unaware of the problems, and symptoms and signs are often ignored or attributed to other causes. Patients may also be unaware of the adverse effects of the drugs, especially if they have been taking them since early life. Often they only become fully aware of the effects of the drugs on various functions when they are withdrawn from therapy.

SUBACUTE OR CHRONIC ENCEPHALOPATHY

Many of the early clinical reports following the

introduction of phenytoin in 1938 suggested a positive psychotropic effect of the drug leading to improved alertness, mood, behaviour and sociability (Trimble & Reynolds, 1976). It seems likely that such effects resulted from a reduction of previously large doses of phenobarbitone and from an improved seizure control. Such changes may be seen even if the patients have been treated for many years with phenobarbitone.

Impaired performance on subtests of WAIS has been correlated to the dose of phenobarbitone in a psychometric study of 20 epileptic patients (Tchicaloff & Gaillard, 1970). The role of phenobarbitone in the precipitation or aggravation of the hyperkinetic syndrome in epileptic children is well known (Ounsted, 1955).

In an acute experiment in healthy volunteers Hutt et al. (1968) found a correlation between serum phenobarbitone concentrations and impairment of perceptuo-motor tasks involving sustained attention.

A 'psychotropic' effect has also been described after treatment with carbamazepine, but may be based on a failure to recognise adverse effects on mental processes caused by the previous treatment with drugs such as phenytoin and primidone. Glaser (1972) has summarised and emphasised a syndrome of subacute or chronic phenytoin encephalopathy which may be overlooked. It is usually associated with high serum levels but can occur with therapeutic levels. It is characterised by an insidious deterioration in intellectual function and behaviour. An increase in seizure frequency may be seen (Lascelles et al., 1970), followed by a change in seizure pattern. There may be a moderate increase in cerebrospinal fluid protein and a mild pleocytosis (Rawson, 1968). Examples of this encephalopathy have been stressed particularly in children, in whom many of the normal adverse effects may not occur. With pre-existing brain damage or mental retardation a deterioration in intellectual function may be overlooked.

Sometimes the encephalopathy may be associated with unusual neurologic signs including involuntary movements. Phenytoin, carbamazepine, primidone and phenobarbitone may cause asterixis, but only phenytoin, carbamazepine and ethosuximide cause orofacial dyskinesias, limb chorea and dystonia (Kirschberg, 1975; Chadwick, Reynolds & Marsden, 1976; Jacome, 1979).

These symptoms may be seen in patients with idiopathic epilepsy (Chadhub & DeVivo, 1976), but generally the frequency of organic cerebral damage seems to be high among these patients (Lühdorf & Lund, 1977). The clinical symptoms are reversible. They may be related to dopamine antagonist properties possessed by phenytoin (Chadwick et al., 1976).

Many factors contribute to the development of encephalopathy in epilepsy, including duration of seizures and seizure frequency, the underlying brain lesion, psychological and social factors. However, it is true, as stated by Reynolds (1975), that the contribution of prolonged drug therapy to mental symptoms has been much underrated in the past.

CEREBELLUM

Cerebellar dysfunction with ataxia and nystagmus is a well-known manifestation of acute phenytoin toxicity. The symptoms generally disappear when the dose is lowered or the drug withdrawn, and they are clearly related to the serum level of phenytoin (Kutt et al., 1964).

Several cases of poisoning with excessive doses of phenytoin without permanent sequelae have been reported (Robinson, 1940; Aring & Rosenbaum, 1941; Cattan, Frumusan & Attal, 1947; Nauth-Misir, 1948; Price & Frank, 1950; Putnam & Rothenberg, 1953; Floyd, 1961).

Clinical reports of permanent ataxia following large doses of phenytoin or prolonged treatment with this drug appear now and then in neurological journals (Livingston, 1954; Livingston, 1957; Utterback, 1958; Utterback, Ojeman & Malek, 1958; Hofmann, 1958; Roger & Soulayrol, 1959; Viukari, 1962; Haberland, 1962; Kokenge, Kutt & McDowell, 1965; Höglmeier & Wenzel, 1969; Selhorst, Kaufman & Horwitz, 1972; Ghatak, Santoso & McKinney, 1976).

Experimentally, cerebellar changes have been reported after administration of phenytoin to animals (Utterback, 1958; Utterback et al., 1958; Kokenge et al., 1965; Dam, 1966; Snider & Del Cerro, 1966; Snider & Del Cerro, 1967; Alcala et al., 1978). These findings seem, however, to be the result of fixation artifacts, as many of the experimental animals were not fixated by perfusion fixation. In other studies the changes were hypoxic, as many of the animals were comatose with uncontrolled respiration. Finally the failure to use quantitative methods of Purkinje cell counting may have given the impression of a cell loss, although such a loss could not be substantiated, when using a quantitative method (Dam, 1970a; 1970b; Dam & Nielsen, 1970; Puro & Woodward, 1973).

Alcala et al. (1978) found ultrastructural changes in rats treated with phenytoin, although the serum levels were well below what is suggested to be the 'therapeutic' level in man. Nielsen, Dam and Klinken (1971) were unable to find any changes in the substructure of the Purkinje cells, even though the animals had been treated with toxic but sublethal doses of phenytoin.

In man, epileptic seizures can lead to pathological changes in cerebellum with loss of Purkinje cells, as reported before the introduction of phenytoin in the treatment of epilepsy (Dam, 1972). There is no convincing pathological evidence of cerebellar changes in man attributable to phenytoin. The significant reduction in Purkinje cell count of epileptic patients treated with high doses of phenytoin is the result of frequent seizures, as most of these patients are severely epileptic.

It can thus still be concluded that there is no real loss of Purkinje cells in animals and that it is due to the seizures rather than to phenytoin in patients. The current theory tends to emphasise intrinsic metabolic requirements as the basic explanation for the phenomenon of susceptible nerve cells. The abnormal firing creates a complex critical metabolic demand which the compensatory increase in blood flow cannot always meet (Salcman et al., 1978).

PERIPHERAL NEUROPATHY

Peripheral neuropathy, demonstrated clinically and by electrophysiological studies, has been ascribed to the treatment with phenytoin. The patients seldom complain of symptoms, but significant correlation is found between arreflexia and the development of neuropathy (Lovelace & Horwitz, 1968). The symptoms and signs are related to the duration and dosage of the antiepileptic therapy (Meienberg & Bajc, 1975). A relation between the neuropathy and subnormal serum-folate concentrations has not been demonstrated, and therapy with folic acid does not result in measurable improvement of the condition (Horwitz, Klipstein & Lovelace, 1967).

There is no convincing evidence to show that any of the other commonly used antiepileptic drugs cause peripheral nerve damage (Argov & Mastaglia, 1979).

THE LIVER

Many drugs with different biochemical and biological properties enlarge the liver and cause enzyme induction when used in non-toxic doses for a longer time, e.g. phenobarbitone, phenytoin and methoin (Kunz et al., 1966; Dam, Møller & Petersen, 1969). The inducing effect of phenytoin and phenobarbitone may explain the raised alkaline phosphatases, serum alanine aminotransferase and plasma prothrombin time, which are often observed in patients treated with these drugs (Andreasen, Lyngbye and Trolle, 1973). The dose seems to be important in determining the degree of induction, but a wide variation between patients seems to exist with respect to their response. The consequences of continued therapy with the mentioned antiepileptic drugs are therefore a state of chronically induced hepatic enzymes. The result may be an altered metabolic activity of a wide spectrum of both endogenous and exogenous substances (Richens and Woodford, 1976; Breckenridge and Robert, 1976).

However, liver biopsies from patients treated with antiepileptic drugs for 10–35 years have so far failed to reveal any signs of permanent liver damage (Jacobsen et al., 1976). Enlargement of the liver seems to be related to the enhancement of drug metabolism in patients treated with phenytoin and phenobarbitone (Pirttiaho et al., 1978).

Hepatitis is a rare complication of phenytoin treatment. The clinical course may be one of prompt resolution or fatal hepatic necrosis (38 per cent), even after discontinuing the drug. Occasionally, symptoms recur after apparent recovery. The histologic picture of hepatitis, with or without cholestasis but with eosinophilia, suggests the diagnosis. Most patients are adolescents or young adults, with equal sex distribution. Most often hepatotoxicity develops within one to three weeks of first phenytoin exposure, without apparent relation to dosage or serum level. A rash seems always to be present together with fever. Lymphadenopathy (75 per cent), hepatomegaly (65 per cent), clinical jaundice (55 per cent) and splenomegaly (35 per cent) are common. Haemorrhagic tendencies, ranging from significantly prolonged clotting times to haemorrhage, occur in 40 per cent. The pathogenesis of phenytoin-induced hepatotoxicity remains unexplained, but the eosinophilia, rash, lymphadenopathy, fever and exfoliative dermatitis suggest a hypersensitivity reaction (Parker & Shearer, 1979).

The incidence of hepatotoxicity induced by sodium valproate seems to be greater than previously reported. In a retrospective analysis of 42 patients treated with sodium valproate, 27 had fibrinogen levels less than normal. The decrease was related to valproic acid level. Other abnormal laboratory values were hypoalbuminaemia (33 per cent), raised serum glutamic oxaloacetic transaminase (30 per cent), prolonged partial thromboplastin time (18 per cent) and prolonged prothrombin time (16 per cent) (Sussman, McLain & Leppik, 1979).

There have been undocumented reports of cases of severe hepatotoxicity in patients treated with sodium valproate (Donat et al., 1979). Most patients had received multiple antiepileptic drugs in addition to sodium valproate. Most of them died in hepatic failure.

Suchy et al. (1979) added two cases studied in detail. A five year old boy was treated with sodium valproate (650 mg daily) giving a level of 1170 μmol/(168 μg/ml). On this level he became weak, lethargic and anorexic with slight facial puffiness. In the week before admission, peripheral oedema, abdominal distension and scleral icterus developed. Although sodium valproate, which was the only drug given, as discontinued, he died. In the second patient, an 11½ year old boy, weakness of the legs, ataxia and lethargy developed six weeks after start of treatment with sodium valproate. He was in addition treated with phenytoin, primidone and clonazepam. He became comatose and died.

In both patients, onset of liver dysfunction was subtle and heralded by a change in mental state and increased seizures. Both developed profound jaundice, moderate aminotransferase elevation and severe coagulation defect. The pathological lesions were in both cases interpreted as mixed toxic/cholestatic hepatitis with diffuse hepatocellular injury, terminating in centrilobular microvesicular fatty change and widespread necrosis. There were features of hepatitis due to virus or drug sensitivity and features of direct hepatotoxic damage.

Clinical and experimental investigations are needed to define the role of sodium valproate in the induction of liver disease. Monitoring of hepatic function is recommended during sodium valproate treatment. On recognition of liver disease the drug should be discontinued.

NEONATAL COAGULATION DEFECTS

Infants born to mothers taking either a hydantoin or a barbiturate derivative or both may show clinical signs of bleeding and diminished levels of coagulation factors. These defects usually become apparent within the first 24 hours of life (Solomon, Hilgartner & Kutt, 1972). This syndrome differs from the more 'physiological' haemorrhagic disorder of the newborn in which the bleeding begins two or three days after birth. This effect of antiepileptic drugs is possibly a consequence of liver enzyme induction accelerating the catabolism of coagulation factors. It has, however, also been suggested that the drugs may be competitive inhibitors of vitamin K.

Vitamin K prevents this coagulation defect, and it has been recommended that epileptic mothers receive vitamin K tablets throughout the month before delivery and intravenously during labour (Mountain, Hirsh & Gallus, 1970). It is also recommended to administer phytomenadione intravenously to the infant immediately after birth. If diminished vitamin K–dependent factors are found in cord blood specimens, fresh frozen plasma should be given at a dose of 20 ml/kg over a one to two hour period (Bleyer & Skinner, 1976).

FOLIC ACID DEFICIENCY

Phenytoin and to a lesser extent phenobarbitone and primidone all influence folate metabolism in man. Four hypotheses are under investigation:

1. Induction of enzymes involved in folate metabolism.
2. Malabsorption of folic acid.
3. Competitive interaction between folate co-enzymes and the drugs.
4. Increased demand for folic acid as a co-enzyme either for antiepileptic drug hydroxylation or for other hepatic enzymes induced by the drugs (Reynolds, 1976).

A wide variety of tissues may be affected by folate deficiency, so that a number of clinical lesions may occur. Folate is required in three reactions in DNA-synthesis, one in pyrimidine synthesis and two in purine synthesis (Hoffbrand, 1977).

Macrocytosis may sometimes be related to folate deficiency, but the real megaloblastic anaemia is uncommon during antiepileptic treatment. Rose and Johnson (1978) found only one subject with a macrocytic blood-picture out of 96 patients treated with antiepileptic drugs. Serum-folate measured by two assay methods was subnormal in 83 per cent of the samples, red-cell folate in 40 per cent. They submit that the megaloblastic anaemia sometimes seen in subjects receiving long-term antiepileptic drug therapy is not caused by the drugs, but simply reflects inadequate nutrition.

It has been postulated that a relationship exists between the antifolate and the antiepileptic effects of phenytoin, phenobarbitone and primidone, and it was shown that 50 per cent of folate-deficient epileptic patients treated with folic acid had an increased seizure frequency as folate values returned to normal (Reynolds, 1967).

Similarly a relationship has been suggested between a high incidence of neuropsychiatric illness in patients with antiepileptic treatment and folic acid deficiency (Reynolds et al., 1972). However, it has not been possible in controlled trials to show any effect of folate administration on seizure activity in folate deficiency states. The same conclusion has been reached concerning the effect on personality, even when careful psychometric evaluations were used (Norris & Pratt, 1974).

The suggestion that methyltetrahydrofolate in the brain may be involved in the methylation of catecholamines and indolamines has not been confirmed as a physiological pathway. As yet, no special important role for folate in the central nervous system has been proven (Hoffbrand, 1977).

BONE DISEASE AND VITAMIN D DEFICIENCY

During the last decade reports of biochemical or radiographic features of rickets have drawn attention to the possible adverse effects of antiepileptic drugs on bone metabolism. Antiepileptic drugs seem to derange bone metabolism, both through induction of hepatic catabolism of vitamin D and its biologically active products, as well as by direct effect on membrane cation transport systems (Hahn, 1976). It has recently been suggested that the bone disease resulting from phenytoin therapy may be associated with a deficiency of 25-hydroxycholecalciferol and not of 1-25-dihydroxycholecalciferol, and that reduced gastrointestinal absorption of calcium or changes in parathyroid function may not be necessary for the development of the bone disease (Bell et al., 1978).

Anticonvulsant osteomalacia may be a specific bone disease, different from that of vitamin D deficiency, but induced by abnormalities in vitamin D metabolism or in effects of vitamin D metabolites on receptor cells (Mosekilde et al., 1977).

The significant clinical manifestations include rickets, increased risk of pathological fracture and reduction in serum calcium levels which may, rarely, predispose to increased seizure frequency (Hahn, 1976). Prolonged hypocalcaemia with tetany may be seen in infants born at term, whose mothers have been treated with phenytoin or phenobarbitone (Friis & Sardemann, 1977).

Several factors appear to determine the severity of the clinical manifestations: drug dose, duration of therapy, vitamin D intake, amount of sunlight exposure, degree of physical activity and presence of other concurrent diseases (Hahn, 1976; Mosekilde & Melsen, 1976).

The pathological alterations develop in the

course of a few months and then remain constant (Christiansen, 1976). Overt bone disease from antiepileptic drugs alone is very uncommon (Christiansen & Rødbro, 1977). When diagnosed it requires treatment. The optimal initial dose is 4000 IU of vitamin D2 a day for about four months. The optimal maintenance dose is 1000 IU vitamin D2 a day (Christiansen & Rødbro, 1974). Whether or not subclinical bone disease should be treated is less certain. The present available data are more in favour of withholding prophylactic treatment than giving it (Christiansen & Rødbro, 1977). Any prophylactic programme which leads to the prescribing of relatively large doses of vitamin D needs to be viewed with circumspection and must be based firmly on clinical and not simply bio-chemical benefit (Editorial, 1976).

DUPUYTREN'S CONTRACTURE

There is a strong suspicion that chronic antiepileptic drug therapy may contribute to the development of Dupuytren's contracture. 50 per cent of 190 male patients with epilepsy and 32 per cent of 171 female patients suffered from this disease, according to Lund (1941). The frequency increased with increasing age. Lund considered that phenobarbitone was a possible causative factor. A similar high prevalence has been confirmed in later investigations (Pojer, Radwojevic & Williams, 1972; Critchley et al., 1976). The incidence increased with the duration of epilepsy and contractures were seen equally in those with idiopathic or symptomatic epilepsy. It is suggested that the disease is a sequel to long-term administration of phenobarbitone (Critchley et al., 1976).

IMMUNOLOGICAL DISORDERS

Low IgA levels were found in 25 per cent of sera from 100 adult patients treated for epilepsy for at least six months (Aarli & Tönder, 1975). In untreated epileptic patients IgA values were normal, but they fell during treatment with phenytoin. It has been suggested that epilepsy with constitutional characteristics might predispose to low IgA which only occurs when hydantoins are given

(Fontana et al., 1976). In patients with epilepsy thought to be secondary to traumatic or infectious events, IgA was normal whether or not the patients were treated with hydantoins. Others have not been able to confirm these findings (Aarli, 1976a). Evidence of depressed T cell function was found in patients with low serum IgA levels treated with phenytoin. There was no correlation with the dose or the serum level. A correlation was found, however, with HL-A status, patients with low IgA showing increased frequency of HL-A2. It has been suggested that epileptic patients with HL-A2 status are likely to develop IgA deficiency when given phenytoin (Shakir et al., 1978). Imbalance of the IgG subclasses was often observed with IgG4 being undetectable in 65 per cent of epileptic patients with constitutional factors for seizures and low IgA (Fontana et al., 1978).

Phenytoin-induced deficiency of salivary IgA can result in increased susceptibility to gingival inflammation, which is considered one of the predisposing factors for subsequent development of gingival hyperplasia (Aarli, 1976b). Insufficient mouth hygiene seems to be another factor (Kristensen, 1977).

The changed immunological response in patients treated with phenytoin may be of importance for the development of cancer. Pseudolymphoma has been known for a long time with the characteristic symptoms, fever, rash, and lymphadenopathy. This syndrome has been judged to lack the sinister prognosis of other lymphomas, provided the condition is recognised and the drug withdrawn. Some reports, however, have described the occurrence of true lymphoma in epileptic patients who had received hydantoins for a long time (Editorial, 1971). A study of the survival-time and occurrence of neoplasms of 9136 patients treated with antiepileptic drugs checked against national death files, however, failed to disclose any evidence of an oncogenic effect (Clemmesen, Fuglsang-Frederiksen & Plum, 1974). A more recent study, however, has shown an increased mortality in epileptic patients, some of the excess being accounted for by malignant disease (White, McLean & Howland, 1979). Apart from the brain and central nervous system, no particular site had a significant excess of tumours.

It is known that the administration of sodium valproate in daily doses of 1200 to 3000 mg may be associated with a reduction of the platelet count. Thrombocytopenia without concomitant bleeding abnormalities is uncommon. Platelet counts normally return to baseline levels after withdrawal of the drug (Neophytides, Nutt & Lodish, 1979). Thrombocytopenic purpura may be seen after large doses, with rapid recovery after the discontinuance of the drug (Boutillier et al., 1979). An autoimmune response limited to an IgM antibody occurred in a six year old child treated with sodium valproate 2000 mg daily. The platelet count rose rapidly after halving the dose. It was suggested that sodium valproate was responsible and that, in excess, the drug binds to a macromolecule, producing an immunogenic structure. The antibody is directed against platelets because of their membrane fatty acids, which are chemically and configurationally similar to sodium valproate (Sandler et al., 1978).

THE ENDOCRINE SYSTEM

It has long been known that phenobarbitone and phenytoin accelerate the metabolism of cortisol through enzyme induction in the liver (Burstein and Klaiber, 1965; Werk, McGee & Sholiton, 1964). The increased metabolism of administered corticosteroids is of clinical importance in epileptic recipients of cadaver renal allografts. A decreased allograft survival has been observed in these patients possibly caused by an ineffective immunosuppression (Wassner et al., 1976). After two weeks' treatment with phenytoin or carbemazepine in previously untreated epileptic men, free urinary cortisol excretion increased and urinary 17 ketogenic steroid excretion decreased significantly (Bennet, 1977). Serum testosterone increased slightly and androsterone and etiocholanolone urinary excretion decreased. No difference between the effect of the two drugs was disclosed.

Sex hormone binding globulin was increased in both sexes as was testosterone level in male patients on chronic antiepileptic therapy. It seems, however, improbable that the observed changes by themselves would alter sexual function sig-nificantly (Barragry et al., 1978). Impairment of potency and infertility in patients with epilepsy have been ascribed to the treatment with antiepileptic drugs. A specific action of the antiepileptic drugs on the germinative tissue should be taken into consideration (Christiansen & Lund, 1976).

There is evidence from animal experiments that oestrogens and androgens are metabolised more rapidly when phenobarbitone and phenytoin are administered chronically (Kuntzman, 1969). It has similarly been suggested that patients under antiepileptic medication became pregnant despite regular intake of oral contraceptives (Janz & Schmidt, 1974).

Phenytoin in therapeutic doses displaces thyroxine and, to a lesser extent, triiodothyronine from binding proteins in serum and thus increases peripheral clearance of the hormones (Finucane & Griffiths, 1976).

Hyponatraemia and low plasma osmolality may occur in patients receiving carbamazepine (Rado, 1973; Ashton et al., 1977; Stephens et al., 1977 Perucca et al., 1978). Water intoxication as a side-effect of carbamazepine may occur more often than has been recognised. Some of the common side-effects of carbamazepine are similar to the clinical features of water intoxication. Dizziness, headaches, nausea, and mental confusion may occur with both. It has been suggested that the drug acts by stimulating the release of antidiuretic hormone from the posterior pituitary (Ashton et al., 1977). Perucca et al. (1978) found that hyponatraemia was more frequent in the patients on monotherapy and that plasma sodium and serum carbamazepine correlated more strongly in these patients. Subsequently, these authors have shown that the lower incidence of hyponatraemia in patients on additional phenytoin therapy is due to a pharmacokinetic drug interaction, the serum carbamazepine levels being much lower than in patients on monotherapy (Perucca & Richens, 1980). Twelve subjects given therapeutic doses of carbamazepine showed no change in their plasma electrolyte concentrations (Ashton et al., 1977). Ten had abnormal water metabolism. Plasma arginine vasopressin concentrations fell while the subjects were taking the drug, indicating that the mechanism is unlikely to be increased secretion of antidiuretic hormone. It was suggested that the water-retaining property of carbamazepine is a physiological effect of the drug, mediated by increased renal sensitivity to normal plasma concentrations of plasma arginine vasopressin and resetting of osmoreceptors (Stephens, Coe & Baylis, 1978).

TERATOGENICITY

Since 1964 antiepileptic drugs have been suspected of teratogenic effect. An abnormally high incidence of cleft palate is observed in fetuses of mice treated with phenytoin. Carbamazepine is thought to be equal to phenobarbitone and primidone in producing a lower incidence of defects than phenytoin. Clonazepam and ethosuximide are found to be the least teratogenic antiepileptic drugs in mice (Sullivan & McElhatton, 1976, McElhatton & Sullivan, 1977).

The babies of epileptic mothers have a higher frequency of congenital malformations, a lower birth weight and a higher perinatal mortality rate (Bjerkedal & Bahna, 1973). The incidence of malformations varies between 4 per cent and 15 per cent with an average incidence recorded in nine major surveys of 7 per cent. The increased malformation rate has been related to treatment with antiepileptic drugs during pregnancy. The majority of malformations, facial clefts and heart defects, has occurred in association with the use of phenytoin, phenobarbitone and primidone (Speidel & Meadow, 1972).

It has been suggested that epilepsy *per se* might be a factor in the production of malformations (Shapiro *et al.*, 1976). The same conclusion was reached in a study of 391 live-born infants with facial clefts admitted to treatment. Seven fathers and 11 mothers with epilepsy were identified which gives a prevalence of epilepsy among the parent three times the expected value. Only two of the fathers were treated with antiepileptic drugs suspected of teratogenicity (Friis, 1979). An alternative explanation of the defects, however, may be that damage has been caused by maternal convulsions during embryogenesis. This possibility has not been studied.

It is evident that further prospective investigations are required to resolve these issues.

CONCLUSION

The study of chronic toxicity of antiepileptic drugs is of tremendous importance. The literature of the various aspects of adverse drug reactions is growing rapidly, perhaps a little too often with uncritical enthusiasm for scattered case reports. Clinical impressions have led to hypotheses, which have been published and repeated so often that they now seem to be the truth – although proofs are lacking. What we need are controlled prospective investigations employing quantitative analyses if possible with rating scales of the side-effects, and psychological tests. Through a recording system of all chronic side-effects and their consequences we should be able to select the antiepileptic drug with the smallest risk of adverse reactions to the patients or their offspring.

REFERENCES

Aarli, J.A. (1976a) Drug-induced IgA deficiency in epileptic patients. *Archives of Neurology* (Chicago), **33**, 296.

Aarli, J.A. (1976b) Phenytoin-induced depression of salivary IgA and gingival hyperplasia. *Epilepsia*, **17**, 283.

Aarli, J.A. & Tönder, O. (1975) Effects of antiepileptic drugs on serum and salivary IgA. *Scandinavian Journal of Immunology*, **4**, 391.

Alcala, H., Lertratanangkoon, K., Stenbach, W., Kellaway, P. & Horning, M.G. (1978) The Purkinje cell in phenytoin intoxication; ultrastructural and Golgi studies. *Pharmacologists*, **20**, 240.

Andreasen, P.B., Lyngbye, J. & Trolle, E. (1973) Abnormalities in liver function tests during long-term diphenylhydantoin therapy in epileptic out-patients. *Acta Medica Scandinavica*, **194**, 261.

Argov, Z. & Mastaglia, F.L. (1979) Drug-induced peripheral neuropathies. *British Medical Journal*, **1**, 663.

Aring, C,D. & Rosenbaum, M. (1941) Ingestion of large doses of dilantin sodium. *Archives of Neurology and Psychiatry*, **45**, 265.

Ashton, M.G., Ball, S.G., Thomas, T.H. & Lee, M.R. (1977) Water intoxication associated with carbamazepine treatment. *British Medical Journal*, **1**, 1134.

Barragry, J.M., Makin, H.L.J., Trafford, D.J.H. & Scott, D.F. (1978) Effect of anticonvulsants on plasma testosterone and sex hormone binding globulin levels. *Journal of Neurology, Neurosurgery and Psychiatry*, **41**, 913.

Bell, R.D., Pak, C.Y.C., Zerwekh, J., Barilla, D.E. & Vasko, M. (1978) Effect of phenytoin on bone and vitamin D metabolism. *Annals of Neurology*, **5**, 374.

Bennet, E.P. (1977) Influence of phenytoin and carbamazepine on endocrine function. *Epilepsia*, **18**, 294.

Bjerkedal, T. & Bahna, S.L. (1973) The course and outcome of pregnancy in women with epilepsy. *Acta Obstetrica et Gynecologica Scandinavica*, **52**, 245.

Bleyer, W.A. & Skinner, A.L. (1976) Fatal neonatal hemorrhage after maternal anticonvulsant therapy. *Journal of American Medical Association*, **235**, 626.

Boutillier, L., De Lumley, L., Saura, R. & Boulesteix, J. (1979) Aplasie médullaire transitoire au cours d'un traitement par le dipropylacétate de sodium. *La Nouvelle Presse Médicale*, **8**, 611.

Breckenridge, A.M. & Robert, J.B. (1976) Clinical significance of microsomal enzyme induction. *Pharmacological Research Communication*, **8**, 229.

Burstein, S. & Klaiber, L. (1965) Phenobarbital-induced increase in 6-hydroxycortisol excertion: clue to its significance in human urine. *Journal of Clinical Endocrinology and Metabolism*, **25**, 293.

Cattan, R., Frumusan, P. & Attal, P. (1947) Intoxication aiguë par la diphénylhydantoïne. *Bulletin de Societé Médicine*, **63**, 346.

Chadhub, E.G. & DeVivo, D.C. (1976) Phenytoin-induced choreoathetosis. *The Journal of Pediatrics*, **89**, 153.

Chadwick, D., Reynolds, E.H. & Marsden, C.D. (1976) Anticonvulsant-induced dyskinesias: a comparison with dyskinesias induced by neuroleptics. *Journal of Neurology, Neurosurgery and Psychiatry*, **39**, 1210.

Christiansen, C. (1976) *Knoglemineralindhold hos epilepsipatienter i antikonvulsiv behandling*. Copenhagen: Dansk Undervisningsforlag.

Christiansen, C. & Rødbro, P. (1974) Initial and maintenance doses of vitamin D-2 in the treatment of anticonvulsant osteomalacia. *Acta Neurologica Scandinavica*, **50**, 631.

Christiansen, C. & Rødbro, P. (1977) Anticonvulsant osteomalacia. *British Medical Journal*, **1**, 439.

Christiansen, P. & Lund, M. (1976) In Janz, D. (ed.) *Epileptology*, p. 190. Stuttgart: Georg Thieme.

Clemmesen, J., Fuglsang-Frederiksen, V. & Plum, C.M. (1974) Are anticonvulsants oncogenic? *Lancet*, **1**, 705.

Critchley, E.M.R., Vakil, S.D., Hayward, H.W. & Owen, V.M.H. (1976) Dupuytren's disease in epilepsy: result of prolonged administration of anticonvulsants. *Journal of Neurology, Neurosurgery and Psychiatry*, **39**, 498.

Dam, M. (1966) Organic changes in phenytoin-intoxicated pigs. *Acta Neurologica Scandinavica*, **42**, 491.

Dam, M. (1970a) Number of Purkinje's cells after diphenylhydantoin intoxication in pigs. *Archives of Neurology* Chicago, **22**, 64.

Dam, M. (1970b) The number of Purkinje cells after diphenylhydantoin intoxication in monkeys. *Epilepsia*, **11**, 199.

Dam, M. (1972) The density and ultrastructure of the Purkinje cells following diphenylhydantoin treatment in animals and man. *Acta Neurologica Scandinavica*, suppl. **48**, pp 65.

Dam, M. & Nielsen, M. (1970) Purkinje's cell density after diphenylhydantoin intoxication in rats. *Archives of Neurology* (Chicago), **23**, 555.

Dam, M., Møller, J.E. & Petersen, P. (1969) The effect of diphenylhydantoin and phenobarbital on the liver of the pig. *Epilepsia*, **10**, 507.

Donat, J.F., Bocchini, J.A.Jr., Gonzalez, E. & al. (1979) Valproic acid and fatal hepatitis. *Neurology* (Minneapolis) **29**, 273.

Editorial. (1971) Is phenytoin carcinogenic? *Lancet*, **2**, 1071.

Editorial. (1976) Anticonvulsant osteomalacia. *British Medical Journal*, **2**, 1340.

Finucane, J.F. & Griffiths, R.S. (1976) Effect of phenytoin therapy on thyroid function. *British Journal of Clinical Pharmacology*, **3**, 1041.

Floyd, F.W. (1961) The toxic effects of diphenylhydantoin: A report of 23 cases. *Clinical Proceedings of Childrens Hospital*, **17**, 195.

Fontana, A., Joller, H., Skvaril, F. & Grob, P. (1978) Immunological abnormalities and HLA antigen frequencies in IgA deficient patients with epilepsy. *Journal of Neurology, Neurosurgery and Psychiatry*, **41**, 593.

Fontana, A., Sauter, R., Grob, P.J. & Joller, H. (1976) IgA deficiency, epilepsy and hydantoin medication. *Lancet*, **2**, 228.

Friis, B. & Sardemann, H. (1977) Neonatal hypocalcaemia after intrauterine exposure to anticonvulsant drugs. *Archives of Disease in Childhood*, **52**, 239.

Friis, M.L. (1979) Epilepsy among parents of children with facial clefts. *Epilepsia*, **20**, 69.

Ghatak, N.R., Santoso, R.A. & McKinney, W.M. (1976) Cerebellar degeneration following long-term phenytoin therapy. *Neurology*, (Minneapolis) **26**, 818.

Glaser, G.H. (1972) In Woodbury, D.M., Penry, J.K. & Schmidt, R.P. (eds) *Antiepileptic Drugs*, p. 219. New York: Raven Press.

Haberland, C. (1962) Cerebellar degeneration with clinical manifestation in chronic epileptic patients. *Psychiatria et Neurologia*, **143**, 29.

Hahn, T.J. (1976) Bone complications of anticonvulsants. *Drugs*, **12**, 201.

Hoffbrand, A.V. (1977) Pathology of folate deficiency. *Proceedings of the Royal Society of Medicine*, **70**, 82.

Hofmann, W.W. (1958) Cerebellar lesions after parenteral Dilantin administration. *Neurology* (Minneapolis) **8**, 210.

Horwitz, S.J., Klipstein, F.A. & Lovelace, R.E. (1967) Folic acid and neuropathy in epilepsy. *Lancet*, **2**, 1305.

Hutt, S.J., Jackson, P.M., Belsham, A.B. & Higgins, G. (1968) Perceptual-motor behaviour in relation to blood phenobarbitone level. *Developmental Medicine and Child Neurology*, **10**, 626.

Höglmeier, H. & Wenzel, U. (1969) Zerebellarer Dauerschaden durch vorübergehende Hydantoin-überdosierung. *Deutsche Medizinische Wochenschrift*, **94**, 1330.

Jacobsen, N.O., Mosekilde, L., Myhre-Jensen, O., Pedersen, E. & Wildenhoff, K.E. (1976) Liver biopsies in epileptics during anticonvulsant therapy. Acta Medica Scandinavica, **199**, 345.

Jacome, D. (1979) Carbamazepine-induced dystonia. *Journal of American Medical Association*, **241**, 2263.

Janz, D. & Schmidt, D. (1974) Anti-epileptic drugs and failure of oral contraceptives. *Lancet*, **1**, 1113.

Kirschberg, G.J. (1975) Dyskinesia – An unusual reaction to ethosuximide. *Archives of Neurology* (Chicago), **32**, 137.

Kokenge, R., Kutt, H. & McDowell, F. (1965) Neurological sequelae following dilantin overdose in a patient and in experimental animals. *Neurology* (Minneapolis) **15**, 823.

Kristensen, C.B. (1977) One-sided gingival hyperplasia after treatment with diphenylhydantoin. *Acta Neurologica Scandinavica*, **56**, 353.

Kuntzman, R. (1969) Drugs and enzyme induction. *Annual Review of Pharmacology*, **9**, 21.

Kunz, W., Schaude, G., Schmid, W. & Siess, M. (1966) Lebervergrösserung durch Fremdstoffe.

Naunyn-Schmiedebergs Archiv für Pharmakologie und experimentelle Pathologie, **254**, 470.

Kutt, H., Winters, W., Kokenge, R. & McDowell, F. (1964) Diphenylhydantoin metabolism, blood levels, and toxicity. *Archives of Neurology* (Chicago), **11**, 642.

Lascelles, P.T., Kocen, R.S. & Reynolds, E.H. (1970) The distribution of plasma phenytoin levels in epileptic patients. *Journal of Neurology, Neurosurgery and Psychiatry*, **33**, 501.

Livingston, S. (1954) *The diagnosis and treatment of convulsive disorders in children*. Springfield: Thomas.

Livingston, S. (1957) Drug therapy for childhood epilepsy. *Journal of Chronic Diseases*, **6**, 46.

Lovelace, R.E. & Horwitz, S.J. (1968) Peripheral neuropathy in long-term diphenylhydantoin therapy. *Archives of Neurology* (Chicago), **18**, 69.

Lund, M. (1941) Dupuytren's contracture and epilepsy. *Acta Psychiatrica et Neurologica Scandinavica*, **16**, 465.

Lühdorf, K. & Lund, M. (1977) Phenytoin-induced hyperkinesia. *Epilepsia*, **18**, 294.

McElhatton, P.R. & Sullivan, F.M. (1977) Comparative teratogenicity of six antiepileptic drugs in the mouse. *British Journal of Pharmacology*, **59**, 494.

Meienberg, O. & Bajc, O. (1975) Acute polyneuropathy caused by diphenylhydantoin intoxication. *Deutsche Medizinische Wochenschrift*, **100**, 1532.

Mosekilde, L. & Melsen, F. (1976) Anticonvulsant osteomalacia determined by quantitative analysis of bone changes. *Acta Medica Scandinavica*, **199**, 349.

Mosekilde, L., Melsen, F., Christensen, M.S., Lund, B. & Sørensen, O.H. (1977) Effect of long-term vitamin D2 treatment on bone morphometry and biochemical values in anticonvulsant osteomalacia. *Acta Medica Scandinavica*, **201**, 303.

Mountain, K.R., Hirsch, J. & Gallus, A.S. (1970) Neonatal coagulation defect due to anticonvulsant drug treatment in pregnancy. *Lancet*, **1**, 265.

Nauth-Misir, T.N. (1948) A case of gross overdosage of soluble phenytoin. *British Medical Journal*, **2**, 646.

Neophytides, A.N., Nutt, J.G. & Lodish, J.R. (1979) Thrombocytopenia associated with sodium valproate treatment. *Annals of Neurology*, **5**, 389.

Nielsen, M.H., Dam, M. & Klinken, L. (1971) The ultrastructure of Purkinje cells in diphenylhydantoin intoxicated rats.

Norris, J.W. & Pratt, R.F. (1974) Folic acid deficiency and epilepsy. *Drugs*, **8**, 366.

Ounsted, C. (1955) The hyperkinetic syndrome in epileptic children. *Lancet*, **2**, 303.

Parker, W.A. & Shearer, C.A. (1979) Phenytoin hepatotoxicity: A case report and review. *Neurology*, (Minneapolis) **29**, 175.

Perucca, E., Garratt, A., Hebdige, S. & Richens, A. (1978) Water intoxication in epileptic patients receiving carbamazepine. *Journal of Neurology, Neurosurgery and Psychiatry*, **41**, 713.

Perucca, E. & Richens, A. (1980) Reversal by phenytoin of carbamazepine-induced water intoxication; a pharmacokinetic interaction. *Journal of Neurology Neurosurgery and Psychiatry*, **43**, 540.

Pirttiaho, H.I., Sotaniemi, E.A., Ahokas, J.T. & Pitkänen, U. (1978) Liver size and indices of drug metabolism in epileptics. *British Journal of Clinical Pharmacology*, **6**, 273.

Pojer, J., Radwojevic, M. & Williams, J.F. (1972) Dupuytren's disease. Its association with abnormal liver function in alcoholism and epilepsy. *Archives of Internal Medicine*, **129**, 561.

Price, W.C. & Frank, M.E. (1950) Accidental acute dilantin poisoning. *Journal of Pediatrics*, **36**, 652.

Puro, D.G. & Woodward, D.J. (1973) Effects of diphenylhydantoin on activity of rat cerebellar Purkinje cells. *Neuropharmacology*, **12**, 433.

Putnam, T.J. & Rothenberg, S.F. (1953) Results of intensive (narcosis) and standard medical treatment of epilepsy. *Journal of American Medical Association*, **152**, 1400.

Rado, J.P. (1973) Water intoxication during carbamazepine treatment. *British Medical Journal*, **3**, 479.

Rawson, M.D. (1968) Diphenylhydantoin intoxication and cerebrospinal fluid protein. *Neurology* (Minneapolis) **18**, 1009.

Reynolds, E.H. (1967) Effects of folic acid on the mental state, and fit frequency of drug treated epileptic patients. *Lancet*, **1**, 1086.

Reynolds, E.H. (1975) Chronic antiepileptic toxicity: a review. *Epilepsia*, **16**, 319.

Reynolds, E.H. (1976) In Hoffbrand, A.V. (ed.) *Clinics in hematology*, p. 616.

Reynolds, E.H., Gallagher, B.B., Mattson, R.H. Bowers, M. & Johnson, A.L. (1972) Relationship between serum and cerebrospinal fluid folate. *Nature*, **240**, 155.

Richens, A. & Woodford F.P. (1976) *Anticonvulsant Drugs and Enzyme Induction*. Amsterdam: Elsevier.

Robinson, L.J. (1940) Case of acute poisoning from dilantin sodium with recovery. *Journal of American Medical Association*, **115**, 289.

Roger, J. & Soulayrol, R. (1959) Apropos des accidents neurologiques du traitement de l'épilepsie par les hydantoïnes. *Revue Neurologic*, **100**, 783.

Rose, M. & Johnson, I. (1978) Reinterpretation of the haematological effects of anticonvulsant treatment. *Lancet*, **1**, 1349.

Salcman, M., Defendini, R., Correll, J. & Gilman, S. (1978) Neuropathological changes in cerebellar biopsies of epileptic patients. *Annals of Neurology*, **3**, 10.

Sandler, R.M., Emberson, C., Robert, G.E., Voak, D., Darnborough, J. & Heeley, A.F. (1978) IgM platelet autoantibody due to sodium valproate. *British Medical Journal*, **2**, 1683.

Selhorst, J.B., Kaufman, B. & Horwitz, S.J. (1972) Diphenylhydantoin-induced cerebellar degeneration. *Archives of Neurology* (Chicago), **27**, 453.

Shakir, R.A., Behan, P.O., Dick, H. & Lambie, D.G. (1978) Metabolism of immunoglobulin A, lymphocyte function, and histocompatibility antigens in patients on anticonvulsants. *Journal of Neurology, Neurosurgery and Psychiatry*, **41**, 307.

Shapiro, S., Hartz, S.C., Siskind, V., Mitchell, A.A., Slone, D., Rosenberg, L., Monson, R.R. & Heinonen, O.P. (1976) Anticonvulsants and parental epilepsy in the development of birth defects. *Lancet*, **1**, 272.

Snider, R.S. & Del Cerro, M.P. (1966) Membranous cytoplasmic spirals in dilantin intoxication. *Nature*, **212**, 536.

Snider, R.S. & Del Cerro, M.P. (1967) Drug-induced dendritic sprouts on Purkinje cells in adult cerebellum. *Experimental Neurology*, **17**, 466.

Solomon, G.E., Hilgartner, M.W. & Kutt, H. (1972) Coagulation defects caused by diphenylhydantoin. *Neurology* (Minneapolis) **22**, 1165.

Speidel, B.D. & Meadow, S.R. (1972) Maternal epilepsy and abnormalities of the fetus and newborn. *Lancet*, **2**, 839.

Stephens, W.P., Coe, J.Y. & Baylis, P.H. (1978) Plasma

arginine vasopressin concentrations and antidiuretic action of carbamazepine. *British Medical Journal*, **1**, 1445.

Stephens, W.P., Espir, M.L.E., Tattersall, R.B., Quinn, N.P., Gladwell, S.R.F., Galbraith, A.W. & Reynolds, E.H. (1977) Water intoxication due to carbamazepine. *British Medical Journal*, **1**, 754.

Suchy, F.J., Balistreri, W.F., Buchino, J.J., Sondheimer, J.M., Bates, S.R., Kearns' G.L., Stull, J.D. & Bove, K.E. (1979) Acute hepatic failure associated with the use of sodium valproate. *The New England Journal of Medicine*, **300**, 962.

Sullivan, F.M. & McElhatton, P.R. (1976) A comparison of the teratogenic activity of the antiepileptic drugs carbamazepine, clonazepam, ethosuximide, phenobarbital, phenytoin and primidone in mice. *Toxicology and Applied Pharmacology*, **40**, 365.

Sussman, N.M., McLain, Jr., L.W. & Leppik, I.E. (1979) Hepatotoxicity of valproic acid. *Neurology* (Minneapolis) **29**, 601.

Tchicaloff, M. & Gaillard, F. (1970) Quelques effets indésirables des médicaments anti-épileptiques sur les rendements intellectuels. *Revue de Neuropsychiatrie infantile*, **18**, 599.

Trimble, M.R. & Reynolds, E.H. (1976) Anticonvulsant drugs and mental symptoms: a review. *Psychological Medicine*, **6**, 169.

Utterback, R.A. (1958) Parenchymatous cerebellar degeneration complicating diphenylhydantoin (Dilantin) therapy. *Archives of Neurology and Psychiatry*, **80**, 180.

Utterback, R.A., Ojeman, R. & Malek, J. (1958) Parenchymatous cerebellar degeneration with dilantin intoxication. *Journal of Neuropathology and Experimental Neurology*, **17**, 516.

Viukari, M. (1962) The effects of diphenylhydantoin on the central nervous system. *Duodecim*, **78**, 136.

Wassner, S.J., Pennisi, A.J., Malekzadeh, M.H. & Fine, R.N. (1976) The adverse effect of anticonvulsant therapy on renal allograft survival. *Journal of Pediatrics*, **88**, 134.

Werk E.E., McGee, J. & Sholiton, L.J. (1964) Effect of diphenylhydantoin on cortisol metabolism in man. *Journal of Clinical Investigation* **43**, 1284.

White, S.J., McLean, A.E.M. & Howland, C. (1979) Anticonvulsant drugs and cancer. A cohort study in patients with severe epilepsy. *Lancet*, ii, 458.

PART THREE
DRUG INTERACTIONS

E. Perucca

INTRODUCTION

Epileptic patients are usually maintained on pharmacological treatment for several years and for this reason they are particularly likely to receive multiple drug therapy, either for the control of fits or for the treatment of unrelated intercurrent medical conditions. Interactions between antiepileptic drugs, or between these drugs and other pharmacological agents, may occur for a number of reasons:

1. Many currently used antiepileptic drugs are potent inducers of the hepatic drug-metabolising enzymes resulting in marked stimulation of the metabolism of several therapeutic agents, whose effectiveness may thus be reduced.

2. Phenytoin and valproic acid are highly bound to plasma proteins and may displace or be displaced by other drugs from protein binding sites.

3. The enzymatic system responsible for phenytoin metabolism is easily inhibited by other drugs. Due to the occurrence of saturation kinetics, this may result in a disproportionate increase of the serum concentration of the drug and, consequently, in clinical intoxication.

4. Antiepileptic drugs share with other psychotropic agents a depressant action on the central nervous system. When these agents are used in combination, their effects can be additive and clinical intoxication may occur despite low serum concentration values of the individual drugs.

In recent years the practice of monitoring serum drug levels has greatly improved our understanding of the complex interactions affecting the handling of drugs in the body (pharmacokinetic interactions). Drug interactions at the receptor site (pharmacodynamic interactions) are still incompletely known, due to the lack of adequate techniques for quantifying the action of drugs on the central nervous system in man. In this chapter an attempt has been made to classify antiepileptic drug interactions on the basis of the mechanism involved. Only evidence obtained in patients or normal volunteers is reviewed.

INTERACTIONS AFFECTING HANDLING AND RESPONSE TO ANTIEPILEPTIC DRUGS

Interactions affecting absorption from the gastrointestinal tract

Calcium supplements are sometimes added to the diet of epileptic patients with drug-induced rickets, osteomalacia and/or hypocalcaemia. An early report from Australia providing evidence that calcium sulphate used as an excipient in phenytoin capsules markedly impaired the absorption of the drug was therefore of considerable interest (Bochner et al., 1972). In order to investigate whether a similar effect could be produced by increasing the calcium content of the diet, Herishanu et al. (1976) determined the steady state serum concentration of phenytoin in five normal volunteers given phenytoin (300 mg once daily) for 21 days. The subjects were maintained on a normal diet for ten days, on a calcium-free diet for the following five days and again on a normal diet with the addition of calcium gluconate (1 gm given together with the phenytoin dose) for the remaining six days. In the four subjects who completed the study, the serum phenytoin concentration following administration of calcium gluconate was on average identical to that observed during the calcium-free period but lower than during the control period, possibly due to reduced compliance during the second and third stage of the study. In a separate study (Kulshrestha et al., 1978) administration of therapeutic doses of an antacid suspension containing calcium carbonate also failed to produce any consistent change in the steady state serum concentration of phenytoin in six epileptic patients. Other antacid preparations may, however, impair phenytoin absorption. Kutt (1975) reported that simultaneous administration of phenytoin with an antacid of unspecified composition in three epileptic patients resulted in markedly low serum phenytoin levels; the latter increased two-to-three-fold when the same dose of phenytoin was given two to three hours prior to the ingestion of the antacid. In another study (Kulshrestha et al., 1978), therapeutic doses of a mixture of aluminium hydroxide and magnesium trisilicate slightly but significantly lowered the serum concentration of phenytoin in six patients stabilised on phenytoin therapy. Although O'Brien et al. (1978) were unable to reproduce these results with magnesium and aluminium hydroxide in six normal volunteers, the discrepancy could be attributed to the different experimental conditions used in the latter study, i.e. single dose compared with chronic administration. Since the absorption of barbiturates (Hurwitz, 1977) and benzodiazepines (Shader et al., 1978; Greenblatt et al., 1976) may also be reduced in the presence of magnesium and aluminium hydroxide, it is probably wise to recommend that antiepileptic drugs be administered at least two to three hours before the ingestion of antacids.

In a study by Neuvonen, Elfving and Elonen (1978) activated charcoal completely prevented the absorption of phenytoin only when ingested immediately after the drug; when the same dose of charcoal was given one hour later, phenytoin absorption was less affected, but still considerably reduced.

Acetazolamide has been reported to reduce dramatically the rate and extent of primidone absorption in two patients (Syversen et al., 1977). It was commented that this interaction occurs only in susceptible individuals, and its real incidence is unknown.

Plasma protein binding interactions

Many antiepileptic drugs are extensively bound to plasma proteins. Drugs with high binding affinity may compete for binding sites resulting in increased concentration of free (unbound) drug in plasma. Since only the free drug is available to produce a pharmacological response, displacement from protein binding sites may potentially enhance the therapeutic and the toxic effects of the affected drug. Table 8.20 lists a number of therapeutic agents which have been shown to displace phenytoin and valproic acid from plasma protein binding sites in vitro. Although these interactions are often reported as clinically important, extrapolation of in vitro data to the in vivo situation has to be made cautiously because the displaced drug is available not only to produce pharmacological effects but also to be distributed

Table 8.20 Summary of potential interactions affecting the plasma protein binding of antiepileptic drugs

Drug affected	Interfering drug	Consequences	Reference
Phenytoin	Phenylbutazone	Shift of the therapeutic	Lunde et al. (1970), Neuvonen et al. (1979)
	Sulphafurazole	range towards lower serum	Odar-Cederlof & Borgå (1976)
	Salicylic acid	concentration values	Fraser et al. (1979)
	Diazoxide	Transient potentiation of	Roe et al. (1975)
	Valproic acid	phenytoin activity	Monks et al. (1978)
	Tolbutamide	Transient increase in rate	Wesseling and Mols-Thürkow (1975)
	Halofenate	of phenytoin elimination	Karch et al. (1977)
Sodium valproate	Phenytoin	? Increased metabolic and	Monks et al. (1978)
	Salicylic acid	renal clearance	Schobben et al. (1978)

in tissues and to be eliminated. Figure 8.14 illustrates the effect of a plasma protein binding interaction on the serum concentration and pharmacological activity of a low-clearance drug which, like phenytoin and most other antiepileptic drugs, is characterised by a relatively large distribution volume. Displacement from binding sites following addition of the interfering agent results in a marked fall of the total (free + bound) concentration of the affected drug which is accompanied by a corresponding increase of the free *fraction* in plasma; the actual *concentration* of free drug and the resulting pharmacological effect, however, are only transiently increased and gradually return to baseline levels, as a result of redistribution and increased rate of drug elimination.

The displacement of phenytoin from protein binding sites by valproic acid provides a good example of the important clinical implications of the principles discussed above. An early report largely based on *in vitro* and animal studies suggested that valproic acid could precipitate phenytoin intoxication in epileptic patients by displacing the latter drug from its plasma protein binding sites (Patsalos & Lascelles, 1977). In a subsequent study, however, Mattson et al. (1978) confirmed the very considerable displacing effect of valproic acid on plasma protein-bound phenytoin but failed to detect any marked change in the plasma concentration of unbound drug when 21 epileptic patients were started on valproic acid. In the same patients, initiation of valproic acid therapy

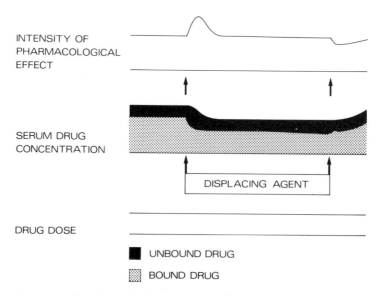

Fig. 8.14 Schematic representation of the effect of a plasma protein-binding interaction on the serum concentration and pharmacological activity of a low clearance highly albumin-bound drug (modified from Koch-Weser & Sellers, 1976)

resulted in a marked decline of the total serum phenytoin concentration; the effect was associated with a 60–100 per cent increase of the unbound *fraction* of phenytoin in plasma while the actual *concentration* of free drug increased by only 10–20 per cent on average. The relative stability of the plasma concentration of free drug following displacement was probably related, at least in part, to a compensatory increase in phenytoin clearance, as suggested by changes in pattern of metabolite excretion in one of the patients, and by the results of a single-dose study in healthy volunteers (Frigo *et al.*, 1979). More recent findings, however, suggest that the interaction may be more complex than it was previously thought and that inhibition of phenytoin metabolism may also occur at the same time, leading to a potentially important rise in the concentration of free drug (Perucca *et al.*, 1980).

An important message that emerges from these studies is that, in the presence of a plasma protein binding interaction, serum levels of total drug may be positively misleading; in some cases, a fall in the concentration of total drug will in fact be accompanied by a concomitant rise in the concentration of free (pharmacologically active) drug. The clinician should remember that any increase in fraction unbound will result in a shift of the therapeutic range towards lower values and that despite the lower concentration of total drug dosage may not need to be increased.

Induction of metabolism

The four main drugs used in the treatment of the adult epilepsies, phenytoin, primidone, phenobarbitone and carbamazepine, are among the most powerful inducers of the hepatic microsomal enzymes (Richens and Woodford, 1976; Perucca, 1978). When these drugs are used in combination, reciprocal stimulation of metabolism may occur resulting in a reduction of the serum concentration at steady state. In most cases the effect is relatively small (probably as a consequence of the already high degree of induction in these patients) and of little clinical significance because of the added therapeutic action of the interfering drug. A possible exception is the marked decline of the serum carbamazepine levels in patients receiving combi-

nation therapy with phenytoin, phenobarbitone and primidone (Fig. 8.15).

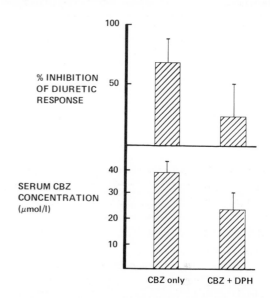

Fig. 8.15 Impairment of excretion of a standard water load (expressed as per cent inhibition of a normal diuretic response) and serum carbamazepine (CBZ) concentration in patients receiving chronic treatment with carbamazepine alone or in combination with phenytoin (DPH). Patients in both groups were matched for carbamazepine dose (n = 6 for each group) (reproduced from Perucca & Richens, 1980b).

Indirect evidence that induction of metabolism is the mechanism responsible for the interaction is provided by the reduction of the ratio of carbamazepine to carbamazepine-10, 11-epoxide in the serum of the same patients (Schneider, 1975; Rane, Hojer & Wilson, 1976). As the epoxide retains part of the pharmacological activity of the parent drug the reduction in therapeutic effectiveness may be smaller than expected from the fall in serum concentration of carbamazepine alone. Another example of an interaction leading to increased rate of formation of an active metabolite is the phenytoin-induced stimulation of the conversion of primidone to phenobarbitone. Phenobarbitone has a longer half-life than primidone, it accumulates and the overall result may be a potentiation rather than a reduction of the pharmacological effect.

A list of interactions resulting in increased elimination (or reduced steady state serum concentration) of other antiepileptic drugs is summarised in Table 8.21. Only in some cases has adequ-

Table 8.21 Summary of potential interactions leading to increased metabolism of some antiepileptic drugs

Affected drug	Interfering drug	Consequences	Reference
Carbamazepine	Phenytoin Phenobarbitone Primidone		Cereghino et al. (1975)
Phenytoin	Carbamazepine Phenobarbitone † Benzodiazepines † Folic acid Nitrofurantoin (?)		Hansen et al. (1971) Kutt (1972) Perucca & Richens (1980a) Makki et al. (1979) Heipertz & Pilz (1978)
Phenobarbitone	Folic acid		Makki et al. (1979)
Primidone	Phenytoin	Reduced serum concentration of the affected drug Clinical consequences negligible in most cases due to the added therapeutic effect of the interfering drug	Fincham et al. (1974) Reynolds et al. (1975)
Sodium valproate	Phenytoin Phenobarbitone Carbamazepine		Perucca et al. (1978a) Bowdel, Levy & Cutler (1979)
Clonazepam	Carbamazepine Phenytoin Phenobarbitone		Lai et al. (1978) Sjö et al. (1975) Nanda et al. (1977)
Diazepam	Phenytoin Phenobarbitone		Viala et al. (1971)
N-desmethyldiazepam	Phenytoin Phenobarbitone		Wilenski et al. (1978)

† Evidence conflicting. References refer to review articles.

ate evidence of induction of metabolism been presented; in other instances, e.g. the stimulation of valproic acid elimination by phenytoin and phenobarbitone, a plasma protein-binding interaction cannot be excluded as a possible cause for the increased elimination.

Among the interactions listed in Table 8.21, those affecting phenytoin metabolism have been most extensively investigated. Induction of phenytoin metabolism by carbamazepine has been clearly demonstrated by Hansen and associates (1971) who described a significant decrease of the serum phenytoin half-life in five patients treated for at least nine days with carbamazepine 600 mg daily. The effect of carbamazepine on steady state serum phenytoin concentration, however, was less consistent and only in three subjects out of seven was a decline of serum phenytoin levels seen after starting carbamazepine therapy.

A fall in the serum concentration of phenytoin has also been described in folate-deficient epileptic patients started on folic acid (Baylis et al., 1971; Mattson et al., 1973), and the suggestion has been made that this effect could be partly responsible for the deterioration in fit control and the simultaneous improvement in mental performance which are occasionally observed in the same patients during folic acid therapy (Viukari, 1968). Makki, Perucca and Richens (1979) administered folic acid 30 mg daily for three months to 40 folate-deficient epileptic patients and noted a significant lowering of the steady state serum concentration of both phenytoin and phenobarbitone; the effect was relatively small (20 and 15 per cent on average respectively) but it tended to be more marked in patients with initially high serum phenytoin levels. A marginal decline in steady state serum phenytoin concentration during folic acid treatment has also been described in normal non-folate deficient volunteers (Furlanut et al., 1978).

Conflicting data have been reported on the effect of phenobarbitone and the benzodiazepines on phenytoin metabolism (see Kutt, 1972 and Perucca & Richens, 1980a for reviews). Elevation, depression or no change in serum phenytoin levels have all been described when these drugs are used as adjunct medication in epileptic patients. A probable explanation for the inconsistent findings is that phenobarbitone may at the same time induce and inhibit phenytoin hydroxylation, the predominant effect being unpredictable in the individual patient.

Although a similar effect has also been proposed

for the benzodiazepines (Houghton & Richens, 1974a), there is no convincing evidence that the latter drugs can stimulate the hepatic drug-metabolising enzymes to any important extent in man.

Inhibition of metabolism

In agreement with predictions based on studies *in vitro*, phenytoin appears to be a particularly poor substrate for the drug metabolising enzymes and inhibition of its metabolism is relatively common when phenytoin-treated patients are exposed to other drugs. Table 8.22 illustrates a list of therapeutic agents which have been shown to increase the steady state serum concentration of phenytoin (or to prolong its half-life) in patients or in normal volunteers. An attempt has been made to include only cases in which reasonable evidence is available, and the list should not be regarded as exhaustive. The clinical importance of the interaction described is likely to vary considerably from one patient to another; interactions are particularly inconsistent in the case of phenytoin, because

Table 8.22 Summary of potential interactions leading to inhibition of metabolism of some antiepileptic drugs

Affected drug	Interfering drug	Consequences	Reference
Phenytoin	Sulthiame	Rise of the serum	Hansen *et al.* (1968)
			Houghton & Richens, (1974b)
	Methsuximide	concentration of	Rambeck (1979)
	Pheneturide	phenytoin and	Houghton & Richens (1974a)
	Phenobarbitone †	precipitation of	Kutt (1972)
	Benzodiazepines †	intoxication in	Perucca & Richens (1980a)
	Sodium valproate	some patients	Perucca *et al.* (1980)
	Isoniazid		Kutt *et al.* (1970)
	Dicoumarol,		Hansen *et al.* (1966); Skovsted *et al.* (1976)
	Phencoupromon		
	Disulfiram		Olesen (1967)
	Chloramphenicol		Christensen & Skovsted (1969)
	Phenyramidol		Solomon & Schrogie (1967)
	Imipramine		Perucca & Richens (1977)
	Chlorpromazine		Bielmann *et al.* (1978)
	Propoxyphene		Kutt (1971)
	Methylphenidate		Kutt & Louis (1972)
			Garettson *et al.* (1969)
	Chlorpheniramine		Pugh *et al.* (1975)
	Sulfaphenazole,		Hansen *et al.* (1979)
	Sulfadiazine,		
	Sulfamethizole, ‡		
	Trimethoprim		
	Phenylbutazone		Neuvonen *et al.* (1979)
Phenobarbitone	Phenytoin		Morselli *et al.* (1971)
	Sodium valproate		Richens & Ahmad (1975)
			Patel, Levy & Cutler (1980)
	Sulthiame		Richens (1976)
	Methsuximide		Stenzel *et al.* (1978); Rambeck (1979)
	Methylphenidate		Garettson *et al.* (1969)
	Chloramphenicol		Koup *et al.* (1978)
	Frusemide		Ahmad *et al.* (1976)
	Dicoumarol		Hansen *et al.* (1966)
Primidone	Sulthiame	Rise in serum	Richens (1976)
	Isoniazid	concentration of the	Sutton & Kupferberg (1975)
Carbamazepine	Triacetyloleandomycin	affected drug and	Dravet *et al.* (1977)
	Propoxyphene	occasionally clinical	Dam *et al.* (1977)
Diazepam,	Disulfiram	manifestations of	MacLeod *et al.* (1978)
chlordiazepoxide		intoxication	
and N-desmethyl			
derivatives			

† Evidence conflicting. References refer to review articles.

‡ Sulfadimethoxine and sulfamethoxypyridazine had no effect.

the consequences of a large interindividual variability in rate of metabolism can be exaggerated by the occurrence of saturation kinetics at serum concentration values commonly encountered in therapeutic practice.

Sulthiame, pheneturide, isoniazid, chloramphenicol, certain sulphonamides, and dicoumarol appear to be the drugs most frequently responsible for causing inhibition of phenytoin metabolism. Among 136 patients admitted to the Chalfont Centre for Epilepsy, 40 per cent of those receiving a combination of sulthiame and phenytoin showed toxic serum phenytoin levels (>100 μmol/1) as opposed to only 13 per cent of the patients not receiving sulthiame, despite similar phenytoin dosages in the two groups; the serum phenytoin concentration was on average 74 per cent higher among the patients receiving sulthiame. Twelve patients were studied both on and off sulthiame therapy (400–600 mg daily). In each case addition of sulthiame caused an elevation of the serum phenytoin concentration, a prolongation of the phenytoin half-life and a reduction in the ratio of pHPPH to phenytoin in the urine, i.e. a change in favour of the unmetabolised drug (Richens & Houghton, 1975). It was suggested that patients with a serum phenytoin level of 50 μmol/1 or greater should be observed carefully and the serum phenytoin measured frequently if sulthiame is prescribed, due to the likelihood of intoxication developing in these patients. Serum levels should be monitored for a prolonged period because there is usually a latent interval of 10–20 days between the addition of sulthiame and the subsequent rise in serum phenytoin concentration.

Pheneturide has also been shown to increase serum phenytoin levels, but the effect is generally less marked than that observed with sulthiame. The time course of the interaction is complex, with a rapid rise of the serum phenytoin levels to peak values and a subsequent slow decline over the next few weeks to steady state values slightly above baseline. This pattern is probably a consequence of initial enzyme inhibition, followed by progressive induction of phenytoin metabolism.

In 1962, Murray reported the occurrence of marked drowsiness and unsteadiness of gait in 70 out of 637 institutionalised epileptic patients who were given isoniazid for the prophylaxis of tuberculosis. These reactions were almost certainly due to phenytoin intoxication, for isoniazid was subsequently found to be a powerful inhibitor of phenytoin metabolism. In a prospective study carried out at Bellevue Hospital, New York, clinical signs of phenytoin toxicity developed in approximately 10 per cent of patients taking phenytoin (300 mg daily) in addition to isoniazid and PAS or cycloserine (Kutt et al., 1970): serum phenytoin levels above 160 μmol/1 (40 μg/ml) were observed in 16 out of the 34 intoxicated patients. Interestingly, the interaction appears to occur mainly in slow acetylators, probably because only the latter subjects achieve hepatic concentrations of isoniazid sufficient to inhibit phenytoin metabolism. The inhibition is of the non-competitive type and it is potentiated in vitro by PAS, which is frequently associated with isoniazid in the treatment of tuberculosis.

The metabolism of primidone, phenobarbitone, valproic acid, carbamazepine and the benzodiazepines is less susceptible to being inhibited by other drugs. The most frequent of these interactions is probably the increase in serum phenobarbitone concentration in patients receiving combined treatment with sodium valproate (Flachs et al. 1977). The effect is often sufficiently marked to have clinical significance, and may account for the drowsiness experienced by some of these patients following initiation of valproate therapy.

A particularly important interaction occurs between propoxyphene and carbamazepine. Drowsiness, dizziness, headache and other adverse effects developed in five out of seven patients when propoxyphene (65 mg t.d.s.) was introduced in addition to carbamazepine therapy (Dam et al., 1977). The serum carbamazepine concentration was monitored in five patients: in each case a marked (45–77 per cent) increase of the serum carbamazepine level was seen after propoxyphene, inhibition of metabolism being suggested by a reduced ratio of the epoxide to parent drug in the serum.

Interactions affecting renal excretion

Alkalinisation of urine greatly enhances the elimination of phenobarbitone by reducing the reabsorption of the drug from the renal tubular epithelium (Waddell & Butler, 1957). The effect can be exploited therapeutically in severe cases of phenobarbitone intoxication.

Pharmacodynamic drug interactions

Interactions between drugs at their site of action in tissues are termed pharmacodynamic interactions. For many years physicians used to prescribe a combination of several antiepileptic drugs in low dosage, on the assumption that their therapeutic effects would be additive whereas the adverse effects would not. Indeed, the reverse may be true. Drowsiness, incoordination and other signs of drug toxicity are frequently seen in patients receiving a large number of antiepileptic and/or other psychotropic drugs in combination, despite low serum levels of the individual agents. In many of these cases toxic signs are probably the result of the summation of the depressing effects of these drugs on the central nervous system. In other cases, the combined effect may be greater than expected by simple addition. A possible example of this type of interaction is provided by the much higher risk of respiratory arrest when intravenous phenobarbitone and diazepam are combined in the treatment of status epilepticus. A further example of pharmacodynamic interaction whose mechanism is less clearly understood is provided by the occasional occurrence of an absence-like status in patients given clonazepam and sodium valproate in combination (Jeavons, Clark & Maheshwari, 1977).

More rarely, drug interactions at the receptor site may result in antagonism of adverse effects. The incidence of the syndrome of water intoxication induced by carbamazepine is much lower in patients receiving combination therapy with phenytoin (Perucca et al., 1978b) and complete reversal of the syndrome has recently been described in a single patient when phenytoin was introduced in addition to carbamazepine (Sordillo et al., 1978). The latter authors suggested that the antagonism of the carbamazepine-induced anti-diuresis by phenytoin is related to the inhibition of the pituitary release of antidiuretic hormone by the latter drug. More recent studies, however, indicate that the mechanism of the interaction is predominantly pharmacokinetic, i.e. secondary to the lowering effect of phenytoin on serum carbamazepine levels (Fig. 8.15).

INTERACTIONS AFFECTING HANDLING AND RESPONSE TO OTHER DRUGS

Interactions affecting absorption from the gastrointestinal tract

The rate and extent of the absorption of griseofulvin from the gastrointestinal tract are reduced by phenobarbitone treatment (Riegelman, Rowland & Epstein, 1970) resulting in therapeutic ineffectiveness of standard doses of the former drug during combined therapy (Busfield et al., 1963). The diuretic response to frusemide is also reduced in patients receiving chronic treatment with antiepileptic drugs (Ahmad, 1974) due to the marked inhibitory action of phenytoin on the absorption of the diuretic (Fine et al., 1977), although reduced renal responsiveness may also occur (Ahmad, 1974) (see below). It has been suggested that phenytoin may also impair folic acid absorption, but this effect is still controversial (Reynolds, 1976).

Only a few other studies have examined the influence of antiepileptic drugs on the absorption of other therapeutic agents. It is likely that some of the interactions resulting in a decreased steady state serum concentration of the affected drug (Table 8.23) are in fact due to inhibition of absorption rather than to enzyme-induction, as generally assumed.

Plasma protein binding interactions

Chloral hydrate may potentiate the anticoagulant effects of warfarin. The interaction is mediated by displacement of warfarin from plasma protein binding sites by trichloroacetic acid, the main metabolite of chloral hydrate in man; potentially fatal clinical consequences have been reported (Sellers & Koch-Weser, 1970). It remains to be determined whether a similar effect occurs with valproic acid, which is highly bound to plasma proteins and has no significant enzyme inducing properties in man. Phenytoin may displace imipramine and other tricyclic antidepressants *in vitro*

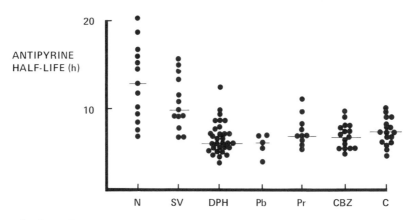

Fig. 8.16 Serum antipyrine half-lives in normal subjects (N) and in patients receiving chronic therapy with antiepileptic drugs, alone or in combination (C). SV = sodium valproate; DPH = phenytoin; Pb = phenobarbitone; Pr = primidone; CBZ = carbamazepine. Horizontal bars indicate the median value for each group.

but the clinical implications of these observations are unclear (Borgå et al., 1969).

Induction of metabolism

Stimulation of the hepatic microsomal enzymes by antiepileptic drugs may dramatically alter the disposition kinetics of many other pharmacological agents which are metabolised by the liver. The magnitude of the effect is clearly illustrated by the marked shortening of the serum antipyrine half-life in patients treated with phenytoin, phenobarbitone, primidone and carbamazepine, either alone or in combination (Fig. 8.16)) (Perucca et al., 1979c). A number of therapeutic agents and other substances whose rate of metabolism is likely to be stimulated in patients treated with antiepileptic drugs are shown in Table 8.23. The clinical significance of the interactions described is largely dependent on the pharmacological properties of the affected drug, being most important for agents characterised by a low therapeutic ratio, e.g. oral anticoagulants. Patients treated with phenytoin, phenobarbitone, primidone or carbamazepine show a reduced response to standard doses of warfarin and/or dicoumarol, and require unusually large doses of these agents for a satisfactory degree of anticoagulation to be achieved. A danger of this phenomenon is the occurrence of a rebound effect when the enzyme-inducing drugs are stopped or their dosage is reduced, because the rate of metabolism of the anticoagulant will slow,

resulting in excessive accumulation and potentially fatal haemorrhage. In one hospital, 14 out of 56 haemorrhagic reactions were possibly due to withdrawal of enzyme-inducing drugs without a modification of the warfarin dose (MacDonald & Robinson, 1968).

The therapeutic response to standard doses of many steroid agents is also reduced in patients treated with antiepileptic drugs. Administration of phenobarbitone 120 mg daily for three weeks to 11 asthmatic patients resulted in an 88 per cent increase of the metabolic clearance of labelled dexamethasone and, in three prednisone-dependent patients, a worsening of the asthma, probably as a consequence of increased prednisone and/or prednisolone metabolism (Brooks et al., 1972). In a similar study, administration of phenobarbitone, 120 mg daily, to patients with rheumatoid arthritis stabilised on prednisolone therapy resulted in marked deterioration of the therapeutic effectiveness of the latter drug, as shown by a significant increase in pain score, articular index and degree of morning stiffness (Brooks et al., 1976). The effect was associated with a 25 per cent reduction of the prednisolone half-life in eight out of the nine patients studied. Induction of steroid metabolism is responsible for the failure of the low-dose dexamethasone test to suppress plasma corticosteroids concentration and urinary 17-hydroxycorticosteroid excretion in phenytoin-treated patients (Jubiz et al., 1970). The therapeutic efficacy of dexamethasone is also reduced in the

Table 8.23 Summary of potential interactions leading to stimulation of metabolism of other drugs

Affecting drug	Interfering drug	Consequences	Reference
Warfarin		Reduced anticoagulant effect	Cucinell et al. (1965)
Dicoumarol		Risk of hemorrhage when interfering drug is withheld	Hansen et al. (1971a, b)
Doxycycline		Reduced antibiotic efficacy	Neuvonen & Penttila (1974) Penttila et al. (1974)
Rifampicin			De Rautlin de la Roy et al. (1971)
Chloramphenicol			Bloxham et al. (1979)
Methylprednisolone			Stiernholm & Katz (1975)
Prednisolone		Reduced therapeutic effect	Petereit & Meikle (1977)
Dexamethasone		Failure of diagnostic tests	Werk et al. (1969)
Cortisol			Werk et al. (1964); Choi et al. (1971)
Metyrapone			Meikle et al. (1969)
Oral contraceptives		Reduced contraceptive efficacy	Hempel & Klinger (1976)
Imipramine	Phenytoin	Reduced therapeutic efficacy but in some cases active	Ballinger et al. (1974); Hewick et al. (1972)
Desmethylimipramine	Barbiturates	metabolites are formed at	Hammer et al. (1967)
Nortriptyline		a faster rate	Alexanderson et al. (1969)
	Primidone		Braithwaite et al. (1975)
Chlorpromazine			Curry et al. (1970); Forrest et al. (1970)
	Carbamazepine		Loga et al. (1975)
Antipyrine		Clearance used as an index	Vesell & Page (1969)
Quinine		of enzyme-induction	Padgham & Richens (1974)
Phenylbutazone			Levi et al. (1968)
			Whittaker & Price-Evans (1970)
Fenoprofen		Reduced therapeutic effect	Helleberg et al. (1974)
Digitoxin			Solomon et al. (1971)
			Jelliffe et al. (1966)
Alprenolol			Alvan et al. (1977)
Quinidine		Reduced therapeutic effect	Data et al. (1976)
Lignocaine			Perucca & Richens (1979b)
Paracetamol		? enhanced hepatoxicity	Perucca & Richens (1979a)
Pethidine		? enhanced CNS toxicity	Stambaugh et al. (1977)
DDT			Davies et al. (1969)
Vitamin D		Rickets and osteomalacia	Hahn (1976)

same patients (McLelland & Jack, 1978) while the response to another test of adrenal function, the inhibition of cortisol biosynthesis by oral metyrapone, fails probably due to induction of metyrapone metabolism during its first passage through the liver (Meikle et al., 1969).

Stimulation of sex hormone metabolism could account for the reduced efficacy of the contraceptive pill in epileptic women, especially when the more recent preparations containing only 20–30 μg of the oestrogen component are used. In one study, phenobarbitone, phenytoin and carbamazepine were the drugs most frequently implicated in causing spotting and breakthrough bleeding in a large population of patients taking various psychotropic drugs in addition to oral contraceptives (Hempel & Klinger, 1976). In the absence of pathological causes, breakthrough bleeding

should be regarded as an index of reduced contraceptive efficacy in these patients.

The implications of microsomal enzyme-induction for many others of the drugs listed in Table 8.23 have not been assessed clinically. In general, a reduction of the therapeutic effectiveness is to be expected except for those agents which are converted to active or toxic metabolites; in the latter case, potentiation of adverse effects may be seen. Genetically predisposed subjects, for example, may convert a small portion of acetophenetidin into the methaemoglobin forming orthohydroxy-metabolite. During phenobarbitone treatment the fraction of the drug that is metabolised through the abnormal pathway is greatly increased and serious methaemoglobinaemic reactions may follow (Shahidi, 1968). Enzyme-inducing agents enhance the toxicity of numerous other drugs in animals and it is possible that some adverse drug reactions seen in epileptic patients are mediated by a similar mechanism. This may indeed be true in cases of paracetamol (Wright & Prescott, 1973) and pethidine (Stambaugh et al., 1977) intoxication.

Pharmacodynamic drug interactions

The inhibitory effect of phenytoin on the absorption of frusemide from the gastrointestinal tract has been discussed above. In patients treated with phenytoin and phenobarbitone the diuretic response to frusemide is reduced even after intravenous administration. Ahmad (1974) postulated the occurrence of a pharmacodynamic interaction at renal level. Another possible exam-

ple of pharmacodynamic interaction is provided by the phenytoin-mediated antagonism of the cytotoxic action of streptozotocin on the beta cells of the pancreas (Koranyi & Gero, 1979).

CONCLUSION

The examples presented above provide sufficient evidence for the complex interactions which may occur in patients receiving antiepileptic drugs. As most drug interactions are potentially adverse, the clinician should always think consciously about the implications of adding a new drug to any therapeutic regime and the possibility of an interaction should be considered whenever unusual symptoms or signs develop in patients receiving multiple drug therapy.

REFERENCES

Ahmad, S. (1974) Renal insensitivity to frusemide caused by chronic anticonvulsant therapy. *British Medical Journal*, **3**, 657.

Ahmad, S., Clarke, L., Hewett, A.J. & Richens, A. (1976) Controlled trial of frusemide as an antiepileptic drug in focal epilepsy. *British Journal of Clinical Pharmacology*, **3**, 621.

Alexanderson, B., Price-Evans, D.A. & Sjöqvist, F. (1969) Steady-state levels of nortryptiline in twins: influence of genetic factors and drug therapy. *British Medical Journal*, **4**, 764.

Alvan, G., Piafsky, K., Lind, N. & von Bahr, C. (1977) Effect of pentobarbital on the disposition of alprenolol. *Clinical Pharmacology and Therapeutics*, **22**, 316.

Ballinger, B.R., Presly, A., Reid, A.H. & Stevenson, I.H. (1974) The effects of hypnotics on imipramine treatment. *Psychopharmacologia*, (Berlin), **39**, 267.

Baylis, E.M., Crowley, J.M., Preece, J.M., Sylvester, P.E. & Marks, V. (1971) Influence of folic acid on blood phenytoin levels. *Lancet*, **1**, 62.

Bielmann, I., Levac, T. & Gagnon, M.A. (1978) Clonazepam: its efficacy in association with phenytoin and phenobarbital in mental patients with generalised major motor seizures. *International Journal of Clinical Pharmacology*. **16**, 268.

Bloxham, R.A., Durbin, G.M., Johnson, T. & Winterborn, M.H. (1979) Chloramphenicol and phenobarbitone – a drug interaction. *Archives of Disease in Childhood*, **54**, 76.

Bochner, F., Hooper, W.D., Tyrer, J.H. & Eadie, M.J. (1972) Factors involved in an outbreak of phenytoin intoxication. *Journal of Neurological Sciences (Amsterdam)*, **16**, 481.

Borgå, O., Azarnoff, D.L., Forshell, G.P. & Sjöqvist, F. (1969) Plasma protein binding of tricyclic antidepressants in man. *Biochemical Pharmacology*, **18**, 2135.

Bowdle, T.A., Levy, R.H. & Cutler, R.E. (1979) Effect of carbamazepine on valproic acid clearance in normal man. *Clinical Pharmacology and Therapeutics*, **25**, 215.

Braithwaite, R.A., Flanagan, R.A. & Richens, A. (1975) Steady-state plasma nortriptyline concentrations in epileptic

patients. *British Journal of Clinical Pharmacology*, **2**, 469.

Brooks, P.M., Buchanan, W.W., Grove, M. & Downie, N.W. (1976) Effects of enzyme-induction on metabolism of prednisolone. Clinical and laboratory study. *Annals of Rheumatic Disease*, **35**, 339.

Brooks, S.M., Werk, E.E., Ackerman, S.J., Sullivan, I. & Thrasher, K. (1972) Adverse effects of phenobarbital on corticosteroid metabolism in patients with bronchial asthma. *New England Journal of Medicine*, **286**, 1125.

Busfield, D., Child, K.J., Atkinson, R.M. & Tomich, E.G. (1963) An effect of phenobarbitone on blood levels of griseofulvin in man. *Lancet*, ii, 1042.

Cereghino, J.J., Brock, J.T., van Meter, J.C., Penry, J.K., Smith, L.D. & White, B.G. (1975) The efficacy of carbamazepine combinations in epilepsy. *Clinical Pharmacology and Therapeutics*, **18**, 733.

Choi, Y., Thrasher, K., Werk, E.E., Sholiton, L.J. & Olinger, C. (1971) Effect of diphenylhydantoin on cortisol kinetics in humans. *Journal of Pharmacology and Experimental Therapeutics*, **176**, 27.

Christensen, L.K. & Skovsted, L. (1969) Inhibition of drug metabolism by chloramphenicol. *Lancet*, ii, 1397.

Cucinell, S.A., Conney, A.H., Sansur, M. & Burns, J.J. (1965) Drug interactions in man I. Lowering effect of phenobarbital on plasma levels of bishydroxycoumarin (Dicoumarol®) and diphenylhydantoin (Dilantin®). *Clinical Pharmacology and Therapeutics*, **6**, 420.

Curry, S.H., Davis, J.M., Janowsky, D.S. & Marshall, J.H.L. (1970) Factors affecting chlorpromazine plasma levels in psychiatric patients. *Archives of General Psychiatry*, **22**, 209.

Dam, M., Kristensen, C.B., Hansen, B.S. & Christiansen, J. (1977) Interaction between carbamazepine and propoxyphene in man. *Acta Neurologica Scandinavica*, **56**, 603.

Data, J.L., Wilkinson, G.R. & Nies, A.S. (1976) Interaction of quinidine with anticonvulsant drugs. *New England Journal of Medicine*, **294**, 699.

Davies, J.E., Edmunson, W.F., Carter, C.H. & Barquet, A. (1969) Effects of anticonvulsant drugs on dicophane (DDT) residues in man. *Lancet*, ii, 7.

De Rautlin de La Roy, Y., Beauchant, G., Breuil, K. & Patte, F. (1971) Diminution du taux sérique de rifampicine par le phenobarbital. *La Presse Medicale*, 79, 350.

Dravet, C., Mesdjian, E., Cenraud, B. & Roger, J. (1977) Interaction between carbamazepine and triacetyloleandomycin. *Lancet*, i, 810

Fincham, R.W., Schottelius, D.D. & Sahs, A.L. (1974) The influence of diphenylhydantoin on primidone metabolism. *Archives of Neurology (Chicago)*, 30, 259.

Fine, A., Henderson, I.S., Morgan, D.R. & Tilstone, W.J. (1977) Malabsorption of frusemide caused by phenytoin. *British Medical Journal*, 2, 1061.

Flachs, H., Würtz-Jørgensen, A., Gram, L. & Wulff, K. (1977). Sodium di-n-propylacetate – its interaction with other antiepileptic drugs. In Vree, T.B. & Van der Kleijn, E. (eds) *Pharmacokinetics and metabolism of the antiepileptic drug sodium valproate (Depakine®, Epilim®)*, p. 61. Utrecht: Bohn, Scheltema and Holkema.

Fraser, D.G., Ludden, T., Evens, R.P. & Sutherland, E.W. III (1979) *In vivo* displacement of phenytoin from plasma proteins with salicylates. *Clinical Pharmacology and Therapeutics*, 25, 226.

Forrest, F.M., Forrest, I.S. & Serra, M.T. (1970) Modification of chlorpromazine metabolism by some other drugs frequently administered to psychiatric patients. *Biology in Psychiatry*, 2, 53.

Frigo, G.M., Lecchini, S., Gatti, G., Perucca, E. & Crema, A. (1979) Modification of phenytoin clearance by valproic acid in normal subjects. *British Journal of Clinical Pharmacology*, 8, 553.

Furlanut, M., Benetello, P., Avogaro, A. & Dainese, R. (1978) Effects of folic acid on phenytoin kinetics in healthy subjects. *Clinical Pharmacology and Therapeutics*, 24, 294.

Garrettson, L.K., Perel, J.M. & Dayton, P.G. (1969) Methylphenidate interaction with both anticonvulsants and ethyl-biscoumacetate. *Journal of the American Medical Association*, 207, 2053.

Greenblatt, D.J., Shader, R.I., Hármatz, J.S., Franke, K. & Koch-Weser, J. (1976) Influences of magnesium and aluminium hydroxyde mixture on chlordiazepoxide absorption. *Clinical Pharmacology and Therapeutics*, 19, 234.

Hahn, T.J. (1976) Bone complications of anticonvulsants. *Drugs*, 12, 201.

Hammer, W., Idestrom, C-M. & Sjöqvist, F. (1967) In Garattini, S. & Dukes, M.N.G. (eds) *Proceedings of the First International Symposium on Antidepressant Drugs, Milan 1966, Minerva Medica International Congress Series*, 122, 301.

Hansen, J.M., Kampmann, J.P., Siersbaek-Nielsen, K., Lumholtz, I.B., Arrøe, M., Abildgaard, V. & Skovsted, L. (1979) The effect of different sulfonamides on phenytoin metabolism in man. *Acta Medica Scandinavica (Supplement)*, 624, 106.

Hansen, J.M., Kristensen, M., Skovsted, L. & Christensen, L.K. (1966) Dicoumarol-induced diphenylhydantoin intoxication. *Lancet*, ii, 265.

Hansen, J.M., Kristensen, M. & Skovsted, L. (1968) Sulthiame (Ospolot®) as inhibitor of diphenylhydantoin metabolism. *Epilepsia*, 9, 17.

Hansen, J.M., Siersbaek-Nielsen, K., Kristensen, M., Skovsted, L. & Christensen, L.K. (1971a) Effect of diphenylhydantoin on the metabolism of dicoumarol in man. *Acta Medica Scandinavica*, 189, 15.

Hansen, J.M., Siersbaek-Nielsen, K. & Skovsted, L. (1971b) Carbamazepine induced acceleration of diphenylhydantoin and warfarin metabolism in man. *Clinical Pharmacology and Therapeutics*, 12, 539.

Heipertz, R. & Pilz, H. (1978) Interaction of nitrofurantoin with diphenylhydantoin. *Journal of Neurology*, 218, 297.

Helleberg, L., Rubin, A., Wolen, R.L., Rodda, B.E., Ridolfo, A.S. & Gruber, C.N. Jr. (1974) A pharmacokinetic interaction in man between phenobarbitone and fenoprofen, a new anti-inflammatory agent. *British Journal of Clinical Pharmacology*, 1, 371.

Hempel, E. & Klinger, W. (1976) Drug stimulated biotransformation of hormonal steroid contraceptives: clinical implications. *Drugs*, 12, 442.

Herishanu, Y., Eylath, U. & Ilan, R. (1976) Effect of calcium content of diet on absorption of diphenylhydantoin. *Israel Journal of Medical Science*, 12, 1453.

Hewick, D.S., Sparks, R.G., Stevenson, I.H. & Watson, I.D. (1977) Induction of imipramine metabolism following barbiturate administration. *British Journal of Clinical Pharmacology*, 4, 399.

Houghton, G.W. & Richens, A. (1974a) The effect of benzodiazepines and pheneturide on phenytoin metabolism in man. *British Journal of Clinical Pharmacology*, 1, 344.

Houghton, G.W. & Richens, A. (1974b) Phenytoin intoxication induced by sulthiame in epileptic patients. *Journal of Neurology, Neurosurgery and Psychiatry*, 37, 275.

Hurwitz, A. (1977) Antacid therapy and drug kinetics. *Clinical Phamacokinetics*, 2, 269.

Jeavons, P.M., Clark, J.E. & Maheshwari, M.C. (1977) Treatment of generalized epilepsies of childhood and adolescence with sodium valproate (Epilim). *Developmental Medicine and Child Neurology*, 19, 9.

Jelliffe, R.W. & Blankenhorn, D.H. (1966) Effect of phenobarbital on digitoxin metabolism. *Clinical Research*, 14, 160.

Jubiz, W., Meikle, A.W., Levinson, R.A., Mizutanic, S., West, C.D. & Tyler, F.H. (1970) Effect of diphenylhydantoin on the metabolism of dexamethasone. *New England Journal of Medicine*, 283, 11.

Karch, F.E., Wardell, W.M., Danably, M. & Gringeri, A. (1977) Effect of halofenate on the serum binding of phenytoin. *British Journal of Clinical Pharmacology*, 4, 625.

Koch-Weser, J. & Sellers, E.S. (1976) Binding of drugs to serum albumin. *New England Journal of Medicine*, 294, 311 & 526.

Koranyi, L. & Gero, L. (1979) Influence of diphenylhydantoin on the effect of streptozotocin. *British Medical Journal*, 1, 127.

Koup, J.R., Gibaldi, M., McNamara, P., Hilligoss, D.M., Colburn, W.A. & Bruck, E. (1978) Interaction of chloramphenicol with phenytoin and phenobarbital. *Clinical Pharmacology and Therapeutics*, 24, 571.

Kulshrestha, V.K., Thomas, M., Wadsworth, J. & Richens, A. (1978) Interaction between phenytoin and antacids. *British Journal of Clinical Pharmacology*, 6, 177.

Kutt, H. (1971) Biochemical and genetical factors regulating Dilantin® metabolism in man. *Annals of the New York Academy of Sciences*, 179, 704.

Kutt, H. (1972) Diphenylhydantoin. Interactions with other drugs in man, In *Antiepileptic Drugs*. ed. Woodbury, D.M., Penry, J.K. & Schmidt, R.P., p. 169. New York: Raven Press.

Kutt, H. (1975) Interactions of antiepileptic drugs. *Epilepsia*, 16, 393.

Kutt, H., Brennan, R., Dehejia, H. & Verebely, K. (1970) Diphenylhydantoin intoxication. A complication of isoniazid therapy. *American Review of Respiratory Disease*, **101**, 377.

Kutt, H. & Louis, S. (1972) Anticonvulsant drugs. II Clinical pharmacological therapeutic aspects. *Current Therapy*, **13**, 59.

Lai, A.A., Levy, R.H. & Cutler, R.E. (1978) Time course of interaction between carbamazepine and clonazepam in normal man. *Clinical Pharmacology and Therapeutics*, **24**, 316.

Levi, A.J., Sherlock, S. & Walker, D. (1968) Phenylbutazone and isoniazid metabolism in patients with liver disease in relation to previous drug therapy. *Lancet*, **ii**, 1275.

Loga, S., Curry, S. & Lader, M. (1975) Interactions of orphenadrine and phenobarbitone with chlorpromazine; plasma concentrations and effects in man. *British Journal of Clinical Pharmacology*, **2**, 197.

Lunde, P.K.M., Rane, A., Yaffe, S.J., Lund, L. & Sjöqvist, F. (1970) Plasma protein binding of diphenylhydantoin in man. *Clinical Pharmacology and Therapeutics*, **11**, 846.

MacDonald, M.G. & Robinson, D.S. (1968) Clinical observations of possible barbiturate interference with anticoagulation. *Journal of the American Medical Association*, **204**, 97.

MacLeod, S.M., Sellers, E.M., Giles, H.G., Billings, B.J., Martin, P.R., Greenblatt, D.J. & Marshman, J.A. (1978) Interaction of disulfiram with benzodiazepines. *Clinical Pharmacology and Therapeutics*, **24**, 583.

Makki, K.A., Perucca, E. & Richens, A. (1980) Metabolic effects of folic acid replacement therapy in folate deficient epileptic patients. In Johannessen, S.I., Morselli, P.L., Pippenger, C.E., Richens, A., Schmidt, D. & Meinardi, H. (eds) *Antiepileptic Therapy: Advances in Drug Monitoring*, p. 391. New York: Raven Press.

Mattson, R.H., Cramer, J.A., Williamson, P.D. & Novelly, R.A. (1978) Valproic acid in epilepsy: clinical and pharmacological effects. *Annals of Neurology*, **3**, 20.

Mattson, R.H., Gallagher, B.B., Reynolds, E.H. & Glass, D. (1973) Folate therapy in epilepsy. A controlled study. *Archives of Neurology (Chicago)*, **29**, 78.

McLelland, J. & Jack W. (1978) Phenytoin/dexamethasone interaction: a clinical problem. *Lancet*, **i**, 1096.

Meikle, A.W., Jubiz, W., Matsukura, S., West, C.D. & Tyler, F.H. (1969) Effect of diphenylhydantoin on the metabolism of metyrapone and release of ACTH in man. *Journal of Clinical Endocrinology*, **29**, 1553.

Monks, A., Boobis, S., Wadsworth, J. & Richens, A. (1978) Plasma protein binding interaction between phenytoin and valproic acid *in vitro*. *British Journal of Clinical Pharmacology*, **6**, 487.

Morselli, P., Rizzo, M. & Garattini, S. (1971) Interaction between phenobarbital and diphenylhydantoin in animals and in epileptic patients. *Annals of the New York Academy of Sciences*, **179**, 88.

Murray, F.J. (1962) Outbreak of unexpected reactions among epileptics taking isoniazid. *American Review of Respiratory Disease*, **86**, 729.

Nanda, R.N., Johnson, R.H., Keogh, H.J., Lambie, D.G. & Melville, I.D. (1977) Treatment of epilepsy with clonazepam and its effect on other anticonvulsants. *Journal of Neurology, Neurosurgery and Psychiatry*, **40**, 538.

Neuvonen, P.J., Elfving, S.M. & Elonen, E. (1978) Reduction of absorption of digoxin, phenytoin and aspirin by activated charcoal in man. *European Journal of Clinical Pharmacology*, **13**, 213.

Neuvonen, P.J. & Penttila, O. (1974) Interaction between doxycycline and barbiturates. *British Medical Journal*, **1**, 535.

Neuvonen, P.J., Lehtovaara, R., Bardy, A. & Elonen, E. (1979) Antipyretic analgesics in patients on antiepileptic drug therapy. *European Journal of Clinical Pharmacology*, **15**, 263.

O'Brien, L.S., Orme, M.l'E. & Breckenridge, A.M. (1978) Failure of antacids to alter the pharmacokinetics of phenytoin. *British Journal of Clinical Pharmacology*, **6**, 176.

Odar-Cederlof, I. & Borgå, O. (1976) Impaired plasma protein binding of phenytoin in uremia and displacement effect of salicylic acid. *Clinical Pharmacology and Therapeutics*, **20**, 36.

Olesen, O.V. (1967) The influence of disulfiram and calcium carbide on the serum diphenylhydantoin. Excretion of HPPH in the urine. *Archives of Neurology (Chicago)*, **16**, 642.

Padgham. C. & Richens, A. (1974) Quinine metabolism: a useful index of hepatic enzyme-induction in man? *British Journal of Clinical Pharmacology*, **1**, 352.

Patel, I.H., Levy, R.H. & Cutler, R.E. (1980) Phenobarbital-valproic acid interaction. *Clinical Pharmacology and Therapeutics*, **27**, 515.

Patsalos, P.N. & Lascelles, P.T. (1977) Effect of sodium valproate on plasma protein binding of diphenylhydantoin. *Journal of Neurology, Neurosurgery and Psychiatry*, **40**, 570.

Penttila, O., Neuvonen, P.J., Aho, K. & Lehtovaara, R. (1974) Interaction between doxycycline and some antiepileptic drugs. *British Medical Journal*, **2**, 470.

Perucca, E. (1978) Clinical consequences of microsomal enzyme-induction by antiepileptic drugs. *Pharmacology & Therapeutics*, **2**, 285.

Perucca, E. & Richens, A. (1977) Interaction between phenytoin and imipramine. *British Journal of Clinical Pharmacology*, **4**, 485.

Perucca, E. & Richens, A. (1979a) Paracetamol disposition in normal subjects and in patients treated with antiepileptic drugs. *British Journal of Clinical Pharmacology*, **7**, 201.

Perucca, E. & Richens, A. (1979b) Reduction of the oral availability of lignocaine by induction of first-pass metabolism in epileptic patients. *British Journal of Clinical Pharmacology*, **8**, 21.

Perucca, E. & Richens, A. (1980a) Antiepileptic drug interactions. In Tyrer, J. (ed.) *The treatment of Epilepsy*. Lancaster: MTD Press (in press).

Perucca, E. & Richens, A. (1980b) Reversal by phenytoin of carbamazepine-induced water intoxication; a pharmacokinetic interaction. *Journal of Neurology, Neurosurgery and Psychiatry*, **43**, 540.

Perucca, E., Garatt, S., Hebdige, S. & Richens, A. (1978b) Water intoxication in epileptic patients receiving carbamazepine. *Journal of Neurology, Neurosurgery and Psychiatry*, **41**, 713.

Perucca, E., Gatti, G., Frigo, G.M., Crema, A., Calzetti, S. & Visintini, D. (1978a) Disposition of sodium valproate in epileptic patients. *British Journal of Clinical Pharmacology*, **5**, 495.

Perucca, E., Hebdige, S., Gatti, G., Lecchini, S., Frigo, G.M. & Crema, A. (1980) Interaction between phenytoin and valproic acid: plasma protein binding and metabolic effects. *Clinical Pharmacology and Therapeutics*, **28**, 779.

Perucca, E., Hedges, A., Makki, K., Hebdige, S., Wadsworth, J. & Richens, A. (1979) The comparative enzyme-inducing properties of antiepileptic drugs. *British Journal of Clinical Pharmacology*, **7**, 414.

Petereit, L.B. & Meikle, A.W. (1977) Effectiveness of

prednisolone during phenytoin therapy. *Clinical Pharmacology and Therapeutics*, 22, 912.

Pugh, R.N.H., Geddes, A.M. & Yeoman, W.B. (1975) Interaction of phenytoin and chlorpheniramine. *British Journal of Clinical Pharmacology*, 2, 173.

Rambeck, B. (1979) Pharmacological interactions of mesuximide with phenobarbital and phenytoin in hospitalized epileptic patients. *Epilepsia*, 20, 147.

Rane, A., Hojer, B. & Wilson, J.T. (1976) Kinetics of carbamazepine and its 10, 11-epoxide in children. *Clinical Pharmacology and Therapeutics*, 19, 276.

Reynolds, E.H. (1976) Neurological aspects of folate and B12 metabolism. *Clinics in Haematology*, 5, 661.

Reynolds, E.H., Fenton, G., Fenwick, P., Johnson, A.L. & Laundy, M. (1975) Interaction of phenytoin and primidone. *British Medical Journal*, 2, 594.

Richens, A. (1976) *Drug treatment of epilepsy*. p. 108. London: Henry Kimpton.

Richens, A. & Ahmad, S. (1975) Controlled trial of sodium valproate in severe epilepsy. *British Medical Journal*, 4, 255.

Richens, A. & Houghton, G.W. (1975) Effect of drug therapy on the metabolism of phenytoin. In Schneider, H., Janz, D., Gardner-Thorpe, C., Meinardi, H. & Sherwin, A.L. (eds) *Clinical Pharmacology of Anti-epileptic Drugs*, p. 87. Berlin: Springer-Verlag.

Richens, A. & Woodford, F.P. (1976) *Anticonvulsant drugs and enzyme-induction*. Amsterdam: Associated Scientific Press.

Riegelman, S., Rowland, M. & Epstein, W.L. (1970) Griseofulvin-phenobarbital interaction in man. *Journal of the American Medical Association*, 213, 426.

Roe, T.F., Podosin, R.L. & Blaskovics, M.E. (1975) Drug interaction: diazoxide and diphenylhydantoin. *Journal of Pediatrics*, 9, 285.

Schneider, H. (1975) Carbamazepine: the influence of other anti-convulsants drugs on its serum level; first results. In Schneider, H., Janz, D., Gardner-Thorpe, C., Meinardi, H. & Sherwin, A.L. (eds) *Clinical Pharmacology of Antiepileptics Drugs*, p. 189. Heidelberg: Springer-Verlag.

Schobben, F., Vree, T.B. & van der Kleijn, E. (1978) Pharmacokinetics, metabolism and distribution of 2-N-propyl-pentanoate (sodium valproate) and the influence of salicylate comedication. In Meinardi, H. & Rowan, A.J. (eds) *Advances in Epileptology*, p. 271. Amsterdam: Swets and Zeitlinger.

Sellers, E.M. & Koch-Weser, J. (1970) Potentiation of warfarin-induced hypoprothrombinemia by chloral hydrate. *New England Journal of Medicine*, 283, 827.

Shader, R.I., Anastasios, G., Greenblatt, D.J., Harmatz, J.S. & Divoll Allen, M. (1978) Impaired absorption of desmethyldiazepam from clorazepate by magnesium-aluminium hydroxide. *Clinical Pharmacology and Therapeutics*, 24, 308.

Shahidi, N.T. (1968) Acetophenetidin-induced methemoglobinemia. *Annals of the New York Academy of Sciences*, 151, 822.

Skovsted, L., Kristensen, M., Hansen, J.M. & Siersbaek-Nielsen, K. (1976) The effect of different oral anticoagulants on diphenylhydantoin and tolbutamide metabolism. *Acta Medica Scandinavica*, 199, 513.

Sjö, O., Hvidberg, E.F., Naestoft, J. & Lund, M. (1975) Pharmacokinetics and side effects of clonazepam and its 7-amino metabolite in man. *European Journal of Clinical Pharmacology*, 8, 249.

Solomon, H.M., Reich, S., Spirt, N. & Abrams, W.B. (1971) Interaction between digitoxin and other drugs *in vitro* and *in vivo*. *Annals of the New York Academy of Sciences*, 179, 362. *Sciences*, 179, 362.

Solomon, H.M. & Schrogie, J.J. (1967) The effect of phenyramidol on the metabolism of diphenylhydantoin. *Clinical Pharmacology and Therapeutics*, 8, 554.

Sordillo, P., Sagransky, D.M., Mercado, R. & Michelis, M.F. (1978) Carbamazepine-induced syndrome of inappropriate antidiuretic hormone secretion. Reversal by concomitant phenytoin therapy. *Archives of Internal Medicine*, 138, 299.

Stambaugh, J.E., Warner, I.W., Hemphill, D.M. & Schwartz, I. (1977) A potentially toxic drug interaction between pethidine (meperidine) and phenobarbitone. *Lancet*, i, 398.

Stenzel, E., Boenigk, H.E. & Rambeck, B. (1978) Methsuximide in the treatment of epilepsy. *Epilepsia*, 19, 114.

Stiernholm, M.R. & Katz, F.H. (1975) Effects of diphenylhydantoin, phenobarbital and diazepam on metabolism of methylprednisolone and its sodium succinate. *Journal of Clinical Endocrinology and Metabolism*, 41, 887.

Sutton, G. & Kupferberg, H.J. (1975) Isoniazid as an inhibitor of primidone metabolism. *Neurology (Minneapolis)*, 25, 1179.

Svendsen, T.L., Kristensen, M.B., Hansen, J.M. & Skovsted, L. (1976) The influence of disulfiram on the half-life and clearance rate of diphenylhydantoin and tolbutamide in man. *European Journal of Clinical Pharmacology*, 9, 439.

Syversen, G.B., Morgan, J.P., Weintraub, M. & Myers, G.J. (1977) Acetazolamide-induced interference with primidone absorption: case reports and metabolic studies. *Archives of Neurology (Chicago)*, 34, 80.

Vesell, E.S. & Page, J.G. (1969) Genetic control of the phenobarbital-induced shortening of plasma antipyrine half-lives in man. *Journal of Clinical Investigation*, 48, 2202.

Viala, A., Cano, J.P., Dravet, L., Tassinari, C.A., Roger, J. & Angeletti-Philippe, A. (1971) Blood levels of diazepam (Valium) and N-desmethyl-diazepam in the epileptic child. A preliminary report. *Psychiatria, Neurologia & Neurochirurgia (Amsterdam)*, 74, 153.

Viukari, N.M.A. (1968) Folic acid and anticonvulsants. *Lancet*, i, 980.

Waddell, W.J. & Butler, T.C. (1957) The distribution and excretion of phenobarbital. *Journal of Clinical Investigation*, 36, 1217.

Werk, E.E., Choi, Y., Sholiton, L., Olinger, C. & Haque, N. (1969) Interference in the effect of dexamethasone by diphenylhydantoin. *New England Journal of Medicine*, 281, 32.

Werk, E.E., McGee, J. & Sholiton, L.J. (1964) Effect of diphenylhydantoin on cortisol metabolism in man. *Journal of Clinical Investigation*, 43, 1284.

Wesseling, H. & Mols-Thürkow, I. (1975) Interaction of diphenylhydantoin (DPH) and tolbutamide in man. *European Journal of Clinical Pharmacology*, 8, 75.

Whittaker, J.A. & Price-Evans, D.A. (1970) Genetic control of phenylbutazone metabolism in man. *British Medical Journal*, 4, 323.

Wilenski, A.J., Levy, R.H., Troupin, A.S., Moretti-Ojemann, L. & Friel, P. (1978) Clorazepate kinetics in treated epileptics. *Clinical Pharmacology and Therapeutics*, 24, 22.

Wright, N. & Prescott, L.F. (1973) Potentiation by previous drug therapy of hepatotoxicity following paracetamol overdosage. *Scottish Medical Journal*, 18, 56.

9

Neuroradiology

B.E. Kendall

INTRODUCTION

The logical application of neuroradiological procedures to the study of epilepsy depends on a clear understanding of the advantages, limitations and potential morbidity of the various tests. The clinical features which influence the probability of demonstrating a causative lesion and its likely nature have been discussed in Chapter 4, and the significance of an underlying structural lesion in management and in assessment of prognosis has been stressed.

Some epileptic patients require no radiological study. These include those who suffer from typical absence seizures in which there are no demonstrable structural changes, and those in which clinical study resolves the nature of the lesion and its treatment as, for example, some cases of tuberous sclerosis and disseminated neoplasm. Ideally, all other patients should have just the radiological study or selection of studies relevant to their particular treatment, preferring always the safest test if there are real alternatives. However, the approach must vary with the clinical problem and when it is evident that a study carrying a risk of morbidity is necessary and that it alone is likely to be sufficient, preliminary time-consuming less invasive tests should be avoided.

Neuroradiological procedures fall naturally into two important groups; firstly, those which cause no significant discomfort to the patient, carry no risk of morbidity and do not require admission to hospital, and, secondly, those which involve injections into blood vessels or into the cerebro-spinal fluid and which are unpleasant and, even in ideal conditions, carry a small risk of permanent morbidity. In the first group skull and chest X-ray,

computer tomography (CT) and isotope encephalography may be relevant to the study of epilepsy. There is no positive contraindication to the use of any or all of these procedures and the extent of their application is primarily a matter of the finance to procure the equipment and to employ a sufficient number of trained personnel to ensure an adequate service. When, even with the best use of available resources, machine time is limited, the study of epileptic patients in the clinical categories which yield a relatively small number of detectable structural lesions has a low priority.

All these neuroradiological studies need skilled radiography; the detection of slight abnormalities and the assessment of borderline normal findings is dependent on excellent technique. It should be understood clearly that worthwhile results can only be achieved when the head is completely immobile which requires co-operating or adequately sedated patients and the clinician should ensure that the patients whom he refers are in a suitable condition for the examination to be performed.

PLAIN X-RAYS

When radiology is indicated it usually starts with plain X-rays of the chest and skull. It may be strongly argued that plain skull X-rays and indeed gamma encephalography are so frequently negative in the presence of significant pathology that they are not useful as screening tests and that any patient with epilepsy requiring radiological study should first be submitted to a plain CT scan. CT increased positive findings from 30 per cent to 55 per cent and the number of tumours detected from 5 per cent up to 10 per cent when compared with all other studies (Gastaut & Gastaut, 1976) and is therefore the best screening test. Where the facilities are available this approach is both logical and economical.

Nevertheless plain films are frequently made prior to referral or at some time during the study and they may reveal significant abnormalities. When skull films are abnormal, some change is usually visible on the lateral projection, and because of the importance of alterations in the pituitary fossa in the recognition of intracranial hypertension, the film should be centred on the sella. On a good quality film there is an intact cortex over the sella in all normal cases.

Raised intracranial pressure

Raised intracranial pressure causes erosion of the inner table of the skull, which is usually first recognised by loss of part of the cortex of the sella, most frequently at the junction of the posterior wall and floor. Erosion of the tip of the dorsum may occur, especially when a dilated third ventricle extends into contact with it. But it should be noted that suprasellar tumours may cause similar change. The incidence of erosion in patients with tumours remote from the sella varies, but it is present in over 25 per cent reaching 44 per cent in

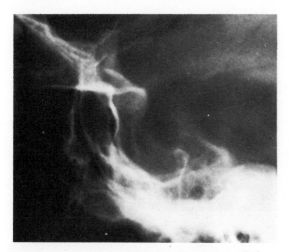

Fig. 9.1 Lateral view of sella turcica. The dorsum sella is short. The anterior wall of the sella is elongated. The appearances indicate chronic hydrocephalus with enlargement of the IIIrd ventricle, often due to aqueduct stenosis.

those studied by Mahmoud (1958); about 20 per cent of such patients have no papilloedema or other clinical evidence of raised intracranial pressure.

Aqueduct stenosis, which may present with fits, is the commonest cause of changes in the sella characteristic of chronic hydrocephalus with enlargement of the third ventricle. There is shortening of the dorsum sellae with elongation of the anterior wall of the sella; the anterior clinoid processes tend to be large (Fig. 9.1).

When intracranial hypertension has been present since before the age of ten years the sutures may be wider than 2 mm or have elongated interdigitations. These changes are most reliably assessed on a basal projection on which the coronal and sagittal sutures are close to the film.

Physiological calcification

Calcification in the pineal body and/or habenular commissure is visible on the lateral film in about 60 per cent of European adults; it is much less frequent in African and Asiatic races and in children. It is more difficult to visualise on the antero-posterior projection due to the relatively greater thickness of the frontal and occipital bones but with careful attention to technical factors, about 75 per cent of those shown in the lateral view can be identified. Deviation of more than 2.5 mm from the midline on a straight film is usually due to displacement by a contralateral mass though rarely it is due to ipsilateral atrophy.

Calcification in the choroid plexus of the lateral ventricles is visible in about 10 per cent of normal adults. Though most usual in the trigone region, it can occur elsewhere and is not infrequently unilateral or asymmetrical. Displacement can only be diagnosed definitely when the calcification is outside the range of the normal curve of the choroid plexus.

Plaques of ossification commonly occur in the dura lining the vault, in the falx and the tentorium. Curvilinear or circular calcified opacities are frequent in the walls of the intracavernous segments of the internal carotid artery in elderly patients. The typical shape and position of these densities facilitates recognition and they should not be mistaken for significant lesions.

Pathological calcification

This occurs in many conditions which may cause epilepsy. Frequently, calcification is not specific but its appearance in a particular position may be diagnostic or it may be associated with other plain film changes making a diagnostic combination.

Care should be taken to ensure that any abnormal density is within the cranium and not a superimposed artefact such as EEG paste on the scalp; tangential projections may be necessary to confirm its position.

Tumours

Calcification visible on skull X-ray is present in 10–15 per cent of meningiomas, sometimes outlining the whole of their extent. When a considerable part of the tumour is involved, the appearance and the position of the calcification, which is usually close to the dura, suggests the diagnosis (Fig. 9.2). There are often other abnormalities on the plain X-ray, such as hyperostosis at the tumour attachment or enlarged meningeal grooves leading up to it (Gold *et al.*, 1969).

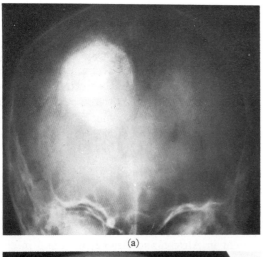
(a)

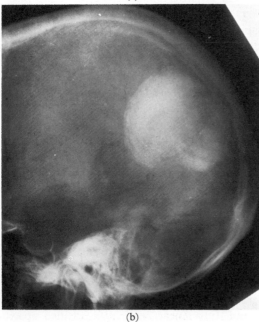
(b)

Fig. 9.2 Plain X-rays of skull. (a) Antero-posterior, (b) lateral projections. A well defined cloud of calcification is present in the right posterior parietal parafalcine region. A prominent meningeal vascular groove ascends towards the lesion. The appearances are typical of a meningioma with calcification in psammoma bodies.

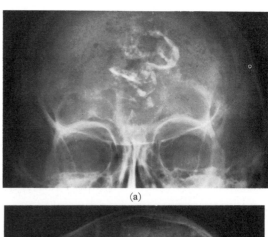
(a)

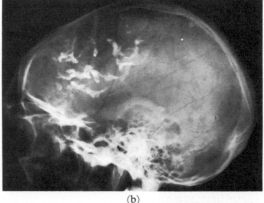
(b)

Fig. 9.3 (a) Antero-posterior, (b) lateral projections. Gyriform curvilinear calcification is shown in the medial frontal region on both sides of the midline but extending further to the left. The appearances are typical of a glioma. This was an oligodendroglioma but an astrocytoma can cause similar findings.

Calcification is visible in only 5.5 per cent of gliomas (Kalan & Burrows 1961), being more frequent in the relatively benign ones. Its extent varies from one or two tiny dots or larger nodules to an irregular conglomeration of nodules or an amorphous aggregate. The most typical appearance is of one or more curvilinear streaks, suggesting gyri, which occurs in both astrocytomas and the less common oligodendrogliomas (Fig. 9.3).

When calcification is found in more aggressive gliomas it suggests that malignant change has occurred in a more benign tumour. Hamartomas which occur most commonly in the temporal lobe may show non-specific calcification, which is usually mistaken for a glioma until histology is obtained.

Tuberous sclerosis

The dysplastic lesions of tuberous sclerosis often undergo progressive calcification in older children causing nodular and curvilinear densities, which are most frequently adjacent to the ventricular system and in the basal ganglia, though they may also occur in other sites (Fig. 9.4). The tubers may obstruct the ventricular system and cause hydrocephalus, but raised intracranial pressure should arouse suspicion of a giant cell astrocytoma, which also occurs in tuberous sclerosis and CT should be performed.

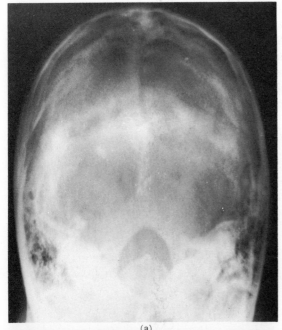

(a)

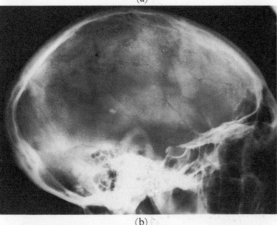

(b)

Fig. 9.4 (a) Antero-posterior, (b) lateral projections. Nodular calcification is present in the region of the basal ganglia on the right side and near the inferior surface of the right cerebellar hemisphere. Several sclerotic areas are present in the bones of the vault. The combination is typical of tuberous sclerosis.

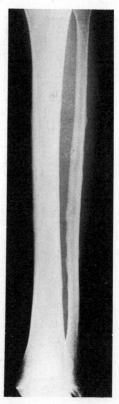

Fig. 9.5 Nodular cortical thickening is shown on the tibia and fibula due to the typical periosteal nodes of tuberous sclerosis.

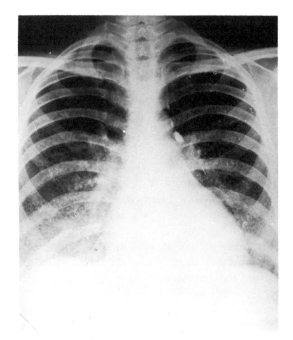

Fig. 9.6 Chest X-ray. There is dense, fine nodular and reticular shadowing, most marked towards the bases due to smooth muscle infiltration in tuberous sclerosis.

Although a family history, typical skin manifestations or associated mental retardation has usually suggested the diagnosis, these features are sometimes absent. Further plain film evidence of the associated mesodermal dysplasia may occur in any of the bones, but especially in those of the hands and feet, which may show subperiosteal cysts or nodular cortical thickening (Fig 9.5), and sclerotic areas, as well as pressure erosion from subungual fibromas. In a small number of patients the lungs are infiltrated by smooth muscle, which causes a honeycomb appearance on chest X-rays (Fig. 9.6). Spontaneous pneumothorax is a not infrequent complication. Multiple renal hamartomas, which are usually bilateral, can be shown by intravenous pyelography or computed tomography. Intestinal polyps have also been described.

Inflammatory disease

Non-specific calcification occurs occasionally in necrotic tissues such as old abscesses and multiple nodules may be present in dead parasites. The his-

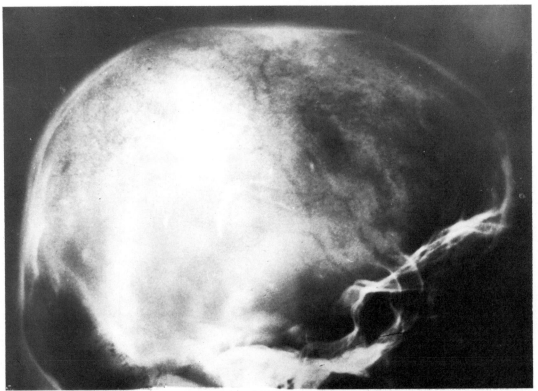

Fig. 9.7 Lateral X-ray of skull. There are multiple nodular calcified lesions. Curvilinear calcification is present in one of the basal ganglia. The dorsum sella is shortened due to erosion by an enlarged IIIrd ventricle secondary to aqueduct obstruction caused by the disease. The appearance is typical of toxoplasmosis.

tory and examination will usually have suggested the diagnosis and the radiological findings are merely confirmatory.

Combined linear cortical and curvilinear basal ganglia calcifications occur in about 40 per cent of cases of congenital toxoplasmosis and are diagnostic in the clinical context (Fig. 9.7). Hydrocephalus, due to occlusion of the aqueduct or outlets of the fourth ventricle, or microcephaly secondary to destruction of brain substance occur in about 50 per cent of patients.

Cysticercosis may be confirmed by showing calcified cysts in the skeletal muscles. They may be recognised incidentally in neck and shoulder girdle muscles on films of the skull (Fig. 9.8) and chest, but are usually searched for in soft tissue films of the thighs (Fig. 9.9). They are typically about 3 mm in diameter and 12 to 15 mm in length and lie parallel to the axis of the muscle fibres. Calcification is much less frequent in the cerebral cysts and is usually only present in the scolices, showing as nodules about 3 mm in diameter. Racemose cysticerci may obstruct the ventricles and cause signs of raised intracranial pressure.

Tuberculomas, which are the commonest intracranial masses in India, may also show non-specific nodular calcification. A very rare but typical calcification occurs in the walls of cysts, which are usually in the parietal regions, in cases infected with the cerebral form of paragonamiasis. It is

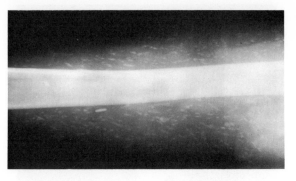

Fig. 9.9 Right thigh. A large number of fusiform calcified lesions due to cysticerci in the muscles.

endemic in the far east and may be found in visitors from Korea, China and Formosa.

Vascular lesions

Fine curvilinear or nodular calcification is present on X-rays in about 15 per cent of intracranial arterio-venous malformations (Fig. 9.10). It usually occurs in the walls of the abnormal veins; which are sometimes aneurysmal and may then cause large ring shadows, but it can also be deposited within old haemorrhages. Meningeal arteries may contribute to the blood supply of the malformation; enlargement of foraminae transmitting vessels and of vascular grooves and channels in the cranial vault may further support the diagnosis.

In the Sturge-Weber syndrome, characteristic sinuous double lines of calcification are laid down in superficial layers of the atrophic cortex underly-

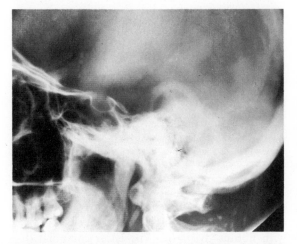

Fig. 9.8 Lateral skull. Fusiform nobular shadows of calcified cysticerci are present in the neck and facial muscles. Nodular calcification is also present in the frontal and parietal lobes in the scolices of intracerebral cysticerci.

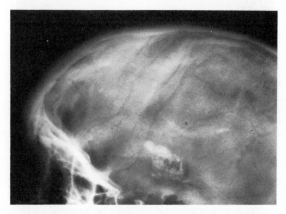

Fig. 9.10 Lateral projection of skull. Aggregates of nodular calcification are shown in the inferior frontal region. These were shown by angiography to be in an angiomatous malformation.

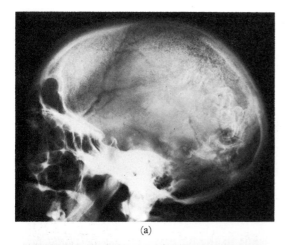

(a)

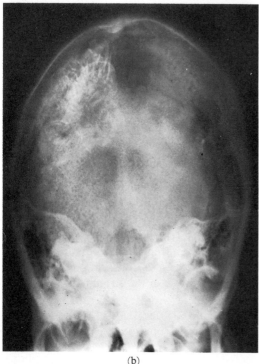

(b)

Fig. 9.11 Plain X-rays of skull. (a) Lateral, (b) antero-posterior. Typical gyriform calcification in the Sturge-Weber syndrome is shown in the right posterior parietal and occipital regions. The right side of the vault is considerably smaller than the left due to associated hemi-atrophy.

ing the meningeal angioma, which is usually in the occipital and posterior parietal regions (Fig. 9.11). Calcification is only evident on skull X-ray in 50–60 per cent of cases. It may be seen as early as 18 months of age but often increases in density up to adult life.

New bone formation

Localised thickening of the inner table of the skull is commonly present at the site of attachment of a meningioma arising near bone. It is sometimes associated with sclerosis of the adjacent diploe and less frequently with bone formation on the outer table of the skull also. Enlarged and tortuous meningeal vascular channels extending to the hyperostosis, and pits in the bone where small branches from the meningeal and scalp arteries perforate the bone to supply the tumour are useful confirmatory signs (Fig. 9.12). Diploic vascular channels may also be prominent but their significance is more difficult to assess because of considerable normal variation. Bone reaction to solitary metastases from carcinoma of the prostate or breast may simulate a meningioma but extension of sclerosis into the facial bones and signs of the disease elsewhere may be present and help to differentiate.

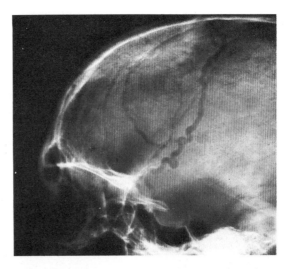

Fig. 9.12 Lateral X-ray of skull. Localised sclerosis is evident in the superior frontal region. The groove of the middle meningeal artery is enlarged and tortuous and branches of the vessel extend to the abnormal bone. Large diploic vascular shadows are also shown. The changes are diagnostic of a frontal convexity meningioma.

Meningioma-en-plaque (Fig. 9.13) typically produces a more diffuse and extensive sclerosis of bone, usually at the base, which can be confused with fibrous dysplasia. The latter condition does not cause epilepsy and would only be an incidental finding. In its sclerotic form the bone is thick-

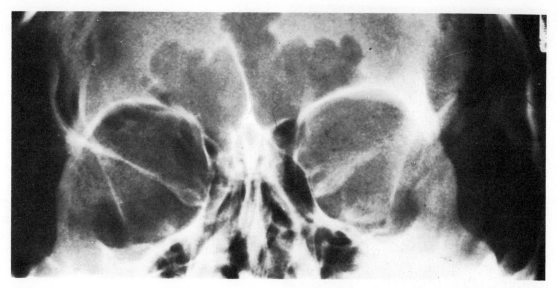

Fig. 9.13 Antero-posterior X-rays of skull. There is sclerosis of the left lesser and greater wings of the sphenoid due to a meningioma.

ened and has a more homogeneous chalky density without trabecular structure.

Bone erosion

Meningioma causes erosion alone much less frequently than sclerosis and hyperostosis. Such erosion is usually ill-defined but, more extensive on the inner aspect of the vault and is usually accom-

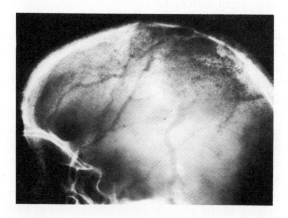

Fig. 9.14 Lateral X-ray of skull. There is a large area of diminished density high in the right parietal and frontoparietal regions. Enlarged meningeal vascular channels extend towards the lesion and large diploic venous changes drain away from it. The changes are diagnostic of a meningioma but lysis is much less common than sclerosis in these tumours.

panied by enlarged meningeal channels. This combination strongly suggests the diagnosis (Fig. 9.14).

Metastases and the rarer primary tumours of bone are a most unusual cause of fits. They usually commence within and cause more extensive destruction of the diploe, which is generally evident on tangential projections.

Pressure from any sub-adjacent mass such as a superficial glioma, a meningioma or a porencephalic or arachnoid cyst may cause smooth corticated erosion of the inner table or localised expansion of the overlying vault. This may be apparent on the routine views but it may be necessary to confirm it by tangential projections.

Cerebral hypoplasia or atrophy

Much stress has been placed on the role of plain films in the diagnosis of cerebral hypoplasia or atrophy of early onset. Because growth of the skull is secondary to that of the underlying brain, which takes place mainly in the first two years of life, radiological findings are most marked when the lesion occurs early in this period. Less marked changes may be seen with severe damage occurring later but before puberty.

When a lesion is unilateral the capacity of the

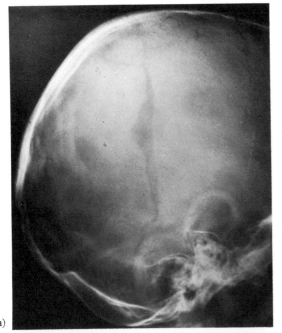

(a)

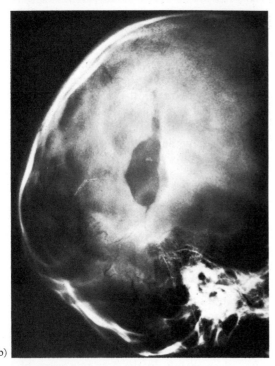

(b)

Fig. 9.15 Lateral X-rays of skull. (a) A linear cleft is shown extending vertically in one of the parietal bones. It is wider than a fresh fracture and trauma had occurred three months previous to the present X-ray. (b) Seven months later. The fracture is considerably wider. At surgery a tear in the dura and arachnoid was found associated with lepto-meningeal cyst formation.

skull over the smaller hemisphere or lobe is less than that of the corresponding region on the normal side. This may be recognised by flattening of the vault, elevation of the base with enlargement of the air cavities in the sinuses or mastoids and deviation of the falx or superior sagittal sinuses towards the affected side. The skull overlying the atrophic lobe is usually thickened but, if there is a wide fluid-filled space between the atrophic lesion and the vault, it may be thinned and smooth. Such changes are obvious when marked, but the borderline between minor degrees of relative asymmetry, such as a short and narrow temporal fossa, and the limits of normal variation are not clearly defined. CT has reduced the importance of such secondary signs by assessing atrophic lesions more directly.

Post-traumatic epilepsy

Linear fractures, especially in young patients, usually heal without trace. In depressed fractures, deformity remains and occasionally bone fragments may be shown projecting medially from the edge; these are commonly associated with scarring in the adjacent brain. When the dura is torn the fracture line may widen (Fig. 9.15). In adults this is associated with lepto-meningeal cyst formation which causes bevelled thinning of the inner table beyond the limits of the fracture, over the area of the cyst. In children erosion may occur due to brain, often with cystic change, or to an overlying cyst in direct contact with the bone. The cyst sometimes herniates through the fracture line and expands under the scalp, causing erosion of the outer table. Widening fractures, especially in children, are usually associated with underlying brain damage.

A meningo-cerebral cicatrix may result in expansion of the ventricle or formation of an arachnoid cyst and, even in the absence of fracture, trauma may cause sufficient contusion and haemorrhage to form an intracerebral cyst. Any of these conditions may incite thinning or lateral bulging of the adjacent inner table; in all of them the pathology is well shown by CT.

CHEST X-RAYS

The importance of the lungs as a mirror of systemic disease needs no emphasis. Bronchial carcinoma is by far the commonest tumour metastasising to the brain. When other primary neoplasms are responsible, secondary deposits are also frequently present in the lungs. Occasionally, evidence of unsuspected cardiac lesions or of chronic lung disease is first revealed on routine chest films.

A specific diagnosis which requires no further radiological investigation may be possible from the plain X-rays of skull and chest. They may show, for example, a primary bronchial carcinoma or evidence of metastases or of calcified parasites, extensive glioma, tuberous sclerosis or Sturge-Weber's syndrome. They may show a specific abnormality which needs further elucidation prior to curative surgery or suggest a focal lesion requiring further study to determine its nature by nonsurgical means or to display it in more detail prior to biopsy or excision. In such cases it may be evident that angiography will be required and it may be reasonable to use it as the next study.

In the large proportion of patients in which plain X-rays are normal or have quite reasonably been omitted as a first test as well as those with evidence of raised intracranial pressure and many others with non-specific abnormalities, computed tomography is the procedure of choice.

In practice, if there is no clinical evidence of a focal lesion and the plain X-rays are normal, it is so unusual to find an abnormality that it is reasonable not to perform a further study in such circumstances in children and in those in whom seizures have been present without personality changes since childhood.

COMPUTED TOMOGRAPHY (CT)

On plain X-rays it is only possible to recognise four densities equivalent to bone or calcification, soft tissue or water, fat and air. CT (Hounsfield, 1973) gives quantitative readings of tissue density, with resolution sufficient to distinguish between the various intracranial soft tissues. Clinical evaluation (Ambrose, 1973; Paxton & Ambrose, 1974; Gawler et al., 1974) left no doubt that CT would radically alter the scope and practice of cranial neuroradiology.

The method requires that the patient lies completely still for periods of between a few seconds and a minute, varying with the type of machine, while a series of contiguous sections of the head are scanned through their edges from a large number of directions, by a finely collimated beam of X-rays with a thickness of 8–13 mm. The intensity of the beam is measured before and after transmission through the head, and many readings are taken in each direction from different angles. A computer assembles the data from each section and, using a mathematical method, reconstructs it as a matrix of cells (pixels) between 0.75 and 1.5 mm square. A number approximating to within 0.5 per cent of the average absorption coefficient of the tissue volume (voxel) represented in each pixel is printed on it. This results in a format corresponding to the shape of the original

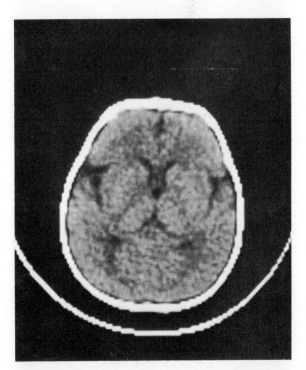

Fig. 9.16 Normal plain computed tomogram taken at level of foramen of Monro. The cerebral spinal fluid in the ventricular system and cerebral subarachnoid spaces is of lowest attenuation (0–6 H) and outlines the anterior horns and the trigones of the lateral ventricles, the upper part of the third ventricle and the Sylvian and interhemispheric fissures in this section. The hemispheric and capsular white matter (20–38 H) is easily distinguised from the grey matter (36–56 H) in the cerebral cortex, basal ganglia and thalami.

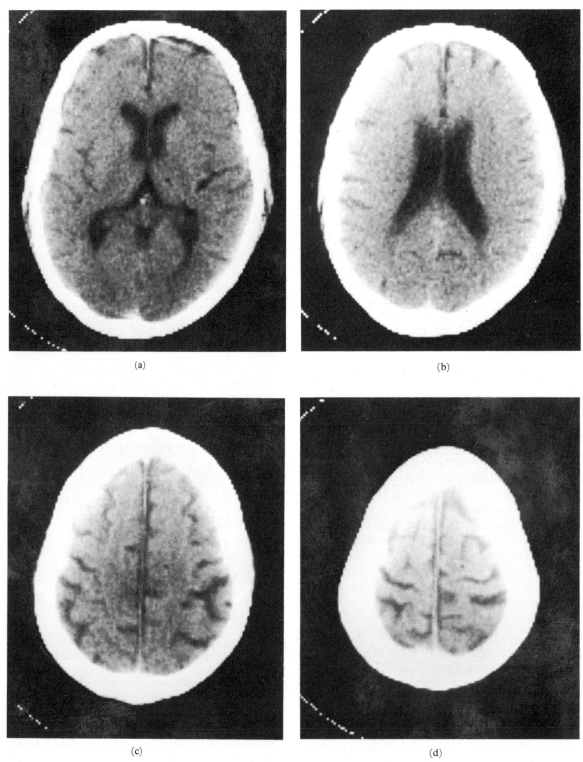

(a)

(b)

(c)

(d)

Fig. 9.17 Diffuse cerebral atrophy. Plain CT. Section level (a) third ventricle (b) upper parts of lateral ventricles (c,d) near vertex. The lateral ventricles and cortical sulci are enlarged. The cerebral substance is normal.

section. An image with corresponding points of variation of light intensity is simultaneously displayed on a cathode ray tube and can be recorded on film.

The most radiopaque tissue normally encountered in the skull is compact bone and the least is air; these have been made the extremes of a scale of absorption, of which water has been given a zero value and they have been placed arbitrarily at +1000 and −1000 Hounsfield units (HU) respectively. Most of the normal intracranial soft tissues fall into the narrow range of 0 to +60 HU. The grey matter of the cortex, caudate nucleus and thalamus has a value of +36 to +56 HU and can be distinguished (Fig. 9.16) from white matter which ranges between +20 and +38 HU with an average value of +24 HU. The pineal gland is always shown and the glomeri of the choroid plexuses are usually outlined due to calcification which is frequently insufficient to be shown on the plain films. Cerebro-spinal fluid with an absorption value of between 0 and +10 HU is shown, giving a close approximation to the configuration of the ventricles and intracranial subarachnoid space (Synek *et al.*, 1979). However, because of their small height relative to the depth of the section, the normal temporal horns may be averaged out by the brain tissue constituting the bulk of the section. Intravenous contrast media do not cross the blood-brain barrier, so that the attenuation of the normal brain is only increased by a relatively small amount (up to 5 HU) by them and this is due to the contrast medium within the bloodstream.

Repeat scanning following intravenous injection of contrast medium causes an increase in the attenuation of some lesions (Fig. 9.26) which is sometimes related to vascularity but more commonly to interstitial extravasation of contrast medium within the lesion or to abnormalities induced in the blood-brain barrier. Enhancement is of great value in detecting tumours which are of similar attenuation to adjacent normal or oedematous brain and it may be useful in other cases also to obtain the maximum information from CT. Cystic or necrotic regions, which do not increase in attenuation are more evident when surrounding tumour or abscess capsule is enhanced by contrast (Fig. 9.24).

Pathological findings

Atrophy and hydrocephalus

Generalised atrophy (Fig. 9.17), hemi- (Fig. 9.18) and focal atrophy, cortical and cerebellar atrophy (Fig. 9.19), hydrocephalus (Fig. 9.20) and cystic expansions of the ventricles or subarachnoid space are all clearly shown. The more minor degrees of dilatation of these structures including the atrophy associated with temporal sclerosis is not usually sufficient for detection (Polkey, 1978).

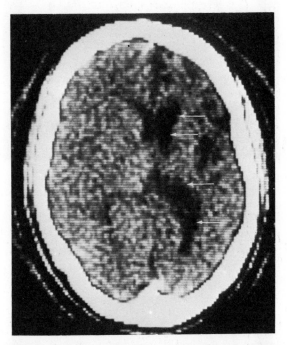

Fig. 9.18 Left hemiatrophy. CT at level just below bodies of lateral ventricles. The left lateral ventricle (arrows) is enlarged and displaced towards the left side. There is dilatation of insula and of cortical sulci over the left hemisphere.

Vascular lesions

A typical infarct (Fig. 9.21) shows as a low attenuation region involving both the white and cortical grey matter, sometimes wedge-shaped when in the distribution of a cortical artery and without displacement of adjacent structures. In a recent infarct however, oedema may cause the lesion to appear ill defined and may produce swelling which may suggest the possibility of a tumour. Repeat study may distinguish by showing a tendency of the infarct to resolve towards a more typical pic-

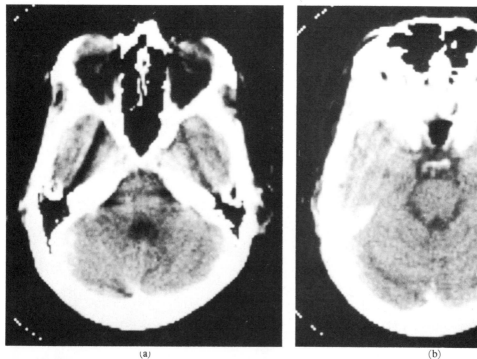

(a)   (b)

Fig. 9.19 Cerebellar cortical atrophy. Plain CT sections (a) level of fourth ventricle (b) including superior surface of cerebellar hemisphere. The fourth ventricle is prominent. The curvilinear dilated superior cerebellar sulci are evident in (b).

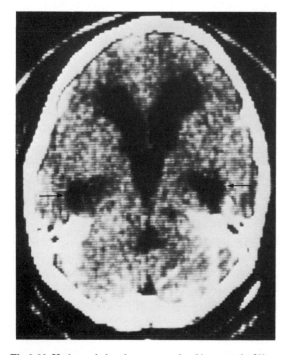

Fig 9.20 Hydrocephalus due to stenosis of lower end of the aqueduct. The dilated lateral and third ventricles and aqueduct are evident. The dilated posterior ends of the temporal horns are shown (arrows). The basal cisterns and cortical sulci are not dilated.

ture within a few days. The blood-brain barrier is damaged by infarction and enhancement may occur until recovery has taken place, which usually takes less than one month after the stroke, but can take up to ten weeks.

Sometimes infarction is patchy and shows as multiple regions of decreased attenuation in the distribution of the occluded vessel. An old infarct may eventually form a cyst which causes a sharply defined region of low attenuation, or a scar, associated with focal atrophy.

The attenuation of clotted blood (+56 to +80 HU) which increases as serum is expressed is sufficiently characteristic to allow recognition of a recent haematoma (Fig. 9.22). Angiography is necessary if details of a causative lesion need to be defined, but large aneurysms and angiomas can be identified by re-examination by CT after intravenous injection of contrast medium. As a clot is absorbed its density diminishes and eventually a cyst or scar, indistinguishable from an old infarct may remain.

Tumours

Neoplasms show as masses with varying degrees of

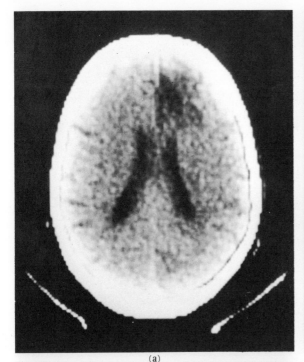

(a)

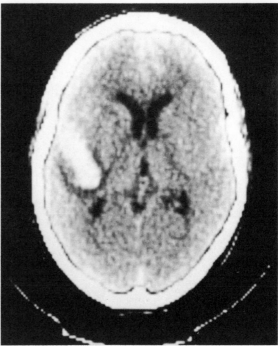

Fig. 9.22 Intracerebral haematoma. Plain CT. There is a region of homogeneously increased attenuation in the posterior part of the left temporal lobe with well demarcated surrounding low attenuation blood clot from a recent haemorrhage. There is also subarachnoid blood which accounts for the increased attenuation around the interhemispheric fissure anteriorly.

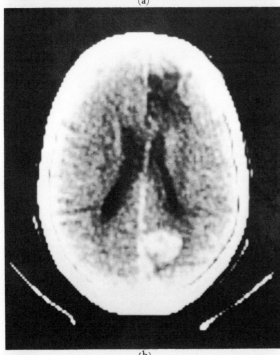

(b)

Fig. 9.21 Cerebral infarcts right frontal and parieto-occipital regions. (a) Plain scan: low attenuation lesions with no mass effect (b) after intravenous contrast medium. There is enhancement of the low attenuation parieto-occipital region and of the surrounding brain indicating injury to the blood-brain barrier and that the infarct is recent. There is no enhancement in the frontal infarct which is probably mature.

space occupation, causing displacement and deformity of normal structures due to compression and/or invasion. The attenuation of tumour tissue itself varies markedly with the cellular structure; it may be higher, similar to or less dense than the adjacent brain. Calcified, haemorrhagic, cystic, necrotic and oedematous regions in or adjacent to tumours may cause superadded variations in the basic attenuation due to the tumour tissue. Grade I and II gliomas (Fig. 9.23) are mainly of diminished attenuation apart from calcified foci which may be revealed when they are not dense enough to show on plain X-rays. Higher grade gliomas (Fig. 9.24) tend to be heterogeneous, usually of diminished but with areas of similar or greater attenuation than the normal white matter. Fluid in cystic and necrotic parts, recognised by very low absorption values, is common in malignant tumours. The edges of gliomas are commonly poorly demarcated although occasionally they may be well defined.

Metastases (Fig. 9.25) usually show as relatively

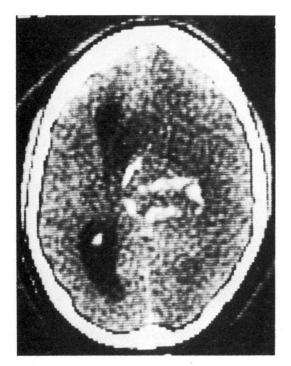

Fig. 9.23 CT at level of frontal horns. There is an extensive area of decreased density deep in the right cerebral hemispheres with thick bands of calcification in its medial part extending across the midline. The lateral ventricles are displaced to the left. Histologically a low grade glioma.

well defined masses which may vary from diminished to increased attenuation relative to normal brain. Not uncommonly they have irregular central necrosis and there may be extensive oedema of the adjacent white matter. If a solitary lesion is revealed, repeating the examination after intravenous contrast injection may show further metastases and is especially important if surgery is contemplated.

Meningiomas (Fig. 9.26) show as peripheral well-defined enhancing masses of greater attenuation in most instances, but sometimes iso-dense with brain. Associated cerebral oedema is not uncommon and if the section does not pass through a small meningioma, this oedema may be mistaken for a primary intrinsic pathology.

Other lesions

The dysplastic lesions of tuberous sclerosis are usually evident by the second year of life. The typical subependymal partly calcified tubers, which

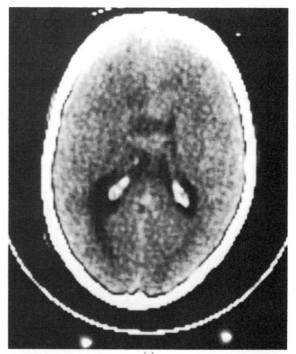

(a)

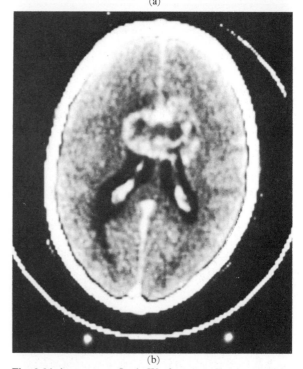

(b)

Fig. 9.24 Astrocytoma Grade IV of corpus callosum. (a) Plain scan: mass of brain attenuation enclosing a low attenuation region in the body of the corpus callosum, which is deforming the anterior horns and bodies of the lateral ventricles. (b) After intravenous contrast medium irregular ring enhancement around the low attenuation region, which was necrotic.

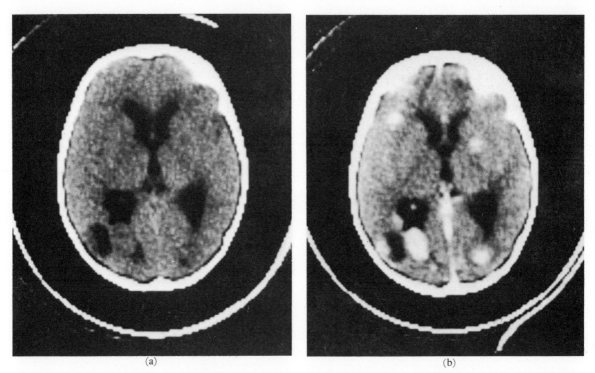

(a)   (b)

Fig. 9.25 Multiple metastases (a) plain scan (b) same section after intravenous contrast medium. There are masses of both low and brain attenuation most of which enhance. One in the left occipital region remains of low attenuation centrally and is likely to be cystic. There is low attenuation due to oedema around most of the lesions, but this is rather less than is usual with metastases. There is moderate hydrocephalus, which was caused by further metastases in the posterior fossa partially obstructing the fourth ventricle.

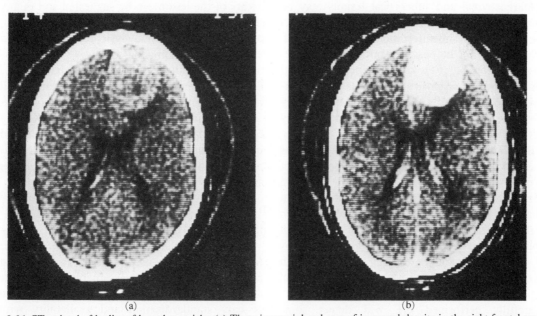

(a)   (b)

Fig. 9.26 CT at level of bodies of lateral ventricles (a) There is a peripheral area of increased density in the right frontal region due to a meningioma. There is a region of diminished density due to intracerebral oedema posterior to it, and the anterior horns of the lateral ventricles are displaced posteriorly. (b) Following intravenous Conray injection there is marked increased in the density of the meningioma.

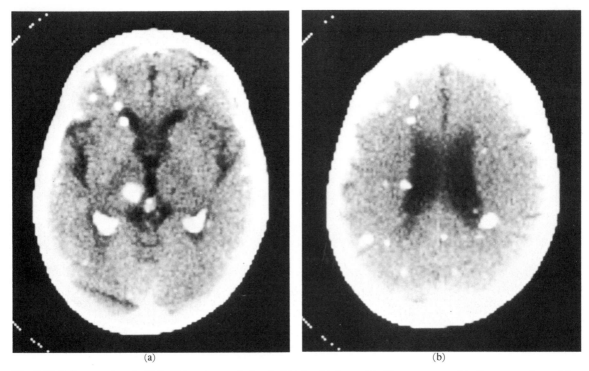

(a)   (b)

Fig. 9.27 Tuberous sclerosis. Plain CT sections at the level of (a) the third ventricle (b) upper parts of bodies of lateral ventricles. There are multiple calcified paraventricular and intraparenchymal tubers. There is also physiological calcification in the pineal gland and the choroid plexuses of the lateral ventricles.

may enhance are most frequent (Fig. 9.27). Intraparenchymal and subcortical lesions may be of low attenuation or less well defined. When these are solitary manifestations a definite CT diagnosis may not be possible, but should be recognised as consistent in the presence of clinical signs of tuberous sclerosis. All lesions which contain calcification can be shown on CT before they are sufficiently dense to be visible on skull X-ray (Figs. 9.28 and 9.29).

Though primary generalised epilepsy was associated with CT abnormality in 10 per cent of cases in one series (Gastaut & Gastaut 1976), in other series the CT, as expected, has differed from a matched control series in only two respects. Firstly, patients who had suffered episodes of status had a higher incidence of cerebral atrophy and, secondly, prolonged therapy with phenytoin was occasionally associated with cerebellar cortical atrophy (Weisberg, Nice & Katz, 1978).

Carefully performed CT will detect some abnormality in about 98 per cent of supratentorial tumours, infarcts and intracerebral haemorrhages and in most atrophic lesions. In most cases the nature of the lesion can be suggested and in a considerable proportion its exact pathology can be predicted. In a recent analysis, 6.5 per cent of cases diagnosed as glioma on CT were proven to be benign (Kendall *et al.*, 1979) so that when CT findings favour a malignancy, their compatibility with a benign lesion should always be considered.

If no abnormality is shown on plain X-ray and computed tomography, it is unlikely that other investigations will show a significant lesion in patients suffering from well controlled epilepsy and no other symptoms.

ISOTOPE ENCEPHALOGRAPHY

Most departments use a simple technique, employing a modern gamma camera and the isotope technetium $^{99}Tc^{m}$, which combines the advantages of easy standardisation and availability with a half-life of six hours. Both lateral, anterior and posterior views are necessary to obtain images in

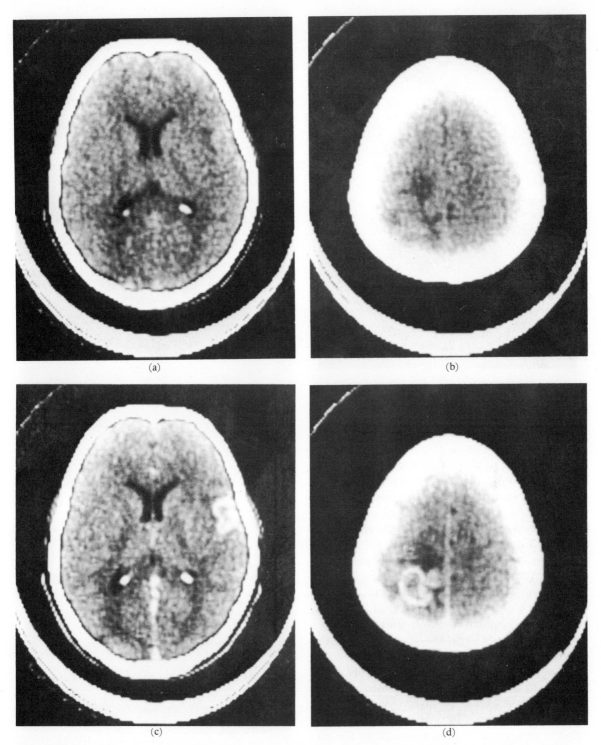

Fig. 9.28 Tuberculomas. Plain CT sections (a) at level of frontal horns (b) at the vertex. (c,d) Same sections after intravenous contrast medium. There are multiple lesions in the right frontotemporal and left parietal regions. Some are iso-dense with brain and others of slightly higher attenuation; all show ring enhancement. The patient is an Asian with pulmonary tuberculosis and the lesions responded to anti-tuberculous chemotherapy.

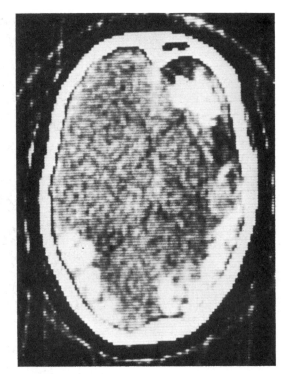

Fig. 9.29 There is extensive calcification around the periphery of the right cerebral hemisphere and of the left posterior parietal and occipital lobes. The appearances are due to the Sturge-Weber syndrome but the calcification was not yet visible on the skull X-ray. There is right-sided hemi-atrophy.

both planes of all regions of the brain and for scanning purposes these are commonly taken at about 30 minutes after intravenous injection of the isotope. Abnormal uptake is recognised in virtually all abscesses, in over 90 per cent of meningiomas and malignant gliomas, 85 per cent of metastases and about 30 per cent of benign gliomas. Abnormal uptake is not usually detected until lesions reach a critical size of about 2 cm and they may be obscured by superimposition of the normal uptake in large venous sinuses, mucous membrane and the large muscles attached to the skull base.

In most cases the appearance of the uptake is non-specific but consideration of its intensity, size, shape and position can be highly suggestive of a particular pathology. Multiple areas of uptake in patients with a known primary neoplasm are virtually diagnostic of metastases (Fig. 9.30) though abscesses and infarcts can also be multiple. The butterfly distribution of a corpus callosum glioma

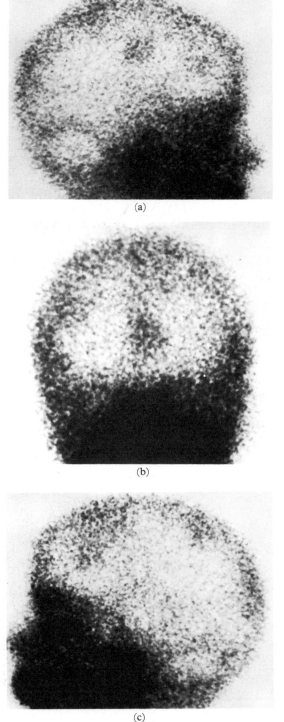

Fig. 9.30 Gamma encephalogram. (a) Right lateral view. (b) Antero-posterior view. (c) Left lateral view. There are multiple areas of increased uptake due to metastases.

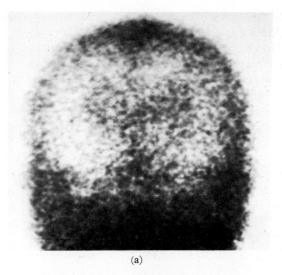

(a)

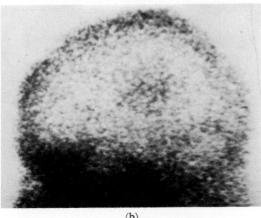

(b)

Fig. 9.31 Gamma encephalogram. (a) Antero-posterior view. (b) Lateral view. There is bilateral parietal uptake, more extensive on the left, joined across the midline. This is typical of a glioma of the corpus callosum.

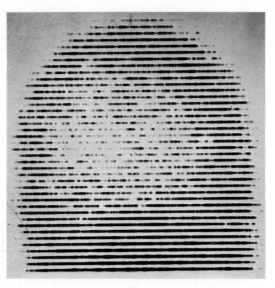

Fig. 9.32 Gamma encephalogram. Antero-posterior view. There is diffuse peripheral uptake over the left hemisphere due to a subdural haematoma.

(Fig. 9.31) and diffuse peripheral uptake in a subdural haematoma (Fig. 9.32) leave little doubt about these diagnoses. High intensity, well demarcated peripheral uptake is usual in meningiomas (Fig. 9.33) and the diagnosis is often confirmed by plain film changes, which are sometimes only recognised on re-examination of the skull films after viewing the isotope study.

Rapid serial filming immediately after injection of technetium gives further information about the nature of the lesions. Angiomatous malformations show very early (Fig. 9.34) and fade quickly as the isotope is rapidly carried into the veins. Sometimes an irregular serpiginous shape giving a vague outline of the vascular pattern of the malformation is evident. Very vascular tumours such as some meningiomas also show early uptake but this increases and is retained as the circulation clears. Malignant gliomas and some metastases have a slower build-up of uptake through the capillary and venous stages of transit which then persists. Most metastases are not shown until 40–70 seconds after the injection and then progressively retain more of the isotope. The real value of early filming is in the detection of angiomatous malformations, which may not be shown by other non-invasive studies including CT without enhancement.

In gliomas and metastases the ratio of uptake between abnormal and normal tissues increases up to about four hours after injection; if early filming gives negative or equivocal findings a later or serial study may be more reliable when such lesions are suspected.

Isotope accumulates in infarcts and haemorrhages when cellular reaction is occurring about 7–10 days from their onset and it persists for several weeks or even months, gradually diminishing; the progression on serial studies is typical.

It should be noted that occasionally abnormal uptake is found after repeated focal seizures in the absence of any demonstrable pathology. It is pre-

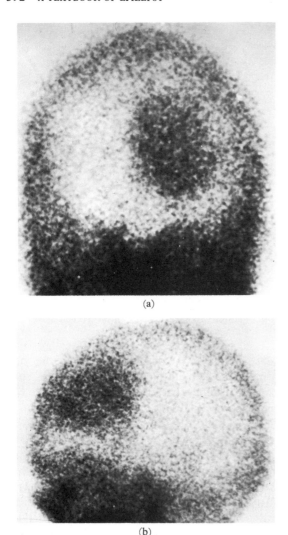

(a)

(b)

Fig. 9.33 Gamma encephalogram. (a) Anterior view. (b) Left lateral view. There is a peripheral area of dense increased uptake in the frontal region due to a meningioma.

In some instances a positive gamma encephalogram alone, or considered with plain film studies, is diagnostic and gives sufficient information for management. More frequently, other studies are necessary to decide the diagnosis or confirm that biopsy is necessary. Unfortunately many of the more benign gliomas and virtually all the atrophic processes will not be revealed by gamma

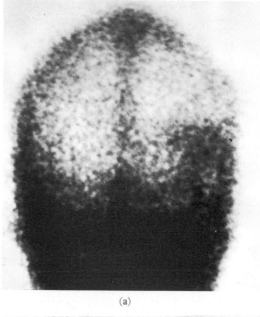

(a)

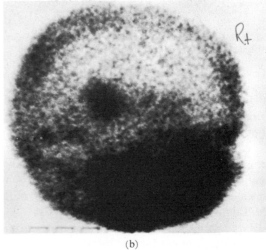

(b)

Fig. 9.34 Gamma encephalogram. (a) Anterior view. (b) Right lateral view, taken immediately after injection of isotope. There is marked increased density in an angiomatous malformation. Increased uptake is shown extending from it in the draining veins.

sumably due to alteration in the blood-brain barrier since it returns to normal on subsequent examinations.

Computed tomography gives more exact localisation and more specific information in a wider range of conditions than isotope encephalography. It is a simpler routine than detailed gamma encephalography performed over a period of hours and consequently, where CT is available it has almost replaced the former. When CT is not available isotope encephalography is a useful screening test for those important conditions usually associated with increased uptake.

encephalography so that a negative study is virtually of no value. Usually these conditions will give rise to more disturbance than well-controlled grand mal epilepsy alone and they will be selected for further studies on clinical grounds when indicated.

CONTRAST STUDIES

The use of pneumo-encephalography and cerebral angiography has diminished as non-invasive studies have become more reliable in the diagnosis and exclusion of structural lesions associated with epilepsy. Both investigations cause unavoidable discomfort which makes the patient's co-operation unpredictable. Since absence of movement is essential, heavy sedation or general anaesthesia must usually be employed. The latter is preferable because it allows control of respiration. In pneumo-encephalography this should be maintained at normal volume so that the pCO_2 remains within the normal range and changes in the size of the cerebral sulci are not induced. Hyperventilation, by depressing the pCO_2 into the lower part of the normal range or slightly below, causes constriction of normal cerebral arteries and slowing of the circulation. This helps to achieve optimum radiographic contrast on angiograms and accentuates pathological circulation through vessels, such as those in malignant tumours, which do not respond normally to physiological stimuli.

Some conditions cause slight and subtle changes which can only be recognised by using special techniques. Since these conditions cannot be foreseen it is desirable that apparatus in routine use should be capable of these techniques. The machine for pneumo-encephalography should perform tomography preferably with complex motion. Automatic serial changers and facilities for magnification and subtraction are routine requirements for modern angiography. With modern facilities and skilled technique the risks attached to contrast procedures are very small, but they have not been completely eliminated; there should be a definite indication for performing these studies, and the techniques adopted should ensure that the maximum amount of information is obtained from them.

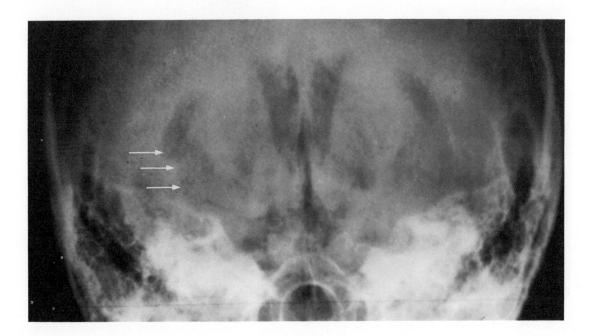

Fig. 9.35 Brow-up Townes' projection air encephalogram. The tip of the right temporal horn is dilated and there is an irregular filling defect in its lateral part (arrows). This was the only abnormal radiological finding. The anterior half of the right temporal lobe was resected and contained a Grade II astrocytoma.

Pneumo-encephalography

Positive findings on CT or on gamma encephalo-graphy usually make pneumo-encephalography redundant. It is very occasionally indicated when CT is negative in cases of temporal lobe epilepsy in which surgery is being considered for the control of intractable seizures. Small infiltrating gliomas (Fig. 9.35) may cause only minimal distortion, narrowing or enlargement of the temporal horn and with hamartomas also compression or displacement may be slight. Dilatation or distortion of the horn may be caused by atrophy (Katada *et al.*, 1978) due to mesial temporal sclerosis or scarring associated with trauma, inflammation or vascular disease which has caused infarction or haemorrhage.

Where CT is not available and the other non-invasive studies are negative, pneumo-encephalography is indicated in cases of epilepsy of recent onset, of changing or intractable nature or associated with dementia, in which there are neither lateralising signs nor any indication of raised intracranial pressure. Generalised, hemi- or focal atrophy (Fig. 9.36) may be disclosed, as may some mass lesions, especially slightly space-occupying gliomas. The latter usually show minor displacements of the ventricles, which do not give a specific indication of the nature of the lesion unless there is also local invasion or local encroachment into the wall of the ventricle or thickening of the septum pellucidum.

Unsuspected cases of tuberous sclerosis (Fig. 9.37) may be recognised when small subependymal nodules, which have not developed calcification, are visible anywhere along the ventricular system. Heterotopic grey matter can give a similar appearance around the lateral ventricles but does not affect the third or fourth ventricles.

Epilepsy following trauma is frequently associated with meningo-cerebral scarring which may be recognised by focal ventricular dilatation or

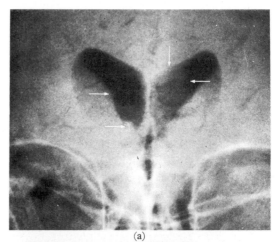

(a)

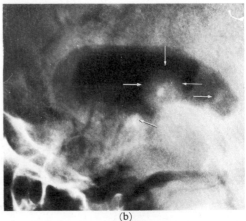

(b)

Fig. 9.37 Air encephalogram. Brow-up (a) antero-posterior and (b) lateral projections. Tuberous sclerosis. There is a large tuber containing a calcified nodule projecting into the medial half of the anterior part of the body of the left lateral ventricle. Two small tubers project into the right lateral ventricle; one from the floor just antero-lateral to the foramen of Monro containing a little calcification and the other from the lateral wall of the posterior part of the body (arrows).

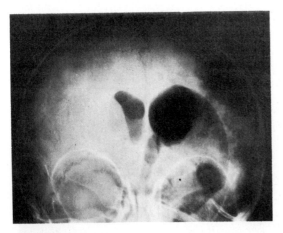

Fig. 9.36 Air encephalogram. Brow-up antero-posterior projection. The capacity of the vault on the left side is diminished. There is dilatation of the subarachnoid space over the left cerebral hemisphere. The left lateral ventricle is dilated and the septum pellucidum and third ventricle are deviated towards it. The appearances indicate left hemi-atrophy.

porencephalic cyst formation. Any more diffuse atrophy will be shown; which may be a factor in deciding against surgery.

Occasionally, cysts with a narrow connection to the main cerebro-spinal fluid spaces may fill late. In post-traumatic cases a film taken several hours after injection of the air may be of value in showing such cysts.

Cerebral angiography

Intracranial masses may be accurately localised from the stretching and splaying of cerebral vessels around the periphery of the swelling (Fig. 9.38). The gyral pattern may also be distorted and the circulation locally delayed in the region of the mass. Intracerebral masses, which compress the surface vessels towards the skull, may be distinguished from extra-axial masses which displace the vessels away from it.

The nature of a lesion may be suspected if changes in vessels are evident on the angiogram. The vascular bed of a tumour may show an abnormal pattern. This tends to be more florid in the more malignant tumours (Fig. 9.39), in which the vessels are composed of sinusoids lined by tumour cells, through which arterio-venous shunting occurs; irregular dilatations are formed where cells have undergone necrosis. Such a pattern occurs in about half of malignant gliomas and patients with metastases. Much less often malignant tumours have fine irregular vessels or a capillary blush which tends to be patchy in gliomas and more homogeneous in metastases.

The vasculature of benign tumours tends to have a radiating or reticular basis with distal tapering, like that of normal tissues. When circulation is increased, as is typical of most meningiomas, such tumours may have a capillary circulation which shows as a prolonged blush. It should be noted that in about half the malignant and a greater proportion of benign intracerebral tumours

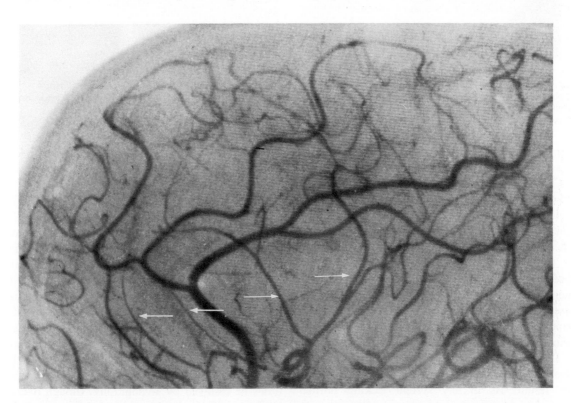

Fig. 9.38 Left internal carotid angiogram – lateral projection. Ascending frontal branches of the middle cerebral artery (arrows) are splayed apart due to a swelling sub-adjacent to them. It was proved at surgery to be a solid astrocytoma but there is no positive angiographic evidence of its nature.

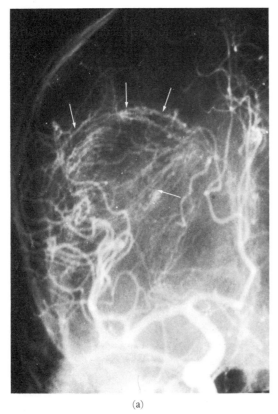 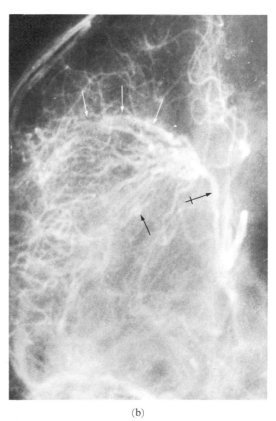

(a)   (b)

Fig. 9.39 Right carotid angiogram – antero-posterior projection. (a) Early arterial phase. (b) Late arterial phase. There is displacement of the anterior cerebral artery and of the internal cerebral vein to the left. Pathological vessels (arrow) are shown extending from the cortical branches of the middle cerebral artery medially through the white matter to drain into the thalamo-striate vein (crossed arrow). The appearances are typical of a malignant glioma.

vascular changes are either absent or minor and non-specific.

Extracerebral tumours especially meningiomas (Fig. 9.40) usually obtain a blood supply from meningeal arteries which often become enlarged and tortuous. This not a pathognomonic feature since intracerebral masses, which invade or adhere to the dura may acquire a meningeal supply, though it is usually less pronounced than that of meningiomas. Intracerebral lesions may be recognised with certainty when they receive blood from penetrating arteries or drain to subependymal veins.

The capsules of intracerebral abscesses contain small vessels which may be seen as a blush ringing the lesion. As in any system lacking normal arteriolar resistance, arterio-venous shunting may occur in the capsule.

Arterio-venous malformations (Fig. 9.41) and

occlusions of moderate sized vessels (Fig. 9.42), which are not infrequent causes of focal epilepsy, are shown directly.

It has been emphasised that plain films and CT considered together frequently suggest a specific diagnosis or give sufficient information for management. Virtually all tumours, infarcts and haemorrhages, and most inflammatory lesions are recognised and in some cases, where swelling is slight or absent, a lesion is obvious on CT whereas angiography reveals either minimal non-specific changes or is normal. The nature of avascular masses without angiographic evidence of their pathology may also be resolved by CT. On the other hand, ambiguous findings on CT may sometimes be resolved by angiography, though overall it gives positive evidence of the nature of the pathological process in only about 30 per cent of the unusual cases in which an equivocal or inaccu-

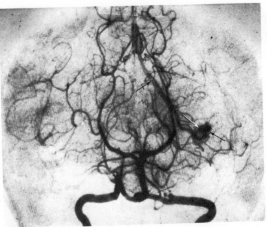

Fig. 9.41 Antero-posterior projection arterial phase of vertebral angiogram. Small angiomatous malformation lying medially in the anterior part of the left temporal lobe is outlined (arrows). There is early drainage to the basal vein (crossed arrow).

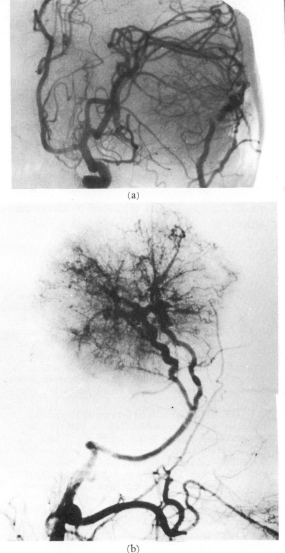

Fig. 9.40 (a) Antero-posterior projection left common carotid angiogram. The trunk of the middle cerebral artery is elevated. Its branches over the insula are displaced medially and those in the lateral ramus of the Sylvian fissure are elevated and splayed apart by an extracerebral mass which is supplied with a rich abnormal circulation from the middle meningeal artery. (b) Lateral projections of left external carotid angiogram. The middle meningeal artery is enlarged. It gives a large number of small branches radiating from the point of attachment to supply the meningioma which is delineated by a capillary blush.

rate diagnosis of glioma is suggested by the CT appearances.

Some information helpful in planning surgery can only be obtained by angiography. For exam-ple, the relationship of major vessels to the lesion, including the presence or absence of tumour cuf-fing or of invasion of the venous sinuses by meningiomas, which may be important in this respect. When CT reveals a small infarct or focal atrophy, especially in a middle-aged or elderly patient with sudden onset of seizures, angiography of the appropriate neck vessels may be indicated to search for an ulcerating or stenosing atheromat-ous plaque in which treatment may prevent a major stroke. Focal atrophy may also be due to arterio-venous malformations. Small ones may not produce abnormalities on the non-invasive studies and constitute a tenable reason for per-forming angiograms on selected epileptics with focal features when such studies are negative.

When CT is not available the role of angiogra-phy is extended. Abnormal uptake of isotope shown on isotope-encephalography is often non-specific and angiography of the appropriate vessel may be helpful in deciding the nature of the pathological process or underlying lesion. When isotope encephalography is negative the appropri-ate angiograms should be performed if there are unexplained focal features. When there is clinical or radiological evidence of unexplained raised intracranial pressure, a non-dominant carotid angiogram should be performed. This will reveal

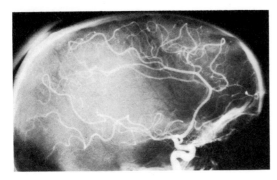

Fig. 9.42 Female aged 55 who presented with left-sided focal fits of recent onset. Right carotid angiogram – arterial phase lateral projection. There is marked delay of filling of the ascending frontal and anterior parietal branches of the middle cerebral artery which was due to occlusion of the trunk supplying them.

the presence of any supratentorial mass; the subependymal veins allow the size of the lateral ventricles to be assessed and, if they are dilated, any deformity of the deep veins may be a useful indicator of the cause. Venous occlusion may also be recognised either directly or by slowing of venous flow towards the obstructed region and the filling of collateral veins.

Following focal status epilepticus, capillary dilatation may occur in the affected region of the brain, and rarely show as a blush on angiography, associated with early venous filling. This returns to normal on follow-up angiography. Failure to consider this possibility may lead to an erroneous diagnosis of significant pathology.

REFERENCES

Ambrose, J. (1973) Computerised transverse axial scanning (Tomography). Part 2: Clinical application. *British Journal of Radiology*, **46**, 1023.

Gastaut, H. & Gastaut, J.L. (1976) Computerised transverse axial tomography in epilepsy. *Epilepsia*, **17**, 325.

Gawler, J., Bull, J.W.D., du Boulay, G.H. & Marshall, J. (1974) Computer assisted tomography (EMI Scanner). Its place in investigation of suspected intracranial tumours. *Lancet*, **2**, 419.

Gold, L.H., Kieffer, S.A. & Peterson, H.O. (1969) Intracranial meningiomas. A retrospective analysis of the diagnostic value of plain skull films. *Neurology* (Minneapolis), **19**, 873.

Hounsfield, G.N. (1973) Computerised transverse axial scanning (Tomography). Part 1: Description of system. *British Journal of Radiology*, **46**, 1016.

Kalan, C. & Burrows, E.H. (1962) Calcification in intracranial gliomata. *British Journal of Radiology*, **35**, 589.

Katada, K., Kanno, T., Sano, H., Shebata, T., Tocla, T. & Koga, S. (1978) Ammon's horns sclerosis on pneumo-encephalography. *Neuroradiology*, **16**, 335.

Kendall, B.E., Jakubowski, J., Pullicino, P. and Symon, L.

(1979) Difficulties in diagnosis of supratentorial gliomas by CAT scan. *Journal of Neurology, Neurosurgery and Psychiatry*, **42**, 485.

Mahmoud, M.S. (1958) The sella in health and disease; value of the radiographic study of the sella turcica in morbid anatomical and topographic diagnosis of intracranial tumours. *British Journal of Radiology*, Supplement 8.

Paxton, R. & Ambrose, J. (1974) The EMI Scanner. A brief review of the first 650 patients. *British Journal of Radiology*, **47**, 530.

Polkey, C.E. (1978) Correlation between EMI scan and pathologic findings in anterior temporal lobectomy for intractable epilepsy. In Wüllemueber, R., Wender, H., Brock, M. & Klinger, M. (eds) *Advances in Neurosurgery 6*, p. 98. Berlin: Springer-Verlag.

Synek, V., Reuben, J.R., Gawler, J. & du Boulay, G.H. (1979) Comparison of the measurement of the cerebral ventricles obtained by C.T. scanning and pneumoencephalography. *Neuroradiology*, **17**, 149.

Weisberg, L.A., Nice, C. & Katz, M. (1978) *Cerebral computed tomography*, p. 282. Philadelphia, London, Toronto: W.B. Saunders & Co.

10

Neurosurgery

PART ONE
C.E. Polkey

INTRODUCTION

Epileptic seizures are familiar in general neurosurgical practice as a symptom of underlying disease, or occasionally as a consequence of neurosurgical interference, but when they are the main symptomatology, and the underlying cause is initially obscure, then they constitute a disease in their own right. It is with the neurosurgical treatment of this situation that this chapter is concerned. There is a large volume of animal experimental work on the neurophysiological basis of epilepsy, but little of this can be shown to be relevant to the surgical treatment of the disease. For this reason this aspect will not therefore be covered in detail, but touched upon as and where it seems appropriate. Details of the neurophysiology relating to electro-corticography are provided by Blume and Girvin (p. 422). It should also be remembered that epilepsy in broad terms results from the interaction between some cerebral disease process, whether identifiable or not, and the individual brain; the identical disease process in the same location in different patients will not necessarily give rise to the same severity of epilepsy or even necessarily the same manifestations. For this reason, therefore, the realistic achievement of surgical treatment must be to control the disease rather than to eradicate it and although the long follow-up periods available for the early and now

classical procedures indicate that in many cases this control is almost perfect, it is possible for patients, even years after a successful operation, to experience further epileptic attacks.

The physician who wishes to decide whether a patient with chronic epilepsy would benefit from surgery is faced with the multitude of techniques used to assess such patients, together with a number of different operative procedures apparently available to treat the same condition. The purpose of this chapter is to resolve some of this confusion and give a rational account of the scope of surgery in this situation. With modern practice the mortality and morbidity of the neurosurgical techniques used in the treatment of epilepsy is acceptably low. By contrast it is agreed by all authorities that chronic epilepsy, especially when poorly controlled, or as part of an underlying cerebral pathology, leads to a decreased life expectancy. Thus, Penning, Muller and Ciompi (1969), noted that the average life expectancy of 202 patients they studied was about 50 years and that the life expectancy was diminished by 43.6 per cent in men and 51.4 per cent in women. They quote similar figures by other authors.

Operations have been used in the treatment of epilepsy since neurosurgery first became practicable and the work of some of the early pioneers is very impressive (Talairach *et al.*, 1974). However, the first rational approach came from the Montreal Neurological Institute where Wilder Penfield, expanding the ideas he had worked on in collaboration with Foerster, began to try to demonstrate that possible epileptogenic zones, identified when stimulated at surgery, could be resected with benefit to the patient. The addition of electrical recording from the surface of the brain at operation and then from the deep structures together with very careful observational and surgical techniques and a bountiful flow of patients, enabled this group to build up an unrivalled experience of resective surgery described in their numerous publications.

However, as the Montreal group was being established, it became clear that this approach of local resection was not suitable for all types of chronic epilepsy and so in other centres different philosophies and means of treatment were developed. The identification of the 'limbic system' and the Papez circuit outlined a system of widespread connections shown experimentally to be especially vulnerable to epileptic type discharges. Also the description of 'kindling' (Goddard, 1967) demonstrated experimentally that repeated electrical stimulation of the same neurophysiological pathway could cause a permanent change in its electrical properties. These observations suggested that chronic epilepsy might alter the electrical activity of the brain in such a way as to increase or even perpetuate the problem. It was then reasoned that if these mechanisms could be modified in circumstances where the basic cause of the epilepsy was either unidentifiable, or untreatable by direct surgery, then some relief from chronic seizures might follow.

With the advent of human stereotactic surgery the principles of which are described later, a number of workers began to explore this approach. Until recently this consisted of causing, by various means, destructive lesions in appropriate parts of the brain. Since the early seventies another technique, introduced by Cooper (1973), and still in its infancy, namely chronic cerebellar stimulation, has been available and is dealt with on page 430.

Because the number of centres carrying out surgical treatment for epilepsy is small, and the number of patients that each centre treats is also small, there has been a tendency for each centre to rely on a few techniques, each well known to them, and so patients with basically the same problem would be treated with functional surgery in one centre and resective surgery in another. Further confusion is introduced by the claims that the personality problems which frequently accompany chronic epilepsy, and temporal lobe epilepsy

in particular, may be alleviated by stereotactic procedures which have then been applied to some patients who present without epilepsy. This has tended to blur the margins of the reports of some workers, making assessment of their value difficult. Finally, in many of the earlier reports of the results of surgery the period of follow-up is rather brief. For these reasons in preparing this review I have tended to refer to reports in which the period of follow-up is five years or more, and the surgical techniques used are clearly defined. Especially valuable are reports from workers such as Talairach and his group or Vaernet where both types of surgical techniques have been used.

The plan adopted will be to outline the principles of assessment of patients for surgery, then the techniques first of resective surgery and then stereotactic surgery will be reviewed and also the results of these procedures. Finally, there will be a brief closing summary.

PRINCIPLES OF ASSESSMENT OF PATIENTS FOR SURGERY

In all cases it must first be established that the patient's epilepsy is both chronic and drug-resistant. This, of course, includes the patient's record of drug compliance. The frequency of fits which is regarded as disabling will vary from centre to centre, and even from patient to patient. Also most patients do not have attacks at regular intervals, but an average of one at least noticeable attack per week seems reasonable. It must also be established that relieving the patient of his epilepsy will be of measurable benefit to him or those who care for him and that there is only the minimal possibility of producing an adverse side effect from the operation which would be more disabling than the original epilepsy. A complete and careful psychiatric history is also of importance. An attempt should be made to distinguish clearly between those psychiatric complaints which are known to be associated with chronic epilepsy, and those of independent conditions, since the association of epilepsy with psychoses can affect the prognosis after surgery. Finally, what the surgeon hopes to accomplish in terms of seizure relief, together with the possible hazard, should be conveyed realistically to the patient, his relatives and the referring physician. In order to produce the best results, and also avoid false optimism or pessimism, it is therefore better that such surgery should be carried out in a few centres with a reasonable turnover, rather than occasionally in general neurosurgical practice. In the case of resective surgery it is now generally established that the success of surgery depends upon demonstrating that the seizures originate in one part of the brain and that frequently one can attribute them to some structural change in that part of the brain. Secondary to these considerations is the necessity to show that the remainder of the cerebral hemisphere is healthy, and that resecting the affected part, large or small, will have minimal effect. The assessment therefore will be described in two parts, clinical and investigative.

Clinical

History

This is taken in the traditional manner with care for detail and with perseverance. Independent corroboration should be obtained both from relatives and previous hospital case notes. Two themes should be sought in such history-taking, the first being an attempt to establish that all the patient's attacks have a common source; the second being to look for evidence of a reason or structural abnormality in the appropriate part of the brain.

In the first case a careful history of the type of attack which the patient suffers must be obtained. It would seem unnecessary to remind readers that in trying to locate the origin of the fit, attention should be paid to the aura, to any focal features in the attack as well as its nature, and to any postictal phenomena such as Todd's palsy. Any inconsistencies must be carefully accounted for or taken as evidence of multiple origins of the attacks. It should be borne in mind that attacks may progress to generalised attacks from a focal origin. Particular difficulty may be experienced with speech phenomena for two reasons. First it may be difficult to establish precise hemisphere dominance, and secondly certain phenomena may arise from the non-dominant hemisphere as described by Falconer (1967a). A good description of the

localising features of various epileptic phenomena is to be found in Penfield and Jasper (1954). It is essential to get a good description of the seizures in layman's terms, avoiding the acceptance of terms such as petit mal or minor fit. Witnesses, especially relatives, may display a kind of mirror description in which they attribute the patient's focal features to the opposite side of their own body, but this can usually be clarified by careful questioning (M.A. Falconer – unpublished observation). For purposes of careful follow-up the frequency of fits should be accurately established. As already noted, such attacks are seldom regular and therefore it seems fairly reasonable to establish, for the year before referral, the average frequency of attacks together with the greatest number in one day and the longest period free of fits, and make a note of any obvious clustering.

The second point to be established from the history is whether there is any possible cause for structural change. In an elegant monograph (1966) Ounsted and his co-workers showed that in 66 out of 100 childdren with temporal lobe epilepsy a definite history could be obtained of birth injury or infantile febrile convulsions and that in the remainder, where the age of onset was later, miscellaneous lesions such as small tumours were found. In a similar vein, Falconer (1974) clearly demonstrated that in patients whose temporal lobectomy specimens showed the changes of mesial temporal sclerosis, there was a high incidence of previous febrile convulsions, whereas patients with other lesions did not show this. Careful documentation of the first appearance of physical signs, such as facial palsy, may likewise be indicative of a small tumourous lesion.

Such history-taking may require several hours, perhaps even several sessions, and considerable background research, but will amply repay the time spent.

Physical signs

Except in cases of obvious previous brain damage, or in patients with rapidly expanding lesions, physical signs during the interictal period are rare, and when present tend to be soft and solitary. In a small series of our own cases, physical signs have only been found in patients with small temporal tumours, but their absence does not exclude the presence of such a lesion.

Examination in the immediate post-ictal period should always be carried out whenever possible, and special weight placed on physical signs found at this time. On several occasions when there has been a doubt as to laterality, the matter has been clarified and allowed successful surgery. This is especially so in the fronto-temporal regions where bilateral frontal EEG abnormalities may occur and lead to doubts which are resolved by the appearance of post-ictal phenomena relating to one or other Rolandic region.

Observation

It is well known that when these patients are admitted to hospital for observation they often go into a seizure-free period. Since it is necessary, for a number of reasons, to see the patient's attacks, it would seem to be reasonable to reduce the patient's antiepileptic medication. It is unwise to remove it altogether, but a reduction, usually to one or two drugs, may be safely made. In this respect, in the case of an adult, either phenytoin 100 mg or primidone 250 mg three times daily are usually safe and with this regime over the past few years we have had only a few cases of status out of several hundred investigations, and none of them serious. Direct clinical observation of the attacks by suitably instructed medical and nursing staff is of considerable value alone and its place in relation to EEG studies will be discussed below.

Although this discussion of clinical observations has been chiefly in relation to resective surgery, it can be seen that the same principles can establish the possibility of functional surgery helping the patient. A period of at least two weeks clinical assessment is therefore necessary pre-operatively, and on some occasions this may need to extend to several weeks.

Investigations

Neurophysiological studies

This volume naturally includes chapters on neurophysiology and this account is therefore written from a neurosurgeon's point of view. It is emphasised that close co-operation with an experienced clinical neurophysiologist is essential for the management of these patients. The purpose of EEG studies in these patients is to demonstrate the presence of a focal abnormality, or of equal importance, the converse. Secondly, they are extremely valuable in the post-operative period and are thought by some to be a good prognostic indicator (Van Buren *et al.*, 1975; Brazier, Crandall & Jann Brown, 1975). The EEG itself is of course a dynamic phenomenon which changes with circumstances and age and it is therefore important to review previous records whenever possible.

Although routine EEG may be helpful, it is frequently without focal features and so further studies are usually necessary, preferably after a reduction in the antiepileptic medication as we have already discussed. This manoeuvre tends to allow the basic abnormalities to emerge and also removes any confusing features due to drug effects. It is known that sleep will increase or produce abnormalities in the record and so we have taken advantage of natural sleep or drowsiness during long records. We have only rarely used sleep deprivation as a means of inducing sleep. It is known that certain sedatives are useful in this respect and we have used quinalbarbitone in a dose of 200 mg in adults. Other workers describe the use of diazepam (Brazier, Crandall & Walsh, 1976) and short-acting barbiturates (Wilder, 1971). When examining records obtained under these circumstances, one is looking for the appearance of or an increase in spikes or sharp waves; and of equal importance when drugs are used to induce sleep, the absence of the induced fast activity to be expected from normal cerebral cortex. The use of stimulants such as bemegride (Megimide) to provoke attacks is a technique we have used less than most centres. The test itself is unpleasant and cannot be repeated more than once or twice, consequently the relevant answer may not be forthcoming. In addition attacks produced in this way may not be the patient's habitual fits so that it then becomes difficult to use the results of this test as a basis for surgery. Wieser *et al.* (1979) have recently shown that chemically induced seizures have the least correlation with spontaneously occurring seizures in depth recordings from patients using the Paris stereo-electroencephalographic technique described in more detail later. It should be mentioned that it is of great value to record during one of the patient's habitual seizures, especially if a visual record of the seizure can be made at the same time.

Up to this point we have been discussing scalp recordings, but certain parts of the cerebral cortex are poorly served by such electrodes, and this is especially true of the inferior surface of the temporal lobes. However, a number of techniques have been evolved to give extra-cranial access to the base of the skull in order to obtain better recordings from these areas. Each centre has its own preferred method, but the use of small wires inserted under the zygoma and coming to rest under the sphenoid bone is the one used at the Maudsley. This is often combined with thiopentone sodium (Pentothal) narcosis and will be referred to hereafter as Pentothal-sphenoidal recording.

If an even more detailed assessment of intracerebral electrical activity is needed, as in certain cases of frontal or motor epilepsy, then it may be necessary to place a large number of electrodes, some passing through the cerebral substance in order to reach either deep structures or medial cerebral cortex. In order to achieve this, suitable electrodes have to be inserted under stereotactic control. Recording in this fashion may be acute or chronic and is conveniently referred to as stereo-electroencephalography or stereo-EEG (SEEG). There are a number of methods of doing this, but a good account is that of the French school (Talairach et al., 1974). They state that with SEEG they can outline a 'zone-épileptogéne' in 85 per cent of cases and in these cases the results of surgery are very good. They do, however, note that 428 patients have been investigated using SEEG and as a result they have carried out 236 surgical procedures, 160 of which were resective operations (Talairach et al., 1974). Finally, it is possible with modern methods to have an electrode array which can be implanted at open craniotomy, used for a short period of chronic recording, and then removed prior to definitive surgery (Goldring, 1979). Electrocorticography is used chiefly at the time of open surgery, and will therefore be discussed in relation to that topic.

Finally, mention should be made of the intra-carotid injection techniques first described by Wada (1949). These can be used for two purposes. The first is to try to determine hemispheric dominance for speech, and in this respect may be combined with tests of memory and other psychometric functions. This latter we have not found very useful, but for a detailed description Milner (1975) should be consulted. The second purpose is to discover whether bilateral discharges originate from independent foci or are due to secondary synchrony. These tests are both uncomfortable and carry some risk, and should therefore only be carried out with good reason.

Neuroradiological studies

The object of these studies is to seek evidence of a focal organic lesion. The plain radiograph of the skull can be helpful. Asymmetry of the hemicranium or of lesser parts of the skull, may indicate atrophy or underdevelopment of one hemisphere as in infantile hemiplegia, or of the temporal lobe as when a small middle fossa is associated with mesial temporal sclerosis. The occurrence of abnormal calcification may reveal the presence of small tumours, arterio-venous malformations, tuberous sclerosis etc. Especial care in radiological techniques and appropriate tomography may be necessary to reveal such abnormalities (see Ch. 9). The use of CT scanning requires no detailed comment, neither would it be useful to catalogue the lesions which this technique may find. There is no doubt that when a population of epileptic patients at large is scanned, as in the series collected by Gastaut and Gastaut (1976), the number of patients with abnormal scans is about twice those in whom abnormalities would have been revealed by previous radiological techniques. In particular they found that the number of tumours or 'tumour-like' lesions doubles from 5 per cent to 10 per cent. Our experience in a small group of patients is given in Table 10.1. It should be noted that in only 50 per cent of these patients, all of whom subsequently underwent surgery, was the scan positively abnormal. It has, however, been our experience that with enhancement scanning none of the tumourous lesions have failed to show up.

The lumbar air encephalogram (AEG) remains an important investigation in these patients. In

Table 10.1 Comparison of CT scan appearances and pathology in 21 cases of 'en bloc' temporal lobetomy

Pathological Findings	Abnormal Radiological Findings			Structural Lesion Found
	Skull X-Ray	CT Scan	AEG or Carotid	
Mesial temporal sclerosis (5 pts)	1	0 (2)	5	5
Tumours and hamartomas (8 pts)	4 (calcification)	7 (1)	8	8
Other lesions (5 pts)	1 (calcification)	3 (2)	5	5
Non-specific (3 pts)	0	0	1	0
Total 21 pts	6	10	19	18

1. Figures in brackets indicate additional patients with visible temporal horns
2. Other lesions were, one infarct, one scar, one arterio-venous malformation, one cortical dysplasia and one astrocytosis

cases of temporal lobe epilepsy due to mesial temporal sclerosis this may be the only neuroradiological study to reveal any abnormality. Also it is important to know, for technical reasons, the precise shape of the temporal horn and other parts of the ventricular system. A good summary of the neuroradiological findings in a group of patients undergoing temporal lobectomy was given by Newcombe and Shah (1975). Especially since the advent of CT scanning, the usefulness of carotid arteriography in assessing epileptic patients for surgery is much diminished. It is, however, an important technique in SEEG to ensure that the electrodes do not penetrate any major vessels during insertion (Talairach et al., 1974). In circumstances where CT scanning is not available, a normal carotid arteriogram on the side of an EEG focus should not be taken as evidence of the absence of a surgically treatable lesion.

Psychometric studies

These are devoted both to seeking a specific defect which may be related to an organic brain lesion, and assessing the degree of any more widespread brain damage which might be a limiting factor in the scale of any planned resection. The chief areas of interest are in relation to speech function and memory function. This latter is especially useful in trying to determine whether temporal lobe disease is unilateral or bilateral. Such studies of course are also useful in gauging the extent and duration of any post-operative defect. The data on these mat-

ters are chiefly in relation to temporal lobe operations and to a lesser degree to hemispherectomy and will be dealt with in more detail in discussing these procedures.

The first requisite in assessing the results of surgery is of course to have the solid base of a good postoperative assessment. There should be a follow-up period of at least five years, since the number of patients remaining fit-free diminishes with time (see Van Buren et al., 1975). Where possible, the pathology of any resection carried out should be known. Finally, although for reasons already given it is desirable that such surgery should be carried out in a few centres, nevertheless, the description of the technical details of this surgery should be such that it can be repeated by an adequately trained neurosurgeon, otherwise the procedure dies with its originator. In general, however, it is reasonable to assert that the success of such surgery tends to rest upon selection techniques rather than the technical details of the surgery.

The purpose of this introduction has been to set out the principles which must be considered before surgery is contemplated. Clearly the final decision with regard to surgery in any particular case will depend upon the result of the foregoing investigations in a way which will emerge later. Because temporal lobe epilepsy is still the commonest type for which surgical assistance is asked, and also because it has been treated with both stereotactic and resective surgery, it will be convenient to discuss first the details of surgical management in relation to this condition.

RESECTIVE SURGERY

Temporal lobectomy

Temporal lobectomy is the commonest and most widely reported surgical procedure for temporal lobe epilepsy. Thus Jensen (1975a) was able to assemble data on 2282 published temporal lobe resections. She points out quite correctly, that the results of these operations vary, but that those surgeons who have included the deep structures of the temporal lobe in their resection have obtained better relief of seizures and this is confirmed by Van Buren *et al*. (1975), who noted that there were only 20 per cent failures with complete operations compared with 50 per cent with topectomies, gyrectomies etc.

Assessment and investigation

The clinical features in the selection of such patients have already been outlined. They should have had complex partial seizures for at least five years in the case of an adult. The history should be such as to establish the nature of the attacks and also where possible to lateralise their origin.

It should be recalled that the auras of complex partial seizures can be very bizarre, and to some extent their nature has a predictive value. Falconer and Taylor (1968) found that an aura was more likely to be present in patients whose temporal lobe, when resected, showed mesial temporal sclerosis and that it was more likely to have a somato-sensory content, for example a rushing cephalic or a rising epigastric sensation rather than taste or smell, which were usually associated with other lesions, such as hamartomas. The attacks themselves, in addition to the recognised features of mumbling, lip-smacking, swallowing, fumbling etc. may have more bizarre components such as rushing about, trying to hide and so on, and finally, frequently terminate in automatisms. Serafetinides and Falconer (1963) made a careful study of speech disturbances in 100 patients and divided them into (i) paroxysmal dysphasia, consisting of the inability of the patient to express himself during a period of awareness and usually associated with subsequent left temporal lobectomy and (ii) speech automatisms consisting of identifiable words and phrases for which the patient is subsequently amnesic, and these were associated with subsequent right temporal lobectomy.

The occurrence of other kinds of attacks in addition to complex partial seizures has not been considered by most authors as a bar to operation. It was noted by Falconer and Serafetinides (1963) that the results of operation in patients who suffered grand mal attacks were no different from those obtained in patients with temporal lobe attacks alone. Van Buren *et al*. (1975) also notes that 50 per cent of his series suffered grand mal attacks. However, Jensen (1976a), analysing 74 cases operated upon by Vaernet, sees grand mal epilepsy as a bad prognostic indicator.

The inter-ictal history is also of importance in these patients. Many of them have personality, social and behavioural difficulties. The proportion of such patients varies between one series and another, presumably because of variation in referral sources and Jensen (1975a) in surveying the world literature states that the proportion varies between 15 per cent and 56 per cent. In the majority of patients the disorder corresponds to that described by Pond (1974) consisting of irritability, unpredictable mood variation, quarrelsome behaviour and so forth. This has been linked by the Boston Group, on slim evidence (Mark & Ervin, 1970) with amygdalar disease, causing loss of impulse control which they call the 'dyscontrol syndrome'. It can certainly be observed in some of these patients that they may manifest a cycle between very poor behaviour and relatively few fits and the reverse. Such 'aggressive' behaviour is not a bar to operation and may well improve as a result of surgery. By contrast only a small number of these patients exhibit frank psychosis. The occurrence rate is about 12 per cent (Falconer, 1973) and this seems general for the epileptic population seen in psychiatric hospitals and clinics (Fenton, 1978). However, in a large population of patients with unselected temporal lobe epilepsy (Currie, *et al*. 1971), the proportion was much lower, being of the order of 2 per cent. The majority of these psychoses are of a paranoid type being schizophreniform, but lacking some of the cardinal features of schizophrenia. There is a tendency for this kind of psychosis to be associated with left, i.e. dominant, hemisphere lesions (Flor-Henry, 1969) and with the presence of alien tissues within the temporal lobe (Taylor, 1975). Even when the surgery is successful in relieving the fits, the psychosis tends to be unaffected, although on the whole they tend to mellow or burn out with time.

Finally, the previous medical history is of importance in looking for possible causes of structural brain damage to account for the epilepsy. In this respect the association between mesial temporal sclerosis and a previous history of severe febrile convulsions is now well accepted, and the evidence of this, together with some possible mechanisms of its pathogenesis, is well summarised by Falconer (1974). The relationship between this lesion and the 'incisural sclerosis' described by the Montreal group, remains obscure, but it seems likely that they are basically the same lesion. As suggested by the work of Ounsted (1967) the absence of a history of birth trauma or febrile convulsions, together with a later onset of epilepsy and the preservation of normal intelligence, suggest the presence of a small 'tumour-like' lesion in the temporal lobe. Although these kinds of guidelines are fairly loose, they are of value in the overall prediction of aetiology.

The question of operating upon children arises. It has been our experience that if chronic drug-resistant epilepsy is established prior to puberty, especially if there is a structural abnormality to account for it, then it seldom remits with age and this is a constant feature in taking the histories of patients coming for consideration of surgery in their late teens and early twenties. Although it is agreed that EEG abnormalities may change with age in children, and especially that a posterior temporal focus may migrate anteriorly, nevertheless Falconer and Davidson (1974), showed that the results of temporal lobectomy in children were similar to those in adults provided that criteria similar to those used for adults were fulfilled, including a predominantly unilateral, anterior temporal EEG focus. Jensen (1976a) noted in the Danish series that early operation was associated with a good prognosis.

To come now to the investigation of such patients. We have already outlined the importance of psychometric testing. In general it is thought that a full scale IQ score of 70 or more is necessary so that the patient shall benefit from temporal lobectomy. Using the appropriate tests a disparity between the verbal IQ and the performance IQ may be found, although it is admitted by Milner (1975) that such differences do not have a high reliability. In addition, the explanation for them lies between a functional deficit, due to electrical disorder, and a deficit due to structural damage and cannot be resolved in practice. However, when the deficit corresponds to the other data it is useful additional evidence. When it is contrary to other evidence then one or two explanations should be sought. It could either be due to mixed hemispheric dominance, a relatively rare phenomenon, or to bilateral brain damage, which is more likely since it is frequently seen in patients where mesial temporal sclerosis is suspected. Of equal importance is the assessment of memory function and here poor performance in either the Wechsler logical memory (dominant temporal lobe) or the Rey-Osterreith test (non-dominant temporal lobe) is well accepted as evidence of appropriate damage. In order to avoid a global amnesic syndrome in which the patient is totally unable to absorb new material, patients with bilateral damage should be approached with caution, especially if it is worse on the side opposite to the proposed resection. In a smaller series of patients we have been unable to use the carotid-amylobarbitone test as effectively as Milner (1975).

As far as the neuroradiological data is concerned, the investigations in the form of plain skull radiographs, CT scans, and AEGs have already been discussed. If the results of these are all normal, then the decision regarding operation has to be made on other grounds. As Newcombe and Shah (1975) pointed out, contra-lateral dilatation of the temporal horn was found in 13 per cent of patients and operation was then carried out on the basis of the EEG studies. Care should, however, be exercised since, if there is also a psychometric deficit corresponding to this dilatation one may be dealing with a situation in which there is more damage on the electrically silent side. One further problem has arisen with the advent of the CT scanner, namely the finding of a discrete lesion on the CT scan in association with a widespread abnormality in the EEG record. For reasons outlined below, my personal opinion is that such lesions should be operated upon, although it will be some time before sufficient cases accrue to justify this course of action.

Electroencephalographic studies, as previously stated, are of paramount importance. The Maudsley custom has been to carry out suitable scalp recordings together with Pentothal-sphenoidal recordings, on more than one occasion if necessary, and usually as inter-ictal recordings. If recordings can be obtained during a fit, this is clearly helpful and if the findings are doubtful then further recordings are carried out until the question is resolved within the limits of these methods. The indications for surgery were considered to be the demonstration in the medial part of the temporal lobe of a unilateral, or predominantly unilateral, spike focus (ratio of spikes no worse than 4:1). If this unilateral focus is accompanied by an ipsilateral deficit of barbiturate-induced fast activity suggesting structural change, then this is also favourable. Engel, Driver and Falconer (1975) analysed the relationship between EEG criteria and pathological findings in 59 patients undergoing temporal lobectomy. They defined medial temporal foci as those showing phase reversal at the sphenoidal electrode; lateral temporal foci showed phase reversal at the appropriate scalp electrode. Independent contra-lateral temporal foci were also seen. Non-spike phenomena were also considered, chiefly induced barbiturate fast activity. They found a good correlation between medial temporal foci and medial temporal pathology. As far as the results of surgery were concerned, certain findings carried a poor prognosis and these included, diffuse spikes, nasal midline spikes and repetitive spikes. With regard to contra-lateral spiking, they assert that when the surgery includes the deep structures, and they review other series besides their own, then these are not of bad import. This has to be seen against the previous statement that the contra-lateral spikes should not exceed the ratio of four to one. As already mentioned, it is possible to demonstrate a discrete CT scan lesion in the presence of widespread EEG abnormalities. In a small number of cases of medial temporal tumours, differing in location from those described by Cavanagh (1958), the EEG records have tended to show extra-temporal abnormalities usually confined to the appropriate hemisphere, although in one case the evolution over some years from a discrete unilateral temporal abnormality to bilateral abnormalities was clearly seen. Removal of this offending lesion has had a good result.

The use of stereo-electroencephalography (SEEG) has already been mentioned. Although in some respects similar cases are equally well investigated by both techniques there is no question that in patients who show equal and bilaterally independent temporal spikes the implantation of depth electrodes may help to resolve the matter. Such electrodes can be accurately implanted in the deep structures of the temporal lobes and chronic recordings made from them in combination with video-recording thus giving a complete record of the patient's fits. In this way one can document the spread of electrical abnormalities and their relationship to aura experiences and so on. Wieser et al. (1979), noted that in only two-thirds of their patients did the inter-ictal SEEG record correspond with the electrical focus seen when spontaneous seizures were recorded. Crandall (1975) states that whereas with scalp recording only 30 per cent of his patients could be shown to have a unilateral temporal focus, such a focus could be identified in 73 per cent after depth recording. A fascinating account of the use of this method in individual cases is given by Walter (1973).

If careful consideration is given to all the factors mentioned, then it is possible to form a shrewd idea of the pathology in the temporal lobe to be resected before operation. In Table 10.2 the accuracy of prediction in a small series of cases is shown.

Operative methods and techniques

It should be said at the outset that it is not appropriate in this text to give a detailed technical account of the surgery involved, but rather to indicate its nature and extent. References to the surgical technique are given below.

The view could be taken that having demonstrated a probable antero-medial temporal abnormality by the pre-operative assessment, the object of the operation is to seek and remove this abnor-

Table 10.2 Pre-operative prediction of pathology in 21 temporal lobectomies

Pathology	EEG		Radiology		Psychometry		History		Predicted	Found
	Pos.	Neg.	Pos.	Neg.	Pos.	Neg.	Pos.	Neg.		
Mesial temporal sclerosis (5)	3	2	5	0	3	1	3	2	3	5
Tumour or hamartoma (8)	4	4	7	1	2	2	8	0	7	8

Other lesions (5)	Predicted	Found
	Tumour	Cortical dysplasia
	Tumour	Small angioma
	Mesial temporal sclerosis	Old encephalitis
	Mesial temporal sclerosis	Severe gliosis and cortical scarring
	Mesial temporal sclerosis	Astrocytosis
Non-specific (3)	In these patients a positive pre-operative diagnosis was not possible and the pathological changes were non-specific	

mality. The standard Falconer 5–6 cm 'en bloc' resection, with appropriate modification on the dominant side, performed under general anaesthetic with current techniques of general neurosurgical practice would suffice to deal with the situation. It is therefore necessary to justify the use of both electrocorticography (ECoG) and local anaesthesia.

Electrocorticography was originally used as a means of defining the area of electrical abnormality in order to delineate the area to be resected. However, it became clear over the years that excision of brain tissue on these grounds alone could have serious consequences without great additional benefits. In particular 'spike chasing' in the insula region leads to increased post-operative hemipareses. Recently, doubt has been cast on the value of ECoG, especially in temporal lobectomy (Gloor, 1975). In analysing some of Falconer's patients, Engel *et al.* (1975) noted that the only positive result of ECoG recording was that the absence of spontaneous discharges from 'depth electrodes' inserted into the amygdala and hippocampus suggested chronic damage to those areas. Most authors agree that ECoG is not a factor in determining the extent of resection in temporal lobectomy.

The use of local anaesthesia for temporal lobectomy is also declining. Originally employed when it was necessary to use cortical stimulation to find the epileptogenic focus and continued when ECoG was added, its use in temporal lobectomy is now almost academic except under a few well-defined

circumstances. It is to be admitted that the ECoG recorded after basal sedation (we use papaveretum (Omnopon) and hyoscine (Scopolamine) with the operative procedures performed under local anaesthesia) is probably nearer to the situation in the awake brain than when inhalation anaesthetic agents are used.

There are two circumstances under which local anaesthesia may have considerable advantages. The first relates to hemispheric dominance for speech. The majority of patients are right-handed and therefore left hemisphere dominant. It is helpful when operating upon the left temporal lobe, to be able to define the limit of the speech area in that temporal lobe by stimulation of the superior temporal gyrus. However, if this is not possible, provided that no more than the anterior 1–1.5 cm of the superior temporal gyrus is resected, then any post-operative dysphasia will be both slight and transient. By contrast, when operating upon the right temporal lobe of a person with mixed hemispheric dominance it may be necessary to be more cautious but again the speech area can be defined by stimulating the superior temporal gyrus whilst under local anaesthesia. The second circumstance under which the use of local anaesthesia is an advantage is when the fit pattern or EEG abnormalities suggest that supra-sylvian areas may be involved requiring an extension of the standard temporal lobectomy. In this case it may be necessary to define the motor areas more accurately so as to avoid or minimise any post-operative deficit. It should be emphasised that when operating upon other cortical areas the need to use local anaesthesia may be more pressing.

The methods used by most centres are similar. The choice of basal sedation may vary. If general anaesthesia is used then generally non-barbiturate agents are employed together with controlled respiration and the patient is kept as light as possible during the corticography. It is not usually necessary to use diuretics or mannitol during these operations. If local anaesthesia is used then infiltration is carried out with 0.5 per cent lignocaine with adrenaline at a dilution of 1:200 000. Details of this technique are to be found in Van Buren et al. (1975). After the corticogram, which is activated with 100–150 mg of thiopentone, the anaesthesia is supplemented with additional thiopentone during the resection and closure. If necessary the skin may be re-infiltrated at the very conclusion of the procedure. We have not found blind endotracheal intubation necessary during this part of the procedure.

The technique of resection by the 'en bloc' method, in which the pathology is preserved, is well described by Falconer (1971a). His account can be followed by any well trained neurosurgeon. The operation is technically easier when some atrophic process is present. In performing the craniotomy it is important to get right down on to the floor of the middle fossa and to within 1–2 cm of the temporal pole, otherwise subsequent manoeuvres become more difficult. In carrying out the resection several points are important. First, the appropriate part of the superior temporal gyrus must be preserved on the dominant side. Second, care is necessary in dissecting the temporal cortex off the insula so as to avoid damage to the branches and main trunk of the middle cerebral artery — in this respect the subpial technique described by Falconer is excellent. Third, it is necessary to remove the anterior 1–2 cm of the hippocampus without encroaching on the medial structures in the tentorial hiatus. The closure is performed in the usual way, as following any other craniotomy, and we do not routinely use antibiotics or steroids. The patient is usually maintained on two antiepileptic drugs, primidone and phenytoin or carbamazepine are useful. If the patient remains free of attacks for two or three years after operation, then after appropriate EEG studies,

withdrawal of this antiepileptic medication can be considered. The usual post-operative complications of craniotomy rarely occur, but can be effectively treated and have no effect on the eventual outcome of the surgery (Falconer & Serafetinides, 1963).

Neuropathology

It is impossible to discuss the resective surgery of epilepsy without reference to the pathology and in this respect the data is greatest and most crisp in relation to temporal lobectomy. Also because the results of operation are related to the pathology this is an appropriate place to discuss it. Murray Falconer, collaborating with Professor J.A.N. Corsellis, who had already carried out important independent studies on autopsy material, produced the largest and most comprehensive series of temporal lobectomy specimens in which the resection included the anterior 1–2 cm of the hippocampus. As described by Falconer (1971b), the pathological material divided itself into four groups. Gross lesions which would have been treated on their own account, e.g. meningiomas, were of course excluded. The four groups, together with their relationship to the results of surgery are shown in Table 10.3, taken from Falconer and Serafetinides (1963). The pathological groups consist of the following.

Mesial temporal sclerosis. Classically this lesion consists of a loss of neurones from the hippocampus in the H_1 or Sommer sector, together with a lesser degree of loss from the end-folium, (H_3 and H_4), but with sparing of the resistant or H_2 sector. This pathology was originally described by Bouchet and Cazauvieihl (1925). Both Sano and Malamud (1953) and Margerison and Corsellis (1966) described this lesion in the brains of chronic epileptic patients dying in psychiatric institutions and noted that the lesion was frequently either unilateral or markedly more pronounced on one side. In the Margerison and Corsellis study a good correlation was found between the clinical and EEG features and the pathological findings. This lesion of mesial temporal sclerosis formed 50 per cent of the material in Falconer's series. Similar findings have been reported by others, although the proportion of this

Table 10.3 Pathological findings (Reproduced from Falconer & Serafetinides, 1963)

	Group A (free or almost free of seizures: 53 cases)	Group B (Worthwhile improvement: 30 cases)	Group C (Remaining patients: 17 patients)	Total
Mesial temporal sclerosis	28	15	4	47
Small focal tumours or angiomas	14*	8‡	2	24*†
Miscellaneous lesions (scars, infarcts, etc.)	7†	3	3	13†
Equivocal changes	8	6	8	22
Total	53	30	17	100

* Includes one patient with mesial temporal sclerosis
† Includes three patients who also had mesial temporal sclerosis
‡ Includes two patients who also had mesial temporal sclerosis

lesion varies: Jann Brown (1973) gives 65.6 per cent; Mathieson (1975) about 10 per cent; Talairach *et al.* (1974) give 56 per cent; and Van Buren *et al.* (1975) give 53 per cent.

Hamartomas and small cryptic tumours. Although this kind of material was found in 20–25 per cent of the surgical material, it was absent from the autopsy material studies by Margerison and Corsellis (1966). It has been suggested that these lesions, with the passage of time, become frank glial tumours (Falconer, 1967b). There is no definite evidence for this and with the CT scanner we are now occasionally seeing small calcified lesions in the medial part of the temporal lobes of older patients. The lesions seen in the surgical specimens are usually of a glial nature, although occasionally mixed lesions classified as ganglion-gliomas are seen. In addition a small number of other lesions are seen such as angiomas or a 'forme fruste' of tuberous sclerosis described as cortical dysplasia by Taylor *et al.* (1971).

Scars and infarcts. These were less common, accounting for 10 per cent or less of the total.

Non-specific lesions. These formed about 25 per cent of the Falconer material and similar proportions are quoted by other centres. The use of the term 'non-specific' is deliberate in that this group do show some neuropathological changes in the form of astrocyte proliferation and some subpial gliosis but without anything more discrete. It is difficult to compare these results with those of other centres in detail, because similar systems of pathological grouping are not used. However, basically the authors already quoted present similar results with about 20–25 per cent of their material lacking a discrete pathology.

Results of temporal lobectomy

These have been well summarised by Jensen (1975a), and her bald statement remains basically true, that 'two-thirds of the patients were either free or almost free of seizures and over half of these patients who were mentally abnormal before operation were normalised or had obtained a marked improvement'. If we make use of her figures for the three centres each with over 100 resections namely, the Montreal Neurological Institute, Murray Falconer's figures from the Maudsley, London, and those from the Salpetrière in Paris, then we obtain the results shown in Table 10.4. The results of operation with regard to seizure control are grouped according to the scheme proposed by Jensen (1975a), in which the divisions are; Group I, free from seizures, Group II; marked improvement in frequency, meaning at least 75 per cent better, Group III some improvement, and Group IV no improvement. It should be noted that this grouping relates only to seizure control. These three series contain 831 patients and it will be seen that 42 per cent were completely free of seizures and a further 22 per cent fell into Group II giving a worthwhile result from operation in 64 per cent of cases. The mortality rate is extremely small, being 0.5 per cent and ever declining.

Neurological sequelae do occur and their documentation varies from series to series. The

Table 10.4 Results of unilateral temporal lobectomy for chronic epilepsy (Data taken from Jensen, 1975a)

Centre	Number	Worthwhile improvement		Remainder		Operative Deaths
		Group I	Group II	Group III	Group IV	
Guy's – Maudsley, London	152	69 (45.4%)	25 (16.4%)	28 (25%)	24 (15.8%)	2 (1.3%)
Salpetriere, Paris	110	32 (29.1%)	40 (36.4%)	20 (18.2%)	17 (15.5%)	1 (0.9%)
Montreal Neurological Institute	569	249 (34.8%)	120 (21%)	200 (35.1%)		1 (0.2%)
Total	831	350 (42.2%)	185 (22.3%)	299 (36%)		4 (0.5%)

'neighbourhood fits' described by Falconer and Serafetinides (1963) in 45 per cent of their patients which consist of twitching of the contra-lateral face and arm and are invariably transient, occur in the first post-operative week and have no effect on the ultimate outcome. In our hands the chief neurological complications from the most minor to the most serious have been: visual field defects, usually an upper quadrantanopia, homolateral third nerve palsy, speech disturbance when operating upon the dominant hemisphere and hemipareses. It is difficult to know the extent of these problems in the published series, because assessment of them is clearly dependent upon how long they persist and the accuracy of observations. Jensen (1975a) pointed out that there is a great disparity in the recording of visual field defects between different centres. If resections are greater than 6.0– 6.5 cm from the temporal pole in adults then a complete homonymous hemianopia is more likely to result, becoming almost certain beyond 7.0 cm. When the resection lies between 5.0 and 6.0 cm then the chance of a complete homonymous hemianopia occurring is only about 5 per cent or less is due to the vagaries of Meyer's loop (Falconer & Wilson, 1958). The upper quadrantanopia appears in about 60 per cent of patients, normally recedes in many of them over one year, and does not seriously incommode those in whom it persists. Similarly, although homolateral third nerve palsies occurred in 15 per cent of Falconer's material, they were usually of short duration disappearing in less than six months. Likewise, if

patients are carefully observed during the first week after a dominant temporal lobe resection they invariably show some degree of expressive dysphasia. However, even patients who have been virtually aphasic for up to four weeks have regained social speech within three to six months. The incidence of dysphasia of 5 per cent given by Jensen (1975a) seems reasonable. Any hemiparesis again is usually transient and an incidence of 2 per cent for permanent hemiparesis suggested by Jensen (1975a) is consistent with our experience.

In summary, the neurological sequelae of temporal lobectomy, although they occur, are not so frequent or permanent as to be a serious deterrent to the operation.

The intellectual sequelae of temporal lobectomy have already been hinted at.

In general, psychometric scores one month after operation show a slight decline, but by one year after operation there is generally an improvement on the pre-operative scores. The dangers of producing a disabling amnesic syndrome when both temporal lobes have been damaged is well known, and the autopsy findings under such circumstances have been described by Penfield (1974). The auditory learning deficit described by Blakemore and Falconer (1967), which may follow left temporal lobectomy, is known to recede in the majority of cases over two or three years. Jones (1974) found that patients who had undergone a left temporal lobectomy needed mnemonic aids to overcome their learning difficulties, whereas those patients who had had a right temporal lobectomy did not need these aids. The subject is well reviewed by Milner (1975).

The assessment of the psychiatric consequences of the operation are made difficult by the relatively high proportion of patients with psychiatric abnormalities among those selected for surgery. In the Copenhagen series of 74 patients, only 8.5 per cent were considered psychiatrically normal (Jensen, 1976b) and in the series of 100 patients described by Taylor and Falconer (1968) only 13 per cent could be considered psychiatrically normal. As we have already mentioned, the chief abnormalities observed were social maladjustment and aggression. In some rare cases a murderous impulse may form part of an ictal pattern, and Falconer certainly had one case in which such attacks ceased completely after temporal lobectomy and a similar case is described by Hamlin and Delgado (1977). It is the experience of all those who have been concerned with these matters that social adjustment is improved by operation (Taylor & Falconer, 1968; Jensen, 1976b) so that more than 50 per cent of these patients can live independently and be employed afterwards. Needless to say, those patients who did best in that respect also showed a good relief of seizures. Jensen (1976b) states that an improvement in personality problems was associated with good seizure relief, normal intelligence and operation undertaken before the age of 15 years. As far as frank aggression is concerned, Falconer (1973) surveying one hundred patients noted that 27 were aggressive prior to surgery, and that 10 of these were improved by temporal lobectomy, and in seven of these 10 cases the pathology in the resected temporal lobe was mesial temporal sclerosis. With regard to psychoses, we have already seen that these usually failed to improve if they were schizophreniform, indeed, we have seen these made worse after operation. Serafetinides and Falconer (1962) describing 12 cases noted that when there was a confusional psychosis, directly related to the epilepsy (see Fenton, 1978) this usually disappeared, that paranoid delusional psychosis accompanied by depression might improve and that schizophrenic-like states usually persisted. The overall effect upon the psychiatric state, summarised by Jensen (1975a), is that only 35.6 per cent of 323 patients surveyed either failed to improve or deteriorated following temporal lobe resection.

The long term fate of these patients has been studied. Jensen (1975b), surveying the long term mortality in 820 patients surviving operation, found a late mortality of 4.76 per cent; one-third of these patients died of epilepsy, one-third of suicide and the remaining one-third of natural causes. Taylor and Marsh (1977) made a detailed study of the cause of death of 37 patients out of 193 operated upon by Murray Falconer. Eight of these deaths were due to persisting epilepsy, nine were due to suicide, three of these patients had been free of seizures since operation, 11 of the deaths were clearly due to natural causes, including recurrent tumours, and the remaining nine deaths occurred in unclear circumstances. Although, as Jensen (1975b) notes, the death rate observed in these patients is in excess of that for an equivalent Danish population aged 10–59 years (47.6/1000 for the former compared with 2.9/1000 for the latter) it is still better than the rate of 59.4/1000 for a representative group of Danish epileptic patients described by Brink Henriksen Juul-Jensen and Lund (1970).

Frontal lobectomy and other cortical resections

The remainder of the resective procedures fall into two groups: first, frontal lobectomy and resection of other parts of the cortical mantle, usually central and parietal since it was rare for the occipital regions to be the site of epileptogenic foci; and secondly, really major resections amounting to total or sub-total hemispherectomies. With the exception of the Montreal Neurological Institute the experience of most centres with these operations is quite small. Thus in the Maudsley Unit where over 300 operations for epilepsy were carried out in 25 years, only 21 were focal resections and about 20 were hemispherectomies. The material of this section therefore derives chiefly from experience of the Montreal group as published by Rasmussen, together with the lesser experience of Talairach et al. (1974) in Paris, a small series by Bhatia and Kollevold (1976) from Scandinavia and our own small series.

The principles of assessment are similar to those already described for temporal lobectomy, but in frontal lobectomy the decisions are more difficult for a number of reasons. The first is that although the typical adversive seizure is common enough, it tends to occur in association with other kinds of seizures which are of more prognostic significance than in temporal lobe epilepsy. According to Rasmussen (1975a) frontal lobe seizures may begin in one of six ways, which include: immediate unconsciousness followed by a tonic-clonic phase (non-lateralising); immediate unconsciousness accompanied by adversion of the head and eyes (anterior third of the frontal lobe); initial adversion of the head and eyes with preserved consciousness (intermediate frontal convexity); posturing of the body, elevation of the contralateral arm, and adversion of the head and eyes (medial hemisphere surface, intermediate part of the frontal lobe); and a vague cephalic sensation or a brief thought disorder consisting of 'forced thinking' (non-lateralising).

The second difficulty is that of localising EEG abnormalities within the frontal lobes by scalp EEG especially when these abnormalities may be near the midline. The prevalence of apparent bi-frontal abnormalities in these patients makes selection difficult even if special tests to try to differentiate between secondary and primary bilateral synchrony are used (Rasmussen, 1975a). The impressive results described with SEEG by Talairach et al. (1974) if adopted more widely might improve this situation. A similar philosophy is adopted by Rossi et al. (1978) who suggest that SEEG may improve the overall failure rate of 30 to 40 per cent in epilepsy surgery which they attribute to inability to define accurately the epileptogenic zone.

In their series of 91 patients, Bhatia and Kollevold (1976) carried out 22 frontal lobectomies as against 36 temporal lobectomies, in the Paris series (Talairach et al., 1974) there were 24 frontal lobectomies compared with 68 temporal lobectomies and in the Montreal material (Rasmussen, 1975a) 760 temporal lobectomies were performed and 244 frontal lobectomies. The pathology found in frontal lobe resections is less well defined than with temporal resections. Rasmussen (1975a) describes the pathological findings in their 244 cases of non-tumourous frontal lobe resections in which 68 per cent were cicatricial or anoxic, 10

per cent miscellaneous and 21 per cent were unknown. The other groups do not give a separate analysis.

The technique of operation in the frontal lobe is similar to that used elsewhere, and provided that a reasonable posterior limit to the resection is observed the neurological sequelae are less than in temporal lobectomy. If the procedure is performed with local anaesthesia then ECoG and cortical stimulation may be used to plan the resection, especially in the dominant hemisphere where speech may be at risk. The results of operation are good though not as good as for temporal lobectomy. In Rasmussen's series of 236 patients (Rasmussen, 1975a) the operative mortality was four (1.7 per cent) and of the remainder, 23 per cent were in Group I (free from seizures), and 32 per cent in Group II (marked improvement in frequency); giving a worthwhile improvement in 55 per cent but with a greater proportion in Group II. In the Paris series, (Talairach et al., 1974) a success rate of 54.2 per cent (equivalent to Groups I and II), was obtained in 24 cases of frontal lobe resection.

The surgery of other parts of the cortex is equally rare and here reliance must be placed almost totally on the results from Montreal, of whose material this group forms 30 per cent (Rasmussen, 1975b). In the lesions in the central area the attacks are more stereotyped and virtually always have a somato-motor or somato-sensory component. These patients also presented with either focal status or epilepsia partialis continua more frequently than other groups. Because many of the causative lesions were gross and acquired early in life, a higher proportion of these patients had a pre-existing neurological deficit, and came to operation at an earlier age than other groups. In these cases also, whenever possible, local anaesthesia, ECoG and cortical stimulation are employed and these techniques become most useful. These matters are dealt with in more detail by Blume and Girvin (p. 422). The surgical technique should be meticulous with excision taken to the gyral margins where possible and down to the underlying white matter. Although the question of post-operative neurological deficit is of course a thorny one in these particular areas, Rasmussen's experience in this respect is fairly encouraging

(Rasmussen, 1975b). He states that complete removal of the motor face area leaves a persisting deficit in only half of the patients, that the post-central leg area can be removed with only a slight decrease in proprioception in the foot, and that the pre-central leg area should only be removed if it is already damaged but that on those rare occasions when it has been thought necessary a flaccid paralysis of the leg has resulted, which may show some recovery over three to four months. Although portions of the arm area may be removed, there will always be some deficit even if it is only slight.

The results of surgery in these areas are quite good with 31 per cent of the patients in Group I and 26 per cent in Group II giving a worthwhile improvement in 57 per cent. In the French series, (Talairach et al. 1974) a success rate of 60 per cent was obtained in resections from central cortex. Details of parietal and occipital resections can be found in the same review (Rasmussen, 1975b).

At the Maudsley, a group of 21 patients had undergone resections in areas other than the temporal lobe for non-tumourous lesions. These consisted of seven frontal resections, 12 from the central area and two from other areas. Except in two patients the variety of epileptic attacks which the patient suffered had no effect on the outcome of surgery. In these two cases there were a wide variety of seizures including focal, minor, and major, probably associated with generalised cerebral disease. The neurophysiological findings were variable but a specifically focal EEG was not necessarily associated with a good surgical result. Corticography was used to define the limits of resection. Resection at the medial border of the hemisphere was less successful than elsewhere. The overall results in these 21 patients were: Group I, six cases; Group II, eight cases; and Group III, seven cases. All the patients in Group I had positive pathology in the specimen and the incidence of abnormalities in the AEG was higher in Group I than in the other groups, and this was also true of the Scandinavian material (Bhatia & Kollevold, 1976).

In summary, resective surgery in these other parts of the cortex can also be rewarding. The investigation of such patients, especially the neurophysiological investigations, is more difficult than with temporal lobe epilepsy, particularly in the absence of a discrete CT scan abnormality, although the use of SEEG may improve this aspect. The side effects of these operations are minor and except when operating in areas where a calculated risk has to be taken, they are relatively infrequent. The results of operation in terms of epilepsy relief are reasonable; Rasmussen (1975b) has 64 per cent in Groups I and II, Talairach et al. (1974) obtained 67 per cent in Groups I and II, and in our small series there was 64 per cent in these categories. But Bhatia and Kollevold (1976) had only 30 per cent in these groups. In general this degree of seizure relief is worthwhile and with better selection procedures may improve.

Major resective procedures

Major resective procedures in the form of total or subtotal hemispherectomy have in recent years lacked popularity because of the late complications and also a natural aversion to such major procedures; this is unfortunate because these operations are in many ways very successful. The indications for operation are as follows. The subject should of course suffer with intractable epilepsy and in addition have a complete infantile hemiplegia usually accompanied by a complete homonymous hemianopia although if there is a partial field defect its conversion to a complete hemianopia would be justified in exchange for the benefits of operation. It is debatable as to whether a progressive hemiparesis rendered almost complete by the Todd's paresis of an intractable focal epilepsy is effectively the same thing as a complete hemiplegia. In addition there should be evidence that only one hemisphere is involved, the degree of mental deficiency should be acceptable and parental collaboration should be good. The onset of progressive dementia, preferably supported by psychometric data, should be regarded as an indication for urgent action if all the other parameters are right (Griffith, 1967). Otherwise, the situation may become irretrievable. These patients often have a behaviour disorder and this is not a bar to operation but may indeed be improved by surgery. This group may experience a number of different seizures, although Wilson (1970), reviewing 50 hemispherectomies carried out by McKissock, notes that major seizures occurred in

56 per cent of the patients but predominated in only 40 per cent. Minor seizures occurred as the sole form of epilepsy in only 12 per cent, but occurred in all of the mixed group which comprised 38 per cent of the total. Exclusively focal or unilateral seizures were uncommon (10 per cent of the series). In the same series 72 per cent of the patients had a behaviour disorder, sometimes episodic, which was sufficiently severe to disrupt home, institutional or working life.

Generally, there is a clear cut cerebral insult early in life to account for the hemiplegia and Wilson (1970) describes two main causes. The first was an episode of perinatal trauma or hypoxia which occurred in 54 per cent of the patients. The other cause was an acute febrile illness between the ages of one year and four years, accompanied or followed by convulsions which were frequently focal or unilateral, and during the convalescent phase of the illness the hemiplegia was noticed. These cases constituted 30 per cent of that series. In a small number of cases the aetiology is different, thus two of Wilson's patients suffered with Sturge-Weber Syndrome. On other occasions it has been expedient to perform hemispherectomy on children with intractable epilepsy due to progressive hemisphere disease who otherwise fulfil the indications for the operation.

We have already noted that these patients show a severe hemiplegia in spite of which all of them are able to walk pre-operatively, and many of them will have undergone orthopaedic procedures to try to help their walking. Psychometric studies usually show a low level of function. In the cases described by Wilson (1970), 66 per cent of the patients had an IQ score less than 65 points. Fortunately, the fate of speech after hemispherectomy is not a problem, it is usually present before operation and preserved. In the series described by Wilson (1970), there was no alteration in speech in 84 per cent of the patients as a result of operation. However, post-operative dysphasia or aphasia did occur in six patients (12 per cent of the total); in five of these the left hemisphere was removed, and in the other patient the right hemisphere was removed and the patient was reputed to be right-handed. In three of these patients, including the last, the deficit persisted, although the author states that accurate assessment was difficult because of the degree of mental retardation. The available literature on the subject is unhelpful. There are certainly reports in the literature of adult patients surviving dominant hemispherectomy for glioma and regaining some speech function (Smith, 1966). The data about the age at which speech transference to the opposite hemisphere can occur is sparse and based upon poor observation. It seems to be true that if the hemisphere damage occurs before speech acquisition then there will be no problem. After that it can be assumed that in the majority of cases speech will reappear and from our own experience this seems to be true, at least up to the age of six or seven years.

Plain skull radiographs usually show the changes of hemiatrophy. Encephalography usually demonstrates unilateral ventricular dilatation sometimes with a porencephaly which is frequently in the territory of the middle cerebral artery. Anything other than minimal damage to the opposite hemisphere on radiological investigation should be regarded as a contra-indication to operation. With CT scanning these changes can be demonstrated very elegantly. The use of arteriography is purely an adjunct to the technical aspects of the surgery. Even in cases where examination of the resected hemisphere subsequently shows an arterial lesion as the definitive pathology the pre-hemispherectomy angiograms often fail to demonstrate such a lesion (Till & Hoare, 1962). However, pre-operative angiography is necessary because often both anterior cerebral arteries are fed from the internal carotid artery of the affected side, which affects the technique of operation. The EEG changes in these patients at first sight seem contrary in that there are frequently more abnormalities to be seen over the 'good' hemisphere whereas the record over the affected hemisphere may be relatively flat. However, it is known that these changes respond well to surgery, indeed it was in part the progressive deterioration over the 'good' hemisphere which led Krynauw (1950) to propose the operation and he was gratified to find these changes reversible.

The operative technique is well known. The practice is to carry out a hemicorticectomy in which all the neocortex and the hippocampus is removed leaving the pallium. With experience this is a relatively safe procedure to perform and details may be found in the appropriate references (Rasmussen, 1975b; Kempe, 1968). Because of the problem of delayed haemorrhage described below the Montreal group have suggested that a buttress of cortex should be left on the affected side. This prevents small movements of the falx which they assert are the origin of this complication. In order to determine whether this remnant should be frontal or occipital, we use ECoG to find out which area is electrically more innocuous. Rasmussen (1975b) calls this procedure subtotal hemispherectomy and stated that he has carried it out on 48 patients since 1937 with no cases of delayed haemorrhage. In a few cases the hemispherectomy has subsequently been 'completed' without further complication.

In modern times, the operative mortality of these operations is low; both Rasmussen (1975b) and Wilson (1970) report only one such death, although two more of the Montreal patients died within a year as a result of a progressive encephalopathy. In the early post-operative period, in spite of very careful attention to haemostasis at the operation, it is common to see a form of aseptic meningitis characterised by irritability, drowsiness, headache, fever and meningism. It occurred in 28 per cent of the cases described by Wilson (1970). It usually resolves in one to two weeks, is best treated by daily lumbar puncture, or if severe by washing out the cavity through a separate trephine hole. It may also respond to steroids. The possible neurological sequelae have already been discussed. After the period of aseptic meningitis has passed, the patient is mobilised and may require a period of three to four weeks to relearn his walking. The late morbidity of total hemispherectomy has already been alluded to. In a few cases there was progressive hydrocephalus of the remaining ventricle without clear evidence of an acute cause or bleeding. However, the commonest complication was the late delayed haemorrhage which occurred in one-third to one-quarter of most series and could occur up to 20 years after the original operation. This eventually leads to superficial haemosiderosis of the brain, spinal cord and the remaining ventricle as first described by Oppenheimer and Griffith (1966). Clinically this is

seen as headache, sometimes sudden in onset so as to mimic sub-arachnoid haemorrhage, accompanied by vomiting and followed by intellectual and sometimes neurological deterioration.

The possible pathogenesis of the condition is discussed in detail by Wilson (1970). This complication accounted for death in one third of the Montreal cases (Rasmussen, 1975b) and in 20 per cent of the cases described by Wilson (1970). However, it is possible that with early and energetic treatment the condition can be ameliorated and Falconer and Wilson (1969) described how the complication occurred in four of their 18 cases and was successfully treated in three of these patients.

The results of both total and sub-total hemispherectomy are good, although the results obtained with the sub-total procedure are slightly inferior to those described from the total procedure. In the cases described by Rasmussen (1975b) there were 69 per cent of cases in Group I after total hemispherectomy with 85 per cent of cases showing a marked improvement, whereas the corresponding figures for patients undergoing sub-total hemispherectomy were 45 per cent in Group I and 70 per cent showing a marked improvement. In the total hemispherectomies described by Wilson (1970) the results are similar to those described by Rasmussen for that procedure with 68 per cent of patients in Group I and 82 per cent showing a marked improvement. A similarly gratifying result was obtained for behaviour disturbance with 53 per cent becoming normal and a further 40 per cent improved.

In view of the major surgery involved and the problem of late delayed haemorrhage, alternatives to hemispherectomy have been sought. Lesser degrees of cortical resection have usually proved ineffective. Griffith has used a combination of anterior callosal section and section of the internal capsule from within the dilated ventricle with some success (personal communication). Another alternative is suggested by Balasubramanian and Kanaka (1975), who described the effect of stereotactic amygdalectomy, carried out in the affected hemisphere on ten patients with epilepsy, behaviour disorder and hemiplegia. They reported relief of epilepsy in all the patients and improvement in behaviour in seven of these children who were followed up for between two and nine years.

If similar experiences were obtained by other people then this could be the solution to the disadvantages of hemispherectomy. If, however, this approach should prove disappointing, then the use of the 'subtotal' hemispherectomy would seem to be justified in properly selected patients.

STEREOTACTIC PROCEDURES

The application of the techniques of stereotactic neurosurgery to chronic epilepsy is a superficially attractive idea. The basis of such surgery is well known in its application to the treatment of movement disorders such as Parkinson's disease, and to a lesser extent to the treatment of chronic psychiatric illness. The original method was developed by Horsley and Clarke for experimental use, but was subsequently adapted by others for use in the human brain. In essence it depends upon the fact that if an accurate map in three dimensions can be made of the brain with reference to fixed points, then a needle inserted through a small drill hole in the skull can be guided under X-ray control using co-ordinates from the fixed points in three planes, to any particular structure known as the target. This target can then be made the subject of neurophysiological investigation, including stimulation, as has already been described under the topic of SEEG. But in addition it is possible to destroy such targets using a variety of means. Making these small intra-cerebral lesions, provided that they are reasonably accurate, is likely to have less morbidity and mortality than major open surgery.

The idea that the persistence of chronic epilepsy may be equally attributable to the electrical properties of the neural paths over which the seizure discharge travels and to whatever basic pathology is responsible, gathers some support from experimental work. If we accept this, then the bulk of the clinical and experimental evidence would be in favour of a subcortical midbrain origin for such pathways, occurring in reverberating circuits between the reticular formation, thalamus and cerebral cortex. Such a concept was that of 'centrencephalic epilepsy' from the Montreal school. It was therefore suggested that interruption of some of these 'circuits' by judiciously placed stereotactic

lesions would help to control generalised epilepsies which were not otherwise amenable to surgical treatment. Earlier methods used to achieve the interruption of these pathways involved the use of open surgery and these will be dealt with briefly at the end of this section. But using stereotactic techniques, this reasoning suggested targets in various subcortical structures including the internal capsule, thalamus, basal ganglia and hypothalamus.

By contrast the use of targets in the deep structures of the temporal lobe emerged as a side product of placing of stereotactic lesions in these areas to try to control aggressive behaviour, as pioneered by Narabyashi et al. (1963). It was noted that if such patients had poorly controlled epilepsy, which a significant proportion did, then if the lesion was successful in controlling their behaviour it would also frequently ameliorate their epilepsy. Since it was also known that poorly controlled psychomotor epilepsy was often associated with structural lesions in one or both temporal lobes, this seemed an added reason to feel that targets in these areas would be rewarding. Finally, there was theoretical justification from the properties of the 'Papez' circuit and the basolateral components of the limbic system (Livingston & Escobar, 1972), for supposing that such lesions would be effective. Likewise, McLardy (1969) had for many years suggested that the interruption of neural connections between the amygdala and the CA two part of the hippocampus was the effective part of all temporal lobe surgery.

Technique

The nature of the lesion-making process does not seem to be important and various methods have been used including warm wax and lipiodil, radio-frequency currents and radioactive seeds. Also the particular variety of stereotactic technique used in setting up the target does not seem to be critical. However, three factors influence the use and assessment of stereotactic surgery in the treatment of epilepsy. The first is that because most of these procedures are free of mortality, direct verification of the placing of these lesions is almost impossible and their size at present makes them difficult to detect with routine CT scanning techniques. Therefore, if there is an error in the placing of these lesions this may either result in a good target being mis-reported, or vice versa. Secondly, when experimental results from animal work are looked at they are not sufficiently consistent to serve as a valid model for human lesions. Thirdly, the diversity of clinical disease, placing of lesions and description of results in published reports make any attempt to utilise specific targets for any particular patient almost impossible. In recent reviews, both Talairach *et al*. (1974) and Ojemann and Ward (1975) state that this method of surgery, even in the best reported series, is much less effective than resective surgery and largely empirical.

Stereotactic lesions in subcortical structures

As we have already noted, the targets in this group have included the internal capsule, pallidum, thalamic nuclei, fields of Forel and the hypothalamus. There is little to be gained from a catalogue of the papers in this field, most of which relate to a diversity of lesions in a small number of patients. A good review is to be found in Ojemann and Ward (1975) and a few examples of this work will suffice. Thus, Spiegel, Wycis and Baird (1958) report the effect of pallidal lesions and in their later papers they note that the combination of these with amygdala lesions is particularly effective. Typically, however, of their nine patients, three only were free of seizures and three others 'improved'. Likewise, Pertuiset *et al*. (1969) describe the effect of stereotactic thalamotomy on ten patients with 'grand mal' but note that the results are inconclusive. Jelsma *et al*. (1973) describe how various capsular lesions will improve primary focal epilepsy, but not primary or secondary centrecephalic epilepsy. Finally, lesions made in the fields of Forel are also disappointing in their results (Jinnai, Mukawa & Kobayashi, 1976) although this may depend in part on the accuracy of placing of the lesion (Jinnai & Mukawa, 1970).

Because of the considerable variation in the case and target selection when subcortical lesions are used, these must still be regarded as largely speculative without clear indications which can be perceived by those not directly concerned in this work.

Stereotactic lesions in temporal structures

Here the prospect seems more hopeful, a greater number of cases are described and the effect of the lesions seems more evident. In most series, lesions were made in the amygdala but these were often combined with other targets including the anterior commisure and the fornix.

Narabayashi and Shima (1973) recently summarised the results of stereotactic amygdalotomy upon 47 children, and notes that 44 of these had poorly controlled epilepsy. As a result of this procedure, 22 of the children were improved, both in respect of their seizures and their behaviour. Likewise Umbach (1966) describes 25 cases where unilateral or bilateral fornicotomy was combined, in some patients with lesions of the amygdala, lamella medialis or hypothalamus. In 18 cases with good follow-up, five were completely free of epilepsy. They felt that it might be possible in difficult cases with bilateral temporal abnormalities, to combine an open resection on one side with a stereotactic procedure on the other. Adams and Rutkin (1969), however, found only one patient free of epilepsy out of 16 treated with amygdalectomy. By contrast 15 of 36 patients treated by Bouchard, Kim and Umbach, (1975) were improved. It is significant that the best results were found in patients with psychomotor epilepsy requiring only unilateral lesions, precisely the group which might be expected to benefit from resective surgery. Mundinger *et al*. (1976) noted the same kind of results in 33 cases, treatment of unilateral foci being twice as successful as that of bilateral foci. They found that the best combination of lesions was fornicotomy and anterior commissurotomy. The results of other groups are equally scattered. Balasubramanian and Kanaka (1976) obtained complete relief in 36 out of 76 cases using limbic lesions, and Flanigan and Nashold (1976) had four out of 16 patients who would have been in Groups I and II. Barcia-Solario and Broretta (1976) followed up 42 patients who had fornicotomy over eight years and 43 per cent had an improvement in their epilepsy and 58 per cent in their behaviour.

Particular attention should be paid to the results reported by Vaernet (1972) who carried out amygdalectomies on 45 patients. When unilateral lesions were necessary, five out of 27 patients were fit-free, or virtually so, and with bilateral lesions three out of 18. Significantly, eight of 12 patients with unilateral foci who did not do well with this method were subsequently treated with temporal lobectomy with a good result in all cases. Also Talairach *et al*. (1974) describing their results in 44 patients, note that only 23 per cent of patients obtained complete relief of their seizures. They felt that this method of treatment was less successful than open resection and were also anxious about possible memory defects in patients with bilateral disease, having encountered some problem in three of their patients. A final warning is given by Narabayashi and Mizutani (1970) who note that psychomotor attacks are especially prone to return after six to 12 months.

How can one summarise this work? It is clear that both the selection procedures used and the multiplicity of lesions produced makes a comparison between the results of the various groups difficult. The kind of patient treated by Narabayashi is clearly quite different from those treated by Vaernet. In spite of these differences, a number of common themes may be discerned. As the selection criteria approach those for open surgery the results of stereotactic intervention improve. However, it is clear that some patients who do not fulfil the strict criteria for open surgery may be helped by stereotactic lesions. Other workers do not report the memory problems which have been mentioned by the Paris group and indeed many of them positively record the absence of such problems. It is reasonable to suggest that a combination of lesions of the type proposed by Mundinger *et al*. (1976) namely, amygdalotomy combined with fornicotomy and possibly anterior commissurotomy, should be performed.

Other procedures

Brief mention should be made of two other procedures. The first described by Turner (1963) and unique to him, consists of cutting either unilaterally or bilaterally deep temporal fibre connections. When originally reported the operation seemed to have been moderately successful. The second procedure was section, at open operation, of the corpus callosum, so called commissurotomy. The object was to prevent the spread of seizure discharges from one hemisphere to the other. This was first reported by Van Wagenen and Herren (1940). Although the seizures were modified, their frequency was not reduced. Other exponents of this procedure, such as Gorden, Bogen and Sperry (1971) and Luessenhop, de la Cruz and Fenichel (1970) report some reduction in seizure frequency with modifications of this procedure. Complex neuropsychological defects can be demonstrated following these operations, although opinions vary as to their practical importance.

Summary

The history of stereotactic surgery in epilepsy is much shorter than that of resective surgery, and the case material is of necessity more heterogenous. Therefore, the indications for these procedures are less crisp, and because they lack easily identifiable success they have been used more sparsely. However, they are not without some success and it would seem therefore reasonable to continue to explore the possibilities that they present so that eventually we may arrive at more definite indications for their use.

CONCLUSION

This review, after a brief historical introduction, summarises the factors used to select patients for the classical resection procedures used to treat chronic drug-resistant epilepsy. Since the beginning of Penfield's work in 1930, over a period of almost 50 years, it has become possible to predict the value of these procedures to individual patients, achieving freedom from seizures in 30 per cent or more, with a further worthwhile improvement in at least the same proportion, leaving only about 20 per cent unaffected. Over the same period the mortality has dropped to 1 per cent or less and the incidence of serious side effects is in the region of 10 per cent or less, with many of the patients better adjusted to their social environment. Although the results of stereotactic surgery are less impressive they can still bring about a cessation of seizures in 20 per cent of patients, with a lower risk of side effects or fatality.

If we recall that the classical resection techniques were considered novel at the time of their introduction, and that the neurophysiological and pathological grounds on which they were based have shifted and expanded since that time, then it seems reasonable to expect that the extension of our present imperfect techniques in stereotaxy and chronic stimulation will in time yield equally good results provided that their use is carefully documented and observed with the same care that has been applied to the development of resective surgery.

REFERENCES

Adams, J.E. & Rutkin, B.B. (1969) Treatment of temporal lobe epilepsy by stereotactic surgery. *Confinia Neurologica*, **31**, 80.

Balasubramanian, V. & Kanaka, T.S. (1975) Why hemispherectomy? *Applied Neurophysiology*, **38**, 197.

Balasubramanian, V. & Kanaka, T.S. (1976) Stereotactic surgery of the limbic system in epilepsy. *Acta Neurochirugica*, Supplement 23, 225.

Barcia-Solario, J.L. & Broretta, J. (1976) Stereotactic fornicotomy in temporal lobe epilepsy: indications and long term results. *Acta Neurochirugica*, Supplement 23, p. 167.

Bhatia, R. & Kollevold, T. (1976) A follow-up study of 91 patients operated on for focal epilepsy. *Epilepsia*, **17**, 61.

Blakemore, C.B. & Falconer, M.A. (1967) Long-term effects of anterior temporal lobectomy on certain cognitive functions. *Journal of Neurology, Neurosurgery and Psychiatry*, **30**, 364.

Bouchard, G., Kim, Y.K. & Umbach, W. (1975) Stereotaxic methods in different forms of epilepsy. *Confinia Neurologica*, **37**, 232.

Bouchet & Cazauvieihl (1925) De l'épilepsie considerée dans ses rapports avec l'alienation normale. *Archives Generales de Medecine*, Paris, **9**, 510.

Brazier, M.A., Crandall, P.H. & Jann-Brown, W. (1975) Long term follow-up of EEG changes following therapeutic surgery in epilepsy. *Electroencephalography and Clinical Neurophysiology*, **38**, 495.

Brazier, M.A., Crandall, P.H. & Walsh, G.O. (1976) Enhancement of EEG lateralising signs in temporal lobe epilepsy: a trial of diazepam. *Experimental Neurology*, **51**, 241.

Brink-Henriksen, P., Juul-Jensen, P. & Lund, M. (1970) The mortality of epileptics. In Brackenridge R.D.C. (ed.) *Life Assurances Medicine*, p. 139. Proceedings 10th. International Congress Life Assurance Medicine. London: Pitman & Co. Ltd.

Cavanagh, J.B. (1958) On certain small tumours encountered in the temporal lobe. *Brain*, **81**, 389.

Cooper, I.S., (1973) Effect of chronic stimulation of anterior cerebellum on neurologic disease. *Lancet*, **1**, 1321.

Crandall, P.H., (1975) Post-operative management and criteria for evaluation. In Purpura, D.P., Penry, J.K., & Walter, R.D. (eds) *Neurosurgical Management of the Epilepsies* advances in neurology, Vol. 8, p. 265. New York: Raven Press.

Currie, S., Heathfield, K.W.G., Henson, R.A., and Scott, D.F. (1971) Clinical course and prognosis of temporal lobe epilepsy. A survey of 666 patients. *Brain*, **94**, 173.

Engel, J., Driver, M.V., and Falconer, M.A. (1975) Electrophysiological correlates of pathology and surgical results in temporal lobe epilepsy. *Brain*, **98**, 129.

Falconer, M.A. (1967a) Brain mechanisms suggested by neurophysiologic studies. In *Brain Mechanisms Underlying Speech and Language*. p. 185. Grune & Stratton Inc.

Falconer, M.A. (1967b) Surgical treatment of temporal lobe epilepsy. *New Zealand Medical Journal*, **66**, 539.

Falconer, M.A. (1971a) Anterior temporal lobectomy for epilepsy. In Logue, V. (ed.) *Operative Surgery*, Vol. 14, Neurosurgery, p. 142. London: Butterworths.

Falconer, M.A. (1971b) Genetic and related aetiological factors in temporal lobe epilepsy. *Epilepsia*, **12**, 13.

Falconer, M.A. (1973) Reversibility by temporal-lobe resection of the behavioural abnormalities of temporal-lobe epilepsy. *New England Journal of Medicine*, **289**, 451.

Falconer, M.A. (1974) Mesial temporal (Ammon's Horn) sclerosis as a common cause of epilepsy, aetiology, treatment and prevention. *Lancet*, **2**, 767.

Falconer, M.A. and Serafetinides, E.A. (1963) A follow-up study of surgery in temporal lobe epilepsy. *Journal of Neurology, Neurosurgery and Psychiatry*, **26**, 154.

Falconer, M.A., & Taylor, D.C. (1968) Surgical treatment of drug-resistant epilepsy due to mesial temporal sclerosis. Etiology and significance. *Archives of Neurology* (Chicago), **19**, 353.

Falconer, M.A., & Davidson, S. (1974) The rationale of surgical treatment of temporal lobe epilepsy with particular reference to childhood and adolescence. In Harris, P., & Mawdsley, C. (eds) *Epilepsy Proceedings of the Hans Berger Centenary Symposium*, p. 209. Edinburgh: Churchill, Livingstone.

Falconer, M.A., & Wilson, J.L. (1958) Visual field changes following anterior temporal lobectomy: their significance in relation to 'Meyer's Loop' of the optic radiation. *Brain*, **81**, 1.

Falconer, M.A., & Wilson, P.J.E. (1969) Complications related to delayed haemorrhage after hemispherectomy. *Journal of Neurosurgery*, **30**, 413.

Fenton, G.W. (1978) Epilepsy and psychosis. *Journal of the Irish Medical Association*, **71**, 315.

Flanigan, H.F., & Nashold, B.S. (1976) Stereotactic lesions of the amygdala and hippocampus in epilepsy. *Acta Neurochirugica*, Supplement **23**, 235.

Flor-Henry, P. (1969) Psychosis and temporal lobe epilepsy: a controlled investigation. *Epilepsia*, **10**, 363.

Gastaut, H., & Gastaut, J.L. (1976) Computerised transverse axial tomography in epilepsy. *Epilepsia*, **17**, 325.

Gloor, P. (1975) Contributions of electroencephalography and electrocorticography to the neurosurgical treatment of the epilepsies. In Purpura, D.P., Penry, J.K., & Walter, R.D. (eds) *Neurosurgical Management of the Epilepsies* advances in neurology, Vol. 8, p. 59. New York: Raven Press.

Goddard, G.V. (1967) Development of epileptic seizures

through brain stimulation at low intensity. *Nature*, **214**, 1020.

Goldring, S. (1979) A method for the surgical management of focal epilepsy, especially as it relates to children. *Journal of Neurosurgery*, **49**, 344.

Gordon, H.W., Bogen, J.E., & Sperry, R.W. (1971) Absence of deconnexion syndrome in two patients with partial section of the neocommissures. *Brain*, **94**, 327.

Griffith, H.B. (1967) Cerebral hemispherectomy for infantile hemiplegia in the light of late results. *Annals of the Royal College of Surgeons*, **41**, 183.

Hamlin, H., & Delgado, J.M.R. (1977) Case report; juvenile psychomotor epilepsy and associated behaviour disorder – 20-year follow-up of temporal lobectomy. In Sweet, W.H., Obrador, S. & Martin-Rodriguez, J.G. (eds) *Neurosurgical Treatment in Psychiatry, Pain and Epilepsy*, p. 596. Baltimore: University Park Press.

Jann-Brown, W. (1973) Structural substrates of seizure foci in the human temporal lobe. In Brazier, M.A. (ed.) *Epilepsy; Its Phenomena in Man*. U.C.L.A. Forum in Medical Sciences. No. 17, p. 339. New York: Academic Press.

Jelsma, R.K., Bertrand, C.M., Martinez, S.N., & Molina-Negro, P. (1973) Stereotaxic treatment of frontal-lobe and centrencephalic epilepsy. *Journal of Neurosurgery*, **39**, 42.

Jensen, I. (1975a) Temporal lobe surgery around the world. *Acta Neurologica Scandinavica*, **52**, 354.

Jensen, I. (1975b) Temporal lobe epilepsy – late mortality in patients treated with unilateral temporal lobe resections. *Acta Neurologica Scandinavica*, **52**, 374.

Jensen, I. (1976a) Temporal lobe epilepsy. Types of seizures, age and surgical results. *Acta Neurologica Scandinavica*, **53**, 335.

Jensen, I. (1976b) Temporal lobe epilepsy: social conditions and rehabilitation after surgery. *Acta Neurologica Scandinavica*, **54**, 22.

Jinnai, D., & Mukawa, J. (1970) Forel-H-Tomy for the treatment of epilepsy. *Confinia Neurologica*, **32**, 307.

Jinnai, D., Mukawa, J., & Kobayashi, K. (1976) Forel-H-Tomy for the treatment of intractable epilepsy. *Acta Neurochirugica*, Supplement **23**, 159.

Jones, M.K. (1974) Imagery as a mnemonic aid after left temporal lobectomy: contrast between material-specific and generalised memory disorders., *Neurophyschologia*, **12**, 21.

Kempe, L.G. (1968) Hemispherectomy. In *Operative Neurosurgery*, Vol. 1, p. 180., New York: Springer-Verlag.

Krynauw, R.A. (1950) Infantile hemiplegia treated by removing one cerebral hemisphere. *Journal of Neurology, Neurosurgery and Psychiatry*, **13**, 243.

Livingston, K.E., & Escobar, A. (1972) The continuing evolution of the limbic system concept. In Hitchcock, E., Laitinen, L., & Vaernet, K. (eds) *Psychosurgery*, Ch. 2., p. 25. Springfield: Charles C. Thomas.

Luessenhop, A.J., de la Cruz, T.C., & Fenichel, G.M. (1970) Surgical disconnection of the cerebral hemisphere for intractable seizures, results in infancy and childhood. *Journal of the American Medical Association*, **213**, 1630.

Margerison, J.H., & Corsellis, J.A.N. (1966) Epilepsy and the temporal lobes: a clinical, electro-encephalographic and neuropathological study of the brain in epilepsy, with particular reference to the temporal lobes. *Brain*, **89**, 499.

Mark, V.H., & Ervin, F.R. (1970) *Violence and the Brain*. New York: Harper and Row.

Mathieson, G. (1975) Pathological aspects of epilepsy with special reference to the surgical pathology of focal cerebral seizures. In Purpura, D.P., Penry, J.K., & Walter, R.D. (eds) *Neurosurgical Management of the Epilepsies* Advances in neurology Vol. 8, p. 107. New York: Raven Press.

McLardy, T. (1969) Ammons horn pathology and epileptic dyscontrol. *Nature*, **221**, 877.

Milner, B. (1975) Psychological aspects of focal epilepsy and its neurosurgical management. In Purpura, D.P., Penry, J.K., & Walter, R.D. (eds) *Neurosurgical Management of the Epilepsies* Advances in neurology, Vol. 8., p. 299. New York: Raven Press.

Mundinger, F., Becker, P., Grolkner, E., & Bachschmid, G. (1976) Late results of stereotactic surgery of epilepsy predominantly temporal lobe type. *Acta Neurochirugica*, Suppl. **23**, 177.

Narabayashi, H., Nagao, T., Saito, Y., Yoshida, M., & Nagahata, M., (1963). Stereotactic amygdalotomy for behaviour disorders. *Archives of Neurology* (Chicago). **9**, 1.

Narabayashi, H., & Mizutani, T. (1970) Epileptic seizures and the stereotaxic amygdalotomy. *Confinia Neurologica*, **32**, 289.

Narabayashi, H., & Shima, F. (1973) Which is the better amygdala target, the medial or lateral nuclei? (for behaviour problems and paroxysm in epileptics). In Laitinen, L.V., & Livingston, K.E. (eds) *Surgical Approaches in Psychiatry*, Ch. 19, p. 129. Lancaster, U.K.: M.T.P.

Newcombe, R.L., & Shah, S.H. (1975) Radiological abnormalities in temporal lobe epilepsy with clinico-pathological correlations. *Journal of Neurology, Neurosurgery and Psychiatry*, **38**, 279.

Ojemann, G.A., & Ward, A.A. (1975) Stereotactic and other procedures for epilepsy. In Purpura, D.P., Penry, J.K., & Walter, R.D. (eds) *Neurosurgical Management of the Epilepsies* Advances in neurology Vol. 8, p. 241. New York: Raven Press.

Oppenheimer, D.R., & Griffith, H.B. (1966) Persistent intracranial bleeding as a complication of hemispherectomy. *Journal of Neurology, Neurosurgery and Psychiatry*, **29**, 229.

Ounsted, C. (1967) Temporal lobe epilepsy: the problem of aetiology and prophylaxis. *Journal of the Royal College of Physicians of London*, **1**, 273.

Ounsted, C., Lindsay, J., & Norman, R. (1966) *Biological Factors in Temporal Lobe Epilepsy*. London: Heinemann.

Penfield, W.D. (1974) Autopsy findings and comments on the role of hippocampus in experiental recall. *Archives of Neurology* (Chicago), **31**, 145.

Penfield, W., & Jasper, H. (1954) *Epilepsy and the Functional Anatomy of the Human Brain*. Boston: Little Brown & Co.

Penning, R., Miller, C., & Ciompi, L. (1969) Mortalité et Cause de Décés des épileptiques. *Psychiatrica Clinica* (Basel), **2**, 85.

Pertuiset, B., Hirsch, J.F., Sachs, M., & Landau-Ferey, J. (1969) *Selective Stereotactic Thalamotomy in 'Grand Mal' Epilepsy*. Excerpta Med. Amst. I.C.S. No. 193, p. 72, Item 190.

Pond, D.A. (1974) Epilepsy and personality disorders. In Vinken, P.J., & Bruyn, G.W. (eds) *Handbook of Clinical Neurology*, Vol. 15, p. 576. Amsterdam: North Holland Publishing Company.

Rasmussen, T. (1975a) Surgery of frontal lobe epilepsy. In Purpura, D.P., Penry, J.K. & Walter, R.D. (eds) *Neurosurgical Management of the Epilepsies* Advances in neurology. Vol. 8, p. 197. New York: Raven Press.

Rasmussen, T. (1975b) Surgery for epilepsy arising in regions other than the temporal and frontal lobes. In Purpura, D.P.,

Penry, J.K., & Walter, R.D. (eds) *Neurosurgical Management of the Epilepsies* advances in neurology Vol. 8., p. 207. New York: Raven Press.

Rossi, G.F., Colicchio, G., Gentilomo, A., & Scerrati, M. (1978) Discussion on the causes of failure of surgical treatment of partial epilepsies. *Applied Neurophysiology*, **41**, 29.

Sano, K., & Malamud, N. (1953) Clinical significance of sclerosis of the cornu ammonis. *Archives of Neurology and Psychiatry*, **70**, 40.

Serafetinides, E.A., & Falconer, M.A. (1962) The effects of temporal lobectomy in epileptic patients with psychoses. *Journal of Mental Science*, **108**, 584.

Serafetinides, E.A., & Falconer, M.A. (1963) Speech disturbances in temporal lobe seizures: a study in 100 epileptic patients submitted to anterior temporal lobectomy. *Brain*, **86**, 333.

Smith, A. (1966) Speech and other functions after left (dominant) hemispherectomy. *Journal of Neurology, Neurosurgery and Psychiatry*, **29**, 467.

Spiegel, E.A., Wycis, H.T., & Baird, H.W. (1958) Long-range effects of electropallidoansotomy in extrapyramidal and convulsive disorders. *Neurology* (Minneapolis), **8**, 734.

Talairach, J., et al (1974) Approche Nouvelle de la Neurochirugie de l'épilepsie. *Neurochirugie*, **20**, Suppl. 1.

Taylor, D.C. (1975) Factors influencing the occurrence of schizophrenia-like psychoses in patients with temporal lobe epilepsy. *Psychological Medicine*, **5**, 249.

Taylor, D.C., & Falconer, M.A. (1968) Clinical, Socio-economic and psychological changes after temporal lobectomy for epilepsy. *British Journal of Psychiatry*, **114**, 1247.

Taylor, D.C., Falconer, M.A., Bruton, C.J., & Corsellis, J.A.N., (1971) Focal dysplasia of the cerebral cortex in epilepsy. *Journal of Neurology, Neurosurgery and Psychiatry*, **34**, 369.

Taylor, D.C., & Marsh, S.M. (1977) Implications of long-term follow-up studies in epilepsy: with a note on the cause of death. In Penry, J.K. (ed.) *Epilepsy. The Eighth International Symposium*, p. 27. New York: Raven Press.

Till, K., & Hoare, R.D. (1962) Cerebral angiography in investigation of acute hemiplegia in childhood. Little Club. *Clinics in Developmental Medicine*, **6**, 69.

Turner, E. (1963) A new approach to unilateral and bilateral lobotomies for psychomotor epilepsy. *Journal of Neurology, Neurosurgery and Psychiatry*, **26**, 285.

Umbach, W. (1966) Long term results of fornicotomy for temporal epilepsy. *Confinia Neurologica*, **27**, 121.

Vaernet, K., (1972) Stereotaxic amygdalotomy in temporal lobe epilepsy. *Confinia Neurologica*, **34**, 176.

Van Buren, J.M., Ajmone-Marsan, C., Mutsuga, N., & Sudowsky, D. (1975) Surgery of temporal lobe epilepsy. In Purpura, D.P., Penry, J.K. & Walter, R.D. (eds) *Neurosurgical Management of the Epilepsies* Advances in neurology Vol. 8., p. 155. New York: Raven Press.

Van Wagenen, W.P., & Herren, R.Y. (1940) Surgical division of commissural pathways in the corpus callosum. *Archives of Neurology and Psychiatry*, **44**, 740.

Wada, J. (1949) A new method for the determination of the side of cerebral speech dominance. A preliminary report on the intra-carotid injection of sodium amytal in man. *Medicine and Biology*, **14**, 221.

Walter, R.D., (1973) Tactical considerations leading to surgical treatment of limbic epilepsy. In Brazier, M.A. (ed.) *Epilepsy; Its Phenomena in Man*. U.C.L.A. Forum in Medical Sciences, No. 17, p. 99. New York: Academic Press.

Wieser, H.G., Bancaud, J., Talairach, J., Bonis, A., & Szikla, G. (1979). A comparitive value of spontaneous and chemically and electrically induced seizures in establishing the lateralisation of temporal lobe seizures. *Epilepsia*, **20**, 47.

Wilder, B. (1971) Electroencephalogram activation in medically intractable epileptic patients: activation technique including surgical follow-up. *Archives of Neurology* (Chicago), **25**, 415.

Wilson, P.J.E. (1970) Cerebral hemispherectomy for infantile hemiplegia; a report of 50 cases. *Brain*, **93**, 147.

PART TWO

ASSESSMENT FOR NEUROSURGERY, WITH REFERENCE TO CORTICOGRAPHY

W.T. Blume
J.P. Girvin

INTRODUCTION

In this section consideration will be given to those patients who are potentially able to be treated satisfactorily by some type of surgical intervention. The discussion of such treatment will cover the theoretical physiological basis for such surgery, the criteria which must be satisfied before a patient can be considered a surgical candidate, and some of the more important considerations involved in the surgical protocol and intraoperative cortical recording (electrocorticography). Constraints of space limit the depth of discussion. Selected references are available to those readers wishing to probe further (Penfield & Jasper, 1954; Jasper, Ward & Pope, 1969; Brazier, 1973; Purpura, Penry & Walter, 1975; O'Leary & Goldring, 1976).

This discussion excludes any consideration of progressive lesions such as neoplasms which on their own merits may require neurosurgical intervention. Walter (1973) recently discussed concisely some of the more subtle clinical features of epileptic patients who harbour tumours.

PATHOPHYSIOLOGICAL CONSIDERATIONS FOR EPILEPSY SURGERY

From both clinical and experimental observations it is known that any damage to the central nervous system results in some type of structural abnormality, or 'scar'. The histological characteristics of such a scar contain varying proportions of two primary alterations:

1. Neuronal loss and/or morphological change
2. An increase in glial cells (gliosis)

Under normal physiological conditions cortical neurones discharge at relatively low rates and patterns of discharge may vary from one neuronal population to another. Moreover, widely synchronous repetitive bursts of discharge at rates of 10–100 times normal which characterise the epileptogenic region are not seen normally. These altered discharge patterns have been investigated extensively by Ward and his colleagues (Schmidt, Thomas & Ward, 1959; Ward, 1969, 1975; Calvin, Ojemann & Ward, 1973). Whether this epileptogenic discharge is due to alterations in synaptic function or to intrinsic abnormalities of the neuronal membrane, or both, remains an open question (Prince, 1978).

The characteristic EEG interictal abnormality of epilepsy is the 'spike', and its cellular counterpart is a large amplitude, prolonged membrane depolarisation which was initially termed the *paroxysmal depolarisation shift* (PDS) by Matsumoto and Ajmone-Marsan (1964; see also Prince, 1968; 1978; Ayala *et al.*, 1973; Ajmone-Marsan & Gumnit, 1974).

The hyperpolarisation which follows the interictal PDS is lost during the transition from this interictal spike to the ictus, being replaced by depolarisation. When the involvement of a critical mass of cells showing such abnormal behaviour occurs, then the neuronal population exhibits the property of spontaneous and self-sustaining prop-

agation. This creates the symptoms of a clinical seizure.

From the above it becomes obvious that lesions which result in a widespread disturbance of neuronal function do not give rise to a discrete epileptogenic focus. Such situations exist particularly in those individuals who clinically exhibit bi-hemispheric impairment of behaviour and/or cognitive function, such as mental subnormality and/or bilateral neurological deficit. In these patients significant multifocal epileptogenic regions are common.

Patients with very focal lesions are likely to have an associated seizure disorder which would be amenable to surgical excision. This being the case, it is really this 'focal' (partial), as opposed to 'general', epilepsy which is the primary subject of this section.

Kindling

Goddard (1967) found that daily bursts of subthreshold stimulation within the limbic system of the rat gave rise eventually to the production of seizures. This phenomenon has become known as 'kindling'. Much subsequent experimental evidence has demonstrated that extralimbic structures can also be 'kindled' (see Wada, 1976). By this phenomenon, secondary foci can be produced which continue to discharge after ablation of the primary focus (Racine, 1972).

To date, there is no concrete evidence that kindling can occur in human patients. If, however, it should turn out that humans can in fact be kindled, then one would have to look at the interictal spikes as potentially representing continual subthreshold stimulation which in time might give rise to secondary kindled, or fixed, epileptogenic foci. Thus, the removal of such inter-ictal discharge foci, either prophylactically by drugs (Ward, 1975) or surgically would have to be considered more seriously.

CRITERIA FOR SELECTION OF PATIENTS FOR SURGICAL TREATMENT

The actual selection of the patient for surgical treatment is probably no less important than the excision itself and in the hands of the experienced surgeon is probably even more important than the surgical resection. The basis for this statement of course resides in the ability to localise with reasonable certainty the site of the epileptogenic discharge. In selecting patients as potential surgical candidates, the assimilation of many data is required, data which originate from many different neuroscientifically oriented areas. Thus, the decision is not that of one person, but rather that of a 'team'. The importance of this team concept has been repeatedly emphasised. For example, McNaughton and Rasmussen (1975) indicate that such a decision '... requires a team effort ... with a broad experience in every aspect of epilepsy...' or as Walter (1975) states, a team with '... more than a casual interest in seizure disorders' and such responsibility should be '... the province of fairly specialised centres.' Such a team includes the neurosurgeon, neurologist, electroencephalographer, neuropsychologist, neuroradiologist, and the neuropathologist who provides such important feedback from the clinico-pathological correlation.

The criteria for selection vary to some degree from one centre to another. However, within the group of selection criteria there are those which are relatively absolute, in that there is relative unanimity of opinion with respect to their importance. On the other hand there are some in which such uniformity of opinion does not exist and these will be referred to as relative criteria.

Absolute criteria

Incapacitating disorder

The disorder must significantly interfere with the patient's life. The judgement of the 'incapacitating' nature of the disorder is really multifactorial, depending at least to some degree upon occupation, age, psychological make-up and personal goals and responsibilities. For example, exactly the same habitual seizure disorder might exist in two individuals but only prove to be incapacitating to one.

Intractable seizures

Good medical management using individual and combinations of antiepileptic drugs must have been satisfactorily tried and have failed. This includes, of course, the use of drug levels for assessing possible variations in drug absorption and metabolism and for checking the compliance of the patient.

Localised focus

The lesion giving rise to the epilepsy must be 'focal' in nature. Several lines of investigation should ideally implicate the same part of the brain as giving rise to the seizures. Although the electroencephalographic, neuropsychological, and neuroradiological investigations are essential, the patient's own description of the seizure pattern remains the most significant factor. In this regard, it is well to emphasise repeatedly that it is the very beginning of the seizure (whether one wishes to call this an 'aura' or not) which is most important. This indicates either the area of seizure onset or the first clinically 'functional' area to which spread from a 'silent' area has occurred. It should be recognised that there will be variations in the extent of the spread from this focus which will give rise to variations in the clinical seizure pattern, even to the point of generalisation. This rarely represents an additional focus of origin.

Amenability of focus to surgical removal

The focus cannot be in an area the removal of which would result in a significant neurological deficit. At first glance many seizure patterns would appear to implicate origins in areas which cannot be removed. However, in our experience, these patterns nearly always reflect spread from origins in adjacent surgically resectable areas (see above). This principally applies to patients without a neurological deficit appropriate to the area in question. This type of resection can only be carried out safely under local anaesthesia when the accurate boundaries of these important functional areas can be delimited by electrical stimulation.

Relative criteria

These include factors which may vary either from one centre to another or from one team member to another – a grey area within which clinical judgement plays a major role.

Improved quality of life

During the process of considering surgery for an epileptic patient the team continually asks itself 'If the surgery satisfactorily controls the seizures, will the patient's quality of life definitely be measurably improved?' Nowhere is the answer to this question more controversial than in the group of patients on or near the borderline of socioeconomic dependence. For example, there are very cogent arguments for at least considering patients in whom improved seizure control would achieve the following:

1. Avoidance or termination of institutionalisation
2. Conversion of a totally dependent existence to one of some independence (special school classes, sheltered workshop)
3. The reduction or abolition of an associated behavioural abnormality.

Age of the patient

Several factors have led traditionally to a reluctance to operate upon children for epilepsy except in the case of hemispherectomy for infantile hemiplegia. Firstly, in some children the seizure disorder spontaneously improves with age. Secondly, with the exception of the primary generalised epilepsies, children with uncontrolled seizure disorders have multiple epileptogenic foci. With maturation the characteristic inconstancy of such foci in the younger child diminishes and is replaced by more stable foci; the relative prominence among these foci tends to become fixed. Finally, there is a greater likelihood of being able to use local anaesthesia in the older, more mature child.

Falconer (1970) has argued that if children are left until they become post-adolescent, their seizure disorders may have given rise to an accompanying behaviour disorder of such severity as to become a fixed disability even though seizures may be controlled. Because of this, he suggested that these children should be considered for surgical treatment earlier than they had been previously.

Drug intoxication

Control at the expense of intoxication by anti-epileptic medication is obviously not satisfactory. The availability of serum levels of antiepileptic drugs has refined considerably the medical management of seizure disorders. However, it is becoming increasingly apparent that two or more drugs maintained in the high therapeutic range may dull the intellect and flatten the affect. If seizure control can only be achieved at the expense of significant toxicity, then these patients become candidates for surgical treatment when other criteria pertain.

SURGICAL PROTOCOL

Psychological preparedness of the patient

Teams who manage epileptic patients appreciate that there is a necessary psychological 'preparedness' of the patient for surgery; many features of this are intangible. We assess this 'readiness' for operation at one or more interviews which involve a thorough explanation of the rationale for surgery and its procedure. Such preparedness includes the behavioural maturity of the patient, a genuinely appreciated disability from the seizures, and a clear understanding of both the potential benefits and the potential risks of the proposed operation. These interviews also serve to impart confidence in the team, particularly the surgeon. Such confidence is particularly crucial when local anaesthesia is used. A surgical procedure for the relief of seizures must never be 'sold' to the patient or to the relatives of a mentally subnormal patient. Any misgivings unearthed during the interview which remain after thorough discussion should lead to postponement of the surgery.

Anaesthesia

The role of the anaesthetist, especially with the use of local anaesthesia, cannot be over-emphasised. Compassion, patience, and expertise in the selection of anaesthetic agents and particularly the newer neuroleptanalgesic agents,★ charac-

★Dr. George Varkey is the primary anaesthetist for epilepsy surgery at the University Hospital, London, Ontario and from a broad experience with a wide variety of drugs he has arrived at the use of a combination of droperidol, fentanyl, and dimenhydrinate in a continuous intravenous drip.

terise such an individual. This was emphasised specifically from the experience of the Montreal Neurological Institute (Penfield & Jasper, 1954; Penfield, 1954; Pasquet, 1954).

The use of local anaesthesia will depend in large part upon the behavioural maturity of the patient. All intellectually competent patients over 16 years of age can be operated upon under local anaesthesia and neuroleptanalgesia. Behaviourally mature patients can be operated upon quite readily as young as 12 years.

Combined local anaesthesia and neuroleptanalgesia is preferred because it, alone, has no discernible effect upon the electrocorticogram (ECoG). Moreover, it allows the surgeon to map motor, sensory, and speech areas by electrical cortical stimulation. In the young child or uncooperative adult, general anaesthesia is required. In order to minimise its effect on the ECoG, the anaesthetic must be maintained as light as possible. This is facilitated by the use of local anaesthetic infiltration of the scalp and dura.

Surgical resection

An incision in the cerebral cortex in itself will give rise to a 'scar' of some type which is potentially epileptogenic. The aim, therefore, of the surgery is not only to remove an already existing scar but also to reduce to a minimum any damage inflicted upon the intact cortex by the resection.

Surgically induced scarring is minimised by the use of *subpial resection* of the cortex, a method of resection the principles of which were recognised by Horsley (1886). Operations on awake epileptic patients were carried out in the early part of this century by Foerster (1925; 1926) but the protocol of the surgical procedure as practised today was brought to its present degree of refinement at the Montreal Neurological Institute under the impetus of Drs. Penfield and Rasmussen (Rasmussen, 1975; 1977).

The method of subpial resection allows removal of epileptogenic cortex with the least interference with the blood supply and the efferent and afferent connections of the remaining adjacent (intact) cortex. Utilising sulcal boundaries for the resection line, wherever possible, gyri are removed subpially so that the resection line is at the depths of the sulci. Bipolar coagulation is particularly helpful in reducing damage over those portions of the resection line which must cross gyri perpendicularly.

Aside from any general neurosurgical complication, the postoperative course with respect to neurological deficit will be determined in large part by the area resected. If the resection line immediately adjoins an important functional area, then it is not unusual to observe development of altered function of this area (e.g. dysphasia, paresis, sensory apraxia). This usually begins between six and 36 hours postoperatively, reaches a maximum within two to four days, and nearly always clears within a matter of five to ten days. This transient postoperative deficit under such circumstances is presumably the result of swelling within the area as a result of manipulation or ischemia and its duration is shortened by the use of steroids post-operatively.

PREOPERATIVE ELECTROENCEPHALOGRAPHY

The role of serial preoperative EEGs is to confirm the region of seizure origin indicated by clinical data; its function is particularly crucial when such data would be compatible with more than one site of origin. Interictal epileptiform discharges give valuable clues, but an adequate EEG recording of three or more typical seizures is essential. This may be accomplished by scalp and sphenoidal or nasopharyngeal recording, or by the addition of chronic leads implanted in the brain (depth recording). Which method is chosen depends on the clinical problem and to a considerable extent upon the experience and expertise of the centre. Familiarity with the ictal and principal interictal EEG discharges allows a more immediate interpretation of the ECoG. The final preoperative EEG is done the day before surgery to check for any unexpected change.

ELECTROCORTICOGRAM (ECoG)

Close cooperation between the electroencephalographer and the neurosurgeon is essential for success of the ECoG.

The electroencephalographer should have a clear view of the operative field and the surgeon should directly see the corticogram. This is best achieved, in our experience, by the presence of recording equipment and personnel near the operative site in the operating room. In this way communication between these two 'principals' can be immediate.

Recording equipment

To assure proper recording characteristics, corticography electrodes should be nonpolarisable, manoeuvrable, and sufficiently flexible to accommodate a pulsating brain. The procedure also requires electrodes which can be placed on unexposed or hidden surfaces of the brain. In addition, a depth probe for infero-mesial temporal lobe recording is necessary.

The electrodes are mounted on a holder which should be readily adjustable and easily stabilised to the skull.

A standard fully transistorised EEG machine has a sufficient frequency response to record the ECoG adequately. 16 channels are a minimum while 18 channels are preferred.

Procedure

The technologist places a full array of electrodes on the contralateral scalp (ear excluded) after the head is shaved. One of these scalp electrodes serves as a reference to the ECoG. In selecting this reference, we avoid any position which had moderately active preoperative spiking and any position homologous to the region of the corticography. One or two other scalp electrodes serve as linkages for bipolar control of this reference, e.g. in identifying artefacts or physiological reference contamination. The remainder are applied in case the ECoG picture is confused by suspected generalised or bisynchronous epileptiform discharges.

For the initial survey run, electrodes should be placed in a semi-equidistant array to cover the full dorsal lateral surface exposed by the craniotomy. In addition, mobile 'snake' electrodes are placed in other areas implicated in the ictal mechanism such as the inferior and mesial surfaces, and portions of the adjacent lobes beyond the craniotomy.

Almost all of our recording is monopolar, usually referred to an uninvolved contralateral scalp electrode or rarely to an electrically silent cortical electrode. There are several advantages to referential recording of ECoGs. Multifocal spiking, polyphasic potentials and dipoles are common events at corticography, and create an excessively complex pattern on bipolar runs. The origin of widely synchronous spikes is more easily discerned with referential recording. Finally, instances of confusion between physiological and artefactual cancellation of potentials are reduced.

Most artefacts with referential recording can be eliminated by an adequate grounding system. The following grounds are applied: EEG machine, corticogram electrode holder bar, scalp for scalp leads, and the patient's leg for cautery. These grounds should be led to a single grounding point serving the operating room, or ground loops with their attendant interference will occur.

Because the cortical potentials exceed scalp potentials by a factor of five to ten, the sensitivity setting is usually between 20 and 50 $\mu V/mm$.

Each montage should be carefully annotated on printed brain maps for a permanent record of its relationship to anatomical and lesional landmarks. This annotation should be done by the neurosurgeon or under his direct supervision. Copies of these maps form part of the ECoG report. Positions of the most significant abnormalities are indicated by symbols. The maps are supplemented by photographs of the operative site on which sterile numbered paper tickets indicate the sites of the most significant ECoG abnormalities.

Reading the ECoG

Artefacts

Three classes of artefacts which may resemble abnormal patterns occur commonly. Brief spike-like potentials with a rise time of only a few milliseconds may represent cortical spikes (unlike scalp recordings) or artefactual electrostatic potentials. Differentiating clues include the presence or absence of an aftercoming slow wave, as would occur with a real spike, the field distribution of the potential which may be bizarre in an artefactual situation, and its production or elimination by manipulation of surgical instruments or other devices. ECG potentials (which could mimic spikes) should not occur if the ground is placed cephalad to the heart. Secondly, delta activity should be viewed with suspicion as it may represent several conditions in addition to cortical dysfunction: pulsating vessel, respiration, movement of electrically charged objects (including people), irrigation of cortex, and temperature changes. Finally, very low voltage activity may be recorded when an electrode is placed in a pool of fluid or over minimally active cortex. Visual inspection should resolve many of these difficulties.

Normative data

ECoGs are distinguished from scalp recordings by:

1. Five to ten times greater voltage
2. Greater inter-regional differences when the patient is awake
3. Relative prominence of the higher frequency rhythms.

Alpha activity predominates over the occipital, parietal and posterior temporal regions in an awake patient with the eyes closed. Beta is the principal frequency in the Rolandic region, particularly over the pre-central gyrus. It may combine with a mu rhythm to create sharply contoured waves which can be confused with spikes. Beta gradually diminishes with distance from the motor strip.

Theta and delta activity predominate in the temporal lobes, mixed with alpha posteriorly. Beta is normally absent. Insular and rhinencephalic temporal regions have 14–16 Hz activity with occasional delta activity superimposed.

Sleep potentials resemble those of the scalp recordings; vertex waves must not be interpreted as abnormal sharp waves.

Abnormal potentials

Spikes are the most common form of paroxysmal discharge seen in the area of cortical epileptogenic lesions (Penfield & Jasper, 1954; Ajmone-Marsan, 1973). ECoG spikes are commonly polyphasic and are briefer than EEG spikes. As on the scalp, they are usually followed by a wave. The ECoG may demonstrate multifocal spiking in a region where the EEG recorded only unifocal discharges. This finding is particularly common over the temporal lobe (Magnus et al., 1962). Nevertheless, the localisation of principal ECoG foci usually correlates well with scalp findings. In situations where several foci are of approximately equal prominence, an on-line computer spike recognition programme (Vera & Blume, 1978) serves as a useful 'second opinion' for the electroencephalographer in assessing their relative quantity.

Differentiation between epileptiform potentials arising from an epileptogenic region and those projected to relatively normal cortex from a distance is obviously of enormous importance. Spikes arising from an epileptogenic region are usually of higher voltage and shorter duration than transmitted spikes, and arise from a more abnormal background. A grossly abnormal cortex would confirm this impression. The spike recognition programme also assists in this differentiation by detecting the earliest-occurring of roughly synchronous spikes.

ECoG-recorded electrographic seizures resemble those recorded on the scalp except for more prominent high frequency waves which traverse the scalp with difficulty.

Factors affecting the incidence of inter-ictal and ictal discharges

With the exception of rapidly expanding lesions, absent or minimal epileptiform potentials on the pre-resection ECoG can usually be attributed to an improper type and/or quantity of medication given pre- or intra-operatively. Benzodiazepines as antiepileptic drugs, hypnotics, or preoperative medications should be omitted. We usually reduce antiepileptic medication by 50 per cent over the five to ten pre-operative days although we are unaware of any clinically controlled study which shows an effect of such reduction.

The relative effects of neuroleptanalgesia and general anaesthesia on the corticogram have been discussed earlier.

The quantity of spike discharges may be augmented by allowing a patient to fall into a light sleep or by hyper-ventilation.

Post-excision electrocorticography

After resection, the ECoG should be repeated under the same conditions to determine whether or not a very significant reduction of epileptiform activity has occurred. Studies by Jasper, Arfel-Capdeville and Rasmussen (1961) and Bengzon *et al.* (1968) have demonstrated a good correlation between the amount of post-resection epileptiform activity and ultimate seizure control. Because of this, the persistence of active significant spiking may necessitate further resection if surgically feasible. A fortunate exception to this correlation is the insula where persistence of spikes or sharp waves appears to have no adverse prognostic significance (Bengzon *et al.*, 1968). The post-excision recording should last a sufficient length of time as an initial absence of spikes may be consequent to a relatively transient upset in cortical metabolism due to surgical trauma.

The value of electrocorticography

Some experienced epileptologists (Falconer *et al.* 1958; Bates, 1962) have questioned the value of electrocorticography on the basis that the nature and extent of the resection is already determined pre-operatively. However, improved medical management has shifted the spectrum of surgical candidates to ever more complex cases. Thus, with the possible exception of certain temporal lobe operations, 'standard' ablations are becoming less and less common. Instead, the corticographer is asked, intra-operatively, to resolve crucial questions sometimes unanswered by pre-operative studies, such as: the inter-relationship of epileptogenic areas in adjacent lobes, and the origin of roughly synchronous discharges. Moreover, the prognostic significance of post-resection findings (see above) help decide whether further resection is indicated.

REFERENCES

Ajmone-Marsan, C. (1973) Electrocorticography. In Remond, A. (ed.) *Handbook of Electroencephalography and Clinical Neurophysiology, 1971–1978*, Vol. 10, Part C. Amsterdam: Elsevier.

Ajmone-Marsan, C. & Gumnit, R.J. (1974) Neurophysiological aspects of epilepsy. In Vinken, P.J. & Bruyn, G.W. (eds) *Handbook of Clinical Neurology: The Epilepsies*, Vol. 15, p. 30. Amsterdam: North-Holland Publishing Co.

Ayala, G.F., Dichter, M., Gumnit, R.J., Matsumoto, H. & Spencer, W.A. (1973) Genesis of epileptic inter-ictal spikes: new knowledge of cortical feedback systems suggests a neuro-physiological explanation of brief paroxysms. *Brain Research*, 52, 1.

Bates, J.A.V. (1962) The surgery of epilepsy. In Williams, D. (ed.) *Modern Trends in Neurology*. Vol. 3, p. 125. London: Butterworths.

Bengzon, A.R.A., Rasmussen, T., Gloor, P., Dussault, J. & Stephens, M. (1968) Prognostic factors in the surgical treatment of temporal lobe epileptics. *Neurology* (Minneapolis), 18, 717.

Brazier, M.A.B. (1973) (Ed) *Epilepsy: its phenomena in man*. New York: Academic Press.

Calvin, W.H., Ojemann, G.A. & Ward, A.A. (1973) Human cortical neurons in epileptogenic foci: comparison of inter-ictal firing patterns to those of 'epileptic' neurons in animals. *Electroencephalography and Clinical Neurophysiology*, 34, 337.

Falconer, M.A., Hill, D., Meyer, A., & Wilson, J.L. (1958) Clinical, radiological and EEG correlations with pathological changes in temporal lobe epilepsy. In Baldwin, M. & Bailey, P. (eds) *Temporal Lobe Epilepsy*. Springfield, Ill: Thomas.

Falconer, M.A. (1970) Significance of surgery for temporal lobe epilepsy in childhood and adolescence. *Journal of Neurosurgery*, 33, 233.

Foerster, O. (1925) Zur pathogenese und chirurgischen behandlung der epilepsie. *Zentralblatt fur Chirurgie*, 52, 531.

Foerster, O. (1926) Zur operativen behandlung der epilepsie. *Deutsche Zeitschrift fur Nervenheilkunde*, 89, 137.

Goddard, G.V. (1967) Development of epileptic seizures through brain stimulation at low intensity. *Nature*, 214, 1020.

Horsley, V. (1886) Brain-Surgery. *British Medical Journal*, 2, 670.

Jasper, H:H., Arfel-Capdeville, G., & Rasmussen, T. (1961) Evaluation of EEG and cortical electrographic studies for prognosis of seizures following surgical excision of epileptogenic lesions. *Epilepsia*, 2, 130.

Jasper, H.H, Ward, A.A. Jr., & Pope, A. (1969) *Basic Mechanisms of the Epilepsies*. Boston: Little, Brown and Company.

Magnus, O., de Vet, A.C., van der Marel, A., & Meyer, E. (1962) Electrocorticography during operations for partial epilepsy. *Developmental Medicine and Child Neurology*, 4, 35.

Matsumoto, H., & Ajmone-Marsan, C. (1964) Cortical cellular phenomena in experimental epilepsy: inter-ictal manifestations. *Experimental Neurology*, 9, 286.

McNaughton, F.L., and Rasmussen, T. (1975) Criteria for selection of patients for neurosurgical treatment. In Purpura, D.P., Penry, J.K. & Walter, R.D. (eds) *Neurosurgical Management of the Epilepsies*. Advances in Neurology Vol. 8, p. 37. New York: Raven Press.

O'Leary, J.L., & Goldring, S. (1976) Role of neurological surgery in the treatment of epilepsy. In *Science and epilepsy: Neuroscience gains in epilepsy research*, p. 227. New York: Raven Press.

Pasquet, A. (1954) Combined regional and general anaesthesia for craniotomy and cortical exploration. Part II. Anaesthetic

considerations. *Current Researches in Anaesthesia &*
Analgesia, 33, 156.

Penfield, W. (1954) Combined regional and general anaesthesia
for craniotomy and cortical exploration. Part I.
Neurosurgical considerations. *Current Researches in*
Anaesthesia & Analgesia, 33, 145.

Penfield, W., & Jasper, H. (1954) *Epilepsy and the functional*
anatomy of the human brain. Boston: Little, Brown and
Company.

Prince, D.A. (1968) The depolarization shift in 'epileptic'
neurons. *Experimental Neurology*, 21, 467.

Prince, D.A. (1978) Neurophysiology of epilepsy. *Annual*
Review of Neuroscience, 1, 395.

Purpura, D.P., Penry, J.K., & Walter, R.D. (1975) eds.
Neurosurgical management of the epilepsies. Advances in
Neurology, Vol. 8. New York: Raven Press.

Racine, R.J. (1972) Modification of seizure activity by
electrical stimulation. II. Motor seizure.
Electroencephalography and Clinical Neurophysiology, 32, 281.

Rasmussen, T. (1975) Cortical resection in the treatment of
focal epilepsy. In Purpura, D.P., Penry, J.K. & Walter,
R.D. (eds) *Neurosurgical Management of the Epilepsies*
Advances in Neurology Vol. 8, p. 139. New York: Raven
Press.

Rasmussen, T.B. (1977) Surgical treatment of epilepsy.
Canadian Medical Association Journal, 116, 1369.

Schmidt, R.P., Thomas, L.B., and Ward, A.A. Jr. (1959) The
hyper-excitable neurone. Microelectrode studies of chronic
epileptic foci in monkey. *Journal of Neurophysiology*, 22, 285.

Vera, R.S., & Blume, W.T. (1978) A clinically effective spike
recognition program: its use at electrocorticography.
Electroencephalography and Clinical Neurophysiology, 45, 545.

Wada, J.A. (1976) Ed. *Kindling*. New York: Raven Press.

Walter, R.D. (1973) Tactical considerations leading to surgical
treatment of limbic epilepsy. In Brazier, M.A.B. (ed.)
Epilepsy: its phenomena in man, p. 99. New York: Academic
Press.

Walter, R.D. (1975) Principles of clinical investigation of
surgical candidates. In Purpura, D.P., Penry, J.K. &
Walter, R.D. (eds) *Neurosurgical Management of the*
Epilepsies Advances in Neurology Vol. 8, p. 49. New York:
Raven Press.

Ward, A.A. (1969) The epileptic neuron: chronic foci in
animals and man. In Jasper, H.H., Ward, A.A. Jr. & Pope,
A. (eds) *Basic Mechanisms of the Epilepsies*, p. 263. Boston:
Little, Brown and Company.

Ward, A.A. (1975) Theoretical basis for surgical therapy of
epilepsy. In Purpura, D.P., Penry, J.K. & Walter, R.D.
(eds) *Neurosurgical Management of the Epilepsies Advances in*
Neurology Vol. 8, pp. 23. New York: Raven Press.

PART THREE
CEREBELLAR STIMULATION

A.R.M. Upton

INTRODUCTION

For over 50 years there have been clinical observations indicating a relationship between cerebellar pathology and epilepsy (Hodskins & Yakovlev, 1930) but much of our knowledge about the effects of cerebellar stimulation in epilepsy is based on the results of animal studies.

ANIMAL STUDIES

Risien Russel (1894) showed that unilateral cerebellar ablation in dogs aggravated ipsilateral limb movements during generalised convulsions but subsequent animal experiments yielded conflicting results. Studies in rats (Dow, Fernadez-Guardiola & Manni, 1962), cats (Cooke & Snider, 1955;

Iwata & Snider, 1955; Mutani, Bergamini & Doriguzzi, 1969; Hutton, Frost & Foster, 1972) and monkeys (Cooper & Snider, 1974) indicated that low rates of stimulation of the cerebellar cortex may inhibit seizures. Studies of spinal seizures indicated that high rates of stimulation decreased spinal tetanus whereas low rates increased tetanus (Terzuolo, 1954; Shapovalov & Arushanyan, 1963). However, the most obvious effect of cerebellar stimulation has been on the EEG concomitants of epilepsy rather than ictal events (Boone, Nashold & Wilson, 1974; Dow, 1974; Meyers & Bickford, 1974; Soper *et al.*, 1977; Lockard *et al.*, 1979) and other workers have found either little or no effect (Black *et al.*, 1976; Strain, Van Meter & Brockman, 1977; Banlti, Bloedel & Tolbert, 1978) or even an increase in seizures after cerebellar stimulation (Bantli, Bloedel & Tolbert, 1976). Lockard *et al.* (1979) thought that cerebellar stimulation acted mainly on group II neurons which are cells at the periphery of the epileptogenic focus still having considerable afferent input (Wyler, Fetz & Ward, 1975) whereas group I neurons which are deafferented or partially deafferented cells in the epileptogenic focus may be bursting more frequently. Lockard *et al.* (1979) felt that this would explain the inverse relationship between clinical seizures and EEG interictal bursts that they observed during cerebellar stimulation in monkeys made epileptic by alumina-gel lesions.

TECHNIQUE OF CCS IN PATIENTS

Basic aspects

The subject of basic aspects of cerebellar stimulation has been reviewed by Girvin (1978). Previous studies of electrical stimulation of the visual, motor and cerebellar cortex would indicate that pulse widths of 0.1 to 0.5 ms at 50 to 150 Hz produce optimal results, but the total charge and the current density are important. Brown *et al.* (1977) showed that a charge density of $7.4\,\mu C/cm^2$ per phase was safe over 205 hours of stimulation and such charge levels are about five times those required to elicit cerebellar efferent activity. Higher charge levels produced damage beneath the electrodes but not the generalised damage reported by Gilman *et al.* (1975).

The optimal area of electrodes or the optimal area of cerebellum to be stimulated has not been established but there is evidence that stimulation of a larger area of cerebellar surface results in greater physiological effects (Larson *et al.*, 1976; Upton & Cooper, 1976).

Electrodes

The cerebellar electrodes are platinum discs or slabs that may be placed in arrays of four or eight electrodes. Eight platinum electrodes have an area of $32\,mm^2$. The electrodes are embedded in a silicone mesh and they are placed over the anterior and posterior surface of the cerebellum through posterior burr holes. Up to four arrays have been used (Cooper, 1978). The electrode leads are carried out through the burr hole and then they are carried subcutaneously to the receiver placed inferior to the clavicles. Stimulation is achieved by transcutaneous induction of a radiofrequency signal from a power pack carried by the patient but fully implantable and programmable units will soon be available (Fischell, Shulman & Cooper, 1978).

Stimulation

Monopolar, biphasic capacitively coupled stimuli may be more effective than bipolar, monophasic, capacitively coupled pulse waves. Rates of 10 Hz to 200 Hz may produce therapeutic effects in a single patient and there has been no clear evidence that faster frequencies are preferable to slow frequencies of stimulation (Upton & Cooper, 1976). Stimulating voltage, and therefore stimulating charge and charge density, are set by 'biocalibration'. The threshold level of stimulation required to produce a reduction in amplitude of cortical or subcortical somatosensory-evoked responses can be used to set the voltage of the stimulator but there is less evidence on this point in epileptic patients in comparison with patients suffering from cerebral palsy. The mean setting of the stimulators has been 5.18 ± 3.51 volts at 200 Hz for two electrode arrays or four electrode arrays of a square area of $64\,mm^2$.

CLINICAL RESULTS

Cooper, Amin and Gilman (1973) reported a reduction in seizure frequency in epileptic patients after chronic stimulation of the cerebellar surface and later studies (Cooper *et al*, 1976) indicated improvement in a majority of patients after chronic cerebellar stimulation (CCS). In the most recent report of 32 patients, 18 were considered to demonstrate a good clinical response to CCS. In these patients seizures were reduced by at least 50 per cent. Nine of the 32 patients were rated as therapeutic failures, one died at operation and four subsequently died during sleep (Cooper *et al.*, 1978). Follow-up of these patients was 13 to 53 months, but statistical analysis was limited by the small number of patients in each seizure category. However, it was possible to demonstrate on/off effects of CCS on the EEG of three patients who showed a more than 50 per cent reduction in their seizures. One patient, a 16 year old boy, developed recurrence of seizures four months after insertion of the electrodes and it was found that the leads had broken. After surgical repair seizure control was never re-established.

These results can be compared with those of Dow, Smith and Maukonen (1977) who reported improvement in seizures in three patients undergoing CCS but they observed a spontaneous remission in one patient for 18 months after surgical implantation of the electrodes but before CCS was started. Six further cases were reported by Levy and Auchterlonie (1979). These patients were between 17 and 55 years old and all had intractable seizures. Four had generalised major convulsions. Stimulation was instituted after the patient had a post-operative seizure. Two patients were greatly improved and they managed to hold employment whereas they had been unemployed prior to surgery. One patient felt better but seizure frequency seemed unchanged and another thought there had been no improvement despite a 50 per cent reduction in seizures. One patient committed suicide and another drowned. One prosthesis had to be removed because of infection.

Fenton *et al.* (1977) reported a single patient who seemed to have improved with CCS.

However, Correll (1977) reported disappointing results in psychomotor and generalised convulsive seizures. Seven patients were followed for one to several years and only two showed any degree of improvement. In an attempt at a double-blind controlled assessment of CCS, Van Buren *et al.* (1978) studied five patients over the course of two years. Trained observers and a hospital setting were employed but there was no decrease in seizure frequency and there was a tendency for seizure frequency to increase over a 21 month period in the absence of CCS. Unfortunately, Van Buren *et al.* chose to set the cerebellar stimulator at a level which was just below the charge levels required to produce a headache and there is good evidence that such stimulating levels are well above the therapeutic threshold so that 'paradoxical effects' might be expected (Upton & Cooper, 1976; Upton, 1978; Cooper & Upton, 1978).

DISCUSSION

Problems in assessment of seizure frequency

One of the major problems in the assessment of any treatment of epilepsy is the difficulty of measuring the true frequency of seizures. Seizure charts, observations of family members and patient reports may not provide an accurate indication of the number of seizures, particularly if the attacks are brief or if the patient is amnesic for the episodes. The electroencephalogram may show frequent bursts of abnormal activity without clinical correlates, but special procedures such as tests of reaction times or a continuous motor task (Upton, LeBlanc & Longmire, 1976) may demonstrate clinical disturbances during brief electrical bursts in the EEG. Admission of the patient to hospital usually alters seizure frequency and seizures may fluctuate in severity over hours, days or weeks. Split-screen videomonitoring may provide a more accurate measure of the frequency of observable seizures, but the procedure requires unusual conditions for the patient and observation times are limited. In addition, it is becoming increasingly apparent that psychological factors play an important part in the development and inhibition of seizures (Upton, 1978) so that belief in a procedure, response to attention, improved compliance of drug therapy and desire to please the investigator may be associated with a reduction in seizure frequency. Since cerebellar stimulation has been tried in patients with intractable seizures there has been previous failure of standard therapies, particularly medications. It is unlikely that any treatment will produce total resolution of the seizure disorder and a reduction in seizure frequency will be difficult to quantify in a statistical manner. Double blind studies of cerebellar stimulation are limited by the fact that patients may experience feelings of relaxation during stimulation so that the patient may become aware of the stimulation even if it is not therapeutic. Quantitative assessment of the effects of cerebellar stimulation on the EEG (Upton, 1978) may not correlate with clinical changes and clinical improvement may not be reflected in the EEG.

Paradoxical effects of CCS

In addition to these difficulties we must add the special problems associated with electrical stimulation of the nervous system. Neurophysiological studies have demonstrated that threshold levels of stimulation can be assessed by measurement of evoked potentials or EEG changes (Upton & Cooper, 1976; Upton, 1978). Subthreshold stimulation may have no clinical or neurophysiological effects but excessive stimulation may have 'paradoxical' effects involving an increase in EEG discharges or frequency of seizures; there is good reason to believe that such paradoxical effects contributed to the results of Van Buren et al. (1978) who adjusted the stimulators to a level just below that required to produce a headache. A similar mechanism may explain some of the disappointing results of animal studies. Wada (1975) stimulated the cerebellum of kindled monkeys but the stimulation was associated with movement, cranial nerve effects and vocalisation which would indicate that the stimulating charge was well above threshold and paradoxical effects might be expected.

Rebound effects of CCS

Neurophysiological studies have demonstrated 'rebound' increases in interictal manifestations of seizures after cerebellar stimulation in animals (Dow, 1965; Fernandez-Guardiola et al., 1962; Payan Levine & Strebel, 1966) and in man (Upton & Cooper, 1976; Upton, 1978; Cooper & Upton, 1978 a & b). More recently Lockard et al. (1979) published charts of seizure frequency in epileptic monkeys who had received cerebellar stimulation and a number showed increases in seizure frequency after cessation of a few weeks of cerebellar stimulation. These rebound effects may be seen within minutes of cessation of chronic cerebellar stimulation in man (Upton, 1978) and they would complicate any assessment of average seizure frequency in patients undergoing periods on and off cerebellar stimulation. Such results would also raise doubts about the ethics of double blind crossover studies of CCS since the increase in seizures off CCS might increase the overall mean seizure frequency.

Prolonged effects of CCS

Neurophysiological effects of CCS have been demonstrated for more than half an hour after cessation of stimulation (Upton, 1978). Measurement of reflexes, V_1 and V_2 responses, somatosensory evoked potentials after median nerve or peroneal nerve stimulation, subcortical (short latency) somatosensory evoked responses (Cracco &

Cracco, 1976), EEG discharges and quantitative studies of movement have demonstrated prolonged effects of CCS (Upton & Cooper, 1976; Upton, 1978; Milner et al., 1978) and these results have been confirmed by animal studies which demonstrated rebound increases in seizure frequency lasting for about four weeks after cessation of CCS (Lockard et al., 1979).

Mechanism of action of CCS

Since there are conflicting animal and human studies of the effects of CCS in epilepsy it may be premature to discuss the probable mechanisms of action of the procedure. However, there is good evidence about the effects of cerebellar stimulation on EEG discharges (Upton, 1978), evoked responses (Upton & Cooper, 1976), movements (Milner et al., 1978), and psychological measurements (Riklan et al., 1978) in man. Animal studies have indicated that stimulation of the cerebellar surface may activate neurones in the cerebellar nuclei and ascending reticular formation of the brainstem (Bantli et al., 1976). More recent studies indicate that stimulation of the cerebellar surface may inhibit the discharge of Purkinje cells (Dauth, Dell & Gilman, 1978) and Johnson et al. (1979) thought that cerebellar stimulation acted mainly to depress the thalamocortical system. Johnson et al. thought that cerebellar stimulation had a far greater capacity to control excitability and threshold responsiveness of the thalamocortical system in comparison with anticonvulsant medication.

Studies of evoked responses in patients undergoing CCS led to the hypothesis that cerebellar stimulation depressed thalamic excitability (Upton & Cooper, 1976). Since then it has been possible to record the thalamic component of the short latency somatosensory evoked responses after median nerve stimulation. These potentials have been recorded from surface and deep electrodes, and such studies have validated the conclusions reached after surface or 'far field' recordings (Cracco & Cracco, 1976; Upton, 1978; Cooper & Upton, 1978a & b). Cerebellar stimulation at or above threshold levels produces depression of the amplitude of the thalamic component of the somatosensory evoked responses after electrical stimulation of the median nerve. The reduction in the amplitude of the thalamic component is usually associated with depression of the cortical somatosensory evoked responses. In a study of 87 patients undergoing CCS (Upton *et al.*, 1979) (age 24 ± 9; 35 women 52 men; cerebral palsy, 69; epilepsy, 18) it was found that the subcortical (short latency) somatosensory evoked responses were reduced in amplitude in 35 and the cortical somatosensory response was reduced in 44; one or both responses were reduced in amplitude in 55. Evoked responses showed significant reductions (*p* <0.05) in only three patients who did not show clinical improvement. Hence, it is reasonable to believe that CCS does depress the thalamocortical system and this may explain some of the effects of CCS.

Biocalibration and CCS

Since there is a correlation between the clinical effects of CCS and the changes in somatosensory evoked responses, measurement of the amplitude of these evoked responses would provide a practical method of adjustment of the stimulating charge for CCS. Subthreshold levels of stimulation may not yield therapeutic effects although we have seen clinical improvement in the absence of any change in evoked responses in 13 of 87 patients. However, the biocalibration technique provides a method of avoiding paradoxical effects of CCS and controlled trials of CCS in epilepsy should include such physiological checks on the levels of stimulation.

Safety of CCS

There is a mortality and morbidity of any surgical procedure and the original technique for insertion of cerebellar electrodes involved a posterior fossa craniotomy. However, the electrodes can be placed through posterior burr holes and this has reduced the risk considerably, although haemorrhage (Cooper *et al.*, 1976) and infection (Levy & Auchterlonie, 1979) may still occur.

The main concern about cerebellar stimulation was raised by the work of Gilman and his colleagues (Gilman *et al.*, 1975) on the basis of the results from a single monkey. Continuous stimulation of human electrodes in a 3.2 kg monkey

resulted in extensive cerebellar damage. Intermittant stimulation, as in humans, produced some local damage under the electrodes (Dauth *et al.*, 1977). Larson *et al.* (1976) showed that cerebellar lesions under the electrodes did not occur in all animals. Brown *et al.* (1977) showed that there may be local damage under the electrode but this depends on the stimulating charge that is employed. A study of 30 biopsies of the cerebellum taken at the time of implantation of cerebellar electrodes demonstrated that 11 out of 12 epileptic patients showed a significant loss of Purkinje cells prior to any electrical stimulation and this loss was 50 per cent or greater in all the abnormal biopsies (Urich *et al.*, 1978). These authors concluded that cerebellar stimulation did not produce generalised damage of the cerebellum and there is no significant cerebellar damage as a result of electrical stimulation at therapeutic levels. All the clinical evidence indicates that cerebellar stimulation does not produce significant or progressive cerebellar damage and this has now been acknowledged by Gilman (1977). However, patients with intractable epilepsy may die spontaneously for no apparent reason (Hirsch & Martin, 1971) and since cerebellar stimulation has been applied to patients who have been incapacitated by uncontrolled seizures, it is important to distinguish between deaths that are attributable to the epilepsy and to cerebellar stimulation.

CONCLUSION

It can be seen that CCS has not been established as a treatment for epilepsy. Some of the conflicting results of CCS in epilepsy in animals can be explained by differences in the settings of the stimulators and by differences between animal models. Human studies of CCS have been hampered by the problems of assessment of seizures and by differences in techniques of stimulation. Clinical studies employing 'biocalibration' have indicated that CCS may have promise as a treatment for epileptic patients but acceptance of any surgical treatment for epilepsy must depend on the results of controlled trials. The development of fully programmable, rechargeable and totally implantable stimulators, careful measurement of electrode impedances and stimulating charge at the time of implantation of the electrodes and later, biocalibration of stimulating charges by evoked potential techniques, objective assessments of seizure frequency and quantitative evaluation of EEG changes may well allow assessment of the value of CCS and other forms of neurostimulation as a treatment for intractable epilepsy in man.

REFERENCES

Babb, T.B., Soper, H.V., Leib, J.P., Brown, W.J., Ottino, C.A. & Crandall, P.H. (1977) Electrophysiological studies of long-term electrical stimulation of the cerebellum in monkeys. *Journal of Neurosurgery*, **47**, 353.

Bantli, H., Bloedel, J.R., Anderson, G., McRoberts, R. & Sandberg, E. (1978) Effects of stimulating the cerebellar surface on the activity in penicillin foci. *Journal of Neurosurgery*, **45**, 539.

Bantli, H., Bloedel, J.R. & Tolbert, O. (1976) Activation of neurons in the cerebellar nuclei and ascending reticular formation by stimulation of the cerebellar surface. *Journal of Neurosurgery* **45**, 539.

Black, P., Fischell, R.E., Markowitz, S. & Powell, W.R. (1976) Cerebellar stimulation: comparison of effect on electrically induced and spontaneous alumina seizures. *American Epilepsy Society*, Dearborn, Michigan, Oct. 1–2, p. 21.

Boone, S.C., Nashold, B.S. & Wilson, W.P. (1974) The effects of cerebellar stimulation on the averaged sensory evoked responses in the cat. In Cooper, I.S., Riklan, M. & Snider, R.S. (eds) *The Cerebellum, Epilepsy and Behaviour*, p. 257. New York: Plenum Press.

Brown, W.J., Babb, T.L., Soper, H.V., Lieb, J.P., Ottino, C.A. & Crandall, P.H. (1977). Tissue reaction to long-term electrical stimulation of the cerebellum of monkeys. *Journal of Neurosurgery*, **47**, 366.

Cooke, P.M. & Snider, R.S. (1955). Some cerebellar influences on electrically induced cerebral seizures. *Epilepsia* **4**, 19.

Cooper, I.S. (1978) Some technical considerations of cerebellar stimulation. In Cooper, I.S. (ed.) *Cerebellar Stimulation in Man*, p. 13. New York: Raven Press.

Cooper, I.S. & Snider, R.S. (1974) The effect of varying the frequency of cerebellar stimulation upon epilepsy. In Cooper, I.S., Riklan & Snider, R.S. (eds) *The Cerebellum, Epilepsy and Behaviour*, New York: Plenum Press.

Cooper, I.S. & Upton, A.R.M. (1978a) Effects of cerebellar stimulation on epilepsy, the EEG and cerebral palsy. In Cobb, W.A. & van Duijn, H. (eds) *Contemporary Clinical Neurophysiology*, EEG Supplement **34**, p. 349.

Cooper, I.S. & Upton, A.R.M. (1978b) Use of chronic cerebellar stimulation for disorders of disinhibition. *Lancet*, i, 595.

Cooper, I.S., Amin, I. & Gilman, S. (1973). The effect of chronic cerebellar stimulation upon epilepsy in man. Transactions of the American Neurological Association. **98**, 192.

Cooper, I.S., Riklan, M., Amin, I., & Cullinan, T. (1978) A long-term follow-up study of cerebellar stimulation for the control of epilepsy. In Cooper, I.S. (ed.) *Cerebellar Stimulation in Man*, p. 19. New York: Raven Press.

Cooper, I.S., Amin, I., Riklan, M., Waltz, J.M. & Poon, T.P. (1976). Chronic cerebellar stimulation in epilepsy. *Archives of Neurology* (Chicago) **33**, 559.

Correll, J. (1977) Cerebellar stimulation. Panel presentation to the American Association of Neurological Surgeons. April 24–28.

Cracco, R.Q. & Cracco, J.B. (1976) Somatosensory evoked potential in man: far field potentials. *Electroencephalography and Clinical Neurophysiology* **41**, 460.

Dauth, G.W., Defendini, R., Gilman, S., Tennyson, V.M. & Kremzner, L.T. 1977. Long-term surface stimulation in the monkey. 1. Light, microscopic, electrophysiologic and clinical observations. *Surgical Neurology* **7**, 377.

Dauth, G.W., Dell, S. & Gilman, S. (1978) Alteration of Purkinje cell activity from transfolial stimulation of the cerebellum in the cat. Neurology (Minneapolis). **28**, 659.

Dow, R.S. (1965) Extrinsic regulatory mechanisms of seizure activity. *Epilepsia* **6**, 122.

Dow, R.S. (1974) Experimental cobalt epilepsy and the cerebellum. In Cooper, I.S., Riklan, M. & Snider, R.S. (eds) *The Cerebellum, Epilepsy and Behaviour*, p. 97. New York: Plenum Press.

Dow, R.S., Fernandez-Guardiola, A. & Manni, E. (1962) The influence of the cerebellum on experimental epilepsy. *Electroencephalography and Clinical Neurophysiology* **14**, 383.

Dow, R.S., Smith, W. & Maukonen, L. (1977) Proceedings of the Western EEG Society *Electroencephalography and Clinical Neurophysiology* **43**, 906.

Fenton, G.W., Fenwick, P.B.C., Brindley, G.S., Falconer, M.A., Polkey, C.H. & Rushton, D.N. (1977) Chronic cerebellar stimulation in the treatment of epilepsy: a preliminary report. In Penry, J.K. (ed.) Epilepsy: *The Eighth International Symposium*, p. 333. New York: Raven Press.

Fernandez-Guardiola, A., Manni, E., Wilson, J.H. & Dow, R.S. (1962) Microelectrode recording of cerebellar and cerebral unit activity during convulsive after discharge. Experimental Neurology **6**, 48.

Fischell, R.E., Schulman, J.H. & Cooper, I.S. (1978) An intracorporeal system for cerebellar stimulation. In Cooper, I.S. (ed.) *Cerebellar Stimulation in Man*, p. 195. New York: Raven Press.

Gilman, S. (1977) Cerebellar stimulation. *Neurology* (Minneapolis), **27**, 998.

Gilman, S., Dauth, G.W., Tennyson, V.M. & Kremzner, L.T. (1975) Chronic cerebellar stimulation in the monkey: preliminary observations. *Archives of Neurology* (Chicago). **32**, 474.

Girvin, J.P. (1978) A review of basic aspects concerning chronic cerebral stimulation. In Cooper I.S. (ed.) *Cerebellar Stimulation in Man*, p. 1. New York: Raven Press.

Hirsch, C.S. & Martin, D.L. (1971) Unexpected death in young epileptics. *Neurology* (Minneapolis), **21**, 682.

Hodskins, M.B. & Yakovlev, P.I. (1930) Anatomico-clinical observations on myoclonus in epileptics and on related symptom complexes. *American Journal of Psychiatry*. **9**, 827.

Hutton, J.T., Frost, J.D. & Foster, J. (1972) The influence of the cerebellum in cat penicillin epilepsy. *Epilepsia* **13**, 401.

Iwata, K. & Snider, R.S. (1955) Cerebello-hippocampal influences on the electroencephalogram. *Electroencephalography and Clinical Neurophysiology* **11**, 439.

Johnson, R.N., Charton, J.S., Englander, R.N., Brickley, J.J., Nowak, W.J. & Hanna, G.R. (1979) Cerebellar stimulation: regional effects on a thalamocortical system. *Epilepsia*. **20**, 247.

Larson, S.J., Sances, A., Cusick, J.F., Myklebust, J., Millar, E.A., Boehner, R., Hemmy, D.C., Ackman, J.J. & Swiontek, T.J. (1976) Cerebellar implant studies. I.E.E.E. Trans. Biomedical. Engineering. **23**, 319.

Levy, L.F. & Auchterlonie, W.C. (1979) Chronic cerebellar stimulation in the treatment of epilepsy. Epilepsia. **20**, 235.

Lockard, J.S., Ojemann, G.A., Congdon, W.C. & DuCharme, L.L. (1979) Cerebellar stimulation in alumina-gel monkey model: inverse relationship between clinical seizures and EEG interictal bursts. *Epilepsia*. **20**, 223.

Meyers, R.R. & Bickford, R.G. (1974) Modulation of spontaneous and evoked chloralose myoclonus by cerebellar stimulation in the cat. In Cooper I.S., Riklan, M. & Snider, R.S. (eds) *The Cerebellum, Epilepsy and Behaviour*, p. 217. New York: Plenum Press,

Milner, M., Herschler, C., de Bruin, H., Baker, R.S., Upton, A.R.M. & Cooper, I.S. (1978) Preliminary investigation of influence of cerebellar stimulation on gait by analysing angle-angle diagrams. In Cooper, I.S. (ed.) *Cerebellar Stimulation in Man*, p. 123. New York: Raven Press.

Mutani, R., Bergamini, L. & Doriguzzi, T. (1969) Experimental evidence for the existence of an extrarhinencephalic control of the activity of the cobalt rhinencephalic epileptogenic focus. 2. Effect of palaeo-cerebellar stimulation. *Epilepsia*, **10**, 351.

Payan, H., Levine, S. & Strebel, R. (1966) Inhibition of experimental epilepsy by chemical stimulation of cerebellum. *Neurology* (Minneapolis) **16**, 573.

Riklan, M., Halgin, L., Shulman, M., Cullinan, T. & Cooper, I.S. (1978) Behavioural alterations following acute, shorter-term, and longer-term cerebellar stimulation in humans. In Cooper, I.S. (ed.) *Cerebellar Stimulation in Man*, p. 161. New York: Raven Press.

Russel, J.S.R. (1894) Experimental researches into the functions of the cerebellum. *Philosophical Transactions of the Royal Society of London*. **185**, 819.

Shapovalov, A.T. & Arushanyan, E.B. (1963) The effect of strychnine on the activity of the motor and interneurons of the spinal cord in stimulation of the anterior lobe of the cerebellum. *Bulletin of Experimental Biology and Medicine* **51**, 3.

Soper, H.V., Lieb, J.P., Babb, T.L., Strain, G.M. & Crandall, P.H. (1977) Experimental epilepsy and cerebellar stimulation in monkey. *Abstracts of the Society of Neurosciences* **3**, 146.

Strain, G.M., Van Meter, W.G. & Brockman, W.H. (1977) Effects of cerebellar stimulation on seizure thresholds. *ibid*. **3**, 147.

Terzuolo, C. (1954) Influences supraspinales sur le tétanus strychnique de la moelle épinière. *Archives International de Physiologie*. **62**, 179.

Upton, A.R.M. (1978) Neurophysiological mechanisms in modification of seizures. In Cooper, I.S. (ed.) *Cerebellar Stimulation in Man*, p. 39. New York: Raven Press.

Upton, A.R.M. & Cooper, I.S. (1976) Some neurophysiological effects of cerebellar stimulation in man. *Canadian Journal of Neurological Sciences* **3**, 237.

Upton, A.R.M., Cooper, I.S., Amin, I. & Rappaport, Z.H. (1979) Correlation of clinical and physiological effects of cerebellar stimulation. IV Meeting of the European Society for Stereotactic and Functional Neurosurgery. Paris, France. July, 1979. Acta Chirurgia. In Press.

Upton, A.R.M., LeBlanc, M. & Longmire, D. (1976) Bilateral motor task (BMT) in assessment of seizures. *ibid* **3**, 146.

Urich, H., Watkins, E.S., Amin, I. & Cooper, I.S. (1978) Neuropathologic observations on cerebellar cortical lesions in patients with epilepsy and motor disorders. In Cooper, I.S. (ed.) *Cerebellar Stimulation in Man*, p. 145.

Van Buren, J.M., Wood, J.H., Oakley, J. & Hambrecht, F. (1978) Preliminary evaluation of cerebellar stimulation by double blind stimulation and biological criteria in the treatment of epilepsy. *Journal of Neurosurgery* **48**, 407.

Wada, J.A. (1975) Progressive seizure recruitment in subhuman primates and effect of cerebellar stimulation upon developed versus developing amygdaloid seizures. *Boletin de Estudios Medicos y Biologicos* (Mexico) **28**, 285.

Wyler, A.R., Fetz, E.E. & Ward, A.A. Jr. (1975) Review article: firing patterns of epileptic and normal neurons in neocortex of undrugged monkeys during different behavioural states. *Brain Research*. **98**, 1.

11

Pathology and pathophysiology

PART ONE
PATHOLOGY
G. Mathieson

INTRODUCTION

Morphological studies have made a modest but well-defined contribution to our knowledge of the dynamic disorder of epilepsy in man. With increasing awareness of the focal origin of seizures in many patients and the efficacy of surgical therapy in some, there has been a growing need and opportunity to study the tissue changes associated with seizures of focal onset. In contrast, pathological studies of patients with cortico-reticular epilepsy have been rather barren. In a third broad group of patients, those with endogenous metabolic encephalopathies, his-topathological investigation has delineated some distinct diseases which are almost invariably associated with some form of epilepsy.

Since there are no specific histopathological criteria to determine definitively whether or not any particular pattern of cerebral lesion will give rise to seizure discharges, our knowledge depends in large part on implication by association. We must therefore distinguish:

1. Lesions which, directly or indirectly, cause epileptic neuronal discharges
2. Lesions which result from repeated seizures, i.e. ictal brain damage. These secondary lesions may in their turn be potentially epileptogenic

3. Lesions sharing an aetiology with epileptogenic lesions but not themselves epileptogenic
4. Incidental lesions in the brains of habitual epileptics not causally related to the seizure tendency

The concept of epileptic threshold, applying to the brain as a whole, and to various structures and cortical regions in the brain, clearly implies that the patient's morphological lesion is only one factor in determining if and when cerebral seizures will occur. Brain lesions may therefore be regarded as predisposing to epilepsy and determining the site of origin of abnormal discharges in susceptible subjects.

By common consent, the proximate cause of an epileptic event is an abnormal pattern of discharge in a neuronal pool. Structural abnormalities of individual neurones or, more frequently, an alteration in their number and arrangement are observed in some epileptic lesions, but in many patients non-neural elements dominate the morphological picture – for example vascular malformations, scars, glial neoplasms. These obscure the neuronal component of the lesion, but indicate, to a first approximation, its pathogenesis. Thus many of the lesions described in this chapter are at least once removed from the essential predisposing mechanism of the patient's epilepsy. Their demonstration, however, is essential in elucidating intermediary pathogenetic steps; they may also provide valuable clues in the clinical and laboratory investigation of patients with epilepsy.

CATEGORIES OF EPILEPTOGENIC LESIONS

A systematic aetiological classification is the ultimate aim of an account of the pathology of epilepsy. Our present knowledge does not as yet allow this. The range of response of the brain to injury is limited so that, in the long term, the results of various noxious processes may be very similar (pathogenetic convergence). The state of maturation of the brain at the time of initial insult is important. In retrospective assessment of an adult epileptic patient, the age at which the presumed causal event occurred is often more reliably ascertained than the exact nature of the event.

The classification of lesions offered here (Table 11.1) is heterogeneous, being based partly on the stage of development at which the initial cerebral insult occurred, and partly on standard pathological concepts of aetiology.

Table 11.1 Outline classification of epileptogenic lesions

Lesions originating during intrauterine life
Lesions associated with childbirth
Lesions resulting from febrile convulsions of childhood
Inflammatory lesions and their residua
Lesions resulting from head injury
Acquired vascular lesions of adults
Neoplasms
Subtle dendritic lesions
Endogenous metabolic encephalopathies
Metabolic encephalopathies of extra-cerebral origin.

Epileptogenic lesions originating during intrauterine life

Disturbances of the complex sequence of events by which the embryonic neural tube becomes the neonate brain give rise to a wide spectrum of neurological abnormalities. Some are incompatible with extrauterine survival; others, e.g. dysraphic states, do not concern us here. Lilienfeld and Pasamanick (1954) and Pasamanick and Lilienfeld (1955), in a retrospective survey with controls matched for age, and for maternal age, showed that mothers of epileptic patients had a significantly ($p < 0.05$) higher incidence of complications of pregnancy and delivery in general. In particular, the incidence of maternal bleeding and toxaemia of pregnancy was increased over controls. Their epileptic patient records were clinical, and histopathological evidence was not available to them.

The formal origin of some of these developmental abnormalities is known in general terms. Clues

to aetiology may be available in the maternal history: placental abnormality, anoxic episodes, radiation, viral infection and undernutrition have all been implicated. An appropriate gestational age at the time of the noxious event appears to be essential for the development of certain anomalies e.g. polymicrogyria. Diffuse and morphologically more subtle abnormalities may occur with undernutrition during the brain growth spurt (Dobbing & Sands, 1973; Dobbing & Smart, 1974), but it is speculative whether these increase the liability to the development of life-long epilepsy, as distinct from impaired motor skills and mentation. Our main concern here is with certain distinctive patterns of anomalous development readily recognised histologically and known to be associated with habitual epilepsy. They are listed in Table 11.2.

Table 11.2 Epileptogenic lesions originating during intrauterine life

A. *Disorders of cellular migration and differentation*
   Heterotopias
   Polymicrogyria
   Megalencephaly
   Focal cortical dysplasia
   Tuberous sclerosis and formes frustes
   Hamartomas
   Meningio-angiomatosis
   Neuro-cutaneous melanosis
   Dermoid and epidermoid cysts
B. *Disorders of vascular organisation*
   Cavernous haemangioma
   Arterio-venous malformation
   Sturge-Weber disease

Heterotopias

Occasional neurones scattered in the subcortical white matter are a common finding of no significance. Larger ectopic clusters of neurones and glia forming grey masses occur in two patterns: laminar within the centrum ovale, and nodular at the angles of the lateral ventricles (Fig. 11.1). Some people with heterotopias are free from any neurological disability; others have seizures and some degree of mental retardation. The lesions are commonly bilateral and roughly symmetrical. In the unilateral case reported by Layton (1962), there was close correlation between the site of the lesion and its clinical and electrographic manifestations. Cortical gyral pattern and lamina-

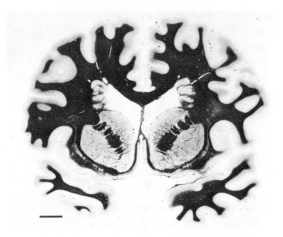

Fig. 11.1 Nodular heterotopias at the angles of the lateral ventricles. From a mildly retarded girl; seizures of varying pattern began in early adolescence; death at 19 years in status epilepticus. Heidenhain's method for myelin. Scale marker 1 cm.

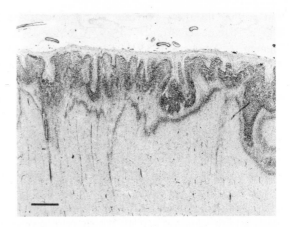

Fig. 11.3 Polymicrogyria. Four layered cortex in a neonate with disseminated cytomegalovirus infection. Haematoxylin and eosin. Scale marker 1 mm.

tion are usually normal. However cases also occur in which heterotopias are but one component of a complex cerebral maldevelopment. Crome (1952) has reported occipital heterotopia in a case of extensive polymicrogyria, and Kirschbaum (1947) and Norman (1958) in association with agenesis of the corpus callosum and megalencephaly.

Polymicrogyria

This distinctive lesion is characterised by many small gyrus-like formations without formed sulci.

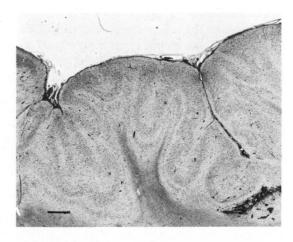

Fig. 11.4 Polymicrogyria. Patient began having seizures characterised by an aura of 'buzzing' followed by automatism at 12 years of age. Left temporal lobectomy at 23 years. Focal polymicrogyria is readily apparent histologically but was inconspicuous on naked eye examination. Luxol fast blue-cresyl violet. Scale marker 1 mm.

The surface of the involved brain presents rather wide gyri with wrinkled surfaces. The lesion may be fairly extensive and bilateral, but in adults isolated patches of this malformed cortex are more commonly encountered. The opercula of the insula are frequent sites of predilection (Fig. 11.2). Cortical lamination is typically four layered (Fig.11.3). Small foci of this lesion may be quite inconspicuous in surgically excised specimens (Fig. 11.4).

Neonates succumbing to cytomegalovirus infec-

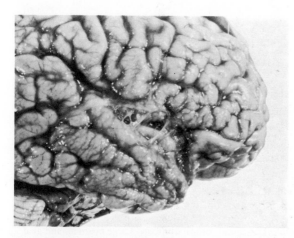

Fig. 11.2 Polymicrogyria. Right frontal and temporal gyri adjacent to the Sylvian fissure are involved.

tion frequently show polymicrogyria in extreme degree (Crome & France, 1959; Crome, 1961; Bignami & Appicciutoli, 1964). It is reasonable to suppose that less severe brain involvement with survival into adult life may result from intrauterine infection by this and possibly other viruses. A range of nonspecific noxious events, e.g. coal gas poisoning, occurring at a critical stage of cortical maturation, usually in the fifth month of intrauterine life, can produce an identical lesion. Polymicrogyria is, then, generally regarded as resulting from a disturbance of the orderly pattern of differentiation and migration of neuroblasts into the cerebral mantle. An alternative point of view is that the four layered cortical lamination is due to post-migratory destruction. This has received support from a serial section study (Richman, Stewart & Caviness, 1974) of a 27 week fetus in whom the cell sparse zone of the polymicrogyric cortex was shown to be in continuity with layer V of the intact cortex. The outer cellular layer may thus be formed by layers II, III and IV and the inner cellular layer by layer VI. However, this post-migrational encephaloclastic concept does not account for the abnormality of convolutional pattern. Polymicrogyria may accompany other major malformations. Extensive, usually bilateral, porencephaly was recorded by Dekaban (1965) in 11 patients with profound neurological deficits, including epilepsy; fields of polymicrogyric cortex lay adjacent to these pallial defects. Peach (1965) observed a four layered cortex type of microgyria in 11 of 20 cases of Arnold-Chiari malformation.

Megalencephaly

The term megalencephaly is properly applied only when the brain is large, not hydrocephalic, and storage diseases such as lipidosis have been rigorously excluded. It is not to be equated with the clinical descriptive term macrocephaly. Essentially the cerebral cortex is unduly thick and heterotopias are absent. Laurence (1946a) reported a patient with unilateral involvement and persistent seizures leading to death at 5½ months of age; both neurones and glia contributed to the enlarged hemisphere. In another unilateral example, Bignami, Palladini and Zapella (1968) using quantitative histochemical techniques showed a three fold

increase in neuronal nuclear volume and suggested heteroploidy as the basic disorder. Laurence (1964b) in a brief review stressed the frequency of seizures in children with this lesion.

Focal cortical dysplasia

This lesion, while often inconspicuous on naked eye examination, presents prominent histopathological features. Lamination of the involved cortex is lost. Abnormally large neurones are scattered throughout the cortex in a disorderly fashion (Fig. 11.5) and may extend in small clus-

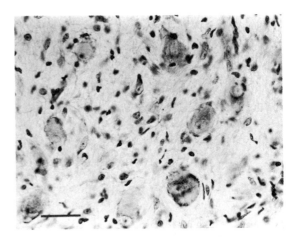

Fig. 11.5 Focal cortical dysplasia. Cortical architecture is disorganised by scattered large neurones and glial proliferation. Luxol fast blue-cresyl violet. Scale marker 50　m.

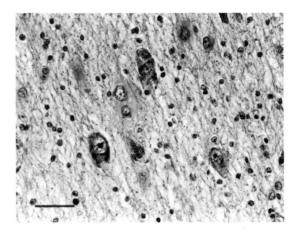

Fig. 11.6 Focal cortical dysplasia. Large neurones and glial cells are clustered in the subcortical white matter. Haematoxylin and eosin. Scale marker 50 μm.

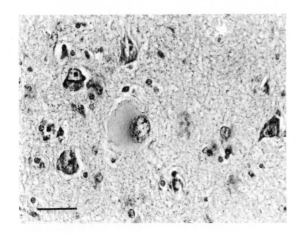

Fig. 11.7 Focal cortical dysplasia. A large astrocyte with voluminous cytoplasm is in the centre of the field. Several small binucleate astrocytes are also present. Haematoxylin and eosin. Scale marker 50 μm.

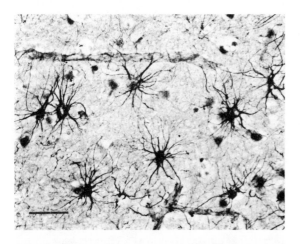

Fig. 11.8 Focal cortical dysplasia. Astrocytic fibre formation in dysplastic cortex. Cajal's gold sublimate impregnation. Scale marker 50 μm.
Figs 11.5 to 11.8 are from the second temporal gyrus of a 26 year old woman whose complex partial seizures began at age 15 years. Her birth and early life were normal and she had no features suggesting tuberous sclerosis.

ters into the subjacent white matter (Fig. 11.6). There is an overall reduction in neuronal population in the affected cortex, which is sharply demarcated from adjoining normal cortex. Astrocytes with abundant cytoplasm, lobulated or multiple nuclei, and fibre formation are frequent (Figs. 11.7 & 11.8). These features are reminiscent of tuberous sclerosis but cortical nodularity, calcification, subependymal lesions and the

cutaneous and visceral manifestations of tuberous sclerosis do not occur in patients with focal cortical dysplasia.

One of the three cases described by Crome (1957) had an extensive, although unilateral, lesion accompanied by cortico-spinal tract degeneration. His patients were under three years of age, and had intractable focal seizures, retarded development and motor deficits. Two were siblings. The patient reported by Cravioto and Feigin (1960), a 21-year-old woman, had seizures with focal onset beginning at six months of age. She had permanent interictal neurological deficits but these are not invariable.

The status of this entity was firmly established by Taylor *et al.* (1971) in a detailed account of ten patients operated upon for intractable seizures; one subsequently died in status epilepticus. These authors give convincing reasons for regarding this disease as distinct from tuberous sclerosis and its formes frustes. A remarkable clinical feature reported by them is the range of age at first seizure of from two to 31 years. This latency is interesting in view of the undoubtedly intrauterine developmental origin of the lesion.

Tuberous sclerosis and formes frustes

The pathology of tuberous sclerosis is systematically described by Urich (1976). Our present concern is with patients whose disease is limited, in whom mental retardation and/or cutaneous manifestations are lacking, so that diagnosis is uncertain in the absence of histopathological evidence. Such partial forms of tuberous sclerosis are being increasingly recognised. The three patients reported in detail by Duvoisin and Vinson (1961) were of superior intelligence although all had radiological evidence of cerebral involvement as well as lesions of tuberous sclerosis elsewhere. Lagos and Gomez (1967) reviewed the records of 71 patients with tuberous sclerosis studied at the Mayo Clinic; 26 of the 69 patients on whom there were records of intellectual capacity had normal intelligence; 18 of these 26 had seizures. Surgical excision of cortical lesions for the relief of seizures in such patients, as carried out by Perot, Weir and Rasmussen (1966), allows histopathological confirmation of the diagnosis. The essential

pathological features distinguishing oligosymp-
tomatic tuberous sclerosis from focal cortical dysplasia, which undoubtedly resemble each other, are
given in the section above.

Hamartomas

These lesions are tumour-like malformations. On
microscopic examination, many bear a strong
resemblance to neoplasms but they lack the property of progressive growth and expansion. Penfield
and Ward (1948) directed attention to this lesion
as a rare anatomical substrate of temporal lobe
seizures. Twenty years later, hamartomas (and
closely related lesions) were reported as the essential pathological finding in 22 of 100 consecutive
epileptic patients treated by anterior temporal
lobectomy (Falconer & Taylor, 1968). In the
Penfield-Rasmussen-Feindel series from Montreal
(reported by Mathieson, 1975a), a diagnosis of
hamartoma was made in 14 of 202 discrete focal
lesions, in a series of 857 patients undergoing surgical excision for epilepsy. This three-fold discrepancy of incidence in the two series may be a consequence of lack of uniform histopathological
criteria and terminology, as well as patient selection.

The exact nature of these lesions is thoroughly
discussed by Cavanagh (1958), whose paper
remains the definitive account and should be consulted for detailed histopathology. Most such
hamartomas occur in the amygdaloid nucleus,
medial occipito-temporal (fusiform) gyrus or less
frequently in the hippocampus. Occurrence in the
frontal and parietal lobes has been recorded
(Mathieson, 1975b, Table 5, p. 114). Any combination of astrocytes, oligodendrocytes and
neurones may occur. Calcification is frequent.

An interesting clinical correlation of hamar-
tomatous lesions has emerged from Falconer's
(1973) review of patients operated on by him.
Patients with a psychosis accompanying their
epilepsy were statistically more likely to have a
hamartoma than an atrophic temporal lobe lesion.
Furthermore, although relief of seizures occurred
in patients with both types of lesions, aggressive
behaviour or a schizophrenia-like illness were
more likely to persist in patients who had a
pathological diagnosis of hamartoma. The reason

for this rather surprising finding remains speculative (Geschwind, 1973).

Meningio-angiomatosis

Strictly this lesion should be considered under the
above heading of hamartoma, for such it is. However, it is non-glial and predominantly composed
of cellular elements which normally lie outside the
pia mater. Meningio-angiomatosis is not to be confused with examples of multiple meningiomas
such as sometimes occur in Von Recklinghausen's
disease, nor with meningioma-en-plaque. In
meningio-angiomatosis a portion of cerebral cortex
is replaced by tissue having the structure of
meningioma but lacking its propensity to grow.
Large neurones are scattered within the lesion
(Fig. 11.9). These were present in case 1 of
Worster-Drought, Dickson and McMenemy (1937)
who gave the first clear account of the lesion
and established its association with central
neurofibromatosis. This disease probably belongs
to that large group of conditions referred to as
neurocristopathies by Bolande (1974).

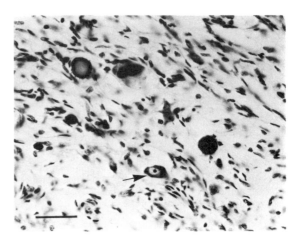

Fig. 11.9 Meningio-angiomatosis. The meningioma-like
structure contains psammoma bodies and occasional neurones
(arrow). From the insular cortex of an adolescent girl with focal
cerebral seizures. Haematoxylin and van Gieson. Scale marker
50 μm.

Neuro-cutaneous melanosis

This striking complex comprises a 'garment type'
pigmented lesion of the skin and an excessive

accumulation of melanocytes in the lepto-meninges. Additionally, in some cases, melanin of both cutaneous and neuronal type is found in neurones, melanocytes and macrophages within certain brain structures. These include the amygd-aloid nuclei and dentate nuclei of the cerebellum (Fox *et al.*, 1964; Slaughter *et al.*, 1969). The development of primary malignant intracranial melanomata bring these patients to the attention of pathologists. In some, however, focal seizures clearly arise from causes other than intracranial neoplasm. In a patient studied personally in con-junction with Dr. F. Andermann, seizures began at three years of age, had a consistent stereotyped pattern and occurred infrequently. Electro-physiological evidence indicated an origin in one amygdaloid nucleus. The appropriate tem-poral lobe, resected at 26 years of age, showed intense melanosis of the amygdala. There has been no seizure recurrence or evidence of tumour dur-ing a three year follow up.

Dermoid and epidermoid cysts

The features of dermoid and epidermoid cysts are too well known to require detailed description here. Most are basally situated. Intracerebral examples are more likely to have epilepsy as a prominent, or occasionally the sole clinical feature (Tytus & Pennybacker, 1956).

Disorders of vascular organisation

The extensive remodelling that the cerebral vascu-lature undergoes during embryogenesis occasion-ally results in malformations. Those that concern us here are cavernous haemangioma, arterio-venous malformation and Sturge-Weber disease.

Cavernous haemangiomas are usually static les-ions and are certainly not neoplastic despite their terminology. Composed essentially of endothelial lined channels with thick collagenous walls, they often have a surrounding zone of gliosed brain and scattered haemosiderin pigment. Calcification is common. The lesions reported as haemangioma calcificans by Penfield and Ward (1948) in the temporal lobes of five patients with longstanding seizures belong in this category. The frequent incidence of focal motor seizures associated with cavernous haemangiomata in the region of the cen-tral fissure is stressed by Russell and Rubinstein (1977). Familial occurrence has been reported by Clark (1970).

In contrast, the shunting of arterial blood into much altered venous channels in arterio-venous malformations produces a dynamic lesion with profound local, and occasionally systemic, altera-tions in cerebral blood flow. Widespread zones of anomalous patterns of epicerebral blood flow and regional cortical blood flow have been demons-trated by Feindel, Yamamoto and Hodge (1971). Regional autoregulation of cerebral blood flow is lost. Fluctuating hypoxia of nearby cortex may play a role in the genesis of seizures which occur so commonly in patients with this lesion. An over-view of these and related lesions is given by McCormick (1966).

The well known triad of facial naevus flam-meus, seizures and intra-cerebral calcification which forms Sturge-Weber disease or encephalo-facial angiomatosis is the subject of an extensive literature. The monograph by Alexander and Norman (1960) and the systematic account by Urich (1976) should be consulted. The extent of the pial venous angioma varies considerably; corti-cal atrophy is often more extensive than the vascu-lar abnormality. The site or sites of most active epileptic cortical discharge may be some distance away from the mossy carpet of abnormal pial blood vessels as displayed at operation. Surgical aspects of therapy and the light they shed on pathology are considered by Falconer and Rush-worth (1960) and by Rasmussen, Mathieson and LeBlanc (1972).

Lesions associated with childbirth

By long tradition, birth injury is believed to give rise to lesions causing habitual epilepsy. That prematurity, excessive moulding, precipitate delivery and neonatal asphyxia may give rise to intracranial lesions is not in dispute. Some lesions, such as subependymal cell plate haemorrhages with secondary ventricular rupture are not com-patible with prolonged survival. Others, such as periventricular leukomalacia and basal ganglia lesions are not associated with epilepsy. Lesions identified as being related to habitual epilepsy are listed in Table 11.3

Table 11.3 Lesions associated with childbirth

Neonatal asphyxia
    Laminar cortical necrosis
    Ulegyria
    Lobular cerebellar sclerosis
Perinatal arterial occlusion
    Cerebral infarct
Excessive moulding
    Medial temporal lobe lesions ('incisural sclerosis')
    Inferior temporal and medial occipital lobe infarction

The early stages of laminar cortical necrosis in neonatal asphyxia are illustrated by Banker (1967) and Friede (1975). The selective involvement of the depths of sulci compared with the crowns of gyri is clear and consistent, but why this pattern should occur remains unknown.

Ulegyria, often in the boundary zones of major cerebral arteries, can readily be visualised as evolving from these earlier stages by resorption of necrotic tissue and gliosis to form the unmistakable mushroom-like gyri. Hypotension complicating hypoxia is believed to determine the distribution of ulegyria in these cases (Norman, Urich & McMenemey, 1957). In some early accounts of the surgical treatment of epilepsy (e.g. Penfield & Humphries, 1940; Penfield & Jasper, 1954) these lesions are referred to as focal microgyria, although it is clear from their illustrations that they are entirely different from the lesion termed microgyria by Crome (1952) and described above under the now more customary term of polymicrogyria.

Circumscribed lobular cerebellar sclerosis is discussed and illustrated in a later section of this chapter.

Large, well-defined, destructive lesions occurring in recognised arterial territories in the brains of patients with seizures and often with fixed neurological deficits are readily recognised as old infarcts. Clinical data in some of these patients indicate that the lesion occurred in the perinatal period. The patients with temporal lobe epilepsy and homonymous hemianopia reported by Remillard, Ethier and Andermann (1974) undoubtedly belong in this category; some of the 85 patients reviewed by Rasmussen and Gossman (1963) under the term gross destructive brain lesions probably had neonatal infarcts; a case is illustrated by Mathieson (1975a). Autopsy accounts in neonates by Clark and Linell (1954) and by Banker (1961) confirmed the occurrence of perinatal arterial cerebral infarcts. In the infantile cases reported by Cocker, George and Yates (1965) there was excellent correlation between the regions of brain infarcted and the sites of arterial lesions; these occurred at arterial bifurcations, suggesting lodgement of an embolus. The cause of arterial occlusion is often obscure although in some cases there is evidence of embolism from the placenta, fetal placental veins, or mural cardiac thrombus. In patients who develop epilepsy in later infancy or childhood and are found to have a cerebral infarct, the aetiology of the perinatal arterial occlusion usually remains tentative and dependent on analogy with cases studied carefully at an earlier stage of their evolution.

Increasing recognition of the frequency of a temporal lobe origin of habitual seizures and the demonstration of atrophic lesions in therapeutic excisions led Earle, Baldwin and Penfield (1953) to formulate a hypothesis about their origin. In essence, they postulated that transtentorial herniation of medial temporal structures resulting from excessive moulding of the skull vault during delivery might compress the anterior choroidal and posterior cerebral arteries with resultant ischaemic lesions in their territories. Hence their term incisural sclerosis. With our increasing knowledge of temporal lobe pathology, this mechanico-vascular hypothesis has proved to be untenable in the many cases of sclerotic temporal atrophy which are now attributed to other causes. The term incisural sclerosis has thus generally lapsed. The distribution of the temporal atrophy, which could not be mapped in the earlier limited therapeutic excisions, is not consistent with anterior choroidal or posterior cerebral occlusion (Falconer, Serafetinides & Corsellis, 1964; Falconer & Taylor, 1968). However, some unusual cases with extensive inferior temporal and medial occipital infarction may be a consequence of posterior cerebral artery compression at the incisura tentorii.

Lesions resulting from febrile illness of childhood

Convulsions due to pyrexial illness, not primarily

involving the brain, are reported to occur in from 19 to 48 per thousand children, mostly between the ages of six months and five years (Miller *et al.*, 1960; Costeff, 1965; Schuman & Miller, 1966; Van den Berg & Yerushalmy, 1969; Rose *et al.*, 1973). The tendency for a child to convulse when febrile appears to be genetically determined (Lennox, 1949a; Ounsted, 1952; Schuman & Miller, 1966; Ounsted 1955). Furthermore the evidence indicates that this tendency is inherited in an autosomal dominant fashion (Ounsted, Lindsay & Norman, 1966; Frantzen *et al.*, 1970). The tendency becomes manifest only when febrile provocation occurs within the appropriate age range in childhood (Ounsted, 1971). The whole subject of febrile convulsions is discussed in detail by Lennox-Buchthal (1973), and in Chapter 3 of this book.

During the age of susceptibility to febrile convulsions, the brain is in a phase of active growth and maturation. On general grounds, therefore, it might be supposed that excessive neuronal discharge and hypoxia occurring during prolonged and/or recurrent convulsions might be particularly likely to cause brain damage. The evidence is that this is so. Zimmerman (1938) described cortical neuronal necrosis, sometimes widespread, occasionally laminar, and often most evident in the walls and depths of sulci in 11 children (age range five months to six years) who died within 1 to 13 days of the onset of severe febrile convulsions. This type of lesion is illustrated in Figure 11.10. Destruction of neurones of Sommer's sector of the hippocampus was prominent in Zimmerman's cases. Cerebellar lesions occurred in some patients. The five patients under three years of age reported by Fowler (1957) were previously healthy but, following convulsions associated with fever, had extensive brain lesions with neuronal necrosis and loss. The distribution of lesions included cerebral cortex, hippocampus, amygdaloid nucleus, thalamus and basal ganglia. In one case the hippocampi were normal. Cortical lesions, where not complete, tended to be laminar, with layer III most frequently involved. Inflammatory lesions of meninges or brain were not present.

Necropsy studies such as these and others in the literature necessarily describe lethal and therefore exceptionally severe instances of insult to the

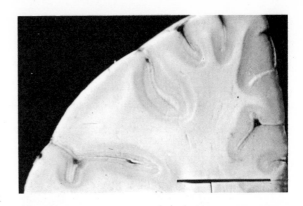

Fig. 11.10 Laminar cortical necrosis. U-shaped involvement of walls and depths of sulci of convexity. From an 18 month old male infant whose persistent febrile convulsions terminated in death on the 3rd day. Scale marker 2 cm.

brain. Their relevance to long-lasting habitual epilepsy is by extrapolation to patients with lesser degrees of cerebral damage. Thom (1942) quotes figures to indicate that children with a history of febrile convulsions are twelve times more likely to have epilepsy than children without such a history. This theme has been further developed with examples by Lennox (1949b).

Viewed retrospectively, patients with established temporal lobe epilepsy have a greater than normal probability of having had febrile convulsions in early life (Ounsted, Lindsay & Norman, 1966; Ounsted, 1967; Mathieson, 1975b). Furthermore, patients with temporal lobe epilepsy and a preceding history of febrile convulsions are more likely (at a high degree of statistical significance) to have siblings who have also had febrile convulsions (Ounsted, 1967). Of 100 patients treated by temporal lobectomy, those shown histologically to have gliosis of medial temporal structures had a significantly ($p<0.01$) more frequent onset with status epilepticus than those with other lesions such as hamartomas or cryptic tumours (Falconer & Taylor, 1968).

The pathogenetic sequence of events, for which the evidence has been given above, is summarised in Figure 11.11. This is probably not the only aetiology of sclerotic atrophy of the temporal lobe, nor are the lesions resulting from febrile status invariably temporal in distribution. An example of widespread destruction with ulegyria and accentuation in arterial watershed

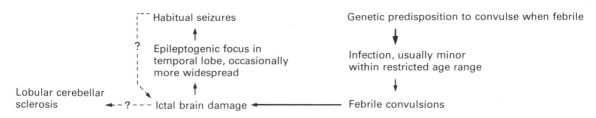

Fig. 11.11 Suggested sequence of events in some patients following prolonged or repeated febrile convulsions. See text for evidence.

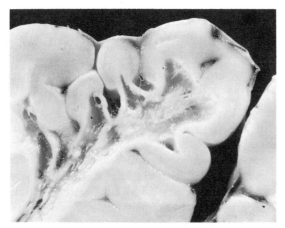

Fig. 11.12 Ulegyria. Birth and early development entirely normal. Severe febrile convulsions at two years. Frequent seizures of variable pattern, resistent to medication. Death following epileptic status at 10 years. Autopsy showed widespread ulegyria mainly in arterial watershed distribution.

zones is shown in Figure 11.12. The tendency for less severe lesions, especially those in the temporal lobe, to be predominantly unilateral is not yet fully understood; possible operative factors include greater seizure discharge on one side (Aicardi & Chevrie, 1970) and a hypothesis regarding differential maturation rates of the cerebral hemispheres (Taylor, 1969; Taylor & Ounsted, 1971).

Evidence derived from animal experimentation relevant to this problem is discussed in a subsequent section of this chapter.

Inflammatory lesions and their residua

Established and essentially static epileptogenic lesions may follow bacterial meningitis and cerebral abscess. In some patients with epilepsia partialis continua and progressive neurological deficit an encephalitic histopathology has been found.

In patients with pyogenic meningitis, several pathogenetic mechanisms may be operative. Although fibrino-purulent exudate is usually confined to the leptomeninges, microscopic changes are observed in the superficial cortical layers even in the early stages. These comprise microglial infiltration and astrocytic hypertrophy which may be surmised to affect dendritic arborisations in these layers. Selective neuronal necrosis occurs in some patients (Smith & Landing, 1960). More obvious ischaemic lesions, taking the form of patchy infarcts, result from endarteritis obliterans, with or without supervening thrombosis of leptomeningeal vessels, especially in patients who have received inappropriate or delayed antibiotic therapy and have passed into a subacute phase. A third pathogenetic mechanism, that of convulsions consequent upon fever, may operate in genetically susceptible children of appropriate age. Dodge and Swartz (1965) reported four of 99 patients as having seizures as a late sequel of pyogenic meningitis.

Cerebral abscesses with their attendant granulation tissue, fibrosis and progressive surrounding zone of gliosed brain form potent epileptogenic foci, as a voluminous literature attests. Legg, Gupta and Scott (1973) recorded epilepsy as occurring in 51 of 70 patients with supratentorial abscesses, with a mean latency of 3.3 years; latency was shorter in patients with a temporal site than in those with a frontal site. Carey, Chou and French (1971) reported a 32 per cent incidence of seizures in 40 patients surviving surgical therapy; seizures in children were more frequent and more resistent to anticonvulsant medication than in adults. Morgan, Wood and Murphey (1973) found a 55 per cent incidence of seizures in 31 patients with supratentorial abscesses; onset was within two years of operation in all but one patient.

Other published series confirm that one-third to one-half of patients surviving cerebral abscess develop epilepsy, no matter how treated. These figures bear eloquent witness to the potent epileptogenicity of this lesion.

Seizures are a prominent clinical feature of various forms of encephalitis of known or suspected viral aetiology. Of special interest are those patients in whom epilepsia partialis continua or recurrent seizures with focal onset are accompanied by a slowly progressive neurological deficit. A histopathological picture of encephalitis, still apparently active many months after onset, has been described in some such patients by Rasmussen, Olszewski and Lloyd-Smith (1958) and by Aguilar and Rasmussen (1960). The syndrome occurs mainly in the first decade of life (Mathieson, 1975a). While inflammatory features are impressive, inclusion bodies are rarely found. Serological evidence of viral infection is lacking and attempts to demonstrate virus by electronmicroscopy and culture have not as yet yielded convincing results, despite a number of preliminary published reports, unfortunately unconfirmed. Clinically there is some resemblance to the syndrome of hemiconvulsions, hemiplegia and epilepsy discussed by Gastaut et al., (1959) but this latter usually has an abrupt onset and is believed to result from vascular occlusion in most instances, although Coxsackie A9 viral infection causing focal vasculitis or encephalitis has been described (Roden et al., 1975; Chalhub et al., 1977).

Parasitic infestation of the brain in the form of cysticercosis cerebri is generally limited to certain geographical regions.

Lesions resulting from head injury

Convulsions occurring contralateral to severe head injury have been observed since early times (Hippocrates, cited by Temkin, 1971). More recent accounts of post-traumatic epilepsy have been concerned, inter alia, with the probability of its occurrence following varying degrees and types of injury (see Ch. 4). Caveness and Liss (1961) and Caveness (1963) in studies of Korean war veterans found an incidence ranging from 8.5 per cent after mild closed injury to over 50 per cent after dural and brain penetration. Jennet (1975) in a long term statistical study of epilepsy following non-missile injuries reported an overall incidence of 5 per cent. This risk was greatly increased by acute intra-cranial haematoma, by early epilepsy and by depressed skull fracture. In pathological terms, these factors reflect laceration of the brain, as occurs inevitably in penetrating injury. Breach of the pial barrier and mechanical damage to the cortex are therefore important determinants of post-traumatic epilepsy.

Morphologically, the focal residual lesions of trauma comprise saucer-shaped defects with smoothly scalloped borders, occurring most frequently on the crests of the orbital frontal and lateral temporal gyri. Lesions extending into the depths of sulci may result from transient interference with the epicerebral circulation and consequent infarction. Histopathologically the superficial or all cortical layers are destroyed; a variable amount of collagenous fibrosis intermingled with glial proliferation forms a meningo-cerebral cicatrix. A narrow bordering zone of partially depopulated cortex is usual.

The more obvious lesions may not be the only important ones. Microscopic lesions, widely scattered throughout the cerebral hemispheres and brain stem, were recorded by Oppenheimer (1968) as occurring in about three quarters of fatal head injuries; not all brain injuries were severe in the conventional sense, as death in some patients was due to non-neurological causes. Essentially these lesions seem to stem from stretching and tearing of axons and subsequent cellular reaction. They are considered to be the precursors of the more extensive lesions described by Strich (1956; 1961) in patients with profound neurological deficits following closed head injury. It may be postulated that these predominantly subcortical abnormalities cause partial deafferentation of the cortex and predispose to the development of post-traumatic epilepsy. The evidence from therapeutic cortical resection, however, at least in selected cases of post-traumatic epilepsy (Rasmussen, 1969), suggests that the local cortical lesion is of paramount importance in the genesis of seizures; the role of possible subcortical damage in the 33 per cent of patients whose seizures were not ameliorated by cortical excision remains speculative.

Another factor possibly contributing to seizures in head injured patients is anoxic encephalopathy consequent upon systemic hypoxia from thoracic and other injuries.

Acquired vascular lesions of adults

Some patients develop epilepsy following a stroke. Louis and McDowell (1967) recorded seizures in 77 of 1000 patients surviving a cerebral infarct; 29 patients had long term seizures as a sequel of their infarcts. Richardson and Dodge (1954) reported a 12.5 per cent incidence of seizures in a consecutive series of 104 stroke patients. The importance of occlusive cerebro-vascular disease in the genesis of epilepsy in the population as a whole is heavily age dependent. In a study of 1008 adult epileptics, roughly representative of the population at risk, seizures were attributed to cerebro-vascular disease in 8.7 per cent. In patients with onset of seizures after age 40, the proportion attributed to cerebro-vascular disease rose to 44.5 per cent (Juul-Jensen, 1963).

What determines whether or not a stroke patient develops seizures is not clear. Involvement of the cerebral cortex appears to be essential (Dodge, Richardson & Victor, 1954). The responsible infarcts are often small and consequent upon small branch occlusion in the epicerebral circulation (Richardson, 1958; Waddington, 1970). Nevertheless patients with medium to large infarcts and associated fixed neurological deficits do occasionally have recurrent seizures. The infarcts and the morphological changes in the brain surrounding them differ in no discernable way from those seen in nonconvulsing patients. Patients surviving massive stroke rarely have persistent seizures.

Neoplasms

Brain tumours as a cause of adult onset epilepsy are so well known as to require little description here. Some general conclusions can be drawn from the large published series of cases, for example those of White, Liu and Mixter (1948), Penfield and Jasper (1954) and Wyke (1959). Almost any supratentorial intracranial tumour can cause brain changes giving rise to seizures. The tendency of different tumours to do so depends partly on their site, but also to a considerable degree on their growth rate as determined by their histopathology. Whether the tumour impinges on the cerebral cortex from without (e.g. meningioma) or infiltrates the brain substance from within (e.g. astrocytoma) appears to make little difference to epileptogenicity. Proximity to the Rolandic motor strip or, more generally, a frontal situation increases the probability of seizures. Chronicity of the lesion is a major factor in epileptogenicity. Thus well-differentiated tumours with low biological growth potential and a course running for several years rather than months are more likely to be associated with epilepsy. Small indolent gliomas with seizures as their sole clinical manifestation are sometimes distinguished with difficulty, if at all, from glial hamartomas (Cavanagh, 1958; Mathieson, 1975b).

In the case of extrinsic tumours, the essential morphological change appears to be an area of pressure atrophy of the cortex characterised by neuronal loss and gliosis. Intrinsic tumours produce a peripheral zone of infiltrated, but incompletely destroyed, brain tissue. This zone, with engulfed but viable neurones, is characteristically prominent in oligodendrogliomas and well differentiated astrocytomas; these lesions are associated with a high incidence of seizures.

For detailed pathological descriptions of nervous system tumours, the reader is referred to standard monographs such as those of Russell and Rubinstein (1977) and Rubinstein (1972).

Subtle dendritic lesions

The arrangement and structure of dendrites are poorly displayed by the staining methods customarily used in light microscopy. Electron microscopy presents difficulties in sampling and the availability of adequately fixed tissue. Morphological observations on dendrites in naturally occurring epileptogenic foci in man are therefore regrettably sparse despite the importance of the dendritic tree in the electrophysiological status of neurones. This is in sharp contrast to extensive accounts of dendritic changes in experimental models of epileptogenic foci.

Using Golgi techniques, the Scheibels have

described a constellation of dendritic changes in the hippocampal neurones of patients with temporal lobe epilepsy (Scheibel, Crandall & Scheibel, 1974; Scheibel & Scheibel, 1973). Loss of dendritic spines, nodularity of the dendritic shaft and fusiform swellings of apical dendrites occurred in a patchy fashion in neurones of the pyramidal cell layer. Changes in the neurones of the gyrus dentatus were less consistent but included a 'windswept' appearance of dendrites and narrowing of the dendritic field giving a 'closed parasol' appearance. These changes were not thought to result from deafferentation or remote anoxic injury; in only 50 per cent of the patients reported was there a history of difficult birth or febrile convulsions in childhood. Paucity of dendritic spines has been corroborated by electron microscopic studies, but the fine structure of dendritic nodularity has not been observed (Brown, 1973). It is not clear whether the changes described by these investigators form a part of the customary hippocampal sclerosis or are a distinct abnormality selectively involving dendritic spines such as has been described by Marin-Padilla (1972) in infants with established chromosomal anomalies. The authors considered that they constituted a continuing process of neuronal destruction.

Endogenous metabolic encephalopathies

A host of diseases due to endogenous metabolic abnormality (inborn errors of metabolism) give rise to seizures. They defy brief description. Reference should be made to standard texts, such as that of Blackwood and Corsellis (1976), which give access to primary sources. Some of these diseases are readily recognised clinically and have a chemically characterised storage product and enzymatic deficiency, for example Tay-Sachs disease, GM2 gangliosidosis and hexosaminidase deficiency. Others, such as neuronal ceroid-lipofuscinosis (Zeman et al., 1970; Boehme et al., 1971) await full biochemical elucidation. Yet others remain to be segregated from the so-called degenerative diseases.

Clinical manifestations of many endogenous metabolic encephalopathies begin in childhood but some are asymptomatic until well into adult life, for example adult ceroid-lipofuscinosis or Kufs'

disease. Some of the non-gangliosidotic storage diseases may be diagnosed by histochemical and electron-microscopic examination of sweat glands obtained by skin biopsy (Carpenter, Karpati & Andermann, 1972; Carpenter et al., 1973) or of lymphocytes (Noonan, Desousa & Riddle, 1978). Lafora's disease, in which myoclonic and generalised seizures are prominent clinical features, may be diagnosed by cerebral biopsy and demonstration of characteristic neuronal inclusions; a detailed description is given by Van Heycop ten Ham (1974). Increasing knowledge of the biochemical abnormalities in the endogenous metabolic encephalopathies should lead to their more precise diagnosis by non-invasive methods.

Metabolic encephalopathies of extra-cerebral origin

Foremost in frequency and importance amongst these is anoxic encephalopathy which is increasingly encountered among general hospital patients following cardio-pulmonary resuscitation. Persistent myoclonic jerks and occasional generalised seizures occur in some patients. Typically at autopsy there is laminar cortical necrosis with accentuation in sulcal depths. An arterial watershed distribution is sometimes encountered or superimposed on a more widespread abnormality.

A morphologically similar encephalopathy may follow profound hypoglycaemia.

ATROPHIC LESIONS OF THE TEMPORAL LOBE

Alike from their frequency, amenability to surgical therapy, and possible prevention, atrophic lesions of the temporal lobe merit our special attention. Sano and Malamud (1953) observed hippocampal sclerosis in 29 of 50 long term epileptics at autopsy; 16 of the 18 with normal mentation had what we would now term complex partial seizures. Corsellis (1957) reported Ammon's horn sclerosis in 15 of 32 patients. Margerison and Corsellis (1966) found hippocampal sclerosis at autopsy in 36 of 55 unselected epileptic patients. Most early descriptions of temporal lobe pathology stressed hippocampal lesions (see Falconer, 1970, for a historical review) but other temporal lobe structures are involved in patients with temporal lobe epilepsy. Neuronal loss and gliosis in the amygdaloid nucleus and uncus of the parahippocampal gyrus occur in a substantial proportion of cases (Meyer & Beck, 1955; Margerison & Corsellis, 1966). In tabulating severe and often widespread lesions in the temporal lobe, Cavanagh and Meyer (1956) recorded involvement of the fusiform gyrus and the inferior and middle temporal gyri in about half the cases with hippocampal sclerosis. These considerations led Falconer, Serafetinides and Corsellis (1964) to introduce the term mesial temporal sclerosis as descriptive of the diffuse lesion found in a large proportion of their patients operated upon for temporal lobe epilepsy. In view of the laterally situated lesions in some cases, and the pan-temporal atrophy in severe examples, sclerotic temporal atrophy has been suggested as a synonym (Mathieson, 1975b). Niceties of terminology aside, the important fact is that atrophic lesions extend beyond the hippocampus and other mesial structures to involve both cortex and white matter of the temporal convolutions. They lie beyond the territories of irrigation of both choroidal and posterior cerebral arteries and we must look to mechanisms other than impaired circulation in any single vessel for their genesis. Indeed the laminar cortical cell loss involving mainly the second and third layers with accentuation in the depths of sulci (Meyer, Falconer & Beck, 1954) is unlikely to be the result of infarction, either arterial or venous. While opinions remain to some extent open, there is a general trend towards the view that most cases of sclerotic temporal atrophy result from severe and/or recurrent febrile convulsions in early childhood; that pre-existing cerebral damage from perinatal asphyxia increases the risk; and that some patients develop this lesion solely as a consequence of birth anoxia. The magnitude of the problem is indicated by the study of Nelson and Ellenberger (1976): 2 per cent of 1706 children who had had one or more febrile convulsions developed epilepsy by the seventh year of life. Children known or suspected of having some neurological abnormality before the febrile convulsive episode had a higher than average incidence of subsequent afebrile seizures. The prophylactic measures indicated are,

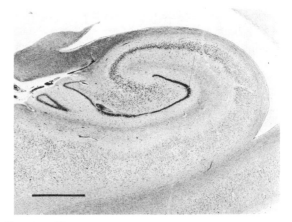

Fig. 11.13 Normal hippocampus. For comparison with Figure 11.14. Cresyl violet. Scale marker 2 mm.

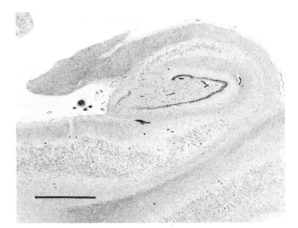

Fig. 11.14 Hippocampal sclerosis. Neuronal loss in hl (Sommer's) sector and in end plate. The hippocampus is shrunken. Cresyl violet. Scale marker 2 mm.

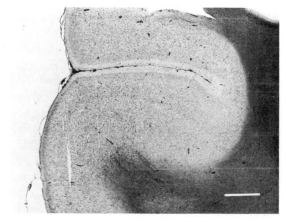

Fig. 11.15 Normal temporal neocortex. For comparison with Fig. 11.16. Luxol fast blue-cresyl violet. Scale marker 2 mm.

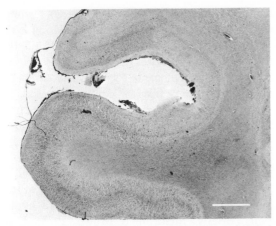

Fig. 11.16 Temporal neocortex. Cortical atrophy especially in depth of sulcus. The flask-shaped dilatation of the sulcus is the most readily apparent feature. From a 42 year old man who had had focal seizures since 20 years of age. Early history not available. Luxol fast blue-PAS. Scale marker 2 mm.

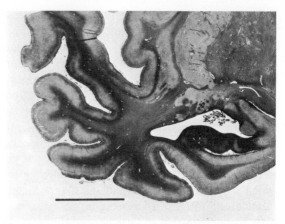

Fig. 11.17 Sclerotic temporal atrophy. There is intense gliosis of the pes hippocampi and diffuse gliosis of gyral white matter. Cortex of all gyri shows patchy thinning and gliosis, especially in walls and depths of sulci. Long history of temporal lobe epilepsy. Holzer's method for glial fibres. Scale marker 1 cm.

in principle, clear (Mathieson, 1975b; Meldrum, 1975). Whether the maturing lesion can be influenced in respect of its potential epileptogenicity following the initiating events is another matter. Evidence derived from animal experimental models is discussed by Meldrum in this chapter.

The range of severity of lesions found, and their histopathological pattern is illustrated in Figures 11.13 to 11.18.

Lesser degrees of presumed abnormality in resected temporal lobes sometimes make it difficult for the surgical pathologist to give a clear opinion. In patients operated upon in middle life some degree of subpial (Chaslin's) gliosis and perivascular atrophy of the white matter are not unexpected. The gyral pattern of the temporal lobe is variable. Studies by Geschwind and Levitsky (1968), Witelson and Pallie (1973) and

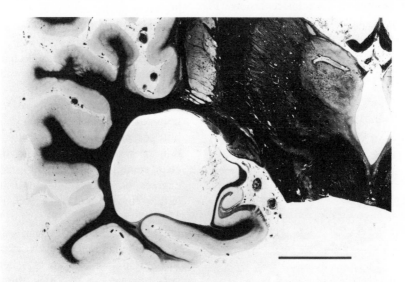

Fig. 11.18 Sclerotic temporal atrophy. Ulegyria of lateral and basal temporal gyri, extending to floor of insula. Hippocampal atrophy. Dilatation of temporal horn of lateral ventricle. Patient had a history of difficult birth and convulsions in infancy. Habitual seizures of varying pattern began at nine years; episodes of status epilepticus; death from unrelated causes at 50 years of age. Heidenhain's method for myelin. Scale marker 1 cm.

Yeni-Komshian and Benson (1976) indicate that there are systematic anatomical differences between right and left temporal lobes. There are thus formidable difficulties in the path of morphometric investigation of resected temporal lobes. Additionally, Crome (1955) has pointed out that many of the histopathological features seen in temporal lobe epilepsy occur in non-epileptic subjects including some of normal intelligence. Equally disturbing are the approximately 20 per cent of therapeutically excised temporal lobes which show little or no morphological abnormality (Mathieson, 1975a). Increasing experience suggests that recognition of flask shaped dilatation of sulci indicating local cortical atrophy will reduce this percentage. Those remaining emphasise the need for studies of dendritic and synaptic morphology and for biochemical collaboration.

CEREBELLAR LESIONS IN PATIENTS WITH EPILEPSY

These take the form of either a diffuse cortical atrophy with Purkinje cell loss, gliosis of the molecular layer and sometimes granular cell layer involvement, or a rather well-circumscribed lobular cerebellar sclerosis. This latter lesion (Fig. 11.19) is commonly bilateral and in the posterolateral cerebellar hemispheres suggesting a border zone hypoxic-ischaemic pathogenesis. Lobular cerebellar sclerosis is most often observed in

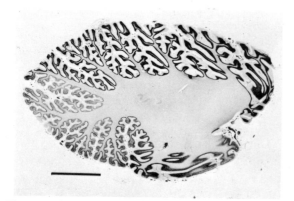

Fig. 11.19 Cerebellum. Lobular cerebellar sclerosis involving posterolateral parts of hemispheres bilaterally. Frequent generalised seizures began at 11 years; early history uncertain; erratic and antisocial behaviour. Death at 25 years due to aspiration pneumonia following seizure. Cresyl violet stain. Scale marker 1 cm.

institutionalised patients with severe seizures, making it tempting to assume that the lesion is the cumulative effect of ictal brain damage. While this may be so in some cases, the alternative view that the cerebral epileptogenic foci and the cerebellar lesions both stem from a common episode of perinatal anoxia or febrile convulsions (such as cause ulegyria of watershed distribution) is more attractive. The concepts are not mutually exclusive. The Purkinje and basket cells are known to be selectively vulnerable to hypoxia; boundary zone lesions occur either when there is an abrupt fall in blood pressure or sudden severe hypoxaemia (Brierly, Meldrum & Brown, 1973). Cerebellar lesions in epileptic patients were recognised before the introduction of phenytoin and are probably not attributable to its use.

IATROGENIC LESIONS IN PATIENTS WITH EPILEPSY

These lesions include gingival hypertrophy, a peculiar form of lymphadenopathy, and, arguably, cerebellar cortical abnormalities, all relating to phenytoin therapy.

The gum changes, histologically, consist of proliferation of the submucosal connective tissue with plasma cell infiltration and acanthosis of the epithelium (Van der Kwast, 1956). Symmers (1978) regards the essential change as hyperplasia of connective tissue, but secondary inflammatory features are usually present.

Hydantoin lymphadenopathy most frequently involves cervical nodes which become enlarged but not matted. Histologically there is proliferation of reticulum cells, formation of binucleate cells, some loss of nodal architecture, and variable degrees of eosinophilic infiltration and necrosis (Saltzstein & Ackerman, 1959; Krasznai & Györy, 1968; Symmers, 1978). The major differential diagnosis is that of Hodgkin's disease. Regression of nodal enlargement on withdrawal of the drug is the best demonstration of a benign reactive process. In very rare cases the lymphadenopathy progresses to malignant lymphoma, even following initial regression (Gams, Neal & Conrad, 1968).

While an ataxic syndrome is well recognised clinically following phenytoin intoxication, its morphological basis, if any, has proved to be something of a mirage. Purkinje cell loss following phenytoin administration to experimental animals has been described (Utterback, 1958 and other investigators) but morphometric studies by Dam (1972) do not confirm any such cell loss in rats, pigs or monkeys. Furthermore Dam (1970) has shown that a diminished Purkinje cell population in patients with major seizures is related to the frequency of seizures rather than prolonged large doses of phenytoin. Fine structural changes in Purkinje cell dendrites in rats subject to near lethal doses of phenytoin were described by del Cerro and Snider (1967), but Nielsen, Dam and Klinken (1971) found normal Purkinje cell ultrastructure in rats subject to intoxicating but sublethal doses of this drug.

CONCLUSION

The outstanding feature of any review of the pathology of epilepsy is the range and diversity of lesions which can give rise to seizures. It is clear that the obvious and readily categorised lesions are several steps removed from the essential local abnormality which is causative of seizures. Our inability to find consistent changes in patients with cortico-reticular seizures emphasises this problem. Whether the lesions are discrete and focal, or diffuse and subtle, the abnormal discharges take place in remaining viable neurones. Their environment has been changed not only in structure but also physiologically and biochemically. These aspects are considered in the ensuing section of this book.

REFERENCES

Aguilar, M.J. & Rasmussen, T. (1960) Role of encephalitis in pathogenesis of epilepsy. *Archives of Neurology*, 2, 663.

Aicardi, J. & Chevrie, J.J. (1970) Convulsive status epilepticus in infants and children. A study of 239 cases. *Epilepsia*, 11, 187.

Alexander, G.L. & Norman, R.M. (1960) *The Sturge-Weber Syndrome*. Bristol: Wright.

Banker, B.Q. (1961) Cerebral vascular disease in infancy and childhood. I occlusive vascular disease. *Journal of Neuropathology and Experimental Neurology*, 20, 127.

Banker, B.Q. (1967) The neuropathological effects of anoxia and hypoglycaemia in the newborn. *Developmental Medicine and Child Neurology*, 9, 544.

Bignami, A. & Appicciutoli, L. (1964) Micropolygyria and cerebral calcification in cytomegalic inclusion disease. *Acta Neuropathologica*, 4, 127.

Bignami, A., Palladini, G. & Zappella, M. (1968) Unilateral megalencephaly with nerve cell hypertrophy. An anatomical and quantitative histochemical study. *Brain Research*, 9, 103.

Blackwood, W. & Corsellis, J.A.N. (1976) (eds) *Greenfield's Neuropathology*, 3rd edn. Edinburgh: Edward Arnold.

Boehme, D.H., Cottrell, J.C., Leonberg, S.C. & Zeman, W. (1971) A dominant form of neuronal ceroid-lipofuscinosis. *Brain*, 94, 745.

Bolande, R.P. (1974) The neurocristopathies. A unifying concept of disease arising in neural crest maldevelopment. *Human Pathology*, 5, 409.

Brierly, J.B., Meldrum, B.S. & Brown, A.W. (1973) The threshold and neuropathology of cerebral 'anoxic-ischemic' cell change. *Archives of Neurology*, 29, 367.

Brown, W.J. (1973) In Brazier, M.A.B. (ed.) *Epilepsy. Its Phenomena in Man*, New York: Academic Press.

Carey, M.E., Chou, S.N. & French, L.A. (1971) Long-term neurological residua in patients surviving brain abscess with surgery. *Journal of Neurosurgery*, 34, 652.

Carpenter, S., Karpati, G. & Andermann, F. (1972) Specific involvement of muscle, nerve and skin in late infantile and juvenile amaurotic idiocy. *Neurology*, 22, 170.

Carpenter, S., Karpati G., Wolfe, L.S. & Andermann, F.

(1973) A type of juvenile cerebromacular degeneration characterized by granular osmiophilic deposits. *Journal of the Neurological Sciences*, 18, 67.

Cavanagh, J.B. (1958) On certain small tumours encountered in the temporal lobe. *Brain*, 81, 389.

Cavanagh, J.B. & Meyer, A. (1956) Aetiological aspects of Ammon's horn sclerosis associated with temporal lobe epilepsy. *British Medical Journal*, 2, 1403.

Caveness, W.F. (1963) Onset and cessation of fits following craniocerebral trauma. *Journal of Neurosurgery*, 20, 570.

Caveness, W.F. & Liss, H.R. (1961) Incidence of post-traumatic epilepsy. *Epilepsia*, 2, 123.

Chalhub, E.G., Devivo, D.C., Siegal, B.A., Gado, M.H. & Feigin, R.D. (1977) Coxsackie A9 focal encephalitis associated with acute infantile hemiplegia and porencephaly. *Neurology*, 27, 574.

Clark, J.V. (1970) Familial occurrence of cavernous angiomata of the brain. *Journal of Neurology, Neurosurgery and Psychiatry*, 33, 871.

Clark, R.M. & Linell, E.A. (1954) Case report: prenatal occlusion of the internal carotid artery. *Journal of Neurology, Neurosurgery and Psychiatry*, 17, 295.

Cocker, J., George, S.W. & Yates, P.O. (1965) Perinatal occlusion of the middle cerebral artery. *Developmental Medicine and Child Neurology*, 7, 235.

Corsellis, J.A.N. (1957) The incidence of Ammon's horn sclerosis. *Brain*, 80, 193.

Costeff, N. (1965) Convulsions in childhood. Their natural history and indications for treatment. *New England Journal of Medicine*, 273, 1410.

Cravioto, H. & Feigin, I. (1960) Localized cerebral gliosis with giant neurons histologically resembling tuberous sclerosis. *Journal of Neuropathology and Experimental Neurology*, 19, 572.

Crome, L. (1952) Microgyria. *Journal of Pathology and Bacteriology*, 64, 479.

Crome, L. (1955) A morphological critique of temporal lobectomy. *Lancet*, 1, 882.

Crome, L. (1957) Infantile cerebral gliosis with giant nerve cells. *Journal of Neurology, Neurosurgery and Psychiatry*, **20**, 117.

Crome, L. (1961) Cytomegalic inclusion – body disease. *World Neurology*, **2**, 447.

Crome, L. & France, N.E. (1959) Microgyria and cytomegalic inclusion disease in infancy. *Journal of Clinical Pathology*, **12**, 427.

Dam, M. (1970) Number of Purkinje cells in patients with grand mal epilepsy treated with diphenylhydantoin. *Epilepsia*, **11**, 313.

Dam, M. (1972) The density and ultrastructure of the Purkinje cells following diphenylhydantoin treatment in animals and man. *Acta Neurologica Scandinavica*, 48 Supplement **49**, 3.

Dekaban, A. (1965) Large defects in cerebral hemispheres associated with cortical dysgenesis. *Journal of Neuropathology and Experimental Neurology*, **24**, 512.

Del Cerro, M.P., Snider, R.S. (1967) Studies on Dilantin intoxication. *Neurology (Minneapolis)* **17**, 452.

Dobbing, J. & Sands, J. (1973) Quantitative growth and development of human brain. *Archives of Diseases in Childhood*, **48**, 757.

Dobbing, J. & Smart, J.L. (1974) Vulnerability of developing brain and behaviour. *British Medical Bulletin*, **30**, 164.

Dodge, P.R., Richardson, E.P. & Victor, M. (1954) Recurrent convulsive seizures as a sequel to cerebral infarction: a clinical and pathological study. *Brain*, **77**, 610.

Dodge, P.R. & Swartz, M.N. (1965) Bacterial meningitis – a review of selected aspects. II Special neurological problems, postmeningitic complications and clinicopathological correlations. *New England Journal of Medicine*, **272**, 1003.

Duvoisin, R.C. & Vinson, W.M. (1961) Tuberous sclerosis. Report of three cases without mental defect. *Journal of the American Medical Association*, **175**, 869.

Earle, K.M., Baldwin, M. & Penfield, W. (1953) Incisural sclerosis and temporal lobe seizures produced by hippocampal herniation at birth. *Archives of Neurology and Psychiatry*, **69**, 27.

Falconer, M.A. (1970) Historical review. The pathological substrate of temporal lobe epilepsy. *Guy's Hospital Reports*, **119**, 47.

Falconer, M.A. (1973) Reversibility by temporal-lobe resection of the behavioural abnormalities of temporal-lobe epilepsy. *New England Journal of Medicine*, **289**, 451.

Falconer, M.A. & Rushworth, R.G. (1960) Treatment of encephalotrigeminal angiomatosis (Sturge-Weber disease) by hemispherectomy. *Archives of Disease in Childhood*, **35**, 433.

Falconer, M.A. & Taylor, D.C. (1968) Surgical treatment of drug-resistant epilepsy due to mesial temporal sclerosis. *Archives of Neurology*, **19**, 353.

Falconer, M.A., Serafetinides, E.A. & Corsellis, J.A.N. (1964) Etiology and pathogenesis of temporal lobe epilepsy. *Archives of Neurology*, **10**, 233.

Feindel, W., Yamamoto, Y.L. & Hodge, C.L. (1971) Red cerebral veins and the cerebral steal syndrome. Evidence from fluorescein angiography and microregional blood flow by radioisotopes during excision of an angioma. *Journal of Neurosurgery*, **35**, 167.

Fowler, M. (1957) Brain damage after febrile convulsions. *Archives of Diseases in Childhood*, **32**, 67.

Fox, H., Emery, J.L., Goodbody, R.A. & Yates, P.O. (1964) Neuro-cutaneous melanosis. *Archives of Disease in Childhood*, **39**, 508.

Frantzen, E., Lennox-Buchthal, M., Nygaard, A. & Stene, J. (1970) A genetic study of febrile convulsions. *Neurology*, **20**, 909.

Friede, R.L. (1975) *Developmental Neuropathology*, Ch. 6. New York – Wien: Springer-Verlag.

Gams, R.A., Neal, J.A. & Conrad, F.G. (1968) Hydantoin induced pseudo-pseudolymphoma. *Annals of Internal Medicine*, **69**, 557.

Gastaut, H., Poirier, F., Payan, H., Salamon, G., Toga, M. & Vigouroux, M. (1959) H.H.E. syndrome. Hemiconvulsions, hemiplegia, epilepsy. *Epilepsia*, **1**, 418.

Geschwind, N. (1973) Effects of temporal lobe surgery on behaviour. *New England Journal of Medicine*, **289**, 480.

Geschwind, N. & Levitsky, W. (1968) Human brain: left-right asymmetries in temporal speech region. *Science*, **161**, 186.

Jennett, B. (1975) *Epilepsy After Non-missile Head Injuries*, 2nd edn. London: Heinemann.

Juul-Jensen, P. (1963) Epilepsy. A clinical and social analysis of 1020 adult patients with epileptic seizures. *Acta Neurologica Scandinavica*, **40**, Supplement 5, 1.

Kirschbaum, W. (1947) Agenesis of the corpus callosum and associated malformations. *Journal of Neuropathology and Experimental Neurology*, **6**, 78.

Krasznai, G. & Györy, Gy. (1968) Hydantoin lymphadenopathy. *Journal of Pathology and Bacteriology*, **95**, 314.

Lagos, J.C. & Gomez, M.R. (1967) Tuberous sclerosis: reappraisal of a clinical entity. *Mayo Clinic Proceedings*, **42**, 26.

Laurence, K.M. (1964a) A case of unilateral megalencephaly. *Developmental Medicine and Child Neurology*, **6**, 585.

Laurence, K.M. (1964b) Megalencephaly (Annotation) *Developmental Medicine and Child Neurology*, **6**, 638.

Layton, D.D. (1962) Heterotopic cerebral gray matter as an epileptogenic focus. *Journal of Neuropathology and Experimental Neurology*, **21**, 244.

Legg, N.J., Gupta, P.C. & Scott, D.F. (1973) Epilepsy following cerebral abscess. A clinical and EEG study of 70 patients. *Brain*, **96**, 259.

Lennox, M.A. (1949a) Febrile convulsions in childhood. A clinical and electroencephalographic study. *American Journal of Diseases of Children*, **78**, 868.

Lennox, M.A. ((1949b) Febrile convulsions in childhood: their relationship to adult epilepsy. *Journal of Pediatrics*, **35**, 427.

Lennox-Buchthal, M.A. (1973) *Febrile Convulsions. A Reappraisal. Electroencephalography and Clinical Neurophysiology Supplement No 32*. Amsterdam/London/New York: Elsevier.

Lilienfeld, A.M. & Pasamanick, B. (1954) Association of maternal and fetal factors with the development of epilepsy. 1. Abnormalities of the prenatal and paranatal periods. *Journal of the American Medical Association*, **155**, 719.

Louis, S. & McDowell, F. (1967) Epileptic seizures in nonembolic cerebral infarction. *Archives of Neurology*, **17**, 414.

Margerison, J.H. & Corsellis, J.A.N. (1966) Epilepsy and the temporal lobes. A clinical, electroencephalographic and neuropathological study of the brain in epilepsy with particular reference to the temporal lobes. *Brain*, **89**, 499.

Marin-Padilla, M. (1972) Structural abnormalities of the cerebral cortex in human chromosomal aberrations: a Golgi study. *Brain Research*, **44**, 625.

Mathieson, G. (1975a) Pathologic aspects of epilepsy with special reference to the surgical pathology of focal cerebral seizures. In Purpura, D.P., Penry, J.K. & Walter, R.D. (eds) *Advances in Neurology* Vol 8, *Neurosurgical Management of the Epilepsies*, Ch. 6. New York : Raven Press.

Mathieson, G. (1975b) Pathology of temporal lobe foci. In

Penry, J.K. & Daly, D.D. (eds) *Advances in Neurology Vol II, Complex Partial Seizures and Their Treatment*, Ch. 8. New York: Raven Press.

McCormick, W.F. (1966) The pathology of vascular ('arteriovenous') malformations. *Journal of Neurosurgery*, **24**, 807.

Meldrum, B.S. (1975) Present views on hippocampal sclerosis and epilepsy. In Williams D. (ed.) *Modern Trends in Neurology*, Vol. 6, Ch. 12. London: Butterworths.

Meyer, A. & Beck, E. (1955) The hippocampal formation in temporal lobe epilepsy. *Proceedings of the Royal Society of Medicine*, **48**, 457.

Meyer, A., Falconer, M.A. & Beck, E. (1954) Pathological findings in temporal lobe epilepsy. *Journal of Neurology, Neurosurgery and Psychiatry*, **17**, 276.

Miller, F.J.W., Court, S.D.M., Walton, W.S. & Knox, E.J. (1960) *Growing up in Newcastle upon Tyne: a Continuing Study of Health and Illness in Young Children Within Their Families*. London: Oxford University Press.

Morgan, H., Wood, M.W. & Murphy, F. (1973) Experience with 88 consecutive cases of brain abscess. *Journal of Neurosurgery*, **38**, 698.

Nelson, K.B. & Ellenberger, J.H. (1976) Predictors of epilepsy in children who have experienced febrile seizures. *New England Journal of Medicine*, **295**, 1029.

Nielsen, M.H., Dam, M. & Klinken, L. (1971) The ultrastructure of Purkinje cells in diphenylhydantoin intoxicated rats. *Experimental Brain Research*, **12**, 447.

Noonan, S.M., Desousa, J. & Riddle, J.M. (1978) Lymphocyte ultrastructure in two cases of neuronal ceroid-lipofuscinosis. *Neurology*, **28**, 472.

Norman, R.M. (1958) Malformations of the nervous system, birth injury and diseases of early life. In Greenfield, J.G. (ed.) *Neuropathology*, London: Arnold.

Norman, R.M., Urich, H. & McMenemey, W.H. (1957) Vascular mechanisms of birth injury. *Brain*, **80**, 49.

Oppenheimer, D.R. (1968) Microscopic lesions in the brain following head injury. *Journal of Neurology, Neurosurgery and Psychiatry*, **31**, 299.

Ounsted, C. (1952) The factor of inheritance in convulsive disorders in childhood. *Proceedings of the Royal Society of Medicine*, **45**, 865.

Ounsted, C. (1955) Genetic and social aspect of the epilepsies of childhood. *Eugenics Review*, **47**, 33.

Ounsted, C. (1967) Temporal lobe epilepsy: the problem of aetiology and prophylaxis. *Journal of the Royal College of Physicians of London*, **1**, 273.

Ounsted, C. (1971) In Gairdner, D. & Hull, D. (eds) *Recent Advances in Paediatrics*, Fourth edn. Ch. 11. London: Churchill.

Ounsted, C., Lindsay, J. & Norman, R. (1966) *Biological Factors in Temporal Lobe Epilepsy. Clinics in Developmental Medicine No. 22*. London: Heinemann.

Pasamanick, B. & Lilienfeld, A.M. (1955) Maternal and fetal factors in the development of epilepsy. 2. Relationship to some clinical features of epilepsy. *Neurology*, **5**, 77.

Peach, B. (1965) Arnold-Chiari malformation. Anatomic features of 20 cases. *Archives of Neurology*, **12**, 613.

Penfield, W. & Humphreys, S. (1940) Epileptogenic lesions of the brain. A histologic study. *Archives of Neurology and Psychiatry*, **43**, 240.

Penfield, W. & Jasper, H. (1954) *Epilepsy and the Functional Anatomy of the Human Brain*, Ch. 7. Boston: Little, Brown.

Penfield, W. & Ward, A. (1948) Calcifying epileptogenic

lesions. Haemangioma calcificans; report of a case. *Archives of Neurology and Psychiatry*, **60**, 20.

Perot, P., Weir, B. & Rasmussen, T. (1966) Tuberous sclerosis. Surgical therapy for seizures. *Archives of Neurology*, **15**, 498.

Rasmussen, T. (1969) Surgical therapy of post traumatic epilepsy. In Walker, A.E., Caveness, W.F. & Critchley, M. (eds) *The Late Effects of Head Injury*, Ch. 26. Springfield: Thomas.

Rasmussen, T. & Gossman, H. (1963) Epilepsy due to gross destructive brain lesions. *Neurology*, **13**, 659.

Rasmussen, T., Mathieson, G. & LeBlanc, F. (1972) Surgical therapy of typical and a forme fruste variety of the Sturge-Weber Syndrome. *Schweizer Archiv für Neurologie, Neurochirurgie und Psychiatrie*, **111**, 393.

Rasmussen, T., Olszewski, J. & Lloyd-Smith, D. (1958) Focal seizures due to chronic localised encephalitis. *Neurology*, **8**, 435.

Remillard, G.M., Ethier, R. & Andermann, F. (1974) Temporal lobe epilepsy and perinatal occlusion of the posterior cerebral artery. *Neurology*, **24**, 1001.

Richardson, E.P. (1958) Late life epilepsy. *Medical Clinics of North America*, **42**, 349.

Richardson, E.P. & Dodge P.R. (1954) Epilepsy in cerebral vascular disease. *Epilepsia (3rd series)*, **3**, 49.

Richman, D.P., Stewart, R.M. & Caviness, V.S. Jr. (1974) Cerebral microgyria in a 27-week fetus. An architectonic and topographic analysis. *Journal of Neuropathology and Experimental Neurology*, **33**, 374.

Roden, V.J., Cantor, H.E., O'Connor, D.M., Schmidt, R.R. & Cherry, J.D. (1975) Acute hemiplegia of childhood associated with Coxsackie A9 viral infection. *Journal of Pediatrics*, **86**, 56.

Rose, S.W., Penry, J.K., Markush, R.E., Radloff, L.A. & Putnam, P.L. (1973) Prevalence of epilepsy in children. *Epilepsia*, **14**, 133.

Rubinstein, L.J. (1972) *Tumors of the Central Nervous System*. Atlas of Tumor Pathology, Second Series, Fasicle 6. Washington: Armed Forces Institute of Pathology.

Russell, D.S. & Rubinstein, L.J. (1977) *Pathology of Tumours of the Nervous System*. London: Arnold.

Saltzstein, S.L. & Ackerman, L.V. (1959) Lymphadenopathy induced by anti-convulsant drugs and mimicking clinically and pathologically malignant lymphomas. *Cancer*, **12**, 164.

Sano, K. & Malamud, N. (1953) Clinical significance of sclerosis of the cornu Ammonis. *Archives of Neurology and Psychiatry*, **70**, 40.

Scheibel, M.E., Crandall, P.H. & Scheibel, A.B. (1974) The hippocampaldentate complex in temporal lobe epilepsy. A Golgi study. *Epilepsia*, **15**, 55.

Scheibel, M.E. & Scheibel, A.B. (1973) In Brazier, M.A.B. (ed.) *Epilepsy. Its Phenomena in Man*, New York: Academic Press.

Schuman, S.H. & Miller, L.J. (1966) Febrile convulsions in families: findings in an epidemiological survey. *Clinical Pediatrics*, **5**, 604.

Slaughter, J.C., Hardman, J.M., Kempe, L.G. & Earle, K.M. (1969) Neurocutaneous melanosis and leptomeningeal melanomatosis in children. *Archives of Pathology*, **88**, 298.

Smith, J.F. & Landing, B.H. (1960) Mechanisms of brain damage in H. influenzae meningitis. *Journal of Neuropathology and Experimental Neurology*, **19**, 248.

Strich, S.J. (1956) Diffuse degeneration of the cerebral white matter in severe dementia following head injury. *Journal of Neurology, Neurosurgery and Psychiatry*, **19**, 163.

Strich, S.J. (1961) Shearing of nerve fibres as a cause of brain damage due to head injury. *Lancet*, **2**, 443.

Symmers, W. StC. (1978) In Symmers, W. StC. (ed.) Systemic Pathology, 2nd edn. Vol 2, Ch. 9. Edinburgh: Churchill Livingstone.

Taylor, D.C. (1969) Differential rates of cerebral maturation between sexes and between hemispheres. Evidence from epilepsy. *Lancet*, **2**, 140.

Taylor, D.C. & Ounsted, C. (1971) Biological mechanisms influencing the outcome of seizures in response to fever. *Epilepsia*, **12**, 33.

Taylor, D.C., Falconer, M.A., Bruton, C.T. & Corsellis, J.A.N. (1971) Focal dysplasia of the cerebral cortex in epilepsy. *Journal of Neurology, Neurosurgery and Psychiatry*, **34**, 369.

Temkin, O. (1971) *The Falling Sickness*, 2nd edition, p. 35. Baltimore: The Johns Hopkins Press.

Thom, D.A. (1942) Convulsions of early life and their relation to the chronic convulsive disorders and mental defect. *American Journal of Psychiatry*, **98**, 574.

Tytus, J.S. & Pennybacker, J. (1956) Pearly tumours in relation to the central nervous system. *Journal of Neurology, Neurosurgery and Psychiatry*, **19**, 241.

Urich, H. (1976) In Blackwood, W. & Corsellis, J.A.N. (eds) *Greenfield's Neuropathology*, Ch. 10. London: Arnold.

Utterback, R.A. (1958) Parenchymatous cerebellar degeneration complicating diphenylhydantoin (Dilantin) therapy. *Archives of Neurology and Psychiatry*, **80**, 180.

Van den Berg, B.J. & Yerushalmy, J. (1969) Studies on convulsive disorders in young children. 1 Incidence of febrile and nonfebrile convulsions by age and other factors. *Pediatric Research*, **3**, 298.

Van der Kwast, W.A.M. (1956) Speculations regarding the nature of gingival hyperplasia due to diphenylhydantoin-sodium. *Acta Medica Scandinavica*, **153**, 399.

Van Heycop ten Ham (1974) Lafora disease. A form of progressive myoclonus epilepsy. In Vinken, P.J. & Bruyn, G.W. (eds) *Handbook of Clinical Neurology*, Vol. 15, Ch. 22. Amsterdam: North Holland Publishing Company.

Waddington, M.W. (1970) Angiographic changes in focal motor epilepsy. *Neurology*, **20**, 879.

White, J.C., Liu, C.T. & Mixter, W.J. (1948) Focal epilepsy. A statistical study of its causes and the results of surgical treatment I Epilepsy secondary to intracranial tumours. *New England Journal of Medicine*, **238**, 891.

Witelson, S.F. & Pallie, W. (1973) Left hemisphere specialisation for language in the newborn. Neuroanatomical evidence of asymmetry. *Brain*, **96**, 641.

Worster-Drought, C., Dickson, W.E.C. & McMenemy, W.H. (1937) Multiple meningeal and perineural tumours with analogous tumours in the glia and ependyma (neurofibroblastomatosis). *Brain*, **60**, 85.

Wyke, B.D. (1959) The cortical control of movement. A contribution to the surgical physiology of seizures. *Epilepsia (4th series)*, **1**, 4.

Yeni-Komshian, G.H. & Benson, D.A. (1976) Anatomical study of cerebral asymmetry in the temporal lobe of humans, chimpanzees and rhesus monkeys. *Science*, **192**, 387.

Zeman, W., Donahue, S., Dyken, P. & Green, J. (1970) The neuronal ceroidlipofuscinoses (Batten-Vogt Syndrome). In Vinken, P.J. & Bruyn, G.W. (eds) *Handbook of Clinical Neurology*, Vol. 10, Ch. 25. Amsterdam: North Holland Publishing Company.

Zimmerman, H.M. (1938) The histopathology of convulsive disorders in children. *Journal of Pediatrics*, **13**, 859.

PART TWO
PATHOPHYSIOLOGY

B.S. Meldrum

An ideal account of the pathophysiology of epilepsy would provide an explanation for the clinical phenomena of epilepsy in terms of events described at the cellular or molecular level. A great deal is known about abnormal patterns of electrical activity that can be recorded at the cellular level during ictal or inter-ictal activity, in both focal and generalised epilepsy. Some of this information is summarised in Chapter 5; a review is provided by Ward (1969). However, most of the clinical phenomena of epilepsy cannot yet be described in terms of molecular or cellular events.

In this chapter the action of physiological and pathological processes in epileptic phenomena will be described under four headings:

1. Systemic factors, physiological and pathological, that influence the occurrence of seizures

2. Epileptogenesis at the cellular level

3. Physiological events that occur as a result of seizures

4. Pathological changes that occur in the brain as a result of seizures.

1. SYSTEMIC FACTORS

That physiological or pathological changes involving the whole body can increase the excitability of the brain and thus favour the occurrence of fits in predisposed subjects has been appreciated since the time of Galen. Fits occurring subsequent to systemic disturbances can be considered in three categories. Firstly, patients with epilepsy sometimes find that their usual type of seizure is apt to occur under certain physiological circumstances (e.g. on awakening, premenstrually, during overbreathing, or hypoglycaemia). Secondly, fits may occur in subjects with an appropriate predisposition only during a specific stress (e.g. febrile convulsions in a genetically predisposed child). Thirdly, in subjects with no neurological abnormality, and no special predisposition to seizures, certain severe stresses (including profound hypoglycaemia and a wide range of poisonings) may induce focal or generalised seizures.

The factors discussed under the headings below are all quantifiable and their effects on seizures have been demonstrated in both clinical and experimental studies. Many patients and their physicians believe that emotional stress can favour the occurrence of fits and there is evidence for a clinical group where seizures occur only after stress (Friis & Lund, 1974). Emotional stress is often accompanied by some of the physiological changes discussed below, such as overbreathing and, most important, the lack of sleep. However, it is possible that psychological factors can modify cerebral excitability irrespective of systemic changes.

Water and electrolyte disturbances

If the quantity of water, sodium, calcium or magnesium in the extracellular or intracellular compartments of the body is abnormal, seizures may be facilitated in epileptic and non-epileptic subjects. Table 11.4 summarises data on critical variations in plasma composition. Systemic disturbances of potassium balance tend not to alter susceptibility to seizures. Reviews of disturbances of hydration and electrolytes in relation to epilepsy are provided by Teglbjaerg (1936), Reynolds (1970) and Millichap (1974).

Overhydration, hyponatraemia

The experimental induction of seizures by overhydration was described by Rowntree (1923, 1926). Subsequently, a pitressin water load test was devised (McQuarrie & Peeler, 1931) to confirm or eliminate the diagnosis of epilepsy. The habitual type of attack was reliably induced in

epileptic children given pitressin and an oral water load (2–5 ml per kg per hour). Seizures did not occur in non-epileptic children.

However, children with no neurological abnormality may experience generalised seizures during the course of rehydration following a severe dehydrating illness or after hypernatraemia (Melekian, Laplane & Debray, 1962; Friis-Hansen & Buchthal, 1965).

Overhydration is usually associated with a reduction in the osmolarity of plasma and with hyponatraemia, i.e. a plasma sodium concentration below 125 mEq/1. Hyponatraemia with coma, or more rarely convulsions, can occur in anterior hypopituitarism and in Addison's disease. It is more commonly the result of inadequate management of an acute illness. Hyponatraemia seizures are not uncommon in psychiatric patients as a result of self-induced water intoxication (Jose, Barton & Perez-Cruet, 1979).

Seizures due to overhydration or to hyponatraemia respond poorly to anticonvulsant drugs. The slow administration of hypertonic saline is usually required (e.g. 3 per cent NaCl). Potassium or calcium depletion may also require correction.

Experimentally, generalised seizures can be induced by administering a massive water load to normal rats, rabbits or cats (Funck-Brentano, Lossky-Nekhorocheff & Altman, 1960; Waltregny & Mesdjian, 1969). Such seizures can be prevented if sodium chloride is given with the water load. During a rapid reduction in plasma osmolarity the brain swells, because of an increase in intracellular water. This so-called *vasogenic* cerebral oedema occurs also after local ischaemia (Klatzo, 1967) and favours the initiation of epileptic activity. In water-intoxicated rats the potassium content of the brain (on a dry weight basis) is reduced by 20 per cent. This ion shift probably serves to limit brain swelling. Coma and convulsions appear to arise from the increase in intracellular water rather than the decrease in potassium content (Rymer & Fishman, 1973).

Dehydration, hypernatraemia, hyperosmolal coma

Illnesses associated with severe dehydration are not uncommonly complicated by seizures. Melekian *et al.* (1962) saw convulsions in 48 out of

Table 11.4 Deviations in plasma composition and seizure activity

	Normal range	Deviation	'Epileptogenicity' in man — No epilepsy	'Epileptogenicity' in man — With epilepsy	Seizures in animals	References
Arterial PO$_2$	11–14 kPa (85–105 mm Hg)	<4kPa (30mm Hg)	+gm (++ts)	+pm	++	Luft & Noell, 1956; Passouant et al., 1967
		>300kPa	++		+++	Wood, 1972
Arterial PCO$_2$	4.7–6.0 kPa (35–45 mm Hg)	<4 kPa (30 mm Hg)	0	++ pm + gm	++	Lennox, Gibbs & Gibbs, 1936; Toman & Davis, 1949
		>32kPa (240mm Hg)	0		++	Woodbury et al., 1958
Glucose	2.5–10 mmol/l (45–180 mg/100 ml)	<1.2 mmol/l (22 mg/100 ml)	+++ my +gm	+		Poiré, 1969
		>40mmol/l (720mg/100ml)	+		+	Maccario, 1968
Sodium	132–142 mmol/l	<125mmol/l	+		+++	Rymer & Fishman, 1973; Funck-Brentano et al., 1960
		>150mmol/l	++	+		Morris-Jones, Houston & Evans, 1967
Calcium	2.25–2.65 mmol/l (9–10.6 mg/100 ml)	<1.7 mmol/l (6.5 mg/100 ml)	++my or ts +gm		+++	Frame & Carter, 1955; Corriol et al., 1969; Glaser & Levy, 1960
Magnesium	0.7–0.9 mmol/l (1.4–1.8 mEq/l)	<0.6 mmol/l (1.2 mEq/l)	+		++	Suter & Klingman, 1955; Kruse, Orent & McCollum, 1932
Urea	2.5–7.5 mmol/l	>25mmol/l	+		++	Prill, Quellhorst & Scheler, 1969; Zuckerman & Glaser, 1972
Ammonia	23–41 µmol/l	>500µmol/l	+		+ or ++	Hindfelt & Siesjö, 1971; Gastaut et al., 1968
Osmolarity	285–295 mosmol/kg	>340mosmol/kg	+		+	Kurtz et al., 1971; Singh, Gupta & Strobos, 1973

Values are given in SI Units (with traditional units in parenthesis).
'Epileptogenicity' is graded as:

+ = 0.33%
++ = 33–67%
+++ = 67–100%
pm = petit mal; gm = grand mal
f = focal seizure; my = myoclonus
hs = habitual pattern of seizure; ts = tonic spasm.

324 children with acute dehydration, an incidence of 15 per cent. However, a high proportion of the children with convulsions were pyrexial, and in two-thirds of the cases convulsions occurred during rehydration. The incidence of convulsions during rehydration can be reduced by infusing saline and calcium as well as glucose. Hypernatraemia (i.e. plasma sodium concentration above 150 mEq/l) usually accompanies dehydration, but it may also occur in the absence of dehydration, sometimes as a complication of focal cerebral disorders involving the hypothalamus or frontal lobe (Lascelles & Lewis, 1972). Seizures may accompany hypernatraemia. They are very apt to occur during its correction even when this is performed cautiously so as to avoid overhydration or hyponatraemia.

Hyperosmolal coma may occur when the combined osmotic effect of plasma electrolytes and glucose exceeds 340 mosmol/kg. It usually takes the form of non-ketotic diabetic coma, in which blood glucose concentrations of 33–66 mmol/l (600–1200 mg/100 ml) are found. Generalised or focal convulsions sometimes complicate such comas, indeed epilepsia partialis continua is the presenting symptom in 6 per cent of cases (Singh, Gupta & Strobos, 1973). That convulsions are a direct consequence of the hyperosmolality is suggested by the high incidence of convulsions in hyperosmolal coma induced in experimental animals by loading glucose, saline, mannitol or urea (Maccario, 1968; Zuckerman & Glaser, 1972).

In rats perfusion with hypertonic mannitol leads to focal opening of the blood-brain barrier associated with a marked increase in local glucose utilisation, which probably indicates focal seizure activity (Pappius et al., 1979) Osmotically-induced shrinkage of the brain can modify the blood-brain barrier and permit more ready access to the brain of substances normally partially or totally excluded. It can also cause subdural haemorrhages through venous ruptures (Luttrell, Finberg & Drawdy, 1959).

It has frequently been claimed that cellular dehydration or plasma hyperosmolality has a protective action against seizures. Clearly, in cases where generalised or focal cerebral oedema is a contributory cause of the seizures, cellular dehydration might well diminish the probability of seizure activity.

Several American authors had difficulty repeating the initial successful results with dehydration therapy described by Fay (1929, 1931). Teglbjaerg (1936) in two relatively large trials of epileptic in-patients found that a dehydrating diet reduced the incidence of generalised seizures in 68 per cent of men and 80 per cent of women. However, most of the patients were receiving barbiturates and dehydration might have been effective through an elevation of the plasma barbiturate content.

Experiments originally considered to show that cerebral dehydration protects rodents against chemically-induced convulsions (Defeudis & Elliott, 1967) should probably be explained by a different mechanism (Meldrum & Stephenson, 1975).

Hypocalcaemia

Ionised calcium 'stabilises' nerve and muscle cell membranes, preventing spontaneous or mechanically triggered oscillations in membrane potential. Movement of calcium ions across the nerve cell membrane plays an important role in synaptic transmission. Approximately half the 2.25–2.65 mmol calcium/litre serum is protein-bound, the proportion depending on the serum protein concentration. Tetany and seizures are not unusual when the ionised calcium concentration falls below 0.6 mmol/l (2.4 mg/100 ml). Such hypocalcaemia may be seen following parathyroidectomy, in rickets and neonatal tetany, in steatorrhoea or in the therapy of severe dehydration. Tetany and seizures due to hypocalcaemia respond promptly to the administration of calcium gluconate.

Hypomagnesaemia

In some cases of tetany and seizures the serum levels of both magnesium and calcium are low and a clear therapeutic response is obtained following the administration of magnesium sulphate. Such treatment raises plasma ionised calcium concentration (Zimmet, Breidahl & Nayler, 1968). Magnesium depletion has been described in the course of various nutritional and metabolic disorders and is sometimes associated with seizures (Suter & Klingman, 1955).

Hypoglycaemia

We can distinguish three types of seizure which occur during hypoglycaemia. Firstly, in a minority of patients with epilepsy mild to moderate hypoglycaemia sometimes precipitates their habitual type of seizure, which may therefore be an absence or a focal Jacksonian fit, a temporal lobe seizure or a generalised seizure. Fits triggered in this way occur well before the stage of hypoglycaemic coma is reached; usually only mild signs and symptoms of hypoglycaemia are present (increased pulse pressure, sweating, hunger).

The second type of seizure is seen most clearly in patients at or after the transition from precoma to coma in the course of profound insulin-induced hypoglycaemia (as in insulin therapy for schizophrenia, but also in brittle diabetics and the newborn). Initially there is irregular and fragmentary myoclonus, commonly involving the muscles of the face or of one limb. It becomes progressively more rhythmic, generalised and sustained, and is associated with rhythmic spikes and waves on the EEG. This generalised myoclonus may lead to a tonic seizure associated with the usual EEG picture of fast rhythmic activity of augmenting amplitude, followed by a phase of slow generalised myoclonus, and then post-ictal depression with an isoelectric EEG record. In a series of over 20 000 insulin comas in schizophrenic patients (Poiré, 1969), myoclonus was seen in 90 per cent of comas, but generalised tonic-clonic seizures in only 3 per cent. Although patients with tonic-clonic seizures were not known to suffer from epilepsy, most of them showed EEG signs of epilepsy during stroboscopic stimulation. Myoclonus, or seizures following myoclonus, can be aborted within seconds by the intravenous administration of glucose. The mechanism linking cerebral glucose metabolism with seizure activity is uncertain; brain energy state is unchanged at this stage in experimental hypoglycaemia (Lewis et al., 1974a) but the concentration of amino acids and tricarboxylic acid cycle intermediates is altered (Lewis et al., 1974b).

Thirdly, during profound hypoglycaemic coma tonic spasms sometimes appear while the EEG shows generalised high amplitude delta activity. This phenomenon occurs irrespective of any epileptic predisposition and is apparently a release phenomenon arising in subcortical centres and thus comparable to anoxic spasms. Experimentally it occurs when derangement of cerebral energy metabolism is demonstrable. The brain is undoubtedly at risk of hypoglycaemic brain damage.

Clinical significance Except in petit mal, hypoglycaemia is only rarely a cause of fits. There is experimental evidence that moderately severe hypoglycaemia makes some types of epileptic activity less likely (Naquet et al., 1970). This may explain the observation that patients with epilepsy are not more likely than non-epileptics to show generalised convulsions during therapeutic insulin coma.

The weak focal myoclonus that may be the only sign of sustained epileptic activity during profound hypoglycaemia in the newborn, is not always recognised as the urgent signal for therapy that it is. Hypoglycaemia in the absence of seizure activity can produce brain damage (Ingram, Stark & Blackburn, 1967; Meldrum, Horton & Brierley, 1971; Brierley, Brown & Meldrum, 1971a & b) and the presence of seizure activity exacerbates the crisis by augmenting the energy demand, but sometimes also leads to an increase in blood glucose (see p. 475).

Blood gases and pH

That a reduction in atmospheric pressure can induce seizures in animals was demonstrated by Boyle (1660). The use of over-breathing to reduce the partial pressure of carbon dioxide and trigger epileptic activity is routine in electroencephalography. However, seizure susceptibility is often unchanged during severe changes in plasma pH occurring during metabolic acidosis or alkalosis.

As with the disturbances of water, electrolytes and glucose, we must consider both the possibility of triggering seizures in patients with epilepsy and of convulsions in patients with no chronic neurological disorder.

Cerebral oxygenation

Moderate cerebral hypoxia may occasionally facilitate epileptic activity in patients with epilepsy, especially petit mal. With sudden severe hypoxia as in sudden atmospheric decompression a small number of susceptible subjects (not necessarily having epilepsy) show grand mal seizures at the moment of transition to unconsciousness. During profound unconsciousness when scalp EEG records indicate that cortical activity is suppressed, tonic spasms may be observed. Oxygen is essential for the energy metabolism that sustains epileptic activity. In experimental drug-induced convulsions the cortical epileptic discharges can be suppressed by systemic hypoxia (Gellhorn & Ballin, 1950; Caspers & Speckmann, 1972).

The seizures directly related to impaired cerebral oxygenation that provide the most important clinical problem are those which occur during the course of recovery. After severe cerebral anoxia, however caused (e.g. asphyxia, cardiac arrest, cerebral air embolism, vascular obstruction, head injury, atmospheric decompression) restoration of cerebral blood flow and oxygenation is commonly complicated by seizures. These first appear one to four hours after the anoxic episode at the time that cerebral oedema is also first evident and when ischaemic cell change becomes histologically apparent. Status epilepticus carries a particularly bad prognosis; it is common when the stress has led to brain damage and it may itself damage the brain. Lesions that result from cerebral hypoxia or ischaemia may become the focal source of seizures later in life (see below).

Hyperbaric oxygen Partial pressures of oxygen in the blood produced by breathing pure oxygen at 3–6 atmospheres pressure (300–600 kPa) induce generalised tonic-clonic seizures in animals and man. Although diving accidents of this kind are now rare, the situation is of considerable theoretical and experimental interest. Oxidation occurs in SH groups that play a critical role in certain enzymes (either in the active centre or by maintaining the tertiary structure of the enzyme). Among the enzymes affected is glutamic acid decarboxylase which synthesises γ-aminobutyric acid (GABA), a major inhibitory neurotransmitter within the brain. A correlation has been demons-

trated between the fall in brain GABA content and the onset of seizures during hyperbaric oxygenation (Wood, 1972).

Carbon dioxide

Changes in the partial pressure of carbon dioxide in the arterial blood dramatically modify cerebral blood flow (reviewed by Purves, 1972). The reduction in $PaCO_2$ following hyperventilation reduces cerebral blood flow to 40 per cent of normal; breathing air containing 7 per cent of carbon dioxide doubles cerebral blood flow (Kety & Schmidt, 1948). The reduced availability of oxygen to the brain during hyperventilation can be demonstrated by polarographic measurements (Cooper, 1974). This cerebral hypoxia is thought to be partially responsible for the diffuse frontal slow waves and for the activation of epileptic activity (especially of bursts of spikes and waves associated with motor signs of petit mal) seen during hyperventilation. There is also evidence from clinical and experimental studies that the $PaCO_2$ modifies cerebral activity and excitability independently of any effect on cerebral oxygenation (Wyke, 1963). Thus, when the activating effect of hyperventilation on EEG signs of epilepsy was first reported (Lennox, Gibbs & Gibbs, 1936) suppression of such signs by raised respiratory carbon dioxide was also described. Experimentally the threshold for electroconvulsive shock rises in animals breathing carbon dioxide mixtures containing up to 15 per cent CO_2. However, very high concentrations of CO_2 (30–40 per cent) may facilitate convulsions and coma (Brodie & Woodbury, 1958; Woodbury *et al.*, 1958). Convulsions induced in monkeys or small mammals can be suppressed by the inhalation of 9–40 per cent CO_2 (Meyer, Gotoh & Tazaki, 1961; Caspers & Speckmann, 1972). In rats inhalation of 25–35 per cent CO_2 induces seizures (Woodbury *et al.*, 1958; Withrow, 1972).

Activation of epilepsy by respiratory alkalosis and inhibition by acidosis is probably related to changes in intracellular pH. Acidosis favours the synthesis of the inhibitory transmitter GABA; alkalosis favours its further metabolism by GABA-transaminase (Meldrum, 1975b).

Temperature

Febrile convulsions (seizures associated with pyrexia, believed to result from infection not involving the brain) are common in infants and young children, affecting 29–72 per 1000 (Lennox-Buchthal, 1973) The incidence is maximal between 9 and 20 months of age. There is a strong genetic element controlling susceptibility to febrile convulsions. In general, the severity of the pyrexia, not the nature of the illness, determines the occurrence of a fit; in 75 per cent of children the temperature is above 39.2 °C (Herlitz, 1941). Hyperthermia induced artificially in the absence of infection in rats, rabbits and kittens leads to generalised convulsions (Millichap, 1968).

The clinical features of febrile convulsions are described in Chapter 3. Seizures are usually isolated or brief. Prolonged or repetitive seizures are sometimes followed by behavioural disorders, neurological deficits and later established epilepsy (Ounsted, Lindsay & Norman, 1966; Aicardi & Chevrie, 1970; Lennox-Buchthal, 1973). This commonly takes the form of temporal lobe seizures, but petit mal is seen in 10–20 per cent of children developing epilepsy after febrile convulsions (Lennox-Buchthal, 1973). The occurrence of a unilateral Ammon's horn sclerosis as a result of prolonged febrile convulsions is discussed below (page 479).

A separate phenomenon is that of pyrexia secondary to seizures. This may arise as a result of the increased energy consumption by the brain, heart and muscles during the seizure, or because of disturbance in the temperature regulating mechanisms. It is difficult to evaluate these phenomena clinically, but the effect of sustained myoclonic activity is evident in experimental studies (Meldrum & Horton, 1973a; Meldrum, Vigouroux & Brierley, 1973). The raised cerebral temperature increases the probability of sustained seizure activity, and by raising cerebral metabolic rate (Nemoto & Frankel, 1970) increases the likelihood of epileptic brain damage (Meldrum & Brierley, 1973).

Sleep

The complex and important relationships between seizures and the sleeping-waking cycle have been reviewed by Janz (1974). Four phenomena can be differentiated:

a. The traditional observation that in many patients seizures occur predominantly at a particular time of day was analysed quantitatively by Langdon-Down and Brain (1929), and a synthesis of more recent studies is given by Janz (1974). Adults with major seizures can be classified as *random epilepsies*, not contingent upon the phase of the sleeping-waking cycle (23 per cent); *sleep epilepsies*, generalised, often originating in the temporal lobe, occurring predominantly just after falling asleep or in the early morning sleep period (44 per cent); and *waking epilepsies*, grand mal seizures occurring after waking or during the late afternoon (33 per cent). Over the years some waking epilepsies and some sleep epilepsies become random epilepsies. The majority of random epilepsies are symptomatic whereas only about 10 per cent of waking epilepsies are. The shift towards sleeping and random epilepsies during the course of the illness probably reflects the development or progression of brain damage related to the seizures (see Section 4 of this chapter).

b. Inter-ictal EEG signs of epilepsy appear preferentially in certain phases of sleep and wakefulness; the distribution between the phases is different according to the kind of seizure (this is discussed in Ch. 5). Not surprisingly, background slowing and dysrhythmias are commoner during waking in waking epilepsy than in sleeping epilepsy (Christian, 1960).

c. Abnormalities of sleep patterns are found in patients with epilepsy. An excess of the deeper phases of sleep is found in patients with sleep epilepsy, particularly in patients with generalised seizures that originate in the temporal lobe. An excess of light sleep occurs in patients with waking epilepsy (Jovanovic, 1967).

d. Perhaps related to the above, sleep deprivation increases the likelihood of certain types of seizure, especially waking epilepsy (grand mal) and pykno-epilepsy (very frequent absences). Sleep deprivation can be used as a specific precipitant for diagnostic purposes in the latter two syndromes (Christian, 1960; Bennett, 1963). Deprivation of rapid-eye movement sleep in rats or cats leads to lowering of the electroshock seizure threshold (Owen & Bliss, 1970; Cohen, Thomas & Dement, 1970).

In the pathophysiology of epilepsy the phenomena relating to the sleep-waking cycle have a two-fold significance. Firstly, they indicate an important biological difference between sleeping and waking epilepsies. Secondly, they challenge the research worker to identify the physiological features of sleep and wakefulness that are responsible for the changes in seizure susceptibility. These may include endocrine or metabolic factors as numerous hormones show circadian rhythms, most notably cortisol (Dixon, Booth & Butler, 1974) but also growth hormone (Sassin *et al.*, 1969). There are changes in body temperature, water and electrolyte excretion. Wakefulness and the different phases of sleep are associated with altered activity in the serotoninergic and catecholaminergic systems that ascend from the brain stem (Jouvet, 1972) and there is much experimental evidence linking changes in seizure threshold to changes in activity in aminergic systems (Meldrum, Anlezark & Trimble, 1975). Changes in background EEG rhythms are associated with altered seizure susceptibility and incidence of EEG signs of epilepsy.

Nutrition

Food intake can modify the tendency to seizures either because of a specific deficiency (e.g. vitamin B_6, magnesium) or an excess (e.g. water, lipids).

An intake of lipids that is very high relative to protein and carbohydrate forms the basis of the 'ketogenic diet' which has some therapeutic action in childhood epilepsy (Wilder, 1921; Huttenlocher, Wilbourn & Signore, 1971; Livingston, 1972). The mechanism of this is not understood; the metabolic acidosis itself is probably not antiepileptic; there may be some degree of cerebral dehydration involved. It has recently been shown that the brain in young animals and in starving people is capable of utilising ketone bodies (acetoacetate and β-hydroxybutyrate) for energy metabolism (Owen *et al.*, 1967; Hawkins, Williamson & Krebs 1971) and this metabolic shift might change seizure susceptibility.

The plasma concentrations of acetoacetate and β-hydroxybutyrate rise in rats fed on a high fat diet. The cerebral sodium content also increases and the electroconvulsive shock threshold is elevated (Appleton & DeVivo, 1974).

The possibility is currently being explored that the concentration of inhibitory transmitter substances in the brain can be raised by dietary treatments. GABA (γ-aminobutyric acid) and taurine are putative central inhibitory neurotransmitter compounds (Curtis & Johnston, 1974), but experimental studies indicate that they enter the brain only to a very limited extent following systemic administration.

However, it is possible to raise the cerebral concentration of serotonin and noradrenaline by administration of the precursors L-tryptophan and tyrosine. The effect on seizures in man of changes in brain amine content has yet to be defined (Chadivich *et al.*, 1978).

Dietary deficiency of vitamin B_6 can give rise to seizures in infants fed deficient milk preparations (Coursin, 1954). Vitamin B_6 forms pyridoxal phosphate, a coenzyme essential for numerous cerebral enzymes, including glutamic acid decarboxylase, which synthesises the inhibitory transmitter GABA (reviewed by Meldrum, 1975b).

Endocrine changes

As already indicated hormones influencing plasma osmolarity or content of glucose or ionised calcium can modify seizure susceptibility. Hormones with other primary actions that have been shown clinically and experimentally to influence the course of fits include glucocorticoids, thyroxine, oestrogen and progesterone. Pituitary dysfunction, because of its influence on the other systems, may also be a factor affecting seizure susceptibility. A review of experimental studies on the role of hormones is given by Timiras (1969).

Adrenal steroids and ACTH

Mineralocorticoids have an anti-epileptic action in several test systems. An anaesthetic-like action of desoxycorticosterone acetate was described by Selye (1941), and it was subsequently reported to give therapeutic benefit to some patients with grand mal seizures (Aird & Gordan, 1951). Woodbury and numerous colleagues (reviewed

Woodbury, 1958) demonstrated a raised threshold for electroshock seizures in animals treated with desoxycorticosterone.

Glucocorticoids (cortisol and related 11-oxosteroids) when given to rats increase brain excitability and lower the electroshock seizure threshold (Woodbury & Vernadakis, 1966). An acute seizure-enhancing effect of the administration of cortisone has been demonstrated in baboons with photosensitive epilepsy (Ehlers & Killam, 1979). That a similar effect may operate in man is suggested by the occurrence of convulsions in Cushing's syndrome (Starr, 1952). The mechanism is unknown. The turnover of adrenaline in the rat brain is increased by dexamethasone treatment (Moore & Phillipson, 1975) but this is not likely to increase seizure susceptibility.

The synthesis of glycerolphosphate dehydrogenase, a cerebral enzyme concerned in both phospholipid synthesis and the regulation of carbohydrate metabolism is controlled by cortisol or other glucocorticoids (De Vellis & Inglish, 1968).

Animal experimental studies with the anterior pituitary hormone, ACTH, corticotrophin have given varied results.

In man, although petit mal may be benefited by ACTH or steroids (Miribel & Poirier, 1961), the syndrome that responds most decisively to ACTH or adrenal steroids is hypsarrhythmia, infantile spasms (Sorel & Dusaucy-Bauloye, 1958; Jeavons & Bower, 1964). This effect is probably unrelated to any electrolyte shifts produced by mineralocorticoids. Commonly the brain shows diffuse pathological changes in hypsarrhythmia and the adrenal steroids may act directly on the pathological process. Alternatively they could be modifying the rate of synthesis of cortical enzymes such as glycerolphosphate dehydrogenase. Prompt treatment may diminish the intellectual deterioration which accompanies hypsarrhythmia (Jeavons, Bower & Dimitrakoudi, 1973).

Thyroid disorders

Both myxoedema and thyrotoxicosis can be complicated by epilepsy and return to a euthyroid state may cure the epilepsy (Evans, 1960; Skanse & Nyman, 1956). Acute thyrotoxicosis not uncommonly (perhaps 9 per cent of cases) presents with seizures (Jabbari & Huott, 1980). There is animal experimental evidence for a therapeutic action of thyroxine administration in photosensitive epilepsy (Serbanescu & Balzamo, 1974) and for increased cerebral excitability (reduced threshold for electroshock seizures) following thyroxine (Timiras & Woodbury, 1956). Sound-induced seizures in DBA/2 mice are associated with high serum thyroxine levels and can be suppressed by antithyroid drugs (Seyfried, Glaser & Yu, 1979). The mechanism of these effects is not clear but thyroxine modifies ionic distribution as well as altering metabolic rate.

Oestrogens, progesterone and testosterone

Oestrogens have been shown to be epileptogenic by systemic administration to rats and rabbits, by local cortical application in animals, and by systemic injection in man (Woolley & Timiras, 1962a & b; Marcus, Watson & Goldman, 1966; Marcus, 1972). This is probably because oestrogens reduce glutamic acid decarboxylase activity and hence produce a fall in GABA synthesis in the brain (Wallis & Luttge, 1980).

Progesterone can, like desoxycorticosterone, act as a general anaesthetic (Selye, 1941) and has been shown to have a protective action against convulsions in two animal test systems (Costa & Bonnycastle, 1952; Woolley & Timiras, 1962a).

These effects of sex hormones may explain the phenomenon of catamenial epilepsy. Among 50 women in a hospital for epileptics, analysing 33 468 fits in 939 patient-years, Laidlaw (1956) found that the fits occurred in relation to the phase of the menstrual cycle in 72 per cent. There was a reduction in fit frequency during the luteal phase and an exacerbation the day before menstruation and subsequently up to the sixth day of the cycle. In rats the phase of the oestrus cycle influences both the threshold to electroshock seizures (Woolley & Timiras, 1962b) and the local seizure susceptibility within the limbic system (Timiras, 1969). High doses of testosterone and related androgens lower seizure threshold in animals (Selye 1941; Heuser & Eidelberg, 1961).

Hormonal effects

As well as the potential mechanisms of action already mentioned, endocrine changes may modify seizure susceptibility by altering sleep patterns, or by acting on protein synthesis in the brain. Specifically, a decrease in adrenal steroids is associated with reduction in sleep phases III and IV (Gillin et al., 1974) and an increase in sleep stages III and IV is associated with hyperthyroidism (Dunleavy et al., 1974). Adrenal steroids can induce enzymes involved in the metabolism of neurotransmitters (Moore & Phillipson, 1975).

Endogenous toxic states

Endogenously derived toxic compounds may accumulate in relation to liver failure, renal failure or certain inborn errors of metabolism. The mechanism leading to seizures in these situations may not, however, be different from some already discussed under previous headings.

Liver failure

Hepatic coma is not usually associated with seizures in spite of the high blood ammonia levels. Comparable blood and brain ammonia levels induced acutely by the administration of ammonium salts may be associated with generalised seizures (Gastaut et al., 1968).

Renal failure

Seizures are relatively common in the various syndromes of renal insufficiency (chronic renal failure following glomerulonephritis, eclampsia of pregnancy etc). They are usually primarily generalised grand mal seizures, and in most cases there is evidence of some antecedent cerebral pathology. Correlative EEG and metabolic studies have been described by Prill, Quellhorst and Scheler (1969). These authors and Gastaut et al. (1971), considered that the severity of uraemia was not a critical determinant of seizure onset. Urea infusions given to cats produce initially facial then generalised myoclonus, associated with reticular spikes, and ultimately status epilepticus (Zuckerman &

Glaser, 1972). Hypocalcaemia and overhydration probably play a role in some cases of renal failure. A common finding is a primary metabolic acidosis leading to a compensatory reduction in arterial pCO_2 (which increases cerebral excitability) and, when corrected, a reduction in ionised calcium.

During dialysis, grand mal seizures and sometimes status epilepticus occur because of the disequilibrium syndrome. Brain and plasma share hyperosmolarity (urea, creatinine, electrolytes) during renal failure and rapid correction of the plasma composition may lead to intracellular overhydration. This is usually prevented by dialysis with a hyperosmolar fluid.

Inborn errors of metabolism

Seizures are a major feature in a number of these syndromes, and in some the accumulation of an unusual metabolite appears to be responsible. Commonest among the aminoacidurias is phenylketonuria in which the inability to hydroxylate phenylalanine to tyrosine leads to the accumulation of metabolites of phenylalanine not usually detectable in blood or urine. It is not certain whether it is deficiency of the compounds normally derived from tyrosine (such as the catecholamine transmitter substances) or the excess of abnormal metabolites (such as phenyllactic acid which is known to inhibit the enzyme synthesising GABA) that is primarily responsible for the seizure tendency. Other inborn errors associated with seizures are described by Crome and Stern (1972).

Exogenous toxins

It is not possible here even to classify the vast range of toxic substances that can produce seizures. A restricted list is given in Table 11.5. Of great theoretical interest are the compounds that compete with inhibitory transmitter substances for receptor sites. The best established experimentally is the competition between strychnine, or related alkaloids, and glycine for sites on spinal motoneurones. Two toxins of plant origin, bicuculline and picrotoxin block inhibition due to GABA in many parts of the brain including the

Table 11.5 Exogenous toxins producing seizures

	Source or 'category'	Action	Convulsant dose (mg/kg) IV in animals	Type of seizures	References
Strychnine / *Brucine*	Plant alkaloids	Block inhibition due to glycine	2–3	'Spinal', tonic extension	Everett & Richards, 1944; Pylkko & Woodbury, 1961
Picrotoxin / *Bicuculline*	Plant toxins	Block GABA-mediated inhibition	1–2; 0.2–0.6	Sustained Generalised	Meldrum & Horton, 1974; Meldrum & Horton, 1971
Benzyl-penicillin / *Pentylene tetrazol*	Antibiotic; Synthetic	—	400 000 units/kg; 20–80	'Myoclonic'; Tonic-clonic	Gloor & Testa, 1974; Goodman et al., 1953; Chusid & Kopeloff, 1969
Isoniazid / *Thiosemicarbazide* / *Allylglycine* / *3-mercaptopropionic acid* / *4-deoxypyridoxine*	Tuberculostatic hydrazides; Amino acid; Pyridoxine analogue	Inhibits GABA synthesis	100–150; 7–10; 200–400; 25–70; 100–150	Tonic-clonic	Meldrum et al., 1970; Meldrum et al., 1970; Horton & Meldrum, 1973; Horton & Meldrum, 1973; Meldrum & Horton, 1971
Fluorothyl / *Bemegride* / *Thujone* / *Catechol*	Volatile ether; Analeptic; Absinthe	—; —; —	(Vapour); 5–9; 5–7; 8	Myoclonus	Krantz, 1963; Chusid & Kopeloff, 1969; Opper, 1939; Angel & Lemon, 1974
Imipramine / *Amitriptyline* / *Desmethylimipramine*	Tricyclic antidepressants	—	25–50	Clonic-tonic	Wallach et al., 1969; Trimble, 1977
Cocaine / *Lignocaine*	Local anaesthetic		50; 7–14	Limbic seizures; Tonic-clonic	Eidelberg, Lesse & Gault, 1963; Munson & Wagman, 1969; Wagman, DeJong & Prince, 1968; Chusid, Kopeloff & Kopeloff, 1956
Diphenhydramine	Antihistamine		20	Tonic-clonic	Folbergrova et al., 1969
Methionine dl-sulphoximine	Agenized flour	Alters amino acid metabolism	300	Long latency Repetitive	Folbergrova, 1975
Homocysteine	Amino acid	Alters ammonia metabolism	700–1400 i.p.; 700–1400 i.p.		
Dieldrin / *Lindane*	Chlorinated hydrocarbon insecticides		6; 12	Tonic or tonic-clonic	St Omer, 1971
Di-isopropylfluorophosphate / *Tetra-ethylpyrophosphate* / *parathion*	Organophosphorous insecticides	Irreversible inhibitors of cholinesterase	2 i.m.; 1–2 i.m.; 6 i.m.		Grob, 1963; Stone, 1957
Fluoroacetate / *iodoacetate*	Metabolic poisons	Inhibits aconitase; Inhibits glycolysis at phosphoglyceraldehyde dehydrogenase	2; 180 i.p.	Tonic-clonic	Peters, 1963; Samson & Dahl, 1957
Cyanide		Inhibits cytochrome oxidase	2–4	Myoclonus	Wheatley, Lipton & Ward, 1947
2-deoxyglucose		Impairs glycolysis	1000–30 000		Meldrum & Horton, 1973a

cerebral cortex, and benzyl penicillin probably acts in the same way (Curtis & Johnston, 1974). A vast range of enzyme inhibitors produce generalised seizures. These include anticholinesterases such as 'nerve gases' and organophosphorus insecticides, and pyridoxal phosphate antagonists that inhibit glutamic acid decarboxylase (Meldrum, 1975b). Compounds that interfere with cerebral energy metabolism (such as cyanide or 2-deoxyglucose) also produce seizures (Meldrum & Horton, 1973a).

Clinically, the most significant exogenous toxins are drug overdoses, particularly of drugs used in psychiatry, including the tricyclic antidepressants (Wallach *et al.*, 1969). Many drugs given therapeutically, not necessarily in an overdose, can precipitate seizures. Thus generalised fits occurring during status asthmaticus are commonly due to aminophylline (Holmgren & Kraeplin, 1953; Schwartz & Scott, 1974). Seizures due to the administration of penicillin directly into the CSF have long been recognised, but high doses of penicillin given intravenously can also be epileptogenic.

Seizures due to withdrawal of barbiturates or drugs of addiction may take the form of status epilepticus. Such seizures may follow the emergency hospitalisation of a patient whose intake of addictive drugs is not known to the medical staff.

Summary

When a patient suffers his first fit, it is necessary for the physician to consider the possible role of systemic factors. He must distinguish between factors that might be precipitants in a subject likely to have further seizures and factors which are causal, and which, if prevented, would remove the likelihood of further fits. The distinction is not absolute. Seizures triggered by sleep deprivation, overbreathing or overhydration or mild hypoglycaemia, are often the fore-runners of seizures occurring without evident contributory factors, whereas a drug overdose or severe hypoglycaemia will provoke fits in subjects who are unlikely to experience seizures in the absence of such severe insults.

2. EPILEPTOGENESIS AT THE CELLULAR LEVEL

The gross cerebral pathology giving rise to epilepsy is described in Part One of this chapter. It is natural to look for common cellular mechanisms that may provide links between different primary lesions and epilepsy (Table 11.6). Several features in the clinical history (e.g. latent period and family history of epilepsy) are common to focal or generalised seizures following a tumour, cerebral abscess or penetrating head injury. This suggests that all three pathologies induce similar critical cellular changes. Similarly, one looks for a single cellular or focal neuropathology that is common to the diffuse disorders producing myoclonic syndromes. Infantile spasms, or West's syndrome (Jeavons & Bower, 1964) also provide a very distinctive clinical syndrome suggesting there must be specific changes in the brain that can follow numerous primary pathologies.

Table 11.6 'Unifying' hypotheses of the basic pathology of epilepsy

---

a. Meningocerebral cicatrix
   Vascular abnormality leading to focal ischaemia
b. Blood or iron as epileptogens
c. Cytological mechanisms
   1. Loss of inhibitory interneurones
   2. 'Deafferentation'
      (i) Supersensitivity
      (ii) Loss of dendritic spines
   3. 'Overloading' of excitatory synapses
   4. Proliferation of fibrous astrocytes
      (? inadequate regulation of extracellular potassium concentration)
d. Enzymic defects
   1. Synthesis of inhibitory transmitter substances
   2. Sodium-potassium activated ATPase deficiency

Meningocerebral cicatrix

Penfield & Jasper (1954) have claimed that scar tissue vascularised by both cerebral and meningeal arteries plays a critical role in focal epileptogenesis following purulent meningitis, cerebral abscess and penetrating brain injury. They suggested that the vessels of extracerebral origin might show abnormal or inappropriate vasoconstrictive responses, that, within and around the scar, capillaries were abnormal or deficient, and that, with progressive shrinkage of the scar, the surrounding capillaries could become obstructed thus creating new ischaemic lesions. Following Penfield's advocacy many neurosurgeons selected operative procedures designed to minimize the formation of meningo-cerebral anastomotic vessels. Proof that this practice has significantly altered . the post-operative incidence of epilepsy is lacking.

The cellular changes around a scar include loss of neurones and proliferation of glial elements – initially microglial (rod) cells, subsequently reactive astrocytes and fat-laden phagocytes. Such changes are not confined to meningo-cerebral scars but are found in almost all the disorders discussed in this section.

Blood, haemoglobin and iron

Experimental studies provide strong evidence for blood or iron as factors causing focal epileptogenesis. This indicates a probable mechanism for induction of post-traumatic epilepsy, but could also be relevant to seizures after cerebrovascular accidents, vascular malformations or invasive tumours.

Haemolysed blood applied to the cat cortex was initially shown to produce spike discharges (Levitt, Wilson & Wilkins, 1971). Subsequently the injection of ferrous or ferric chloride into the cortex was shown to have both an acute and a chronic epileptogenic effect (Wilmore et al., 1978). Studies of the time course of the development of focal discharges after blood or haemoglobin application suggest that release of iron during the course of haemoglobin breakdown could be the critical step in epileptogenesis (Rosen & Frumin, 1979; Hammond et al., 1980).

Selective loss of neurones

The normal functioning of the nervous system depends on the interplay of inhibitory and excitatory activity (see Eccles, 1964, 1969; Tebecis, 1974). Although the action of some transmitter substances varies according to the specificity of the post-synaptic receptor site, some compounds, such as glycine and gamma-aminobutyric acid (GABA) have an important inhibitory action almost everywhere they are found in the vertebrate brain or spinal cord (Curtis & Johnston,

1974). Reduction in the efficiency of such inhibitory transmission leads to seizures in many experimental situations (Meldrum, 1975b). Thus, if ischaemic or other pathological processes can produce a destruction of neurones that is at least partially selective for inhibitory interneurones, their epileptogenicity can be explained. The selective vulnerability to hypoxia of different areas of grey matter and of different neuronal populations within those areas is well established (Schadé & McMenemy, 1963; Brierley, Meldrum & Brown, 1973), and there is substantial evidence for a relatively greater involvement of neurones that can be identified on biochemical or physiological criteria as inhibitory interneurones.

Arterial occlusion producing spinal cord ischaemia for one hour can be shown by chemical measurements to destroy with partial selectiveness neurones containing the inhibitory transmitter glycine (Werman, Davidoff & Aprison, 1968). This lesion produces spasticity and sometimes myoclonic limb jerks but not epileptic seizures.

In the cerebellum, hypoxia, arterial hypotension or hypoglycaemia selectively destroy the Purkinje cells and basket cells (Brierley et al., 1973); these neurones are inhibitory in function and contain high concentrations of GABA (Curtis & Johnston, 1974; Tebecis, 1974). Other regions showing selective vulnerability (third and fifth layers of neocortex; hippocampus, basal ganglia and thalamus) have a relatively high content of GABA and of glutamic acid decarboxylase, the enzyme synthesising GABA (Lowe, Robins & Eyerman, 1958; Fahn & Côté, 1968; Perry et al., 1971). In the motor cortex the large pyramidal neurones which initiate motor activity are relatively insensitive whereas the small inter-neurones are highly sensitive to hypoxia or ischaemia. Biochemical measurements in brain samples from epileptic patients have not given decisive results (Van Gelder, Sherwin & Rasmussen, 1972; Perry et al., 1972) although an apparent fall in cortical GABA content has been described (Van Gelder et al., 1972). Using an immunocytochemical method that stains terminals containing glutamic acid decarboxylase, Ribak et al. (1979) have demonstrated a reduction in the number of such inhibitory endings in the cortex adjacent to an epileptic focus (induced in monkeys by alumina gel).

It thus appears appropriate to seek biochemical changes related to GABA in the brains of patients having developed epilepsy after known episodes of cardiac arrest or asphyxia. The action myoclonus in such patients is known to respond therapeutically to oral or intravenous administration of 5-hydroxytryptophan, the precursor of serotonin (Lhermitte, Marteau & Degos, 1972). Experimental studies with lesions or biochemical manipulations suggest that there is an interaction of GABA and serotonin mediated transmission in the brain stem and basal ganglia (Hassler, 1972) so that a therapeutic action of 5-hydroxytryptophan is not incompatible with a deficit in availability of GABA being responsible for the myoclonus. However, it does raise the possibility that a selective destruction of the serotoninergic systems originating in the brain stem might be responsible for the syndrome. Changes in seizures and myoclonic responses following manipulation of serotoninergic transmission have been extensively described in animal models of epilepsy (Meldrum et al., 1975). Additionally, measurement of the concentration of serotonin and of 5-hydroxyindoleacetic acid (a metabolite of serotonin) in the cerebrospinal fluid of children and adults with epilepsy has suggested that the synthesis and turnover of serotonin are reduced (Papeschi et al., 1972; Shaywitz, Cohen & Bowers, 1975).

A very marked regional deficiency in the concentration of glutamic acid decarboxylase and of GABA has been demonstrated in the basal ganglia of brains from patients with Huntington's chorea (Perry, Hansen & Kloster, 1973; Bird & Iversen, 1974). Generalised seizures occur in up to 50 per cent of cases of Huntington's chorea. A small but significant fall in the GABA content of occipital cortex was measured (Perry et al., 1973). The selective loss of GABA-containing neurones in the basal ganglia probably contributes to the chorea, and the smaller changes elsewhere in the brain may contribute to the occasional generalised seizures.

Studies on the amino acid content of focal areas of epileptogenesis in man and experimental animals have indicated that the concentration of taurine is sometimes lowered (Van Gelder et al., 1972; Van Gelder & Courtois, 1972; Craig & Hartman, 1973). Physiological evidence that taurine is an inhibitory transmitter substance in the cortex is less definitive for taurine than for GABA and glycine (Curtis & Johnston, 1974) but it does have an inhibitory action when applied iontophoretically.

Deafferentation and loss of dendritic spines

Physiological and morphological studies suggest that there are mechanisms by which neuronal loss could favour epileptogenesis without being selective for inhibitory neurones. Thus, when neocortex which has been 'deafferented' by undercutting (Halpern, 1972) is given a brief electrical stimulus it shows a sustained after-discharge which has many properties resembling those of a focal cortical discharge. The mechanism of this change is not understood, but the time course of its development suggests that a process occurs which resembles the denervation supersensitivity that can be demonstrated in skeletal muscle or autonomic effector organs when peripheral nerves are cut (Sharpless, 1969).

Morphological studies employing Golgi impregnations (Globus & Scheibel, 1966) reveal a structural correlate of deafferentation of cortical neurones, namely, a loss of dendritic spines. These are specialised sub-synaptic structures lying along apical and other dendrites.

A loss of dendritic spines has been seen in temporal lobectomy specimens removed from patients undergoing neurosurgery for temporal lobe epilepsy (Scheibel & Scheibel, 1973; Scheibel, Crandall & Scheibel, 1974). The hippocampal pyramidal neurones and dentate granular cells also showed shrinkage or simplification of the apical dendritic system and the appearance of nodular deformities on the dendritic extremities. The Scheibels interpret these changes as indicative of a progressive process. Such appearances in Golgi preparations are not confined to the hippocampus and temporal lobe epilepsy. They were, in fact, first described in epileptic neocortex by DeMoor in 1898. They can also be found in and around epileptogenic foci created in the neocortex of monkeys by the application of alumina cream (Westrum, White & Ward, 1965; Ward, 1969). Electrophysiological studies of the behaviour of single neurones in such experimental foci have led to the identification of so-called *epileptic neurones* which show firing activity of an abnormal pattern with repetitive bursts. The abnormal neurones identified in Golgi preparations may provide the structural correlate of these *epileptic neurones* (Ward, 1969).

The primary loss of neurones can occur in brain areas anatomically distant from the area in which the deafferentation and loss of dendritic spines occurs provided that there are sufficient afferent connections. Such a mechanism operating on subcortical centres could lead to seizures of generalised onset following focal cortical lesions.

Demoor (1898) also described a loss of dendritic spines and nodular degeneration in patients with mental retardation and tertiary syphilis. This observation has recently been repeated in mentally retarded children (Purpura, 1974). Such pathological synaptic morphology could be the basis of abnormal excitability in a variety of generalised cerebral degenerative disorders.

The age at which a particular lesion occurs influences the subsequent risk of epilepsy. Experimental studies involving deafferentation suggest a possible mechanism. A few months after the stereotaxic destruction of specific neuronal systems providing afferents to the septal nuclei in young rats, new synapses may be formed that appear anatomically and physiologically inappropriate (Raisman, 1969). Such pathological regeneration, if it occurs in man, could contribute to seizures of delayed onset following brain injury.

Overloading of excitatory synapses

In two experimental models of epilepsy an abnormal pattern of electrical activity apparently contributes to the creation of an epileptic focus. In the *mirror focus* phenomenon (Wilder, 1969) a primary focus created by a destructive neocortical lesion (e.g. from cobalt, penicillin, freezing or alumina cream) gives rise to a secondary focus in the contralateral hemisphere. In the *kindling* phenomenon repeated *subthreshold* focal electrical stimulation of the amygdala or other nuclei modifies the threshold for seizure induction so that ultimately spontaneous seizures may occur (Goddard, McIntyre & Leech, 1969; Wada, Sato & Corcoran, 1974). In neither of these phenomena can

degenerative phenomena be excluded (Westmoreland, Hanna & Bass, 1972). However, electron-micrographic studies of projected foci in the rat and measurements of the localisation and density of synaptic vesicles in somatosensory cortex suggest that there is a concentration of such vesicles close to the presynaptic membrane (Fischer, 1973) which would have the effect of enhancing transmission.

Proliferation of fibrous astrocytes

One cytological change that is almost universally identifiable in the brains of patients dying with epilepsy is the proliferation of fibrous astrocytes. Such gliosis is seen in and around all chronic focal lesions and it occurs incidentally in a large number of the diffuse *degenerative* pathologies that may lead to epilepsy. It also occurs patchily or diffusely in the most superficial layer of the cortex (sub-pial or marginal gliosis) as first described by Chaslin (1891). Gliosis is also seen in the hippocampus, amygdala and temporal gyrus in *mesial temporal sclerosis* the most characteristic pathology of temporal lobe epilepsy (see Section 4 below). Fibrous or reactive astrocytes differ in morphology and staining reactions from normal astrocytes. The latter have end-feet that terminate in relation to capillaries or to neurones. They are believed to transport metabolic substrates and other materials to and from neurones, and to regulate the composition of extracellular fluid (Trachtenberg & Pollen, 1970; Henn, Haljamae & Hamberger, 1972). Changes in the ionic composition of extracellular fluid modify the excitability of neurones – in particular an increase in the extracellular content of potassium can induce epileptic discharges, especially in the hippocampus (Zuckerman & Glaser, 1970).

These observations have led to the hypothesis that faulty regulation of extracellular potassium concentration by reactive astrocytes could be responsible for epileptogenesis in gliotic lesions (Pollen & Trachtenberg, 1970). However, direct measurements of intracellular potentials and membrane properties in reactive glial cells in a focus created by injury show high resting potentials and a high *glial safety factor*, and thus fail to confirm the presence of impaired regulation of extracellular potassium concentration in gliosis (Grossman & Rosman, 1971; Glötzner, 1973).

Enzyme defects

It is possible that the final common path by which various pathological processes create the tendency to seizures is to be found not at the level of the cell but at that of the protein molecule. The activity of particular enzymes could be impaired by diverse mechanisms, ranging from genetically-determined deficiency to lack of a co-factor or trace metal or the presence of toxic factors.

It is natural to consider first the enzymes involved in the synthesis of transmitter substances. Early reports suggested that there was an alteration in the metabolism of acetylcholine in the epileptogenic focus (Tower & Elliott, 1952). More recently interest has centred on the metabolism of glycine, GABA, taurine, serotonin, dopamine and noradrenaline, as these compounds are believed to act as inhibitory transmitters. A reduction in the brain GABA content due to dietary deficiency of pyridoxine (required as the co-factor of glutamate decarboxylase) is associated with seizures (Coursin, 1964). There is also a rare genetically determined epileptic syndrome (pyridoxine dependency) that responds dramatically to sustained administration of high doses of vitamin B6 (Hunt et al., 1954; Tower, 1969). A reduction in the concentration of GABA in CSF of patients with epilepsy (receiving drug therapy) has been reported (Wood et al., 1979).

The possible involvement of taurine in epilepsy is discussed by Barbeau and Donaldson (1974). In some animal experimental models of epilepsy depletion of brain amines (as by reserpine, or by inhibition of tyrosine hydroxylase) is associated with a lowered threshold for seizures (Meldrum et al., 1975). Measurements of amines and their metabolites in cerebrospinal fluid (mentioned above under *loss of inhibitory interneurones*) suggest that there may be an abnormality of amine metabolism in epilepsy – however, enzyme studies are lacking.

The possibility also exists of an abnormality in receptor molecules (for inhibitory transmitters) or in the mechanism of inactivation of excitatory transmitters. Here also appropriate data are not available.

The intracellular-extracellular concentration ratios of sodium and potassium critically determine resting, action and synaptic potentials (Eccles, 1964) and the maintenance of these ratios depends on a magnesium dependent, sodium-potassium activated ATPase found in neuronal and glial membranes. Evidence of various kinds suggests that abnormalities in the functioning of this enzyme may be important in seizures. Compounds known to inhibit the membrane ATPase, such as ouabain, when applied locally to the cortex or hippocampus induce seizure discharges (Bignami & Palladini, 1966; Baldy-Moulinier, Arias & Passouant, 1973). A diminished cerebral ATPase activity was described by Abood & Gerard (1955) in the genetically-determined syndrome of audiogenic seizures found in DBA 2 mice. Recently it has been shown that this decrease is specifically in the sodium-potassium activated ATPase and that it shows an age dependence that corresponds to the age dependence of the seizure susceptibility (Hertz et al., 1974).

Epilepsy occurs incidentally in numerous inborn errors of metabolism, such as phenylketonuria, maple syrup urine disease and homocystinuria. Genetic studies of epilepsy (reviewed by Metrakos & Metrakos, 1974) show a familial incidence of *centrencephalic epilepsy* (with three per second spike and wave discharges on the EEG) that is consistent with autosomal dominant transmission. Simple febrile convulsions show a similar pattern of transmission but with an even more pronounced age-dependence in the expression of the disorder (Lennox-Buchthal, 1973). Non-epileptic subjects may show spikes or spikes and waves on the EEG in response to stroboscopic stimulation. This syndrome is age and sex dependent and also shows a familial incidence consistent with autosomal dominant transmission. As these three syndromes are non-fatal and do not require neurosurgical intervention studies of the underlying biochemical abnormalities are lacking.

3. PHYSIOLOGICAL CHANGES ASSOCIATED WITH SEIZURES

Changes that are secondary to seizures include (1) metabolic changes in the brain that are a direct

Table 11.7 Physiological changes in generalised seizures (tonic-clonic or status epilepticus)

Transient or early (0–30 minutes)	'Late' (after 30 minutes)
Arterial hypertension	Arterial hypotension
Cerebral venous pressure (CVP) raised	CVP raised or normal
Arterial PO_2 low or normal	Arterial PO_2 low or normal
Arterial PCO_2 high	Arterial PCO_2 normal
CV PO_2 normal (or low or high)	CV PO_2 normal or low
CV PCO_2 high	CV PCO_2 normal (or high)
Cerebral blood flow (CBF) increased	CBF increased normal or decreased
Hyperglycaemia	Normoglycaemia, hypoglycaemia
Hyperkalaemia	Hyperkalaemia
Hemoconcentration	
Lactacidosis	Hyperpyrexia (secondary)

result of the abnormal activity and (2) systemic changes. The latter are summarised in Table 11.7. They arise in two ways. Firstly, there are physiological and metabolic changes secondary to the motor component of the seizure (i.e. changes in blood gases and pH, a rise in body temperature). Their dependence on the motor activity can be demonstrated in experiments employing peripheral muscular paralysis (by curare-like agents) and artificial respiration. Secondly, there are autonomic and endocrine changes which, although they may be influenced by the motor activity, appear to arise primarily through the direct effect of neuronal discharges impinging on the hypothalamus and other controlling centres.

The significance of the physiological changes accompanying seizures is best understood when they are considered in relation to data summarised elsewhere in this chapter. Thus, some changes will tend to prolong seizure activity, whereas others will facilitate its termination (Section 1). Epileptic brain damage (described in Section 4) is the result of the interaction of systemic factors and local metabolic changes, and may be diminished or prevented if these are appropriately manipulated. A more obscure problem is the refractory period, or increase in seizure threshold that follows a generalised seizure. This is presumably the result of metabolic or physiological changes that accompany and follow the seizure.

Cardiovascular changes

a. Blood pressure

A dramatic increase in systolic and diastolic blood pressure is usually seen at the onset of a generalised tonic seizure, whether it occurs spontaneously or is induced by electroshock or drugs in man or animals (White et al., 1961; Magnaes & Nornes, 1974; Meldrum & Horton, 1973b; Meyer, Gotoh & Favale, 1966; Posner, Plum & Poznak, 1969; Plum, Posner & Troy, 1968). There is initially a marked tachycardia but sometimes when the pressure reaches its peak the heart slows. With brief seizures the mean arterial pressure remains elevated throughout the seizure and returns to normal in the first few minutes of the post-ictal period.

The arterial hypertension and tachycardia are the results of enhanced sympathetic activity. They can be abolished by ganglionic blockade (or a spinal section in animals).

Several factors interact to produce the phenomena associated with more prolonged seizures. Comparison of the blood pressure changes in experimental primates with and without peripheral muscular paralysis (Meldrum & Horton, 1973b; Meldrum, Vigouroux & Brierley, 1973) shows that the initial rise in blood pressure is similar. However, in the paralysed, ventilated animal, this increase is transient and the blood pressure returns to normal levels and remains relatively stable even when cerebral seizure activity continues for many hours. In the non-paralysed animal the initial rise in blood pressure is sometimes more sustained (up to 20–30 minutes) indicating that the excessive motor activity is raising the blood pressure perhaps partially through the improved venous return, but more probably reflexly through changes in blood gases and pH acting on the chemoreceptors in the aortic arch and carotid body. Late in status epilepticus, both experimentally and in man, there is commonly a drop in the mean arterial blood pressure below normal, and this arterial hypotension may persist in the post-ictal period (Meldrum & Horton, 1973b). The peripheral vascular resistance drops in muscle, skin and brain and the heart is unable to sustain the increase in output necessary to maintain mean arterial pressure.

The massive sympathetic and vagal discharges reaching the heart early in a seizure are probably responsible for a significant proportion of unexpected deaths in young epileptic patients (Hirsch & Martin, 1971). Ventricular tachycardia, conduction block or asystole apparently result from the sudden excessive autonomic bombardment early in the seizure.

Another consequence of excessive motor activity that affects the heart is hyperkalaemia. This initially produces characteristic disturbances of the cardiac rhythm and electrocardiogram. If untreated the blood pressure may suddenly collapse and cardiac arrest and death follow.

b. Cerebral blood flow

A marked increase in cerebral blood flow (up to three or even five times normal) occurs within one to two seconds of the onset of generalised seizure activity, and a comparable focal increase in blood flow accompanies focal seizures (Penfield, Von Santha & Cipriani, 1939; White et al., 1961; Meyer, Gotoh & Favale, 1966; Ingvar, 1973; Magnaes & Nornes, 1974; Meldrum & Nilsson, 1976). This focal or general increase in blood flow arises as much or more from a decrease in cerebral vascular resistance as from the increase in arterial pressure. It is still seen in the absence of any change in arterial pressure.

The decrease in cerebral vascular resistance is attributed by many authors (Brodersen et al., 1973; Kety, 1964; Meyer et al., 1966; Plum & Duffy, 1975) to a direct effect on the vessels of a local increase in PCO_2 and lactic acid or hydrogen ion concentration. It is evident that this explanation is not quantitatively adequate. The increase in blood flow is often more than sufficient to compensate for the increased metabolic demand of the brain during the seizure. Thus the oxygen tension

in the cerebral venous blood often rises during seizures (Plum et al., 1968; Meldrum & Horton, 1973b), and the rise in cerebral venous PCO_2 is often small and slow. Yet the cerebral blood flow increases at, or slightly before, the onset of the tonic seizure (Plum et al., 1968). The possibility of direct neuronally mediated vasodilatation deserves consideration. The existence of a cerebral vasodilator mechanism that runs in the VIIth cranial nerve, can be reflexly activated, and is more powerful than the sympathetic vasoconstrictor mechanism demonstrated by Ponte and Purves (1974). Thus the early dilatation of the peripheral resistance vessels in the brain could be a consequence of the autonomic discharge triggered by the seizure. Rises in arterial PCO_2 might, at a later stage, sustain the cerebral vasodilatation through an action on the normal reflex mechanism, i.e. chemoreceptors in the aortic arch and carotid sinus, vagal afferents and outflow via the VIIth nerve (James, 1975).

Clearly, the normal mechanisms for autoregulation that ensure a uniform cerebral blood flow in spite of variations in cerebral perfusion pressure cease to be effective during a generalised seizure. The presence of dilated cerebral vessels in the presence of a normal or reduced arterial pressure can lead to focally or generally inadequate cerebral perfusion.

c. Cerebral venous pressure

During a tonic seizure the cerebral venous pressure rises dramatically; values above 10 kPa (1000 mm H_2O) are seen in experimental animals (Hendley, Spudis & de la Torre, 1965; Meldrum & Horton, 1973b). The increase in muscle tone and intrathoracic pressure makes an important contribution to this. Thus transient rises accompany whole body jerks during a myoclonic seizure. That the cerebral vasodilatation is also an important factor is shown by the reduced but still substantial rise in cerebral venous pressure seen in paralysed, artificially-ventilated animals.

In paralysed, ventilated volunteers receiving pentylenetetrazol, cerebrospinal fluid pressure rose on average by 5.5 kPa (549 mm H_2O) during the seizure (White et al., 1961).

The small haemorrhages occurring subpially

and elsewhere (see Section 4) may result from the excessive venous pressure.

d. Haemoconcentration

Early in generalised seizures haemoconcentration as shown by a rise in haemotocrit or haemoglobin content of the blood of about 5 per cent is seen. This is part of the autonomic response. Release of splenic reserves of red cells may play a part, but a sudden increase in the rate of fluid secretion is probably more important.

Respiratory changes

The effects of seizures on respiration are complex and vary with the type of seizure and the phase of the individual fit. Tachypnoea and/or a transient apnoea are nearly always seen in relation to a tonic seizure. A change in respiratory rate or pattern is sometimes the most notable motor sign in a petit mal attack.

There are three mechanisms by which cerebral seizure activity leads to respiratory embarrassment:

1. Brain stem centres regulating respiration may be directly influenced by the cerebral seizure activity. There is evidence for this not only in most types of generalised seizure, but also in some partial seizures such as temporal lobe epilepsy.

2. Abnormal motor activity may directly impair normal mechanical respiration, and additionally by greatly increasing whole body oxygen consumption and carbon dioxide production may overload the respiratory exchange capacity of the lungs.

3. Peripheral autonomic components of the seizure may have a dramatic influence on gas exchange in the lungs. This is the explanation for the drop in arterial PO_2 and rise in PCO_2 seen during drug-induced seizures in paralysed, artificially-ventilated animals (Meldrum et al., 1973). The excessive glandular out-pouring, not only of the salivary glands, but more importantly of the tracheo-bronchial secretions, is the most evident factor and gives rise to the classical foaming at the mouth. However, parasympathetically-mediated bronchial constriction and haemodynamic factors leading to less efficient alveolar gas exchange may also be important. In experimental animals haemorrhagic consolidation of the lungs has been described after pentylenetetrazol or high-pressure oxygen convulsions (Bean, Zee & Thom, 1966; Harris & Van den Brenk, 1968).

The net effect of these three factors during generalised tonic or clonic seizures can be a severe impairment of respiratory function. It is usually only transient; a severe degree of hypoxia rarely lasts more than two or three minutes.

Autonomic events

Reference has been made to the autonomic components of seizures in the discussion of cardiovascular and respiratory changes. A massive activation of both the sympathetic and parasympathetic systems occurs in generalised tonic seizures (see Table 11.8). One sign of this is the rise in serum dopamine-β-hydroxylase activity that is seen one to five minutes after electroconvulsive shock in man and experimental animals (Lamprecht et al., 1974). Some of the autonomic manifestations are reflexly operated, but it is likely that local spread of abnormal activity to diencephalic and brain stem centres is the critical factor in most cases. It is through the connections of the amygdala and hippocampus with hypothalamic and other centres controlling autonomic function that temporal lobe seizures provoke autonomic changes. However, the greater emphasis on autonomic changes in clinical descriptions of temporal lobe seizures compared with generalised seizures should not lead to the conclusion that such changes are greater or occur more frequently in temporal lobe seizures. The reverse is the case,

Table 11.8 Autonomic components of seizures

Sympathetic	Parasympathetic
Tachycardia	Bradycardia
Arterial hypertension	Cerebral vasodilation
Skin vasoconstriction	Bronchial constriction
	Exocrine secretion
Mydriasis	Miosis
Galvanic skin response	Bladder detrusor contraction
Sweating	
Adrenaline release	
Glucagon release	

but subjectively, autonomic symptoms are more important in temporal lobe epilepsy because they occur while consciousness is preserved. Events corresponding to the epigastric aura appear variable, but oesophageal peristalses and inhibition of gastric contraction have been recorded (Van Buren & Ajmone-Marsan, 1960). In petit mal, changes in heart rate and a galvanic skin response are sometimes seen about two seconds after the clinical signs of an attack (Johnson & Davidoff, 1964). They are probably the result of awareness of an attack.

The autonomic events may pursue a characteristic sequence of parasympathetic and sympathetic components, as in some cases of temporal lobe epilepsy, some pure tonic seizures and some experimental models (Van Buren & Ajmone-Marsan, 1960; Huot, Radouco-Thomas & Radouco-Thomas, 1973). In some seizures they may be the only or the predominant signs. However, in most generalised tonic-clonic seizures, a variety of sympathetic and parasympathetic responses occur more or less simultaneously, and where the two systems act in opposition it appears that the most powerful system predominates. Sympathetic activity produces tachycardia, arterial hypertension, mydriasis, a falling skin resistance, sweating and adrenaline release. Parasympathetic activity produces exocrine secretion (sialorrhoea, tracheo-bronchial and gastrointestinal secretion), bladder contraction, miosis (which sometimes precedes or follows mydriasis) and cerebrovascular vasodilatation.

Cerebral arterioles receive an adrenergic innervation via the superior cervical ganglion, which has a vasoconstrictor action (James, 1975; Owman & Edvinsson, 1978). This system is potently activated during seizures (Mueller, Heistad & Marcus, 1979). It produces a marked reduction in blood volume in the face at the onset of seizures (Ancri et al., 1979). Denervation experiments indicate that sympathetic activity diminishes the increase in cerebral cortical blood flow during seizures by about 10 per cent (Mueller et al., 1979).

The parasympathetic vasodilator mechanism is poorly understood in anatomical and pharmacological terms. Cholinergic nerves have been identified in extracerebral vessels, but not significantly in the vertebral artery system (Owman & Edvinsson, 1978). There is immunocytochemical evidence for a peptidergic, vasodilator system, utilising vasoactive intestinal peptide (Owman & Edvinsson, 1978). This has a higher density in the forebrain than in the hindbrain. Prostaglandins may also play a role.

There is no experimental evidence that allows a quantitative assessment of the relative importance of parasympathetically induced vasodilation compared with that of local factors (PCO_2, pH, $[K^+]$) in the increased cerebral blood flow during seizures.

Endocrine events

There is little quantitative data about the endocrine consequences of seizures although there is much indirect evidence that such consequences are complex and highly important.

Staining the hypothalamus of cats and baboons to reveal neurosecretory granules has indicated an activation of neurosecretion following pentylenetetrazol seizures in cats (Seite, Picard & Luciani, 1964) or photically-induced myoclonus in *Papio papio* (Luciani et al., 1969; Riche, 1973).

Hyperglycaemia in man follows generalised seizures induced by electroshock or pentylenetetrazol (Georgi & Strauss, 1938) and an increased concentration of adrenaline in the blood has been demonstrated (Weil-Malherbe, 1955).

A comparable hyperglycaemia is observed in a wide variety of animal test systems (Feldman, Cortell & Gellhorn, 1940; Kessler & Gellhorn, 1941; Belton, Etheridge & Millichap, 1965; Naquet et al., 1970; Meldrum & Horton, 1973b; Chapman, Meldrum & Siesjö, 1977). Cutting the splanchnic nerves or removing adrenal glands (Feldman, Cortell & Gellhorn, 1940) markedly reduces the hyperglycaemia in rats and rabbits suggesting adrenaline release is mainly responsible. In primates a release of glucagon from the pancreas also contributes (Meldrum et al., 1979).

The peak blood glucose can be moderately high (over 200 mg/100 ml) 15–30 minutes after seizure onset (Meldrum & Horton, 1973b). In man and experimental primates the hyperglycaemia is sometimes followed by hypoglycaemia, which is primarily due to the action of insulin but increased glucose consumption may play a part (Meldrum & Horton, 1973b; Meldrum et al., 1979).

In adrenalectomised rats pentylenetetrazol seizures evoke a hypoglycaemia which can be prevented by prior vagotomy (Feldman, Cortell & Gellhorn, 1940). Presumably, parasympathetic activity leads to insulin release. In bicuculline-induced seizures in baboons, the major increase in plasma insulin occurs in response to the early increase in blood glucose (Meldrum et al., 1979).

Adrenocortical activation also occurs in generalised seizures, with a marked rise in plasma cortisol (Meldrum et al., 1979).

Plasma prolactin levels increase a few minutes after ECT in depressed patients (Öhman et al., 1976) or following spontaneous or drug-induced seizures (Trimble, 1978; Meldrum et al., 1979).

Metabolic changes in the brain

Changes in the brain occur during seizures (a) as a consequence of the other physiological changes described in this section and (b) as a direct result of the abnormal neuronal activity. Such changes may influence the continuation, or cessation, of seizure activity. They are also a critical factor in the inception of ischaemic neuronal damage (see next Section).

a. Cerebral metabolic rate

The usual procedure for estimating cerebral metabolic rate is to determine the cerebral blood flow (in ml blood/100 g brain/min) and the arterial and cerebral venous oxygen content and from these values to derive the oxygen consumption, CMR O_2. It is remarkably constant in man at 3.3 ml O_2/100 g brain/min (147 μmol/100 g/min). Quantitative studies in man of the change in metabolic rate during seizures are not available.

In monkeys, Schmidt, Kety and Pennes (1945) found cerebral metabolic rate was increased by 0–80 per cent during picrotoxin or pentylenetetrazol seizures. A 60 per cent increase in CMR O_2 was reported for dogs receiving pentylenetetrazol (Plum et al., 1968). Gilboe and Betz (1973) found no increase in CMR O_2 for the isolated canine brain during pentylenetetrazol seizures. For vari-

ous technical reasons these three studies have probably underestimated the maximum increases occurring during seizures. Recently, a sustained 2–3 fold increase in cerebral oxygen consumption has been demonstrated (Chapman, Meldrum & Siesjö, 1975; Meldrum & Nilsson, 1976) throughout 2 hours of status epilepticus (induced in rats by bicuculline).

By measuring the rate of change in the concentration of energy metabolites (see below) in mouse brain in the first few seconds of seizures induced by electroshock or pentylenetetrazol, King et al. (1967) and Collins, Posner and Plum (1970) were able to show a three- to four-fold increase in the rate of energy utilisation.

b. Energy metabolites

The energy derived from the oxidation of glucose and required for the active transport of sodium and potassium is stored in the form of adenosine triphosphate and creatine phosphate. The concentrations of these high-energy phosphate compounds in the brain are remarkably stable in normal physiological circumstances. They decline progressively in total anoxia or ischaemia. They decline as fast or faster in the first few seconds of a generalised seizure in mice (Sacktor, Wilson & Tiekert, 1966; King et al., 1967). If the mice are paralysed and ventilated with air the decline in high-energy phosphates is smaller, and if they are ventilated on oxygen it is absent (Collins, Posner & Plum, 1970). Thus, in the presence of adequate oxygenation the brain is able to increase the rate of oxidative metabolism to compensate for the increased energy requirement.

When the oxygen supply is insufficient the rate of glycolysis is speeded up but lactate accumulates instead of being further metabolised. This and the increase in PCO_2 produce a marked acid shift in the intracellular pH.

The most marked changes in concentration of energy metabolites occur within the first 30 seconds of generalised seizures. After 60–90 seconds stable levels are reached and even if seizure activity continues, further changes in creatine phosphate, adenosine triphosphate and glucose concentrations occur extremely slowly (Sacktor et al., 1966; King et al., 1970; Chapman et al., 1977). It is probable that in prolonged seizures or status epilepticus further falls in concentration occur but exact data are not available.

c. Other metabolic changes

Changes in the cerebral concentrations of a wide variety of other compounds can be detected during or after seizures. Ionic shifts between extracellular and intracellular compartments are a direct consequence of the neuronal activity. Evidence from arteriovenous differences in man suggests that the brain gains sodium and loses potassium during generalised seizures (Meyer et al., 1966). An increased brain sodium content has been observed in rats following electroconvulsive shock (Woodbury, 1955). By utilising ion-specific micro-electrodes it is possible to measure the extracellular concentration of potassium in the cerebral cortex (Prince, Lux & Neher, 1973). During seizure activity or local after-discharges potassium concentration rises to 8–10 mmol/1 but falls during prolonged activity, and shows an underswing to below normal values post-ictally (Lux, 1974; Sypert & Ward, 1974). The membrane ATPase is apparently activated by the change in ionic distribution. The onset of discharges showed no relation to extracellular potassium concentration in acute penicillin foci (Futamachi, Mutani & Prince, 1974), but a threshold elevation of potassium concentration is required for propagated seizure activity (Sypert & Ward, 1974).

Brain ammonia concentration is raised following convulsions induced by electroshock, pentylenetetrazol (Richter & Dawson, 1948) or bicuculline. Complex changes in the concentrations of amino acids and tricarboxylic acid cycle intermediates include increases in alanine and glutamine and decreases in glutamate and aspartate concentration (Chapman, Meldrum & Siesjö, 1977).

A variety of effects on amine metabolism follow electroshock (reviewed by Essman, 1973). Thus there is a sustained increase in the rate of synthesis of noradrenaline in the rat brain (Kety et al., 1967). The activity of the enzyme tyrosine hydroxylase is enhanced (Musacchio et al., 1969). Electroshock also increases the forebrain concentration of serotonin in the rat, rabbit and other animals (Garattini, Kato & Valzelli, 1960; Bertaccini, 1959; Essman, 1973).

Changes in brain amine metabolism could be responsible for a wide range of post-ictal phenomena, such as the resistance to fits (Herberg & Watkins, 1966), alterations in sleep, feeding behaviour and mood.

4. PATHOLOGICAL CHANGES IN BRAIN RESULTING FROM SEIZURES

The apparently clear, logical distinction between (a) cerebral pathology which is a direct or indirect consequence of fits, (b) cerebral pathology which is a cause of fits, and (c) pathology which occurs coincidentally in the brains of epileptic patients, is not easily made in practice (Meldrum, 1975a). Some of the problems posed by the differentiation between (b) and (c) are presented in Section 3 above. The difficulty in distinguishing group (a) is that pathology arising as a direct consequence of seizures is of an anoxic-ischaemic kind and may therefore be indistinguishable from pathology arising from, say, perinatal asphyxia or later cardiac or cerebrovascular disorders. This problem is most severe for chronic lesions in the brains of patients who have had epilepsy for the greater part of their lives. It is less severe in patients dying a few hours or days after an episode of status epilepticus and showing only acute lesions in the brain.

Physiological changes during seizures as causes of epileptic brain damage

Evidently lesions found in the brains of patients dying after status epilepticus or chronic epilepsy may be a cause of the seizures or indeed be unrelated to the seizures. However, in the case of ischaemic or hypoxic brain damage of the type described under Status Epilepticus there are reasons for thinking that the lesions are the result of events occurring during or directly after the episode of status. In individual cases viral infections may contribute directly to the pathology, as suggested by Wallace & Zealley (1970). However, the similarity of the lesions in the presence of diverse primary factors (such as abrupt drug withdrawal, a frontal tumour or an acute febrile dehydrating illness) implicates events directly related to the prolonged seizure. The similarity of the cerebral lesions after status epilepticus, after chronic epilepsy and after known episodes of cerebral hypoxia or ischaemia (e.g. cardiac arrest) led Spielmeyer (1927) and Scholz (1951) to conclude that the epileptic brain damage was the result of cerebral hypoxia or ischaemia occurring immediately before, during, or after the seizure. Because *vasospasm* or *angiospasm* was then believed to play a role in the initiation of seizures, they thought it likely that arterial constriction might also be important in the aetiology of brain damage. This hypothesis was abandoned when it became clear from studies in man and animals that vasodilatation was the predominant vascular reaction during seizures. Lindenberg (1955) drew attention to the occurrence of ischaemic lesions in the inferior and medial aspect of the temporal lobe, resulting from compression of branches of the posterior cerebral artery at the tentorial edge, in patients with severe elevation of supratentorial pressure, as in acute intracranial haemorrhage. Scholz (1959) and Gastaut *et al.* (1960) subsequently suggested that cerebral oedema resulting from a prolonged seizure could lead to a similar compression of cerebral arteries and secondary ischaemic lesions. The moderate or severe systemic hypoxia occurring during the tonic phase of a generalised seizure is commonly presumed to lead to cerebral hypoxia. Similarly, post-ictal electrical silence or depression has been widely (but erroneously) supposed to be a manifestation of cerebral hypoxia developing during the course of a seizure. It has not been possible in man to demonstrate quantitative correlations between physiological changes during seizures and subsequent brain damage.

Animal experiments have led to some conclusions about the causes of epileptic brain damage (Meldrum, 1978). In adolescent baboons physiological changes can be closely monitored during status epilepticus induced with bicuculline, and then correlated with the focal incidence and severity of ischaemic neuronal changes in the brain (Meldrum & Horton, 1973b, Meldrum & Brierley, 1973). The total duration of seizure activity is important in determining brain damage;

less than 90 minutes of sustained epileptic activity did not cause brain damage in the baboons. Several other animal studies have also shown an absence of pathological changes after up to 90 minutes of seizure activity (Schwartz, Broggi & Pappas, 1970; Brennan, Petito & Porro, 1972). The possible greater vulnerability of very young animals has not yet been investigated. Among systemic changes the events occurring after 30 minutes of seizure activity correlate most clearly with brain damage. These include arterial hypotension, hyperpyrexia secondary to the motor activity and hypoglycaemia (see Table 11.7). These changes are themselves capable of producing ischaemic neuronal changes under experimental conditions. Cerebral metabolic rate is greatly increased during a seizure; hyperpyrexia further increases it (Nemoto & Frankel, 1970) and the effects of hypoglycaemia or oligaemia would be additive in producing a failure of cerebral energy metabolism. Secondary systemic changes are much reduced in paralysed, ventilated animals, thus permitting an evaluation of their importance (Meldrum, Vigouroux & Brierley, 1973). Their contributory role is shown by the longer duration of seizure activity required to produce neocortical, thalamic or hippocampal damage in paralysed animals. Hyperpyrexia and arterial hypotension appear to be significant causes of cerebellar damage (which fails to occur in baboons when these changes are absent).

Marked transient rises in cerebral venous pressure are probably responsible for the small subarachnoid haemorrhages seen after experimental seizures (Krushinsky, 1962, Meldrum & Horton, 1973). More sustained rises in cerebral venous pressure, focal venous obstruction or venous thrombosis could contribute to the development of focal or more generalised cerebral oedema (Gastaut *et al.*, 1960; McLardy, 1974). Experimentally, epileptic brain damage can occur when oedema is not macroscopically evident. Radiological studies in children show that focal or hemispheric oedema can be severe a few days after generalised or unilateral status epilepticus (Isler, 1971). Evidence has been presented showing that such oedema can cause herniation of the medial aspect of the temporal lobe (parahippocampal gyrus) over the tentorial edge, compressing the

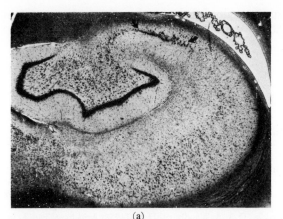

(a)

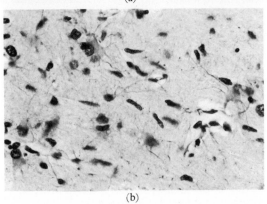

(b)

Fig. 11.20 Microscopical appearance of right hippocampus in an adolescent baboon, whose brain was fixed by perfusion three weeks after an eight hour-long sequence of 34 brief seizures induced by the intravenous injection of allylglycine. (For experimental details see Meldrum et al., 1974.) (a) The h2 zone lies between the arrows. A loss of pyramidal neurones is evident in the Sommer sector, and is most severe at its junction with the h2 zone. There is also a loss of neurones in the h3 Sommer sector, showing loss of neurones and dense gliosis, comprising microglia and fibrous (reactive) astrocytes. (Paraffin section stained with phosphotungstic acid haematoxylin, magnification × 600.)

branches of the anterior choroidal and posterior cerebral arteries and producing a secondary cerebral ischaemia (Gastaut et al., 1960).

Experimentally pathological changes confined to or predominating in the hippocampus can follow a sequence of brief generalised seizures, not associated with severe systemic changes (Meldrum, Horton & Brierley, 1974), or sustained seizures involving only the limbic system (Baldy-Moulinier, Arias & Passouant, 1973). Such lesions, examined one to six weeks after a seizure sequence (see Fig. 11.20), show a striking resem-

blance to lesions found in the hippocampi of patients with chronic epilepsy. The marked loss of neurones within the Sommer sector tends to be unilateral, whereas the changes in the endfolium occur symmetrically, thus conforming to the pattern described by Margerison and Corsellis (1966). A microglial response with neuronophagia is evident after one week; subsequently the proliferation of fibrous astrocytes predominates.

A swelling of astrocytic end-feet within the vulnerable areas of the hippocampus can be identified during seizure activity (De Robertis, Alberici & De Lores Arnaiz, 1969; Meldrum et al., 1973). Presumably the uptake function of astrocytes is overloaded by the excessive local release of potassium and amino acids. The changes within the astrocytes will impair the exchange and transport of metabolites for neurones and will also lead to an impaired capillary circulation. Thus intraneuronal metabolism will be unable to meet the energy demand of seizure activity, and ischaemic neuronal changes will follow.

Conclusions

In considering the pathophysiology of epilepsy we are constantly seeking, with variable success, to separate causes and effects. It is not difficult to demonstrate that changes in blood gases, plasma glucose, electrolyte or hormone levels can influence the occurrence of seizures, or that seizures themselves can modify all these factors. However, we do not know what factors lead to the spontaneous termination of a seizure, or cause a prolonged seizure to become self sustaining. In a high proportion of patients we cannot even give an account of the seizures that explains why the patient is epileptic and why seizures occur at some times and not at others. The same problems occur in relation to the pathological changes in the brain. We can describe the diverse lesions within the brain that may cause epilepsy, but why one such lesion is epileptogenic and another similar one is not remains unknown.

Undoubtedly, more could be done on the basis of existing knowledge to reduce the incidence of epilepsy in Europe and North America, and vastly more could be achieved in the tropical countries. However, additional basic knowledge is required before we can specify the medical and social measures that will reduce the incidence of epilepsy

substantially below its current prevalence of 1 in 200 in the Western world.

REFERENCES

Abood, L.G. & Gerard, R.W. (1955) A phosphorylation defect in the brains of mice susceptible to audiogenic seizure. In *Biochemistry of the Developing Nervous System*, p. 467. New York: Academic Press.

Aicardi, J. & Chevrie, J.J. (1970) Convulsive *status epilepticus* in infants and children. A study of 239 cases. *Epilepsia*, **11**, 187.

Aird, R.B. & Gordan, G.S. (1951) Anticonvulsive properties of desoxycorticosterone. *Journal of the American Medical Association*, **145**, 715.

Ancri, D., Naquet, R., Basset, J.Y., Menini, C., Lonchampt, M.F., Meldrum, B.S. & Stutzmann, J.M. (1979) Correlation entre volume sanguin regional et crise d'épilepsie chez le *Papio Papio*. *Bull. Académie Sciences (Paris)*, **3**, 343.

Angel, A. & Lemon, R.N. (1974) An experimental model of sensory myoclonus produced by 1,2-dihydroxybenzene in the anaesthetized rat. In Harris, P. & Mawdsley, C. (eds) *Epilepsy*, p. 37. Edinburgh: Churchill Livingstone.

Appleton, D.B. & DeVivo, D.C. (1974) An animal model for the ketogenic diet. *Epilepsia* (Amsterdam) **15**, 211.

Baldy-Moulinier, M., Arias, L.P. & Passouant, P. (1973) Hippocampal epilepsy produced by ouabain. *European Neurology*, **9**, 333.

Barbeau, A. & Donaldson, J. (1974) Zinc, taurine and epilepsy. *Archives of Neurology* (Chicago) **30**, 52.

Bean, J.W., Zee, D. & Thom, B. (1966) Pulmonary changes with convulsions induced by drugs and oxygen at high pressure. *Journal of Applied Physiology*, **21**, 865.

Belton, N.R., Etheridge, J.E. & Millichap, J.G. (1965) Effects of convulsions and anticonvulsants on blood sugar in rabbits. *Epilepsia* (Amsterdam), **6**, 243.

Bennett, D.R. (1963) Sleep deprivation and major motor seizures. *Neurology* (Minneapolis), **13**, 953.

Bertaccini, G. (1959) Effect of convulsant treatment on the 5-hydroxytryptamine content of brain and other tissues of the rat. *Journal of Neurochemistry*, **4**, 217.

Bignami, A. & Palladini, G. (1966) Experimentally produced cerebral *status spongiosus* and continuous pseudorhythmic electroencephalographic discharges with a membrane-ATPase inhibitor in the rat. *Nature*, **209**, 413.

Bird, E.D. & Iversen, L.L. (1974) Huntington's Chorea. Post-mortem measurement of glutamic acid decarboxylase, choline acetyltransferase and dopamine in basal ganglia. *Brain*, **97**, 457.

Boyle, R. (1660) New experiments: Physico-mechanical. Touching the spring of air and its effects. Oxford: H. Hall.

Brennan, R.W., Petito, C.K. & Porro, R.S. (1972) Single seizures cause no ultrastructural change in brain. *Brain Research*, **45**, 574.

Brierley, J.B. (1971) The neuropathological sequelae of profound hypoxia. In Brierley, J.B. & Meldrum, B.S. (eds) *Brain Hypoxia*, p. 147. London: William Heinemann Medical Books.

Brierley, J.B., Brown, A.W. & Meldrum, B.S. (1971a) The neuropathology of insulin-induced hypoglycaemia in the primate: topography and cellular nature. In Brierley, J.B. & Meldrum, B.S. (eds) *Brain Hypoxia. Clinics in Developmental Medicine*, No. 39/40, p. 225. London: William Heinemann Medical Books.

Brierley, J.B., Brown, A.W. & Meldrum, B.S. (1971b) The nature and time course of the neuronal alterations resulting from oligaemia and hypoglycaemia in the brain of Macaca mulatta. *Brain Research*, **25**, 483.

Brierley, J.B., Meldrum, B.S. & Brown, A.W. (1973) The threshold and neuropathology of cerebral 'naoxic-ischaemic' cell change. *Archives of Neurology* (Chicago) **29**, 367.

Brodersen, P., Paulson, O.B., Bolwig, T.G., Rogon, Z.E., Rafaelsen, O.J. & Lassen, N.A. (1973) On the mechanism of cerebral hyperaemia in electrically-induced epileptic seizures in man. *Stroke*, **4**, 359.

Brodie, D.A. & Woodbury, D.M. (1958) Acid-base changes in brain and blood of rats exposed to high concentrations of carbon dioxide. *American Journal of Physiology*, **192**, 91.

Caspers, H. & Speckmann, E.J. (1972) Cerebral pO_2, pCO_2 and pH: Changes during convulsive activity and their significance for spontaneous arrest of seizures. *Epilepsia* (Amsterdam) **13**, 699.

Chadwick, D., Trimble, M., Jenner, P., Driver, M.V., & Reynolds, E.H. (1978) Manipulation of cerebral monoamines in the treatment of human epilepsy: A pilot study. *Epilepsia*, **19**, 3.

Chapman, A.G., Meldrum, B.S. & Siesjö, B.K. (1975) Cerebral blood flow and cerebral metabolic rate during prolonged epileptic seizures in rats. *Journal of Physiology* (London) **254**, 61.

Chapman, A.G., Meldrum, B.S., & Siesjö, B.K. (1977) Cerebral metabolic changes during prolonged epileptic seizures in rats. *Journal of Neurochemistry*, **28**, 1025.

Chaslin, P. (1891) Contribution à l'étude de la sclérose cérébrale. *Archives Med. Exp. Anat. Pathol.*, **3**, 305.

Christian, W. (1960) Biolektrische Charakteristik tages-periodisch gebundener Verlaufsformen epileptischer Erkrankungen. *Deutsch Zeit Nervenheilk*, **181**, 413.

Chusid, J.G. & Kopeloff, L.M. (1969) Use of chronic irritative foci in laboratory evaluation of antiepileptic drugs. *Epilepsia* (Amsterdam) **10**, 239.

Chusid, J.G., Kopeloff, L.M. & Kopeloff, N. (1956) Convulsant action of antihistamines in monkeys. *Journal of Applied Physiology*, **9**, 271.

Cohen, H., Thomas, J. & Dement, W.C. (1970) Sleep Stages, REM deprivation and electroconvulsive threshold in the cat. *Brain Research*, **19**, 317.

Collins, R.C., Posner, J.B. & Plum, F. (1970) Cerebral energy metabolism during electroshock seizures in mice. *American Journal of Physiology*, **218**, 943.

Cooper, R. (1974) Influence on the EEG of certain physiological states and other parameters. In Rémond, A. (ed.) *Handbook of Electroencephalography and Clinical Neurophysiology*, Part B, **7**, 1.

Corriol, J., Papy, J-J., Rhoner, J.J. & Joanny, P. (1969) Electroclinical correlations established during tetanic manifestations induced by parathyroid removal in the dog. In Gastaut, H., Jasper, H.H., Bancaud, J. & Waltregny, A. (eds) *Physiopathogenesis of the Epilepsies*, p. 128. Illinois: Springfield. C.C. Thomas.

Costa, P.J. & Bonnycastle, D.D. (1952) The effect of DCA, compound E, testosterone, progesterone and ACTH in modifying 'agene induced' convulsions in dogs. *Archives Internationales Pharmacodynamie*, **91**, 330.

Coursin, D.B. (1954) Convulsive seizures in infants with pyridoxine-deficient diet. *Journal of the American Medical Association*, **154**, 406.

Coursin, D.B. (1964) Vitamin B₆ metabolism in infants and children. *Vitamins and Hormones* (New York) 22, 755.

Craig, C.R. & Hartman, E.R. (1973) Concentration of amino-acids in the brain of cobalt-epileptic rat. *Epilepsia* (Amsterdam), **14**, 409.

Crome, L.C. & Stern, J. (1972) The pathology of mental retardation, 2nd edn. London: Churchill Livingstone.

Curtis, D.R. & Johnston, G.A.R. (1974) Amino acid transmitters in the mammalian central nervous system. *Ergebnisse der Physiologie*, **69**, 97.

DeFeudis, F.V. & Elliott, K.A.C. (1967) Delay or inhibition of convulsions by intraperitoneal injections of diverse substances. *Canadian Journal of Physiology and Pharmacology*, **45**, 857.

Demoor, J. (1898) Le mécanisme et la signification de l'état moniliforme des neurones. *Annales de la Société Royale des Sciences Médicales et Naturelles de Bruxelles*, **7**, 205.

De Robertis, E., Alberici, M. & De Lores Arnaiz, G.R. (1969) Astroglial swelling and phosphohydrolases in cerebral cortex of metrazol convulsant rats. *Brain Research*, **12**, 461.

De Vellis, J. & Inglish, D. (1968) Hormonal control of glycerolphosphate dehydrogenase in the rat brain. *Journal of Neurochemistry*, **15**, 1061.

Dixon, P.F., Booth, M. & Butler, J. (1914) The Corticosteroids. In Gray, C.H. & Bacharach, A.L. (eds) *Hormones in Blood*, 2, 305. London & New York: Academic Press.

Dunleavy, D.L.F., Oswald, I., Brown, P. & Strong, J.A. (1974) Hyperthyroidism, sleep and growth hormone. *Electroencephalography and Clinical Neurophysiology*, **36**, 259.

Eccles, J.C. (1964) *The physiology of synapses*, p. 316. Berlin: Springer-Verlag.

Eccles, J.C. (1969) *The inhibitory pathways of the central nervous system*. Springfield, Illinois: C.C. Thomas.

Ehlers, C.L. & Killam, E.K. (1979) The influence of cortisone on EEG and seizure activity in the baboon, Papio papio. *Electroencephalography and Clinical Neurophysiology*, **47**, 404.

Eidelberg, E., Lesse, H. & Gault, F.P. (1963) An experimental model of temporal lobe epilepsy. Studies of the convulsant properties of cocaine. In Glaser, G.H. (ed.) *EEG and Behaviour*, p. 272. New York: Basic Books.

Essman, W.B. (1973) *Neurochemistry of cerebral electroshock*, p. 181. Flushing, New York: Spectrum Publications.

Evans, E.C. (1960) Neurologic complications of myxoedema convulsions. *Annals of Internal Medicine*, **52**, 434.

Everett, G.M. & Richards, R.K. (1944) Comparative anticonvulsive action of 3 5, 5-trimethyl-oxazolidine-2,4-dione (Tridione), Dilantin and phenobarbital. *Journal of Pharmacology and Experimental Therapeutics*, **81**, 402.

Fahn, S. & Côté, L.J. (1968) Regional distribution of γ-aminobutyric acid (GABA) in brain of the rhesus monkey. *Journal of Neurochemistry*, **15**, 209.

Fay, T. (1929) Factors in 'mechanical theory of epilepsy', with especial reference to influence of fluid, and its control, in treatment of certain cases. *American Journal of Psychiatry*, **8**, 783.

Fay, T. (1931) Convulsive seizures, their production and control, with especial reference to the probable mechanism of the seizure itself. *American Journal of Psychiatry*, **10**, 551.

Feldman, J., Cortell, R. & Gellhorn, E. (1940) On the vago-insulin and sympathetico-adrenal system and their mutal relationship under conditions of central excitation induced by anoxia and convulsant drugs. *American Journal of Physiology*, **131**, 281.

Fischer, J. (1973) Change in the number of vesicles in synapses of a projected epileptic cortical focus in rats. *Physiologia Bohemoslovaca*, **22**, 537.

Folbergrova, J. (1975) Changes in glycogen phosphorylase activity and glycogen levels of mouse cerebral cortex during convulsions induced by homocysteine. *Journal of Neurochemistry*, **24**, 15.

Folbergrova, J., Passonneau, J.V., Lowry, O.H. & Schulz, D.W. (1969) Glycogen, ammonia and related metabolites in the brain during seizures evoked by methionine sulphoximine. *Journal of Neurochemistry*, **16**, 191.

Frame, B. & Carter, S. (1955) Pseudohypoparathyroidism. Clinical picture and relation to clinical seizures. *Neurology* (Minneapolis) 5, 295.

Friis-Hansen, B. & Buchthal, F. (1965) EEG findings in an infant with intoxication and convulsions incident to hypernatraema. *Electroencephalography and Clinical Neurophysiology*, **19**, 387.

Friis, M.L. & Lund, M. (1974) Stress convulsions. *Archives of Neurology* (Chicago) 31, 155.

Funck-Brentano, J.L., Lossky-Nekhorocheff, I. & Altman, J. (1960) Étude expérimentale des manifestations cérébrales de l'intoxication par l'eau. *Electroencephalography and Clinical Neurophysiology*, **12**, 185.

Futamachi, K.J., Mutani, R. & Prince, D.A. (1974) Potassium activity in rabbit cortex. *Britain Research*, **75**, 5.

Garattini, S., Kato, R. & Valzelli, L. (1960) Biochemical and pharmacological effects induced by electroshock. *Psychiatrica Neurologica* (Basel) 140, 190.

Gastaut, H., Papy, J.J., Toga, M., Murisasco, A. & Dubois, D. (1971) Epilepsie de l'insuffisance rénale et crises épileptiques accidentales survenant au cours de l'épuration extra-rénale (rein artificiel). *Revue EEG Neurophysiologie*, **1**, 151.

Gastaut, H., Saier, J., Mano, T., Santos, D. & Lyagoubi, S. (1968) Generalised epileptic seizures, induced by 'non-convulsant' substances. Part 2. Experimental study with special reference to ammonium chloride. *Epilepsia* (Amsterdam) **9**, 317.

Gastaut, H., Poirier, F., Payan, H., Salamon, G., Toga, M. & Vigouroux, M. (1960) HHE Syndrome. Hemiconvulsions, Hemiplegia, Epilepsy. *Epilepsia* (Amsterdam), **1**, 418.

Gellhorn, E. & Ballin, H.M. (1950) Further investigations on effect of anoxia on convulsions. *American Journal of Physiology*, **162**, 503.

Georgi, F. & Strauss, R. (1938) The problem of convulsions and insulin therapy. II. Special comment on the method described by Meduna. *American Journal of Psychiatry*, **94**. Supplement, 76.

Gilboe, D.D. & Betz, A.L. (1973) Oxygen uptake in the isolated canine brain. *American Journal of Physiology*, **224**, 588.

Gillin, J.C., Jacobs, L.S., Snyder, F. & Henkin, R.I. (1974) Effects of decreased adrenal corticosteroids: changes in sleep in normal subjects and patients with adrenal cortical insufficiency. *Electroencephalography and Clinical Neurophysiology*, **36**, 283.

Glaser, G.H. & Levy, L.L. (1960) Seizures and idiopathic hypoparathyroidism. *Epilepsia* (Amsterdam), **I**, 454.

Globus, A. & Scheibel, A.B. (1966) Loss of dendritic spines as an index of presynaptic terminal patterns. *Nature*, **212**, 463.

Gloor, P. & Testa, G. (1974) Generalised penicillin epilepsy in the cat: effects of intracarotid and intravertebral pentylenetetrazol and amobarbital injections. *Electroencephalography and Clinical Neurophysiology*, **36**, 499.

Glotzner, F.L. (1973) Membrane properties of neuroglia in epileptogenic gliosis. *Brain Research*, **55**, 159.

Goddard, G.V., McIntyre, D. & Leech, C. (1969) A permanent change in brain function resulting from daily electrical stimulation. *Experimental Neurology*, **25**, 295.

Goodman, L.S., Grewal, M.S., Brown, W.C. & Swinyard, E.A. (1953) Comparison of maximal seizures evoked by pentylenetetrazol (Metrazol) and electroshock in mice, and their modification by anticonvulsants. *Journal of Pharmacology and Experimental Therapeutics*, **108**, 168.

Grob, D. (1963) Anticholinesterase intoxication in man and its treatment. In *Handbuch der experimentellen Pharmakologie*. Supplement *15*, 989. Cholinesterases and Anticholinesterase Agents. Berlin: Springer-Verlag.

Grossman, R.G. & Rosman, L.J. (1971) Intracellular potentials of inexcitable cells in epileptogenic cortex undergoing fibrillary gliosis after a local injury. *Brain Research*, **28**, 181.

Halpern, L.M. (1972) Chronically isolated aggregates of mammalian cerebral cortical neurons studied *in situ*. In Purpura, D.P., Penry, J.K., Tower, D.B., Woodbury, D.M., & Walter, R.D. (eds) *Experimental Models of Epilepsy*, p. 197. New York: Raven Press.

Hammond, E.J., Ramsay, R.E., Villarreal, H.J. & Wilder, B.J. (1980) Effects of intracortical injection of blood and blood components on the electrocorticogram. *Epilepsia*, **21**, 3.

Harris, J.W. & van den Brenk, H.A.S. (1968) Comparative effects of hyperbaric oxygen and pentylenetetrazol on lung weight and non-protein sulfhydryl content of experimental animals. *Biochemical Pharmacology*, **17**, 1181.

Hassler, R. (1972) Physiopathology of rigidity. In Siegfried, J., Hawkins, R.A., Williamson, D.H. & Krebs, H.A. (eds) (1971) *Parkinson's Disease*, **1**, 20. Vienna: Hans Huber.

Hawkins, R.A., Williamson, D.H. & Krebs, H.A. (1971) Ketone body utilisation by adult and suckling rat brain *in vivo*. *Biochemical Journal*, **122**, 13.

Hendley, C.D., Spudis, E.V. & De la Torre, E. (1965) Intracranial pressure during electroshock convulsions in the dog. *Neurology* (Minneapolis) **15**, 351.

Henn, F.A., Haljamae, H. & Hamberger, A. (1972) Glial cell function: Active control of extracellular K^+ concentration. *Brain Research*, **43**, 437.

Herberg, L.J. & Watkins, P.J. (1966) Epileptiform seizures induced by hypothalamic stimulation in the rat: Resistance to fits following fits. *Nature*, **209**, 515.

Herlitz, G. (1941) Studien uber die sogenannten initialen Fieberkrampfe bei Kinden. *Acta Paediatrica Scandinavica*, **29**. Supplement *1*, 142.

Hertz, L., Schousboe, A., Formby, B. & Lennox-Buchthal, M. (1974) Some age-dependent biochemical changes in mice susceptible to seizures. *Epilepsia* (Amsterdam) **15**, 619.

Heuser, G. & Eidelberg, E. (1961) Steroid-induced convulsions in experimental animals. *Endocrinology*, **69**, 915.

Hindfelt, B. & Siesjö, B.K. (1971) Cerebral effects of acute ammonia intoxication. The influence on intracellular and extracellular acid-base parameters. *Scandinavian Journal of Clinical and Laboratory Investigation*, **28**, 353.

Hirsch, C.S. & Martin, D.L. (1971) Unexpected deaths in young epileptics. *Neurology* (Minneapolis) **21**, 682.

Holmgren, B. & Kraeplin, S. (1953) Electroencephalographic study of asthmatic children. *Acta Pediatrica*, **42**, 432.

Horton, R.W. & Meldrum, B.S. (1973) Seizures induced by allylglycine, 3-mercaptopropionic acid and 4-deoxypyridoxine in mice and photosensitive baboons, and different modes of inhibition of cerebral glutamic acid decarboxylase. *British Journal of Pharmacology*, **49**, 52.

Hunt, A.D., Stokes, J., McCrory, W.W. & Stroud, H.H. (1954) Pyridoxine dependency: report of a case of intractable convulsions in an infant controlled by pyridoxine. *Pediatrics*, **13**, 140.

Huot, J., Radouco-Thomas, S. & Radouco-Thomas, C. (1973) Qualitative and quantitative evaluation of experimentally-induced seizures. In Mercier, J. (ed.) *Anticonvulsant Drugs*, **1**, 123. Oxford: Pergamon Press.

Huttenlocher, P.R., Wilbourn, A.J. & Signore, J.M. (1971) Medium chain triglycerides as a therapy for intractable childhood epilepsy. *Neurology* (Minneapolis) **21**, 1097.

Ingram, T.T.S., Stark, G.D. & Blackburn, I. (1967) Ataxia and other neurological disorders as sequels of severe hypoglycaemia in childhood. *Brain*, **90**, 851.

Ingvar, D.H. (1973) rCBF in focal cortical epilepsy. *Stroke*, **4**, 359.

Isler, W. (1971) Acute hemipelgia and hemisyndromes in childhood. *Clinics in Developmental Medicine*, **41–42**, 314. London: William Heinemann.

Jabbari, B. & Huott, A.D. (1980) Seizures in thyrotoxicosis. *Epilepsia*, **21**, 91.

James, I.M. (1975) Autonomic control of the cerebral circulation. In Meldrum, B.S. & Marsden, C.D. (eds) *Primate Models of Neurological Disorders*, p. 167. New York: Raven Press.

Janz, D. (1974) Epilepsy and the sleeping-waking cycle. In Vinken, P.J. & Bruyn, G.W. (eds) *Handbook of Clinical Neurology. The Epilepsies*, **15**, 311. Amsterdam: North Holland Publishing Co.

Jeavons, P.M. & Bower, B.D. (1964) Infantile spasms. A review of the literature and a study of 112 cases. *Clinics in Developmental Medicine*, No. 15. London: William Heinemann Medical Books.

Jeavons, P.M., Bower, B.D. & Dimitrakoudi, M. (1973) Long-term prognosis of 150 cases of 'West syndrome'. *Epilepsia* (Amsterdam) **14**, 153.

Johnson, L.C. & Davidoff, R.A. (1964) Autonomic changes during paroxysmal EEG activity. *Electroencephalography and Clinical Neurophysiology*, **17**, 25.

Jose, C.J., Barton, J.L. & Perez-Cruet, J. (1979) Hyponatraemic seizures in psychiatric patients. *Biological Psychiatry*, **14**, 839.

Jouvet, M. (1972) The role of monoamines and acetylcholine-containing neurons in the regulation of the sleep-waking cycle. *Ergebnisse Physiologie*, **64**, 166.

Jovanović, U.J. (1967) Das schlafverhalten der epileptiker. I. Schlafdauer, schlaftiefe und bensonderheiten der schlafperiodik. *Deutsche Zeitschrift für Nervenheilkunde*, **190**, 159.

Kessler, M. & Gellhorn, E. (1941) Effect of electrically-induced convulsions on vago-insulin and sympathetico-adrenal systems. *Proceedings of the Society for Experimental Biology & Medicine*, **46**, 64.

Kety, S.S. & Schmidt, C.F. (1948) The effects of altered arterial tensions of carbon dioxide and oxygen on cerebral blood flow and cerebral oxygen consumption of normal young men. *Journal of Clinical Investigation*, **27**, 484.

Kety, S.S. (1964) The cerebral circulation. In Field, V. (ed.)

Handbook of Physiology. I. Neurophysiology, **3**, 1751. Washington: American Physiological Society.

Kety, S.S., Javoy, F., Thierry, A-M., Julou, L. & Glowinski, J.A. (1967) A sustained effect of electroconvulsive shock on the turnover of norepinephrine in the central nervous system of the rat. *Proceedings of the National Academy of Science*, **58**, 1249.

King, L.J., Lowry, O.H., Passoneau, J.V. & Venson, V. (1967) Effects of convulsants on energy reserves in the cerebral cortex. *Journal of Neurochemistry*, **14**, 599.

King, L.J., Webb, O.L. & Carl, J. (1970) Effects of duration of convulsions on energy reserves of the brain. *Journal of Neurochemistry*, **17**, 13.

Klatzo, I. (1967) Neuropathological aspects of brain oedema. *Journal of Neuropathology and Experimental Neurology*, **26**, 1.

Krantz, J.C. (1963) Volatile anaesthetics and Indoklon. *Journal of Neuropsychiatry*, **4**, 157.

Kruse, H.D., Orent, E.R. & McCollum, E.V. (1932) Studies on magnesium deficiency in animals, I. Symptomatology resulting from magnesium deprivation. *Journal of Biological Chemistry*, **96**, 519.

Krushinsky, L.V. (1962) A study of pathophysiological mechanisms of cerebral haemorrhage provoked by reflex epileptic seizures in rats. *Epilepsia* (Amsterdam), **3**, 363.

Kurtz, D., Micheletti, G., Tempe, J.D., Brogard, J.M., Girardel, M. & Fletto, R. (1971) Etude électroclinique des comas hyperosmolaires. *Revue EEG et Neurophysiologie* (Paris), **I**, 353.

Laidlaw, J. (1956) Catamenial epilepsy. *Lancet*, **2**, 1235.

Lamprecht, F., Ebert, M.H., Turek, I. & Kopin, I.J. (1974) Serum dopamine-Beta hydroxylase in depressed patients and the effect of electroconvulsive shock treatment. *Psychopharmacologia*, **40**, 241.

Langdon-Down, M. & Brain, W.R. (1929) Times of day in relation to convulsions in epilepsy. *Lancet*, **I**, 1029.

Lascelles, P.T. & Lewis, P.D. (1972) Hypodipsia and hypernatraemia associated with hypothalamic and suprasellar lesions. *Brain*, **95**, 249.

Lennox, W.G., Gibbs, F.A. & Gibbs, E.L. (1936) Effect on the electroencephalogram of drugs and conditions which influence seizures. *Archives of Neurology & Psychiatry* (Chicago), **36**, 1236.

Lennox-Buchthal, M.A. (1973) Febrile convulsions. *Electroencephalography and Clinical Neurophysiology*. Supplement *32*, 1.

Levitt, P., Wilson, W. & Wilkins, R. (1971) The effects of subarachnoid blood on the electrocorticogram of the cat. *Journal of Neurosurgery*, **35**, 185–191.

Lewis, L.D., Ljunggren, B., Norberg, K. & Siesjö, B.K. (1974a) Changes in carbohydrate substrates, amino acids and ammonia in the brain during insulin-induced hypoglycaemia. *Journal of Neurochemistry*, **23**, 659.

Lewis, L.D., Ljunggren, B., Ratcheson, R.A. & Siesjö, B.K. (1974b) Cerebral energy state in insulin-induced hypoglycaemia, related to blood glucose and to EEG. *Journal of Neurochemistry*, **23**, 673.

Lhermitte, F., Marteau, R. & Degos, C.F. (1972) Analyse pharmacologique d'un nouveau cas de myoclonies d'intention et d'action post-anoxiques. *Revue Neurologique*, **126**, 107.

Lindenberg, R. (1955) Compression of brain arteries as pathogenetic factor for tissue necroses and their areas of predilection. *Journal of Neuropathology and Experimental Neurology*, **14**, 223.

Livingston, S. (1972) *Comprehensive management of epilepsy in infancy and childhood*. Springfield, Illinois: C.C. Thomas.

Lowe, I.P., Robins, E. & Eyerman, G.S. (1958) The fluorimetric measurement of glutamic decarboxylase and its distribution in brain. *Journal of Neurochemistry*, **3**, 8.

Luciani, J., Riche, D., Lanoir, J. & Seite, R. (1969) Modifications de la neurosécrétion hypothalamique sous l'influence de manifestations épileptiformes par photo stimulation chez le Papio papio. *Comptes Rendues du Sociétés Biologiques*, **163**, 1167.

Luft, V.C. & Noell, W.K. (1956) Manifestations of brief instantaneous anoxia in man. *Journal of Applied Physiology*, **8**, 444.

Luttrell, C.N., Finberg, L. & Drawdy, L.P. (1959) Hemorrhagic encephalopathy induced by hypernatraemia. II. Experimental observations on hyperosmolarity in cats. *Archives of Neurology* (Chicago) **1**, 153.

Lux, H.D. (1974) The kinetics of extracellular potassium: relation to epileptogenesis. *Epilepsia*, **15**, 375.

Maccario, M. (1968) Neurological dysfunction associated with non-ketotic hyperglycaemia. *Archives of Neurology* (Minneapolis), **19**, 525.

Magnaes, B. & Nornes, H. (1974) Circulatory and respiratory changes in spontaneous epileptic seizures in man. *European Neurology*, **12**, 104.

Marcus, E.M., Watson, C.W., & Goldman, P.L. (1966) Effects of steroids on cerebral electrical activity: epileptogenic effects of conjugated oestrogens and related compounds in the cat and rabbit. *Archives of Neurology* (Chicago), **15**, 521.

Marcus. E.M. (1972) Experimental models of petit mal epilepsy. In Purpura, D.P., Penry, J.K., Tower, D., Woodbury D.M. & Walter, R. (eds) *Experimental Models of Epilepsy*, p. 113. New York: Raven Press.

Margerison, J.H. & Corsellis, J.A.N. (1966) Epilepsy and the temporal lobes – a clinical, electroencephalographic and neuropathological study of the brain in epilepsy, with particular references to the temporal lobes. *Brain*, **89**, 499.

McLardy, T. (1974) Pathogenesis of epileptic-hypoxic Ammon's horn sclerosis: contribution of basal vein constriction by looped posterior cerebral artery. *IRCS Anatomy: Neurology*, **2**, 1574.

McQuarrie, I. & Peeler, D.B. (1931) The effects of sustained pituitary antidiuresis and forced water drinking in epileptic children. A diagnostic and etiologic study. *Journal of Clinical Investigation*, **10**, 915.

Meldrum, B.S. (1975a) Present views on hippocampal sclerosis and epilepsy. In Williams, D. (ed.) *Modern Trends in Neurology*, **6**, 223. London: Butterworths.

Meldrum, B.S. (1975b) Epilepsy and γ-amino butyric acid-mediated inhibition. *International Review of Neurobiology*, **17**.

Meldrum, B.S. (1978) Physiological changes during prolonged seizures and epileptic brain damage. *Neuropädiatrie*, **9**, 203.

Meldrum, B.S. & Brierley, J.B. (1973) Prolonged epileptic seizures in primates: ischaemic cell change and its relation to ictal physiological events. *Archives of Neurology* (Chicago) **28**, 10.

Meldrum, B.S. & Horton, R.W. (1971) Convulsive effects of 4-deoxypyridoxine and of bicuculline in photosensitive baboons (*Papio papio*) and in rhesus monkeys (*Macaca mulatta*). *Brain Research*, **35**, 419.

Meldrum, B.S. & Horton, R.W. (1973a) Cerebral functional effects of 2-deoxy-D-glucose and 3-O-methylglucose in rhesus monkeys. *Electroencephalography and Clinical Neurophysiology*, **35**, 59.

Meldrum, B.S. & Horton, R.W. (1973b) Physiology of *status epilepticus* in primates. *Archives of Neurology* (Chicago) **28**, 1.

Meldrum, B.S. & Horton, R.W. (1974) Neuronal inhibition mediated by Gaba, and patterns of convulsions in photosensitive baboons with epilepsy (Papio papio). In *The Natural History and Management of Epilepsy*. Edited by P. Harris & C. Mawdsley, p. 54. Edinburgh & London: Churchill Livingstone.

Meldrum, B.S. & Nilsson, B. (1976) Cerebral blood flow and metabolic rate early and late in prolonged epileptic seizures induced in rats by bicuculline. *Brain*, **99**, 523–542.

Meldrum, B.S. & Stephenson, J.D. (1975) Enhancement of picrotoxin convulsions in chicks and mice by the prior intraperitoneal injection of hypertonic GABA or mannitol. *European Journal of Pharmacology*, **30**, 368.

Meldrum, B.S., Anlezar, G. & Trimble, M. (1975) Drugs modifying dopaminergic activity and behaviour, the EEG and epilepsy in Papio papio.

Meldrum, B.S., Horton, R.W. & Brierley, J.B. (1971) Insulin-induced hypoglycaemia in the primate: relationship between physiological changes and ultimate neuropathology. In *Brain Hypoxia*. Edited by J.B. Brierley & B.S. Meldrum, *Clinics in Developmental Medicine*, No. 39/40, p. 207. London: William Heinemann Medical Books.

Meldrum, B.S., Horton, R.W. & Brierley, J.B. (1974) Epileptic brain damage in adolescent baboons following seizures induced by allylglycine. *Brain*, **97**, 407.

Meldrum, B.S., Vigouroux, R.A. & Brierley, J.B. (1973) Systemic factors and epileptic brain damage. Prolonged seizures in paralysed artificially ventilated baboons. *Archives of Neurology* (Chicago) **29**, 82.

Meldrum, B.S., Balzano, E., Gadea, M. & Naquet, R. (1970) Photic and drug-induced epilepsy in the baboon (Papio papio). The effects of isoniazid, thiosemicarbazide, pyridoxine and amino-oxyacetic acid. *Electroencephalography and Clinical Neurophysiology*, **29**, 333.

Meldrum, B.S., Balzano, E., Horton, R.W., Lee, G. & Trimble, M. (1975) Photically-induced epilepsy in Papio papio as a model for drug studies. In Meldrum, B.S. & Marsden, C.D. (eds) 'Primate Models of Neurological Disorders', *Advances in Neurology*, **10**. New York: Raven Press.

Meldrum, B.S., Horton, R.W., Bloom, S.R., Butler, J. & Keenan, J. (1979) Endocrine factors and glucose metabolism during prolonged seizures in baboons. *Epilepsia*, **20**, 527.

Melekian, B., Laplane, R. & Debray, P. (1962) Considérations cliniques et statistiques sur les convulsions au cours des déshydrations aiguës. *Annales de Pédiatrie*, **34**, 1494.

Metrakos, K. & Metrakos, J.D. (1974) Genetics of epilepsy. In Vinken, P.J. & Bruyn, G.W. (eds) *Handbook of Clinical Neurology*, **15**, 429. Amsterdam: North Holland Publishing Co.

Meyer, J.S., Gotoh, F. & Tazaki, Y. (1961) Inhibitory action of carbon dioxide and acetolamide in seizure activity. *Electroencephalography and Clinical Neurophysiology*, **13**, 762.

Meyer, J.S., Gotoh, F. & Favale, E. (1966) Cerebral metabolism during epileptic seizures in man. *Electroencephalography and Clinical Neurophysiology*, **21**, 10.

Millichap, J.G. (1968) *Febrile Convulsions*. New York: Macmillan.

Millichap, J.G. (1974) Metabolic and endocrine factors. In Vinken, P.J. & Bruyn, G.W. (eds) *Handbook of Clinical Neurology. The Epilepsies*, **15**, 311. Amsterdam: North Holland Publishing Co.

Miribel, J. & Poirier, F. (1961) Effects of ACTH and adrenocortical hormones in juvenile epilepsy. *Epilepsia* (Amsterdam) **2**, 345.

Moore, K.E. & Phillipson, O.T. (1975) Effects of dexamethasone on phenylethamolamine N-methyltransferase (PNMT) and adrenaline (A) in the brains of adult and neonatal rats. *British Journal of Pharmacology*, **53**, 453.

Morris-Jones, P.H., Houston, I.B. & Evans, R.C. (1967) Prognosis of the neurological complications of acute hypernatraemia. *Lancet*, **2**, 1385.

Mueller, S.M., Heistad, D.D. & Marcus, M.L. (1979) Effect of sympathetic nerves on cerebral vessels during seizures. *American Journal of Physiology*, **237**, H178–H184.

Munson, E.S., & Wagman, I.H. (1969) Acid-base changes during lidocaine-induced seizures in Macaca mulatta. *Archives of Neurology* (Chicago), **20**, 406.

Musacchio, J.M., Julou, L., Kety, S.S. & Glowinski, J. (1969) Increase in rat tyrosine hydroxylase activity produced by electroconvulsive shock. *Proceedings of the National Academy of Sciences*, **63**, 1117.

Naquet, R., Meldrum, B.S., Balzano, E. & Charrier, J.P. (1970) Photically-induced epilepsy and glucose metabolism in the adolescent baboon (Papio papio). *Brain Research*, **18**, 503.

Nemoto, E.M. & Frankel, H.M. (1970) Cerebral oxygenation and metabolism during progressive hyperthermia. *American Journal of Physiology*, **219**, 1784.

Öhman, R., Walinder, J., Balldin, J., Wallin, L. & Abahamsson, L. (1976) Prolactin response to electroconvulsive therapy. *Lancent*, **2**, 936.

Opper, L. (1939) Pathologic picture of thujone and monobromated camphor convulsions. *Archives of Neurology and Psychiatry*, **41**, 460.

Ounsted, C., Lindsay, J. & Norman, R. (1966) Biological factors in temporal lobe epilepsy. *Clinics in Developmental Medicine* No. 22. London: William Heinemann Medical Books Ltd.

Owen, O.E., Morgan, A.P., Kemp, H.G., Sullivan, J.M., Herrera, M.G. & Cahill, G.F. (1967) Brain metabolism during fasting. *Journal of Clinical Investigation*, **46**, 1589.

Owen, M. & Bliss, E.L. (1970) Sleep loss and cerebral excitability. *American Journal of Physiology*, **218**, 171.

Owman, C. & Edvinsson L. (1978) Histochemical and pharmacological approach to the investigation of neurotransmitters, with particular regard to the cerebrovascular bed. In *Cerebral vascular smooth muscle and its control*. CIBA Foundation Symposium, **56**, 275–304.

Papeschi, R., Molina-Negro, P., Sourkes, T.L. & Erba, G. (1972) The concentration of homovanillic and 5-hydroxyindoleacetic acids in ventricular and lumbar CSF: Studies in patients with extrapyramidal disorders, epilepsy and other diseases. *Neurology*, (Minneapolis) **22**, 1151.

Pappius, H.M., Savaki, H.E., Fieschi, C., Rapoport, S.I. & Sokoloff, L. (1979) Osmotic opening of the blood-brain barrier and local cerebral glucose utilisation. Annals of Neurology, **5**, 211.

Passouant, P., Cadilhac, J., Pternitis, C. & Baldy-Moulinier, M. (1967) Epilepsie temporale et décharges ammoniques provoquées par l'anoxie exprive. *Revue Neurologique*, **117**, 65.

Penfield, W. & Jasper, H. (1954) *Epilepsy and the Functional Anatomy of the Human Brain*. Boston, Massachusetts: Little, Brown & Co.

Penfield, W., Von Santha, K. & Cipriani, A. (1939) Cerebral blood flow during induced epileptiform seizures in animals and man. *Journal of Neurophysiology*, **2**, 257.

Perry, T.L., Berry, K., Hansen, S., Diamond, S. & Mok, C. (1971) Regional distribution of amino acids in human brain obtained at autopsy. *Journal of Neurochemistry*, **18**, 513.

Perry, T.L., Hansen, S., Sokoi, M. & Wada, J.A. (1972) Amino acids in brain biopsies of epileptic foci. *Clinical Research*, **20**, 949.

Perry, T.L., Hansen, S. & Kloster, M. (1973) Huntington's chorea: deficiency of γ-aminobutyric acid in brain. *New England Journal of Medicine*, **288**, 337.

Peters, R.A. (1963) *Biochemical lesions and lethal synthesis*. Oxford: Pergamon Press.

Plum. F. & Duffy, T.E. (1975) The couple between cerebral metabolism and blood flow during seizures. In *Alfred Benzon Symposium 8: The Working Brain*. Copenhagen: Munksgaard.

Plum, F., Posner, J.B. & Troy, B. (1968) Cerebral metabolic and circulatory responses to induced convulsions in animals. *Archives of Neurology* (Chicago) **18**, 1.

Poiré, R. (1969) Hypoglycaemic epilepsy: Clinical, electrographic and biological study during induced hypoglycaemia in man. In Gastaut, H., Jasper, H., Bancaud, J. & Waltregny, A. (eds) *The Physiopathogenesis of the Epilepsies*, Ch. 8, p. 75. Springfield, Illinois: C.C. Thomas. *Archives of Neurology* (Chicago), **20**, 388.

Pollen, D.A. & Trachtenberg, M.C. (1970) Neuroglia: Gliosis and focal epilepsy. *Science*, **167**, 1252.

Ponte, J. & Purves, M.J. (1974) The role of the carotid body chemoreceptors and carotid sinus baroreceptors in the control of cerebral blood vessels. *Journal of Physiology*, **237**, 315.

Posner, J.B., Plum, F. & Poznak, A.V. (1969) Cerebral metabolism during electrically-induced seizures in man. *Archives of Neurology* (Chicago) **20**, 388.

Prill, A., Quellhorst, E. & Scheler, F. (1969) Epilepsy: Clinical and electroencephalographic findings in patients with renal insufficiency. In Gastaut, H., Jasper, H., Bancaud, H. & Waltregny, A. (eds) *The Physiopathogenesis of the Epilepsies*, Ch. 6, p. 60. Springfield, Illinois: C.C. Thomas.

Prince, D.A., Lux, H.D. & Neher, E. (1973) Measurement of extracellular potassium activity in cat cortex. *Brain Research*, **50**, 489.

Purpura, D.P. (1974) Dendritic spine 'dysgenesis' and mental retardation. *Science*, **186**, 1126.

Purves, M.J. (1972) *The physiology of the cerebral circulation*. Cambridge: Cambridge University Press.

Pylkko, O.O. & Woodbury, D.M. (1961) The effect of maturation on chemically-induced seizures in rats. *Journal of Pharmacology & Experimental Therapeutics*, **131**, 185.

Raisman, G. (1969) Neuronal plasticity in the septal nuclei of the adult rat. *Brain Research*, **14**, 25.

Reynolds, E.H. (1970) Water, electrolytes and epilepsy. *Journal of the Neurological Sciences*, **11**, 327.

Ribak, C.E., Harris, A.B., Vaughn, J.E. & Roberts (1979) Inhibitory GABAergic nerve terminals decrease at sites of focal epilepsy. *Science*, **205**, 211.

Riche, D. (1973) L'hypothalamus du singe Papio papio (Desm): stéréotaxie, cytologie et modifications neurosecretoires liées aux crises d'épilepsie induites par la lumière. *Journal für Hirnforschung*, **14**, 527.

Richter, D. & Dawson, R.M.C. (1948) The ammonia and glutamine content of the brain. *Journal of Biological Chemistry*, **176**, 1199.

Rosen A.D. & Frumin, N.V. (1979) Focal epileptogenesis after intracortical hemoglobin injection. *Experimental Neurology*, **66**, 277.

Rowntree, L.G. (1923) Water intoxication. *Archives of Internal Medicine*, **32**, 157.

Rowntree, L.G. (1926) The effects on mammals of the administration of excessive quantities of water. *Journal of Pharmacology & Experimental Therapeutics*, **29**, 135.

Rymer, M.M. & Fishman, R.A. (1973) Protective adaptation of brain to water intoxication. *Archives of Neurology* (Chicago), **28**, 49.

Sacktor, B., Wilson, J.E. & Tiekert, C.G. (1966) Regulation of glycoloysis in brain, *in situ*, during convulsions. *Journal of Biological Chemistry*, **241**, 5071.

Samson, F.E. & Dahl, N.A. (1957) Cerebral energy requirement of neonatal rats. *American Journal of Physiology*, **188**, 277.

Sassin, J.F., Parker, D.C., Mace, J.W., Gotlin, R.W., Johnson, L.C. & Rossman, L.G. (1969) Human growth hormone release: relation to slow-wave sleep-waking cycles. *Science*, **165**, 513.

Schadé, J.P. & McMenemy, W.H. (1963) *Selective vulnerability of the brain in hypoxaemia*. Oxford: Blackwell Scientific.

Scheibel, M.E. & Scheibel, A.B. (1973) Hippocampal pathology in temporal lobe epilepsy. A Golgi survey. In *Epilepsy: its Phenomena in Man. UCLA Forum in Medical Sciences*, **17**, 311.

Scheibel, M.E., Crandall, P.H. & Scheibel, A.B. (1974) The hippocampal-dentate complex in temporal lobe epilepsy. *Epilepsia* **15**, 55.

Schmidt, C.F., Kety, S.S. & Pennes, H.H. (1945) The gaseous metabolism of the brain of the monkey. *American Journal of Physiology*, **143**, 33.

Scholz, W. (1951) Die Krampfschadigungen des Gehirns. *Monographien aus dem Gesamtegebiete der Neurologie und Psychiatrie*. Heft 75. Berlin: Springer-Verlag.

Scholz, W. (1959) The contribution of patho-anatomical research to the problem of epilepsy. *Epilepsia* (Amsterdam) **1**, 36.

Schwartz, I.R., Broggi, G. & Pappas, G.D. (1970) Fine structure of cat hippocampus during sustained seizures. *Brain Research*, **18**, 176.

Schwartz., M.S. & Scott, D.F. (1974) Aminophylline-induced seizures. *Epilepsia* (Chicago) **15**, 501.

Seite, R., Picard, D. & Luciani, J. (1964) In Bargmann & Schadé (eds) *Progress in Brain Research*, **5**, 171. Amsterdam: Elsevier.

Selye, H. (1941) Anaesthetic effect of steroid hormones. *Proceedings of the Society of Experimental Biology and Medicine*, **46**, 116.

Serbanescu, T. & Balzano, E. (1974) The influence of thyroxine in photosensitive baboons, *Papio papio*. *Electroencephalography and Clinical Neurophysiology*, **36**, 253.

Seyfried, T.N., Glaser, G.H. & Yu, R.K. (1979) Thyroid hormone influence on the susceptibility of mice to audiogenic seizures. *Science*, **205**, 598.

Sharpless, S.K. (1969) Isolated and deafferented neurons: Disuse supersensitivity. In Jasper, H.H., Ward, A.A. & Pope, A. (eds) *Basic Mechanisms of the Epilepsies*, p. 299. London: Churchill.

Shaywitz, B.A., Cohen, D.J. & Bowers, M.B. (1975) Reduced cerebrospinal fluid 5-hydroxyindoleacetic acid and homovanillic acid in children with epilepsy. *Neurology* (Minneapolis) **25**, 72.

Singh, B.M., Gupta, D.R. & Strobos, R.J. (1973) Non-ketonic

hyperglycaemia and epilepsia partialis continua. *Archives of Neurology* (Chicago) **29**, 187.

Skanse, B. & Nyman, G.E. (1956) Thyrotoxicosis as a cause of cerebral dysrhythmia and convulsive seizures. *Acta Endocrinologica* (Kobenhavn) **22**, 246.

Sorel, L. & Dusaucy-Bauloye, A. (1958) Á propos de 21 cas d'hypsarhythmia de Gibbs. Traitement spectaculaire par l'ACTH. *Revue Neurologique* (Paris) **99**, 136.

Spielmeyer, W. (1927) Die pathogenese des epileptischen krampfes. *Zeitschrift fúr die gesamt. Neurologie und Psychiatrie*, **109**, 501.

St Omer, V. (1971) Investigations into mechanisms responsible for seizures induced by chlorinated hydrocarbon insecticides: The role of brain ammonia and glutamine in convulsions in the rat and cockerel. *Journal of Neurochemistry*, **18**, 365.

Starr, A.M. (1952) Personality change in Cushing's syndrome. *Journal of Clinical Endocrinology*, **12**, 502.

Stone, W.E. (1957) The role of acetylcholine in brain metabolism and function. *American Journal of Physical Medicine*, **36**, 222.

Suter, C. & Klingman, W.O. (1955) Neurologic manifestations of magnesium depletion states. *Neurology* (Minneapolis) **5**, 691.

Sypert, G.W. & Ward, A.A. (1974) Changes in extracellular potassium activity during neocortical propagated seizures. *Experimental Neurology*, **45**, 19.

Tebecis, A.K. (1974) *Transmitters and Identified Neurons in the Mammalian Central Nervous System*. Bristol: Scientechnica Publishers.

Teglbjaerg, H.P.S. (1936) Investigations on epilepsy and water metabolism. *Acta Pyschiatrica et Neurologica* (Copenhagen). Supplementum 9.

Timiras, P.S. & Woodbury, D.M. (1956) Effect of thyroid activity on brain function and brain electrolyte distribution in rats. *Endocrinology*, **58**, 181.

Timiras, P.S. (1969) Role of hormones in development of seizures. In Jasper, H.H., Ward, A.A. & Pope, A. (eds) *Basic Mechanisms of the Epilepsies*, p. 727. London: Churchill.

Toman, J.E.P. & Davis, J.P. (1949) The effects of drugs upon the electrical activity of the brain. *Journal of Pharmacology & Experimental Therapeutics*, **97**, 425.

Tower, D.B. & Elliott, K.A.C. (1952) Activity of acetylcholine system in human epileptogenic focus. *Journal of Applied Physiology*, **4**, 669.

Tower, D.B. (1969) Neurochemical Mechanisms. In Jasper, H.H., Ward, A.A. & Pope, A. (eds) *Basic Mechanisms of the Epilepsies*, p. 611. Boston, Massachusetts: Little, Brown & Co.

Trachtenberg, M.C. & Pollen, D.A. (1970) Neuroglia: Biophysical properties and physiologic function. *Science*, **167**, 1248.

Trimble, M.R. (1978) Serum prolactin in epilepsy and hysteria. *British Medical Journal*, **2**, 1682.

Trimble, M., Anlezark, G. & Meldrum, B.S. (1977) Seizure activity in photosensitive baboons following antidepressant drugs and the role of serotoninergic mechanisms. *Psychopharmacologia*, **51**, 159.

Van Buren, J.M. & Ajmone-Marsan, C. (1960) A correlation of autonomic and EEG components in temporal lobe epilepsy. *Archives of Neurology* (Chicago) **3**, 683.

Van Gelder, N.M. & Courtois, A. (1972) Close correlation between changing content of specific amino acids in epileptogenic cortex of cats, and severity of epilepsy. *Brain Research*, **20**, 949.

Van Gelder, N.M., Sherwin, A.L. & Rasmussen, T. (1972) Amino acid content of epileptogenic human brain. Focal *versus* surrounding regions. *Brain Research*, **40**, 385.

Wada, J.A., Sato, M. & Corcoran, M.E. (1974) Persistent seizure susceptibility and recurrent spontaneous seizures in kindled cats. *Epilepsia* (Amsterdam) **15**, 465.

Wagman, I.H., DeJong, R.H. & Prince, D.A. (1968) Effects of lidocaine on spontaneous cortical and subcortical electrical activity. *Archives of Neurology* (Chicago) **18**, 277.

Wallace, S.J. & Zealley, H. (1970) Neurological, electroencephalographic and virological findings in febrile children. *Archives of Disease in Childhood*, **45**, 611.

Wallach, M.B., Winters, W.D., Mandell, A.J. & Spooner, C.E. (1969) A correlation of EEG, reticular multiple unit activity and gross behaviour following various antidepressant agents in the cat. IV. *Electroencephalography and Clinical Neurophysiology*, **27**, 563.

Wallis, C.J. & Luttge W.G. (1980) Influence of estrogen and progesterone on glutamic acid decarboxylase activity in discrete regions of rat brain. *Journal of Neurochemistry*, **34**, 609.

Waltregny, A. & Mesdjian, E. (1969) Convulsive seizure and water intoxication. A polygraphic study. In Gastaut, H., Jasper, H., Bancaud, J. & Waltregny, A. (eds) *The Physiopathogenesis of the Epilepsies*, p. 69. Springfield, Illinois: C.C. Thomas.

Ward, A.A. (1969) The epileptic neurone: Chronic foci in animals and man. In Jasper, H.H., Ward, A.A. & Pope, A. (eds) *Basic Mechanisms of the Epilepsies*, p. 263. London: Churchill.

Weil-Malherbe, H. (1955) The concentration of adrenaline in human plasma and its relation to mental activity. *Journal of Mental Science*, **101**, 733.

Werman, R., Davidoff, R.A. & Aprison, M.H. (1968) Inhibitory action of glycine on spinal neurons in the cat. *Journal of Neurophysiology*, **31**, 81.

Westmoreland, B.F., Hanna, G.R. & Bass, N.H. (1972) Cortical alterations in zones of secondary epileptogenesis: a neurophysiologic, morphologic and microchemical correlation study in the albino rat. *Brain Research*, **43**, 485.

Westrum, L.E., White, L.E. & Ward, A.A. (1965) Morphology of the experimental epileptic focus. *Journal of Neurosurgery*, **21**, 1033.

Wheatley, M.D., Lipton, B. & Ward, A.A. (1947) Repeated cyanide convulsions without central nervous pathology. *Journal of Neuropathology & Experimental Neurology*, **6**, 408.

White, P.T., Grant, P., Mosier, J. & Craig, A. (1961) Changes in cerebral dynamics associated with seizures. *Neurology* (Minneapolis) **11**, 354.

Wilder, B.J. (1969) Projection phenomena and secondary epileptogenesis-mirror foci. In Purpura, D.P., Penry, J.K., Tower, D., Woodbury, D.M. & Walter, R. (eds) *Experimental Models of Epilepsy*, p. 85. New York: Raven Press.

Wilder, R.M. (1921) The effect of ketonuria on course of epilepsy. *Mayo Clinic Proceedings*, **2**, 307.

Willmore, L.J., Sypert, G.W., Munson, J.B. & Hurd, R.W. (1978) Chronic focal epileptiform discharges induced by injection of iron into rat and cat cortex. *Science*, **200**, 1501.

Withrow, C.D. (1972) Systemic carbon dioxide derangements. In Purpura, D.P., Penry, J.K., Woodbury, D.M. & Walter, R. (eds) *Experimental Models of Epilepsy*, p. 477. New York: Raven Press.

Wood, J.D. (1972) Systemic carbon dioxide derangements. In Purpura, D.P., Penry, J.K., Woodbury, D.M. & Walter, R.

(eds) *Experimental Models of Epilepsy*, p. 459. New York: Raven Press.

Wood, J.H., Hare, T.A., Glaeser, B.S., Ballenger, J.C. & Post, R.M. (1979) Cerebrospinal fluid GABA reductions in seizure patients. *Neurology* (Minneapolis), **29**, 1203.

Woodbury, D.M. (1955) Effects of diphenylhydantoin on electrolytes and radiosodium turnover in brain and other tissues of normal, hyponatraemic, and post-ictal rates. *Journal of Pharmacology*, **74**, 115.

Woodbury, D.M. (1958) Relation between the adrenal cortex and the central nervous system. *Pharmacological Reviews*, **10** 275.

Woodbury, D.M. & Vernadakis, A. (1966) Effects of steroids on the central nervous system. In Dorfman, R.J. (ed.) *Methods in Hormone research*, Vol. 5, p. 1. New York: Academic Press.

Woodbury, D.M., Rollins, L.T., Gardner, M.D., Hirschi, W.L., Hogan, J.R., Rallison, M.L., Tanner, G.S. & Brodie, D.A. (1958) Effects of carbon dioxide on brain excitability and electrolytes. *American Journal of Physiology*, **192**, 79.

Woolley, D.E. & Timiras, P.S. (1962a) The gonad-brain relationship: effects of female sex hormones on electroshock convulsions in the rat. *Endocrinology*, **70**, 196.

Woolley, D.E. & Timiras, P.S. (1962b) Estrous and circadian periodicity and electroshock convulsions in rats. *American Journal of Physiology*, **202**, 379.

Wyke, B. (1963) *Brain function and metabolic disorders*. London: Butterworths.

Zimmet, P., Breidahl, H.D. & Nayler, W.G. (1968) Plasma ionised calcium in hypomagnesaemia. *British Medical Journal*, **1**, 622.

Zuckerman, E.C. & Glaser, G.H. (1970) Slow potential shifts in dorsal hippocampus during epileptogenic perfusion of the inferior horn with high-potassium CSF. *Electroencephalography and Clinical Neurophysiology*, **18**, 236.

Zuckerman, E.G. & Glaser, G.H. (1972) Urea-induced myoclonic seizures. *Archives of Neurology* (Chicago) **27**, 14.

12

Epilepsy in developing countries

B. Chandra

One of the most important health problems facing developing countries, has been epilepsy. First of all because of its incidence and prevalence, which for instance in Indonesia is of the same magnitude as tuberculosis (both have an incidence of 7 per 1000). A second reason is that leading causes of epilepsy like birth injury, childhood infections, febrile seizures and head injuries because of traffic accidents are all very frequent in developing countries. The third reason is that because of lack of paramedical personnel, physicians and funds it is often difficult to diagnose and treat the patient with epilepsy. Many developing countries face the same problem as Indonesia, how to reach with few doctors and nurses epileptic patients in a population of 135 million people spread over a distance equal to that from London to Turkey. Finally, in the future these problems will increase as most of the world population increase will occur in developing countries, especially in Asia (Tower, 1978).

In this chapter epilepsy in developing countries will be discussed under five headings:

1. Identifying patients
2. Aetiological factors
3. Clinical management
4. Prevention
5. Rehabilitation

IDENTIFYING PATIENTS

Every doctor working in a village in a developing country knows, that one of the main problems is how to identify the epileptic patient. Some factors which need to be considered are as follows.

The belief, that epilepsy is always hereditary and cannot be cured

Several foreign physicians, whom I invited to visit some rural areas, were astonished to hear the negative answer given by the people in the village to a simple question like: 'Do you suffer from convulsions?' Nearly everyone answered this question with a firm no.

If however the question was phrased: 'Did you ever suffer an attack of *twitchings* and *cramps* of your arms and legs followed by unconsciousness and sometimes urinary incontinence?' To this question many people responded with an affirmative yes.

The reason for this behaviour was, that for most people in the village, convulsions (*ayan* in Indonesian) meant a hereditary incurable disease, which is a disgrace for the family.

Shortage of local paramedical and medical personnel

As in many other developing countries, one of the problems is how to reach the epileptic patient, with few physicians and nurses. Much help was received with the inauguration of the new Indonesian health care system in 1974. In this system every district (with approximately 20 000 inhabitants on Java and 10 000 inhabitants outside Java) has at least one health centre, with one nurse and one doctor. These district health centres feed into regional hospitals (C. hospitals) which are staffed by one surgeon, one internist, one gynaecologist and one pediatrician and which are capable of dealing with the common medical and surgical problems. The regional hospitals (C. hospitals) in turn will feed into provincial hospitals

(B. hospitals), which are fully staffed and usually connected with a medical school. In these B hospitals there is usually a department of neurology, with an EEG. At the top of this health referral system are the two teaching hospitals in Jakarta and Surabaya (A hospitals), which can offer all the facilities of modern neurology. Since this system was established, the staff of the department of neurology has frequently visited and given postgraduate lectures and demonstrations for the doctors working in the regional hospitals and the district health centres. The rationale behind this scheme was that excellent neurological health care could only be given if the doctors manning these hospitals were sufficiently and regularly upgraded on the advances and capabilities of modern epileptology.

The use of teachers in helping identify patients

In Indonesia every child between 6 and 12 years is obliged to attend an elementary school. As there is at least one school in every district, which is usually used in two shifts (one in the morning and one in the afternoon) it was easy to ask the help of the teachers in identifying epileptic patients, as was done by Edoo (1978). As each school was visited at least once a month by the district physician, he could examine and treat if necessary the suspected epileptic patients. After four years experience it could be observed that elementary school teachers were a reliable and fruitful source of referral of epileptic children.

AETIOLOGICAL FACTORS

From clinical surveys done in rural areas and in big towns like Surabaya, it is evident that several factors play an important role in the pathogenesis and causation of epilepsy.

Birth injury

Especially in rural areas birth injury to the brain was a leading cause of epilepsy. This was especially the case in areas in which a health centre had only recently been established and where deliveries formerly were done by non-medically

trained witch-women (*dukun*). With the establishment of district health centres, which offer better obstetrical and prenatal care, I am sure we could prevent this cause of seizures. During discussions with local physicians it was stressed repeatedly, that by simply offering better obstetrical and prenatal care and thereby preventing anoxia, we could prevent epilepsy in many children.

Meningoencephalitis

As in many other developing countries, both in rural and urban areas meningitis is frequently seen. During the acute phase, but more often as a sequella, convulsions do appear. It was therefore repeatedly stressed to general physicians that they should be aware of meningitis and treat it as rapidly and vigorously as possible to prevent convulsions and hydrocephalus. We made an appeal to the paediatricians to do a lumbar puncture in children who were suspected of having meningitis. With these measures we hope to suppress the incidence of these post-meningial fits.

Post-traumatic fits

Year by year the number of traumatic brain injuries is rising and with it the number of post-traumatic convulsions. In Indonesia most of the casualties are caused by collisions and falls of motor cycle drivers, because they are not wearing helmets (as in most other countries). We have therefore stressed and emphasised to students and doctors alike that they should use helmets and give an example to the layman how to protect the brain.

Alcohol is luckily not an important factor in Indonesia, because drinking alcohol is forbidden by the Islamic religion.

Febrile seizures (Chandra, 1978)

As in many other developing countries, infectious diseases are very frequent and, because of this, febrile seizures are so common that many parents don't pay much attention to them. This fact combined with the large distances between the patient's home and the doctor's office or health centres is the reason why prolonged convulsions are often not adequately treated (diazepam by intravenous injection). With these frequent prolonged convulsions the danger of complex partial seizures (psychomotor) later in life is significant and cannot be ignored. We have therefore stressed to paediatricians and general practitioners alike that if the parents are living far from a health centre or the doctor's office and the child has more than two febrile seizures, if he is younger or older than the usual age for febrile convulsions, or if the child has already a neurological defect, then he should be treated with prophylactic phenobarbitone because of the difficulty in suppressing rapidly these prolonged convulsions. These prolonged febrile fits are more frequent, because many parents in Indonesia lack medical knowledge and do not suppress quickly a rising body temperature with alcohol, tepid water or aspirin, but instead cover the child in a thick woollen blanket. Even in large towns it is still a common sight to see a child with high fever coming into the doctor's office wrapped in a thick blanket.

CLINICAL MANAGEMENT

Clinical management of epileptic patients may be divided into three sections:

Diagnosis

Ideally every new patient with seizures should be seen and examined by a neurologist (Aird & Woodbury, 1974; see also Ch. 4). This is difficult to realise in developing countries because of the large number of patients and the lack of neurologists. The following scheme has been used with success in East Java. The diagnosis may be considered under three headings:

1. Is it epilepsy?

As the diagnosis of epilepsy is made mainly on clinical grounds, it should be possible to give the responsibility of managing this section to the general practitioner, who has followed a special course on epileptology. This course should be given before the general practitioner departs for his health centre. It should be stressed that taking an extensive history (from the patient, from his family friends, fellow students or workers) is a prerequisite of establishing a good diagnosis.

A. Periodic attacks of neurological symptoms without diminishing consciousness are usually not epilepsy. For instance transient ischaemic attacks, tetany and migraine can be differentiated by detailed questioning. Also the often encountered hyperventilation syndrome can be easily recognised.

B. If the attacks are accompanied by a lowering of consciousness then a differential diagnosis should be made with syncope, by observing the following points:

1. Did the patient collapse after a strong emotional stress or did it happen in a room filled with people to a patient who had not eaten sufficient breakfast?
2. How long was the duration of the attack? Syncope usually lasts some seconds, while the duration of an epileptic attack is between 5 to 15 minutes.
3. Did the attack begin with a cry? Grand mal attacks sometimes begin with a cry, syncope never.
4. Was there urinary incontinence? Convulsions often are accompanied by incontinence, syncope never.
5. Was there tongue biting? Epilepsy often shows tongue biting, syncope never.
6. How was the patient's face? During convulsions the patient's face is often flushed, in syncope the patient is pale.
7. Was the patient lying in bed when the attack began? Syncope, while the patient is lying, is rare. A grand mal attack can occur anywhere.
8. How was the patient after the convulsion? An epileptic patient is often confused and sleepy after a convulsion, a patient with a syncope is alert.
9. Carry out an EEG in cases of doubt. The record of a grand mal patient often shows spikes, while the record of a pateint with syncope is normal.

C. Generalised seizures have to be differentiated from psychogenic fits. In this respect the following points are worth observing:

1. How long was the duration of the attack? Psychogenic seizures may last hours or even days, a grand mal attack usually lasts between 5 to 15 minutes, except in patients with status epilepticus.
2. Was there urinary incontinence? In grand mal epilepsy incontinence is rather common, in hysterical seizures it is never seen.
3. In generalised seizures injuries caused by tongue biting or falling are frequent, in psychogenic pseudoseizures they are never seen.
4. In grand mal attacks the movements follow a certain (constant) pattern, while in hysterical seizures the movements are bizarre and inconsistent.
5. An 'unconscious' patient because of an hysterical seizure can be aroused by pain, a grand mal patient will remain unconscious.
6. Generalised seizures may occur anywhere, psychogenic seizures often occur in circumstances where they may attract a large audience.
7. After the convulsion, the grand mal patient is confused and sleepy (post-ictal phase), the patient with pseudo-seizures is fully alert.

D. In children the differential diagnosis of convulsions with breath-holding attacks may be difficult.

In breath-holding spells the child usually does not move his arms or legs as during convulsions, but cries loudly and then stops breathing in the expiration phase. Because of this an anoxaemia develops and the child becomes unconscious. The child then becomes flaccid, starts breathing regularly and falls asleep. The good observer will note that there are no real convulsions in breath-holding attacks.

2. *Which type of epilepsy?*

It is the duty of a neurologist to distinguish between the various types of epilepsy. Points worth observing are:

A. Some neurologists working only in the big cities have the impression that absences (pure petit mal attacks) are rare in developing countries. Like Edoo (1978) the author has the experience that, if a persistent search is made for patients with absences, by surveying the schools (with the help of the teachers) and testing the suspected children with an EEG, it will show that the frequency of petit mal in developing countries is the same as in Europe or the United States.

B. Because of clouding of consciousness, patients with psychomotor epilepsy are often referred to psychiatrists. To help these patients it is recommended that regular courses are given to general practitioners and psychiatrists about the symptoms of temporal lobe epilepsy. It must be stressed in these courses, that patients with lowered consciousness, who do seemingly purposeful movements, who smack their lips or chew repeatedly, should be referred to a neurologist, who by arranging an EEG can establish the right diagnosis. Often only a sleep record will reveal the temporal lobe seizure.

3. *Aetiology*

A. In Indonesia and in other South East Asian countries, focal seizures are often caused by arterio-venous malformations. Therefore in any unexplained focal seizure arteriography is often necessary to establish the right diagnosis.

B. Compared with Europe or the United States, meningoencephalitis is still one of the main causes of convulsions. In developing countries, fever and convulsions are always an indication for a lumbar puncture to exclude an inflammatory disease.

Section 1 should be the responsibility of the general practitioner in the local health centre. The few cases, in which the general practitioner cannot decide whether it is epilepsy or not, he should refer to the neurologist in the hospitals. Sections 2 and 3 should be in the hands of the neurologist, who has an EEG machine.

Treatment

In general the principals of treatment are similar to that in other countries, except for some constraints.

A. *The shortage of doctors and nurses.* The lack of physicians and paramedical personnel in developing countries makes effective treatment of prolonged convulsions often difficult. Intravenous injections with diazepam have to be administered by nurses or physicians. Until now, no other drug is known which is as effective as diazepam in stopping prolonged convulsions, but which can be injected intramuscularly. Because phenobarbitone cannot be given at the same time as diazepam (respiration difficulties) we have warned the general practitioners not to use phenobarbitone to stop a prolonged convulsions or status epilepticus.

B. In most developing countries the so-called front-line drugs like diazepam, phenytoin, carbamazepine and phenobarbitone are available. The newer drugs like clonazepam or sodium valproate are often not available or difficult to get.

C. Estimation of serum drug levels is often not possible. In Indonesia only the top-referral hospitals (A hospitals) have facilities for monitoring serum drug levels, but the B hospitals where most of the epileptic patients are treated cannot do serum level monitoring.

D. In most developing countries health insurance is still in an embrionic stage or non-existent. Because most of the epileptic patients are poor and antiepileptic therapy lasts several years, the doctors have to choose not only the most effective drug for the seizure type, but also have to consider the price of the drug the patient can afford to pay.

E. In Indonesia, like in many developing countries, liver diseases are frequent. Therefore every doctor treating epileptic patients has to realise the influence of the liver metabolism on the pharmacokinetics of antiepileptic drugs, before adjusting the dosage.

F. As most of the patients visiting an epileptic clinic are simple village people, extra effort and time is required to educate these patients regarding the long term nature of antiepileptic therapy. For good results in the management of epilepsy, intelligent co-operation of the patient is required.

Treatment of status epilepticus

As in other developing countries, status epilepticus is often seen in Indonesia. In my experience status epilepticus often occurs because of:

1. Sudden discontinuance of antiepileptic therapy
2. Meningoencephalitis
3. Subarachnoid or intracerebral bleeding
4. Acute electrolyte disturbances

As in other unconscious states, the first task of a doctor, when confronted with a patient in status epilepticus should be to maintain an open airway with sufficient respiratory ventilation. After that, a slow intravenous injection of diazepam (10 mg) should be given, which may be repeated after two hours if necessary. A combination of diazepam and phenobarbitone should be avoided to prevent respiratory difficulties. Immediately after control of the convulsions, phenytoin should be given to ensure better control, because diazepam is a short acting drug. After the convulsions have ceased, the patient should be admitted to hospital for a complete work-up.

Inter-ictal antiepileptic treatment

The inter-ictal treatment of patients with epilepsy will be discussed under three headings:

1. When to start antiepileptic treatment
2. The technique of treatment
3. When to stop treatment

When to start antiepileptic treatment. In developing countries the decision to start antiepileptic treatment should be taken by a neurologist because:

1. Antiepileptic treatment is a long term treatment, which means a heavy burden for the usually uninsured patient.
2. The epileptic patient needs regular supervision, which again means loss of time and more expense.
3. The treatment of the different types of epilepsy is not the same and therefore before starting the treatment the physician should first determine the electro-clinical type of epilepsy, from which the patient is suffering. This means an EEG is required and a neurologist to read the record.

In the department of neurology, Airlangga University, we have decided not to give antiepileptic drugs to a patient:

1. Who has had only one attack
2. Who has less than one seizure a year, provided the inter-ictal EEG is normal

The technique of treatment. Once it has been

decided to start treatment, the following rules should be used:

1. Always start with one drug. Because in developing countries serum levels of the anti-epileptic drug cannot be estimated, the drug used is usually increased in dosage until the convulsions are controlled or until signs of intoxication develop. If more than one drug is used, observation of these signs will be more difficult. Monotherapy will also be of advantage if a drug allergy develops. The third reason, why monotherapy is advised, is that if we use more than one drug, one has to take into account the drug interactions.

2. *Always start with a low dose.* Many antiepileptic drugs will give side-effects at first. By starting with a low dose these side-effects will be less.

3. Increase the dosage of the drug slowly, and only change the dosage after there is a stabilisation of the serum drug level. As the serum drug level only becomes stable after four times the half-life of the drug used, the half-life of each antiepileptic drug should be known. Phenobarbitone with a half-life of 96 hours, will only reach a stable serum level after 16 days.

4. Every neurologist is advised to use only the antiepileptic drugs with which he has had experience. Because in developing countries estimation of drug levels is often not possible, one should increase the dosage slowly until the convulsions cease or until toxic complications develop. Therefore every physician working with antiepileptic drugs should know these complications and he should only work with the drugs with which he is familiar.

5. As most of the patients are people living in the villages, who are busy all day and do not pay enough attention to the regular intake of the antiepileptic drugs, one has to instruct the patient and his family to put the day dosage in a small box. This box should be filled each evening to diminish errors because of forgetting.

6. In developing countries control of patients' compliance cannot be done by measuring drug levels. Instead the doctor has to advise his patients to bring to the doctor's office all tablets which are left, when they come for their monthly physical examination.

7. As most of the developing countries have a tropical climate, it is advisable not to prescribe antiepileptic drugs in the form of a suspension or syrup, as the concentration may change because of evaporation. It is much better to use capsules or tablets.

8. In grand mal patients the first choice of an epileptic drug should be phenytoin. If it does not help it may be combined with carbamazepine. The same choice should be made in case of focal motor attacks. In case of absences the first choice should be ethosuximide. If it does not help one should search for clonazepam or sodium valproate, which are both difficult to get in developing countries. In minor motor attacks, one should try first sodium valproate and clonazepam as a second drug if sodium valproate does not decrease the attacks. In temporal lobe epilepsy the first drug used should be carbamazepine.

9. As there is a wide variation in body weight between people living in rural and urban areas, it is advisable to administer antiepileptic drugs on a mg/kg basis.

When to stop treatment. When the patient has been free of attacks for three years, one may decrease the dosage of the antiepileptic drug slowly and try to stop it after six months. In cases of grand mal attacks usually no recurrence of convulsions is seen, but in complex partial seizures one often has to continue giving drugs for a longer time.

Prognosis

The prognosis depends upon the following factors.

The aetiology

In cases of infections (meningoencephalitis) the prognosis is often better than in cases of trauma, neoplasms or vascular disease.

The type of epilepsy

For instance myoclonic epilepsy is difficult to control.

The age of the patient

Attacks of secondary generalised epilepsy in early childhood are often resistent to therapy.

PREVENTION

As in many other diseases, prevention is very important. In developing countries many factors can be corrected easily, if the patient pays enough attention. Several factors which may be improved are as follows.

Better obstetrical care

In many infants, convulsions are caused by cerebral bleedings, which develop during parturition. In breech presentation of the baby it is often better to deliver the baby by the abdominal route than by the vaginal one. Vaginal delivery may cause more lacerations to the cerebral bloodvessels. The aim of every doctor should not only be to deliver a living baby but a healthy baby.

Combat meningoencephalitis

Every physician working in a developing country should be aware that infections are still frequent. Especially in children, he should diagnose and treat meningitis by doing a lumbar puncture in every suspected case. Only this aggressive approach will decrease the post-encephalitic convulsions which are so common in developing countries.

Decrease the incidence of traumatic brain injuries

The incidence of traumatic brain injuries, with its consequent rise in post-traumatic convulsions, is increasing faster in developing countries than in the United States. In three years the incidence of traumatic brain injuries in the general hospital in Surabaya, which is the only hospital which receives emergency traffic accidents, has risen by 100 per cent. Although it is not entirely the duty of the doctor to lower this extremely high figure, he should try to advise the authorities regarding the following points:

1. As most of the head injuries occur to motor bike riders, who do not use a helmet, everyone riding one should be strongly advised to use a helmet. Doctors and medical students should set an example.
2. Decrease the speed limit.
3. Make separate lanes for rapid moving cars and the slower traffic, consisting of bicycles, oxcarts etc.
4. Persuade the general public, not to drive a motor vehicle, when they feel ill.

Febrile convulsions

This factor has been explained in the section on aetiology.

REHABILITATION

As a physician, one should be aware, that besides treating the patient with drugs, one should always try to restore the patient to society. This vocational rehabilitation is usually not present in developing countries, although it is needed more than in Europe or the United States. The large professional workshops, who do this rehabilitation so efficiently in Europe, usually are non-existent and the neurologist has to ask the help of volunteers to arrange small programmes. What one can do is usually to help in the placement of the patients.

School problems in epilepsy

Because of misinformation children with epilepsy are often refused admittance in schools. To alter this, courses were given to the school-teachers with the purpose of changing their attitude. In these courses explanation was given in simple terms regarding the nature of epilepsy. It was stressed that the epileptic child needed a normal school and not a special school, where overprotection easily developed.

Marriage problems in epileptic patients

More than in advanced countries, the belief is widely held in developing countries that epilepsy is a hereditary disease and that marriage with an epileptic patient should be avoided. We have tried to change this ignorance, by:

1. Giving courses to district doctors, in the hope that they in turn explain to teachers and district chiefs the modern concepts of epilepsy.
2. Distributing leaflets explaining in simple terms the fundamental aspects of epilepsy.
3. Playing cassette-recorders in waiting rooms of hospitals with essential information regarding the nature of epilepsy.

It is hoped that in this manner superstition and confusion regarding epilepsy and convulsions will decrease.

Employment problems in epileptic patients

In developing countries, more than in the U.S.A. and Europe it is very difficult for an epileptic patient to get work. First of all because jobs even for normal people are not abundant, but also because of wrong public attitudes based upon poor information. We have tried to overcome this by giving leaflets to big firms and important business men and we have tried to stimulate hospitals and medical schools to set an example by using epileptic patients for jobs, whenever possible.

SUMMARY

In this chapter we have tried to highlight the importance of epilepsy in developing countries and the problems facing a neurologist when working with epileptic patients. We have advocated a health referral scheme which may be used in developing countries to treat epilepsy on a wide basis with the limited resources available. Much still needs to be done, but we are convinced that by hard work and the intelligent use and distribution of doctors, nurses and facilities, we will after some time get the same results with antiepileptic treatment as in more affluent countries.

REFERENCES

Aird R.B. & Woodbury D.M. (1974) *The management of epilepsy*, p. 239. Springfield: Charles C. Thomas.
Chandra B. (1978) Management of febrile convulsions. In Meinardi, H. & Rowan, A.J. (eds) *Advances in epileptology*, p. 308. Amsterdam: Swets & Zeitlinger.
Edoo B.B. (1978) Absences in Ghanaian children – The problem of diagnosis in a developing country. In Meinardi, H. & Rowan, A.J. (eds) *Advances in epileptology*, p. 420. Amsterdam: Swets & Zeitlinger.
Tower D.B. (1978) Epilepsy: a world problem. In Meinardi, H. & Rowan, A.J. (eds) *Advances in epileptology*, p. 2. Amsterdam: Swets & Zeitlinger.

13

Epilepsy and work

E.A. Rodin

For the overwhelming majority of human beings meaningful employment is essential not only for a livelihood, but also for the maintenance of self-esteem. Yet, all too often the epileptic patient faces seemingly insurmountable hurdles in obtaining or maintaining this goal. Until a few years ago, it was felt that the unpredictable occurrence of seizures and the attitudes of employers were the main factors in a patient's problems with work. Recent investigations have shown, however, that these are only two facets and not necessarily the most important ones in the difficulties experienced by many patients in the employment market. Our own work (Dennerll *et al.*, 1966; Rodin *et al.*, 1972; Rodin, Shapiro and Lennox, 1977) as well as that of de Torres (1963), Juul-Jensen (1961) and Sillanpää (1973) has demonstrated that motivation to work, good intelligence, especially Verbal I.Q., and absence of major psychiatric difficulties provided the best criteria whether or not a given patient will be employed. The fact that seizure frequency or seizure type did not correlate with employment status in several of our own multivariate statistical studies (Rodin, 1968) was rather surprising, and led us subsequently to a more detailed look at the data. When the sample was considered as a whole, there was no statistically significant difference between employed and unemployed patients with respect to frequency of seizures. However, when a group of patients who had seizures less than once a year was compared with those who had seizures more frequently, employment status indeed became statistically significant, as Table 13.1 shows. This is an important observation because it points to the necessity for total seizure control rather than being satisfied with only 'improvement' of seizure frequency. While it is clear that this goal is not going to be achieved in every instance, it needs to be emphasised because the epilepsy specialist, unfortunately, sees patients whose treatment all too often has been neglected initially by the physician and subsequently by the patient. Under- or over-medication with concomitant seizures or side effects is unfortunately still rather common and so is the use of improper medication for the seizure type(s) the patient presents. For a patient to have maximum opportunity to achieve a meaningful life

Table 13.1 114 males with completed education

Seizure frequency	Employed	Unemployed	Seizure frequency	Employed	Unemployed
Less than once a year	21	5	Less than once a year	21	5
About once a year	3	3	Once a year or more	41	47
2 to 3 a year	4	9			
4 to 6 a year	5	7			
7 to 12 a year	4	3	Total	62	52
Once a month	5	4			
2 to 3 a month	10	5	$X^2 = 9.45$		
Once a week	0	3	$P < 0.01$		
Several a week	10	12			
Total	62	52			

$t = 1.68$, not significant

in spite of the illness, several conditions have to be met:

1. A supportive family situation
2. A physician who acts not only as diagnostician and dispenser of medication, but also as adviser as to what is and what is not possible
3. A patient who is willing to take advice and is determined to minimise the impact of the disorder on his life.

To achieve the needed reduction of seizure frequency mentioned above, all three of these conditions have to be fulfilled unless the illness is very mild.

Since our previous studies had shown that motivation, intellect and intact personality structure were the most important variables for the success or failure on the employment market, we subsequently divided our population into four groups:

1. Patients who had seizures but were intact in all other respects – 'epilepsy only'
2. Patients who had associated intellectual or organic mental changes
3. Patients who had associated behavioural disturbances
4. Patients who had associated other handicaps such as hemiplegia, blindness, or severe ataxia.

Of 369 patients who had undergone comprehensive evaluation at the Epilepsy Center of Michigan (ECM) between 1970 and 1974, only 23 per cent fell into the 'epilepsy only' category. 48 per cent had epilepsy with associated intellectual disturbances, 54 per cent had associated psychiatric problems and 10 per cent, other organic handicapping conditions. When one subsequently compared the 'epilepsy only' group with the other three groups combined, calling them 'epilepsy associated with other handicaps', it became apparent that the 'epilepsy only' population had done very well in regard to work, as shown in Table 13.2. If the total population involved in the study is considered (N 369), the percentage of those having no appreciable work impairment is 67.5 per cent. Accurate statistics from other sources are difficult to obtain, but a recent study carried out in the United Kingdom is notable in this context (MacIntyre, 1976). It dealt with a work force of

Table 13.2 Employment characteristics of patients with epilepsy only and those who have additional other handicaps

Intensity of work impairment	Epilepsy only N86	Epilepsy with other handicaps N283 percentages
None	92.3	42.8
Minimal	0	5.7
Mild	2.5	14.2
Moderate	0	16.1
Marked	5.1	20.9
	F 26.8	P 0.01
Usual occupation		
Habitually unemployed	0	32.9
Unskilled or semiskilled	32.0	45.7
Skilled or lower white collar	44.0	15.9
Upper white collar	24.0	5.3
Professional or executive	0	0
	F 24.8	P 0.01

150 000 people supervised by 29 industrial physicians, in which there were 177 epileptic individuals, 150 or 89 per cent of whom had no employment difficulty. While this figure is quite impressive, it needs closer scrutiny. The overall prevalence for epilepsy was assumed to be 0.5 per cent, which is probably a somewhat conservative estimate. On the basis of this estimate, it was stated that there are about 300 000 persons in Britain who have epilepsy and at least 100 000 are in the work force. If one-third of all epileptic patients are in the work force, then the prevalence of the epileptic patients found in the sample should have been 0.16 when in fact it was 0.11. It appears therefore that some patients may have been missed. What is also important is the observation that 61 per cent of the patients had less than one attack a year and only 9 per cent had more than five episodes a year. 91 per cent of these patients had therefore a relatively mild seizure disorder which undoubtedly contributed to their successful employment. This can be contrasted with the rather unsatisfactory outcome of rehabilitation services reported on by Freeman and Gayle (1978), where 70 per cent of the patients had active seizure disorders. Sillanpää (1973) found likewise that frequent seizures were detrimental to employment. Since intractable seizures are more commonly found in brain-damaged individuals who also show associated intellectual and/or psychiatric problem, employment difficulties would be expected for

these reasons, even if seizure frequency was not a relevant variable.

If our own figure, that 67.5 per cent of all epilepsy patients have no appreciable employment problems, were to be representative for the epilepsy population at large, it would be quite respectable. The figure, regardless of its accuracy does not, however, take into account the type of work the patients are doing and as our studies as well as those of Sillanpää have shown, a disproportionate number of patients with epilepsy are employed in unskilled and poorly paid jobs. This underemployment can cause psychological problems for the patient and was the reason why the term 'meaningful employment' was used in the opening sentence of this chapter.

How then can the employment situation of the patient be improved further? The problem can be divided into several distinct but interrelated categories:

a. Efforts required by the physician
b. Efforts required by the family
c. Efforts required by the patient
d. Efforts required by the rehabilitation counsellor
e. Efforts required by society at large

a. Physician's efforts

Until recently, the physician was quite handicapped in his treatment efforts because there was no way of knowing whether a patient was indeed taking the drugs as prescribed. Routine determinations of antiepileptic drug levels have obviated this problem and it has been demonstrated that compliance with a given drug regime improved markedly when a patient was seen frequently and the antiepileptic drug levels monitored. This is important at any stage of the illness, but especially so at the beginning. There seems little doubt now that each seizure tends to pave the way for the next one with its physiological and psychological consequences and there is an increasing literature on such kindling and secondary epileptogenesis.

It is therefore necessary for the physician to take this into account when confronted with a new patient so that, together with family and patient, an optimal regimen can be achieved. While this regimen is usually based primarily on drugs and

advice as to appropriate living habits, it should not be unduly prolonged in cases of temporal lobe epilepsy, especially when a unilateral focus is present. A patient with this type of epilepsy who continues to have frequent, pronounced complex partial seizures with associated behavioural automatisms should, after one to two years of intensive drug treatment, be referred to a surgical centre for evaluation of the feasibility of anterior temporal lobectomy. In well-selected cases, the results are excellent not only in improved seizure control, but also in the overall functioning of the patients, including employment (Taylor & Falconer, 1968; Jensen, 1976). They also emphasised that patients operated on surgically under 18 years of age had a better social prognosis than those who underwent the surgery later in life. This may well be related to the factor of secondary epileptogenicity, as well as to faulty social and academic learning. This is emphasised because although it is commonly agreed that the attitudes of the patients and society towards epilepsy have to be changed, it is equally necessary for us, as physicians, to re-evaluate our own attitudes in order to be of most benefit to our patients by keeping abreast with results of treatment other than with drugs.

The physician also has an important duty to provide the lay public with accurate information on the nature and consequences of the illness so that realistic rather than Utopian legislation can be enacted.

b. Family efforts

Since approximately 80 per cent of all seizure disorders start before the age of majority, a considerable proportion of the responsibility for early successful management rests on the shoulders of parents. The family plays a vital role in determining to what extent the patient's illness will be compounded by social effects. If the family shows reasonable but not undue concern, enforces good medication habits, sees to it that regularly scheduled medical appointments are kept and is accepting rather than rejecting or overprotecting, then a solid foundation will have been laid for the patient's future behaviour, when he is left on his own. If the family is having problems in coping with the patient's illness, they must have counselling available from someone with a knowledge of epilepsy.

c. Patient's efforts

Whatever else is being done, it is most important to obtain the full co-operation of the patient in the total treatment regimen. All too often, one is confronted with the proverbial horse which can be led to water, but which won't drink. The causes are multiple and may be related to rejection or denial of the illness, adolescent rebellion against authority, or to a more severe personality disorder. For treatment to be successful, it is essential that the role of the patient be outlined at the initial evaluation and subsequently reinforced on each return visit. The physician must not be lulled into a false sense of security by reassuring statements from the patient that everything is all right, when he will continue to prescribe drugs without checking serum levels and the EEG when indicated. Young patients, especially when unaccompanied by family members, usually minimise their problems in order to obtain relaxation of strictures, particularly in regard to obtaining a driver's licence. They may also hide poor school performance which can subsequently lead to failure on the employment market. The patient needs to be confronted with this so that he realises it is not the physician he is fooling, only himself. Sometimes it even takes the occurrence of a grand mal seizure to bring the patient face to face with the potential seriousness of his disorder. The following case report illustrates this aspect:

The patient was first seen at ECM in 1975 at the age of 12. During the previous year, he had suffered from episodes which were regarded as day-dreaming. He stopped talking in mid-sentence, lost track of the conversation, had a blank facial expression, was unresponsive and subsequently scratched his sides for a few seconds. There were no aftereffects. Initially he had been placed by his physician on 250 mg of ethosuximide a day which was subsequently increased to 500 mg. The attacks, although improved, still occurred several times per day. The rest of the past history was unremarkable. He came from a stable family, was well behaved and an intelligent, good student. On psychological testing at ECM he scored a Verbal IQ of 103, Performance IQ of 118 and Full Scale IQ of 111. He was regarded as an overachiever, very motivated at school, no signs of organic central nervous system disturbance were found and he was felt to be emotionally intact. The EEG showed high voltage atypical spike-wave activity, maximal in the left hemisphere.

As a result of his visit to ECM, ethosuximide was

increased to 1g a day and further improvements was noted within one month, although he still continued to have attacks. It was therefore increased to 1.25g a day, but, at that dosage, the ethosuximide level of 1505 μg/1 (212 μg/ml) was in the toxic range and he experienced considerable dizziness. It was reduced again to 1g a day. For two months he had no further attacks. Since the parents were concerned about the possibility of grand mal seizures occurring, 200 mg of phenytoin were added but the patient became too drowsy and the parents reduced the phenytoin to 100 mg.

Six months later, he was seen at follow-up. He had not experienced any further attacks. The phenytoin level was 36 μmol/1 (9 μg/ml), ethosuximide 646 μmol/1 (91 μg/ml) on a dosage of 1g of ethosuximide and 100 mg of phenytoin. Two years later, he was seen again in re-evaluation. Clinically he was intact, the EEG showed only quite minor non-specific changes and he had been seizure-free for two and a half years. It was decided therefore to take him off drugs, especially since the phenytoin level at that time was only 16 μmol/1 (4 μg/ml) and ethosuximide 426 μmol/1 (60 μg/ml). It seemed likely that he had been neglecting his treatment régimen but because school was still in session, his drugs were continued until the summer vacation. He returned six months later on 22.6.78. He was again clinically intact but the phenytoin level had dropped to 8 μmol/1 (2 μg/ml) and ethosuximide 114 μmol/1 (16 u g/ml) in spite of supposedly continued regular doses. On this occasion the EEG showed several atypical spike-wave discharges and a sensitivity to photic stimulation. The results of the test were explained to the mother and the patient with the advice that the antiepileptic drugs could not be discontinued at this time because of the danger of a grand mal seizure occurring. Phenytoin was increased to 300 mg. He was also given a return appointment in 14 days. On 10.7.78, clinically he was still doing well but the phenytoin level had only risen to 32 μmol/1 (8 μg/ml) and ethosuximide 227 μmol/1 (32 μg/ml). The EEG showed again spike-wave activity. The need for adequate drugs was re-emphasised to the patient and his mother and phenytoin was increased to 350 mg by adding a 50 mg dose in the morning. A return appointment was scheduled in three weeks for another blood level but on 28.7.78 a phone call was received from the mother reporting that he had had a grand mal seizure in the morning. She was told to bring him to ECM for an immediate blood level. On that occasion, phenytoin was 12 μmol/1 (3 μg/ml) and ethosuximide 57 μmol/1 (8 μg/ml). He had a second grand mal seizure while at the Center. Although he had previously insisted that his drugs were being taken regularly, he now admitted to having neglected them. Within one week, he showed clinical toxicity on the previously mentioned phenytoin dose of 350 mg and the level was 128 μmol/1 (32 μg/ml). Phenytoin was therefore reduced to 325 mg, toxicity cleared up and the level dropped to 112 μmol/1 (28 μg/ml). At follow-up on 19.10.78 there had been no further seizures and the phenytoin level had again dropped to 44 μmol/1 (11 μg/ml) in spite of a supposed intake of 325 mg. To rule out laboratory error, another level was obtained within 48 hours which was only 56 μmol/1 (14 μg/ml) The mother and patient were again confronted with the necessity for adhering to the prescribed treatment. Three months later, the phenytoin level was 92 μmol/1 (23 μg/ml) and the ethosuximide 327 μmol/1 (46 μg/ml). There had been no seizures and the EEG was normal. At his most recent visit on 5.3.79 he was still seizure-free and the phenytoin level was 96 μmol/1 (24

μg/ml), ethosuximide 298 μmol/1 (42 μg/ml) on the same doses. The EEG was again normal.

This patient clearly has a good prognosis if his drugs are taken regularly and he should not become a problem to society, and should be capable of finding work on his own. He will be followed on a three-monthly basis so that he knows his treatment is under scrutiny. If there are no further seizures within a five-year period from December, 1978, another attempt can be made to reduce and discontinue his antiepileptic drugs provided the EEG remains normal.

If patients reject their treatment altogether, they need to be referred for psychotheraphy but, at this stage, the prognosis must already be quite guarded because negativistic patients do not make good candidates for psychotherapy.

d. Role of the rehabilitation counseller

Sooner or later the majority of unemployed epileptic patients will have some contact with a rehabilitation agency. Although frequently a great deal of honest effort is expended, the results are not encouraging at present, as has been shown in the previously mentioned study by Freeman and Gayle (1978) which will be discussed in more detail later. Apart from the problems presented by the patient, there are additional ones because frequently rehabilitation counsellers receive inadequate training in the field of epilepsy. All too often, the counseller is not aware of modern treatment, its relative effectiveness, the side-effects of antiepileptic drugs, the common behavioural changes which may occur and the need for a close liaison with a specialised unit which will treat the patient with up-to-date methods while the rehabilitation programme is going on.

Counsellers are recommended strongly to study the book 'Epilepsy Rehabilitation' Wright (1975) and the paper 'Rehabilitation and the Client with Epilepsy: A Survey of the Client's View of the Rehabilitation Process and its Results' Freeman and Gayle (1978).

e. Role of society at large

While the previous comments apply, in theory at least, to most countries around the world, the role of society in helping the individual with epilepsy will vary from culture to culture. Within the Western world, the United States has set and is still setting an example for a progressively more humane approach toward minorities and the handicapped. Regardless of the faults and failures that accompany this drive, it is important to recognise that the goal towards a 'barrier free' society has been expressed and gradually is being put into practice. Barriers are beginning to fall in this country and attitudes are changing as evidenced by a number of judicial and legislative decrees.

The National Rehabilitation Act of 1973 prohibits discrimination on the basis of physical or mental handicap. Although it does not require an employer to 'hire the handicapped', it was designed to assure a handicapped person an equal chance of employment if he is as competent as an able-bodied applicant. This Act has no official binding force on private industry, but it does apply to federal agencies and those private companies receiving federal contracts in excess of $2500. The definition of handicapped in the federal law is 'any person who (1) has a physical or mental impairment which substantially limits one or more of such person's major life activities, (2) has a record of such impairment, or (3) is regarded as having such an impairment'. While the intent is admirable, implementation has been lagging intermittently and injustices still persist. Nevertheless, the diligent and persevering individual now has an opportunity, through consumer advocates, to set legal machinery in motion to right a perceived wrong. The following is a recent example:

A patient was first seen at ECM in February, 1978, because he had been refused admission to qualifying examinations as a state trooper on the basis of his past history of epilepsy. He was 22 years old, intelligent, in good physical and mental health and had been seizure-free for 11 years. Antiepileptic drugs had been discontinued by his physician two and a half years before. The past history was negative apart from the fact that he had developed petit mal absences when he was 11 years old. Initial treatment was inadequate, and, after a series of petit mal seizures, one morning he had a grand mal attack. He was then placed on a combination of phenytoin and phenobarbitone and has never had a recurrence of either type of seizure.

At ECM, his neurological examination was negative and so was the EEG. Psychiatric evaluation revealed no evidence of emotional disturbance and he was regarded as being a well balanced, emotionally mature person. As a result of this evaluation, reports were sent to the medical consultant of the State Police Department giving these facts and concluding that 'the past history of his attacks should not be held against him for obtaining employment with the State Police'. In spite of this, the patient was again denied admission to the qualifying examinations because of a rule that prohibits employment by the State Police of individuals with a history of epilepsy. With the help of attorneys of the Protection and Advocacy Service for Developmentally Disabled Citizens, legal action was brought against the State Police Department citing Section 504 of the Federal Rehabilitation Act of 1973, which makes it illegal for any agency receiving federal funds to discriminate against a handicapped person solely on the basis of the person's handicap. A federal judge ruled in favour of the patient who was then admitted to and passed the required entrance examinations. He enrolled in the police academy during the Spring, 1979.

This case has implications which extend beyond the individual concerned because an attempt is now being made to remove the stigmatising rule from the books altogether. Medical testimony during the hearing stressed that while it was not possible to give an absolute assurance that the patient would never again have a seizure, it did appear unlikely and so he should at least be given a chance to show whether or not he was capable of performing the work, strenuous as it might be. It was furthermore argued that a blanket rule which automatically excluded any individual with epilepsy from a given job was unjust and that each case had to be decided on its own merits. It was fortunate that the patient found a sympathetic judge who resolved the issue promptly in his favour. This case is also important because it shows what can be accomplished in today's society towards overcoming stigmata, if the patient, the medical and the legal profession are united in their efforts.

As an expression of the growing concern about epilepsy, its consequences and possible prevention, the United States Senate established in 1975 The Commission for the Control of Epilepsy and its Consequences. The final report is now available and the salient pertinent features are as follows: In addition to other factors, two major barriers to employment were felt to be 'firstly the attitude of the employers who are often reluctant to hire people with epilepsy because they do not understand epilepsy; and secondly, the attitude of people with epilepsy themselves. Many seem insecure and defensive, possibly because of repeated rebuffs by potential employers, and many have behavioural, psychological and social problems'. 'Other important difficulties were: inadequate education, lack

of particular skills, poor efforts in seeking work, inadequate diagnosis and treatment, difficulty in getting to and from work for those who are not permitted to drive, failure by vocational rehabilitation agencies to deal with educational or medical problems, failure to match interest and potential with actual training or to match training with existing job opportunities. Lowly paid jobs can be a disincentive to work because of loss of Medicaid and other unemployment benefits. Such employment actually results in a lower income than when not working.' To overcome these problems, 73 specific recommendations were made which need not be repeated here, but can be found in the original document (U.S. Department of Health, Education and Welfare, 1978). Looking at the magnitude of the whole problem and considering the present state of the world's economy, the objectives quoted below read rather optimistically, especially when one considers the timetable involved:

> Assuring that by 1980 individualised education plans for all pre-school and school age children with epilepsy are available.
>
> Achieving by 1982 a reduction by half of the presently estimated 25 per cent unemployment rate among those with epilepsy and doubling the number of persons with epilepsy placed through rehabilitation programmes by improved vocational education, vocational rehabilitation, job training and placement services.
>
> Achieving by 1982 an increase in the number of severely handicapped persons with epilepsy in non-competitive employment from the currently estimated 4000 in sheltered workshops to 16 000 either in sheltered workshops or in equivalent non-competitive employment in industry.

While these objectives reflect what should be done, it is doubtful that they can be achieved in the near future and furthermore, the unemployment rate is probably closer to 33 per cent rather than 25 per cent.

A much greater effort by the schools is required to train adequately epileptic children to the maximum of their abilities. At this point, however, marked economic problems are being encountered. As mentioned in my previous report, 'epilepsy is not a popular cause and probably never will be. Only a relatively small proportion of the total population is affected and it is, therefore, unrealistic to hope for public funds to come pouring in to help with the educational needs' (Rodin *et al.*, 1972). Except for the passage of some Laws and Acts, nothing has changed to invalidate these statements. School Boards throughout the United States are still forced to cut back on their regular programmes rather than being able to expand services. When special programmes are indeed provided, as required by law, to multiple-handicapped epileptic patients, they are usually of a token variety rather than genuine educational efforts.

The feasibility of the objective to cut the unemployment rate to half by increasing rehabilitation efforts is also open to some doubt. It assumes that the majority of unemployed epileptic persons really want to work, an assumption that, as has been shown previously, is not necessarily valid. Our own experience is most enlightening in this respect. From October, 1974, to September, 1975, ECM participated in a joint project with the state Bureau of Rehabilitation and Jewish Vocational Service in order to ascertain how many chronically unemployed, multiple-handicapped epileptic patients could be successfully placed into the competitive job market when maximum resources were made available to them. The term 'multiple-handicapped' refers to patients who had epilepsy associated with other handicaps, as defined earlier in the chapter. Patients with 'epilepsy only' do not, in general, require rehabilitation because they are able to find jobs through their own resources. The results of this study are quite discouraging when viewed numerically and can be summarised as follows: 91 patients were identified for the project, but 33 either dropped out or were screened out prior to having had contact with ECM; 58 were evaluated and staffed by ECM for the programme, but only 44 of them were found to be suitable candidates. Patients with severe neurologic disability, e.g. spastic triplegia, were excluded. Of these 44, 25 completed the programme and 19 found employment subsequently. One year later, only 11 were still working and the number dropped to eight after two years. The successful rehabilitation rate from the total group of 91 unemployed was only 9 per cent; of those who were deemed able to benefit, it was 19 per cent and of those who completed the programme 32 per cent. The latter figure corresponds reasonably well to other reports published in the literature: Porter 59 per cent, Firestein 36 per cent and Juul-Jensen 31 per cent. It needs to be re-

emphasised, however, that these figures are inflated because they are derived only from individuals who found themselves able to complete a structured programme of several weeks duration and thus they represent a minority of the multiple-handicapped epileptic population. The true figure is probably much closer to 10 per cent when all unemployed epileptic patients are taken into account.

The previously cited report by Freeman and Gayle (1978) supports our experience. These investigators took a random sample of 183 people with epilepsy who were in the active files of the Maryland Division of Vocational Rehabilitation (DVR) for the fiscal year of 1974. They were all contacted by mail requesting their agreement to participate in a survey dealing with effectiveness of services provided by DVR. 67 agreed to be reviewed, but 20 could not be reached and only 47 surveys were completed. From this sample, four individuals were not accepted for training, twelve were still in training and 31 had completed training. Of these 31, 17 had obtained a job within six months of completion of training and, at the time of the survey, twelve were still on the same job. A major and probably unexpected finding was that of these 17 individuals, only three said that the Vocational Rehabilitation Counseller had found them a job. Ten had done so on their own, three were employed at their place of training and one had been employed through an agency. It is therefore clear that the number of epileptic patients who derive major profit from current day rehabilitation services is, unfortunately, quite small.

While this low success rate is disappointing, it should be pointed out that for successfully rehabilitated patients, a 'total push' programme of the type carried out in Detroit can indeed make a great deal of difference. One person with a long history of institutionalisation had, at the time of this report, been employed in the same job for three years and so was another who had previously been unemployed for twenty years. The follow-up period is still quite short and some of the patients who are working now may no longer be doing so in five or ten years time. One of the critical flaws in the published results on rehabilitation of epileptic patients is that the follow-up duration is either not mentioned at all or it is so short that the results are bound to decay in time.

The following example is that of a successfully rehabilitated patient.

A 47-year-old man was first seen at ECM in 1974 as part of the previously mentioned Vocational Rehabilitation study. He had suffered from non-focal grand mal seizures since the age of 17 years. Initially they had occurred once a month, but later on, in spite of inadequate treatment, they occurred only two to three times a year. With the onset of his seizure disorder, he was placed on phenytoin, 100 mg twice a day, but this was later reduced to 100 mg at bedtime.

His past medical history was negative and only his social history is of importance. He had been working until the age of 27 in a variety of unskilled jobs but, after having been laid off because of a seizure which had occurred while working in a department store, he no longer sought further work. He lived with his 73 year old widowed mother and he helped to look after the apartment. He described himself as a loner who led a quiet, socially restricted life. He had always had very few friends and at the time of his visit to the Center, he had none. However, both he and his mother were keen to take part in the project. As an example of his conscientious attitude, it may be mentioned that during a major snowstorm which practically paralysed the city, he telephoned the Epilepsy Centre to state that he would keep his laboratory appointment that day. The laboratory was closed as a matter of fact because personnel were unable to drive in and he was therefore advised to remain at home. Clinical neurological examination was normal and so were the routine laboratory tests. The EEG was also normal in spite of the fact that the patient had a phenytoin level of only 4 mol/l (1 g/ml), which was related to an extremely low intake and a weight of 93 kilograms. On psychiatric evaluation, it was noted that he was an extremely isolated and probably schizoid person, but that there was no appreciable suspiciousness. It was felt that if some type of unskilled employment could be found, where he would not be required to interact a great deal with others, he might be able to function quite well. On psychological testing, he achieved a Verbal IQ of 97, Performance IQ of 96, with a resultant Full Scale IQ of 96, which placed his ability within the average intellectual range. During testing, he was pleasant and co-operative but not verbally spontaneous. He had difficulty with the neuropsychological test battery in regard to visual-motor and pure motor speed. On the Minnesota Multiphasic Personality Inventory (MMPI) he showed repression and denial. He also appeared quite rigid in his thinking and it was felt that he could not adequately deal with stress and pressure. Although he was somewhat anxious in the testing situation, his self-confidence appeared to be within normal limits. The psychologist commented that he would be employable in a situation which did not require a great deal of decision making or motor speed.

As a result of his visit to the Center, his phenytoin dose was raised initially to 300 and subsequently 400 mg per day which resulted in a low therapeutic level of 40 mol/l (10 µg/ml). Since his seizure disorder was quite mild, the dose did not need to be increased any further. He was enrolled in a work evaluation programme and subsequently employed in the stockroom of one of the local hospitals. In the three and a half years up to the time of this report, he has risen to a supervisory position and has remained seizure-free.

This case demonstrates that a basically mild seizure disorder which would readily respond to treatment was neglected by the physician, leading to loss of employment and subsequently to complete social isolation. Nevertheless, the patient had a sufficiently sound personality to overcome two decades of unemployment and settle in a job that was appropriate for his abilities.

The following case vignette reflects a failure of efforts at rehabilitation because of the patient's lack of motivation.

A 28-year-old patient first seen in 1974 at the Epilepsy Center of Michigan, was referred by Michigan Employment Security Commission in order to assess his rehabilitation potential. Seizures of the non-focal grand mal variety had started at the age of 21. These occurred initially once a year, thereafter increased to five to six per year and for several months before being seen at the Center, they had occurred nearly every month. As a result of the increase in seizure frequency, he lost his job as an offset printer. When seen at the Center, he was being treated with phenytoin, 100 mg four times a day, phenobarbitone, 32 mg, three times a day, phenobarbitone spansule, 100 mg at bedtime, diazepam, 5 mg twice a day, troxidone, 300 mg, three times a day. He was on troxidone because of episodes when for a few moments he could not find the right answers to questions, although he had not been told of having associated staring or eye-blinking episodes.

His past history was negative apart from abuse of alcohol. However, he had cut down his alcohol intake after his last seizure three months ago and had not had a recurrence of seizures since then. Neurological examination was negative. The EEG showed diffuse, generalised spike-wave discharges with some atypical petit mal features. On psychiatric evaluation, it was felt that he was an inhibited schizoid type person, but that there was not sufficient indication to warrant psychiatric treatment. On psychological testing, he achieved a Verbal IQ of 94, Performance IQ of 86 with a resultant Full Scale IQ of 90 which placed his ability at the low end of the average range of intelligence. His personality structure showed mild depression, anxiety and poor self-esteem. The levels for phenytoin and phenobarbitone were 52 µmol/l (13 µg/ml) and 82 µmol/l (19 µg/ml) respectively. Diazepam and troxidone could not be measured. As a result of his visit to the Center, diazepam and phenobarbitone spansules were stopped but, in view of the EEG, troxidone was increased to 1.2 g a day. He was also placed in a work evaluation programme. There he was found to be perfectionistic, to show considerable rigidity, to be forgetful and unable to cope well with quick changes. Mathematics was one of his major areas of difficulty. After work exposure, he was trained in watchmaking and in spite of having had several attacks during the programme, he was hired by the training company. However, he was fired three months later because of an inability to get on with others on the job. Since he remained unemployed, he was seen by Vocational Rehabilitation Services but his continuation in that programme was made contingent on his receiving some counselling. This he refused. He continued to be followed subsequently at Lafayette Clinic and in view of increasing seizure frequency in spite of adequate antiepileptic drug levels, he was admitted for a five month period where further attempts were made to assess his work potential. He continued to have seizures during the first three months of hospitalisation but was seizure-free during the last two months. In the hospital, he was found to be quite demanding, frequently asking for changes in his anti-epileptic drugs which consisted of phenytoin, sodium valproate and subsequently carbamazepine. He complained of various side effects from sodium valproate and when this was changed to carbamazepine, he complained of side effects from that drug also and wanted to go back on phenobarbitone. Although pleasant and co-operative on the ward, he showed no appreciable motivation for work. After discharge, he relapsed into having major seizures with some post-ictal automatisms at a rate of one to two per month and he failed to follow through with any recommendations for vocational rehabilitation.

This patient has a moderately severe seizure disorder which, however, would have responded to adequate antiepileptic drugs had he been willing to put up with minor subjective side effects. However, his employment prospects will be non-existent unless he develops some motivation for work. His social situation is also quite undesirable because his elderly mother, with whom he lives, drinks alcohol to excess. Although intellectually intact, the patient is not sufficiently motivated to seek separate living arrangements outside the home. Unless and until he shows a change in his attitude towards employment, no rehabilitation efforts will be of any use.

It has been mentioned repeatedly that patient and employer attitudes towards epilepsy still constitute major employment barriers and the problem of disclosure has to be considered. Should the patient tell a prospective employer voluntarily that he has a history of epileptic attacks or should he hide the fact? A blanket answer covering each patient's situation cannot be given. It depends on the frequency, severity and time of occurrence of the attacks, as well as the nature of the job being applied for. Patients whose attacks occur exclusively in the sleeping or awakening state theoretically would not pose a problem, even if they worked as overhead crane operators. If there are frequent daytime attacks, it is likely that one will happen on the job and unless the patient is an exemplary employee, he may be laid off even if he has a desk job. The employer is within his rights to do this if the patient denied the fact that he has epilepsy on the application form and in so doing, forfeited his chance for any legal recourse. On the other hand, if the patient admits to his disorder, he may not be hired in the first place. My personal approach has always been to discuss the situation with the individual patient, informing him that if the job is not dangerous and he is not asked about having had epilepsy (or passing-out spells) he is under no obligation to mention it. However, if specifically confronted with this question, he must tell the truth, but he should also emphasise his skills and assets. Furthermore, I tell him that regardless of what happens legally, the illness will always be held against him by someone. He is urged to develop exceptional skills and a positive personality to reduce his chances of getting fired at the first opportunity. While an intact patient will understand these conditions, it is sometimes very difficult to explain to a multiple-handicapped person who has intellectual limitations, psychomotor slowing or dysphoria, or even paranoid traits.

As a part of the non-discrimination drive in the United States which I have mentioned, job application forms are actually being rewritten omitting any reference to epilepsy. Instead, strictly job-related terms have been used, for example: 'Do you have any physical handicaps or illnesses which might interfere with or be aggravated by your work?' A simple change of this type, if adopted throughout the world, would be a major step forward in helping patients gain and keep employment.

Especially in the United States patients are presented with another barrier which is frequently insurmountable. Inadequate public transport as well as long distances to work make the legal use of a car a necessity rather than a luxury. Laws differ between the various states of the Union, as shown in a recent survey by The Epilepsy Foundation of America (1976). Some states mandate a fixed period of freedom from seizures ranging from six months to three years; others require a physician's certificate indicating that the person is 'free from seizures while under medication' or the person 'can safely operate a motor vehicle'. The latter statement is a potentially hazardous one for the physician to make because a patient may well have a recurrence of seizures at some unpredictable time, resulting in a serious accident. The physician may then be sued for having declared it was 'safe' for the patient to drive. To protect everyone concerned, it would probably be best to follow the example set by the State of Wisconsin, namely, issuing a permit after a six month period free of seizures, renewable every six months until there has been a two year period free of attacks. A regular licence can then be issued. In addition to this general rule, there should be some mechanism for individual appeal in special cases. Restricted permits might also be issued which are limited to driving to and from work and the nearest shopping centre. This would cut down on driving time, thereby reducing the risks while allowing the patient to lead a reasonably normal life.

Finally, the problem of workman's compensation should be mentioned and the fear that many employers have that an epileptic patient's seizure will result in a serious injury which, in turn, would lead to exorbitant insurance costs. Several states in the United States have created a 'second injury fund' which would cover these contingencies. Although undoubtedly of benefit, it does not at present operate throughout the country. In order to qualify, however, a patient has to declare that he suffered from epilepsy prior to employment. A similar procedure is required if a patient wants to be protected by the anti-discrimination statutes. However, since the employer is under no obligation to hire a handicapped worker, disclosure may jeopardise a patient's chances of getting a job.

For all these reasons it is essential that decisions are made by the individual patient and his family, with the physician merely acting as an adviser giving the most accurate possible prognosis in regard to the likelihood of seizures occurring on the job. Knowledge of the following points will allow a reasonable prediction:

1. The duration of the illness

2. The seizure type(s)
3. The frequency and timing of attacks
4. Possible precipitating factors
5. The presence or absence of pronounced seizure patterns in the EEG when serum drug levels are in the therapeutic range.

Once a prognosis has been established and the patient and his family realise the limitations of prognostications, the final decision about disclosure rests with them.

Gaining and keeping employment will remain a problem for a considerable number of people with epilepsy. It is advisable that those having difficulties should have a comprehensive medical, social, psychological and psychiatric evaluation. Once completed, team members in charge of the multi-disciplinary work-up should meet in conference (as is done at ECM) with the rehabilitation specialist so that suitable employment recommendations can be made. The attempts at rehabilitating the multiple-handicapped epileptic patient, which have been discussed, show conclusively that 'follow-along' rather than 'follow-up' is essential to achieve lasting results. Members of the team have to be prepared to continue helping the patient wherever problems exist lest the initial efforts be wasted within a few months. Although evaluations of this sort are expensive, the cost will repay itself if the patient is eventually integrated into the work force. If the evaluation shows that a patient is clearly unsuitable and would be better off drawing disability benefits, further rehabilitation expenses are avoided. Nevertheless, since appropriate employment is of great significance to most people, anyone unable to find a job on his own deserves a chance to receive the type of evaluation described.

REFERENCES

Dennerll, R.D., Rodin, E.A., Gonzalez, S., Schwartz, M.L. & Lin, Y. (1966) Neurological and pyschological factors related to employability of persons with epilepsy. *Epilepsia*, **7**, 318.

de Torres, T. (1963) Employment problems of epileptics. Research and Demonstration Grant No. 382, Office of Vocational Rehabilitation, Washington, D.C.: Department of Health, Education and Welfare.

Epilepsy Foundation of America (1976) *The Legal Rights of Persons with Epilepsy*. Washington, D.C.: Epilepsy Foundation of America.

Freeman, J.M. & Gayle, E. (1978) Rehabilitation and the client with epilepsy: A survey of the client's view of the rehabilitation process and its results. *Epilepsia*, **19**, 233.

Jensen, I. (1976) Temporal lobe epilepsy: Social conditions and rehabilitation after surgery. *Acta Neurologica Scandinavica*, **54**, 22.

Juul-Jensen, P. (1961) Vocational training of epileptics. *Epilepsia*, **2**, 291.

MacIntyre, E. (1976) Epilepsy and employment. *Community Health*, **7**, 195.

Rodin, E.A. (1968) *Prognosis of Patients with Epilepsy*. Springfield, Illinois: Charles C. Thomas.

Rodin, E., Rennick, P., Dennerll, R. & Lin, Y. (1972) Vocational and educational problems of epileptic patients. *Epilepsia*, **13**, 149.

Rodin, E., Shapiro, H. & Lennox, K. (1977) Epilepsy and life performance. *Rehabilitation Literature*, **38**, 34.

Sillanpää, M. (1973) Medico-social prognosis of children with epilepsy: Epidemiological study and analysis of 245 patients. *Acta Paediatrica Scandinavica*, Supplement No. 237.

Taylor, D.C. & Falconer, M.A. (1968) Clinical, socio-economic and psychological changes after temporal lobectomy for epilepsy. *British Journal of Psychiatry*, **114**, 1247.

U.S. Department of Health, Education and Welfare (1978) *Plan for Nationwide Action on Epilepsy*, Vol. II, Part 1, by The Commission for the Control of Epilepsy and its Consequences. DHEW Publication No. (NIH) 78.

Wright, G.N. (ed.) (1975) *Epilepsy Rehabilitation*. Boston: Little, Brown & Co.

14

Dental problems in epilepsy

P. Westphal

An attractive smile means a good deal for the individual while he is growing up, especially as a teenager. Beautiful teeth are a symbol for youth and beauty, whereas loss of the teeth is a sign of aging. A pathological dentition can be fateful for anybody and this is especially true for someone who is already handicapped. Every defect leads to indirect, often emotional, consequences beyond the local, direct effect of the defect. These emotional consequences make adjustment as a whole more difficult. There is no reason to maintain that oral status is more important than anything else, but it is certainly as important.

There is an essential difference in certain aspects of the dental problems of the person with epilepsy as compared to those of other handicapped groups. Although only a few systematic studies have been conducted, it has been shown that dental care is considerably neglected in the former; there is a high incidence of caries, periodontal disease and oral hyperplasia. These problems are the combined result of the patient's medication, poor oral hygiene, incorrect diet, and infrequent dental treatment. As a rule, dental care for the person with epilepsy is available only when an acute problem arises, and the usual therapy is extraction. Conservative dentistry is less often embarked upon because of the fear that the patient may have a seizure in the dentist's chair or because painstaking work may be irrepairably destroyed in a subsequent fit (Westphal, 1972a).

PROBLEMS IN CONNECTION WITH MEDICATION

It is well known that certain antipsychotic drugs, soporifics and tranquillisers influence the teeth, periodontium, other oral mucous membranes and surrounding tissue.

Teeth

Probably the most common side-effect of medication is hyposialosis, which leads to an increasing quantity of plaque and thus higher caries frequency. Other contributing factors to this higher caries rate are an increased intake of sweetened drinks, altered dietary habits, and inadequate oral hygiene.

Several of the drugs within the categories of tranquillisers, antiepileptic drugs, spasmolytics, antipsychotics and antidepressants have such a strong depressant effect on salivation that the patient treated with these drugs ought to be encouraged to contact his dentist in order to institute an adequate caries prevention programme, which may include medication for increasing saliva flow.

Within the group of antipsychotics there are also a relatively large number of drugs which, because of their sucrose content, are unfavourable for long-term use from a cariological point of view.

Root abnormalities

Richens and Rowe (1970) noticed a disturbance in calcium metabolism as a result of antiepileptic drug therapy. This appears to be the result of vitamin D deficiency (Silver *et al.*, 1974). The teeth in epileptic patients, however, often show root abnormalities which resemble the changes found in hypoparathyroidism, and Harris and Goldhaber

(1974) postulated that phenytoin might block the peripheral effects of this hormone.

Periodontium

The use of phenytoin in the treatment of epilepsy creates an important adverse effect which must be dealt with, i.e. gingival hyperplasia. There have been many reports concerning the extent and frequency of this type of hyperplasia. Some authors claim that it occurs chiefly in children. Others have observed different age relationships (Aas, 1963; Babcock, 1965; Klar, 1973). Differences relating to the size of the daily dosage of phenytoin and to the duration of treatment have been described by other authors such as Esterberg and White (1945), Staple (1953), Yahr and Merritt (1956) and Klar (1973). Our experience, based on the observations of a larger number of patients, leads us to conclude that gingival hyperplasia is unrelated to age and sex. Neither is it related to the daily amount of phenytoin administered nor the duration of the treatment. Some patients on phenytoin manifest clinically observable gingival hyperplasia only after many years, while others develop symptoms after only a short time. We have also shown that even in patients without clinically observable hyperplasia it is possible to find excessive collagen growth histologically (Westphal & Melin, 1968). The mechanism by which the adverse effect of phenytoin is brought about is not understood. It has a proliferating effect primarily on the basal cell layer of the oral epithelium, thus increasing the epithelium-connective tissue interface. The oral epithelium may have an inducing effect on the underlying fibroblasts in which alkaline phosphates may be involved. Effects of a two-day exposure to phenytoin have been described by Benveniste (1979). Phenytoin concentrations not exceeding 20 μmol/l did not alter the rate of protein synthesis, the percentage of collagenous protein or the DNA content of normal fibroblasts. At concentrations of 20–40 μmol/l, however, fibroblast cultures contained higher quantities of DNA, incorporated ^{3}H-leucine into protein more rapidly and produced a higher percentage of collagen. Phenytoin stimulation of the fibroblasts occurred only when the cells were in the log phase of growth. At concentrations of 40 μmol/l or more, phenytoin inhibited all growth and protein synthesis.

It is suspected that a metabolite of phenytoin might be responsible for gingival hyperplasia, not the parent molecule itself. Hassell (1979) performed gas-liquid chromatographic analysis of human hyperplastic gingiva and demonstrated the presence of 5-(parahydroxyphenyl)-5-phenylhydantoin (pHPPH) in concentrations of up to 12 μmol/l. Subba Rao (1979) observed covalent binding of phenytoin to gingival proteins which appeared to involve an arene oxide metabolite of the drug.

Significant *in vivo* protein binding occurred in the gingiva of rats treated with phenytoin. When compared with extra-oral tissues such as liver and kidney, it was found that the highest rate of protein binding took place in the gingival tissues.

The role of saliva in the development of hyperplastic disorders in the gingiva has been discussed by a number of researchers. Steinberg (1979) proposed that phenytoin or one of its metabolites was secreted with the saliva where it was subsequently concentrated in the dental plaque. The gingival inflammation usually accompanying plaque accumulation may thereby increase the diffusion and retention of phenytoin by the sulcular tissues. However, Westphal (1969) demonstrated that in two groups of guinea pigs treated with phenytoin, those with the parotid glands removed did not show any difference from the other group with the glands remaining. This would seem to indicate that the salivary glands do not have effect on the development of gingival hyperplasia. The finding of an increased growth of connective tissue in the lungs of these animals supports this conclusion.

Vitamin C deficiency resulting from phenytoin medication has been described by Kimball (1939), Frankel (1940) and Drake, Gruber and Haurg (1941). Angelopuolos (1968) believes that phenytoin has a direct effect upon the gingival mast cell. Van der Kwast (1956) suspected that an allergic reaction is the cause of gingival hyperplasia.

Despite the scientific work of many authors, it can be said that the aetiology and pathogenesis of gingival hyperplasia are not well understood. At a clinical level what is of importance is to identify correctly the cause of hyperplasia. Angelopuolos

(1975) has paid great attention to differential diagnosis, and recommends consulting the following list of generalised gingival enlargements from which phenytoin-induced hyperplasia must be differentiated:

1. Simple hyperplastic gingivitis – general irritation
2. Hereditary gingival fibromatosis – elephantiasis gingivae
3. Idiopathic gingival fibromatosis – resembles hereditary gingival fibromatosis
4. Hormonal gingivitis – pregnancy, puberty
5. Scorbutic gingivitis – local irritation
6. Leukaemic gingival enlargement – infiltration of neoplastic blood cells
7. Gingival enlargements in connection with syndromes – e.g. Hurler's and Sturge-Weber syndromes

These hyperplastic alterations are of great inconvenience to the patient. Hyperplastic growth leads to deepening of the gingival sulci, which creates poor hygienic conditions and facilitates gingivitis. The rapid cell growth is very powerful and can lead to deviation of the teeth as much as several millimetres, and cause rotation and protrusion of the teeth. This in consequence leads to malocclusion and faulty articulation, which in turn may cause a number of problems such as temporomandibular joint disturbances, headache, speech and eating difficulties, and clamping. Clamping often goes together with hyperventilation, and may act as a triggering mechanism for an attack. Increased pain may lead to increased general irritability.

Unfortunately, the patient often first presents for dental care when the above problems make themselves felt. It is obvious that treatment must have a greater preventive emphasis. Occlusal therapy for the patient may significantly contribute to his rehabilitation.

Treatment

Discontinuation or change of medication. When phenytoin medication is discontinued or when a different medication replaces it, partial or complete recovery of the gingival tissues occurs in most cases. In long-standing lesions, however, the tissue will remain fibrotic, and surgical correction may be necessary. Withdrawal of phenytoin when gingival hyperplasia occurs depends upon its severity and upon the effectiveness of phenytoin compared with other drugs in controlling the patient's epilepsy.

Surgical removal of hyperplastic tissue. Gingivectomy usually requires an extensive incision, which is often painful to the patient. It is not a final solution to the problem, since the hyperplasia will recur if phenytoin medication is continued. In these cases, however, it is used to promote better results in combination with other methods.

Oral hygiene. A number of studies have established a relationship between the degree of hyperplasia and the state of oral hygiene. Improved oral hygiene eliminates secondary inflammation and perhaps decreases the hyperplasia. It will not produce total regression of the hyperplasia. Meticulous oral hygiene possibly combined initially with surgical correction, will delay or even prevent recurrence of gingival hyperplasia.

Other tissue disorders

Smith (1979) has noted phenytoin effects on prenatal growth and morphogenesis. A growth deficiency involving both nasal and distal digital growth yields a short nose with a low nasal bridge, and small distal phalanges with nail hypoplasia. Major malformations such as cleft lip and palate and cardiac defects are less frequent.

Johnston and Sulik (1979) have studied gene-environment interaction. The A/J mouse strain in their laboratory had a spontaneous 7 per cent incidence of cleft lip, with or without cleft palate. A single oral dose of phenytoin sufficient to raise the plasma phenytoin to human therapeutic levels was administered on gestational day 10. This increased the incidence of cleft lip to 4–5 times that of the vehicle-treated controls. A single dose of 75 mg/kg phenytoin intraperitoneally resulted in an incidence of almost 100 per cent.

Other connective tissue disorders associated with phenytoin medication are Dupuytren's contracture and coarsening of the facial features (Dudley, 1979). Moore (1959) described radiographic changes in the lungs of 81 per cent of 31 epileptic patients treated with phenytoin.

TRAUMA

Soft tissue injuries can either be intra- or extra-oral. They usually are treated quite easily. Facial contusions, fractures of the jaws or other bones of the facial skeleton must be managed with the help of radiographic examination.

Tongue-biting during a tonic-clonic seizure is not unusual. The injury usually heals without any complications in a short time. Infection risk is very low. Sutures may be necessary. It is dangerous to place hard objects between the patient's teeth during a seizure, especially during the convulsive phase because of the risk of mandibular fracture or subluxation of the temporo-mandibular joints. Furthermore, broken teeth do not heal whereas a bitten tongue does. In a survey conducted among 100 policemen and 100 ambulance drivers, Westphal (1972a) found that no fewer than 80 per cent placed something between the teeth of the patient during a seizure.

Hard tissue injuries are of either osseous or dental character. Two types of injuries to the teeth are most common in connection with an epileptic seizure:

1. Enamel injuries when the teeth slam together at the beginning of an attack, including fractures of the crown or root
2. Fractures of the crown, cusps and fillings due to pressing of the teeth during the course of the seizure (bruxism)

In cases of repeated fractures, even if these are only fractures of the teeth, a disturbance of calcium metabolism should be suspected. Teeth which have been knocked out must be immediately removed from the mouth, and very loose teeth extracted, to prevent aspiration.

The study of Besserman (1978), which included 432 patients, showed that a large number of patients had sustained some form of oral injury. In some age groups, up to 100 per cent of the patients had been affected. Apart from soft tissue and enamel injuries, 80 per cent of the patients between the ages of 16–30 had sustained other types of tooth injuries. 1.4 per cent had suffered fractures of the jaw, several of them more than once.

General measures to be adopted in connection with a seizure during dental surgery

During a seizure never use force. Only try to prevent the patient from injuring himself by attempting to guide his movements. Holding the head or extremities too firmly may be injurious. Never try to lift the patient from the chair during a fit. Tilt the chair back, push the instrument tray out of the way and try, if possible, to guide the patient's movements. After the seizure, a period of rest is required, which may vary from several minutes to several hours of sleep. As a rule, no particular measures are called for after awakening.

It must be borne in mind that some patients are photosensitive and the operation-lamp may trigger a fit. The dentist should therefore avoid shining the lamp in the region of the patient's eyes and bring the lamp up towards the oral cavity from below.

Protective devices such as rubber blocks and metal fingers are old-fashioned and psychologically reprehensible. An effective protective measure is to press the patient's cheek gently between the upper and lower teeth.

When administering injections, avoid using glass syringes. If during a sudden, powerful seizure an instrument or drill should become fastened between the patient's teeth, it should never be forcibly removed. Removal is possible when the spasm has subsided. A cusp fracture is easier to treat than a mandibular fracture. When making an impression with alginate or the like, it is of the greatest importance not to panic if the patient has a seizure. Let the tray remain *in situ*, fixate it against the jaw and follow the movements of the head until the compound has hardened. Only then may the tray be removed. In this way the patient avoids aspiration of the liquid compound where it may harden in the respiratory passages and cause suffocation.

Treatment

It is not always possible to reconstruct the bite in an epileptic patient with the help of conservative treatment; for example, crown and bridge therapy. In these patients, partial or complete dentures may be necessary. The great majority are able to manage removable dentures without difficulty. The patient himself will, during the course of a seizure, spit out the dentures with the help of tongue and lips. The dentures may also be pressed against each other during a seizure in such a way as to fix them in place in the patient's mouth. The author has never met a situation in which a removable denture has blocked the respiratory passages during a seizure, with the subsequent risk of suffocation. Obviously, however, it is necessary to check whether the patient is wearing a denture in the event of a fit. The denture must not be removed by force under any circumstances. Removal may be possible at the end of the tonic stage, and when the patient himself opens his mouth during the clonic spasms.

Crown and bridge replacements are made with maximal possible metal reinforcements, sometimes at the expense of aesthetic considerations. Removable or complete dentures should be made of cast metal, and the denture should be reinforced with mesh to prevent scattering, (Baczkowsky, 1969).

Orthodontic therapy may be quite difficult to conduct with patients with frequent grand mal seizures.

The use of lignocaine. A frequently recurring question is whether there is any objection to using lignocaine for local and regional anaesthesia in the dental treatment of epileptic patients. There is nothing to prevent this. On the contrary, lignocaine has been shown to have anticonvulsant activity. Ottosan (1955) showed that small doses of lignocaine injected intravenously were able to shorten the discharges occurring after electro-shock therapy. Bernhard *et al.* (1956) gave an account of the way in which an intravenous injection of 8 mg/kg of lignocaine can prevent photoconvulsive EEG activity. Mosovich and Etchepareborda (1964) described an improvement in the EEG trace for up to 63 minutes after administration of 2–5 mg/kg of lignocaine to patients who had generalised spike-and-wave discharges. There is therefore no reason for withholding lignocaine in treating the epileptic patient.

General anaesthesia. The diagnosis of epilepsy is not alone a sufficient reason for conducting dental care under general anaesthesia. The resources for treating the patient in this way are so limited today that they must primarily be reserved for those handicapped patients who could not be treated otherwise. These are, for example, patients with multiple sclerosis, Parkinson's disease, muscular dystrophy, spinal muscular atrophies and dyskinesias. On the other hand, severely retarded patients can learn to accept conventional treatment with a little perseverance and time. A patient with epilepsy should be treated conventionally, as long as there are no further complicating factors beyond the epilepsy itself.

Co-operation with the physician. When planning dental treatment for the handicapped, it is of great value for the dentist to collaborate closely with the patient's physician. In the case of epilepsy, the dentist needs to be informed of the type and frequency of the fits, possible seizure-triggering factors (e.g. photosensitivity) and the severity and duration of seizures.

Also of importance is a list of the patient's medication and dosage. Additional sedation may be considered for maintaining control during the course of dental treatment.

The dentist in turn should always inform the patient's physician about dental findings, such as alterations in growth and development, hyperplasia, root changes, and seizures during dental treatment. More extensive incisions ought to be discussed with the physician in advance.

As part of the rehabilitation team, the odontologist's contribution is an important one in improving the patient's appearance and self-confidence.

The role of the dental nurse. It is obvious from what has been said that there are a number of measures that should be adopted in connection with an epileptic seizure in the course of dental treatment. The dentist is therefore dependent on a specially trained nurse. Not only should she be familiar with the purely practical problems, but also with the treatment and its aims. Especially when it comes to the treatment of mentally retarded patients, the dental nurse may serve as a good connecting link between the dentist and the patient.

REFERENCES

Aas E. (1963) Hyperplasia gingivae diphenylhydantoinea. *Acta Odontologica Scandinavia*, **21**, Supplement 34.

Angelopoulos A.P. (1968) The role of mast cells in the pathogenesis of diphenylhydantoin gingival hyperplasia. *Journal of Dental Research*, Supplement/ADR, abstract 417.

Angelopoulos A.P. (1975) Aetiology, pathogenesis, differential diagnosis and treatment. *Journal of the Canadian Dental Association*, **5**, 275.

Babcock J.R. (1965) Incidence of gingival hyperplasia in dilantin therapy in a hospital population. *Journal of the American Dental Association*, **7**, 1447.

Baczkowsky T. (1969) Practical remarks on fitting dentures to patients with epilepsy. Protet. Stomatol. Warsawa, **19**, 203.

Benveniste K. (1979) Effects of phenytoin on cultured human gingival fibroblasts. Symposium-University of Carolina 1979. Phenytoin induced teratology and gingival pathology.

Bernhard C., Bohm E., Högberg S. & Melin K.A. (1956) The effect on intravenous xylocain on cortical seizure activity evoked by intermittent photic stimulation in epileptics. *Acta Psychiatrica Scandinavia*, **31**.

Besserman K. (1978) Frequency of maxillo-facial injuries in a hospital population of patients with epilepsy. *NFH Bulletin* Vol. 5, No.1.

Drake M.E., Gruber C.M. & Haury U.G. (1941) Effects of sodium diphenylhydantoin on vitamin C level in tissues and vitamin C excretion in rats. *Journal of Pharmacology and Experimental Therapeutics*, **71**, 268.

Dudley K.H. (1979) Phenytoin Metabolism. Symposium-University of Carolina 1979. Phenytoin induced teratology and gingival pathology.

Estenberg H.L. & White P.H. (1945) Sodium dilantine gingival hyperplasia. *Journal of the American Dental Association*, **32**, 16.

Frankel S.I. (1940) Dilantin sodium in treatment of epilepsy. *Journal of the American Medical Association*, **114**, 1320.

Hassell T.M. (1979) Phenytoin – induced gingival overgrowth in a mongrel cat model. Symposium-University of Carolina 1979. Phenytoin induced teratology and gingival pathology.

Harris M. & Goldhaber P. (1974) Root abnormalities in epileptics and the inhibition of parathyroid hormone induced bone resorption by diphenylhydantoin in tissue culture. *Archive of Oral Biology*, **19**, 981.

Johnston M.C. & Sulik K.K. (1979) Gene-environment interaction in phenytoin induced malformations in mice. Symposium-University of Carolina 1979. Phenytoin induced teratology and gingival pathology.

Kimball O.P. (1939) Treatment of epilepsy with sodium diphenylhydantoin. *Journal of the American Medical Association*, **119**, 1244.

Klar L.A. (1973) Gingival hyperplasia during Dilantin therapy. *Journal of Public Health and Dentistry*, **33**, 180.

Moores M.T. (1959) Pulmonary changes in hydantoin therapy. *Journal of the American Medical Association*, **171**, 1328.

Mosovich A. & Etchepareborda J. (1964) The effect of xylocain upon the burst of paroxymal activity in the EEG of epileptics. *Acta Neurologica Scandinavia*, **40**, 1.

Ottoson J.O. (1955) The effect of xylocaine in electric convulsive treatment. Experentia II, 453.

Richens A. & Rowe D.J.F. (1970) Disturbance of calcium metabolism by anticonvulsant drugs. *British Medical Journal*, **4**, 73.

Silver J., Davies T.J., Kupersmitt E., Orme M., Petrie A. & Vajda F. (1974) Prevalence and treatment of vitamin D deficiency in children on anti-convulsant drugs. *Archives of Diseases in Childhood*, **49**, 344.

Smith D.M. (1979) Fetal hydantoin syndrome: Nature and risk. Symposium-University of Carolina 1979. Phenytoin induced teratology and gingival pathology.

Staple P.H. (1953) Some tissue reactions associated with 5:5 phenylhydantoin sodium therapy. *British Dental Journal*, **95**, 289.

Staple P.H. (1979) Phenytoin-induced gingival overgrowth in the Stump-Tailed Macaque. Symposium-University of Carolina 1979. Phenytoin induced teratology and gingival pathology.

Steinberg A.D. (1979) Phenytoin penetration through sulcular tissues and its possible relationship to phenytoin – induced gingival overgrowth. Symposium-University of Carolina 1979. Phenytoin induced teratology and gingival pathology.

Subba Rao G. (1979) Gingival Metabolism of phenytoin and covalent binding of its reactive metabolites to gingival proteins. Symposium-University of Carolina 1979. Phenytoin induced teratology and gingival pathology.

Thorburn I.O. (1965) Oral lesions due to a drug therapy. *Australian Dental Journal*, **10**, 75.

Van der Kwast, W.A.M. (1956). Speculations regarding the nature of gingival hyperplasia due to diphenylhydantoin sodium. *Acta Medica Scandinavica*, **153**, 399.

Westphal P. (1969) Salivsekretion och gingivalhyperplasi hos försöksdjur behandlade med Difenylhydantoin. *Tadläker Tidning Sweden*, **62**, 8.

Westphal P. (1972a) En kunskapsmätning omkring Epilepsiproblematiken. *Svenska Epilepsia*, **2** Nr, 2.

Westphal P. (1972b) Dental care of epilepsy. *Epilepsia* **3**, 233.

Westphal P. & Melin K.A. (1968) Aspects of dental welfare

Yahr M.D. & Merritt H.H. (1956) Current status of the drug therapy of epileptic seizures. *Journal of the American Medical Association*, **161**, 333.

15

People with epilepsy – living with epilepsy

J. Laidlaw
M.V. Laidlaw

INTRODUCTION

To understand epilepsy and to attempt to treat fits rationally, three questions need to be answered.

1. What happens during a fit?
2. Why do some people and not others have fits?
3. Why do fits occur when they do?

The first two questions can be answered for epilepsy as adequately as for most medical conditions. Electroencephalography, electrocorticography and depth recordings are providing more and more information about the electrical events associated with the ictus. Biochemistry and neuropharmacology are cultivating exciting new fields of knowledge. Although there are still many differences of opinion about the aetiology of epilepsy, there is a good deal that we do know. There are a number of rather rare neurological diseases which are hereditary and which cause fits. There is very probably some inherited proclivity to fits and more certainly to febrile convulsions. There is increasing evidence that severe and prolonged such febrile convulsions can cause brain damage which may later provoke complex partial seizures. There is a whole list of other potentially provocative factors: injuries, infections and neoplasms. Not all brain tumours cause fits but at least it is possible to propose a rational explanation why some do and others do not – the type, site and rate of growth of the tumour or perhaps the proclivity to fits inherited by the brain in which the tumour is growing. There are acute disorders of blood constituents which provoke fits (if not causing epilepsy) such as anoxia, hypoglycaemia or uraemia.

However, if we exclude fits in early infancy, the third question remains unanswered. This unanswered question is the mystery of epilepsy. It is also why the subject has fascinated so many different doctors working in their various disciplines. We might be forgiven for suggesting that in looking back on what has been written in this book we are seeing islands of knowledge in an ocean of ignorance. It is not surprising that in the days before the first two questions could be answered there were many who thought of epilepsy as due either to Divine intervention or to the more sinister intervention of the Devil. Today we know enough to reject these hypotheses and to assert that the proximate cause of a fit must be some alteration in the more profane environments, whether the internal environment of metabolic and biochemical changes and the serum levels of antiepileptic drugs, or the psychosocial environment of the patient's reaction to what is going on around him.

This chapter is based on the premise that the influences of these two environments are mixed inextricably and that the doctor must be concerned with the external as much as with the internal. Therefore, we do not feel we are adding a soft sociological appendage to a book filled with hard science supported by innumerable references. Rather by having the last word, we are taking the opportunity to re-emphasise what medicine, and especially the medicine of epilepsy, is all about: the application of science to people and the lives they live. In particular we want to redefine the role of the doctor. When all the diagnoses have been made and the serum levels estimated; when fits have been controlled as far as is scientifically possible, the patient still has to live with his epilepsy. Even in these days of the multi-disciplinary team, nearly always it is the doctor who carries the final responsibility, and it is to the doctor that the patient turns – or would like to run – for help and advice. As medicine becomes more complicated and sophisticated, many senior doctors must delegate their responsibilities for dealing with day to day problems to their juniors or to valued ancilliaries. We hope that this chapter will remind them how important these day to day problems are to their patients with epilepsy and to the control of their fits, so that, if they need to delegate, they will also guide and their responsibilities will not be abrogated.

The long-term care of people with epilepsy, who are not able to live independent lives in the open community, will be considered at the end of this chapter. However, any proposals for this group of patients must take into account the interaction between the disability and the environments. Many disadvantaged people in need of care have what may be termed static disabilities – the blind, the physically-intact elderly, and the mentally handicapped. Such people need medical supervision and access to specialised medical advice. Nevertheless, it can be argued that they may be helped better to adjust their disabilities to their new environment under the general aegis of specialists in other disciplines, be they social workers, psychologists, educationalists or those experienced in physical re-education. However, unless epilepsy is a marginal secondary disability, the overall management of those with epilepsy needing care must be medical. It is not enough to leave it to ancillary workers with a smattering of medicine, having a doctor to fall back on only in times of crisis. If the responsibility for this small but important group of people with epilepsy was brought into the main stream of the medicine of epilepsy, there would be an improved understanding of icto-environmental reactions and perhaps some reallocation of time and money from the diagnosis of rare and often untreatable causes of fits, to helping those, whose fits cannot be controlled adequately, to live with their epilepsy.

It is a reasonable working hypothesis that epilepsy is due to a combination of two factors: a congenital, and probably inherited, proclivity to fit; and an acquired provocative one which, in most adult patients, is a degree of brain damage.

Furthermore, it often seems to be the case that the less the brain damage the more the epilepsy may be influenced by environmental adjustments, including alterations in the internal environment produced by antiepileptic drugs. Whether or not these hypotheses are wholly true, it is convenient to divide the population of those with epilepsy into three broad groups.

A. Those with little or no evidence of brain damage whose fits can usually be controlled quite easily, often with a single antiepileptic drug in adequate dosage.
B. A large intermediate group with greater or lesser brain damage who are likely to continue to have fits despite the best possible treatment.
C. Those with severe brain damage whose primary problem is likely to be mental handicap but whose management may be made the more difficult by intractable fits.

On the whole Group A are likely to present few problems. Not only will they have few, if any fits, but they are likely to be of average intelligence. If it is accepted that emotional, behavioural and personality problems in those with epilepsy are not due to an epileptic diathesis but rather are secondary to a variety of factors such as brain damage, antiepileptic drugs, and the reactions of the patient himself and others to his fits, it follows that the Group A patient will have few superadded difficulties. By definition the Group A patient has little or no brain damage. His fits being relatively easy to control he will not be subject to excessive doses or a multiplicity of antiepileptic drugs. Because he has few fits, he will be less bothered by the few that he does have, and, if he is lucky, his colleagues may not even need to know that he suffers from epilepsy. However, although these sanguine comments may apply to the majority of those in this group, it is an over-simplification and there will be those who do suffer from the problems peculiar to epilepsy which we will be considering. For example, an intelligent and sophisticated patient may not be worried so much by the fits that he does have as by those that he might have; or, a professional man might find that his skills are marginally but significantly blunted even by modest doses of antiepileptic drugs.

Although patients in Group C cannot be discounted, their problems are likely to be due mainly to their mental handicap and not primarily to their epilepsy. Nevertheless, because of the severity of their brain damage, their fits may be difficult to control, particularly since it has been our experience that brain-damaged patients may be especially sensitive to antiepileptic drugs and liable to become intoxicated at serum levels within the so-called therapeutic range. The majority of these patients will be in hospitals for the mentally subnormal although a minority will be placed inappropriately in mental hospitals, centres for epilepsy, or may even be maintained in the open community with little advantage to themselves and at inordinate cost to their families. However, the correct placement of these patients is more a politico-economic than a medical concern. Until hospitals for the mentally handicapped are upgraded with adequate finance, there will be inevitably strong family pressure for disadvantaged relatives to be looked after elsewhere.

Group B patients are those who have problems because of their epilepsy: partly because they still have fits, and partly because of the psychosocial consequences of having fits. It is a large group with a wide range: from those living and working in the open community, who run into occasional difficulties; through those who only manage to live independently with considerable difficulty and who are often unemployed and socially isolated; and those, who are unable to live without social support, and are only able to work under sheltered conditions; to those who require long-term residential care and can only do limited work adapted to their disabilities. Many Group B patients will suffer from complex partial seizures often arising in the temporal lobe, and, perhaps, due to mesial temporal sclerosis produced by uncontrolled or severe and prolonged febrile convulsions. This important sub-group are especially liable to have problems because of the following factors.

1. The site of the causative lesion. The functions of the temporal lobes and the structures with which they are connected are highly complex and not understood fully. However, it is probable that temporal lobe dysfunction, even in the absence of seizures, may influence emotions, behaviour and higher integrative functions.

2. The nature of their fits. These are often difficult for the observer to understand, and, if consciousness is not lost completely, they may be very distressing to the patient.

3. Although secondary generalisation may be controlled with antiepileptic drugs, the primary attack may not be and so the patient will be more liable to continue to have complex seizures.

4. Since complex partial seizures are relatively unresponsive to antiepileptic drugs, the patient is at greater risk of intoxication with too large doses or too many different drugs.

We will be considering particularly Group B patients. They are also the group in which the interactions between fits and the environments are the most liable to set up a vicious cycle (Fig. 15.1). The more fits a patient has the greater his psychosocial problems. The more psychosocial problems he has, the more fits he will have. Antiepileptic drugs may add to his psychosocial problems. If he has more fits, his drugs may be increased, and his psychosocial problems exacerbated. When his drugs reach toxic levels, his psychosocial problems may become severe and he may even become psychotic: at the same time the drugs may even make his fits worse.

The changing attitudes towards epilepsy over the centuries – a microcosmic history of medicine – have been described in Temkin's classic study (Temkin, 1971). Some hundred years ago the 'epileptic' was still all too often an outcast and epilepsy carried the official stigma of a form of insanity. Later the cult of the *epileptic personality* developed and was nurtured by the segregation of those more disabled into institutions, where what was being observed was the depersonalisation which resulted from people being required to conform to a rigid, uniform, if paternalistic, system which took little account of individual needs let alone aspirations. If there were those who presented an epileptic personality but did not have fits, it was suggested blandly that: 'they were liable to have fits'. To this pre-judgement there was an expected reaction. There were many, perhaps with equal prejudice, who, asserting that the person with epilepsy had been accused wrongly and was beset by ignorance, proposed that epilepsy did not differ qualitatively from any other symptom, – from a cough or a stomach ache – that there were no problems peculiar to

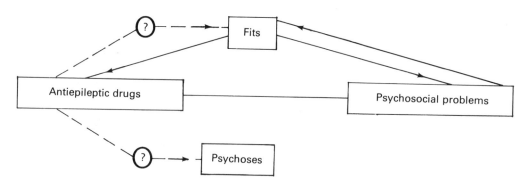

Fig 15.1

epilepsy. It is an interesting paradox that many of these worthy champions busied themselves forming special Epilepsy Associations, and Leagues against and Bureaux for Epilepsy.

We maintain strongly that those with epilepsy, as people, are just like everyone else. However, we would propose that there are *problems peculiar to epilepsy*. Furthermore, if we are to help our patients, this proposition needs to be accepted, and the problems considered carefully and understood; being neither exaggerated nor minimised. In the first part of this chapter we will discuss these problems in general terms. Some may appear trivial and inconsequential: but so often it is the little things that matter, that are so readily overlooked and yet may tip the balance between success and failure. Some, such as popular prejudice and over-protection, may appear to be so obvious that they do not merit inclusion in a textbook. Nonetheless, we feel that they require critical reassessment; too often such concepts are passed on as a part of the currency of accepted opinion. If some of our ideas appear to be quasiphilosophical, this may not be altogether a bad thing. Despite enormous scientific advances, epilepsy remains an enigma. If we evoke criticism, we will have stimulated thought. The problems which we will discuss are, nevertheless, those with which we have been faced when we have tried to help and advise patients. Therefore, as well as presenting the problems, we will try to suggest ways in which we would advise patients to overcome them. We have considered this from the patient's point of view elsewhere (Laidlaw & Laidlaw, 1980) but, since it is to the doctor that the

patient turns when he is in trouble, some of these suggestions may be appropriate to a chapter written for doctors.

When we wrote the corresponding chapter for the first edition of this book, we were responsible for Chalfont Centre for Epilepsy with some 475 beds for the long and short term management of Group B patients. We included ten case histories drawn from this experience. We are retaining these *personal situations* unchanged because we feel that we cannot better them to illustrate not only the functions and usefulness of Epilepsy Centres, but also, more importantly, the problems peculiar to epilepsy, the vicious cycle of the interactions of fits and the environments, and the impossibility of separating the medical and social management of this particular section of the disadvantaged population.

We will conclude by reviewing past and present provisions for those of the epileptic population who have difficulties in living with their epilepsy, and suggest in very general terms a plan for the future.

PROBLEMS PECULIAR TO EPILEPSY

The doctor and the patient

To most patients or their families presented with the diagnosis of epilepsy, it is wrongly rather than rightly a diagnosis of disaster. The same might be said for cancer or impending death but in these cases it is seldom necessary for the doctor to spell out his diagnosis until the patient has a very good idea of it himself. In the case of epilepsy we feel that the doctor should not wrap up his diagnosis in meaningless and confusing euphemisms. Rather it is his responsibility over a period to help the patient to overcome his irrational fears and understand the condition with which he will have to live, very probably for the rest of his life. Epilepsy like diabetes is a condition in which proper management requires the greatest possible co-operation of the patient and/or his family. Nevertheless, although diabetes is probably the more dangerous disease, it is epilepsy that is feared the more. The doctor must appreciate not only that this fear exists, but understand why it exists so that he may help to exorcise it.

When a patient and his family are faced for the first time with the diagnosis of epilepsy, there is almost invariably this feeling of shock; of inevitable disaster. This is probably the worst possible time to try to discuss the implications. Both the patient and his family are likely to be so overwrought that they are unable to absorb anything which is said to them. Long afterwards, the doctor, who may have spent some time trying to help, may hear that he has been accused, altogether unjustifiably, of never having explained anything. It is much more sensible for the doctor to send the patient away with a few soothing words and to make an appointment to see him again in a week or two, telling him in the meantime to think out any questions which he would like to discuss.

Nowadays in developed countries most patients will be referred to a neurological (or neuro-psychiatric) hospital department to confirm the diagnosis and in some cases to exclude a remedial lesion. Again we would like to re-emphasise the importance of the consultant's total responsibility for the management of the patient with epilepsy. In a neurological department any competent second year registrar can cope with 90 per cent of the work involved in excluding gliomas or picking up rare cases of tuberous sclerosis. It is for the more experienced consultant to help the patient adjust to the diagnosis – perhaps on the suggested return visit. He has the knowledge and the authority. So of course do many general practitioners but there are others whose experience with epilepsy may be limited to a few patients and who do not have any special interest in the subject. Hospital Social Workers except in very specialised units are unlikely to have sufficient information about epilepsy and they lack the authority of the consultant. Whoever it is who undertakes to help the patient overcome his initial shock, he will be helped by the national Epilepsy Associations and by pamphlets and books written for the patient (Burden & Schurr, 1976; Laidlaw & Laidlaw, 1980). However, many patients are a bit inarticulate and, particularly when faced with senior hospital doctors, do not voice their fears, and there are some topics which need to be discussed whether or not they have been raised by the patient.

Mental disturbance

Although it is seldom voiced spontaneously, there are many patients who have considerable latent anxiety that having epilepsy means that they are or will become in some way mad or peculiar. The doctor should be prepared to bring this fear out into the open, appreciate how it arose, and explain to the patient that it is without foundation. If he does not, it may well grow, nurtured by gossip and anecdote, and become a belief so firmly held that it is difficult or impossible to eradicate later on. It would be too simple an explanation to suggest that it is left over from the prejudices of the past. It is much more probable that many of the reasons that made our forefathers think that epilepsy was a form of insanity still operate.

A major fit is a dramatic event. All too often it is taken as the common factor of that wide variety of conditions causing fits; termed epilepsy, it carries with it associations with all these conditions. Severe mental deficiency often associated with corresponding physical stigmata is commonly complicated by major convulsions: epilepsy. May not the patient presented with the diagnosis of epilepsy, conjure up, not altogether irrationally if it has not been explained to him, a picture of a convulsing brain-damaged village idiot, in a way that the symptom of a hacking cough, diagnosed as tracheitis, does not evoke fears of the putrefying lung of phthisis or bronchial carcinoma? It is fairly easy for the doctor to explain to his patient that fits are (probably) due to a combination of a congenital brain sensitivity, or liability to fits, and acquired brain damage, which in only the extreme case results in significant mental handicap.

The word *seizure* describes an epileptic attack much more aptly than *fit*. In nearly every case the patient is quite unable to prevent or control his ictus. Literally, he seems to have been seized by something not only outwith his control but which he cannot see or begin to understand. It is all too easy for him to believe that this something is supernatural, or, if he is more sophisticated, that it is something apart from his physical self: something in his mental self – his mind. It is not difficult to understand the basic idea of an EEG recording and patients may often be reassured by seeing a seizure on the EEG.

It is wrong to assume that the patient is always unconscious and therefore is unaware of and never disturbed by what happens during a fit. It is appreciated that simple partial attacks are usually associated with little or no alteration of consciousness. However, a part or the whole of a complex partial seizure may involve alteration without full loss of consciousness. In this case the patient will be aware, dimly and in part, of what is happening, as if in a dream, which may well be a nightmare. Such experiences are the more frightening if he is unable to mobilise his intellect fully to integrate what he is experiencing and feeling into his consciousness. Some aurae and partially appreciated attacks may be indescribably awesome and may be entangled with horrifying thoughts and obscene tastes and smells. Public attitudes may have altered from the days when the *epileptic* was considered as insane, but how often does the patient himself assume or fear that he is going mad? He is frightened. He cannot describe in ordinary language the penumbra of his consciousness, and so he cannot, even if he would, share his fears with his doctor.

Special investigations

Although some may be nervous or embarrassed, most patients find examination by the doctor reassuring. However, special investigations such as the EEG or the CT with complex and formidable equipment can be very frightening. The doctor needs to do more than dismiss them as harmless and painless. An equally important problem is that the patient is often confused as to why they are being carried out. The neurologist will be

quite clear that the EEG may be of some help in arriving at the diagnosis of epilepsy or in determining the type, whereas the CT is only called for if he feels that a potentially remediable lesion needs to be excluded. This is in no way obvious to the patient unless it is explained to him. Particularly at the time of diagnosis, a patient's epilepsy is of paramount importance to him and between his out-patient appointments he and his family are likely to have absorbed a great deal of quasi-information from the library, from friends or from acquaintances who knew someone who had fits and had this that or the other done. If the doctor does not explain fully to his patient why certain tests are necessary, whereas others are not, he may well lose the latter's confidence. It is all too common for the patient, faced with the diagnosis which he considers disastrous, to spend money (which he can ill afford) seeking a real doctor who will do all the proper tests, (which he does not need).

Many patients do not distinguish investigations to exclude a potentially lethal cause from *finding a cure*, and yet this is something which it is so easy to explain. There are even those who confuse investigations with treatment, although we would not recommend serial EEGs for their placebo effect.

Antiepileptic drugs

The scientific aspects of drug treatment and potential side effects have been dealt with very thoroughly earlier in this book. It is hardly necessary to reiterate the general advice which the doctor will give to this patient: the importance of compliance, the dangers of stopping or reducing the dose, and the need to report untoward side-effects. It is perhaps worth mentioning that quite a few patients are worried about the long term taking of drugs and the dangers of addiction and need reassurance on this point. However, it is most important to consider the patient's reaction to the drugs which he is taking to stop his epilepsy. Patients will have been given to understand that there is no dramatic cure for epilepsy and that all that they can hope for is that antiepileptic drugs will control their fits. There is often great pressure from patients and their families to increase the dose or change the tablets in order to deal with a temporary exacerbation of seizures. It needs a good deal of sense of security on the part of the doctor to resist these appeals. Not only is it essential that he should do so but it is important that he should take the time to explain to the patient how vicarious may be the incidence of fits and how essential it is to consider the fit pattern over long periods. Further he must explain that excessive doses of drugs, apart from causing important side-effects, may in fact make fits worse, and he must point out that high doses of drugs, even if they do not produce frank intoxication, may result in a degree of slowing down or minimal inco-ordination which are greater disabilities than the occasional fit.

Popular prejudice

Popular prejudice has become part of the dialect used in talking about epilepsy. Not an adjuvant, all too often it is adduced as the main cause of a patient's problems or his failure. To mention it in a textbook is not superfluous. To consider it carefully is essential.

Prejudice is an emotive word. It raises spectres of apartheid and ghettoes. Almost invariably linked with ignorance, it is inflated to imply brutish stupidity, or even overt brutality. However, the prejudice is always described as popular. But surely the general public is also described as remarkable for its common sense, tolerance and kindness, and, in particular, for its anxiety to help the disabled. The white stick of the blind man evokes almost embarrassing sympathy and desire to help. If, then, epilepsy evokes in the same general public stupid, intolerant and unkind prejudice, this atypical response needs examination. Either it does not exist, or, if it does, there must be some reason. We would suggest that popular prejudice is not nearly as widespread as it is supposed to be, and, that when it does exist, it is not irrational but based on genuine fear.

No longer would anyone maintain that the person with epilepsy was a dangerous fiend, a creature possessed of the devil, but there are ways in which a fit may be fearsome and awesome to the onlooker. The first witness of a friend or a colleague seized by a major convulsion needs com-

ment. We all expect life to be consequential: an action to provoke a reaction. The intense drama of a major fit is the more frightening because it is quite inconsequential. It comes out of the blue: only exceptionally is there any apparent proximate cause. This proposition is to some extent substantiated by the differing reactions to so-called symptomatic and idiopathic epilepsy. An artisan engineer, who fractures his skull in a motor car accident, later develops epilepsy and returns to his firm as a storeman will arouse less unease when he has an occasional fit than an unknown young man with 'idiopathic' epilepsy who is found a job in the same firm by his welfare officer.

However, with adequate treatment major fits should be rare events. Various forms of complex partial seizures are much more difficult to control and are common. After the initial impact of the grotesque and obviously abnormal, it is easier to accept the generalised convulsion than the subtle, often barely perceptible deviations from the usual, which may imbue the lesser attack with an eerie unreality: is he going mad or am I? To awake one morning to find one's garden trampled down by the neighbour's cows would cause shock and horror. To look out to see that some of yesterday's yellow daffodils were blue, would evoke an awesome fear, not of the daffodils, but of one's own sanity.

We would suggest that prejudice is a good deal less widespread than many patients fear and that it is easier to prevent it developing than to remove it once it has become established. The patient should be warned not, himself, to prejudge, not to anticipate non-existent difficulty and adopt a scratchy abrasive mien to those around him. His associates may not be put off by his epilepsy but may be by his own attitude to it and to them. Those around him will reflect the patient's own attitude to his fits and the patient will reflect the attitude of his doctor. It is sensible to advise him to talk quite openly about the seizures – although not of course to the point of obsession since they are of less interest to others than to himself – to give some explanation of when they may occur, describe what form they usually take and what help he may need. If he does so, he is more than likely to meet kindness, understanding and help, which he did not expect, rather than the popular prejudice, which he feared. If he is fortunate enough to be in work, he must be warned in the strongest possible terms against using his epilepsy as a crutch, as an excuse for avoiding difficult jobs or getting special concessions. If others help him out, he must be more than prepared to give them a hand in other ways.

Allowing that there may still be a significant amount of residual prejudice, what then can the doctor do to help to dispel it? The various national Epilepsy Associations offer courses and seminars which are helped greatly by medical contributors. Anything which can be done to remove ignorance and correct misunderstandings will cut at the roots of prejudice, but, sadly, all too often those who attend such meetings are those already converted and the most that can be hoped is to give them facts and arguments to deal with prejudice when they meet it. In the long term it is the patients themselves who will do most to improve the image of epilepsy. If their fits are obvious, by showing how well they can cope with them, and by behaving as the ordinary reasonable people that they are. If their fits are well controlled and so not apparent, to have the courage to admit they have epilepsy and so from their position of strength, and good fortune, give a great deal of help to those less fortunate who have greater difficulty in coping with their disadvantage.

Overprotection

Overprotection is another word, the use of which needs to be examined critically. In the social workers' reports which accompany patients referred for admission to Centres for Epilepsy a high proportion mention over-protective parents as an important factor in causing problems. Doctors seldom do so.

It is a simple biological instinct of parents to protect their young. A young person, who is disabled, requires more protection, and a disability such as epilepsy may call for special precautions. In our experience most parents try hard to approach the hazards of fits in a sensible way and to control their fears. It does not require much imagination to put oneself in the position of someone responsible for a person subject to frequent seizures. It is only reasonable to assert that there is

overprotection when the protection is more than is needed, is exercised stupidly, or in some way harms the patient.

Doctors can do a great deal to guide parents. The general practitioner will be the one to give detailed advice since he should be in closer touch with the family circumstances and personalities. However, the specialist consultant has an important role in guiding the family doctor and offering him the support of his authority. It may be very difficult for even the most sensible parent to know just where to draw the line, and it is really not adequate for the doctor, whether general practitioner or specialist, to dismiss the subject with: 'Treat Johnnie like the other children, but, of course, take reasonable care.' It is essential that he should take the time to discuss the whole position with the family, including the patient if he is old enough and intelligent enough to understand. He must define necessary limitations specifically, and explain why they are necessary. If he does this, he will be able to accept the responsibility for any improbable misfortunes. If he does not, and if something goes wrong, the family will have to bear an intolerable burden of guilt. The doctor in his surgery or in the out-patient clinic is able to make his assessment and give his specific advice in an objective way which is not possible for the family who are involved so personally and subjectively. We have emphasised repeatedly the effect of environment upon fits. There is no situation more epileptogenic than the family whose whole life revolves around the unfortunate patient, the fits which he may have and the disasters which may occur; and consequently the fits which he does have and the disasters which are only too likely to occur. How many patients whose fits are well controlled in hospital or in a Centre for Epilepsy, spend their week-end leave having serial seizures? For that matter how many patients in status asthmaticus recover on admission to hospital without specific treatment? If families are over-protective, it is because they are worried and anxious, and it is their uncertainties which may exacerbate the patient's seizures. Although he may not be certain, there is so much that the doctor with his authority can do to help; by accepting overall responsibility he relieves anxiety and gives confidence.

The doctor can do a great deal to advise parents how to approach the protection of a young person with seizures. As children grow older they need less looking after and they become more independent. It is an easy mistake for parents, because a child needs looking after on account of his fits, to treat him as being much younger than his years, since considering him as a younger child is the only way they understand of exercising the degree of supervision which he needs. Inevitably this approach arouses great resentment: not because his activities are being restricted, but because his dignity has been offended by being treated as a baby. Not only should the parents talk things over with the child as an equal, but, whenever possible he should be included in discussions with the doctor. This applies more particularly to adolescents, who are especially sensitive. The patient should help to work out plans for his own protection. Handled in the proper way, this should not be too difficult because he is often frightened himself by his attacks and the consequences of them. Risks must be taken and they should be explained to the young person. However, we would advise that very great care should be taken of fire. Broken bones usually mend and lacerations heal but many patients with severe epilepsy suffer mutilating burns, which, particularly if they affect the face, cause permanent disfigurement which will have profound psychosocial effects throughout his life on his relationships with other people. In assessing risks it is important to remember that seizures are more likely to occur when patients are relaxed and it may well be more dangerous to browse over a book in front of the fire with the room full of people than it is to cross a busy road on one's own.

Adolescence is always a difficult time. For the person with epilepsy it is especially so. Physiologically, changes are occurring which may exacerbate his fits. It is possible because of a degree of brain damage, frequent fits, or antiepileptic drugs that his maturation was delayed. Unless parents are exceptionally well guided, ordinary adolescent frustrations may be exacerbated to the point of rebellion.

Achievement and approval

Success, a sense of achievement, is one of the strongest stimuli to further effort: a very basic need for a gregarious animal such as man. If we are honest with ourselves, how many of us are not only encouraged by but dependent upon attitudes of approval: applause, private congratulations, spontaneous comment: 'You explained that very well', or 'You do look nice today'.

The average person with epilepsy may have considerable ability but very often his performance is impaired in some measure by the lesion responsible for his fits, by the occurrence of subclinical electro-cerebral disturbances, or by the antiepileptic drugs which he is taking. A patient once described this as, 'Feeling like a powerful motor car with the brakes half on'. He appreciated that he was not stupid, he knew what he wanted to do, but he was frustrated by his inability to achieve his purpose. Within the environments of school, family, social life or at work, these people may never really succeed, never achieve what they expect of themselves, or feel that others expect of them. The great majority are not beset by prejudice or intolerance, they meet sympathy, understanding and support, albeit too often flavoured with patronage. May it not be that what they need even more is the opportunity to achieve even limited success, to merit genuine praise. Without these things, they lack a very real stimulus and are at risk of slipping into disinterested apathy. This problem is often the greater for the children of intelligent and sophisticated families. True, they are more likely to receive enlightened understanding and well-structured support. But is the understanding really enlightened and are they getting the kind of support which they need? It is so much more difficult for them to compete with their more talented brothers and sisters; to play a positive role in the life of the family. When there is conversation, they are talked *at*. They have the sense of being second-class citizens. Perhaps no-one would suggest that they are failures, but they do not feel that they are a success. There is a present tide in Great Britain which would seek to wash all disadvantaged people back into the open community – at all costs. We suggest that this shibboleth needs to be examined most critically to ensure that the person with epilepsy is not called upon to substantiate an ill-founded theory at the price of his self-respect and self-confidence.

Special provision for people with epilepsy is considered at the end of this chapter. It is comparatively easy, under sheltered conditions, to offer the more disadvantaged minority of patients opportunities adapted to their competence, and so to give them the chance to succeed and to receive praise and approval which is properly deserved. Some examples are included in the *personal situations*. It is considerably more difficult to suggest how the large majority of less disabled patients in domiciliary practice may be helped. However, certain suggestions may be helpful. It is most important not to treat the patient as if he was a fool. If his features are coarsened and his responses slowed down by antiepileptic drugs, he is probably a good deal more intelligent than he looks. Behind a mask, perhaps of indifference, perhaps of truculence, he may well be hyper-sensitive and he is very likely to resent deeply being patronised. It is sensible to discuss openly the factors which may limit his opportunities – the nature and frequence of his seizures and the effects of his treatment. Having done so, every effort should be made to identify and encourage the development of the abilities which he has, rather than emphasising what he cannot do. If he feels hemmed in by prohibitions, he is liable to opt out and fall back on the cushion of welfare benefits. If he can see opportunities and possibilities of success, if he can be encouraged to realise that it is worth trying, his desire to prove himself, to achieve, and his need for approval and appreciation may well confound the gloomy estimates of the experts.

It may be suggested that these ideas, which to some may appear banal, apply with equal force to other disabled groups, that they all have a need for a sense of achievement and approval. They do. However, there remain problems peculiar to epilepsy. Unless a patient is permanently handicapped by a significant degree of brain damage, he is for by far the greater part of his life capable and in control of his destiny: but for a tiny percentage of his life, he is seized by ictal and peri-ictal events or by subclinical electrocerebral disturbances; he is almost entirely incapable and there is nothing that he can do about it. Although it may not be possible to validate by formal testing, it would seem probable that, if toxic doses of antiepileptic drugs can impair performance seriously,

even therapeutic doses cannot be wholly without some effect. Cerebral lesions causing epilepsy are seldom global. The normal parts of the brain may find it difficult to appreciate the limitations imposed by those parts which are damaged. For all these reasons the person with epilepsy is in a position different from the person who is globally mentally handicapped. He may at once be at risk of failing to achieve his ambitions and at the same time aware of and frustrated by his failure.

Stress

We have emphasised already the important interrelation between environmental problems and the severity of fits. However, the effect of stress is more complex. It is accepted that most patients are less likely to have fits when they are alert, and that a moderate degree of anxiety may be a useful alerting stimulus. It has been our experience that, when a patient is faced with a single stress with which he is competent to deal, he does not fit. Patients seldom have seizures when they come for a consultation and it is rare for children to have fits during examinations. An exception being that myoclonic jerks often seem to be particularly sensitive to simple stress. It seems probable in other cases that epilepsy is exacerbated by a stress, whether physical or psychological, which is excessive, with which the patient cannot cope. This applies particularly to prolonged stresses and when the patient feels encompassed by an environment which he finds intolerable: when there is a long-term build up of multiple pressures of adverse circumstance. It is as if, when there is no single superable difficulty, he withdraws altogether, and opts out of trying. Out of touch with his environment, unoccupied, unmotivated, he retires into a vegetative hopelessness, devoid of stimuli, and at risk of having a greatly increased number of fits.

If these propositions are accepted, there are various ways in which the doctor can help. It is obvious that he should advise his patient to avoid unnecessary physical or mental stresses with which he is unlikely to be able to deal, but this applies to conditions other than epilepsy and is little more than common sense. However, for the patient with epilepsy it is perhaps especially important, and so the doctor needs to know his patient and his limitations rather better. He needs to do more than put himself in the patient's place, he must see things from the patient's point of view. On no account must the doctor try unnecessarily to advise the patient against any stress. Rather he must try to understand those with which he has to deal and help him to do so, otherwise the patient will be quite unable to live effectively in the ordinary environment which is filled with problems and difficulties. To cite a practical example: a child of ordinary intelligence, but who is still having fits, should be encouraged to work for and take the normal examinations, provided they are well within his competence. However, it is important that he should prepare for them steadily and not find himself faced with a last minute panic and excessive pressure which might well prove disastrous.

It is worth drawing attention to a situation which should not, but sadly all too often does occur. Johnnie starts to have fits, say when he is 11. His parents naturally are anxious to protect him. His doctor, still believing that fits are exacerbated by stress, reinforces this anxiety by injunctions such as: 'You must take care of Johnnie; do not upset him or he might have another of his attacks.' Very often the doctor is not quite clear what he means; he is passing on one of those ideas which he has absorbed rather uncritically, and he does not have the time to discuss the matter thoughtfully with the family. The parents, shocked by the diagnosis, desperately anxious to do everything possible to help, also uncritically are liable to take the doctor's injunction literally, and initiate a dangerous regimen of over-protection and over-indulgence. Johnnie, a nice little boy, who is quite bright, will soon begin to appreciate that he can get his own way when his sisters and brothers cannot. He will learn to manipulate his parents and, if one is more realistic, he will play the other off against the one. Relatively immune from sanction or punishment, he will become increasingly irresponsible because he will not have had the opportunity to learn that action provokes reaction, unacceptable behaviour, unpleasant consequences. He will grow up to be a particularly tiresome and unpleasant adolescent. In some cases, he may even evoke spurious *attacks* as a most effective weapon to oppose the final efforts by exasperated and distracted parents to control behaviour which has become patently intolerable. If the doctor is called in at this stage, there may even be occasions when he will nod his head and comment sadly that his earlier warnings had been justified by events. This is a Cautionary Tale told to make a point, but it is not wholly fictional.

It has been noted that behavioural and personality difficulties are commoner when fits have started in early life. Although the main reasons for this may be other than environmental – a failure of social learning due to brain damage, drug treatment or electrocerebral disturbance – a great deal can be done to minimise or even prevent these problems if there is a sound and sensible family background. Parents need advice and guidance. If the doctor does not have the time or experience of epilepsy to give this, he should arrange for someone else to do so. Within the security of a good family the child will have the chance, which he may never have again, of learning to face up to and deal with difficult situations, so that in later life even minor stresses do not prove too much for him; do not provoke fits. It is probable that, for one reason or another, certain people with epilepsy are hyper-irritable. Fits, their cause, or their treatment, may be the reason for this irritability, but they must not be allowed to be used as an excuse. The doctor must ensure that parents do not condone bad temper in their child 'because he is an *epileptic*'. Rather they must help him to make greater efforts to control it, and if he fails, must make sure, albeit with sympathy and understanding, that he meets the consequences of behaviour which is not socially acceptable. If he does not learn this when he has his family to help him, he will be at risk of being rejected by society when he grows up – and not because he has fits.

The patient beset by multiple long-standing pressures presents a much more difficult problem. He is likely to have relatively poorly controlled epilepsy and a significant degree of brain damage, both of which factors are liable to exacerbate the environmental adversities with which he cannot deal. The best possible efforts of social workers are unlikely to be able to improve his environment more than marginally. For this group of people the best solution is often to remove them altogether from the intolerable environment for a period to the supportive environment of a Centre for Epilepsy (p. 540). However, such centres must be organised properly as therapeutic communities. They must do more than offer temporary asylum. Like a supportive family they must train patients to deal with progressively increasing stress and to be responsible for the consequences of their own actions. This may take quite a long time, but the time can be shortened considerably if the centre is not considered as a last resort, if patients are admitted before their problems have become virtually irremediable. One of the main defects of the Colonies, which in Britain anteceded the present Centres, was that they were designed as long-term refuges. They sought to protect patients from all stresses and to excuse behaviour which was unacceptable as an inevitable consequence of epilepsy. Therefore, few patients were helped so that they could leave. Colonies were the last resort, the end of the road.

Sixteen to eighteen year olds are an important group who may find environmental pressures intolerable. They have left the security of school with the opportunities for achievement and companionship. They may have great difficulty in getting work and, if unemployed, increasingly they become socially isolated. Many may be rather immature and with the added difficulty of fits they are likely to miss out on the boy-friend/girl-friend scene. They are further isolated because they cannot drive. They are at an age when their fits are liable to be rather worse. Because they are working through the normal stage of child-to-adult rebellion, there will be family tensions, which are particularly important since they are rejecting the security of family, a security which they need so badly. The provisions in Britain for this group are inadequate and should be developed. The prognosis is much better for them than for those who need to be admitted to Centres for Epilepsy, since many of the intolerable environmental problems are transient. They need an opportunity to adjust within a new environment in which their problems are understood. If such environments could be established a great many people could be prevented from becoming, as adults, social casualties.

Employment and occupation.

The employment of people with epilepsy has been considered by Dr. Rodin in Chapter 13. The position in the U.K. is somewhat different from that in the U.S. and reference may be made to a valuable comprehensive pamphlet issued by the Department of Employment (1977) and to a leaflet entitled *Epilepsy and getting a job* from the British Epilepsy Association. Some additional points which may be helpful are discussed here.

In Britain disabled people are registered and carry a green card stating their disability. Disablement Resettlement Officers (DROs), who do excellent work in finding jobs for the disabled, meet with particular difficulties in placing those with cards marked *epilepsy*. The majority of the epileptic population is in ordinary employment. Those who are not, and who consequently register as disabled, are often those with associated disabilities such as a degree of mental handicap, or those disorders of personality and behaviour which have accrued over the years as secondary to their epilepsy. It is these associated disabilities which give the green card of epilepsy its bad reputation and make it so much more difficult to place the patient with epilepsy than the one, say, suffering from multiple sclerosis or rheumatoid arthritis. A patient may only be registered after his doctor has filled in the appropriate form. We would suggest very strongly that doctors should not fill in these forms automatically and uncritically, but rather that they should consider very carefully whether a patient's disability is such that his chances of employment will be improved by registration. The doctor must assume the primary responsibility for advising this patient about his work, whatever use may be made of the ancillary services of DROs and social workers in putting this advice into practice. After all, the doctor is the person responsible for his patient, it is to him that he will turn for help when he is totally demoralised, if not potentially suicidal, after having been rejected time and time again when he has applied for *green card* jobs. It is most important that patients should be advised not to apply for jobs which they have only the remotest chance of getting. It is wrong that the responsibility should rest, as it too often does, with a non-medical person working only from the information on a buff-coloured official form. If the doctor does not feel that it is necessary or wise for his patient to be registered as disabled, it is often most helpful for him to give him an open letter addressed to a potential employer, emphasising that he is a perfectly normal average citizen, explaining the nature, severity and frequency of his fits, the effect, if any, which they may have on his work, and offering to give a more detailed report pertinent to any job which a potential employer may consider offering him. The doctor, who shows detailed knowledge of and interest in his patient, still carries a lot of authority, perhaps because he is a proper doctor.

The more someone has to offer the better his chances of employment. This truism is particularly apposite to those with epilepsy who have rather a poor chance of unskilled work, both because of the nature of their disability, and because they are more likely to meet prejudice and intolerance from the least educated section of the community, struggling for survival under conditions of underemployment, when too many people are chasing too few jobs. If it is important that the patient gets the best possible education or training, it is essential that his doctor should guide him as to what is possible. If he attempts more than that of which he is capable, not only will he become frustrated and demoralised, but he will be exposed to stresses with which he cannot cope (p. 522) and his epilepsy may well become worse. It must be accepted that, for an important group of patients, a significant degree of brain damage is a factor contributing to their epilepsy and so militating against training which those not fully informed might advocate.

If there is a reasonable possibility that a patient may have a seizure while at work, in our opinion he must tell his employer that he suffers from epilepsy. Inevitably there will be resistance from the patient, and, if he goes to his interview accepting his doctor's advice, he will feel faced with a most difficult situation. As we have suggested already it will be particularly helpful to him if he can take with him a personal letter from his doctor explaining that in his opinion his patient's epilepsy

should in no way prevent him doing the job for which he is applying. After the first part of the interview is over and if he feels that there is a reasonable chance of his getting the job, the patient should introduce the subject: 'I am keen on this job and feel sure that I can do it. However, I must be frank with you. I suffer from epilepsy and was worried since either this might make it impossible for me to do the work, or, if I told you about it, you would turn me down out of hand. Therefore, I took my doctor's advice. He told me that he thought that the job was fully within my competence, and that my epilepsy should in no way prevent me from working to your satisfaction. He gave me this letter, which I hope will assure you that, if you think I am capable of doing the work, there is no need for you to turn me down on account of my fits.' If your patient is not open with his employer, there are potential hazards. If he has a seizure at work, he is at great risk of losing his job, not so much because of his fits but because he has not been honest. If he starts a job in fear that he will lose it because of fits, he is the more likely to have one. If his livelihood and his future depend on his not having a seizure at work, there is the danger that he and/or his doctor should increase his antiepileptic drug treatment, in an effort to prevent fits at all costs, but at the cost of impairing his performance to an extent which would make it impossible for him to do his job properly.

In small communities the doctor may often be able to guide his patient from local knowledge. Epilepsy is of course very common and an employer or foreman who has himself or has a close relative with epilepsy is likely to be sympathetic. Or again a business which already employs a sensible hard worker with reasonably well-controlled epilepsy is more likly to employ another, whereas a tiresome patient with secondary personality and behavioural problems will close the doors of his place of work quite effectively against anyone else with epilepsy. Another patient may get an entrée to a job through a member of his family or a family friend. He has enough to contend with and should not be too proud to accept such influence. He can satisfy any reservations about nepotism, once he has got his job, by working hard and showing that he is more than entitled to keep it.

It is quite common to have patients referred with the story that they have lost frequent jobs because of their fits. This is very seldom true. Usually they have been discharged because they were not able to do the work properly or even more often because of acquired faulty attitudes to work and to other people. If an employer knows someone has epilepsy and still employs him, he is most unlikely to discharge him unless his fits present a really serious risk either to himself or to others. However, he is likely to dismiss him if he is a source of disturbance to the rest of the workforce. The patient must not only get a job, he must keep it, and keeping it is very much up to him. He should explain to those close to him at work what sort of fit he may have and what, if any, help he may need. On the other hand he must not bore people by talking about his epilepsy all the time. If he is liable to lose time and if other people have to do extra work in consequence, he must be sure to make the opportunity to help them out later on. He must avoid giving any impression that he is using his fits as an excuse for slacking or avoiding unpleasant work. In the event, if he is adjusted to his epilepsy and accepts his fits, others are likely to do so too.

It is easy to appreciate the demoralising effect of unemployment. The erosion of the personality by mis-employment is not considered so often. A person's work must be emotionally, intellectually and socially tolerable as well as providing a weekly wage packet. A patient's ambitions may be inappropriate to his abilities, particularly if the latter have been impaired by brain damage causing late onset epilepsy. He is more likely to accept work within his capabilities if it is something of which he can have some conceit. It is not good enough to condone that the son of a company director, whose sister is a trained nurse and brother an accountant, should apply for a job as a hospital porter or, worse still, that he should work as a labourer, feather-bedded in his father's farm; or to allow that an electronic engineer with post-traumatic epilepsy should sweep the paths of the municipal gardens. In many countries it is policy to try to look after the mildly mentally handicapped in the open community rather than in hospitals or institutions. There is an increasing popula-tion of old people many of whom need a great deal of supervision. It should not be beyond the imagination of welfare authorities to offer certain patients with epilepsy meaningful and satisfying employment helping to look after these and other vulnerable groups.

However, at times of high unemployment it is inevitable that there should be large numbers of those with epilepsy out of work. It is an important part of a doctor's overall management of his patient to advise and guide his attitude to his situation: that he does not see himself as 'idle and unemployed', increasingly frustrated and demoralised, but rather as 'active and occupied' with a good conceit of himself. He should not stay in bed half the day and sit up watching television half the night. He must make a positive effort to structure his day and, within this structure, plan his interests and activities. He must not spend his time feeling sorry for himself because he has epilepsy, building up increasing resentment because his fits prevent him from working. Much the same applies to the man forced to retire at a statutory age after a long active working life. He has the alternative of rotting away in his bedroom slippers in front of the fire or of keeping himself neat and tidy and filling his day with all those alternative activities for which he did not have time when he was working.

Driving a motor car

The regulations restricting a patient with epilepsy from driving vary from country to country and it is not practicable to discuss them all. A summary of the regulations in Britain published by the British Epilepsy Association with recommendations from their Medical Advisory Committee is printed as an Appendix to this chapter. There is one defect which applies to those regulations which require a patient to have been free of fits for a specified period before he can hold a driving licence. It is widely accepted that antiepileptic drugs should be given in the smallest dose necessary to control fits and that, if possible, polypharmacy should be avoided. Many patients, whose fits have been controlled for long enough to qualify for a licence, are taking several different drugs in doses which, if not actually toxic, are unnecessarily high. There is always a risk of rebound fits when drugs are reduced and this applies particularly to phenobarbitone and primidone which are the very drugs which should be reduced if possible because of their obtunding effect. Both doctors and patients, however, are very hesitant about making desirable drug changes in case fits recur and patients are unable to drive for another prolonged period. Some alteration of the law needs to be devised to enable drug changes to be made. Otherwise there is a risk that patients, or even doctors, will ignore that part of the regulations which they consider unreasonable.

It is of course obvious that in modern developed countries the person with epilepsy, who is unable to drive, is at a social and economic disadvantage. Many patients would say that this was the greatest of the problems peculiar to epilepsy. However, it is worth contrasting the plight of two different types of patient. A mature adult develops epilepsy of late onset, perhaps even as a result of a car accident. If his epilepsy can be controlled reasonably well, he can continue his life and adapt to the driving problem from a position of some security. If his job involves a lot of travelling, he will have to ask for a change. His firm are likely to be sympathetic to his acquired disability. He will probably be able to manage reasonably well with his wife driving him to the station and on social occasions. His adaptation is of the same kind as, let us say, that of the patient with severe hypertension or arthritis. His disability is understandable, acceptable, and so readily evokes sympathy and practical help. Consider, on the other hand, a boy of 17 with established epilepsy. All too often he feels desperately insecure. He has left the ordered structure and companionship of school. He may well have been unable to get a job and so his school friends will not have been replaced by acquaintances at work. His features coarsened and his acne exacerbated by antiepileptic drugs, he may be terribly shy and feel that he is unpopular with the girls. Nowadays it is usual for the young to drive about in their own or other people's cars. Even if a motor car is not a sex symbol, at least it is essential equipment in the *mate race*. To be unable to drive increases enormously this patient's feeling of inferiority and social isolation. To him it may appear to be the cause of all his

social failures, and he may well develop deep and long-lasting resentments against his epilepsy. This very real difficulty in living with epilepsy, which affects patients at an age when they are especially vulnerable, needs to be emphasised, and must meet with real sympathy and understanding from those now middle-aged, whether parents or doctors, who would never have dreamed of owning a motor car when they were 17.

Psychic clothes

It may be said that we all wear psychic clothes. These clothes make it possible for us to present ourselves, not as we are, but as we would like to be: kind, intelligent, a good fellow, beautiful, fearless or sophisticated. Most of us are continuously in touch with our environment, affected by it, trying to relate to it, to manipulate or rather to control it. Our psychic clothes are an essential part of our relationships with our environment. Putting them on should not be criticised and dismissed as an empty charade. What we imagine ourselves, or would like to be, is almost invariably better than what we are. It is no better or no worse to adjust the psychic dress than it is to glance in the mirror before going off to work or to shave on the morning of one's execution. As time goes on, we come to fit these clothes better and we are the better for them.

Almost inevitably a seizure involves a loss or significant alteration of consciousness, a break in the continuity of contact with and, therefore, control of environment: the inescapable removal of the psychic clothes. It is difficult to quantify or define the effects of this on the person with epilepsy. The different ways in which patients react will depend on their personalities. Bereft of the security of the protection of his psychic clothes, a patient comes to place less reliance on them. Therefore he has less room for manoeuvre, for subtle adjustments in inter-personal relationships. His reactions will be more direct and may be more extreme. The gregarious extrovert may present as more boisterous, more brash. The timid introvert may creep into a corner to avoid the exposure which he dreads. It must be remembered that the patient subject to complex partial seizures may be very deeply concerned with what he may have done when he lost control of his environment. Apart from reassuring him that the distorted appreciation of sensory input experienced in his state of altered consciousness is not a portent of impending insanity, it is useful to encourage him to discuss his attacks with people who have witnessed them. To surround his seizures with a well-meaning conspiracy of silence often arouses deep-seated fears that his behaviour must in fact have been unspeakable.

When we go home in the evening, we usually take off some of our outer psychic clothes. However, we all need occasions when we can remove them altogether: times when we can be ourselves, when we can walk alone on the moor or the common and, if we so mind, put out our tongues at the birds. All too often the patient with frequent fits is denied the opportunity ever of being alone. Whatever the risk of accident or injury, it is important to appreciate that privacy is an essential human need. Without it anyone will become institutionalised within even the most enlightened and supportive family circle.

We feel that it is so important to think about the possible effects on the person with epilepsy of being denied, on the one hand, the opportunity to present himself in public as he would that he was, and, on the other hand, the right in private to be himself as he is.

PERSONAL SITUATIONS

The following *personal situations* are based on case histories of patients for whom we were responsible when we worked at Chalfont Centre for Epilepsy. A short explanation is needed to explain certain terms which are used. An Epileptic Colony was founded at Chalfont in 1893. By the 1960's there were some 500 'colonists' nearly all of whom were long-term and considered the Colony – albeit an institution – as their home. With a change in policy, many who were able were eventually discharged to live and work successfully in the open community. The Colony became The Chalfont Centre for Epilepsy and the colonists were renamed as residents. Short-term patients were admitted. The experiment proved successful and it developed as the basis of the Special Centre

which was opened officially at the beginning of 1972. In accordance with the Reid Report (Reid, 1969) this was run in association with The National Hospital, Queen Square, London and patients were admitted to the Special Centre for a variety of reasons – control of fits, adjustment of antiepileptic drugs, assessment, rehabilitation, and so on – the criterion for admission being that something useful could be done for them during a limited period of admission. The long-term residents remained in what was called the Main Centre. A Work Centre was established with trained instructors where light industrial work was carried out on a contract basis. An important function of the Work Centre was to assess whether or not Special Centre patients were employable. Later, a Medical Unit was opened. This was a small hospital to deal with ordinary medical problems and to facilitate drug adjustments and the more detailed observation of Special Centre patients.

Personal situation 1 *H.M. (21)*
Hannah lived in a small isolated Midlands mining village. Her father was a miner. She had a married brother and sister, both living away from home. Hers was a close-knit, sensible and very supportive family, although, naturally, her parents were worried by her fits which started when she was 5 years old and were classified as idiopathic. She had both major and minor attacks. During her school years they presented no great problem. She attended a Secondary Modern School where she was described as cheerful, friendly and fond of company. She passed the leaving certificate in art, home economics and social studies.

She began to run into difficulties when she left school. There were few opportunities for work where she lived. She tried, unsuccessfully, for various jobs, but was discouraged by her parents from further efforts because her attacks were becoming more frequent. She helped her mother in the house, but her antiepileptic drugs had been increased, she had slowed down considerably, and her busy mother found it so much quicker to do things herself. Progressively, she lost touch with her school friends whose company she had enjoyed so much. They were not prejudiced against her epilepsy. They were in work, married, or about to be, and involved in the ordinary pursuits of a small village. Hannah was frustrated by her idleness, demoralised by her increasing attacks, and she felt desperately lonely and isolated.

She was referred for admission to the Special Centre for assessment and rehabilitation. Her case had been well worked up. A clinical psychologist estimated her IQ at 56 and suggested that, because of her mental subnormality and uncontrolled epilepsy, she required long-term care in a sheltered environment. Her daily drug treatment was: ethosuximide 750 mg, carbamazepine 600 mg, and diazepam 30 mg. Her general practitioner described her as of average intelligence. She had been investigated fully and no structural lesion had been demonstrated.

She spent 10 months in the Special Centre. Her fits were observed very carefully and, at no time did she suffer from petit mal absences. This was confirmed by repeated EEGs which consistently showed a right-sided spike focus which occasionally spread to give bilateral spike and slow wave discharges. Her antiepileptic drugs were altered gradually so that she was having daily doses of 750 mg of primidone and 300 mg of phenytoin. On this regime her fits were well controlled and she had less than one mild major convulsion a month. Her IQ was reassessed and was found to be within the normal range but to show some evidence of brain damage.

Provided with an environment within which she had the opportunity to rehabilitate herself, this she did most successfully. She had the chance to mix socially and to work with young people. In our Work Centre she was assessed as being employable. It was noted that she was particularly good at getting on with other people although she found repetitive work rather boring. She was transferred to orderly work, at which she did very well.

Although she had been so successful, we advised her to stay on until we had been able to help her organise a residential job in a hospital or caring unit. We felt that she would be unable to *live with her epilepsy* within the village environment where she had failed before. Very naturally, anxious to return to her family, and because she felt so well, she decided that she preferred to go home.

Unhappily, our advice proved correct. Despite a great deal of help from her family, and a most understanding boyfriend, everything went wrong. For some nine months she did part-time voluntary work in a local nursery. This was never really satisfactory and the arrangement broke down through no fault of her own. Her earlier difficulties recurred. Even more isolated and lonely at home, fits became a major problem. There was frequent visits to consultants and several hospital admissions. Finally, she was discharged from hospital on a daily dose of 600 mg of phenytoin and 40 mg of diazepam, her fits uncontrolled and, apparently, uncontrollable. When she reported for her follow-up out-patient appointment she was considered to be 'possibly intoxicated'; her phenytoin was reduced considerably and she was referred back to Chalfont for reassessment, after almost two years of disaster.

When Hannah came up for a pre-admission consultation she had obviously deteriorated pathetically. She was barely able to walk. Her speech was unintelligible. Euphoric, she sat smiling, giggling and making continuous facial grimaces. Every few minutes her trunk would twist and she would make choreoathetoid movements of her arms. Clinically, she was grossly intoxicated and she was admitted immediately. Blood was taken for serum phenytoin estimation and she was taken into the Medical Unit. Her phenytoin was reduced to 150 mg a day. During the first two days she had one major convulsion. She then started to have frequent lesser attacks, always involving the right side of her body. Experienced nursing staff were puzzled by these attacks. Firstly, they did not fit in with the consistent right-sided EEG focus which had been noted during her early admission and, secondly, the attacks seldom occurred when medical or nursing staff were not present. A two-hour EEG was recorded. During this time she had seven of her partial attacks and, although muscle artefact was recorded, there were no EEG signs of cerebral dysfunction. It was decided that these attacks were very probably not epileptic and, after 10 days in the Medical Unit, she was returned to the Special

Centre on the regular dose of phenytoin and primidone which had been found suitable during her earlier admission. Over the course of two weeks, her fits became well controlled. She had no further minor attacks and during the past four months has had only two major convulsions. The signs of intoxication improved very gradually so that only after six months was she almost back to her ordinary self, although still with minimal dysarthria and a slightly awkward gait.

COMMENT

Most of this situation speaks for itself. Some points are, perhaps, worth emphasising.

Particular attention needs to be paid to the time after leaving school, when employment is often difficult and those with epilepsy may become lonely, isolated, frustrated and consequently have an increased number of fits.

It is still all too common for attacks modified by antiepileptic drugs to be classified as petit mal and treated ineffectively with ethosuximide. Furthermore, although diazepam is very useful in the treatment of status epilepticus, our experience has been that its usefulness when given by mouth over long periods is very limited.

IQ assessments can be most valuable as guidelines, but it is surely rather foolish to classify as mentally subnormal a girl, who has completed successfully secondary schooling.

The considerable improvement during Hannah's first admission was due, in part, to adjustment of her antiepileptic drugs but, in greater measure, to environmental change, to giving her the opportunity of living a normal gregarious life, and of achieving success and approval. Since it was not possible materially to effect the environment within which she had failed originally, it was necessary either for her to be helped to establish herself in a different environment, or for her to have a prolonged period at a Special Centre, so that she could acquire sufficient stability and confidence to return to her mining village, perhaps to marry her boy friend. This is the problem, as yet unsolved, with which we are faced.

This case illustrates very well the increase in non-epileptic attacks in patients with epilepsy who are intoxicated. It also shows how very long it may take for the signs of intoxication to subside, although some levels of antiepileptic drugs may return to normal levels. When Hannah was readmitted, her serum phenytoin level was already well below the therapeutic range at 26 μmol/1 (6.5 μg/ml).

Personal situation 2   R.W. (66)

Mr W. had lived a rather ordinary useful and happy life until a few years ago*. He was devoted to his wife and his two children. His daughter, who was the deputy headmistress of a school, had three children of whom he was extremely proud. He had always worked regularly and for 20 years had been a cost clerk dealing with stock control. His health had been reasonably good, although 20 years ago he had had a coronary thrombosis which was said to have left him with a right bundle branch block. About four years before admission his son was killed and soon afterwards his wife, who was diabetic, became gravely ill. He nursed her throughout her terminal illness from which she died some months later.

Mr W. never really got over these tragedies. Soon after, he started to have attacks. Many of these were said to have developed into major convulsions. Living alone, he began to lose all confidence in himself, and withdrew more and more from his usual life because of the attitude of his friends to his fits. Increasingly, he became less and less able to cope. He did not work, and was said to be unwilling even to shave himself or boil a kettle. He was referred as *in need of institutional care*. We explained that he would be most unlikely to be considered as suitable for the Main Centre for long-term care but that we would see him with a view to admission to the Special Centre for assessment. We queried whether he would be able to adapt happily to a community type life with patients very much younger than himself, and asked specifically whether, considering the late onset of his epilepsy, all necessary hospital investigations had been carried out. We were assured that he had been thoroughly investigated and that no organic cause had been found for his fits. However – perhaps to facilitate admission to the Special Centre – it was stated that he was grossly inadequate, attention-seeking and manipulative, and that admission would be justified on the grounds that many of his attacks were considered spurious and it would be important to determine how many *genuine* fits he had.

When he came for consultation, he was a pathetic figure. He broke down, wept, and was greatly embarrassed by his emotions. He was very frightened by his attacks which he said that he did not understand, and he was much puzzled by the way people treated him. To some extent he appeared still to be brooding over his wife's death, but his main problem was the horrifying and inexplicable nature of his fits. We explained to him the difficulties which he might encounter in trying to live in a community of younger people, but he was obviously desperate and begged for admission. He appeared to feel that, even if we were not able to control his attacks, at least we would be able to help him to understand and accept them.

Examination on admission showed minor neurological signs which might well have been due to cerebro-vascular disease. Several EEGs showed variable findings from normal to some excess of bitemporal slow wave activity. At no time were there discharges suggesting subclinical epileptic activity. His fits started with an indescribable feeling on the left side of the thorax, followed by shaking. He would fall and there would be brief generalised jerking and a period of confusion for up to half an hour. He was aware of the earlier part of his attack and found it very frightening. He had these attacks very often and might have as many as 20 in a day. They were not affected by alterations in antiepileptic drugs, nor by the addition of phenothiazines.

Despite our initial reservations, he settled in remarkably well and seemed to appreciate the support that he was given, although we had not controlled his attacks. It is interesting that experienced nursing staff suggested that they were psychogenic. He was referred for psychiatric advice, but a trial of amitriptyline did nothing to help him. Since his attacks were, if anything, becoming more frequent, he was admitted to the Medical Unit for more careful observation. The doctor in change of this unit witnessed one of his attacks and, noticing initial pallor, felt his pulse. He was pulseless. An extended ECG was then carried out during which he had one of his typical attacks which was accompanied by asystole.

Mr W. was immediately referred through the National Hospital to a special cardiac unit. After further investigations, the diagnosis of Stokes-Adams attacks was confirmed and he was fitted with a cardiac pacemaker. Although he had a difficult and somewhat depressed post-operative period, Mr W. has had no further attacks and, 18 months later, is living quietly the perfectly normal life to be expected of an elderly and rather lonely man.

Comment

This story requires little comment. It is obvious that it is unusual and that it is essential for clinical observation to be available to sense the occasional. In the great majority of similar cases except, perhaps, for the extreme distress evoked by the attacks, the history would fit in well with that of an elderly man with generalised vascular disease suffering from fits of arteriosclerotic origin. The failure to arrive at a rare diagnosis may be admissible. To prejudice the admission to a special unit of a man, who has lived and worked successfully for 40-odd years, by describing him as 'grossly inadequate, attention-seeking and manipulative', is not.

Personal situation 3   R.J. (20)

Rhona's father was a mild, rather inadequate man, who was intellectually inferior to his wife. Her parents were divorced when she was quite young and she was looked after in her early years by her maternal grandmother. Her mother, a teacher, worked full-time to keep the family going. Highly intelligent and dominant, she made a great success of her career and became the headmistress of a large school. She remarried, and Rhona's stepfather, who took second place to his wife, never felt secure in the family and, although he always expressed great concern for Rhona's welfare, was never able to accept her fully, or develop any warmth towards her. Her natural father maintained a rather tenuous connection in the face of considerable family opposition.

---

*In many of these Personal Situations, a time scale is referred to. These times were taken as from the time of writing, not of publication.

Rhona's fits started when she was 11 years old. She was fully investigated and no apparent cause was discovered. She had major convulsions followed by a period of confusion. The frequency of the attacks varied and although they were frequent at times, they were never intractable. There were no episodes of status epilepticus. Her drug levels had been carefully monitored and there was no question either of intoxication or inadequate dosage. She was always an intelligent girl and won a bursary to a grant-aided school where she obtained two O-levels. Her IQ at that time was 127. During her adolescence she was described as often sullen and moody; at times withdrawn. She made a suicidal gesture at the time of her school examinations when her results did not keep up with either her own or her family's expectations. On leaving school she had no form of training and, although she had done odd jobs on a voluntary basis, she never had ordinary employment. Increasingly, in the home environment, she became more withdrawn and lost. She was considered as being very difficult and she had more attacks than she had had when she was at school.

She was admitted to the Special Centre 11 months ago, in order to effect a better control of her fits, and for assessment and rehabilitation. On admission, physical examination was negative. Her EEG showed mild non-specific abnormalities. The serum levels of her antiepileptic drugs were within the therapeutic range and their dosage was considered suitable. Her IQ was reassessed and on the WAIS she had a verbal score of 115 and performance of 108. Her fits were as described before admission. During the first two weeks she had 10. Thereafter, they improved, without change in treatment and in over 10 months she only had eight, having had none, at Chalfont, for three months. She presented as an intelligent and well-educated girl, who found it very difficult indeed to get on with other people. At first she worked in the Work Centre where, although she was not particularly happy, her assessments were well above the level considered necessary for open employment. Later, she worked as an orderly in the Medical Unit, where she did exceptionally well and seemed to find it much easier to relate to those who were physically ill and dependant. Potentially rather an attractive girl, she made little effort to improve her appearance. She had settled in remarkably well to the environment of the Centre and appeared to be happy. However, it was notable that although she was a very capable person, she had no ambitions, no plans for her future, showed almost no initiative, and was almost incapable of making up her mind.

We had appreciated that Rhona presented a rather complex problem and so her case was not assessed formally until she had been with us some nine months. It was then agreed:

1. That under conditions at the Centre her fits did not cause any important disability.
2. That she was obviously potentially employable but that it would be difficult to find her a suitable job because her intelligence exceeded the adequacy of her personality.
3. That she had difficulty in adjusting to an apparently supportive family and that, if efforts were to be made to get her established in the open community, it might be better for her to do so away from home.
4. That helping her to plan her future was made much more difficult by her almost pathologically negative attitude.

Soon after this, we discussed our assessment with her and suggested that she might like to think it over and come back to tell us in what way we might help her with her plans.

There was no suggestion that she should be discharged before she felt ready to leave, or before we had had time to help her make suitable arrangements. However, her reaction was catastrophic. Within 24 hours, she had been in touch with her mother, her stepfather, her grandmother and local baggage removers, and had made definitive plans to return home within four days. For the next two days we had repeated telephone calls, independently, from each of these people insisting that we must stop Rhona returning home. We had tried at first to persuade her not to act so hastily but, after hearing her family's reaction, we appreciated the reception should she go home, and tried very hard to persuade her not to go. All efforts were fruitless. She went home for a disastrous week. There was complete family chaos. Rhona had innumerable fits and was nearly admitted to hospital in status epilepticus. We were accused of throwing her out of the Special Centre and after numbers of frantic telephone calls from her mother, her stepfather, her grandmother, and her general practitioner, she was re-admitted, totally demoralised, but very greatly relieved.

Comment

There is no doubt that Rhona suffers from epilepsy. That occurrence of her fits, however, is sensitive to changes in her external environment, and relatively unaffected by antiepileptic drugs.

Overtly, her family took us in by presenting a face of well-bred concern for her welfare. It was only when she made her plans for going home that they panicked and showed their almost total rejection. At the time that she left, her fits had been controlled for several weeks, and she had shown that within the environment at Chalfont, she could work extremely well. Had her family offered her any reasonable support and affection when she arrived home, she would have been able to live a normal life, although it might have taken some time for her to find a suitable job.

We do not know her pre-morbid personality. Perhaps she has always been inadequate and rather indecisive. Certainly, by the time she was admitted, she had a severely scarred personality. She had grown up, possibly unwanted, probably unloved, and considered as an incubus. Since she won her bursary, we doubt whether she had ever had praise or approval, had ever experienced any real sense of achievement until, for a short time, she showed her worth as an orderly in our Medical Unit. It was not surprising that she should have withdrawn more and more into herself and opted out of what appeared to her to be the impossible task of fulfilling her mother's expectations of her.

Her epilepsy was not a burden, it was a crutch, a readily acceptable reason for her failures.

Within the Special Centre, Rhona found it difficult to relate warmly to other people, but she felt happy and secure. Her successes were appreciated and valued. She was incapable of reacting rationally to the suggestion that she should begin to plan her life elsewhere. With hindsight, this suggestion was probably made too soon. Once the suggestion had been made, because she could not face the prospect of leaving, she preferred to get it all over, and made what might almost be considered a *suicidal departure*.

Probably Rhona would be quite content to live on at Chalfont indefinitely and, it might well be that, if she did, she would have a more satisfying and happier life than she would ever be able to find elsewhere. There are a number of the Main Centre residents who were in her position 30 or 40 years ago – before the era of rehabilitation – and whose lives have achieved considerable limited happiness. However, although we realise that it is not for us to make her decisions for her, we feel that we should make further efforts to help her so that she may be rehabilitated to live independently. This is likely to prove very difficult. On the one hand, she needs to succeed, to be seen to succeed, and to have her success valued. On the other hand, her present inadequacy and lack of any sort of drive will make it very difficult for her to cope with the type of work which would satisfy her intelligence. She is not likely to be able to manage on her own, nor will her epilepsy be controlled until, by a series of small advances, she can reach the point when she can face her family and herself and say, 'You see, I can do it.'

Personal situation 4   P.A. (24)
Peter was the elder son of professional parents. His father, a chartered accountant, was very successful and affluent, but he appeared rather rigid and humourless. His mother, tense and anxious, had the intelligence but neither the personality nor the common sense to deal with a complex family situation. His younger brother was a third-year medical student at one of the London teaching hospitals.

Peter's paternal grandfather had suffered from epilepsy. He himself had infantile convulsions and an episode of status epilepticus in early life. At the age of 11 he started to have complex partial seizures which were fairly easy to control. He had two major convulsions. His fits were not a significant disability. When his epilepsy became established, his parents were warned that, since their son was an *epileptic* he might be expected to present behaviour problems. Moreover, they were advised not to treat him too firmly since this might provoke an attack. These warnings were accepted quite uncritically.

He had an IQ of 75. He was devoted to his father, whose totally unrealistic ambitions for him he was quite unable to achieve. He was intensely jealous of his brother. Out of his depth with his family and their friends, increasingly frustrated, he reacted to situations with which he could not cope by outbursts of violent rages. On the one hand, these were accepted as a part of his illness and no serious attempt was made to apply any sanctions. On the other hand, his behaviour evoked more and more exacerbation and rejection. His problem was beyond the understanding of his otherwise intelligent parents. His brother was sympathetic, but his sympathy was the last thing that Peter was prepared to accept. His father tried to exorcise a haunting feeling of hereditary guilt by further rejecting him to an organisation for those with epilepsy, although at this time he was having very few fits. Within a disciplined environment, he seems to have done quite well, although his behaviour was described as rather unpredictable. Certainly he was considered well enough for discharge to open employment. This was a total disaster and Peter returned home, a complete failure. There followed three years, free of fits, but punctuated by referrals to neurologists, psychiatrists and hospital admissions. He settled well in hospital but there was no indication for long-term psychiatric care. When he returned home his behaviour was impossible and he was hopelessly bored. His father, who was a prominent member of the local golf club, gave him some pocket money to act as a supernumerary greenkeeper. Ultimately, he was referred to Chalfont for rehabilitation.

Peter was admitted to the Special Centre nine months ago. He presented as a heavily built healthy young man with no physical signs. Polite and well-spoken, his conversation belied his IQ. His EEG showed only a slight excess of slow activity over the temporal lobes. He had no fits during his admission. He was treated with phenytoin and haloperidol with no evidence of toxicity. His serum phenytoin level was at the lower limit ($40\ \mu mol/l\ (10\ \mu g/ml)$) of the therapeutic range, and his red cell folate level was within the normal range. During the first few months he did much better than we had feared. He was a bit of a bully and was involved in some minor scraps. Initially, he did not do very well in the Work Centre, but his later assessments were only just below the level considered necessary for open employment. Once he had settled, he was desperately anxious to succeed and his overriding ambition was to get a job before he went home for a holiday which had been planned. At first his ambitions were most unrealistic. However, after a lot of discussion, he accepted that the important thing was to get work, even though this might mean accepting something which appeared menial. He showed some interest in kitchen work and he agreed to aim towards a job as a kitchen porter in a hospital.

After five months in the Special Centre, he was transferred to the unit for those patients considered in need of some months' experience in living independently with minimal staff supervision. At the same time he was seconded for special work in the central kitchen. Both of these moves were clearly achievements and they were appreciated by Peter as steps to fulfilling his ambition of becoming an independent wage earner. He responded dramatically. His work in the kitchen was considered as very good and he was assessed by the head cook as being fully employable. He proved a valuable and responsible member of the unit. During three months there were no behaviour problems. Without hesitation we were prepared to give Peter a letter recommending him strongly for a residential job doing kitchen work. (In the interests of the many patients whom we help to get jobs, this recommendation is not given lightly and has become respected.)

It is a pity that this *personal situation* could not end at this point. In the event, Peter applied for three jobs with our maximum support. He was accompanied by the House Warden who spoke strongly and honestly on his behalf. He was rejected three times. In the first case, there was an acceptable hesitation because of his past history of outbursts. In the other two cases the interview should have been cancelled, but wasn't, because an economic recession in this country at the time had made the job virtually redundant before it was offered.

Peter's reaction was predictable. Most of us would be devastated by the collapse, into ruins, of years of hopes and months of effort. Sadly, Peter was not sufficiently intelligent to be able to appreciate reasoned explanations. Once again he was surrounded by a situation which he did not understand and with which he could not cope. He responded in the only way which he knew. His behaviour became impossible. He was dismissed from his work in the central kitchen. Frequent outbursts of violence made it unsuitable that he should stay in the special house. Undoubtedly we have failed – if, perhaps only just – in his rehabilitation. It is difficult to see how we can help him further.

Comment

With a possible inherited proclivity to fits, it would seem probable that, as a result of febrile convulsions and early status epilepticus, Peter acquired a temporal lobe lesion responsible for the epilepsy which later became established. He was handicapped not by his fits but by his behaviour. This behaviour was not determined inevitably by his temporal lobe pathology since it was influenced by his environment. We would like to postulate that some people with temporal lobe epilepsy may find it more difficult, but not impossible, to control their outbursts.

Peter needed so desperately to succeed, to offer to his father an achievement. Surely his doctor might have suggested to the highly intelligent chartered accountant that he might think out something better than offering pocket money for helping at the golf course.

Personal situation 5 B.H. (52)
Mr H. came from a small country village in a prosperous part of rural England. His parents kept the local store and post office. He had a good family and they were comfortably off. He started to have minor attacks when he was 11, possibly petit mal, and major fits when he was 14. However, these were not severe, were accepted, and did not interfere with a normal schooling. When he left school he helped in his father's shop until he was 32. Although never considered brilliant, he was certainly not a dullard. After that, he worked for eight years locally as a gardener, work which he enjoyed and for which he showed an aptitude. However, when he was 40, his mother was no longer able to do much in the shop and he came back to help his father. Two years later his father retired, the shop was sold, and in a country area, Mr H., at 42, found it difficult to get work.

His early medical history was not notable. No cause had ever been demonstrated for his fits, although he had been seen by several specialists. Although never a major problem, great efforts had been made to cure them. There had been frequent changes of treatment and at one stage during his adult life he was having daily doses of 500 mg phenytoin, 180 mg of phenobarbitone, as well as 900 mg of troxidone for the petit mal which had been diagnosed in his youth. There was no history of status epilepticus and, since his fits usually occurred at night, he had had no significant head injuries. At the age of 46, with very elderly parents, having been unoccupied for four years, he was referred to Chalfont. Almost certainly the implicit purpose of the referral was for permanent long-term care. At this time we were making tentative steps towards what is now the Special Centre and, in effect, he was admitted as a short-term patient since we felt that there was a reasonable chance that he could be rehabilitated to live and work independently. Before admission his IQ had been assessed at 119, although it was commented that this appeared rather high.

On admission, six years ago, Mr H. was a sensible, obviously intelligent man, who was well preserved and who looked his age. He was slightly ataxic and slow in speech and reply. This we attributed, on the one hand, to his drugs which were in daily dose; phenytoin 400 mg, phenobarbitone 180 mg, and troxidone 900 mg, and on the other, to four years of inactivity and lack of opportunity. We felt that he was the obvious patient for the embryo Special Centre; one who, with suitable adjustment of drugs and given the opportunity to rehabilitate himself, would be helped to return to the community to live independently, although his elderly parents would no longer be able to offer their support.

At a time before the Work Centre, he worked in our market gardens where most of the patients had little opportunity for other than labouring work under supervision. However, although slow, he stood out from the long-term residents and was given responsibility for greenhouse flowers. He did well.

Six years later, Mr H. is a pathetic figure. He has been for some time in a special unit for patients who need constant nursing care. Grossly ataxic, he is unable to walk without help and cannot stand on his own. Although he is not dysphasic and understands what is said to him, there is considerable dysarthria and his speech and thought processes are so slow that any conversation is very difficult. At 52 he looks 78; he is disorientated in time and space and spends his day slumped in his wheel-chair.

Over six years there has been a slowly progressive deterioration for which no obvious cause could be found. He has had two admissions to specialised neurological units, five years ago and last year. Air encephalograms showed some dilation of the ventricles and cerebellar atrophy. Brain scans were negative and hydrocephalus was excluded. While he was at Chalfont he had major fits lasting about three minutes, which were usually at night and averaged about eight a year. We confirmed that he was not liable to injury. His general health has been moderately good although four years ago he had what was probably a mild attack of cardiac ischaemia. His thyroid function was found to be normal. On admission his folate level was low but he has had regular treatment with folic acid and cyanocobalamin. On clinical grounds his antiepileptic drugs were altered and reduced. There was no indication for troxidone, which was stopped, and he has been maintained on daily doses of 150 mg phenytoin and 750 mg primidone without any increase in his fits. Reports on his EEGs before admission had been variable. Some records had shown only minor abnormalities. Others had been grossly abnormal, dominated by large slow waves with frequent spike discharges. While at Chalfont he had some 30 EEGs. That on admission showed only a mild diffuse abnormality. When it was clear that he was deteriorating rather than improving, further records were carried out. These showed little variation. The main feature was of a gross generalised abnormality with large irregular slow waves with occasional spikes and sharp waves. Some records showed intra-record variability with intervening runs of relative normality. Others were completely dominated by almost continuous gross abnormality. There was no apparent clinical correlation with these variations.

Comment

With a population of some 500 patients at Chalfont, over the past eight years a very few have shown progressive deterioration for no apparent reason. This case is presented to draw attention to the problem, rather than to provide an answer. These patients have been under close medical supervision and have had access to sophisticated ancillary investigations. It would seem to be of great importance to study such extreme cases, in order to consider whether the far commoner examples of lesser degrees of deterioration are due to medical or socio-environmental causes. To consider four rather obvious medical causes which might be relevant to Mr. H.

1. Patients with epilepsy subject to frequent fits involving head injuries, might show progressive deterioration, as in the case of punch-drunk boxers. There is no evidence at all that this might apply to Mr H.

2. Severe fits in infants have been shown to cause brain damage. There is some evidence that prolonged status epilepticus in adults may do so. In this case, fits have been neither particularly severe nor frequent. It would seem highly improbable that Mr H's relatively rapid deterioration was due solely to his fits, when large numbers of other patients, living under similar conditions, who had fits far more severe, did not show such deterioration.

3. Patients suffering from progressive cerebral disease may have fits, and are liable to deteriorate because of the causative lesion. In this case there was no apparent cause for fits which started at the age of 11, nor, 40 years later, was there evidence either from clinical examination or special investigations of anything other than an appreciable degree of cerebral and cerebellar atrophy. There was no therapeutic indication for brain biopsy which was, therefore, not justifiable on ethical grounds. However, it might be reasonable to postulate a very slowly progressive chronic encephalitis. Some support for this hypothesis would be the EEG changes which could not be accounted for by the severity of his fits.

4. The protean effects of antiepileptic drugs are considered scientifically in Chapter 8. Mr H's drugs were reduced, on clinical grounds, during the first year of his admission. During later years when the problems of intoxication had been elucidated further, his serum levels, for example, of phenytoin, were within the therapeutic range. But, at this time he was having 150 mg a day, whereas on admission he was having more than twice this dose, and some years before he had as much as 500 mg a day. Without being able to proffer a definitive explanation for Mr H's pathetic deterioration, it is appropriate to emphasise the potential dangers of antiepileptic drugs, and that the damage they may cause may be irreversible.

Personal situation 6 D.V. (52)
'Of course, I do everything for Daniel.' At the preliminary consultation we met an elderly, obviously unwell, excessively voluble, mid-European professional woman who, in her earlier years, had succoured royalty from the Middle East. It was easy to accept that a highly intelligent woman had been an excellent mother to her only child. Later, when we talked to Daniel, we wondered. Educated abroad in the best schools, he was multi-lingual, but his conversation was monosyllabic. When his mother was present there was no conversation at all. We also found it difficult to get in a word edgeways.

Initially, Madam V. had approached us with a proposition that if we agreed to look after Daniel when she died, we would inherit her considerable possessions. This suggestion was turned down, we hope, politely. We agreed to admit Daniel for assessment and rehabilitation in the hope that he might be enabled to live for the rest of his life as a relatively independent and happy member of a comparatively sheltered community. He was admitted in an emotionally charged atmosphere. His mother pleaded amidst floods of tears to be admitted with her son. She believed, sincerely, that he could not manage without her. After all, he had always slept in her bedroom. We were concerned that she would not be able to manage without him.

Medically, his case is not notable. He had had fits from the age of 2 years. His attacks involved particularly the right side of his body and variable periods of unconsciousness were followed by confusion. There was a mild dilatation of the ventricles and some cortical atrophy. His EEG showed a moderately severe generalised abnormality with spike discharges from the left temporal lobe. There were minimal right-sided signs. He spoke English well and there were no signs of dysphasia on clinical examination. His IQ was 80 on the WAIS. He was known to be hypothyroid and had been treated with thyroxine for some years. On admission he was having 750 mg of primidone and 50 mg of sulthiame a day. During the six weeks that he was at Chalfont, his fits were not an important problem. His sulthiame was stopped without making any difference.

At first, we feared that his mother's suggestions were correct. Daniel was able to do nothing at all for himself apart from dressing, undressing, and going to the lavatory. However, he settled in surprisingly well and made very good progress. He learnt to make tea, make his bed, and played his part in the rota of domestic chores. He seemed to enjoy these minor successes and his personality expanded. Never talkative, he got on well with other patients, had a dry humour and seemed to be happy. He worked in the Work Centre where, although not considered to be employable, he worked steadily and showed appreciable skills. His mother visited frequently. Daniel did not enjoy these visits and was embarrassed much as a small boy might be if his mother wore the wrong hat to School Prize Giving. On one occasion, when she commandeered a local resident to drive her up to the Centre, we had to bear the brunt of an irate telephone call complaining: 'I see that under your new Special Centre you have taken to admitting lunatics.'

Further investigation of his thyroid function showed that he was still hypothyroid despite what should have been adequate treatment. We arranged for his admission to a specialised unit to investigate whether this might not be related to his antiepileptic drugs. The day these investigations were complete Madam V. told the hospital that Chalfont Centre had closed down for a holiday and she would look after him until it opened again. She kept him hidden in a series of local hotels and eventually they returned home. Strenuous efforts by her family doctor, several social workers and ourselves were of no avail. Daniel is still at home.

Comment

This true story is atypical, but it does dramatise a comparatively common problem. That this is a case of over-protection is obvious: moreover, it shows how an intelligent professional woman, at first doing what she felt was the best for her only son, came herself to be dependent upon his dependence and succeeded effectively in reducing him to the state of a cabbage, institutionalised within the tangled skein of her care. We admit a number of patients in middle age who need long-term care, not because of their disability, but because fossilised by well-meaning parents, they are totally incapable of living or working independently. With hindsight, many of these patients could have lived useful independent lives if the correct advice had been given to their parents by their family doctors.

Personal situation 7   M.M. (74)

Mrs M's early history is poorly documented. Before her marriage, at the age of 26, she worked as a seamstress and is said to have been highly skilled. Certainly, her intelligence was, and still is, a good average. Her first fit occurred soon after the birth of her only child and was attributed to the shock of seeing a drowned man retrieved from the sea. Whatever the aetiology, there is no doubt that she suffers from epilepsy and it appears that at one time her fits constituted a problem and, together with a rather awkward personality, resulted in the disintegration of her marriage. She went to live with her elderly widowed father, ostensibly to look after him. In the event, he had the impossible task of coping with her erratic and irresponsible behaviour. By this time, although she had minor and occasional major fits, her epilepsy was not severe. Her social adjustments were. Possibly, inevitably, she spent a number of years in the chronic ward of a mental hospital. She was referred some 20 years ago to Chalfont as being clean, well-spoken, a good worker, occasionally difficult, but not considered to require long-term care in a mental hospital.

From the first, she was treated with caution. After all, she had been admitted from a mental hospital. She was bossy, argumentative, irritable and verbose. If she did not quite fit into the then current concept of the epileptic personality, soon she had this personality wished upon her. Classified as unreliable, she was relegated to closely supervised and totally unskilled jobs more suitable for mentally handicapped patients. Although she worked hard, repeatedly she got into minor trouble, made herself unpopular with other patients and, disturbing the organised torpor of the department in which she worked, she was moved to another where the same thing happened. There were no major crises; Mrs M. could be contained. She was well fed, provided with clothes, and looked after with considerable kindness. She was very unhappy.

At the time when the Colony was becoming the Centre, a great deal of attention was being paid to rehabilitation. In her late sixties, with no interested family, it was clearly impossible to rehabilitate Mrs M. to the open community. However, although she had a few fits, they were no problem, she was physically well, and an intelligent woman. There should be every opportunity to rehabilitate her to live a fuller and happier life within the community which, perforce, had become her home. In her case this was particularly successful. With some qualms, she was given a responsible job in the sewing room. She was in charge of making staff uniforms and played an active part in developing new designs which were being tried out. She appreciated the opportunity, did very well, and was pathetically happy that her success was appreciated. She remained a little bossy, and did not altogether suffer gladly those more disabled, working under her. Perhaps she was not much different from others in their early seventies. Perhaps we had rehabilitated her epileptic personality. Perhaps we were no longer expecting to find it. Certainly, she was a different woman. If not unusually popular, she was much respected by both patients and staff. For five years she had no fits.

Eighteen months ago, for the first time, she began to show

her age. We felt that her work was too much for her. We are still trying, effectively, to retire Mrs M.

Our first efforts resulted in a recurrence of her fits and a degree of despair. She is now called in, from time to time, to give advice and to help out when people are off sick. She is adapting well to her pseudo-retirement, is beginning to feel a little tired, but retains her pride in walking tall.

Comment

A distinction can be made between the ways in which a person with a degree of disability or inadequacy adapts to different types of community. In the *open community*, success, failure or a tenuous existence, is the resultant of the individual and the stresses in his environment. Many so-called failures are so because the environment is unusually difficult. It is important to appreciate that it is usually only possible to alter the environment marginally and often only temporarily. In an *institution*, an individual is required to adapt to a uniform and inflexible environment. However benign the institution , he is at risk either of presenting with exacerbated disorders of personality, or of losing his personality altogether and ceasing to be an individual. In a *therapeutic community*, a person may often be rehabilitated because there is a much greater opportunity to manipulate the environment to meet the needs of the individual. Therefore, it is possible for a person like Mrs M. to be maladjusted and seriously unhappy in an institution but able to live very successfully in a therapeutic community. Had she been younger, whether or not she could have been rehabilitated to the open community would have depended largely upon the particular circumstances of her open environment. This general proposition has the particular relevance to epilepsy in that a vicious circle is liable to develop. Environmental difficulties commonly lead to an increase in fits which may render the difficult, impossible.

Personal situation 8   M.G. (33)
Millicent arrived for preliminary consultation with her husband. A timid little mouse, wearing inexpensive but fashionable clothes, she was carefully and expertly made up, her hands were not very clean, and her finger nails were bitten down to the quick. Mr G. explained that his wife had had a fit earlier in the day and was not really up to answering questions. She hardly spoke a word. We soon discovered that Mr G. was a wholly admirable person. A highly paid car worker with discreetly revolutionary tendencies, he worked on night shift and did as much overtime as possible. This enabled him

to be buying his own house in a very good area, and to be available during the day time to look after their two children, then aged 10 and 8. For the past few weeks he had been on strike and so he had been able to come with his wife.

Millicent had started to have fits when she was 11 years old. She had major attacks and absences often accompanied by myoclonic jerks. She had been well investigated but no cause had been found. Her fits had not been a major disability and she had had a normal although not outstanding, schooling. She came from a good working-class family who appear to have taken her epilepsy in their stride. Before her marriage at the age of 20, she had held successfully a series of jobs as an office cleaner. Her husband accepted her fits and, at first, their marriage went quite well. They had been able to get a council house and her mother had given a hand with the children. Following a miscarriage, she was sterilised on gynaecological grounds. However, as time went on the home situation started to deteriorate. She had had a lot to offer to her young children with whom her husband had not been at ease. As they grew older, he understood them better and became involved in fetching and carrying them from school. Millicent was having rather more fits and her antiepileptic drugs had been increased. She became slower about her household work and used to get into muddles with the housekeeping money, which became a serious matter after they had moved into their new house. The admirable Mr G. assumed, without complaint, more and more of the household duties. Millicent felt more and more inadequate and became acutely depressed because of her apparent inability to look after the husband and children of whom she was so fond. She had advice from psychiatrists and a series of ECTs, which gave her transient relief. Her fits became even more of a problem and she had a number of prolonged admissions to hospital. On her return she was better for a while, although, after her drugs had been increased, she was more confused. Eventually, she was reduced to a condition of being totally incapable of doing anything in her home, with fits now a major problem.

Millicent spent six months at Chalfont during her first admission. Her fits were as have been described, although her major attacks were very brief and she only had two of them. At first she had one or two lesser attacks a month, but they were not an important disability. On admission, her daily dosage of antiepileptic drugs was: pheneturide 600 mg, phenytoin 300 mg, primidone 750 mg, nitrazepam 7.5 mg, and dexamphetamine 10 mg. Although her serum levels were within the normal range, her drugs were reduced progressively, on clinical grounds, and because her EEG, in addition to occasional subclinical epileptic discharges, showed an appreciable generalised abnormality. She was discharged on a daily dose of phenytoin 300 mg, and primidone 750 mg. She had had only two minor attacks in three months on this regimen, her EEG had improved and showed only a slight slowing of the background activity. She was a great deal brighter. Her red cell folate level had been very low on admission and she was given a maintenance dose of folic acid 5 mg a day and cyanocobalamin 1000 μg a month. Her IQ had been tested on the WAIS, and had given a verbal score of 90 with performance 85.

Such medico-scientific details do little justice to her improvement, which was remarkable. She settled in very quickly. Although at first rather slow, she became cheerful and happy and soon made a number of friends. Although well dressed and groomed, she no longer seemed to need to hide behind a mask of elaborate make-up. In the house in which she lived she was said to be quite capable, although she did not show much initiative in organising her work. She was particularly helpful with the more disabled patients. She worked in the Work Centre, and from an early stage was considered to be employable. At first her husband visited her and seemed pleased with her progress. When we suggested that she should go home for the weekend there was initial resistance. She could not travel on her own and her husband could not take time off both to collect and return her. We persuaded her to go home on her own on the condition that her husband brought her back. She made slow progress in re-adapting to home life and when she got back there were reports of attacks although, at this time was fit-free at Chalfont. Eventually, before she left, she had managed two long and comparatively successful weekends having travelled each way on her own. She was discharged with the strong recommendation that she should allow her mother to help with the children and that she should get a part-time job. We also asked her local social workers to keep in touch with the family and to provide support.

Rather over a year later, Mr G. – perhaps coincidentally – was again on strike when he brought his wife up for advice. For a few months after returning home things had gone quite well. Millicent had done about 10 hours office cleaning a week and had welcomed a degree of financial independence. Her husband and her mother had managed to look after the children and the house. At home she never seemed to be able to do anything right, so her husband, who always could, did everything. He advised her to give up her job, which he thought was too much for her. A failure, all too aware of her inability to cope, she sank into a state of depressed torpor, aggravated by frequent minor fits and occasional major ones. She must have expected to be admitted since she had brought her things with her. She was admitted right away.

Once again, within a few days, she had improved dramatically. The seven months of her second admission were similar to the first but there were more problems. She had more fits and quickly slipped into short spells of mild depression. It was much more difficult to persuade her to go home and she did not seem to welcome visits from her husband. Since her fits were more frequent and her serum phenytoin level low, she was given an extra 50 mg a day. Although her serum level was satisfactory, the increased dose did not suit her. She became mildly confused and improved considerably when her dose was brought back to 300 mg. Later, her fits were controlled, without ill effects, by increasing her primidone to 1 g a day.

After about six months, Millicent had got back to the point when we felt that we should try to rehabilitate her back to her family. She had always maintained strenuously that she was devoted to her husband and that he was the best possible man in the world. When her future was discussed with her, she said that all that she wanted to do was to return home, but that she had a lot of pain in her right knee and she would like this put right first as it made sexual intercourse difficult. It soon transpired that for some years she had suffered from dyspareunia which had compounded her sense of guilt and inadequacy. She and her husband were referred for psychiatric counselling. We felt that we had done all that we could for her, unless she was to be offered a long-term admission to a protected therapeutic community, and that the longer she stayed at Chalfont, the more difficult it would be for her to re-adapt to her family life. A month later, she was discharged with our great doubts about her prognosis, but at least with the confidence that she would

have experienced and expert home support, which had not been provided after her first discharge.

Comment

After the first few years of marriage, Millicent found her environment increasingly intolerable. She could not cope with the stresses it imposed on her, and she retreated to the extent that she could not cope with anything. Her epilepsy was not the underlying cause of the trouble and was not blamed for her earlier difficulties. Her husband and her own family had always accepted her fits very sensibly. It was only when they became exacerbated by her despair at her failures that they became an important factor. Cheerful, gregarious, not very bright, she thought the world of her husband and had put him on a pedestal, even before he had built his own. She understood life in their council house. She nursed her young children and felt needed. As her children grew up and her husband began to fulfil his ambitions, she got out of her depth. Perhaps she tried too hard. Never was she able to do things quite as he would have liked. If she had not cleaned the living-room very well, he would clean it again and, being the admirable man that he was, he would clean it very well. Later she failed to meet his sexual needs and a more complex element was added to her feelings of guilt and inadequacy.

Millicent's earlier reaction took the form of depression and attempted suicide. If she had not had epilepsy, it is doubtful whether matters would have been any better. Probably, as time went on, her increasing fits offered her some crutch so that she felt that her failures were not entirely her own fault. The Special Centre offered her an environment within which she could gain a reasonable pride in her achievements. The reduction in her antiepileptic drugs and the addition of folic acid and cyanocobalamin made only a small contribution to her own success in rehabilitating herself. We are in no doubt that Millicent could live a full, useful, and happy life within a therapeutic community. Whether psychiatric and ancillary support will be able to modify adequately her own particular open environment so that she can cope within it, must remain to be seen.

Personal situation 9   W.J. (40)

Winifred (Mrs J.), came from a closely-knit artisan family. She had been devoted to her father and always maintained close contact with her three married sisters. She had had an ordinary schooling and, although she had started to have minor fits at the age of 18, she had been in regular and successful employment in upholstery until shortly after her marriage when she was 22. Her husband, who was 15 years her senior, had had an uncertain childhood and an erratic work record. He had little contact with his family. There was one child of the marriage who was 15 at the time of Winifred's first admission three years ago. Two years before she was admitted, her father became ill and had a number of fits during his terminal illness. At about the same time, Winifred's attacks, which had not been much of a disability, became more severe and she had several major fits with an aura of olfactory hallucinations and tingling in her left hand. More often she had lesser attacks which consisted of an aura only, but which upset her a great deal because she felt unclean. There were also falling attacks without movements, and with quick recovery. Following her father's death, her attacks became more frequent. She was investigated thoroughly. Air pictures, angiograms and a brain scan were normal, but she had a right temporal EEG focus and minimal left-sided signs. Although it had been suggested that she was reacting hysterically, there was no doubt that she suffered from epilepsy, probably based on slight right brain damage. Even before her father's illness, she had been depressed and had been on regular treatment with antidepressants. During the few months before her admission, she had deteriorated markedly. She became more and more withdrawn, felt able to do little in the house, seldom went out, and was having an increasing number of aurae and minor attacks. Her husband gave up work to look after her, although it was doubtful whether he was in employment at the time. She maintained that he was *kindness itself* and that she could not manage without him.

Mrs J. was admitted for control of fits and to be rehabilitated so that she might return to look after her family. During the eight months that she was in the Special Centre, her medical record was uneventful. Her physical signs and fits were as have been described. She was having large, although non-toxic, doses of antiepileptic drugs, and these were reduced with improvement. Her red cell folate level was low, and she had folic acid and cyanocobalamin. A moderate iron-deficiency anaemia was corrected. She complained that her antidepressants made her feel heavy and, when they were reduced progressively, she felt better. Although she had a number of attacks during her first two months, these improved steadily and soon were no disability. She had no major fits.

She responded predictably to the alleviation of environmental stresses and settled very well indeed to community life. She proved herself an efficient, responsible and warm person. She got on well with patients and staff and was a great help, perhaps as a sort of mother figure, to younger patients with emotional problems. As her interests broadened, her depression receded. Altogether, she behaved as an ordinary person very little disabled by fits. Her formal assessments in the Work Centre were well above the level necessary for open employment, although it was appreciated that there was no intention of her seeking industrial work. She had several visits from her husband, which she accepted equably. She never evinced any particular interest to return home for weekends although she had every opportunity to do so. As she appreciated that she was ready for discharge, she became quieter and rather tense. This was attributed to a natural anxiety about leaving a protective environment. She was discharged with a good prognosis. A sensible and stable woman, whose fits had become well controlled, who had a family to whom she said she wanted to return. We felt she had recovered well from the fits and depression reactive to temporary stresses.

A month later, Winifred came to spend a weekend at Chalfont to see her friends. She was quiet and tearful, complained of frequent attacks of which she was both frightened and ashamed, and said that she seemed unable to do anything right at home. Within a week we had arranged for her to be re-admitted and she spent a further five months in the Special Centre. Soon after her return, she improved considerably, although she remained quiet and withdrawn, and it was thought that she might be suffering from an endogenous depression. She was treated with increasing doses of antidepressants with only slight improvement. After reviewing the disparity between her early work record and normal warm personality and her present state of apparent ineffectiveness' and withdrawal, we decided to try an environmental, rather than a pharmacological approach. After discussion with her, she was given, while still remaining a patient, a post of minor responsibility with a group of more disabled patients. She was altogether successful and soon progressed to doing a job which would have merited full staff status. Her depression cleared, although she was by this time on no antidepressants and, although she had occasional attacks in which she might fall or be unsteady, these were not an important disability. She had occasional visits from her husband and kept in touch with her daughter, but she did not return home. We were hesitant about offering her a staff post because of her comparatively recent difficulties and the fact that she would be in charge of patients whom she knew. However, an opportunity arose for a housekeeper in a local Home for Old People. She held this job for three months, while maintaining close touch with both staff and residents at Chalfont.

When a vacancy was advertised for a Domestic Supervisor at Chalfont, she asked our advice as to whether she should apply for it. While it was not within our competence to make the appointment, we told her that, if she felt capable of doing the work, we saw no reason why she should not. She was appointed on merit, without prejudice or charity. Rather over a year later, she is still in the post. Perhaps it is a measure of Mrs J's achievement that, when she has one of her now rare attacks, one of the patients under her authority makes sure that she has a chair, and that the work carries on as usual so that no one notices anything out of the ordinary. Mrs J. keeps in touch with her family and visits them occasionally. She has single staff accommodation with which she is quite satisfied. She is able to make regular contributions to her family's budget. Her daughter, of whom she is very proud, is training to be a hairdresser. Her husband, who is soon due to retire, is not in work.

Comment

This situation may be contrasted with the last one. In each case there is genuine epilepsy which is environmentally determined but is not the major difficulty. Both Millicent and Winifred had marital problems. Both had had periods of depression. Millicent's depression was probably reactive to her realisation of her own inadequacy and inability to achieve the expectations of the admirable husband whom she admired so much. Winifred is a most competent woman and her marital stresses were more likely to have been due to her husband's inadequacy than her own. Her depression was likely to have been reactive to her epilepsy. She had been deeply ashamed of her fits and had felt unclean. It is important to emphasise the nature of her attacks: the olfactory aura, and the frequent abortive fits when she was fully conscious of this aura. A similar aura was described by another patient as 'terrifying because of its obscenity'. The therapeutic community of the Special Centre provided Millicent with the support which her inadequate personality needed, and Winifred, with the opportunity to exorcise the self-imposed stigma of epilepsy in a setting in which epilepsy was so readily accepted as commonplace. Millicent was the sort of person who might have solved her marital problems by leaving her husband. Had she done so she would not have been able to manage on her own, and she probably appreciated this. Winifred would never have considered deserting her husband and daughter. She was fortunate to find a job which offered only single accommodation.

Personal Situation 10 E.R. (30)

Eva was the eldest of three daughters of a properous farmer and an efficient farmer's wife. Hers was a good family with a sound religious background and a sensible approach to helping other people. One of her sisters was a Child Care Officer and the other a teacher of Mentally Handicapped Children. Fairly recently, her parents had adopted a girl from a grossly deprived home. Eva was educated at a private school until her fits started at the age of 13. She was then excluded from school and had rather haphazard further education at home. Later, she helped to look after the calves on her father's farm but she appreciated that this was rather a made-up job with little challenge and she found it boring. She attended evening classes and without much difficulty got an O-level in English. With an ambition to become independent, she obtained a place on a Government Training Course and achieved a certificate in typing. Repeatedly she failed to use her qualification to get a job. Unable to drive a car, she was very isolated. Unable to use her considerable abilities, she became increasingly frustrated, jealous of her more successful sisters, depressed and irritable with her family. In a state of particular exasperation, she made a rather foolish suicidal gesture and had a brief admission to the local mental hospital. She soon returned home. Disinclined to make further attempts to break out of the web of well-meaning sympathy, she slipped into an unstable lethargy, assisted by increased doses of antiepileptic drugs as well as antidepressants, punctuated by fits

which had increased to a degree when admission to an *epileptic colony* was considered as the only resort.

Eva was admitted four years ago for control of fits and rehabilitation, and stayed for just over a year. She was a very pleasant and sensible girl who made friends readily and never caused anyone the slightest trouble. There were no abnormal physical signs, although there was a slight coarsening of her features, and her speech was slow and almost dysarthric. Her IQ on the WAIS was verbal 130, performance 102. She had major fits which were fairly severe and were often followed by up to an hour of stupor and a longer period of mild confusion, and minor absences sometimes associated with slight myoclonic jerking. Both types of attack were worse premenstrually, and when she was worried. The major fits tended to occur in groups which were led into by serial minor attacks. On admission she was having daily doses of phenytoin 400 mg, primidone 1 g, and amitriptyline 150 mg. Her EEG showed a normal, although rather slow, alpha rhythm interrupted by several 15–20 seconds' paroxysms of regular bilateral slow waves and spikes. Her red cell folate level was well below the normal range. Various gradual adjustments were made to her drugs so that on discharge she was having daily doses of phenytoin 250 mg, primidone 750 mg, ethosuximide 500 mg, diazepam 6 mg, and folic acid 5 mg, with 1000 µg of cyanocobalamin a month. After this regimen had been established, her major fits were controlled and she had few observed absences, although during a week's holiday at home a month before her discharge, it was reported that both types of attack were troublesome.

When Eva first came to the Centre she went to work on our farm. We felt that this would give her an opportunity of settling into more or less familiar surroundings while we made a preliminary assessment. She did quite well and appeared reasonably contented. However, as her fits came under control and her abilities became appreciated, it was clear that she might be able to be rehabilitated to the open community and that we should try to find what sort of work might be the most suitable for her. In view of her earlier training, she was moved to do clerical work. She showed skill and a high sense of responsibility but was handicapped by her slowness and by getting easily fussed. We talked it over with her and she agreed to accept the slower pace of domestic work at the same time as attending our basic Domestic Science Course. She found this quite satisfying and gradually regained her self-confidence. At a time when she herself felt that she was ready to leave, we were able to find a job for her helping an elderly Mrs F., who ran a small boarding house in the village.

Eva settled well into the first job which she had ever had. The slow pace suited her. She became close friends with her employer and was popular with the five guests. She visited the Centre regularly and kept in touch with the friends she had made there. She was a prominent and useful member of her Church. Unfortunately, Mrs F. had a mild stroke and, although she made a good recovery, Eva had to assume some responsibility for the work of the daily maid and to do more herself. All this proved to be too much. Two groups of major fits were dealt with quite easily by overnight admissions to our Medical Unit, but she was having so many absences that she could not do her work properly. She appreciated this, was worried, and matters got worse. Mrs F. was loath to lose Eva, of whom she had become very fond, but realised that by keeping her on she was only making her ill. Eva by now was hopeless, and anxious to leave. We agreed with her that it would be more sensible for her not to return to the Special

Centre but that she should go home to see whether she was able to settle down there. We promised that she could come back to Chalfont whenever she felt like it, if things did not work out all right.

Four months later she was re-admitted for a further 17 months. She had been no more successful than before. She felt lonely, despondent and had nothing to do. She said that she had had a full and happy life at Chalfont and wanted to settle down there. Medically there was nothing notable about her second admission. No change was made in her treatment and most of the time her attacks did not bother her much. She re-established herself after a few months and was able to think about her future. On the one hand, she was happy, settled and had plenty of interests. On the other hand, she feared that, at nearly 30, life was passing her by. We advised her very cautiously and waited for her to ask us for help in furthering her plans. An opportunity arose for her to apply for a residential domestic job in a hospital where she would have had a great deal of support. She went up for interview and, despite numerous absences, was offered the job. She returned, extremely uncertain about accepting the offer. Three days later, when she had recovered from a very bad series of major fits, we helped her to make up her mind. *Since her fits had got rather worse, she was not quite ready to leave*. She was very grateful.

She settled back into her work as an orderly in our Medical Unit where her excellent work was much appreciated. Not very long afterwards, the housekeeper in one of our houses left. Eva was asked whether she would like to take on the job while still staying on as a patient. It was rather a difficult decision to make since the work involved exercising a measure of control over other patients. She accepted the challenge with surprising alacrity. At first she was very insecure, apologetic for any minor failures, and she needed a great deal of support from the nursing staff. However, before very long, she established herself, achieved an unassuming authority, and did her work a great deal better than her predecessor, although she had very occasional major fits and times when she was a little absent. Despite reservations from some of the staff, Eva was offered staff status and pay for the job which she was doing. She turned down the offer.

Six weeks later, diffidently, she asked whether the offer was still open. The job was immediately advertised, she applied for it in the normal way, was interviewed by the personnel department and appointed. That was nine months ago and, so far, Eva has been entirely successful. Her improved status seemed to give her just that extra confidence which she needed. She settled into staff quarters and made her own friends among the staff. Perhaps she needs some measure of understanding support. Perhaps she loses a little time through her attacks. Certainly, she has not been patronised; she has been accepted as the pleasant person that she is, and appreciated for the excellent work which she does.

Comment

Eva represents one of those people referred to at the end of this chapter who are, 'very nearly, but not quite' able to manage on their own. Such people may have different disabilities. Eva was not socially deprived, she was not of low intelligence, nor was her personality scarred by adverse attitudes to her epilepsy throughout her life. She was disabled by the stress-sensitivity of her fits, her anxieties and probably because the ambitions and expectations of her superior intellect were limited appreciably by the drugs which she needed to take to control her attacks.

We must emphasise that Eva's job was not created from compassion, nor from the enthusiasm for rehabilitation. She earns her money. Any time lost through attacks, any occasional support, were more than met by her competence, enthusiasm and sense of responsibility. Some of her work is simple, but her involvement with patients offers her opportunity to use her abilities. When she returns for holidays to her family, she has plenty to tell them, and this is more than: 'I washed twenty plates today and only broke two.'

Twenty years ago, Eva might have been admitted to a 'colony', and ultimately have settled to do useful work. Later, she would probably have been cited as an excellent example of an anachronistic system and efforts might well have been made to discharge her to suitable employment. We feel that it is likely that these efforts would have failed. Over the past four years we have tried, not to determine Eva's future, but to help her to make her own decisions. The use which she made of the opportunity with which she was presented is a part of our concept for the future of Centres for Epilepsy which will be considered in the conclusion to the chapter.

CENTRES FOR EPILEPSY

Despite the most sophisticated medical treatment and the most enlightened psychiatric support, there remains an important group of people with epilepsy, who, whether temporarily or permanently, find it difficult or impossible to live with their epilepsy without some help. How should this help be offered?

Some hundred years ago epilepsy was classified as a form of insanity and the only help available was the doubtful privilege of incarceration in a grim Victorian institution, mis-named an asylum since it provided neither sanctuary nor was it a place of refuge. Others in need enjoyed the most tenuous of existences in the community. The group of whom we are writing – those with problems – had little chance of work and added to the population of the beggared poor or were supported but hidden away by ashamed families. The deprivations which they suffered and the depths to which they sank must have confirmed the opinion of the community that they were insane and increased the prejudice that they were a group apart.

The first special hospital for epileptic patients was The National Hospital for the Paralysed and Epileptic, Queen Square, London, opened in 1860. However, the first move in helping people to live with their epilepsy came from Germany with the opening of a Colony at Bethel, near Bielefeld, in 1867. This formed the model for two British Colonies established soon after at Magull and Chalfont. Over the next few decades several other Colonies were started in Europe. Since the *colony system* has been criticised severely over the past 30 years, it is worthwhile looking at it a bit more carefully. When they were founded, Bethel, Magull, Chalfont and others were pioneers, well in advance of their times. They offered true asylum from prejudice, penury and social denigration. They offered the opportunity to enjoy the dignity of working within the limits of disability. Most importantly, they offered a sense of belonging to a community, of mattering, of being a person of importance. There was a community as between staff and colonists – between them they literally built the Colonies – it was an adventure.

As more Colonies were founded and as they became much larger, progressively they underwent an important change, so that they were condemned with some justice by the Cohen Report (1956) and considered to be obsolescent by the Reid Report (1969). Perhaps there are four reasons for this.

1. They had become too large and too impersonal. No longer were they run by dedicated adventurers, but rather by professional career administrators. The community of staff and Colonists had grown into an *us* and *them* institution. An institution does not take account of individual needs or abilities but refrigerates personalities with an ice cube mentality which demands that everyone fits into a compartment designed for the most disabled.

2. With alterations in public attitudes, improvements in the Social Services, and advances in the treatment of epilepsy, the need for asylum in the Colonies had declined progressively. No longer were there people clamouring to get in. Rather, the Colonies, needing to keep up their numbers to cover their overheads, offered succour to distraught social workers faced with social casualties and inadequates, who happened to have fits, and with whom they could not cope. These unfortunates were sent, if not actually transported, to the Colonies: they did not opt to go because they felt that the Colonies offered them a better quality of life. Inevitably the deterioration in the quality of admissions exacerbated the feeling of difference as between staff and colonists. Co-operation gave place progressively to caring, containing and institutionalisation.

3. Most of the Colonies were voluntary, or non-statutory organisations, who felt that they had to keep down their costs, and so their charges, to those statutory authorities upon whom they were dependent to send Colonists. In some cases this concern with their economy laid the Colonies wide open to two very valid criticisms. Firstly, the amenities they provided for their Colonists were sometimes inferior to those considered adequate by the more enlightened statutory authorities. And secondly, all too often little effort was made to rehabilitate to the community those Colonists able to carry out, for a pittance, work essential to the running of the Colony.

4. The deterioration in the quality of the Colonists and the consequences of their institutionalisation gave them a bad name locally. They became isolated within their Colonies and they felt segregated and shunned because they were *epileptics*. There was a further unfortunate effect on the public image of epilepsy. Although the Colonists suffered from epilepsy, in many cases their main disability was related only vaguely to epilepsy: a degree of mental handicap, behavioural disorders, general inadequacy, and, again, the consequences of institutionalisation. And yet these people were to be found in what was termed an Epileptic Colony. It was not surprising that the general picture of epilepsy was drawn very largely from these associated disabilities of those in the Colonies. Even the medical profession, somewhat uncriti-

cally, based their erstwhile definition of the *epileptic personality* on the institutionalised Colony populations.

The Reid Report (1969) advocated the setting up in England of a limited number of Special Centres for Epilepsy. These would have a hospital component with access to all necessary sophisticated investigations, and a residential component for a small percentage of those referred to the hospital, who it was felt would benefit from a longer period of observation and treatment in a setting less artificial than a hospital and at the same time better controlled than at home. It is interesting that the first special hospital for Epilepsy was set up at The National Hospital, Queen Square, London, and that one of the three first Special Centres for Epilepsy was the National Hospitals – Chalfont Special Centre already referred to. Our experience was that this experiment proved particularly successful. As envisaged in the report, the Special Centre provided a focus for training of medical and paramedical staff, for the education of the public and for research. Patients were admitted for a variety of reasons, but the final criterion for admission was that something useful could be done within a limited period. This might be: better control of fits by drug adjustments under environmental conditions as near as possible to those found in domicilliary practice; the reduction of excessive doses of antiepileptic drugs under expert supervision; assessment and advice about the future; and rehabilitation so that they could adjust to the problems peculiar to epilepsy which had made normal living impossible and so that they could learn to live with their epilepsy in the open community.

The Epileptic Colonies of Great Britain have now disappeared and have been re-named Centres for Epilepsy. The change of name has emphasised a change in approach and many of the valid reasons for condemning the Colonies (see above) no longer apply. What then should be the future of these Centres for Epilepsy? Since there is clearly a present need for them and adequate alternative facilities are not available, it would be doctrinaire idiocy to suggest that they should be abolished forthwith. But, are they obsolescent? Should they be allowed to die gracefully? We would like to suggest that the recommendations of

the Cohen (1956) and Reid (1969) Reports were very nearly but not quite right: that if a system which has provided a much needed service for nearly a century has developed serious and obvious faults, this is an argument not for scrapping the system but rather for correcting the faults.

Medicine is about people and not about the science of disease. It seems appropriate to conclude this textbook with some suggestions as to how those people, who have problems in living with their epilepsy, may be helped to do so. Reports notwithstanding, certain special provisions might be helpful to them.

The future

Whenever possible, people with epilepsy should not live in Centres for Epilepsy. Either they should live ordinary lives in the open community, or, if they need to be looked after, in small units for disabled people in their home area. Certainly the latter group should not be segregated because they suffer from epilepsy. The Special Centres should be developed. However, if they are to be centres of excellence, they must attract really good staff and so there should not be too many of them. In addition to their present functions they should be large enough to be able to admit for limited periods people with epilepsy, whether from the open community or from caring units, who run into temporary difficulties. Since these would be short-term admissions, it would not be so important that the Special Centre should be near the patient's home area and three or four Special Centres would be adequate for a country the size of Great Britain.

A larger number of smaller and less specialised Centres for Epilepsy should be established throughout the country so that no patient would be out of reach of his family and friends. The following reasons justify the setting up of separate Centres for patients with one kind of disability.

1. Epilepsy presents peculiar problems, which have been discussed, and staff in an Epilepsy Centre can learn to understand and help with these.

2. The frequency and severity of the disability (seizures) are influenced to an important extent by environment and Epilepsy Centres can be organ-

ised to exercise appropriate environmental control.

3. The patient with epilepsy has a unique disability since, (unless he has a significant degree of brain damage) for, say, 99 per cent of his life he has no disability at all, and yet for the remaining 1 per cent during the peri-ictal period, he is totally disabled, not responsible for his actions and quite unable to look after himself.

4. Epilepsy itself does not cause awkwardness of personality. Nevertheless, for a variety of reasons (the nature of the disability, the part of the brain affected, the effects of antiepileptic drugs, and real or imagined social prejudices) there are a number of people with epilepsy who find it difficult to relate to other people. Without access to experienced counselling, they are liable to run into difficulties at work and loneliness and isolation in ordinary living.

5. There is still (and there is likely to be for a long time) a degree of popular prejudice against epilepsy.

There are three groups of patients for whom the Epilepsy Centres would be particularly suitable.

1. Those patients who have a disability which would require them to be looked after in a hospital (or specialised unit), but who also have fits which could not be coped with easily in hospital.

2. That quite small group who, despite the best medical treatment, continue to have very frequent or severe seizures.

3. A most important group of able and intelligent people, who should be able to earn an ordinary wage and live in the open community, but are just not quite able to do so the 'very nearly but not quites'. This group given the minimum of support, which a suitable community could provide, would be able to live ordinary lives and work economically within such a community.

There are two essential criteria for admission to an Epilepsy Centre.

1. That the Centre should be able to offer a patient a quality of life better than would be available to him elsewhere.

2. That the patient should appreciate what the Centre has to offer him, should want to go there, and should realise that he is joining a community to which he should be willing to give as much support as he receives.

If these criteria are met, the Epilepsy Centres of the future will be true Therapeutic Communities and will not be open to the valid criticisms of the institutionalised Epileptic Colonies. Furthermore, not only will they provide much needed help to individual patients, but they will go a long way to destroy the false image of epilepsy generated in the Colonies, by giving people with epilepsy the opportunity to show that they can overcome and cope with their disability: that they can succeed in Living with their Epilepsy.

EPILEPSY AND DRIVING LICENCES

The Road Traffic Act 1974 allows licences to be granted to those with a history of epilepsy who satisfy certain conditions. For ordinary vehicles the applicant must:

a. be free from epileptic attacks whilst awake, or
b. have had attacks only whilst asleep for at least three years before the date on which the licence is to have effect, and
c. that the driving of a vehicle by the person is not likely to be a source of danger to the public.

The regulations governing licences to drive heavy goods or public service vehicles bar anyone who has had an epileptic attack since the age of three years from obtaining such licences. If there is doubt about whether a solitary seizure since the age of three years was truly epileptic, then relevant medical evidence may be submitted to the Department of Transport for advice from an Honorary Medical Advisory Panel.

Problems of epilepsy and driving are discussed in Chapter 3 of the booklet Medical Aspects of Fitness to Drive. This is published by the Medical Commission on Accident Prevention as a guide for medical practitioners and has the approval of the Medical Advisory Committee of the British Epilepsy Association. Whenever there is any question about an individual's eligibility for a driving licence, he or she should first discuss this with the GP and/or hospital specialist. The British Epilepsy Association will also be pleased to help, and the Medical Adviser at DVLC Swansea is available for advice.

Applicants for a driving licence

Applications should be made on form D1 obtainable from Post Offices and Local Taxation Offices. The applicant has to answer Question 6d 'Have you now or have you ever had epilepsy?' If there is a history of any attacks, however minor, the answer 'Yes' must be given.

The applicant will then be sent a form which asks questions about dates and details of attacks and treatment. He will be asked for the names and addresses of doctors who have treated him and to consent to these being consulted by the Licensing Authority's Medical Adviser.

The applicant's family doctor will be asked by the Licensing Authority's Medical Adviser for information from his records.

If the Medical Adviser is satisfied that the applicant can comply with the regulations he will normally recommend issue of a licence. In cases of doubt he may obtain further specialist opinion and/or refer the papers to the Honorary Medical Advisory Panel set up by the Department.

The intention is to allow driving licences to be granted to those people who, on the basis of medical evidence, have been free from attacks for at least three years with or without treatment. If they have had attacks only during sleep, the history of such attacks confined to sleep must have extended over three years.

Applicants granted a licence after fulfilling the 'three year rule' will receive a licence for a period of one to three years and will not have to pay an additional fee for renewal thereafter.

Advice for successful applicants

For those applicants with a history of epilepsy who are successful in obtaining a driving licence, the following is a summary of the recommendations of the Medical Advisory Committee of the British Epilepsy Association.

1. You should avoid driving when tired or for many hours at a stretch.

2. Employment involving much daily driving as part of the job is not recommended.

3. Take care not to go for long periods without food or enough sleep.

4. The advice to everyone not to drink alcohol before driving is doubly important for you. Alcohol even in small amounts impairs driving ability and is liable to interact with your antiepileptic drugs.

5. If taking antiepileptic treatment, you must continue doing so regularly and as prescribed. If your treatment is changed or stopped, this may interfere with your fitness to drive.

6. If you have minor attacks causing mental switch-off, dizziness or some other strange feelings, these are as important as major fits when it comes to driving.

7. If you have a recurrence of any sort of attack (major or minor) you should stop driving and tell your family doctor and, if confirmed by him, you must inform the licensing authority.

8. When your attacks have previously occurred only in sleep, a recurrence during sleep need not be reported. However, if you should have an attack, either major or minor, whilst awake, you should stop driving and report this to your family doctor and, if confirmed by him, you must inform the licensing authority.

Reproduced by permission of the British Epilepsy Association, New Wokingham Road, Wokingham RG11 3AY.

REFERENCES

Burden, G. & Schurr, B.H. (1976) *Understanding Epilepsy*. London: Crosby Lockwood Staples.

Cohen Report (1956) *Report of the Sub-committee on the Medical care of Epileptics*. London: HMSO.

Department of Employment (1971) *Employing Someone with Epilepsy*. London: HMSO.

Laidlaw, M.V. & Laidlaw, J. (1980) *Epilepsy explained*. Edinburgh: Churchill Livingstone.

Reid Report (1969) *People with Epilepsy*. London: HMSO.

Temkin, O. (1971) *The Falling Sickness*. Baltimore & London: The Johns Hopkins Press.

Index